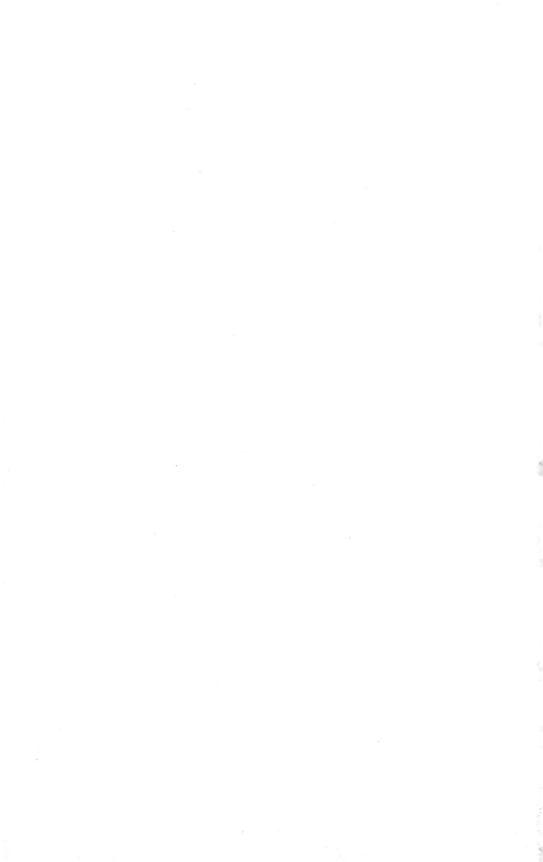

Diagnostic Procedures for Viral, Rickettsial and Chlamydial Infections

DIAGNOSTIC

PROCEDURES *for:*

American Public Health Association
1015 Fifteenth Street NW
Washington, DC 20005

VIRAL, RICKETTSIAL
and CHLAMYDIAL
INFECTIONS

Fifth Edition

Edwin H. Lennette
Nathalie J. Schmidt
Editors

Interdisciplinary Books & Periodicals
For the Professional & the Layman

Fifth Edition

5M9/79
Library of Congress Catalog Number: 79-53720
International Standard Book Number: 0-87553-087-7

Printed and bound in the United States of America
Typography: Byrd PrePress, Inc., Springfield VA
Set in: *Times Roman, Helvetica*
Text and Binding: R. R. Donnelley & Sons Company, Crawfordsville IN

Cover Design: Donya Melanson Assoc., Boston MA

NOTICE

Various products and suppliers are cited throughout this text as ancillary information for the reader. Citation does not constitute endorsement of any product or supplier by the American Public Health Association or the editors and authors involved in the publication of this work.

That level of technical sophistication and nuance which characterizes this highly complex and rapidly growing science requires that we provide the reader as much information as possible, including citation of materials and equipment used in the derivation of data.

Materials and equipment which satisfy criteria for equivalence of performance by definition contribute to reproducible results. Technological improvement in design and usage of materials and equipment is desired and encouraged.

CATEGORIES OF METHODS PREPARED
FOR APHA PUBLICATIONS

The American Public Health Association's Committee on Laboratory Standards and Practices has adopted "Categories of Methods Prepared for APHA Publications." The intention of the Committee in developing this classification scheme is to provide guidelines for the introduction of new methods or techniques that have not been fully evaluated and also to establish as a goal the ideal methods.

While recognizing the state-of-the-art in the rapidly expanding field of virology, it is hoped it will be feasible to incorporate these categories into future editions of this work. Please address comments regarding this proposal to the Committee on Laboratory Standards and Practices, American Public Health Association, 1015 Fifteenth Street NW, Washington, D.C. 20005.

The categories are as follows:

Class O—a method or procedure that has been subjected to a thorough evaluation, has been widely used, and through wide use has demonstrated its utility by extensive application, but has not been formally collaboratively tested. This classification will include methods that are referred to as standard methods in the current APHA publications; essentially it is a grandfather clause.

Class A —a method or procedure that has been subjected to a thorough evaluation, has demonstrated its applicability for a specific purpose on the basis of extensive use, and has been successfully collaboratively tested.

Class B —a method that has been used successfully in research or other disciplines, has been devised or modified explictly for routine examination of specimens, has had limited evaluation, and has not been tested collaboratively.

Class C —(1) a new unproved or suggested method not previously used but one that has been proposed by recognized laboratory workers as useful or gives promise of being suitable; (2) a method that previously has been placed in Classes O, A, or B but which, through technological advances or significant change in numerical level of acceptable exposure or other circumstances, has been rendered not suitable for its intended purpose and presumably has been superseded by a method of a higher classification. In essence C-1 includes proposed new methods and C-2 includes methods no longer recommended.

Except for Class O, the scheme allows for a progression from Class C to Class A thereby permitting a new unproven method or procedure to be made available pending further evaluation (Class C). As the procedure is tested and evaluated it progresses to Class B and, after thorough evaluation and a successful collaborative test, it becomes a Class A method.

The scheme is most readily applied to manuals of methods that are periodically reissued and in which the additions, deletions and changes are a challenge to the user.

TABLE OF CONTENTS

Part One

1. GENERAL PRINCIPLES UNDERLYING LABORATORY
   DIAGNOSIS OF VIRAL INFECTIONS 3

   Introduction   *3*/ Basic Approaches to the Diagnosis of Viral
   Infections   *5*/ Laboratory Organization   *10*/ Equipping the
   Virus Laboratory   *11*/ Diagnostic Approaches   *14*/ Detection
   of Virus or Viral Antigen without Isolation   *29*/ Computation of
   50 Percent Endpoints   *32*/ Complement-Fixation (CF)
   Test   *35*/ Methods of Inoculation of Embryonated Hens'
   Eggs   *42*/ References   *48*

2. PREVENTION OF LABORATORY INFECTIONS 49

   Introduction   *49*/ Recorded Laboratory Infections   *49*/
   Aerosols   *52*/ Some Potentially Hazardous Procedures   *52*/
   Biological Safety Cabinets   *55*/ Experimental Animals and Cell
   Cultures   *56*/ Disposal of Contaminated Materials   *57*/
   Decontamination   *58*/ Oncogenic Viruses   *59*/ Recombinant
   DNA   *60*/ Other Considerations   *61*/ References   *62*

3. CELL CULTURE TECHNIQUES FOR DIAGNOSTIC VIROLOGY   65

   Introduction   *65*/ Preparation of *in vitro* Cell Cultures   *70*/
   Storage, Preservation and Transport of Cell Cultures   *91*/ Virus
   Isolation Attempts in Cell Cultures   *94*/ Titration of Virus in
   Monolayer Cell Cultures, $TCID_{50}$ Endpoints   *100*/ Viral Plaque
   Assays   *100*/ Neutralization Tests in Cell Culture
   Systems   *104*/ Preparation of Viral Serologic Antigens in Cell
   Cultures   *111*/ Mycoplasma Contamination of Cell
   Cultures   *115*/ Detection of Mycoplasma Contaminants   *116*/
   Cell Culture Apparatus   *123*/ Appendix   *127*/
   References   *134*

CONTRIBUTORS

Charles A. Alford, M.D. *(13)**
Meyer Professor of Pediatric Research and Professor of Microbiology
Department of Pediatrics
Room 609, CDLD Building
University of Alabama in Birmingham
University Station
Birmingham, Alabama 35294

Lewellys F. Barker, M.D. *(29)*
Vice President, Blood Services
American Red Cross
1730 E Street N.W.
Washington, D.C. 20006

Marc O. Beem, M.D. *(23)*
Professor of Pediatrics
University of Chicago
School of Medicine
Chicago, Illinois 60637

Denis R. Benjamin, B.Sc., M.D., B.Ch. *(5)*
Associate Director, Department of Laboratories
Children's Orthopedic Hospital and Medical Center
Assistant Professor, Department of Laboratory Medicine and Pathology
University of Washington
4800 Sand Point Way, N.E.
Seattle, Washington 98105

F. Marilyn Bozeman, M.S. *(33)*
Director, Rickettsiology and Cell Biology Branch
Division of Virology
Bureau of Biologics
Food and Drug Administration
8800 Rockville Pike
Bethesda, Maryland 20014

Carl D. Brandt, Ph.D. *(23)*
Research Associate
Research Foundation of Children's Hospital
Associate Professor, Department of Child Health and Development
George Washington University School of Medicine and Health Sciences
111 Michigan Avenue N.W.
Washington, D.C. 20010

Jordi Casals, M.D. *(27)*
Professor of Epidemiology
Department of Epidemiology and Public Health
Yale University School of Medicine
60 College Street
New Haven, Connecticut 06510

Robert M. Chanock, M.D. *(19, 23, 30)*
Chief, Laboratory of Infectious Diseases
National Institute of Allergy and Infectious Diseases
National Institutes of Health
Bethesda, Maryland 20014

Natalie E. Cremer, Ph.D. *(7)*
Research Specialist
Viral and Rickettsial Disease Laboratory
California Department of Health Services
2151 Berkeley Way
Berkeley, California 94704

Chandler R. Dawson, M.D. *(32)*
Professor-in-Residence, Departments of Ophthalmology, Microbiology, and Epidemiology and International Health
Associate Director, Francis I. Proctor Foundation
Co-director, World Health Organization Collaborating Centre for Reference and Research on Trachoma and Other Chlamydial Infections
University of California, San Francisco
San Francisco, California 94143

Walter R. Dowdle, Ph.D. *(18)*
Director, Virology Division
Bureau of Laboratories
Center for Disease Control
Atlanta, Georgia 30333

Bennett L. Elisberg, M.D. *(33)*
Director, Division of Pathology
Bureau of Biologics
Food and Drug Administration
Bethesda, Maryland 20014

Stephen M. Feinstone, M.D. *(29)*
Medical Officer
Hepatitis Virus Section
Laboratory of Infectious Diseases
National Institute of Allergy and Infectious Diseases
National Institutes of Health
Bethesda, Maryland 20014

Bagher Forghani, Ph.D. *(6)*
Research Specialist
Viral and Rickettsial Disease Laboratory
California Department of Health Services
2151 Berkeley Way
Berkeley, California 94704

Anne A. Gershon, M.D. *(22)*
Associate Professor of Pediatrics
New York University School of Medicine
550 First Avenue
New York, New York 10016

Harry B. Greenberg *(30)*
Laboratory of Infectious Diseases
National Institute of Allergy and Infectious Diseases
National Institutes of Health
Bethesda, Maryland 20014

Vincent V. Hamparian, Ph.D. *(16)*
Professor of Pediatrics and Medical Microbiology
The Ohio State University College of Medicine and
Executive Director, The Children's Hospital Research Foundation
333 W. 10th Avenue
Columbus, Ohio 43210

Royle A. Hawkes, B.Sc.Agr., Ph.D. *(1)*
Senior Lecturer, School of Microbiology
University of New South Wales
Box 1, Kensington, N.S.W.
Australia 2221

Gertrude Henle, M.D. *(14)*
Professor of Virology
The Joseph Stokes, Jr. Research Institute at the Children's Hospital of Philadelphia and School of Medicine
University of Pennsylvania
Philadelphia, Pennsylvania 19104

Werner Henle, M.D. *(14)*
Professor of Virology
The Joseph Stokes, Jr. Research
    Institute at the Children's Hospi-
    tal of Philadelphia and School of
    Medicine
University of Pennsylvania
Philadelphia, Pennsylvania 19104

Kenneth L. Herrmann, M.D. *(25)*
Chief, Perinatal Virology Branch
Virology Division
Bureau of Laboratories
Center for Disease Control
Atlanta, Georgia 30333

Hope E. Hopps, M.S. *(20, 21)*
Assistant to the Director for Sci-
    ence
Bureau of Biologics
Food and Drug Administration
8800 Rockville Pike
Bethesda, Maryland 20014

Charles A. Horwitz, M.D. *(14)*
Associate Pathologist
Mount Sinai Hospital and Associ-
    ate Professor of Laboratory
    Medicine
University of Minnesota Medical
    School
Minneapolis, Minnesota 55404

Harald N. Johnson, M.D. *(28)*
Wildlife Viruses Project
Viral and Rickettsial Disease Labo-
    ratory
California Department of Health
    Services
2151 Berkeley Way
Berkeley, California 94704

Anthony R. Kalica, Ph.D. *(30)*
Laboratory of Infectious Diseases
National Institute of Allergy and
    Infectious Diseases
National Institutes of Health
Bethesda, Maryland 20014

Albert Z. Kapikian, M.D. *(24, 30)*
Head, Epidemiology Section
Laboratory of Infectious Diseases
National Institute of Allergy and
    Infectious Diseases
National Institutes of Health
Bethesda, Maryland 20014

Julius A. Kasel, Ph.D. *(9)*
Professor of Microbiology and Im-
    munology
Baylor College of Medicine
1200 Moursund Avenue
Houston, Texas 77030

Alan P. Kendal, Ph.D. *(18)*
Chief, Influenza Laboratory
Respiratory Virology Branch
Virology Division
Bureau of Laboratories
Center for Disease Control
Atlanta, Georgia 30333

Hyun Wha Kim, M.D. *(23, 30)*
Research Associate
Research Foundation of Children's
    Hospital
Associate Professor, Department
    of Child Health and Develop-
    ment
George Washington University
    School of Medicine and Health
    Sciences
111 Michigan Avenue N.W.
Washington, D.C. 20010

Saul Krugman, M.D. (22)
Professor of Pediatrics
New York University School of
  Medicine
550 First Avenue
New York, New York 10016

Joseph L. Melnick, Ph.D. (15)
Distinguished Service Professor of
  Virology and Epidemiology
Baylor College of Medicine
1200 Moursund Avenue
Houston, Texas 77030

James H. Nakano, Ph.D. (10)
Chief, Viral Exanthems Branch
Director, World Health Organiza-
  tion Collaborating Center for
  Smallpox and Other Poxvirus In-
  fections
Virology Division
Bureau of Laboratories
Center for Disease Control
Atlanta, Georgia 30333

Gary R. Noble, M.D. (18)
Chief, Respiratory Virology
  Branch
Virology Division
Bureau of Laboratories
Center for Disease Control
Atlanta, Georgia 30333

Michael B. A. Oldstone, M.D. (8)
Member, Department of Immunopathology
Scripps Clinic and Research Foundation
10666 N. Torrey Pines Road
La Jolla, California 92037

Paul D. Parkman, M.D. (20, 21)
Deputy Director
Bureau of Biologics
Food and Drug Administration
8800 Rockville Pike
Bethesda, Maryland 20014

Robert H. Parrott, M.D. (23)
Director, Children's Hospital Na-
  tional Medical Center and Re-
  search Foundation of Children's
  Hospital
Professor and Chairman, Depart-
  ment of Child Health and Devel-
  opment
George Washington University
  School of Medicine and Health
  Sciences
111 Michigan Avenue N.W.
Washington, D.C. 20010

Luc H. Perrin, M.D. (8)
World Health Organization Re-
  search and Training Center
Geneva Blood Center
Hospital Cantonal
1211 Geneva 4
Switzerland

C. Alan Phillips, M.D. (15)
Professor of Medicine
University of Vermont College of
  Medicine
Given Building
Burlington, Vermont 05401

Robert M. Pike, Ph.D. (2)
Professor Emeritus of Micro-
  biology
The University of Texas Health
  Science Center at Dallas
5323 Harry Hines Boulevard
Dallas, Texas 75235

Robert H. Purcell, M.D. (29)
Head, Hepatitis Viruses Section
Laboratory of Infectious Diseases
National Institute of Allergy and
  Infectious Diseases
National Institutes of Health
Bethesda, Maryland 20014

William E. Rawls, M.D. *(11)*
Professor, Pathology
McMaster University
1200 Main Street
Hamilton, Ontario L8S 4J9
Canada

David W. Reynolds, M.D. *(13)*
Associate Professor of Pediatrics
and Assistant Professor of Microbiology
Department of Pediatrics
Room 609, CDLD Building
University of Alabama in Birmingham
University Station
Birmingham, Alabama 35294

John H. Richardson, D.V.M. *(2)*
Director, Office of Biosafety
Center for Disease Control
Atlanta, Georgia 30333

John L. Riggs, Ph.D. *(4, 7)*
Research Specialist
Viral and Rickettsial Disease Laboratory
California Department of Health Services
2151 Berkeley Way
Berkeley, California 94704

Leon Rosen, M.D., Dr. P.H. *(17)*
Head, Pacific Research Section
Laboratory of Parasitic Diseases
National Institute of Allergy and Infectious Diseases
P.O. Box 1680
Honolulu, Hawaii 96806

Gladys E. Sather, M.P.H. *(26)*
Supervisory Research Microbiologist
San Juan Laboratories
Bureau of Laboratories
Center for Disease Control
GPO Box 4532
San Juan, Puerto Rico 00936

Julius Schachter, Ph.D. *(32)*
Professor of Epidemiology
Acting Director, George Williams Hooper Foundation
Co-director, World Health Organization Collaborating Centre for Reference and Research on Trachoma and Other Chlamydial Infections
University of California, San Francisco
San Francisco, California 94143

Jack H. Schieble, Ph.D. *(24)*
Research Specialist
Viral and Rickettsial Disease Laboratory
California Department of Health Services
2151 Berkeley Way
Berkeley, California 94704

Nathalie J. Schmidt, Ph.D. *(3)*
Research Specialist
Viral and Rickettsial Disease Laboratory
California Department of Health Services
2151 Berkeley Way
Berkeley, California 94704

Robert E. Shope, M.D. *(26)*
Director, Yale Arbovirus Research Unit and Professor of Epidemiology
Yale School of Medicine
333 Cedar Street
New Haven, Connecticut 06510

Sergio Stagno, M.D. *(13)*
Associate Professor of Pediatrics
and Assistant Professor of Microbiology
Department of Pediatrics
Room 609, CDLD Building
University of Alabama in Birmingham
University Station
Birmingham, Alabama 35294

Joel Warren, Ph.D. *(31)*
Director, Leo Goodwin Institute
  for Cancer Research
Nova University
3301 College Avenue
Fort Lauderdale, Florida 33314

Thomas H. Weller, M.D. *(12)*
Richard Pearson Strong Professor
  of Tropical Public Health and
  Chairman, Department of Tropi-
  cal Public Health
Director, Center for the Prevention
  of Infectious Diseases
Harvard School of Public Health
665 Huntington Avenue
Boston, Massachusetts 02115

Herbert A. Wenner, M.D. *(15)*
Professor of Pediatrics
University of Missouri School of
  Medicine
24th at Gilham Road
Kansas City, Missouri 64108

Richard G. Wyatt, M.D. *(30)*
Laboratory of Infectious Diseases
National Institute of Allergy and
  Infectious Diseases
National Institutes of Health
Bethesa, Maryland 20014

Robert H. Yolken, M.D. *(30)*
Laboratory of Infectious Diseases
National Institute of Allergy and
  Infectious Diseases
National Institutes of Health
Bethesda, Maryland 20014

---

*(References to chapters)

PREFACE TO THE FIFTH EDITION

When the present Editors assumed the responsibility, beginning with the Third Edition in 1964, for the preparation and issuance of *Diagnostic Procedures for Viral and Rickettsial Infections*, it was their presumption and expectation that a new edition approximately every five years would serve to keep the compendium up-to-date. This expectation was fulfilled with the publication of the Fourth Edition in 1969 and in that edition we had occasion to mention the truism stated by Dr. Thomas Francis, Jr. in his preface to the Second Edition (1956) that "to attain a completely current status for a book dealing with technical procedures in a field of rapid growth is difficult". This was emphatically brought home to us when preparations were initiated in 1974–1975 to bring out the present edition. A number of factors contributed to a series of postponements of publication. Among these may be mentioned the burgeoning research and consequent rapid accumulation of knowledge on the herpesviruses, especially the Epstein-Barr virus and human cytomegalovirus. Concomitantly, there occurred a number of breakthroughs, with a resultant explosion of research, on viral hepatitis and more recently with respect to viral gastroenteritis. The rapidity with which these developments occurred, and the rate at which new information was acquired, not only in these areas but also in viral immunology, made it obvious that any compendium or handbook such as *Diagnostic Procedures for Viral and Rickettsial Infections* would not only be out-of-date by the time of its publication, but hopelessly so. It was considered prudent and advisable to await a more propitious time for issuing a new edition and this explains the nearly ten-year interval between the last edition and this.

In the case of some diseases and their causal agents, the amount of new information to be added necessitated only a re-writing to incorporate the new data. In other instances, whole new chapters are required as a consequence of the huge amount of in-depth, intensive research that has provided us with so much information on such diseases as viral hepatitis, viral gastroenteritis and Epstein-Barr virus disease. To provide the necessary pages for comprehensive exposition of these subjects, certain other chapters were shortened. Also, the *Mycoplasma* have been dropped from this edition, having found a home in the companion *Diagnostic Procedures for Bacterial, Mycotic and Parasitic Infections*.

Such revisions and shortenings have allowed not only comprehensive presentation of an impressive amount of new information but have also permitted inclusion of new chapters dealing with cell-mediated immunity, immune complexes and immunoglobulin classes and their relationship to viral laboratory diagnosis. In addition to the chapter on fluorescent antibody methods, two new chapters dealing with radioimmunoassay and immunoenzymatic technics have been added to provide a theoretical and practical background for methods and technics described in the various chapters dealing with specific diseases.

Finally, but not least, the increasing emphasis and recognition of the *Chlamydia* as important disease agents has led us to rename this volume *Diagnostic Procedures for Viral, Rickettsial and Chlamydial Infections*.

We take this occasion to express our thanks and appreciation to Mr. Allen Seeber, Publications Office of the American Public Health Association for his assistance in the redactory and manufacturing phases and Mrs. Cheryl Remoy who competently and efficiently carried out the secretarial work and recordkeeping in the office of the Editors.

Edwin H. Lennette
Nathalie J. Schmidt

Part One

CHAPTER 1

GENERAL PRINCIPLES UNDERLYING LABORATORY DIAGNOSIS OF VIRAL INFECTIONS

Royle A. Hawkes

Introduction

Notable advances in both the discovery of "new" viruses and in the development of laboratory technology for viral diagnosis have occurred since the publication of the fourth edition of this book. These advances are incorporated in this edition along with appropriate older techniques so as to provide the laboratory worker with a guide to reliable methods of known reproducibility and established significance. As in previous editions, the emphasis is on acute diseases of humans, but the awareness that certain human infections are zoonotic in origin and that certain viruses are prone to induce chronic disease is also reflected in this volume.

The scope of this chapter is to set the stage for the more detailed chapters which follow by broadly outlining the diagnostic methods employed and their interpretation, and to append some generally used techniques applicable to the study of many viruses and thus not included in later chapters. However, before moving on to these topics, it is necessary to briefly discuss some general issues, mostly of a nonmicrobial nature, which greatly influence the efficiency and smooth running of the virus diagnostic laboratory. Although discussed here from the standpoint of setting up a new diagnostic facility, the issues are pertinent to an established laboratory.

Planning at the local level

Diagnostic virology is done for a variety of reasons, ranging from the etiologic diagnosis of an acutely ill patient's disease at one extreme to retrospective serologic surveys at the other. The ultimate benefit of these diverse diagnostic activities to the community at large is very great indeed. However, in contrast to the activities of diagnostic bacteriology laboratories, they are not usually of direct value to the individual patient, this being chiefly due to the paucity of specific therapy and the long time involved in laboratory diagnosis (there are some notable exceptions). As a consequence, most viral diagnostic laboratories are funded from public sources, and the resultant public accountability makes the efficient running of the laboratory even more important than might otherwise be the case.

This has several aspects. To begin with it dictates that a careful assessment of the needs of the situation be made. This involves consideration of such factors as the types and numbers of patients likely to be investigated, the probable number and nature of specimens likely to be submitted, the location of the laboratory relative to the sources of specimens, facilities for specimen transport, and the presence of existing diagnostic facilities in the area. These considerations determine the level of complexity at which viral diagnosis should be attempted (i.e., which of the various diagnostic approaches should be used). In one situation the correct approach might be to set up a large facility capable of employing a broad range of sophisticated techniques; in another it could be wiser to institute a serologic service as an adjunct to an existing microbiology laboratory; while in a third situation the most fruitful approach could well be to purchase a small number of cell cultures each week, inoculate them, and then forward them to a larger virus laboratory for further observation.

Production or purchase of biologic resources

Another financial aspect to be considered is whether it is more economical to purchase biologic materials such as laboratory animals, cell cultures, sera, antisera, and antigens or whether to produce them in your own laboratory. This decision depends on the local availability and cost of such reagents and the size of the virus laboratory. In many laboratories, especially the medium to small sized ones, it is more economical to purchase some or all of these biologicals, rather than to incur the expense of producing them.

Liaison

It is essential that the virus laboratory maintains effective liaison and consultation with medical (and sometimes veterinary) personnel submitting specimens. This collaboration has several useful effects. From the physicians' standpoint it helps ensure that the appropriate specimens are collected and transported to the laboratory in the correct manner, thus giving the laboratory the best chance of producing useful results. Consultation also promotes realistic expectation in the person submitting specimens as to what the laboratory can and cannot achieve. From the viewpoint of the laboratory, such consultation also permits most intelligent utilization of resources. This is because the nature of diagnostic activities to be undertaken by the laboratory depends to a large degree on clinical and epidemiologic information imparted by the physician submitting the specimens. Such consultation also maintains the morale of laboratory staff by allowing them to relate their laboratory findings to clinical and epidemiologic features. This results in a keener laboratory workforce and has on occasion led to important clinicovirologic correlations being noticed which had not been apparent to either physician or supervising virologist. In addition to verbal collaboration, or in situations (for example regional laboratories) where such conversations are of necessity infrequent, much can be achieved in this respect if the submitting physician includes a resumé of patient's data with the specimen, and if the laboratory sends back provisional and final reports as promptly as possible.

Liaison is also desirable with other sections of diagnostic laboratories carrying out tests on the same patient. This communication can lead to modification or even cessation of diagnostic activities in the various sections concerned, as results in one section are communicated to the other.

Liaison is also important with other workers in the public health field, both laboratory and clinical, medical and veterinary. This can nearly always be achieved at the regional level by periodic meetings, and can sometimes be done by selected individuals at national and international levels. The importance of this activity lies not only in the first-hand sharing of laboratory experiences but also in discussion of the viruses encountered in other areas and perhaps likely to be expected locally. Similarly, publication of frequent and regular lists of specific diagnoses made by virus laboratories is a practice to be commended. Viruses do not respect geographic barriers. Consequently, one role of the diagnostic laboratory is as part of a local, regional, and global surveillance system. Only by collecting information on a global scale can worldwide surveillance be effective. This is especially so in the light of rapid intercontinental travel and its implications in well-known infections like influenza. It is also seen in the occasional emergence of serious viral diseases from enzootic foci in various parts of the world. Incidentally, this latter phenomenon highlights the need for a collaboration between medical and veterinary personnel in the consideration of viral disease—something which has often been lacking in the past.

Basic Approaches to the Diagnosis of Viral Infections

Categories of tests

The methods used to diagnose viral infections have their rationale in the fact that many viruses produce characteristic changes in cells of the host and that most of them induce the production of infectious virus or viral antigen in body tissues, secretions, and excretions. This in turn is usually followed by the production of antibodies which are specific for the virus and its associated antigens. The many diagnostic procedures used can be roughly grouped into 4 categories, each with its particular role, limitations and advantages. These are:

1. Microscopic examination of infected tissues and exudates from the patient for evidence of viral inclusions or other pathologic alterations which may be characteristic of the activity of certain viruses.

2. Isolation (cultivation) and identification of virus from infected tissues or other specimens derived from the patient.

3. Serologic studies carried out to detect the development (or sometimes the presence) of virus-specific antibodies in patient's serum.

4. Tests for the detection of virus or viral antigen in tissues or other specimens from patients, independent of the cultivation of these viruses in the laboratory. Many of the recently developed rapid diagnostic techniques are in this category.

The microscopic examination of fixed and stained tissues for inclusion bodies and other cytologic changes is a rapid means, if positive, of indicating that a clinical condition is of probable viral etiology, and of giving a rough guide in some instances to the *group* of viruses involved. As such, it has value in differentiating between certain critical alternatives (for example herpesvirus etiology versus poxvirus etiology in the provisional diagnosis of smallpox) or allowing for a presumptive specific diagnosis to be made in other clinical conditions (for example Negri bodies in rabies). However it is of no help when significant changes are *not* seen, and furthermore, it does not permit the specific identification of the agent when significant changes *are* seen. In many laboratories histopathologic (microscopic) examination of biopsy and autopsy specimens is traditionally carried out by a department other than the virus laboratory, and liaison with this other department is essential. Electron microscopy is a more recent technique which fits into this category, but it is discussed along with immune electron microscopy under category 4 below.

The isolation of viruses from patients is the traditional viral counterpart of diagnostic bacteriology but differs from it in that a range of *living* host systems of varying complexity must be used. Growth of a virus and its identification usually takes longer than the other approaches but has the great advantage of definitely associating a specific virus with a given clinical condition. As such, virus isolation has long been the cornerstone of diagnostic virology. However, the nature of the association, i.e., causal or otherwise, between virus isolated and patient's clinical condition demands careful interpretation and, conversely, the failure to cultivate virus from a patient does not rule out the viral etiology of the patient's infection.

Serology is of great benefit in viral diagnosis, especially in situations where patients are remote from laboratories, and thus virus isolation from clinical specimens may be unrewarding due to the inactivation of virus during the transit of such specimens to the laboratory. It is also the chief tool used in retrospectively defining the incidence of viral infections in communities and in elucidating the need for, and monitoring the efficacy of, immunization programs. Customarily, the collection of 2 specimens of serum, one in the acute-phase and one in the convalescent-phase of disease, with a 4-fold rise in antibody titer between, has been required to diagnose a patient's infection. However, nowadays the demonstration of virus-specific antibodies in the IgM fraction of a single convalescent-phase specimen of serum is often taken as indicative of recent infection with certain viruses when acute-phase serum is unavailable. It needs to be remembered, that valuable as serology is, it requires the use of *known viral antigens*, and thus can never supplant virus isolation as a discoverer of new viruses. However, once this discovery has been accomplished, viral serology is a powerful tool in assessing the significance of viruses on an individual and community basis.

The detection of virus and viral antigen without prior isolation in laboratory hosts is the category where most progress has occurred in recent years. Insensitive techniques in this area are not new (immunodiffusion and complement fixation for example) but lately there has been an upgrading of the sensitivity of these older methods and the introduction of new ones. Whereas some of these methods, such as electron microscopy (EM), may identify viruses to the morphologic level only, the addition of an immunologic component to the tests enables identification to proceed to the level of the specific virus (for example, immune electron microscopy [IEM]). The advantages of many of these newer methods lie in their rapidity and in the fact that some of them (EM and IEM) permit the detection of viruses currently undetectable by any other means (i.e., unable to be cultivated). Whereas it is conceivable that some of these methods will some day take the place of routine virus isolation for those viruses already discovered, the most sensitive of them depend on the availability of antiserum to known viruses. Thus with the exception of situations where large quantities of antigen are produced and are thus detectable by EM alone (e.g., hepatitis B, rotaviruses), these techniques, like serology, are unlikely to substitute for virus isolation in the discovery of *new* viruses. They will, however, be increasingly used with known viruses to shorten the time required for diagnosis either by application directly to specimens from patients (smears, etc.) or by hastening the process of detection and identification in specimens which are undergoing virus isolation procedures.

Choice of tests employed

As outlined at the beginning of this chapter, the resources devoted to viral diagnosis, themselves determined by consideration of local needs, are one factor determining the range of activities carried out by a laboratory. As a general rule, the microscopic techniques (category 1) are usually capable of implementation either at, or in association with, most virus laboratories— even the smaller ones such as annexes to bacteriology laboratories. Similarly it is often possible for such small laboratories to purchase commercial serologic reagents for those viruses most commonly encountered in that community and to carry out serologic diagnosis for these agents. Virus isolation techniques, require a more substantial investment of resources and are usually performed only by larger laboratories. Finally, the tests in category 4 are usually employed by laboratories of larger size devoted fully to diagnostic virology.

Even in the most sophisticated laboratories, however, the full range of techniques is rarely employed on any given patient. Good stewardship of resources dictates that those methods be used which will lead to the best chance of etiologic diagnosis *at the level required, with the minimal cost, in the shortest reasonable time*. Each of these 3 considerations is important:

Etiologic diagnosis can take place at several levels of specificity. For example, at the beginning of an outbreak of influenza it is important to know whether the agent is a new variant or not. This requires virus isolation from the first few patients and careful characterization of the strain of the virus. Later on in the same epidemic it might be sufficient merely to identify the isolated virus to the level of its antigenic type or even to carry out serologic studies to confirm the clinical diagnosis. Achieving diagnosis at minimum cost is important. Some techniques are inherently more expensive than others without having the capacity to yield additional diagnostic information. From the viewpoint of rapidity of diagnosis, what is reasonable time for one patient may not be so for another. In situations where chemotherapy is available (e.g., severe herpesvirus infections), where speed of diagnosis is

REQUEST FOR VIRUS INVESTIGATION

- -

SURNAME: (Capitals)	Other Names	Age	Sex	Laboratory No.

SPECIMEN	Time Collected	Date	Hospital No.	Ward

THIS SECTION FOR LABORATORY USE ONLY

EXAMINATION REQUESTED: . . . .
DOCTOR SUBMITTING SPECIMEN: . . . .
POSTAL ADDRESS FOR REPORT: . . . .
CLINICAL HISTORY: (i) Onset date . . . . (ii) Virus suspected . . . .
(iii) Clinical findings: . . . .
. . . .
(iv) Other laboratory results relevant to virus studies . . . .
. . . .
. . . .
. . . .
EPIDEMIOLOGIC FACTORS:
PATIENT'S ADDRESS (suburb or town) . . . . . . ANIMAL CONTACTS? . . . .
PATIENT'S OCCUPATION (or that of parent) . . . .
SIMILAR ILLNESS IN FAMILY? . . . . RECENT TRAVEL? . . . .
LOCAL EPIDEMICS? . . . .

VIRAL IMMUNIZATION (specify type, and date of last dose):
    Polio ☐   Smallpox ☐
    Influenza ☐   Others ☐

Figure 1.1A—Example of a form providing essential information to accompany a
specimen. The top half of the form is on carbon-type paper. The results are typed onto it for return to the submitting doctor. The copy,
which is on the same sheet as the relevant information below is retained on the laboratory files. The back of the copy serves as a laboratory worksheet (See Fig 1.1B).

needed for patient management (e.g., maternal rubella in pregnancy), where
etiologic diagnosis has important public health implications (e.g., smallpox,
exotic diseases and new strains of influenza), and in certain life-threatening
and serious infections, the rapidity of diagnosis is paramount and the extra
cost involved in achieving quick results is of secondary importance. In other

LABORATORY USE ONLY

ISOLATION ATTEMPTS:

Host		Passages			Agent Isolated		Identification
		1st	2nd	3rd	No	Yes	
Eggs	Route:						
Mice	Adult						
	Suckling						
Tissue Culture	MK						
	Fibroblasts						
	Others						

SEROLOGIC STUDIES:
Paired Serum Specimens received?   Yes   No

Virus or Antigen	Type of Test	Titer (or other result)

OTHER INVESTIGATIONS (detail):

Figure 1.1B—Reverse side of a request form shown in Fig. 1.1A. Used as a laboratory worksheet to provide a status report of progress of investigations.

situations where no immediate action will ensue as a consequence of diagnosis, cost considerations take precedence over those of rapidity.

The choice of tests is also influenced by the nature of the patient's illness. Where the possible etiology or etiologies can be suggested on clinical, epidemiologic, or other grounds, the selection of viral tests is greatly simplified. For example, sometimes the probable etiology of a severe disease which is a known safety hazard in the laboratory, may mean that there is positive virtue in *not* trying to isolate the agent in a laboratory poorly equipped for high-risk work—but rather carrying out the diagnosis serologically. Similarly, where the clinical and/or biochemical information indicates a group of viruses, with which the usual attempts at cultivation are unlikely to be fruitful (e.g., hepatitis) serologic and antigen detecting methods would be chosen but attempts to routinely isolate virus would not. On the other hand, a situation militating against *serologic* diagnosis is where an illness has a great number of potential causes, each serologic test requiring a separate and unrelated antigen. In such situations, virus isolation is usually attempted as a first approach, serum only being used to assess the significance of any agent isolated. (Sometimes a compromise approach is adopted here, serum being tested for antibodies to the more likely of these agents). Where no possible etiology is suggested for a patient's illness, choice of tests is more difficult. Usually the procedure adopted is to test "likely" specimens for virus isolation and to retain serum for antibody testing against any agent isolated.

From the foregoing it should be evident that the virologist will be severely hampered in his capacity to make appropriate decisions concerning the choice of tests to employ, if he does not have relevant information concerning the patient. Consequently, it is of paramount importance that the communication between physician and laboratory be kept free and open.

Finally, sometimes the *specimens* received themselves dictate the choice of tests. For example, it may be useless to attempt virus isolation from specimens which are obviously contaminated, collected too late in the course of the illness, or inappropriately stored and transported. One may need to resort to serologic diagnosis in such cases. Conversely, there are occasions when serologic diagnosis is inappropriate. A common situation in this regard is where the patient is unable to furnish a convalescent-phase specimen of serum, either because of intervening death, discharge from medical care, or some other reason.

Choice, storage, and transport of specimens

Although each of the diagnostic categories has its own peculiar requirements in these respects, some matters are common to all. The choice and timing of specimens to be submitted depends on the agents suspected. If a brief check-list, based on clinical symptoms, the agents in the area likely to cause the symptoms, and the specimens which should be submitted, can be distributed to medical practitioners, submission of the most profitable types of specimens will be facilitated.

The appropriate conditions of storage and transport of specimens differ depending on the test category and are discussed separately. Common to all is the need to maintain the activity of the feature being sought in the specimen, be it virus, antibody, or antigen. In addition, all require that the specimen be *safely contained* in transit, *clearly labeled*, and *accompanied by relevant information*. An example of an appropriate form for this purpose is seen in Figure 1.1A. It is convenient to use the reverse side of this form as a laboratory "progress sheet" (Fig 1.1B).

Laboratory Organization

Of the virus diagnostic approaches mentioned above, all or only some may be carried out in a given laboratory. Consequently, it is difficult to discuss laboratory organization in a way that embraces all the circumstances which may be encountered in a local situation. The considerations of safety and siting of work areas are pertinent to virus laboratories in general and bear brief mention.

The measures taken to curtail infection of staff in any pathology laboratory are applicable to virus laboratories. In addition, certain aspects of diagnostic virology demand a heightened awareness of the risks involved and corresponding safety measures. These factors include the general lack of antiviral chemotherapy if infection should occur, the slim but distinct possibility that the living host systems used may themselves be infected with a pathogen, and the possibility of aerosol infection during the homogenization procedures which are commonly used to prepare specimens for virus isolation. Methods designed to minimize these risks of infection among personnel are detailed in a subsequent chapter. With respect to laboratory organization, it is imperative that laboratory areas should be quite separate from areas used for glassware preparation, storage, eating, and administration, and that glassware be decontaminated effectively prior to rewashing. If complex and expensive equipment is to be used by another laboratory, as well as the virus laboratory, care must be taken to explain the risks of infection and to educate the personnel of the other laboratory about the procedures to be used.

Unless strict precautions are taken it is possible to unwittingly infect living assay systems such as cell cultures, with the result that they become overtly diseased, or perhaps worse, chronic carriers of contaminating virus. For this reason it is essential that the preparation areas for living hosts (i.e., cell culture preparation area, animal breeding area, and egg incubator) be kept quite separate from those areas where viruses (or viral antigens and human sera) are being used. This requirement also applies to refrigeration facilities. Even within the remainder of the laboratory it is desirable to separate "dirty" (i.e., potentially highly infectious) areas such as virus isolation areas from "less dirty" areas, such as serology.

Equipping the Virus Laboratory

Because of the various combinations in which the diagnostic activities listed above may be engaged and the degree to which they may be integrated with other laboratories, it is difficult to prepare lists of equipment that will be suitable for all situations. A further difficulty is the degree to which numbers of specimens justify the use of automation in a given laboratory. With techniques requiring expensive equipment, such as electron microscopy or radioimmunoassay, it may be necessary to share equipment with other laboratories. With these limitations, the following lists represent a rough guide to the major equipment needed to carry out diagnostic activities of virus isolation, serologic, and antigen detecting categories. (Light microscopy of fixed and stained specimens is not usually the province of the virus laboratory, and the equipment required for this activity is not discussed here).

TABLE 1.1—EQUIPMENT FOR VIRUS ISOLATION AND IDENTIFICATION

ITEM	FUNCTION
ANIMAL INOCULATION	
Holding facilities—uninfected animals —infected animals	
Incinerator/autoclave	Disposal of infected carcases
Instruments (scalpels, scissors, forceps)	Postmortem examination of animals
Needles, syringes	Inoculation of animals
Postmortem facilities (hood, table etc.)	Postmortem examination
Sterilizer (bench)	Sterilization, disinfection of instruments
EGG INOCULATION	
Candling device (fertility tester)	Examination and inoculation of eggs
Dental drill & carborundum disc	Egg inoculation
Egg incubator—uninfected eggs	Development of fertile eggs
Egg incubator—inoculated eggs	Incubation of inoculated eggs
Egg racks	Incubation of inoculated eggs
CELL CULTURE INOCULATION	
Cornwall pipette or pipetting machine	Cell culture preparation
Glassware: Trypsinization flasks, cell culture tubes, beakers, bottles, etc. (or equivalent in sterile plastic)	Cell culture preparation
Incubators (or hot rooms) 37 C 33 C (optional)	Growth of cells and maintenance of infected cells
Incubator (CO_2 humidified)—(optional)	Growth of cells and maintenance of infected cells (with gaseous exchange)
Liquid nitrogen container and controlled rate freezing device	Preservation of cell cultures
Magnetic stirring device	Cell culture preparation
Microscope (binocular) and special tube adaptors	Examination of cell cultures (tubes)
Microscope (inverted)	Examination of cell cultures (bottles)
Millipore filter apparatus and pressure/vacuum pump	Sterilization of heat-labile cell culture media components
Refrigerator 4 C	Storage of cell culture media components
−20 C (deep freeze)	
−70 C (deep freeze)	Storage of stock viruses
4 C	Temporary storage of specimens and viruses etc.
Racks—cell culture—stationary	Growth of cell cultures
Roller drum and motor	Maintenance of inoculated cell cultures
"Sterile" room or laminar flow cabinet	Preparation of cell cultures
Safe working cabinet or hood	Manipulation of viruses and specimens
GENERAL	
Autoclave/Sterilizing oven	Sterilization of solutions and glassware, etc.
Balance—rough	Preparations of media and solutions
—fine	
Centrifuge—bench	Specimen preparation and general laboratory manipulation
—refrigerated	
—ultracentrifuge	Virus purification (and serology)
Distilled water apparatus (high purity)	Solution and media preparation and glass-washing
Homogenizer/blender	Specimen and virus stock preparation
Lyophilization apparatus (optional)	Preservation of virus stocks
pH meter	Preparation of media and solutions
Ultrasonic disintegrator	Preparation of virus stocks or specimens etc.

TABLE 1.2—EQUIPMENT USED IN SEROLOGY

ITEM	FUNCTION
Diluent dispenser (micro and macro)	Pipetting buffer for serum dilution
Fluorescence microscope	Indirect immunofluorescence (especially on IgM fractions of serum)
Microtiter system (manual, semi- or fully automatic) including plates, loops, mirror, shaker)	Performing microtiter serology
Pipette—mechanical—with disposable tips	Preparing initial serum dilution
Serologic racks and tubes	Preparing initial serum dilution and agglutination tests
Storage system for −20 C deep freeze	Storage and retrieval of serum
Water baths—variable setting	Inactivation of serum (56 C) and incubation of antigen-antibody (37 C) etc.

Virus isolation and identification

These activities require equipment for:
Production or maintenance of living host systems
Safe processing and inoculation of specimens
Observation of inoculated hosts for signs of viral infection
Identification of the agents isolated.

If laboratory animals and cell cultures (and media) are commercially available, space and equipment requirements are accordingly reduced. However, even if this is so, some facilities are needed for the maintenance of these hosts after inoculation. Similar reductions in the size of animal-care facilities can be made if commercially produced antiserum is used for virus identification. In the list which follows, a fairly comprehensive laboratory is envisaged, which nevertheless has access to the commercial sources mentioned. An attempt has been made to accompany each item with the purpose for which it is used, but obviously many items have more than a single function (Table 1.1).

Equipment for serology

In addition to the preceding equipment the following items are needed for serologic work. Most of the items concern *in vitro* tests which do not use cell cultures. Materials listed above are also used for serologic tests involving living hosts (animals, eggs, cell cultures) and for serologic tests on serum fractions (ultracentrifuge) (Table 1.2).

Antigen and virus detection

The equipment needed here is dependent on the types of pursuits to be engaged in. Electron microscopy and immune electron microscopy require not only a high quality electron microscope but also the associated equipment needed for fixing, sectioning, and negative staining etc.

Immunofluorescence will utilize a fluorescence microscope, and possibly a cryostat. Radioimmunoassay techniques need a gamma counter. Often these expensive items are shared with other laboratories. Immunoenzyme studies can be carried out with an ordinary visible light microscope, or a simple colorimeter if the color changes are not to be visualized microscopically.

Diagnostic Approaches

Direct microscopic examination of clinical material

For many years histopathologists have recognized that certain abnormalities in fixed and stained cells and tissues of patients are indicative of viral diseases, and that in many instances it is possible to put forward a tentative designation of the viruses involved by the type of changes seen (5). A number of virus groups induce such changes, and the tissues in which they are seen include not only those taken at postmortem examination but also biopsy specimens, urine sediments, scraping from surfaces of the body and bases of vesicles, occular lesions, and aspirates from the body. A variety of changes can be encountered, and these can be either primary manifestations of intracellular viral activity (inclusions and giant cells for example) or secondary changes associated with the inflammatory response.

Histopathologic methods currently play a far less dominant role than they previously did in diagnostic virology. This is chiefly because in only relatively few instances are the changes seen of sufficient specificity to be pathognomonic for a single virus; in addition the absence of significant histologic changes in a specimen is not always indicative of the absence of virus (i.e., the histologic methods are often relatively insensitive). Nowadays histologic methods have been largely superseded by microscopic techniques of greater virus specificity, such as immunofluorescence, electron miscroscopy, and immune electron microscopy.

However, there are circumstances where histopathologic tests have some value; for example, where a presumptive diagnosis of a virus giving a typical histologic picture is required rapidly (for example, Negri bodies in rabies) or where a rapid but presumptive etiologic distinction should be made between 2 agents of greatly different public health significance which have similar clinical symptoms (smallpox and varicella). In both these examples, there are now more virus-specific microscopic tests available (see later), but these are not as widespread in their usage, and some immediate public health action may be required before specimens can be transported to a center where these tests are available. It is important in such circumstances that confirmatory tests of a more virus-specific nature be carried out subsequently. The other situation in which histopathologic study has often been useful is where routine studies of postmortem specimens or blood films have revealed features which have led to successful virus isolation attempts being made on the unfixed portions of such tissues and blood specimens.

Specimens

When smears and films themselves are to be sent to the laboratory, care should be taken to obtain material in the acute phase of the disease, on clean glass slides, clearly labeled, and sent in a way in which the material cannot rub off during transit. In all cases the material on the slide should be regarded as potentially infectious and packed and labeled accordingly. Specimens are best sent air-dried with sufficient clinical information to permit the most appropriate methods of fixing and staining in the laboratory.

It is worthwhile remembering that, with the exception of poxviruses, the virus manifestation looked for is intracellular, and therefore the specimen should contain as large an amount of cellular material as possible. For example, a scraping from the base of a vesicle is generally to be preferred to vesicle fluid for such work.

Portions of biopsy and postmortem specimens should be placed in fixative promptly after collection (Bouin or Zenker acetic acid fixatives are good), and some unfixed material retained for virus-specific studies. Separate sets of instruments and specimen containers for each different tissue should be used to prevent cross-contamination when carrying out autopsy on a case of suspected viral etiology.

Examination and interpretation

Experience is required for meaningful interpretation of the fixed and stained smears. Furthermore, it is desirable that the tentative result obtained by histopathology be confirmed by one or more of the techniques described below. On occasion this confirmation can be obtained by testing smear material itself (e.g., smallpox virus isolation-unfixed smears), but more often separate specimens of a more substantial volume are required. As intimated above, the value of a positive test is somewhat limited and that of a negative test is nil.

Isolation and identification of viruses

Of the several diagnostic approaches, isolation and identification of viruses from clinical material have a unique contribution to make in a number of situations. These are: when confirmation of a tentative diagnosis based on microscopy is required; when the illness being investigated is a previously undescribed one, or is so obscure that serologic investigation is without a "starting point" in terms of choice of antigens; and when the symptoms, though characteristic, may be caused by so many viruses that serology on a routine basis would be impracticable (for example sporadic mild upper respiratory tract infections). From the practical viewpoint, virus isolation is also often able to establish a diagnosis in situations for which serology alone would normally suffice, but for reasons such as death or mobility of patients, only early acute-phase serum is received.

Specimen choice

The choice of specimens to be collected for virus isolation depends on the nature of the symptoms of the patient and a knowledge of the pathogenesis of the agent(s) suspected (if such suspicion exists). Where the index of suspicion for an agent or group of agents is high, appropriate specimens may be determined by reference to later chapters on the viruses concerned.

When no such index exists but symptoms indicate involvement of definite systems of the body ("target organs"), this in itself is a guide—for example throat washings and nasal swabs in upper respiratory tract disease, cerebrospinal fluid (CSF) in disturbances of the central nervous system (CNS) and so on. In geographic localities where the bulk of a certain type of disease tends to be predominantly associated with a group of viruses whose pathogenesis includes other body systems in addition to the target organ, specimens from these sites should be taken as well. When the clinical symptoms are not so distinctive, the general practice is to collect specimens from a variety of materials (feces, urine, nasopharyngeal washings, blood and possibly other sites) and to attempt virus isolation from these. However, for economic reasons, there is a limit to the degree to which laboratories can engage in this type of procedure.

Specimen collection and transport

Infectivity is usually the first property of viruses to be lost in the face of adverse environmental conditions. For this reason it is especially important that specimens for virus isolation be collected from patients at a time when they might be expected to contain virus in highest concentration (i.e., the acute phase) and that they be transported to the laboratory under conditions designed to retain their viral content. As the laboratory staff do not usually collect specimens, this requires education of those who do, and also may necessitate provision of suitable containers for collection and safe transport.

Most of the specimens submitted for virus isolation fall broadly into *excretions* and *exudates* (feces, urine, saliva, sputum, nasopharyngeal aspirates, CSF, vesicle fluid), *tissues* (biopsy and autopsy), and *swabs* (throat, rectal, nasopharyngeal, eye, vesicle). The first 2 groups should be placed in leakproof containers without additives, and the third in small bottles containing a fluid designed to maintain the viability of viruses. Such fluids are usually an isotonic salt solution of some kind with added virus-stabilizing protein such as bovine albumin or antibody-free serum. Dry swabs should *not* be submitted. Specimen-bottle tops should each be screwed on tightly and checked for leakage. They should then immediately be placed in the nonfreezing section of a refrigerator until sent to the laboratory. Specimens may be frozen prior to despatch only if transport is expected to be unavailable for a prolonged period of time (freezing and thawing inactivates some viruses). During transit, which should be as rapid as possible, specimens should be *kept* cold until arrival in the laboratory. In situations where the specimen collection from the patient occurs in close proximity to the laboratory, for example in hospital-based laboratories, specimens may simply be placed upright in a rigid container in such a way that they are unable to topple over. When the distance between the laboratory and collection point is greater, it is wise (and, if sent by mail, legally required) to place the specimen container within a larger leakproof container, wedged with sufficient absorbent material to completely absorb the contents should leakage inadvertently occur during transit. This larger container should itself be placed in a container containing sufficient refrigerant to keep the specimen at the required temperature (frozen or cold only as the case may be) until arrival in the laboratory. If unaccompanied by courier, an advance notice of the parcel's arrival often obviates virus loss due to prolonged standing at post offices pending collection or delivery.

Processing of specimens prior to inoculation

Upon arrival in the laboratory the specimens should be stored either in the cold or frozen state (depending on its temperature at arrival and the expected time lapse before processing), and the details concerning it entered in the laboratory records by laboratory (not clerical) staff. In virus isolation work, when specimens are inoculated into a number of host systems each of which is to be observed on many occasions over many days, it is important to devise a recording system which permits progress reports to be made on specimens and does not allow specimens to become lost in the system.

Before specimens are inoculated, they are treated to get the virions present into suspension, free from nonviral agents (e.g., bacteria, toxins, very high or low pH) which might confuse diagnosis by their effect upon the inoculated hosts. This treatment should have minimal effect on the virus content of the specimen. Some specimens, such as bacteria-free CSF, require no treatment. Others, such as feces and solid tissues, require homogenization in about 10 volumes of fluid (usually a balanced salt solution containing a pH indicator and protein) and low-speed centrifugation to deposit debris and leave viruses in suspension. To the resultant supernatant fluid and other potentially contaminated liquid specimens received, antibiotics are usually added to eliminate any bacterial and fungal flora remaining. If subsequent nonviral infection of the inoculated host reveals that this has not been accomplished, the original suspension is filtered through a 0.4μm pore-size filter to remove such contaminants. If it is obvious that the pH of the suspension is such as might have an adverse effect on the host (especially cell culture) it should be brought to neutrality. Specimens should be retained in the refrigerator until it is certain that nonvirus artefacts have not occurred. A further reason for retaining such specimens is to provide for reisolation should this be necessary.

Two other things are of importance in the processing of specimens for virus isolation. The first is operator safety. For example, manipulations conducive to aerosol formation should be carried out in safety cabinets if possible. Similarly, wherever a "closed system" method can be devised in specimen preparation it is to be preferred. (For example agitation of fecal suspensions with beads in a centrifugable, screw-cap container is preferable to grinding with abrasive in a mortar and pestle). Secondly, specimens must be processed separately, not in batches, to avoid cross-contamination occurring between specimens.

Host inoculation

The host systems used most commonly in the diagnostic laboratory are: laboratory animals, fertile hen eggs, and cell cultures of various types. Each has its virtues and its limitations, and none detect all viruses. As economic considerations preclude inoculating every specimen into every host system, a choice has to be made as to which hosts should be inoculated. Sometimes this choice is comparatively simple. For example in an influenza epidemic for which the host range of the prevailing strain has been established, it is not unusual to restrict the inoculation of specimens from typical cases to the host which has successfully grown the current strain of virus. A similar situation occurs when a characteristic set of symptoms, history, and other laboratory data indicate that a single virus, or group of viruses, are likely to be involved (for example, congenital infections). Here, a knowledge of the host range of the viruses known to cause such infections determines the hosts to be inoculated. In the majority of cases, however, the symptoms of the patient may be caused by many known viral pathogens, and a broader range of hosts must be used. This requires discernment and a good knowledge of the growth characteristics of the candidate agents.

Animals are especially sensitive as detectors of certain groups of viruses (e.g., suckling mice for arboviruses and coxsackie A viruses) but are expensive to produce and maintain. Many species possess their own viruses which are capable of activation by laboratory manipulation and thus of confusing the isolation of the human pathogen inoculated. Furthermore, they are not as susceptible to as wide a range of human viruses as are cell cultures. In this respect the veterinary virologist has an advantage over his medical counterpart in that he can often use for his detector system, animals of the same species as that contributing the specimen. Of the common laboratory animals, only the mouse has found widespread usage for the isolation of human viruses. For many viruses, suckling mice are more susceptible than adults, and thus sucklings are routinely used (an exception here are the arenaviruses). Inoculation is usually by either the intracranial or intraperitoneal routes.

Fertile hen eggs are less expensive than laboratory animals, but once again have a restricted virus range. However, their use is indicated in some situations where they may be especially sensitive, for example with certain strains of influenza and some arboviruses. Eggs may be inoculated at different ages (days postincubation) and by various routes, depending on the virus sought. The most commonly used routes are the amniotic, chorioallantoic membrane (CAM), and yolk sac. The allantoic route is frequently used to propagate large quantities of certain viruses which have been first adapted to growth in eggs by amniotic inoculation. Details of inoculation techniques are given on pages 42–48.

Cell culture inoculation is the most widely used method of virus isolation, and a later chapter is devoted to the use of cell cultures in diagnostic virology. There is no single cell culture which is sensitive to all the viruses likely to be encountered. Choice therefore needs to be made as to which cultures should be kept propagating for routine use in the laboratory and which should be reserved for occasional use (purchased when needed or stored in liquid nitrogen). This choice will vary from laboratory to laboratory. A common practice is to routinely inoculate specimens into 1 primary culture (usually monkey kidney cell cultures), 1 diploid cell strain, and perhaps 1 heteroploid cell line (e.g., HeLa, HEp-2). The latter type of culture is usually kept propagating chiefly for purposes of serology (see later), but is sometimes used as an isolation host as well. Special purpose cell lines, e.g.,

RK13 cells for rubella, are brought into use upon demand. Very rarely, organ cultures are used to facilitate the detection of viruses which cannot be propagated in conventional cell cultures.

Observation of inoculated hosts for evidence of infection

Laboratory animals are observed at daily or twice-daily intervals for 2 weeks or more for signs of infection. These vary with the host inoculated and the agent concerned and may include such obvious things as paralysis, tremors, convulsions, abnormal gait, runting, ruffled fur, and death. Sometimes, however, the evidence of infection may be of a more subtle kind, such as elevated temperature or the development of antibodies to the infecting agent.

In inoculated eggs, death of the embryo, seen by examination with an egg candler sometimes occurs, but more frequently infection is discerned by the examination of fluids and tissues harvested 2–6 days after inoculation, by techniques such as antigen detection (hemagglutinin, complement-fixing antigen), or pock formation.

In cell cultures, low-power microscopic examination over a period of 1–2 weeks or more may indicate the presence of virus in the form of an abnormality, marked or subtle, in cell morphology (cytopathic effect [CPE]). Alternatively, there may be no such effects, with virus being detected by other means. These include the presence of hemagglutinins in cell culture fluid, hemadsorption (the attachment of erythrocytes to infected cells) interference with CPE of viruses normally cytopathic or the presence of viral antigen detected by immunofluorescence, immunoenzyme, and immunoradioisotopic techniques. Electron microscopy of the infected culture may also be carried out.

When no evidence of infection is seen in the inoculated host and in specimens with equivocal evidence of infection, a "blind passage" of material from this host may be inoculated into fresh hosts. This procedure sometimes results in amplification and hence unequivocal detection of virus; in others it does not, probably indicating that the equivocal effect previously seen was caused by toxic substances present in the original specimen. As mentioned previously, residual bacteria and fungi which have resisted treatment during specimen preparation may sometimes cause effects in inoculated hosts. These are best met by filtering the specimen and reinoculating them into fresh hosts.

Virus identification

In experienced hands, useful clues to the identity of the isolated agent may be furnished by the *range* of hosts in which an effect is caused and the *type* of abnormality seen in them. This, together with a consideration of the origin of the specimen and the clinical information received with it, can often allow a provisional identification, to group level, to be made. Even if this is not so, a series of simple tests, such as size estimation and ether sensitivity may lead to the agent being categorized, thus furnishing some basis for more definitive identification. In laboratories with access to EM facilities, negative staining and EM examination of concentrated virus from infected hosts, if positive, provides precise information to the morphologic group into which the agent falls.

The avenues adopted for more specific identification differ according to the tentative grouping assigned to the agent, the level of specificity at which identification is desired, and the haste with which it is needed. Sometimes the nature of the specimen and its characteristics in cell culture, taken together with a typical clinical picture, are sufficient to furnish an identification sufficient for most purposes. Such is usually the case, for example, when the slowly progressing CPE characteristic of cytomegalovirus is seen in human diploid fibroblast cultures inoculated with urine from an infant with cytomegalic inclusion disease.

However, in most circumstances, further tests, usually of a serologic nature or at least employing a serologic component, are needed to specifically identify the isolated agent. These all employ antiserum of known titer and known specificity for members of the group of viruses into which the unknown isolate has been tentatively placed. Most of the techniques discussed in the following section on serologic diagnosis may be used for virus identification. However these immunologic tests differ from one another in sensitivity and specificity and this must be taken into account in choosing the method to be used in serologic identification. Sometimes it is necessary to treat the crude virus preparation obtained from the infected host in order to obtain antigen of the requisite specificity (for example, mouse brain infected with certain arboviruses is treated to obtain hemagglutinin (HA) suitable for use in the broadly reactive hemagglutination inhibition (HAI) test).

Where there is no usable group or subgroup reactive antigen and each member of a morphologic or otherwise designated group is a distinct antigenic entity, it is necessary to employ virus-specific antiserum in a series of individual tests. This is cumbersome if the group is large, especially if there is no way to avoid the use of living host systems (neutralization [Nt] tests). In such situations, it is desirable to employ an antiserum pooling system of some type (see the chapter on picornaviruses).

To optimize the effect of the antiserum used, virus identification tests require the estimation of activity of the unknown virus, by the parameter to be used in the test (infectivity, complement-fixing (CF) activity, HA content). Sometimes, especially in experienced hands, this estimation can be done simultaneously with the identification test, but often it is more economical to do it beforehand (this especially being so in Nt tests). Information on methods of calculating infectivity titers, employed in these situations, is given in the *Appendix*.

Significance of virus isolation

Most viruses are able to infect a proportion of the population without causing symptoms, and some viruses persist for extended periods in the body after infection. It follows that the isolation of a virus from a patient's specimen is not necessarily to be taken as proof that the patient's current disease has been caused by the virus isolated (or for that matter, by any virus). A number of factors are involved in deciding whether the virus isolated actually caused the symptoms exhibited. Among these are the site from which the positive specimen was taken relative to the probable site of the pathologic process (for example the causal role of an enterovirus recovered from a patient with meningitis would be more firmly established if recovered from CSF than from feces). Again, the previously reported capacity of a virus isolated to cause similar disease may strengthen belief in a causal association in the case being investigated, as may the absence of the virus from healthy populations being monitored or from patients with other types of disease. Despite consideration of these factors, situations still arise when the significance of virus isolation is uncertain. This is compounded when 2, or even 3, different viruses are isolated simultaneously from the same patient. The use of serology to determine antibody responses to the viruses often helps unravel such interpretive problems, but in some instances it never becomes possible to be sure that an etiologic relationship exists between virus isolated and symptoms seen. And when newly discovered agents are unearthed, a period always needs to elapse until sufficient cases accumulate to permit evaluation of significance.

On the other hand, *failure* to recover virus from a patient does not necessarily mean that the illness is of nonviral etiology. Not all human viruses are cultivable by even the best existing methods, and failure to cultivate virus may simply reflect the inappropriateness of the cultivation techniques used. Less justifiable causes of failure may be the collection of the wrong specimens, collection of specimens too late in the course of the illness (virus content tends to decline in the body with time after onset), or poor transport and storage techniques. For all these reasons, the appropriate result to be reported after fruitless attempts to isolate virus is "No virus was isolated," rather than "virus was not present."

Reporting of virus isolation attempts

A recording system capable of yielding prompt information on the current progress of isolation attempts on any specimen is a necessity. One useful scheme is to use the back of the form carrying the specimen information as a check list (see Fig 1.1B) and to file these forms alphabetically for ready reference until all tests on the specimen are completed. If all tests prove negative, a copy (photo or carbon) of the front of the form is sent to the physician with "No virus was isolated" thereon, and the back copy with the check list is retained in the laboratory. If a virus is recovered from the specimen, a progress report to that effect is sent to the physician immediately with a provisional designation of the virus *group* involved, based on the host range and cultural properties of the agent. This is followed by a final report (front copy) when the definite identification of the agent has been made.

Serologic diagnosis of viral infections

Most viruses induce the formation of detectable levels of specific antibody following a primary infection and may exhibit a boost in titer following subsequent stimulus (reinfection or sometimes reactivation). With certain exceptions, mentioned below, it is thus the *development* of antibodies at or after illness, not merely their presence, which is diagnostically significant.

The significance lies in the fact that antibody development in an ill patient indicates infection *at about the same time* as the onset of illness. This confluence is unlikely to be merely a coincidence and is thus usually indicative of a causal relationship between disease and virus eliciting the antibody development. Where unavailability of acute-phase serum precludes the demonstration of antibody development, the presence of specific antibody in the IgM fraction of patients' later serum is often indicative of recent or current infection with that agent. Similarly, the possession of very high levels of CF antibody in convalescent-phase serum may sometimes be diagnostically significant.

In addition to its unique epidemiologic role in serum surveys, serology has several great virtues in diagnostic virology. Some of these are economic in nature. Serology is often the least expensive way to establish a diagnosis, especially when a limited range of agents is being considered. The fact that many antigens are now commercially available enables the serologic approach to be adopted for the diagnosis of viral diseases in bacteriology laboratories not equipped to produce viral antigens. The miniaturization of many serologic tests and the automation procedures available have reduced the cost of reagents and labor, and have also enabled testing for a wide range of antibodies in quite small samples of serum.

Economic considerations aside, serology has other advantages. It often enables a diagnosis to be reached when virus isolation either is negative or cannot be attempted. By fixing the approximate time of viral infection, serology may also permit assessment of the significance of virus isolation where otherwise this assessment would be difficult. This is especially pertinent in infections with viruses which persist for long periods after infection. The relative stability of antibody to adverse environmental conditions renders serologic diagnosis particularly useful in those situations where distance from the laboratory usually leads to inactivation of viruses in specimens sent for isolation. Serologic diagnosis is often more rapid than virus isolation, especially of slow growing viruses, and, finally, serology is of particular value when the aim of investigations is to establish that the patient has *not* undergone infection with a given virus. For example, patients regularly develop HAI antibody after rubella infection. Consequently negative *serologic* results can definitely exclude rubella from the differential diagnosis. Failure to isolate virus in this situation, however, could be due to a host of factors (discussed under virus isolation) and may thus constitute a false-negative result.

Specimens

Optimally, 2 specimens of serum are required for testing, the first taken as early as possible in the course of the illness and the other 1–2 weeks later. When speed of diagnosis is important and antibody development is rapid (for example, rubella), serum tested at onset and even a day or two later may exhibit a diagnostic change in titer. Conversely, there may be situations where subsequent specimens of serum need to be collected several weeks or even months after onset if antibody development is to be seen (for example, the anti-HBs antibody of hepatitis B). In suspected congenital infections, serum collected at or shortly after birth may be used. In addition subsequent samples are collected from the child at intervals of weeks or months to trace antibody decline or development. Diagnosis may also be achieved by the detection of virus-specific antibody in the IgM fraction of a single specimen of serum collected at birth (congenital infections) or convalescence (postnatal infections).

Whole blood, collected aseptically and without additives, is the specimen of choice for most investigations. If the laboratory is within reasonable traveling time of the collection point (i.e., 1–2 days) serum is usually separated from the clot by centrifugation when it arrives. If this is not so, serum should be removed from clot at the point of collection and stored at 4 C or frozen until despatched. (If no centrifuge is available at the collection point, settling of the sample overnight will usually provide a cell-free sample if care is exercised in removing serum). On no account should whole blood be frozen as the ensuing lysis of red cells complicates certain serologic tests. Ideally, 10 ml of blood should be collected, thus furnishing sufficient for multiple tests and storage if required. However if 10 ml is unobtainable, lesser volumes are quite adequate for many tests, and neonatal serology is frequently carried out on small samples of capillary blood. Specimens for serology should be regarded as potentially infectious and treated accordingly in all phases of processing and testing. This applies of course for other specimens (such as CSF) which are also occasionally submitted for serology.

Provision needs to be made for the storage of serum. In the short term this is necessary to permit the storage of acute-phase serum pending the arrival of the convalescent-phase sample from each patient. (Both sera of a pair must be tested in the *same* test to ensure the validity of any difference in titer between them). From the wider viewpoint, laboratories testing large numbers of serum samples should try to store aliquots of certain pairs of sera for longer, and perhaps indefinite periods of time. These should include *samples* of serum from those patients clearly diagnosed serologically (future "reference" serum). They should also include serum from patients with documented infections, presumed by symptoms and exclusion of alternative etiology to be viral, but for whom exhaustive investigations have failed to reveal a specific cause. Retrospective testing of such serum has often permitted rapid evaluation of the disease-producing role of agents discovered subsequently (often by many years) to their collection. Serum is usually stored frozen (−20 C) to avoid bacterial and fungal growth, but may be stored at 4 C if an inhibitor of microbial growth, such as 0.08% sodium azide (final concentration), is added.

Whichever temperature is used for storage, a system allowing rapid location and retrieval is necessary. Upright and chest-type deep freezes both have advantages, with the former being perhaps generally preferred because of easier retrieval of specimens from them. A −20 C cold room is a great advantage if it can be acquired. Modern freezers have numbered retrieval systems (at a price). An inexpensive alternative is to bore holes in styrofoam (polyurethane) sheets, of a size to take the serum containers. This material has the added advantage of retaining serum in a frozen state when the rack is out of the cold environment. Some system of numbering, visible from the outside is also necessary.

Serologic tests

It is beyond the scope of this chapter to attempt a description of all the serologic techniques currently used in diagnostic virology. They range from the simple to the exceedingly complex, and most are detailed in subsequent chapters.

From the standpoint of inherent *complexity*, the least complex techniques are those in which the presence of antibody is shown by simple interaction with antigen (precipitation or agglutination tests). Next are those tests in which an indicator system is needed to demonstrate that antigen-antibody interaction has occurred. The indicator may be living cells (Nt tests), erythrocytes (HAI tests) or more complex systems involving complement and erythrocytes (immune adherence hemagglutination [IAHA]) or complement and a hemolytic system (CF tests). Even more complex than these are tests in which the presence of antibody is revealed by adding a second (labeled) antibody (from another species of animal) whose specificity is directed against antibodies of the species under test (i.e., anti-immunoglobulin).

From the standpoint of *laboratory practice*, these tests can be grouped into:

In vitro serology—not involving living host systems,

and

Neutralization tests—in which antibody is detected by its inhibitory effect on viral infectivity.

The older-established *in vitro* serologic tests, (CF, HAI, agglutination, and precipitation) involve only moderate expense and may form an adjunct to a bacteriologic laboratory. Tests involving neutralization of viral infectivity are more specialized and costly (especially those involving animals), and are usually carried out only by laboratories which engage in virus isolation activities as well. Some of the more recent *in vitro* tests—such as those utilizing radioisotopes and immunofluorescence (FA)—also require expensive equipment and have a correspondingly restricted usage.

In vitro *tests*

In recent times there has been a great expansion in the number of tests in this group. Indirect immunofluorescence (IFA) has an established role in some infections (rabies for example), passive hemagglutination (PHA) is routine with others (hepatitis B), IAHA with hepatitis A, and radioimmunoisotopic and enzyme-linked immunoassay (ELISA) techniques are established with some viruses and are being evaluated with others. Many of these newer methods are extremely sensitive. However the commonest tests in use are the CF and HAI tests, in that order, and these are discussed in most detail.

Complement-fixation (CF) tests. Because of its applicability to the vast majority of viruses, a virtue shared by no other single method, the CF test is the most widely used of all the serologic tests. Beyond saying that it is based on complement being bound (fixed) by antigen-antibody complexes and that the test involves the competition of 2 antigen-antibody systems (one an indicator) for a fixed amount of complement, we will go no further here into the theory of the method.

Unnecessary variation in the details of CF methodology between laboratories has been a problem rendering interlaboratory comparisons difficult. Features specific to individual virus groups still require that no uniform procedure can be adopted for the preparation of CF antigens for different viruses. However, an encouraging trend towards widespread acceptance of a single method for carrying out the test properly has led us to include the microtiter CF test previously published in the fourth edition of this book and some comments concerning it which appeared there (see pages 38–42).

Hemagglutination-inhibition (HAI) test. This is an extremely valuable test for serologic diagnosis of infections caused by those viruses possessing the property of hemagglutination, i.e., the property to agglutinate erythrocytes of certain animals. Myxoviruses, paramyxoviruses, poxviruses, arboviruses, reoviruses, adenoviruses, rubella, and some picornaviruses are thus endowed, and elicit antibodies which can be detected by specific inhibition of the hemagglutination reaction. The mechanics of the actual test are simpler than those of the CF test. Serial dilutions of patients' serum are allowed to react with a fixed dose of hemagglutinin (HA) and the residual HA is detected by subsequent addition of the appropriate cells. However the test is often complicated by the need to treat serum prior to testing; firstly to remove nonantibody inhibitors of HA which may masquerade as antibody and thus give false-positive results, and secondly to absorb out naturally occurring substances which agglutinate the test erythrocytes and which if not removed, may mask the inhibiting effect of specific viral antibody. Procedures for serum treatment vary from virus to virus, as do other details of the test and associated manipulations such as the preparation of HA antigen from crude material. Similarly, the *specificity* of the test varies from virus to virus, sometimes being wider than that of the CF test and sometimes narrower. For these reasons, no detailed method is given here, and chapters on individual virus groups should be consulted.

Passive (indirect) hemagglutination. With many viruses, themselves incapable of hemagglutination, a useful serologic technique can be devised by coupling viral antigen to the surface of erythrocytes so that when mixed with specific antibody, the erythrocytes are passively (i.e., by antibody) hemagglutinated. The test is often of a very high order of sensitivity, such as with the antibody for hepatitis B surface antigen (anti-HBs). With some agents, the coupling process is a simple one requiring only simple mixing, whereas with others it requires a coupling agent such as chromic chloride or tannic acid and conditions of rigid control.

Agglutination and precipitation techniques. The traditional agglutination and precipitation tests in which the results of antigen-antibody interaction can be seen with the unaided eye or with ordinary microscopy are not widely used in the serologic diagnosis of virus diseases, although they are still used with rickettsiae. The reasons for this are the relatively insensitive nature of the techniques for *antibody* detection and their requirement for large quantities of viral antigen. (It should be noted that immunodiffusion tests still have an important place in identification of viral *antigen*).

Immune adherence hemagglutination (IAHA). Although not widely used as yet, the proven usefulness IAHA in hepatitis work indicates its potential for other agents. It relies on the propensity of complexes of antigen, antibody, and complement to clump certain species of erythrocytes. It is reported as being very much more sensitive than the CF test for the detection of antibodies to hepatitis A and has the added advantage of being less subject to the effect of the anticomplementary activity of serum than is the CF test.

Serologic tests involving anti-immunoglobulin antibody. Recent years have seen rapid expansion in the number of tests in which the combination of antibody with antigen is detected by the addition to the system of a second antibody directed against immunoglobulins of the species contributing the serum under assay. The anti-immunoglobulin antibody is labeled (fluorescein, radioisotope, enzyme) in such a way that it can be detected by the appropriate means (ultraviolet microscope, gamma counter, or color change on reaction with substrate); the corresponding tests being indirect immunofluorescence, radioimmunoassay, and immunoenzyme techniques. There are many variations in methodology. In principle, however, antigen of known specificity attached to a substrate or in solution, is allowed to react with the serum being tested for antibodies. If specific antibody is present, it binds to the antigen. After removing unattached immunoglobulin the labeled anti-immunoglobulin is added. It attaches to any of the first antibody which bound to the antigen. After a second procedure to remove unattached labeled anti-immunoglobulin, the test is examined for residual label, this being a measure of the presence of antibody in the original specimen.

The radioisotope and immunoenzyme tests are more sensitive for many viral antibodies than are most other serologic tests. In addition, all 3 types of test have two other advantages. Firstly, they can be often used for the detection of antibodies to viruses which do not produce sufficient extracellular virus to enable Nt tests to be carried out, and which do not produce either HA or sufficient quantities of CF antigen to permit extensive use of the latter test. The other advantage is concerned with the detection of virus-specific IgM. These techniques allow the detection of such IgM without the need for prior separation (fractionation) of this immunoglobulin from serum under test. This is achieved by using labeled anti-IgM antiserum instead of anti-immunoglobulin as the second antiserum. On the negative side, the FA test and the immunoradioisotope tests require specialized equipment for their performance.

Neutralization tests

Nt (of infectivity) tests, despite their relative antiquity, are still widely used in diagnostic virology. They depend on the finding that the interaction of virus with specific antibody, prior to its inoculation into a susceptible living host system may prevent infection. The way in which the test is set up varies from virus to virus, depending to a large degree on the ability of the virus to infect different assay systems and the types of effects caused in them. Sometimes the index of infection is obvious (death, CPE, pocks, plaques) but in other systems it may need to be elicited by further manipulations such as hemadsorption, interference, immunofluorescence, or testing of the fluids for HA content. In general one tries to opt for cell cultures as assay systems, because of their cost advantage over animals, and to select a cell culture exhibiting a high degree of neutralization (not all cell cultures are alike, even for the same virus, in this respect).

Both nonspecific inhibitors and potentiators of virus neutralization are sometimes present in serum and are often affected by storage. To minimize the possibility of erroneous effects due to these factors, serum is usually heated at 56 C for 30 min prior to testing. In some systems, it is necessary to then add fresh serum or complement to such heated serum to provide the accessory factors needed before the specific antiviral antibody present can exert its full neutralizing effect. In other systems this step is not necessary. Other variables in methodology include the dose of virus used, the route of inoculation (with animals) and the conditions (time and temperature) at which virus and serum are incubated prior to inoculation. Tests may be of a quantitative type, where local lesions such as pocks or plaques are counted, each indicating the presence of one unneutralized virion, or they can be of a semiquantitative nature. In the latter, a larger number of replicate hosts are inoculated with each virus-serum mixture, and an endpoint is estimated on the basis of the proportion of these exhibiting signs of infection. The conventional endpoint is that in which half the inoculated hosts show such signs (50% endpoint), and two methods of calculating these are given in the Appendix. More precise information is given by quantitative tests, but there are circumstances where miniaturization in cell cultures permits semiquantitative tests to be carried out giving precise results at very reasonable cost.

From the viewpoint of quantities of virus and serum mixed together, there are two alternative ways of carrying out Nt tests. In the first, a constant amount of serum (usually undiluted) is mixed with graded, usually logarithmically spaced, dilutions of virus, and antibody activity is calculated as a "Nt index" (i.e., the logarithmic dose of virus neutralized). This "constant serum-varying virus" method is fairly insensitive in demonstrating small changes in antibody level and uses large quantities of serum. The second method, generally preferred, employs a constant dose of virus mixed with serial dilutions of serum, the endpoint usually being calculated on the basis of that serum dilution which neutralizes half of the virus inoculum. By this "constant virus-varying serum" method, smaller changes in antibody content can be detected, and the serum requirement for the test is less.

Practical considerations

For the reasons discussed above, in all tests in which the titers of acute- and convalescent-phase sera are being compared, it is essential that they be tested in the same test run. The test usually includes a negative serum and a positive serum of known titer as a check on the specificity and reproducibility of the test. Much time is saved if the antigen used in the test system (infectious virus, CF, or HA antigen etc.) is of known titer. This can be achieved by producing many identical aliquots, of sufficient size for one test run, placing in conditions which will maintain activity for a known period (-70 C, liquid nitrogen), thawing a sample to estimate activity, and then thawing other aliquots for use at the appropriate dilution in each future test (with a check antigen titration in the test). For safety reasons, noninfectious antigens should be used wherever possible in all but Nt tests.

Most viral serology is done in miniaturized (microtiter) systems. Equipment is available to automate testing either partially or almost completely. The optimal degree of automation depends on the demand, and this needs to be assessed for each laboratory. An assessment also needs to be made on similar grounds on whether it is better to screen serum at a single dilution and then titrate out those with antibody, or whether to do a complete titration on each serum, without prior screening.

Choice of serologic tests

In choosing the type of test to use in a given situation, the factors to be considered are: specificity, the rapidity and longevity of antibody response, sensitivity, and cost.

Specificity. Viruses often possess multiple antigens, some of which are specific for each strain of virus and some of which are shared by related viruses. To test for antibodies to the former requires the use of multiple tests, each using a strain-specific antigen. Unless there are good reasons for carrying out this procedure, such testing should be discouraged in favor of one which tests for antibody development to the group antigen. Thus, in the serologic diagnosis of the sporadic case of influenza, it is better to test for the development of antibodies to the type-specific nucleoprotein (NP) antigens, using the CF test, than to use multiple strain specific antigens in the HAI test.

Rapidity and longevity of antibody response (time sequence). Even when using antigen preparations of the same specificity, the development and persistence of antibody when tested by two different techniques, may not coincide. In rubella, for example, antibodies detectable by the HAI test develop rapidly after onset and usually persist for life, whereas antibodies detectable by CF testing develop later and decline more quickly. Thus, if appropriate serum is available, the HAI test gives a speedier diagnosis, whereas the CF test is more helpful in demonstrating an antibody response if the first specimen collected is late after onset. And, of course, the HAI test gives a better index of prior infection in tests for immunity.

Sensitivity and cost. That different tests for antibody vary in sensitivity has been already mentioned. Unless factors of specificity and time sequence are concerned, there is no value in using a technique of higher sensitivity if all patients infected by the agent develop antibody clearly detectable by a method of lower sensitivity. The general rule is to use the least expensive technique which detects antibody regularly in all infected persons.

Interpretation

Traditionally 2 sera are not considered to have significantly differing antibody titers unless there is at least a 4-fold difference in endpoint in a test in which serial dilutions of serum are tested (most *in vitro* systems). This is a reflection of practical experience under working conditions and is probably a safe practice which minimizes false-positive diagnoses without contributing too many "missed" diagnoses. In tests employing constant serum—varying virus dilutions, the Nt index considered significant varies from virus to virus and individual chapters should be consulted. However, it is usual to regard a Nt index of less than 10-fold (i.e., log Nt index <1) to be insignificant.

The usual situation leading to a positive diagnosis is when the convalescent-phase (second) serum has a significantly higher titer than the acute-phase (first) serum. However, on occasion a *fall* in antibody level between convalescent-phase serum and one taken some weeks subsequently may also indicate a positive diagnosis. This is more likely to happen when CF is used than with other tests, because of the transience of antibody detected by this method.

High antibody titers alone are not a reliable guide to a recent infection, but often experience will permit a *presumptive* diagnosis to be made on the basis of a single high titer in convalescent-phase serum—when no acute-phase specimen is available. It should be emphasized that the diagnosis is only a tentative one, and even then requires considerable experience with the test in question.

A much more confident approach can be made on the basis of a single convalescent-phase specimen (or that of a neonate), when significant levels of virus-specific antibody are detected in the IgM fraction of serum. Because of the transience of the IgM response in postnatal infections, and the inability of maternal IgM to cross the placenta in the newborn, such findings indicate recent or current infections.

Detection of Virus or Viral Antigen without Isolation

The usefulness of procedures aimed at detecting virus-specific antigen directly in specimens without prior virus multiplication in laboratory hosts has been established for many years, immunodiffusion and CF for smallpox antigen probably being the commonest examples. Unfortunately such tests could be applied to only a few viruses, and their sensitivity, compared to virus isolation, was usually low. In recent years however, a plethora of tests of greater sensitivity has developed, prompted to some degree by the need to develop sensitive techniques for the detection of hepatitis B virus and others unable to be easily cultivated in common laboratory hosts. All of these tests are characterized by their ability to detect virus or viral antigen by some index other than one caused by virus multiplication in a laboratory host.

Broadly, such tests have two important applications. Firstly, when antigen or virus concentration is sufficiently high, such tests can detect it *directly in specimens from the patient*. This permits rapid diagnosis of infection (within hours). Whereas this is often a practical advantage with viruses which can be cultivated in the laboratory, it is an even greater asset with viruses which cannot easily be cultivated (for example, hepatitis A, B, and rotaviruses). The secondary application of these techniques is to supplement virus isolation procedures. Certain viruses replicate in cell culture with slowly developing, minimal, or indeed no CPE. If sensitive tests for the detection of antigen are applied to such cultures, a positive result may shorten the time required to achieve a diagnosis.

Most of these techniques are less sensitive than virus isolation methods for viruses which are cultivable. Consequently, when such methods are being used to hasten diagnosis, it is usual to process specimens concurrently by the more traditional methods as well. This practice is commendable, at least until experience shows that no advantage accrues from using both methods.

Specimens

Depending on the viruses concerned, many types of specimens may be submitted for examination by these rapid diagnostic techniques (postmortem tissues, biopsies, blood, serum, vesicle fluids and scrapings, nasal smears, respiratory tract aspirates, fecal matter, and urine). In general, the specimen submitted for such study should be from the site of the pathologic process, or, from sites known in positive cases to contain large concentrations of the virus in question (e.g., serum in hepatitis B, feces in hepatitis A). If the technique requires microscopic examination (immunofluorescence and immunoenzyme methods), it is essential that the specimen contains a substantial cellular component.

Tests

The tests themselves (often referred to as "rapid diagnostic tests") can be broadly grouped into those *without* an essential immunologic component (EM) and those *with* one (the rest of these techniques).

Electron microscopy (EM). Negative staining of material by the addition of heavy metal salts and subsequent examination with the EM by an experienced microscopist allows visualization and thus characterization of agents to morphologic group level. This may be sufficient in itself. Alternatively, the specificity of identification can be enhanced by addition to the test of specific antiserum and observation of subsequent clumping patterns microscopically (IEM). Although EM is limited in its usefulness by its lack of intrinsic specificity, its relative insensitivity, and its unsuitability for processing large numbers of specimens, it has often proven to be the essential point of entry into the study of, and methodology for, undiscovered viruses when more sensitive detection methods, based on antibody of *known specificity*, cannot initially be applied. In addition it has proven usefulness, even at the morphologic level, in the rapid diagnosis of infections when large numbers of virions are present in the specimen, especially when rapid distinction needs to be made between two critical alternatives (e.g., smallpox and chickenpox) of vastly different significance from a public health or clinical viewpoint.

Rapid techniques with an immunologic basis. Immunodiffusion, crossover immunoelectrophoresis, CF, PHA, IAHA, FA, RIA, enzyme immunoassay, and ELISA techniques are all currently used with one or more viruses in the rapid diagnosis of viral infections. All of these techniques may be used either, as discussed here, to detect and identify viral antigen, (provided that *antibody* of known specificity is used), or to estimate the level of antibody in serum, (if *antigen* of known specificity is used). Some brief comments on the principles of the commonly used methods and their application to serologic diagnosis have been given in the preceding section (Serologic Diagnosis of Viral Infections). A few additional remarks need to be made on the use of these methods for detecting and identifying viral antigen in specimens directly from patients.

With all of these immunologically based methods, a choice obviously has to be made of which antiserum to employ. This is a problem not encountered in virus isolation or EM methods and requires information from the person submitting the specimens which will help select candidate agents, as discussed previously. This need for choice of antiserum, with the consequent possibility of the inappropriate antiserum being selected and a false-negative result ensuing, is a reason for carrying out virus isolation studies concurrently.

Immunofluorescence (FA) is currently the most widely used of the rapid immunologically-based techniques for antigen detection, having been applied to most viral infections where antigen is in an intracellular situation and the infected tissues are accessible. Such cells may be examined either by direct FA, where each virus-specific antiserum being used is separately conjugated with fluorescein before being applied to the specimen. Alternatively IFA may be practiced where unconjugated virus-specific antiserum is applied and when, after washing away unattached antibody, a second, fluorescein-labeled antiserum, directed against the immunoglobulins of the species of animal contributing the virus-specific antiserum, is applied. The indirect method has the advantages of greater sensitivity and economy (fewer individual sera need to be conjugated) but requires slightly more time and more controls on specificity.

Immunodiffusion and tests for CF antigen have been used only in situations in which high concentrations of antigen in the specimens make them sufficiently sensitive. Poxvirus infections (skin lesions and serum) and hepatitis B (serum) lend themselves to these approaches although with the latter, more sensitive tests are now generally used. The capacity of the immunodiffusion test to reveal antigenic differences between subtypes make it a valuable epidemiologic tool in situations where this is important.

RIA methods for antigen detection are well established with some viruses (e.g., hepatitis A, hepatitis B) and are being evaluated with others. Their sensitivity with many agents is very high, approaching that of virus isolation methods, and with the solving of technical problems, their acceptance will probably widen somewhat, when specific agents are being sought and when the laboratory organization lends itself to the use of radioisotopes. However, methods in which enzymes such as peroxidase or alkaline phosphatase are linked to antibody (immunoenzyme methods) may eventually supplant both FA and RIA techniques in many situations. The intrinsic sensitivity of immunoenzyme tests is high, and they have the advantages of being applicable to both microscopic and nonmicroscopic (i.e., serologic) testing, without the need for such equipment as ultraviolet microscope and gamma counters.

Interpretation

In many situations in which rapid diagnostic tests are used, the specimen is from a site at, or close to, that of the pathologic process. Consequently, a positive result has etiologic significance of a high order. When a positive result is from a more distant site (e.g., a positive result for hepatitis B surface antigen (HB$_s$Ag) in serum from a patient with no hepatic involvement), the etiologic significance of a positive result is less clear and requires further investigation.

The significance of a negative result varies from situation to situation, depending on the sensitivity and, when immunologically based methods are involved, the specificity of the methods being used. The time after onset at which specimens are taken must also be taken into account. For example, a negative FA test may often result from a nasal aspirate specimen which yields a virus when cultured. In this case the significance of a negative FA result is low (the reason for doing FA being one of rapid diagnosis). In hepatitis B infections, most acutely ill patients do show HB$_s$Ag in serum if it is collected soon after onset and examined by RIA. Consequently, a negative result in such a situation probably is more significant, and would usually be taken as an indication that such a patient's hepatitis was caused by an agent other than the hepatitis B virus.

Computation of 50 Percent Endpoints

In biological quantitation, the endpoint is usually taken as the dilution at which a certain proportion of the test animals reacts or dies. While a 100% endpoint is frequently used, its accuracy is so greatly affected by small chance variations as to make it the worst type of endpoint. The most desirable endpoint is one representing a situation in which half of the animals react, the other half do not (2). The best method of determining such an endpoint is to use large numbers of test animals at closely spaced dilutions near the value for 50% reaction and then interpolate a correct value. A number of practical factors, however, militate against this approach: 1) the cost of using large numbers of animals on every dilution point; 2) the wide variations in titer between any given tests; and 3) the unjustified application, in most instances, of highly accurate statistical methods to procedures replete with uncontrolled variables.

In titrating viruses, or serum for antibody content, a series of dilutions of the test materials is made, and each dilution is inoculated into a small group of animals; ordinarily 6–8 animals are used on each "point"—thereby employing a large number of animals. Reed and Muench (4) devised a simple method for estimating 50% endpoints based on the large, *total* number of

TABLE 1.3—ARRANGEMENT OF DATA USED IN COMPUTATION OF LD$_{50}$ TITER BY REED-MUENCH FORMULA

Virus Dilution (a)	Mortality Ratio (b)	Died (c)	Survived (d)	ACCUMULATED VALUES		Mortality	
				Died (e)	Survived (f)	Ratio (g)	Percent (h)
10^{-1}	6/6	6	0	17	0	17/17	100
10^{-2}	6/6	6	0	11	0	11/11	100
10^{-3}	4/6	4	2	5	2	5/7	71
10^{-4}	1/6	1	5	1	7	1/8	13
10^{-5}	0/6	0	6	0	13	0/13	0

animals, which gives the effect "of using, at the 2 critical dilutions between which the endpoint lies, larger groups of animals than were actually included at these dilutions. By inclining to equalize chance variations, the method tends to define the point more nearly than would be possible if it were simply interpolated between the 2 bracketing results." Kärber (3) also reported a simple method for computing 50% endpoints; this is described below, along with the Reed-Muench method.

The 50% endpoint can be based on several types of reactions. The most widely used is based on *mortality* and is written LD$_{50}$ (50% lethal dose). ID$_{50}$ indicates the dose which *infects* 50% of the test animals, PD$_{50}$ the dose which *paralyzes* 50% of the animals, and so on. The terminology can also be applied to other host systems—for example, tissue cultures—in which TCID$_{50}$ represents the dose that gives rise to cytopathic changes in 50% of the inoculated cultures.

Both the Reed-Muench and the Kärber methods are applicable primarily to a complete titration series, that is, the whole reaction range, from 0 to 100% mortality (or infectivity or CPE etc.), should be represented in the experimental data. However, the methods can be utilized even when these conditions are not fulfilled, provided the reactions occur in a uniform manner over the range of dilutions employed. If, however, these reactions are erratic (for example, deaths irregularly scattered over a number of dilutions), the endpoint is inaccurate. There are, of course, a number of other statistical methods which may be employed (1), but they are not commonly used in virus computations.

Fifty percent endpoints in virus titrations

Calculation of the LD$_{50}$ titer by the Reed-Muench method. If the laboratory work sheets or cards are provided with an appropriate column at 1 side, the accumulated values (Table 1.3 columns e-h) can be quickly calculated and the endpoint determined as outlined below. Table 1.3 gives an example of data derived from observation of inoculated animals and illustrates the procedure of accumulation.

Accumulated values for the total number of animals that died or survived are obtained by adding in the directions indicated by the arrows. The accumulated mortality ratio (col g) represents the accumulated number of dead animals (col e) over the accumulated total number inoculated (col e plus col f); for example, in the 10^{-3} dilution there were 5 deaths out of a total of 7 animals.

In the example in Table 1.3 the mortality in the 10^{-3} dilution is higher than 50%; that in the next lower dilution, 10^{-4}, is considerably lower. The necessary proportionate distance of the 50% mortality endpoint, which obviously lies between these 2 dilutions, is obtained as follows:

$$\frac{(\% \text{ mortality at dilution next above } 50\%) - (50\%)}{(\% \text{ mortality at dilution next above } 50\%) - (\% \text{ mortality at dilution next below})}$$

$$= \text{Proportionate distance}$$

or

$$\frac{71 - 50}{71 - 13} = \frac{21}{58} = 0.36 \text{ (or } 0.4).$$

Since logarithmically the distance between any 2 dilutions is a function of the incremental steps used in preparing the series, for example, 2-fold, 4-fold, 5-fold, 10-fold, etc., it is necessary to correct (multiply) the proportionate distance by the dilution factor, which is the logarithm of the dilution steps employed. In the case of serial 10-fold dilutions, the factor is 1 (log 10 = 1) and so is disregarded; in a 2-fold dilution series, the factor is 0.3 (log of 2.0), in a 5-fold series, 0.7 (log of 5.0), and so on. In the procedure which follows, the factor is understood to be negative. Therefore,

Negative logarithm of LD_{50} endpoint titer = negative logarithm of the dilution above the 50% mortality plus the proportionate distance factor (corrected for dilution series used)

or

Negative logarithm of the lower dilution (next above 50% mortality) = -3.0
Proportionate distance $(0.4) \times$ dilution factor (log 10) = -0.4

$$LD_{50} \text{ titer} = -3.4$$
$$\log LD_{50} \text{ titer} = 10^{-3.4}$$

Calculation of the LD_{50} titer by the Kärber method. This method gives endpoints which are essentially as accurate as those obtained by the Reed and Muench method. It is not necessary to use accumulated mortality ratios (although these can be used), as the observed mortality ratios suffice. The Kärber formula is as follows:

$$\text{Negative logarithm of } LD_{50} \text{ endpoint titer} = \left[\begin{array}{l} \text{negative logarithm} \\ \text{of the highest virus} \\ \text{concentration used} \end{array} \right]$$

$$- \left[\left(\frac{\text{sum of } \% \text{ mortality at each dilution}}{100} - 0.5 \right) \times (\text{logarithm of dilution}) \right]$$

Using the data in Table 1.3 this becomes:

$$\text{Negative logarithm of LD}_{50} \text{ endpoint titer} = -1.0 - \left[\left(\frac{100 + 100 + 66 + 17}{100} - 0.5 \right) \times (\log 10) \right]$$

$$= -1.0 - [(2.8 - 0.5) \times 1]$$

$$= -1.0 - 2.3$$

$$= -3.3$$

$$\text{LD}_{50} \text{ titer} = 10^{-3.3}$$

Complement-Fixation (CF) Test

The microtiter procedure described here represents the standard method od employed for diagnostic procedures by the Viral and Rickettsial Disease Laboratory of the California State Department of Health. It can be recommended as a relatively simple technique that may be used successfully with a large variety of viral and rickettsial diagnostic antigens.

Reagents

Modified Alsever solution

Dextrose	20.5 g
Sodium chloride (NaCl)	4.2 g
Sodium citrate ($Na_3C_6H_5O_7 \cdot 2H_2O$)	8.0 g
Citric acid ($C_6H_8O_7 \cdot H_2O$)	0.55 g
Distilled water q.s.	1000.0 ml

Sterilize by filtration through Millipore membrane 0.22 μ pore size; pH should be 6.0–6.2. Store at 4 C.

Veronal buffer saline (5X stock solution)

Add to a 2-liter volumetric flask

Distilled H_2O	1500.0 ml
NaCl	83.0 g
Na 5, 5-diethyl barbituate (sodium barbital)	10.19 g
1 N HCl	34.58 ml

Add

$MgCl_2 \cdot 6H_2O$	1.02 g
$CaCl_2 \cdot 2H_2O$	0.22 g

Mix

Distilled water q.s.	2000.0 ml

Sterilize by filtration through a Millipore membrane, 0.22 μ pore size.

For use, dilute 1 part stock buffer with 4 parts distilled water. Final pH should be 7.2–7.4. Prepare diluted buffer each week.

Stock solution of anti-sheep cell hemolysin 1:100

Mix well

Veronal buffer saline (VBS)	47.0 ml
5% phenol in saline (0.85%)	2.0 ml

Add

Hemolysin (preserved in 50% glycerine)	1.0 ml

Store at 4 C, stable approximately 4–6 weeks. Discard if precipitate forms.

Preparation of erythrocyte (RBC) suspension

To prepare a standardized suspension of RBC, the cells can be lysed and the released hemoglobin measured on a spectrophotometer. A preferred method is to convert the released hemoglobin to cyanmethemoglobin (CMG) and then read the concentration of CMG against a standard on a spectrophotometer. The reagent to achieve this conversion contains potassium cyanide and potassium ferricyanide. The ferricyanide oxidizes the hemoglobin from ferrous iron to form methemoglobin in an alkaline medium. Methemoglobin interacts with potassium cyanide to form CMG, a stable hemoglobin pigment. The CMG reagent, since it contains cyanide, should not be pipetted by mouth. The CMG standard contains 80 mg CMG/dl and from this a standard curve with known concentrations of CMG is prepared. The optical density (OD) of the desired cell suspension (target OD) is calculated from the experimentally obtained OD readings of the standard dilutions.

Preparation of standard curve and calculation of the target OD

1. *Construct a standard CMG curve.* Prepare dilutions of CMG in CMG reagent containing 80, 60, 40, 20, 0 mg CMG/dl (blank).

Preparation of Standard Curve

Cyanmethemoglobin (mg/dl)	80	60	40	20	0
Volume of standard (ml)	6.0	4.5	3.0	1.5	0.0
Volume of reagent (ml)	0.0	1.5	3.0	4.5	6.0

Read the OD of the dilutions on a spectrophotometer at 540-nm wavelength. On graph paper, plot the OD on the ordinate and mg CMG/dl on the abscissa. Draw a line through the points. A straight line should be obtained. The OD of the desired RBC suspension will vary with different spectrophotometers. Therefore, for each spectrophotometer, the desired OD or target OD is calculated from the experimentally obtained OD readings of the standard dilutions. The factor to be used in this calculation must be determined for each spectrophotometer.

2. *Calculate the factor to be used in determining target OD*

$$\text{Factor} = \frac{\text{sum of the conc. (mg CMG/dl) of std. dil.}}{\text{sum of OD readings of std. dil.}} = \text{mg CMG/dl OD per unit}$$

Calculate the target OD:

$$\text{Target OD} = \frac{\text{mg CMG/dl of desired suspension}}{\text{factor}}$$

For example: 1.4% sheep RBC suspension is used which corresponds to 16 mg CMG/dl

$$\text{Factor} = \frac{80 + 60 + 40 + 20}{.55 + .41 + .27 + .135} = \frac{200}{1.365} = 146.5 \text{ mg CMG/dl per unit}$$

Hence, target OD of 1.4% sheep RBC suspension $= \dfrac{16}{146.5} = 0.11$

3. The factor and target OD determination can be used for all subsequent cell standardizations made with your spectrophotometer providing the instrument is not moved

or unduly jarred. Recheck the reliability of the instrument before each use by reading the OD of the 40 mg CMG/dl standard.

4. Store CMG reagent in brown bottle at room temperature. (Bottle can be clear if stored in the dark.) Do not use rubber or cork stopper unless covered with parafilm. If reagent becomes cloudy or a precipitate forms, discard. The 40 mg CMG/dl standard will remain stable for several months if kept refrigerated and free of contamination.

Washing of cells

1. Wash sheep RBC preserved in Alsever solution by suspending in 2–3 volumes of VBS and centrifuging 8 min at about 700 × g with a rotating radius of 15 cm 3 successive times.

2. Filter cells through several layers of gauze into a graduated centrifuge tube.

3. Pack by centrifuging for 10 min at about 700 × g. Prepare a 4 suspension of the cells in VBS in a volume sufficient to dilute for the day's test.

4. Store suspension at 4 C.

Preparation of working cell suspension

1. Transfer 1 ml of the 4% suspension to a 25-ml volumetric flask. Fill to the mark with CMG reagent and mix well.

2. Let stand at room temperature until RBC are lysed, approximately 15 min. (If solution is not optically clear, spin for 10 min at 700 × g.)

3. Determine the OD of the resulting CMG solution at 540 nm against the reagent blank set at zero.

4. Calculate the dilution necessary to adjust the 4% suspension to the desired OD

$$\frac{\text{(OD of CMG sol.)} \times \text{(vol of 4\% RBC susp.)}}{\text{Target OD}} = \text{final volume}$$

5. Dilute the 4% suspension with VBS to the final volume determined above.

6. Store at 4 C.

Titration of hemolysin, complement, and antigens

Hemolysin

A titration is performed each time a new 1:100 stock dilution is prepared. Use 13-x 100-mm test tubes.

1. Prepare a 1:60 dilution of complement in cold VBS. Store at 4 C.

2. Make the following dilutions of hemolysin:

Final Dilution	VBS (ml)	Hemolysin to be added	
		Dilution	Volume (ml)
1:1,000	4.5	1:100	0.5
1:6,000	5.0	1:1,000	1.0
1:8,000	7.0	1:1,000	1.0
1:10,000	9.0	1:1,000	1.0
1:15,000	0.5	1:10,000	1.0
1:20,000	1.0	1:10,000	1.0
1:25,000	1.5	1:10,000	1.0

3. Titrate the hemolysin as follows (include a cell control):

Reagent	
Hemolysin dilutions	0.2 ml
(1:6,000 to 1:25,000)	
Complement, 1:60	0.2 ml
Sheep RBC suspension	0.2 ml
VBS	0.4 ml
Cell control	
Sheep RBC suspension	0.2 ml
VBS	0.8 ml

4. Shake and incubate the titration in a 37 C water bath for 30 minutes, then read.
The highest dilution of hemolysin which shows *complete* hemolysis represents 1 unit. Use 2 units in the test.
Example: If the 1:10,000 dilution shows complete hemolysis and the 1:15,000 partial hemolysis, 1 unit would be represented by a 1:10,000 dilution. Therefore, 2 units would be contained in a 1:5,000 dilution of hemolysin.
5. For use in each day's test, prepare the proper dilution of hemolysin in a volume equal to the volume of 1.4% sheep RBC suspension. Hold both at 4 C until cells are sensitized the following morning.

Complement titration in microtiter U plates

As a source of complement use only lots of guinea pig serum shown to be free of viral antibodies. Such serum is available from several commercial sources.

A complement titration with the antigen to be used in the test is performed with each test run.

1. Prepare a 1:100 dilution of complement in cold VBS. Mix gently to avoid foaming. Store at 4 C.
2. Dilute each antigen to be used in the titration to the 2-unit test dilution.
3. Make a series of dilutions in cold VBS from the 1:100 dilution of complement.

Final dilution:	120*	140	160	180	200	220	250
1:100							
Complement, ml	0.5	0.5	0.5	0.5	0.5	0.5	0.5
Cold VBS, ml	0.1	0.2	0.3	0.4	0.5	0.6	0.7

*Reciprocal of complement dilution
Hold at 4 C until VBS and antigen have been added to the titration.
4. Use 1 row of wells for each antigen to be included in the titration. Add reagents to a plate with 0.025 ml droppers as outlined below:

Reagent	Volume (ml) of reagent to be added													
VBS	.00	.025	.00	.025	.00	.025	.00	.025	.00	.025	.00	.025	.00	.025
Diluted antigen	.025	.025	.025	.025	.025	.025	.025	.025	.025	.025	.025	.025	.025	.025
Complement dilution	.025	.025	.05	.025	.05	.025	.05	.025	.05	.025	.05	.025	.05	.025
	1:120		1:140		1:160		1:180		1:200		1:220		1:240	

5. Shake plate, cover, and incubate 4 hr at 4 C.
6. At the end of 4 hr, remove the titration plate from the refrigerator and warm at room temperature 15 min.

7. Sensitize a portion of the working suspension of RBC. Measure 10 ml of RBC suspension into a 50-ml flask. Measure 10 ml of hemolysin diluted for test into another 50-ml flask. While constantly swirling flask of cells, pour hemolysin dilution into the flask, then rapidly pour back and forth several times. Incubate at room temperature for 10–30 min.

8. Add 0.05 ml sensitized cells to all wells. Shake plate and incubate at 37 C for 15 min.

9. Read and record results. The endpoint is that dilution showing no lysis in the well containing 0.025 ml (corresponding to 0.5 unit of complement) and complete or nearly complete lysis in the well containing 0.05 ml (corresponding to 1 unit of complement). Two units in 0.025 ml of complement are used in the test.

Example: If a 1:160 dilution of complement has a 4+ reading in the well containing 0.025 ml and a trace of cells remaining in the well containing 0.05 ml, a 1:40 dilution will contain 2 units in 0.025 ml.

Titration of antigen

Titrate each new lot of antigen by testing serial 2-fold dilutions of antigen against serial 2-fold dilutions of immune serum to determine the optimal dilution of antigen which gives fixation. This procedure, often referred to as a "box" titration, is illustrated by the following example:

Antigen dilution	Immune serum dilutions					Negative serum	Complement control unit of complement			
	1:8	1:16	1:32	1:64	1:128	1:8	2.0	1.5	1.0	0.5
1:2	4*	4	4	0	0	0	0	0	±	4
1:4	4	4	4	1	0	0	0	0	0	4
1:8	4	4	4	2	0	0	0	0	0	4
1:16	4	4	4	2	0	0	0	0	0	4
1:32	4	4	2	0	0	0	0	0	0	4
1:64	1	0	0	0	0	0	0	0	0	4.
Previous lot of antigen	4	4	4	0	0	0	0	0	0	4
Control antigen (uninfected)	0	0	0	0	0	0	0	0		4
Serum control	0	0	0	0	0	0				

*Degree of fixation

1. Prepare the initial dilutions of immune and negative serum in VBS. Inactivate at 56 C for 30 min in a water bath.

2. Prepare serial dilutions of serum in VBS using 0.025 ml microdiluters. Use a range of 5–6 dilutions, including 2 above and 3 below the known titer of the immune serum.

3. Prepare dilutions of the antigen to be titrated and dilute the previous lot of antigen to contain 2 units.

4. Dilute control antigen (uninfected tissue) to the same dilution used for the previous lot of antigen.

5. Dilute complement in cold VBS to contain 2 units. Prepare complement controls containing 1.5, 1.0, and 0.5 units from the 2-unit complement dilution.

TABLE 1.4—SCHEME FOR PERFORMANCE OF THE MICROTITER COMPLEMENT-FIXATION TEST

WELLS	SERUM (ML)	VBS (ML)	ANTIGEN (ML)	CONTROL ANTIGEN* (ML)	COMPLEMENT (ML)		SENSITIZED CELLS (ML)
Serum under test	0.025**	—	0.025	—	0.025		0.050
Serum control (test for AC activity)	0.025†	0.025	—	—	0.025		0.050
Serum antigen (un-infected) control	0.025†	—	—	0.025	0.025		0.050
Reagent controls Complement controls for each antigen (specific and control antigens) *Units*						overnight incubation at 4–6 C followed by 15 min at room temperature	
2.0	—	0.025	0.025)	(0.025	0.025		0.050
1.5	—	0.025	0.025) OR	(0.025	0.025		0.050
1.0	—	0.025	0.025)	(0.025	0.025		0.050
0.5	—	0.025	0.025)	(0.025	0.025		0.050
Hemolytic control	—	0.050	—	—	0.025		0.050
Sheep RBC control	—	0.075	—	—	—		0.050

15–30 min at 37 C

* Uninfected antigen prepared and diluted in same manner as test antigen.

** Series of wells each containing 0.025 ml of a serial dilution of serum.

† Initial serum dilution of 1:4 or 1:8.

AC = Anticomplementary

Complement units	1.5	1.0	0.5
Cold VBS, ml	0.5	1.0	1.5
Complement 2 units, ml	1.5	1.0	0.5

Store at 4 C until used.

6. Beginning with the highest dilution of antigen, add 0.025 ml of each dilution to the appropriate immune serum, negative serum, and complement control wells. Add control antigen and previous lot of antigen to the appropriate wells.

7. Add 0.025 ml VBS to the serum control wells and to the complement control wells.

8. Add 0.025 ml of the appropriate complement dilutions to the complement controls containing 0.5, 1.0, and 1.5 units. To the test proper and the 2-unit complement control, add 0.025 ml of complement diluted to contain 2 units.

9. Mix the contents of the wells by rubbing the bottom of the plate gently. Cover and incubate the plates overnight at 4-6 C.

10. Warm the plates for 15 min at room temperature; add 0.05 ml of the sensitized cell suspension to each well. Mix on a vibrating shaker and then incubate the plates at 37 C for 15-30 min, or until the complement controls show proper clearing.

11. Hold plates at 4-6 C until unlysed cells have settled and tests are ready to read.

The highest dilution of antigen showing 3+ or 4+ fixation with the highest dilution of immune serum is generally regarded as 1 unit (1:16 dilution in the example). Use 2 units of antigen in a volume of 0.025 ml. In some titrations a certain dilution of antigen may show a 3+ or 4+ complement fixation with a higher serum dilution than do dilutions of antigen with 2-fold higher or 2-fold lower. For example, a 1:4 antigen dilution gives 4+ fixation at 1:32 dilution of serum, a 1:8 antigen dilution gives 4+ fixation at 1:64 dilution of serum, and a 1:16 antigen dilution gives 4+ fixation at 1:32 dilution of serum. In such a case 1:16 is considered 1 unit of antigen and 1:8 2 units.

Performance of test

Specimens

Serum. Because a nonspecific reaction may be encountered with high concentrations of serum, an initial serum dilution of 1:4 or 1:8 is used in the test. Inactivate the initial serum dilution for 30 min in a 56 C water bath. Include in every run a serum with a known titer to each antigen as a positive control. Hemolyzed specimens and plasma or serum with visible particles after inactivation must be centrifuged to clarify.

Cerebrospinal fluid (CSF). CSF specimens are diluted 1:2 in VBS and inactivated at 56 C for 30 min. Bloody spinal fluids are unsatisfactory as any antibody detected may be serum antibody.

Addition of reagents (see scheme)

1. Add 0.025 ml VBS to dilution wells.

2. Add 0.05 ml of the initial serum dilution to a well for each test antigen; add 0.025 ml to a well for each control antigen and to a well for the serum (anticomplementary) control.

3. Prepare successive 2-fold serum dilutions for the antigen sets using 0.025 ml microdiluters. Add 0.025 ml of VBS to the serum control wells and complement control wells.

4. Dilute test antigens to contain 2 units; dilute control antigens (uninfected) to same dilution. Add 0.025 ml of test antigen to appropriate wells (see Table 1.4). Add 0.025 ml of control antigen to the appropriate wells.

5. Dilute complement in cold VBS to contain 2 units. Prepare complement controls containing 1.5, 1.0, and 0.5 units from the 2-unit complement dilution as follows:

Complement units	1.5	1.0	0.5
Cold VBS, ml	0.5	1.0	1.5
Complement 2 units, ml	1.5	1.0	0.5

6. Add 0.025 ml of the dilution of complement containing 0.5 unit to the appropriate wells; continue by adding 0.025 ml of the dilutions containing 1.0 and 1.5 units. Add 0.025 ml of the initial complement dilution (2 units) to the 2-unit complement control wells.

7. Add 0.025 ml of the initial complement dilution (containing 2 units) to the remainder of the test.

8. Mix by rubbing the bottom of the plates gently. Cover plates and incubate overnight at 4-6 C.

9. On the following day, warm the plates for 15 min at room temperature; add 0.05 ml of sensitized cells, mix and incubate at 37 C for 15–30 min, or until the complement controls show proper clearing.

Explanation of complement controls

The wells containing 2.0 and 1.5 units of complement should show complete hemolysis. The wells containing 1.0 unit should show complete or nearly complete hemolysis, and the wells containing 0.5 unit of complement should show no hemolysis. If the wells containing 0.5 unit show hemolysis, an excess of complement was used in the test. If those containing 2.0 and 1.5 units do not show *complete* hemolysis, insufficient complement was used.

When the complement controls show the proper degree of hemolysis, remove the plates from the incubator. If the complement controls are insufficiently cleared after the initial incubation period, continue incubation, examining the controls at frequent intervals during the succeeding 15 min. Remove the plates from the incubator when the controls show the proper degree of hemolysis.

10. Hold the plates at 4-6 C until the unlysed cells have settled and the tests are ready to read. The test is not valid for any specimen which shows fixation in the control wells.

Treatment of anticomplementary specimens

If the specimen shows anticomplementary activity, such activity can sometimes be blocked by the following treatment.

1. Pipette 0.15 ml of each serum pair to be treated.
2. Add 0.05 ml of undiluted complement.
3. Incubate in 37 C waterbath 30 min.
4. Add 1.0 ml of VBS to obtain a 1:8 dilution.
5. Inactivate the treated serum for 30 min at 56 C.
6. Prepare dilutions of treated serum for the test antigen, control antigen and serum controls to compare specific antibody titers with the anticomplementary or nonspecific titers.

Methods of Inoculation of Embryonated Hens' Eggs

Preliminary handling of the eggs

Fertile eggs for the cultivation of viruses should be obtained from flocks free of infection with known viral or other microbial agents such as Newcastle disease virus or mycoplasmas. In the early stages of development the chick embryo can be recognized only with difficulty, but at 4-5 days of age it is easily seen; consequently, eggs are incubated for 4–5 days before they are candled to determine which are fertile and which are nonfertile. Incubation should be carried out at 37 C in an atmosphere of 40–70% humidity. Too high humidity leads to overdevelopment of the air sac, whereas humidity too low leads to underdevelopment. In the larger egg incubators, the water level is automatically maintained by valves that control the flow from a direct water supply, but in smaller incubators water must be added periodically to maintain the proper level.

To prevent adhesions of the embryonic membranes and to keep the embryo more or less centralized, the eggs are turned at intervals; in the larger egg incubators, this is done automatically by a clockwork mechanism which turns the eggs approximately every 4 hr, but in the smaller incubators eggs must be turned manually several times a day.

The length of time the embryos are to be incubated before inoculation, that is, the stage of development at which the embryo is inoculated, is determined by the route of inoculation that is to be employed.

Structure of the egg

Immediately under the shell is the shell membrane, a tough fibrous material which lines the entire shell but is readily separable from it; at the blunt end of the egg the shell membrane forms an air sac. The chorioallantois, which is a highly vascular membrane serving as the respiratory organ of the embryo, lies directly under the shell membrane throughout the entire egg. The chorioallantois is separated from the amnion by the allantoic cavity, which contains from 5–10 ml of fluid. The amniotic membrane forms a sac which encloses the embryo; the amniotic cavity, within which the embryo lies, contains approximately 1 ml of fluid, termed the amniotic fluid. Attached to the embryo is the yolk sac containing nutriments for the developing embryo.

Techniques of inoculation

Amniotic route

This route of inoculation is employed primarily for the isolation of viruses from clinical or field materials. Inoculum introduced into the amniotic cavity is swallowed by the embryo and also enters the respiratory tract, thereby enhancing the possibilities of virus propagation through the variety of tissues and cell types made available to viruses with specific cellular predilections. Since the amount of amniotic tissue or amniotic fluid available for harvest is small, viruses isolated by amniotic inoculation are generally passaged by the allantoic route in order to adapt them to growth in the allantoic entoderm.

Inoculation into the amniotic cavity is illustrated in Fig 1.2. Embryos as old as 13 or 14 days of age are suitable, although 10- to 11-day-old embryos are the most commonly used. The blunt, or air sac, end of the egg is painted with tincture of iodine and a puncture is made through the shell with a sharp probe or a trocar. The area of the puncture is repainted with tincture of iodine, the egg is held over a candler and inoculated by means of a tuberculin

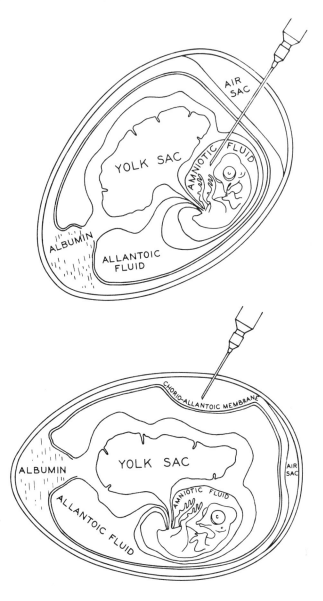

Figure 1.2—Method of inoculation into cavity of amniotic cavity of an 11-day-old
chick embryo (top) and onto chorioallantoic membrane of a 10-day-old
chick enbryo (bottom).

syringe fitted with a 23-gauge needle, 1³/₄ inch (4.5 cm) long. The needle is
aimed toward the shadow of the embryo and enters the amniotic cavity with
a quick stab at the embryo; 0.1 or 0.2 ml of inoculum is deposited in the
cavity. The needle is then withdrawn, the punctured area painted with tincture of iodine, and the hole sealed with a paraffin-vaseline mixture or with

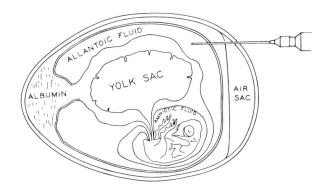

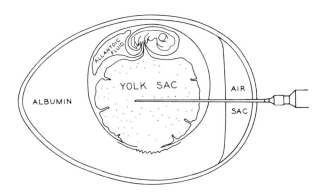

Figure 1.3—Method of inoculation into allantoic cavity of a 10-day-old chick embryo (top) and into the yolk sac of a 6-day-old chick embryo (bottom).

collodion. Inoculated eggs are incubated at 33 C, 35 C or 37 C (depending upon the virus) for 48–72 hr.

   To harvest the infected tissues, the eggs are first chilled at 4 C for 18 hr to induce contraction of the blood vessels. This is particularly important when working with the myxoviruses, since release of RBC into the embryonic fluids may lead to loss of virus through absorption to the cells.

   The chilled eggs are placed in a holder with the blunt end up, and the area over the air sac is painted with tincture of iodine and wiped with 70%

alcohol. The shell over the air sac is broken away with sterile, blunt forceps until the shell membrane lies exposed. The shell membrane is then removed with curved forceps and the chorioallantoic membrane is loosened from the shell membrane; if, however, it is desired to harvest the allantoic fluid, it should be aspirated with a syringe or pipette before the membrane is loosened.

The contents of the egg are carefully decanted into a sterile Petri dish, and the fluid is aspirated from the amniotic sac with a 1-ml syringe to which a 1-1 $^{1}/_{2}$ inch (2.5-4 cm) 26-gauge needle is attached. The amniotic membranes are then harvested. In certain instances the chorioallantoic membranes or the embryos themselves may be harvested, together with the amniotic membranes, in order to increase the virus yield.

Chorioallantoic membrane route

This route is frequently used for the isolation and propagation of viruses which produce plaques or pocks on the chorioallantois, for example, the viruses of vaccinia, variola, herpes simplex and fowlpox. It is also used for titration of these agents, since the number of infected particles can be calculated from the number of pocks or plaques produced; it is also used for the assay of antibody, since the extent to which the plaque count is reduced is related to the concentration of antibody.

This route of inoculation is illustrated in Fig 1.2. Embryos 10-12 days of age are candled and the site of inoculation is marked with a pencil on the side of the egg, the site chosen being an area with well-developed blood vessels. It is necessary to "drop" the chorioallantoic membrane to create a relatively flat surface on which the inoculum can be deposited and evenly distributed. Both the site of inoculation and the air-sac end of the egg are swabbed with tincture of iodine and a perforation is made through the shell into the air sac. At the site of inoculation a mechanical grinder, fitted with a carborundum disk is used to make a slit approximately $^{1}/_{4}$ inch (7-8 mm) long and $^{1}/_{8}$ inch (2-3 mm) wide along the long axis of the shell. The shell membrane is thus exposed but not perforated. The shell membrane is then pierced with a short 23-gauge needle, and with a rubber bulb gentle suction is applied to the hole over the air sac. This causes the membrane to drop, creating a false air sac over the chorioallantoic membrane. The egg is next examined over a candler to ascertain that the air sac has been displaced and that the membrane has dropped. The inoculum (0.1-0.2 ml) is deposited onto the chorioallantoic membrane with a 1-ml tuberculin syringe fitted with a short 23-gauge needle, and the egg is rotated to distribute the inoculum. The hole in the air-sac end is sealed; it is generally unnecessary to seal the slit at the site of inoculation. The inoculated eggs are placed in a horizontal position, covered with plastic wrap, and incubated at 35 C for 48-72 hr.

Before the membranes are harvested, the eggs are candled to determine whether the air sac is still displaced; if not, gentle suction is applied to the puncture in the sac. The shell over the false air sac is painted with iodine; with blunt forceps the shell and shell membrane are broken away to the edge of the false air sac to expose the chorioallantoic membrane to the fullest extent possible. If the membrane shows lesions, it is cut out with sterile scissors and placed in a sterile Petri dish for further examination or for subsequent subinoculation.

Allantoic route

This route is employed for the production of the large quantities of virus required for the preparation of serologic antigens, vaccines, etc. Virus introduced into the allantoic cavity propagates in the entodermal cells of the allantois with subsequent release into the allantoic fluid, so that both the membrane and the fluid can be used as sources of virus.

The allantoic route of inoculation is illustrated in Fig 1.3. Embryos 10–11 days of age are candled; a pencil mark is made in an area over the air sac near the membrane boundary opposite the embryo, where there are few or no major blood vessels. The marked area is painted, with tincture of iodine and a puncture is made through the shell. This area is again swabbed with iodine to remove shell particles, and the egg is inoculated with a tuberculin syringe fitted with a 5/8 inch (1.5 mm) 26-gauge needle. The needle is inserted approximately 1/2 inch into the egg in a direction parallel to the side (see Fig 1.3), the inoculum (0.1–0.2 ml) is then introduced into the allantoic cavity. The puncture is painted with tincture of iodine and sealed as noted above. Inoculated eggs are incubated at 35 C for 24–72 hr, depending upon the virus and the intended use of the harvested material.

For harvest of the infected materials, the eggs are chilled and the air sac and shell membrane are opened as described above for amniotic inoculation. The allantoic fluid is aspirated with a syringe or pipette and the chorioallantoic membranes are harvested with sterile forceps.

Yolk-sac route

This route of inoculation is the route of choice for isolation and propagation of the rickettsiae. It is also used for the isolation and passage of chlamaydiae. These large agents grow readily in the entodermal cells lining the yolk sac, and rickettsiae or elementary bodies can usually be seen after proper staining.

Yolk-sac inoculation is illustrated in Figure 1.3. Young embryos 5–6 days of age are used, because the yolk sacs at this stage are large, are readily entered, and provide a large surface for multiplication of viruses.

The air-sac end of the egg is swabbed with tincture of iodine, and the shell over the air sac punctured with a sharp probe. A 1³/₄ inch (4.5 cm) 23-gauge needle is used for inoculation and, as shown in Fig 1.3, the needle can be passed directly into the yolk sac without concern for appropriate orientation. Since the inoculum generally ranges from 0.5–1.0 ml, a 1 or 2 ml syringe is required. After inoculation the punctured area is repainted with tincture of iodine and sealed; the inoculated eggs are incubated at 35 C for 3–8 days, depending upon the virus or rickettsia inoculated.

To harvest the infected yolk sacs, the eggs are chilled and the shell is broken away from the air sac as described for the harvest of allantoic and amniotic fluids. After removal of the shell membrane, the chorioallantoic membrane is loosened with forceps, and the contents of the egg are decanted into a sterile Petri dish. The yolk sac is then cut away from the embryo and is ruptured to permit the yolk material to drain from the sac; removal of yolk can be facilitated by washing the membrane with sterile saline solution. Membranes free of yolk material are then placed in a sterile Petri dish or beaker for subsequent examination by staining, or for processing for passage.

References

1. BROSS I: Estimates of the LD_{50}: A critique. Biometrics 6:413–423, 1950
2. GADDUM JH: Reports of biological standards. III. Methods of biological assay depending on a quantal response. Medical Research Council (London) Special Report Series No. 183, 1933
3. KÄRBER G: Beitrag zur kollektiven behandlung pharmakologischer reihenversuche. Arch Exp Pathol Pharmakol 162:480–483, 1931
4. REED LJ and MUENCH H: A simple method of estimating fifty per cent endpoints. Am J Hyg 27:493–497, 1938
5. STRANO AJ: Light microscopy of selected viral diseases (morphology of viral inclusion bodies). Patholbiol Annu 11:53–75, 1976

Bibliography

BEHBEHANI AM: Human Viral, Bedsonial and Rickettsial Diseases. A Diagnostic Handbook for Physicians. Charles C. Thomas, Springfield, Illinois, 1972

LABZOFFSKY NA (ED): Virology Manual, Second edition, Ministry of Health, Ontario, Canada, 1974

MADELEY CR: Guide to the Collection and Transport of Virological Specimens (including Chlamydial and Rickettsial Specimens). World Health Organization, Geneva, 1977

SCHMIDT NJ, HAMPARIAN VV, SATHER GE, and WONG YW: In Quality Assurance Practices for Health Laboratories. Inhorn SL (ed) Am Public Health Assoc, Washington, DC, 1977, pp 1097–1144

CHAPTER 2

PREVENTION OF LABORATORY INFECTIONS

Robert M. Pike and John H. Richardson

Introduction

Anyone working with viruses, rickettsiae, or chlamydiae is exposed to the risk of possible infection through an accident or because of failure to observe proper precautions. Careful technique and the use of various protective devices currently available greatly reduce the risk of infection. The purpose of this chapter is to point out the circumstances most likely to lead to accidental infection and to indicate protective measures and available devices that will lessen the risk of laboratory infection.

Recorded Laboratory Infections

An analysis of reported laboratory infections and the circumstances under which they occurred may aid in pointing out preventive measures. To this end, recorded infections have been summarized on several occasions. In 1949, for example, 222 instances of illness due to laboratory-acquired viral infection, of which 21 were fatal, were reviewed (40). Known accidents were responsible for only 27 of these overt infections, and the major sources appeared to be infected animals and tissues. Additional cases were reported in 1951 (41) and in 1965 (27), and by 1974 (26) over 1700 cases of viral, rickettsial, and chlamydial infections with 87 deaths were compiled from published and unpublished records. Since then, an additional number of laboratory infections due to these agents have come to our attention (Table 2.1). Laboratory directors are urged to report instances of overt laboratory-acquired infection to the Office of Biosafety, Center for Disease Control, Atlanta, Georgia 30333, thereby providing a record which may serve as a basis for continued evaluation of the problem of laboratory safety. The increase in viral infections since 1945 (26) is associated with the increased number of persons handling these agents. The potential hazard involved in working with certain agents (8, 16) may not be fully appreciated by persons not specially trained in the use of virus model systems for the study of animal cell biology or by those engaged in tumor research or recombinant DNA research. Such investigators may find it useful to consult appropriate chapters

49

TABLE 2.1—OVERT LABORATORY-ASSOCIATED INFECTIONS*

AGENT OR DISEASE	CASES	DEATHS	NUMBER PUBLISHED
Viruses:			
Hepatitis	268	3	194
Venezuelan equine encephalitis	146	1	85
Lymphocytic choriomeningitis	76	5	66
Kyasanur Forest	67	0	20
Newcastle disease	55	0	46
Influenza	48	1	39
Louping-ill	40	0	37
Yellow fever	40	9	38
Vesicular stomatitis	40	0	39
Marburg disease	31	7	31
Rift Valley fever	28	1	25
Vaccinia and smallpox	28	0	24
Coxsackie	27	0	26
Yaba and Tana viruses	24	0	24
B virus	21	15	18
69 other viruses	239	12	151
Virus Total	1178	56	863
Rickettsiae:			
Q fever	280	1	218
Typhus	237	11	148
Spotted fever	65	13	16
Trench fever	10	0	10
Rickettsialpox	5	0	3
African tick-bite fever	1	0	1
Rickettsia Total	598	25	396
Chlamydiae:			
Psittacosis	116	10	71
Lymphogranuloma venereum	7	0	5
Trachoma	5	0	1
Chlamydia Total	128	10	77
Totals	1904	91	1336

*Cases occurring throughout the world, reported either in the literature or by personal communication to the APHA Committee on Laboratory Infections and Accidents (26, 27, 41) or to the American Committee on Arthropod-borne Viruses Subcommittee on Laboratory Infections (15).

in this volume for recommended techniques employed with certain viruses, and they should be aware of the potential hazards involved in dealing with certain agents. The recently reported cases of lymphocytic choriomeningitis acquired from hamsters infected by a tumor cell line carrying this virus (11) illustrate the potential hazard from an unexpected source.

Of the 1,904 overt infections contracted in the laboratory (Table 2.1), 1,178 were due to viruses, 598 to rickettsiae, and 128 to chlamydiae with 56,

25, and 10 deaths, respectively, attesting to the seriousness of the problem. A significant proportion of these experiences is recorded in various published reports. Hepatitis heads the list in spite of the fact that many cases are probably not recorded. The large number of overt laboratory-associated infections due to arboviruses undoubtedly is a result of the increasing number of studies involving these agents, particularly in recent years (15).

TABLE 2.2—SOURCES OF 1,904 OVERT LABORATORY INFECTIONS, CLASSIFIED ACCORDING TO THE FIRST LISTED SOURCE THAT APPLIED

SOURCE OF INFECTION	NO.
Known accident	233
Contact with animals or ectoparasites	377
Clinical specimens	206
Handling discarded glassware	12
Human autopsy	13
Aerosol	331
Worked with agent	357
Other	10
Unknown or not indicated	365

The sources of these infections, in so far as they can be judged from the information available, are shown in Table 2.2. In many instances it is known only that the person had been working with the agent involved, and it is reasonable to assume that many of these cases resulted from infectious aerosols. A large number of infections resulted from contact with infected animals or ectoparasites. Notable among these are several cases of hepatitis with strong evidence that the disease was contracted from chimpanzees (22). Included also are 31 cases of Marburg disease, with 7 deaths, among laboratory workers in Germany and Yugoslavia handling tissues from African green monkeys imported from East Africa (10, 36). The cases due to known accidents include 24 persons infected with the virus of Venezuelan equine encephalitis (VEE) resulting from a single accident in which ampules of lyophilized mouse brain infected with VEE virus were dropped and broken on a stairway (37).

In the greatest proportion of cases the manner in which the person became infected is not known, but there is substantial evidence that illnesses have occurred in the absence of known accidents or because of poor technique, and that overt laboratory infections do not always follow the pathways of transmission characteristic of naturally occurring disease. It is likely that the respiratory tract can serve as a portal of entry even in infections which are generally arthropod borne, like yellow fever, typhus, rickettsialpox, Rocky Mountain spotted fever, and others.

Table 2.3 lists the types of laboratory accidents which resulted in illness. The distribution of cases suggests that carelessness and human error are more important than the failure of mechanical equipment as a cause of accidents. The fact that the majority of infections occurred in the absence of

TABLE 2.3—TYPES OF ACCIDENTS RESPONSIBLE FOR 233 OVERT LABORATORY INFECTIONS

TYPE OF ACCIDENT	NO.
Spilling or spattering of infectious material	91
Accident involving needle and syringe	64
Bite of infected animal or ectoparasite	34
Pipetting	24
Injury with broken glass or other sharp object	15
Not indicated	5

a known accident indicates that accident prevention alone is only a partial solution to the problem of laboratory infection.

Aerosols

One of the most frequent causes of laboratory infection is the inhalation of an infectious aerosol. An important source of such aerosols is the dried urine or feces of experimental animals inoculated with agents that may be present in these excretions (45). That an aerosol may be unwittingly produced by a variety of common laboratory procedures, such as expelling the last drop from a pipette or removing the plug from a tube that has been shaken, has been convincingly demonstrated (1). A few examples suffice to illustrate the type of manipulation that can result in the aerosolization.

Filtration of infectious material can result in contamination of a vacuum line or pump unless adequate precautions are taken. A trap containing a disinfectant should be placed between the filter flask and the source of vacuum. High efficiency particulate air (HEPA) filters between the filter flask and the source of vacuum will further reduce the escape of an aerosol. The flask should be opened in a biological safety cabinet because foaming or splashing within the flask may produce an aerosol which may contaminate the environment with an infectious aerosol.

Sonication and the maceration of infected tissue by a variety of means may produce an infectious aerosol. Grinding in a mortar or in a Ten Broeck grinder may contaminate the atmosphere unless carried out in a safety cabinet. Mechanical disruption of infected tissue in a Waring Blendor is particularly effective in producing an infectious aerosol. Blenders have been designed to minimize leakage and to provide a means of drawing off fluids without removing the top (31, 38). In addition, if the operation is performed in a biological safety cabinet or other containment system, the hazard will be reduced to a minimum. Other procedures likely to result in aerosol formation are discussed in the next section.

Some Potentially Hazardous Procedures

Egg inoculation and harvesting

The risk of infection resulting from egg inoculation and harvesting is to some extent associated with the dangers inherent in the use of a needle and syringe. The greatest danger lies in the possibility of shell contamination which, in the case of allantoic and yolk sac inoculations, can be reduced by surrounding the needle with a pledget of cotton soaked in 70% alcohol (30). When inoculating the chorioallantoic membrane by the window technique, contamination of the shell can be avoided if care is exercised. Most of the accidential infections among persons working with embryonated eggs occur during harvesting of the infected material, which provides opportunity for the production of aerosols through spattering. This operation should be done in a biological safety cabinet, and within easy reach of the worker should be a receptacle for discarding infectious materials—a jar or preferably a pan for pipettes and another receptacle for contaminated instruments.

Use of syringe and needle

It is good to keep in mind that mishaps with needle and syringe have been among the more frequent types of accident resulting in infection. Careless handling may result in accidental puncture of the operator's skin. Separation of needle from syringe can be prevented by using Luer-Lok syringes. The needle should be shielded with alcohol-soaked cotton if air must be expelled from a syringe. In many or most situations, fluid can be drawn into a syringe without aspirating much air, and it is not necessary to expel the bubble. Although the use of vaccine bottles for making virus dilutions eliminates the hazard of pipetting, it introduces other possibilities of infection. A vaccine bottle cap may be contaminated, and an aerosol may be liberated when a needle is withdrawn unless the needle is surrounded by an alcohol-soaked pledget (30). While animals are being inoculated, accidents can result from an unexpected movement of the animal. If syringes are filled from test tubes, care should be taken not to contaminate the hub of the needle, as this may transfer infectious material to the fingers. The syringe must not be inserted into the test tube, and only the needle shaft (not the hub) should enter the tube.

Lyophilization

The method of drying infectious material from the frozen state creates special situations that are potentially hazardous. The apparatus can become contaminated easily during the drying process, and upon opening ampules containing the dried material, the environment may also become contaminated.

It has been shown that bacteria and viruses present in the material being lyophilized can be recovered from the vapors removed under high vacuum (39). Therefore, the manifolds and condenser should be so constructed that they can be decontaminated after use with infectious material. Contamination of the pump and vacuum gauge can be prevented by inclusion of a suitable biological filter in the vacuum line between the condenser and the pump (39). Manifold outlets become contaminated easily with material being lyophilized and serve as a source of contamination for the operator's hands unless gloves are worn when removing the glass stubs that remain after the ampules are sealed under vacuum (32).

When ampules are opened, some of the dried contents escape into the air unless the point of breakage is surrounded with cotton soaked in 70% alcohol (33). Also, it is advisable to reconstitute lyophilized infectious material in a biological safety cabinet. In addition, the accidental breakage of ampules has been responsible for a number of laboratory-acquired infections (33, 37).

Centrifuging

Although relatively few infections involving the use of a centrifuge have been recorded (41), the potential hazard in centrifugation is obvious. The filling of centrifuge tubes, the removal of caps, or the removal of supernatant fluids can give rise to aerosols (34). These procedures should be carried out in safety cabinets. The use of plastic instead of glass tubes reduces the chance of breakage, but even plastic tubes can break or crack under stress. Tubes should be carefully inspected for cracks which can result in contamination of the carrier cups. Nitrocellulose tubes deteriorate on storage for prolonged periods and should not be used in angle-head centrifuges (20). The routine use of sealable centrifuge safety cups effectively eliminates hazards associated with centrifugation of infectious material. Centrifuge cabinets with filtered exhausts (14) are also effective in controlling aerosols.

Pipetting

The use of pipettes in working with infectious material is a potential source of laboratory infection. Pipetting may be hazardous in at least 3 ways: (a) the contents of the pipette may be accidentally swallowed or aspirated when pipetting by mouth; (b) expelling the contents of the pipette, particularly the last drop, can produce an aerosol; (c) improper disposal of contaminated pipettes can transfer infectious material to personnel subsequently handling them. Contamination of the mouth can be avoided by using a syringe and needle (or preferably a cannula) instead of a pipette, but this technique also requires precautions and is a poor substitute for safety pipetting devices. Mouth pipetting should be prohibited. Observance of this rule not only eliminates the possibility of aspirating infectious or toxic material but also avoids placing in the mouth a pipette that may have been contaminated by hands or aerosols. Hand pipetting devices are extensively used for all pipetting procedures and are available in a variety of sizes and configurations (28). When contaminated pipettes are discarded into a jar containing disinfectant, the disinfectant may not be effectively mixed with the contents of the pipette. Pipettes can be decontaminated by placing them horizontally in stainless steel pans with well-fitted lids, covering them with water, and autoclaving or boiling prior to discard or reuse. Autoclaving soiled pipettes, unless they are submerged in water, greatly increases the difficulty of cleaning them.

Other hazards

Rubber stoppers should not be used in tubes or bottles containing infectious material because of the danger of contaminating hands, the bench, or other objects with the stoppers when they are removed. Screw-cap closures are less hazardous and less likely to become accidentally loosened.

Contamination of the workbench during operations involving infectious material can be avoided by covering the bench with a sheet of plastic-backed paper, plastic side down. When working with large volumes, it is recommended that the work be performed over a tray lined with plastic-backed paper, thereby reducing the chance that spilled material will run off onto the floor or clothing. Upon completion of the operation, the paper should be folded, placed in a waxed-paper bag, and autoclaved.

Food and drink *should not* be brought into a laboratory where infectious agents are handled; nor should food be stored in any part of the laboratory, including the refrigerator. For obvious reasons, smoking should not be permitted. Frequent hand washing should be encouraged.

Protective clothing, appropriate for the work performed, should be provided (20). The minimum requirement is a coat or gown. In the more hazardous situations, gloves, masks, and even plastic head covers and boots may be indicated. The maximum in clothing protection is recommended for work with the most hazardous agents designated in Class 4 (8). After use, such clothing should be autoclaved or properly disposed of and should not be worn outside the laboratory. It is important to remember that protective clothing as well as other means of protection are not substitutes for good laboratory practice and sound judgement.

Biological Safety Cabinets

Laboratories which conduct work on viruses and rickettsiae should be equipped with 1 or more biological safety cabinets, and operations likely to produce aerosols of infectious material should be carried out in the cabinet. Three classes of biological safety cabinets are available which provide varying degrees of protection for the operator and the product (5). The type employed depends upon the level of containment advised for the agent involved according to the hazard category (8) to which the agent has been assigned. Class I biological safety cabinets, which provide for the flow of room air into the cabinet, away from the operator, prevent the dissemination of infectious aerosols if the air exhausted from the cabinet is passed through a HEPA filter. The more recently developed Class II vertical laminar flow cabinets provide a curtain of flowing air between the operator and the work surface, thus protecting both the operator and the work from contamination. Exhaust air and the air bathing the work surface are HEPA filtered. Such cabinets are considered suitable for work involving all but the most hazardous agents (8), provided the cabinets are properly installed, tested, and certified according to recommended standards (23). Work with agents in the highest hazard category (8) requires a Class III gas-tight cabinet in which work is performed through rubber gloves (5).

Experimental Animals and Cell Cultures

Contact with infected animals and ectoparasites is one of the most frequent causes of laboratory infection (Table 2.2). Since circumstances which lead to cross-infection among animals constitute potential opportunities for infection of personnel, these 2 problems are closely related. Attention must be given to the proper housing of animals, disposal of animal carcasses and debris from animal rooms, inoculation of animals, and harvesting of infected tissues. The extent of the precautions necessary depends upon the agent involved. Pertinent information regarding 3 groups of agents frequently associated with laboratory infections, chlamydiae, rickettsiae, and arboviruses, is included in the chapters dealing with these agents.

Rooms where infected animals are kept should be designed to maintain negative pressure with respect to surrounding rooms and corridors. Air from these rooms should ideally be exhausted without recirculation. Air in an animal room can be recirculated within the room provided it is suitably decontaminated (7).

Cross-infection and hazard to personnel can be minimized by using cages with solid sides and screen wire tops arranged under ultraviolet lamps to effect a radiation barrier across the tops of the cages (25) or by using solid cages with filter tops (43). Even more complete isolation is obtained with individually ventilated cages (13, 17); these are particularly useful for animals that have been inoculated by exposure to an aerosol. Animals can also be isolated by enclosing them in plastic isolators originally designed for germ-free animals (13, 42). Air for the animals is supplied by an electric pump; the incoming and effluent air is passed through special filters. Food and water are made available through air locks that afford entrance to the isolator without breaking the air flow or air pressure.

Cages in which infected animals are kept should be autoclaved before the contaminated litter is disturbed. Water bottles frequently become contaminated and thus constitute a potential source of infection.

The possibility that latent infection in animals may be transferred to humans must be considered. Two outstanding examples of concern are B virus *(Herpesvirus simiae)* and hepatitis acquired from monkeys and chimpanzees, respectively. The incidence of B virus infection is low in proportion to the degree of exposure to potentially infected nonhuman primates but, more often than not, the reported disease in man is fatal (Table 2.1). Cases have resulted from monkey bites and from close contact with monkeys and their tissues (9). Since monkey kidney cells are in general use for tissue cultures in viral diagnostic laboratories, and since monkey colonies are maintained for this purpose in some institutions, the safety measures outlined by Davidson and Hummeler (9) are likely to limit the chance of infection. Other viruses that can be acquired from experimental animals are reviewed in detail elsewhere (16).

Access to monkey quarters should be restricted to authorized personnel, and only trained persons should be allowed to handle primates (20). Attendants should wear protective clothing and face masks (20). Aerosol transmission has been implicated in several cases of B virus infection, and every effort should be made to guard against infection with this agent. To prevent animals from biting attendants, cages should be squeeze type for easy capture of the animals they house. Since gloves do not provide absolute protection, the use of short-duration anesthetics or the immobilizing agent, Ketamine, is recommended. All equipment and instruments used to dissect monkeys should be considered contaminated and treated accordingly.

Extreme care in the inoculation of animals is indicated. Several instances of accidental self-inoculation have been recorded, and the precautions already mentioned for the use of syringe and needle should be observed. The materials needed should be conveniently laid out, so that it will be unnecessary to cross the hands or make other awkward motions while holding the syringe. Animals should be anesthetized or properly restrained while being inoculated to avoid accidents resulting from sudden movement of the animals. The utilization of forceps for restraining and handling suckling mice and anesthetized weanling and adult mice for intracerebral inoculation can significantly reduce the hazard of accidental self-inoculation. Infected or potentially infected mice should be handled with forceps. Intranasal inoculation is particularly hazardous and should be performed in a safety cabinet or other suitable containment system. After inoculation by exposure to an infectious aerosol, animals must be housed in ventilated cages until they are externally free of the agent to which they have been exposed.

The increasing use of continuous cell line cultures is likely to reduce the chance of laboratory infections; however, infections have occurred among laboratory workers handling primary tissue cultures prepared from monkey kidneys (9, 10).

Disposal of Contaminated Materials

Contaminated materials to be autoclaved must be handled with precaution to prevent infection of personnel. If contaminated glassware cannot be placed directly in the autoclave, it should be discarded into a deep, covered, metal container for transportation to the autoclave, and it should be the responsibility of the worker using it to see that the container is properly sterilized. Whenever possible, an autoclave should be readily accessible to obviate the transport of contaminated material through other rooms or corridors. Pipettes should be submerged horizontally in water or in disinfectant, then boiled or autoclaved. Disinfectant alone should not be relied upon because it may not be effectively mixed with the contents of the pipettes. Splashing can be avoided if pipettes and instruments are discarded into dry pans and water is carefully poured over them. If needles and syringes are rinsed after use, the point of the needle should be kept under water to prevent production of an aerosol. The use of disposable needles and syringes avoids some of the hazards associated with decontamination.

Care must be taken in the disposal of animal carcasses and infected tissues (38). Small animals and the remains of infected eggs should be placed in wax paper or autoclavable plastic bags and autoclaved in metal containers before discarding. Larger animals should be wrapped in paper or plastic and incinerated. The worker should make sure there is no delay in the disposal of such material. Stainless steel trays are preferable to wooden boards for autopsying animals and should be disinfected after use. The work surface can be covered with a disinfectant-soaked towel and swabbed with disinfectant after the autopsy. Contaminated gowns should be autoclaved.

Chemical germicides are commonly used for the initial decontamination of laboratory glassware and instruments prior to autoclaving. Ideally, a chemical germicide is selected on the basis of known activity against the agent in question. Laundry bleach (approximately 5% hypochlorite solution) is an effective broad-spectrum disinfectant for surface decontamination and for spills in the laboratory. Hypochlorite and other halogen compounds have the undesirable property of corrosiveness to metal, including stainless steel.

Decontamination

Heat, when it can be applied, is of course the most effective means of sterilization. Facilities for autoclaving with steam under 15 lb pressure at 120 C and with dry heat to at least 160 C are basic requirements in infectious disease laboratories. Unfortunately, there are many situations where heat cannot be used.

Delicate instruments, plastics, and other articles that cannot withstand heat can be disinfected with ethylene oxide (ETO). At low temperatures ETO is a liquid, but at room temperature it is a highly flammable and explosive gas requiring special handling. Nonflammable mixtures of ETO and carbon dioxide (Carbide and Carbon Chemical Corp, New York, NY), which must be used under 20 lb pressure, and mixtures of ETO and freon (24), which can be used at atmospheric pressure, are commercially available. An ordinary autoclave can be converted to use these gases; a steel drum can be modified for the purpose; or large polyethylene bags can be used as containers for ETO sterilization (35). Specially made equipment is also available commercially (American Sterilizer Company, Erie, PA, and Wilmot Castle Company, Rochester, NY). Exposure for 6–16 hr has been found to kill vegetative bacteria, spores, fungi, and a number of viruses, although smallpox virus was not completely inactivated (12).

Ultraviolet (UV) light is effective in decontaminating air and surfaces, but its usefulness is limited by its failure to penetrate. Some safety cabinets are equipped with UV lamps: UV lights are also used in air locks, as doorway barriers, and as ceiling installations in laboratories (44). The intensity of the light and the time of exposure are important considerations. For example, with ceiling lights arranged to provide 5–10 μW/cm^2 on exposed floor surfaces, the reduction in bacterial count/ft^3 of air in 1 hr varied from 75–92% (44). UV lights should be installed and shielded so as not to shine directly in the eyes of workers, and personnel should be instructed not to look directly at UV lamps. Ideally the switches for room lighting and UV lights should be interlocked so that both systems cannot be turned on at the same time. To maintain an effective intensity of radiation, UV lamps should be cleaned periodically. A technical report, BL 28, "Use of Ultraviolet Radiation in Microbiological Laboratories," by G. B. Phillips and E. Hanel, Jr., 1960, describing the effectiveness, applications, and installation of UV radiation, can be purchased by order no. PB 147043 from the Library of Congress, Photoduplication Services, Publications Board Project, Washington, D.C. 20540. The efficiency of most UV sources deteriorates with use; a lamp producing a few lumens of blue light may be transmitting relatively small quantities of effective radiation. Therefore, a UV meter (19) should be used to determine when lamps need to be replaced.

For the decontamination of rooms and buildings (12), vaporized formaldehyde has been used most extensively. It is more effective at temperatures above 24 C and at a relative humidity of 70%. It should be vaporized in a concentration of 1.0 ml of 37% formaldehyde/ft^3 of space, held for 4–10 hr, and the space aired at least overnight. Formaldehyde can be disseminated by using commercially available vaporizers, by heating paraformaldehyde in silicone oil, and by vaporizing with steam.

Beta-propiolactone (BPL) has also proven effective (12) for decontaminating spaces when vaporized in a concentration of 1 gal/12,000 ft^3 of space and held for 2–3 hr. However, problems associated with the vaporization of BPL limit its use (24), and the recent classification of BPL as a carcinogen precludes its general use for space decontamination.

Oncogenic Viruses

Up to this point the prevention of laboratory infections has been based on the hazards as demonstrated by observed cases due to certain agents or by the proven tendency of certain procedures to place the worker in contact with infectious agents. In contrast, the subjects of this and the following section are concerned with possible hazards of which the importance has yet to be demonstrated but which suggest such grave potential consequences that every effort should be made to contain the agents involved.

Study of the possible susceptibility of man to viruses that produce tumors in animals has been limited by the fact that experimental inoculation of humans with such viruses is not feasible. The potential health hazards of tumor research are extensively discussed in the report of a conference held in 1973 (16). Although many humans have been accidentally infected with SV40 occurring as a contaminant in poliovirus and adenovirus vaccines, there is no evidence that the virus has any undesirable short-term effect in humans (21), but one cannot yet be certain about possible long-term effects. The observation that serologic conversion to several animal tumor viruses has occurred in laboratory workers (43) indicates that accidental exposure has taken place. The possibilities of crossing species barriers and of virus mutations, and the dangers of working with highly concentrated virus preparations and of contaminating the experimental materials are sufficient reasons to observe the same rigid precautions in work with tumor viruses as are recommended in work with agents of known human pathogenicity (16, 43).

Recombinant DNA

There is as yet no way to evaluate the potential biohazards of work involving recombinant DNA. The many unknowns in this rapidly developing area and the conceivable undesirable consequences of certain combinations of genetic material make it essential to protect the worker and the public (6). To this end, the National Institutes of Health (NIH), with the advice of scientists from various biological disciplines, have prepared guidelines for recombinant DNA research (29), and federal legislation has been proposed to govern both research and the use of recombinant DNA (3). Copies of the guidelines, soon to be revised, are available from the Acting Director, Office of Recombinant DNA Activities, National Institutes of General Medical Sciences, National Institutes of Health, 9000 Rockville Pike, Bethesda, MD 20014. The Board of Directors of the American Society for Microbiology (ASM) has accepted the recommendation of its Task Force to endorse the NIH guidelines (2). The ASM Task Force also pointed out the need for training in the principles of contagion and host-parasite relationships for those engaged in recombinant DNA research who may not be qualified in these areas (3).

The NIH guidelines provide for 4 levels of containment (29), corresponding in general to those established by the Center for Disease Control for containment of human etiologic agents (8). In brief, level P1 requires only standard laboratory practices with work performed on open benches; level P2 requires, among other considerations, limited access to the laboratory and proper decontamination of equipment and discarded materials; level P3, in addition, requires the use of safety cabinets, controlled laboratory air flow, and more stringent policies designed to protect the worker and to prevent the escape of microorganisms into the environment; level P4 requires that work be performed in a separate building or in a controlled area of a building with air locks and the availability of maximum containment (Class III) safety cabinets. In levels P3 and P4, the universal biological hazard sign must be posted on laboratory access doors. The guidelines also prohibit certain types of experiments such as cloning of recombinant DNAs derived from oncogenic viruses classified as moderate risk (8) and other experiments which could create microorganisms with pathogenic properties. These prohibitions and other requirements for work at the 4 levels of containment are detailed in the guidelines (29), which should be consulted before any recombinant DNA work is undertaken.

Most of the research thus far on recombinant DNA has involved *Escherichia coli* K-12, and one engaged only in diagnostic virology is not likely to be concerned with work involving recombinant DNA molecules. The only viral DNAs currently considered to have the properties necessary for safe experimentation are those of polyomavirus and SV40, and then only under the P3 or P4 levels of containment depending on the particular host-vector combination used (29).

Other Considerations

Although not a substitute for good techniques and reasonable pre-cautions, immunization of personnel should be carried out whenever vaccines are available for use against the particular pathogens being handled in the laboratory. Vaccines can be obtained or prepared for certain rickettsiae and many of the viruses (20). Immunization has probably prevented many infections with typhus rickettsiae and yellow fever virus, agents which in the past have frequently infected persons working with them. Immunization with arbovirus vaccines is discussed in the chapter dealing with those viruses. Reliable immunization against psittacosis has not been developed, but antibiotics are effective. Attempts have been made to develop a B virus vaccine (18), but it is not available for general distribution. Although there is no evidence that serum from convalescents or specific immunoglobulin is of any value after symptoms of a virus infection appear, studies in experimental animals, at least with arboviruses, would suggest that passive immunization immediately or soon after an accidental exposure may limit the occurrence of disease. Efforts are being made by the Center for Disease Control (15) and the World Health Organization (4) to stockpile specific immunoglobulins processed from serum of convalescents to use after certain types of accidents in the virus laboratory.

Periodic surveillance and monitoring are recommended for laboratory personnel, and workers exposed to infectious agents should be instructed to seek medical advice whenever they become ill, particularly if the illness is of a febrile nature. Blood specimens should be obtained periodically, and the serum frozen and stored so that preinfection specimens will always be available for serologic tests should an occasion arise for such tests.

Special precautions are indicated for female workers of childbearing age and, in particular, for pregnant women (20). Women of childbearing age should not work in laboratories where rubella virus is used unless they have serologic evidence of past rubella infection or have been successfully immunized to rubella. Likewise, evidence of previous cytomegalovirus infection should be required before permitting such women to work in laboratories where there is possible exposure to this virus. The administration of a live virus vaccine of any sort to a pregnant worker is contraindicated.

A safety manual adapted to the particular circumstances of each laboratory is also recommended. This manual, encompassing the organization's written policy and practices, should state the following: the laboratory is a limited-access area restricted to operational and support personnel; eating, drinking, smoking, and the storing of food in laboratory areas are prohibited; mouth pipetting of infectious or potentially infectious materials or of toxic or corrosive chemicals is prohibited; procedures for proper decontamination and disposal of biological, chemical, and other laboratory wastes should be used. The manual should contain specific instructions for reporting accidents to proper supervisors. A plan should be established to evaluate the situation and to take appropriate action in case of laboratory spills and other emergencies. Instruction in laboratory safety should always be part of the orientation of new employees. Greatest emphasis should be placed on the need for an intelligent and responsible attitude on the part of the worker, because safety rules and mechanical devices do not in themselves prevent laboratory infections.

References

1. ANDERSON RE, STEIN L, MOSS ML, and GROSS NH: Potential infectious hazards of common bacteriological techniques. J Bacteriol 64:473–481, 1952
2. ANONYMOUS: ASM representatives express views on recombinant DNA. Am Soc Microbiol News 43:249–251, 1977
3. ANONYMOUS: Federal legislation on DNA research foreseen. Nat Soc Med Res Bull 28:No. 4, 1977
4. Arboviruses and Human Disease. WHO Tech Rep Ser No. 369, 1967
5. BARKLEY WE: Facilities and equipment available for virus containment *In* Biohazards in Biological Research, Hellman A, Oxman MN, and Pollack R, (eds) Cold Spring Harbor Laboratory, Cold Spring Harbor, NY, 1973, pp 327-341
6. BERG P, BALTIMORE D, BRENNER S, ROBIN RO, and SINGER MF: Summary statement of the Asilomar conference on recombinant DNA molecules. Science 188:991–994, 1975
7. CHATIGNY MA: Protection against infection in the microbiological laboratory: devices and procedures *In* Advances in Applied Microbiology, Vol 3, Academic Press, New York, 1961, pp 131-192
8. CENTER FOR DISEASE CONTROL: Classification of Etiologic Agents on the Basis of Hazard. Center for Disease Control, Public Health Service, US Dept of HEW, Atlanta, Georgia, 1974
9. DAVIDSON WL and HUMMELER K: B virus infection in man *In* Care and Diseases of the Research Monkey. Ann NY Acad Sci 85:970–979, 1960
10. GORDON-SMITH CE, SIMPSON DIH, BOWEN ETW, and ZLOTNIK I: Fatal human disease from vervet monkeys. Lancet 2:1119–1121, 1967
11. GREGG MB: Recent outbreaks of lymphocytic choriomeningitis in the United States of America. Bull WHO 52:549–553, 1975
12. GREMILLION GG, HANEL E JR, and PHILLIPS GB: Practical procedures for microbial decontamination. Technical Report, US Army Chemical Corps, Fort Detrick, Md, 1959
13. GRIESEMER RA and MANNING JS: Animal facilities *In* Biohazards in Biological Research, Hellman A, Oxman MN, and Pollack R, (eds) Cold Spring Harbor Laboratory, Cold Spring Harbor, NY, 1973, pp 316-326
14. HALL CV: A biological safety centrifuge. Health Lab Sci 12:104–106, 1975
15. HANSON RP, SULKIN SE, BUESCHER EL, HAMMON W McD, McKINNEY RW, and WORK TH: Arbovirus infections of laboratory workers. SCIENCE 158:1283–1286, 1967
16. HELLMAN A, OXMAN MN, and POLLACK R: Biohazards in biological research, Cold Spring Harbor Laboratory, Cold Spring Harbor, NY, 1973
17. HORSFALL FL JR and BAUER JH: Individual isolation of infected animals in a single room. J Bacteriol 40:569–580, 1940
18. HULL RN: B virus vaccine. Lab Animal Sci 21:Part II, 1068–1071, 1971
19. JAGGER A: A small and inexpensive ultraviolet dose-rate meter useful in biological experiments. Rad Res 14:394–403, 1961
20. Laboratory Safety at the Center for Disease Control, Center for Disease Control, Public Health Service, US Dept. of HEW, Atlanta, Georgia, 1974.

21. LEWIS AM JR: Experience with SV 40 and adenovirus-SV 40 hybrids *In* Biohazards in Biological Research, Hellman A, Oxman MN, and Pollack R (eds), Cold Spring Harbor Laboratory, Cold Spring Harbor, NY, 1973, pp 96–113

22. McCOLLUM RW: A reappraisal of viral hepatitis in chimpanzees. Mil Med 127:994–996, 1962

23. NATIONAL SANITATION FOUNDATION: Standard No. 49 for Class II (Laminar Flow) Biohazard Cabinets, National Sanitation Foundation, Ann Arbor, Michigan, 1976

24. PHILLIPS CR: Gaseous sterilization *In* Disinfection, Sterilization and Preservation, Lawrence CA and Block SS (eds) Lea & Febiger, Philadelphia, 1968, pp 669–685

25. PHILLIPS GB, REITMAN M, MULLICAN CL, AND GARDNER GD JR: Applications of germicidal ultraviolet in infectious disease laboratories. III. The use of ultraviolet barriers on animal cage racks. Animal Care Panel Proceedings 7:235–244, 1957

26. PIKE RM: Laboratory-associated infections: summary and analysis of 3921 cases. Health Lab Sci 13:105–114, 1976

27. PIKE RM, SULKIN SE, and SCHULZE ML: Continuing importance of laboratory-acquired infections. Am J Public Health 55:190–199, 1965

28. Pipetting Aids and Other Safety Devices for the Biomedical Laboratory. School of Public Health, University of Minnesota, Minneapolis, Minnesota, Rev 1975

29. Recombinant DNA Research Guidelines, DHEW, NIH. Federal Register 41:27902–27943, 1976

30. REITMAN M, ALG RL, MILLER WS, and GROSS NH: Potential infectious hazards of laboratory techniques. III. Viral techniques. J Bacteriol 68:549–554, 1954

31. REITMAN M, FRANK MA, ALG RL, and MILLER WS: Modifications of the high-speed safety blender. Appl Microbiol 2:173, 1954

32. REITMAN M, MOSS ML, HARSTED JB, ALG RL, and GROSS NH: Potential infectious hazards of laboratory techniques. I. Lyophilization. J Bacteriol 68:541–544, 1954

33. REITMAN M, MOSS ML, HARSTED JB, ALG RL, and GROSS NH: Potential infectious hazards of laboratory techniques. II. The handling of lyophilized cultures. J Bacteriol 68:545–548, 1954

34. REITMAN M and PHILLIPS GB: Biological hazards of common laboratory procedures. III. The centrifuge. Am J Med Technol 22:14–16, 1956

35. SCHLEY DG, HOFFMAN RK, and PHILLIPS CR: Simple improvised chambers for gas sterilization with ethylene oxide. Appl Microbiol 8:15–19, 1960

36. SIEGERT R, SHU HL, SLENCZKA W, PETERS D, and MULLER G: Zur Atiologie einer unbekanten, von affen ausgegangen menschlichen Infektionskrankheit. Deutsch Med Wochenschr 51:2341–2343, 1967

37. SLEPUSHKEN AN: An epidemiological study of laboratory infections with Venezuelan equine encephalomyelitis. Probl Virol 4:54–58, 1959

38. SMADEL JE: The hazard of acquiring virus and rickettsial diseases in the laboratory. Am J Public Health 41:788–795, 1951

39. STEIN CD and ROGERS H: Recovery of viable microorganisms and viruses from vapors removed from frozen suspensions of biologic material during lyophilization. Am J Vet Res 11:339–344, 1950

40. SULKIN SE and PIKE RM: Viral infections contracted in the laboratory. N Engl J Med 241:205–213, 1949

41. SULKIN SE and PIKE RM: Survey of laboratory-acquired infections. Am J Public Health 41:769–781, 1951

42. TREXLER PC and REYNOLDS RI: Flexible film apparatus for rearing and use of germfree animals. Appl Microbiol 5:406–412, 1957

43. WEDUM AG, BARKLEY WE, and HELLMAN A: Handling of infectious agents. J Am Vet Med Assoc 161:1557–1567, 1972

44. WEDUM AG, HANEL E JR, and PHILLIPS GB: Ultraviolet sterilization in microbiological laboratories. Public Health Rep 71:331–336, 1956

45. WEDUM AG and KRUSE RH: Assessment of risk of human infection in the microbiological laboratory. Misc Publ 30, Industrial Health and Safety Directorate, Fort Detrick, Frederick, Maryland, 1969

CHAPTER 3

CELL CULTURE TECHNIQUES FOR DIAGNOSTIC VIROLOGY

Nathalie J. Schmidt

Introduction

It has been almost 30 years since the discovery by Enders and his co-workers (24) that polioviruses could replicate in cell cultures of non-neural origin stimulated extensive use of *in vitro* cell cultures for propagation of human and animal viruses. In the ensuing years, cell cultures have provided more economical and easily handled host systems for study of long-recognized viruses such as those of poliomyelitis, measles, and mumps, and have also permitted the recognition of a large number of human enteric and respiratory viruses which are not propagable in eggs or mice. To a large extent cell culture systems have supplanted animal and embryonated egg host systems for use in virus isolation attempts, neutralization (Nt) tests, or for preparation of viral antigens.

The availability of reliable and well-characterized cell cultures and cell culture media from commercial sources, the development of efficient and economical microcell culture techniques, the development of standardized cell culture procedures, the wider availability of viral antisera, and the development of disposable cell culture vessels in both glass and plastic have all facilitated the establishment of cell culture procedures for viral diagnosis in increasing numbers of clinical microbiology laboratories in hospitals and medical centers. The development of more rapid procedures, such as immunofluorescent (FA) or immunoperoxidase (IP) staining, for identification of viruses isolated in cell cultures has made virus isolation and identification a more efficient and rewarding undertaking for the diagnostic laboratory.

Kinds of cell cultures employed in diagnostic virology

In order to achieve greater uniformity and understanding in the use of terms relating to cultivation of cells *in vitro,* the Tissue Culture Association established a committee on terminology which prepared recommendations on the usage of animal cell culture terms (27), and the terminology used in this chapter is based upon these recommendations.

Cell culture is the term used to denote growing of cells *in vitro* under conditions where the cells are no longer organized into tissues. This is the type of culture generally employed in diagnostic virology.

Tissue or organ cultures are terms used to denote maintenance or growth of tissues, organ primordia, or whole or parts of an organ *in vitro,* in a way which allows differentiation and preservation of the architecture and/or function. This type of culture has been valuable for the propagation of certain fastidious respiratory (47) or enteric (128) viruses, but is not widely used due to difficulties in handling the culture and in observing an effect of the virus in the system.

Cells may be cultivated *in vitro* in three different types of systems. In *explant* cultures a fragment of a tissue or organ is used to initiate a culture. In some cases this is embedded into a plasma clot to aid in attachment to the culture vessel. This system is rarely used to prepare host cell cultures for inoculation with virus preparations or clinical materials, but establishment of explant cultures from tissue specimens is sometimes used as a means of recovering viruses from the tissues, and it is generally more sensitive than inoculation of tissue homogenates into prepared cell cultures. *Monolayer* cultures consist of a single layer of cells growing on a surface. These are generally prepared by treating the original tissue, or an established cell culture, with cell-dispersing agents such as proteolytic enzymes or chelating agents, and planting the cell suspension in a glass or plastic culture vessel to which the cells adhere. This is the cell culture system most widely used in diagnostic virology. A *suspension culture* is one in which cells multiply while suspended in fluid medium. With proper manipulation, cells in agitated suspension cultures can be maintained in the logarithmic growth phase and provide a source of cells in a highly reproducible metabolic state. Very large populations of cells can be obtained in this system, and suspension cultures are useful for preparation of large volumes of high-titer virus, as in antigen or vaccine production. Some cell types can not be cultivated in free suspension, but these can be grown in suspension cultures through the use of carrier particles to which the cells adhere and form a monolayer (119).

In vitro cell cultures are also described in terms based upon the characteristics of the cells. A *primary cell culture* is one started from cells, tissues or organs taken directly from the organism; when a primary culture is subcultivated for the first time, it becomes a *cell line.* Cell lines may be of several types. *Diploid cell lines* are those in which at least 75% of the cells have the same karyotype as normal cells of the species from which the cells were originally cultured. These lines do not have the property of indefinite serial passage but tend to die out by the fiftieth passage. In the past, diploid cells in serial passage were frequently referred to as "cell strains," but the term *cell strain* is now applied more specifically to cells derived from either a primary culture or cell line by the selection or cloning of cells having specific properties or markers, and these must persist through subsequent cultivation. A *heteroploid cell line* is one having fewer than 75% of cells with diploid chromosome constitution. This term does not imply that the cells are malignant or are able to grow indefinitely *in vitro.* An *established cell line* is one which has demonstrated the potential to be subcultured indefinitely *in vitro;*

generally, a culture must be subcultured at least 70 times before it can be considered to be established.

Detection of virus replication in cell cultures

Cellular degeneration. Many viruses manifest their presence in susceptible cell cultures by producing degenerative changes in the cells called a cytopathic effect (CPE) which can be observed microscopically (Fig 3.1). Depending upon the virus, CPE may range from a rapid and extensive rounding of the cells which causes their detachment from the surface, to a slowly progressing CPE involving discrete foci of infected cells. Most of the major groups of human viruses produce a characteristic type of CPE, and this may aid the experienced observer in identifying the virus. The diverse types of CPE produced by different viruses are described in the various chapters of this book.

Plaque formation. Cytopathic viruses, and even some viruses which do not produce CPE in cell cultures maintained on a fluid medium, may be detected macroscopically by their ability to form plaques in monolayers under a solid medium. A plaque is a focus of virus-infected cells which does not take up the vital stain, neutral red, and thus appears as a clear area against a background of stained viable cells (Fig 3.2). Plaque formation is further discussed below.

Metabolic inhibition. Infection of cell cultures with cytopathic viruses may be evidenced colorimetrically by metabolic inhibition. Cells metabolizing in a medium containing glucose produce large amounts of acid which converts the phenol red indicator in the medium from red to yellow. If a cytopathic virus is present, however, the cells degenerate before they have an opportunity to produce sufficient acid to convert the indicator. Thus, virus activity (cytopathogenicity) is evidenced by red medium after an appropriate incubation period, while lack of virus activity of specific virus neutralization is indicated by a conversion of the indicator from red to yellow.

For primary isolation of viruses, metabolic inhibition is not a reliable indication of virus replication, since the concentration of virus in clinical specimens is frequently so low that the cultures have an opportunity to produce acid before they are damaged by the virus. Metabolic inhibition tests are employed primarily for virus identification and for Nt-antibody assays in which the virus is established in the particular cell type and conditions of the test are carefully controlled. Figure 3.3 depicts a metabolic inhibition test for assay of coxsackievirus antibodies.

Hemadsorption (HAd). Members of the orthomyxovirus and paramyxovirus groups may fail to produce a clear-cut CPE in infected cell cultures, but the fact that they possess hemagglutinins (sites which combine with erythrocytes [RBC] of certain species) permits their detection by the HAd technique. For this procedure a suspension of guinea pig or chicken RBC is added to the cell culture, and after a suitable incubation period microscopic examination reveals the RBC adhering in clumps to the infected host cell monolayer (Fig 3.4). Not all groups of viruses which agglutinate

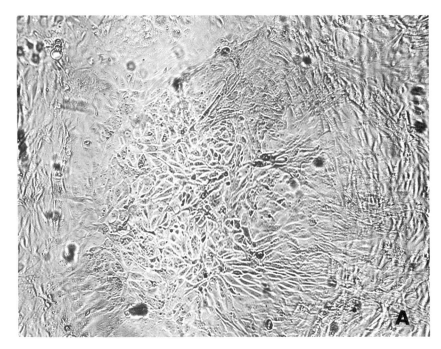

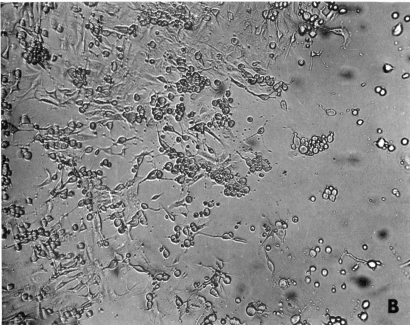

Figure 3.1—Viral CPE: A, uninfected monkey kidney monolayer cell culture; B, monkey kidney monolayer cell culture 4 days after inoculation with 32 TCID$_{50}$ of echovirus type 19.

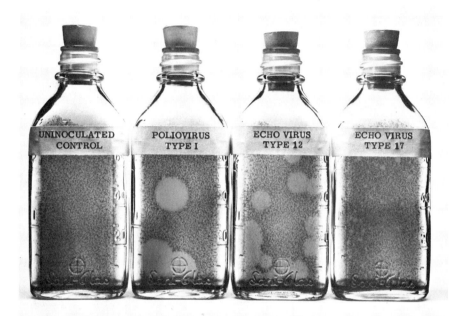

Figure 3.2—Virus plaques in closed bottle cultures. Photographed 5 days after infection of the monkey kidney cell monolayers.

RBC *in vitro* can adsorb them directly onto infected cells in culture; the property of hemadsorption is restricted to those viruses which mature by budding from the host cell surface.

Mixed hemadsorption. A "mixed" HAd technique, quite different in principle from the HAd method, has also been devised for detection of certain viruses which bud from the host cell surface (25, 26). Virus-infected host cells are first treated with viral immune serum produced in rabbits or rats, and the antibodies combine specifically with virus at the cell surface. When the cells are next treated with sheep RBC coated with anti-rabbit or anti-rat globulins, the RBC are adsorbed to the infected cells by virtue of the combination between the rabbit or rat immune globulins (viral antibody) and the antispecies globulins coating the RBC.

Immunofluorescent or immunoperoxidase staining. Another way to detect virus replication in the absence of CPE is by use of FA or IP staining. Chapters 4 and 5 in this volume are devoted to these procedures.

Interference. Some noncytopathic viruses may be detected in cell cultures by the reduced ability of the cultures to support the growth of a challenge virus, i.e., by interference. The test virus is first inoculated into cell cultures, and after several days' incubation a standard dose of a known cytopathic (or hemadsorbing) challenge virus is introduced into the cultures. After further incubation the cultures are observed for presence or absence of CPE or hemadsorption of the challenge virus. This technique has found its widest application in work with rubella virus.

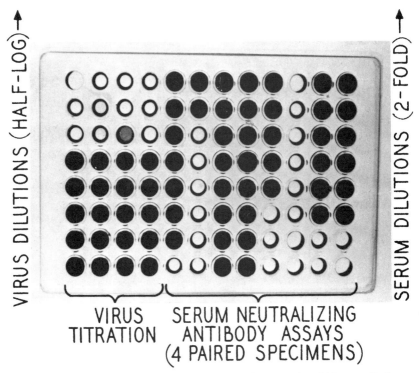

VIRUS DILUTIONS (HALF-LOG)⟶

SERUM DILUTIONS (2-FOLD)⟶

VIRUS   SERUM NEUTRALIZING
TITRATION   ANTIBODY ASSAYS
(4 PAIRED SPECIMENS)

Figure 3.3—Metabolic inhibition test in BS-C-1 grivet monkey kidney cells for coxsackievirus type B5. View of top of plate. The pH of the medium in the
dark wells indicates viral CPE and that of the medium in the light wells
indicates lack of viral effect (in the virus titration) or virus neutralization
(in the antibody assays). Virus is titrated in half-log dilutions using 4
wells for each dilution. Acute- and convalescent-phase sera are titrated
in 2-fold dilutions using a single well for each dilution; these are tested
against approximately 100 $TCID_{50}$ of virus. (See text for further details of
test.)

Evidence of viral infection in organ cultures. Certain viruses multiplying in organ cultures may be detected by subculture of the nutrient fluids
into monolayer cultures where the virus exerts a CPE or hemadsorption.
Others are evidenced by the fact that they cause cessation of ciliary activity
and eventual degeneration of the epithelial cells, some are demonstrable by
means of electron microscopy (EM) or FA staining, and others only by inoculation of human volunteers (47).

Preparation of *in vitro* Cell Cultures

In handling cell cultures, laboratory personnel must be concerned not
only with preventing microbial contamination of the cultures, but also with

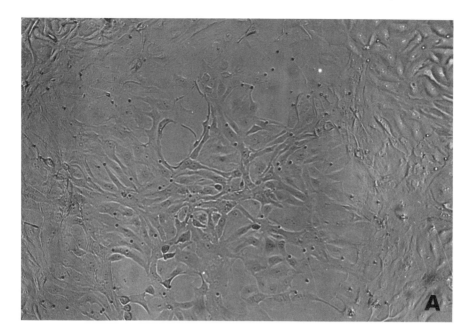

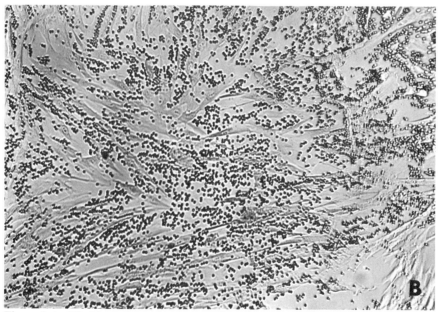

Figure 3.4—Viral hemadsorption: A, uninfected monkey kidney cell culture after addition of guinea pig RBC suspension; B, monkey kidney cell culture infected with parainfluenza type 3 virus after addition of RBC suspension;
the guinea pig RBC are adsorbed to the virus-infected monkey kidney
cell monolayers.

preventing contamination of the working environment with cell culture materials. Cells from any source may be infected with latent viruses or other agents, and therefore uninoculated, as well as inoculated, cultures must be considered potentially hazardous. Cultures should be prepared under strict aseptic conditions, and all cultures, culture fluids, or materials coming in contact with the cultures should be decontaminated by autoclaving before they are discarded.

It is also important to handle cell cultures so as to avoid cross-contaminating different cell types. A recent study has illustrated how readily this can occur (81). Cultures of different cell types should never be prepared or handled at the same time, and working areas should be thoroughly decontaminated between preparation of different cell types.

Cell culture media

Cell culture media employed in virology can be divided into two broad categories, growth media and maintenance media. These contain various combinations of natural or synthetic ingredients.

Growth media are used for initiation of the cultures and are composed of ingredients which promote rapid cellular proliferation, usually serum in combination with a synthetic medium. Prior to inoculating cell cultures with virus, the growth medium is removed and the cultures are washed with a balanced salt solution to remove antibodies or other virus-inhibiting substances which may be present in the serum. However, fetal and agamma calf sera are usually free from virus-inhibiting substances, and if these are used for outgrowth, it is not necessary to wash the cultures before using them for virus propagation.

Maintenance media are intended to keep the cell cultures in a slow, steady state of metabolism during the time of virus replication, and they are less rich than growth media in substances promoting rapid cellular metabolism and proliferation. Maintenance media for virus propagation should be serum-free if possible, but for long maintenance of cultures or for certain types of cells, serum is required. In these cases fetal or agamma calf serum is most suitable. Other sera should be pretested to establish that they are free of inhibitory activity for the viruses being studied.

Biological materials

The biological substances used as components for cell culture media include sera, bacteriological media, skim milk, and embryo extracts.

Although intensive efforts have been made over the past two or more decades to devise chemically defined media for cell culture, none of these has been entirely satisfactory for propagation of cells for growth of mammalian viruses, and the media must be supplemented with serum, at least for outgrowth of the cell cultures. Problems associated with the use of sera in cell culture media are several, including the variable composition of sera which makes standardization impossible, variability in the growth-promoting properties of different lots of sera, and the fact that sera may be contaminated with mycoplasmas, animal viruses, or bacteriophages.

Since the nutritional requirements of cells used in different laboratories can vary widely, it is important to check the growth-promoting qualities of new lots of serum by comparing them to lots previously shown to be satisfactory. In this laboratory, new lots of fetal bovine serum are assessed by carrying cells through 3 serial passages in parallel in medium supplemented with the new serum and in the same medium supplemented with a known satisfactory serum lot, and comparing the cell counts obtained with the 2 sera at each passage level. Other methods have been described based upon comparative cell counts or protein content after a single passage (88) or upon comparative plating efficiency of primary hamster embryo cells (38). It has been noted that fetal bovine serum that is collected aseptically and is not subjected to sterilization by filtration has greater growth-promoting properties than does filtered serum (8), and it is also free from bacteriophage contaminants; however, the cost of producing it is usually very high.

Serum sold by most commercial firms for use in cell culture is pretested for mycoplasma, bovine viruses and, in some instances, bacteriophage contaminants.

The use of bacteriological media as components of cell culture media provides a relatively inexpensive, easily prepared source of many essential nutrients, free from antibody or other virus-inhibiting substances. Lactalbumin hydrolysate, yeast extract, tryptose phosphate, and peptones are the bacteriological media most commonly employed for this purpose. Skim milk has also been utilized as a protein component of cell culture media and similarly possesses the advantage of being inexpensive and free from virus-inhibiting substances.

It was early noted that the *in vitro* growth of cells could be accelerated by addition of embryonic tissue extracts to the nutrient medium. Chick embryo and bovine embryo extracts have been used in cell culture media for virology, but neither is used extensively at this time.

Chemically defined media

A wide variety of synthetic media has been devised for use with mammalian cell cultures, and many of these have been modified based upon specialized needs or upon newer findings on the nutritional requirements of cells in culture. In order to provide a basis for standardization of cell culture media, Morton performed a survey for the Standards Committee of the Tissue Culture Association and in 1970 published the correct formulations for the media most widely used in cell culture procedures (77). A supplement to the survey giving corrected formulas for certain media was published in 1974 (92). Exact adherence to these formulations assures greater uniformity in the commercial production of cell culture media and also aids laboratories in preparing their own cell culture media.

For propagation of cells *in vitro* it is necessary to maintain physiological conditions of osmotic pressure and pH, as well as adequate concentrations of the essential inorganic ions. This is accomplished through the use of a balanced salt solution (BSS) which is the basis of all chemically defined cell culture media. Some BSS also contain glucose as an energy source. The BSS most commonly employed by the virologist are Hanks BSS (41) and

Earle BSS (23), the latter possessing the greater buffering capacity. Detailed instructions for preparing 10X stock solutions of these reagents are given in the Appendix of this chapter.

Most BSS contain a CO_2-bicarbonate-buffering system, and therefore the cultures must be incubated in tightly closed containers or in a 5% CO_2 atmosphere to prevent loss of CO_2 with a resultant increase in pH above the toxic level. However, organic buffers, and particularly HEPES, are being used increasingly in cell culture media (37, 110, 127), and media with a HEPES-buffering system are now available from commercial sources. The organic buffers have greater buffering capacity than bicarbonate buffers in the physiological pH range, and another advantage to their use is the fact that cultures in HEPES buffer need not be incubated in sealed containers or a CO_2 atmosphere. In some instances bicarbonate is used in combination with a HEPES buffer, as the bicarbonate ion is known to be an essential metabolite for certain cell lines. However, it is generally not necessary to supplement HEPES-buffered media with bicarbonate, since sufficient bicarbonate is apparently supplied by serum used in the media or is generated by the CO_2 in the atmosphere. HEPES buffer is used in cell culture media at concentrations of 10 mM–25 mM. The substitution of galactose for glucose in the medium also eliminates the need for a CO_2-buffering system (61), as less acid is produced from the former substrate.

Phenol red indicator, which is active in the physiologic pH ranges, is usually incorporated into cell culture media to indicate decreases in pH produced by cellular metabolism, signaling the need for replenishment of the medium. It is used at concentrations of 15–20 mg/liter; higher concentrations may be toxic.

BSS have been supplemented with various amino acids, vitamins, and other chemically-defined nutrients to produce the many synthetic media which are in use today. Although numerous chemically defined media have been introduced over the past 3 decades, those most commonly used by the virologist are medium No. 199 (76), Eagle basal medium (BME) (20) or minimum essential medium (MEM) (21), Leibovitz medium No. 15 (L-15) (61), and the Roswell Park Memorial Institute (RPMI) series of media devised for cultivation of leukocytes (75, 77). All of these are available from commercial sources, and updated and corrected formulations are given elsewhere (77, 92).

Some of the early cell culture media were extremely complex, containing large numbers of amino acids, vitamins, nucleic acid constituents, intermediary metabolites, and accessory growth factors. However, when it was shown that addition of increasingly large numbers of components to synthetic media might contribute enough trace metals to be toxic to the cells (46), attention was focused upon more exact determination of the nutrients essential for *in vitro* proliferation of cells. Out of some of these studies evolved Eagle BME, which contains minimal requirements of vitamins and amino acids essential for growth of mammalian cells, and Eagle MEM, which is considered to contain optimal concentrations of these components. MEM is more widely used in virology than is BME, and it has been modified by various investigators for specialized purposes (77). For certain cell types the concentrations of amino acids and vitamins are increased 2-fold or 4-fold to give "fortified" MEM. For propagating cells in suspension, the calcium is omitted and the concentration of NaH_2PO_4 is increased 10-fold for more effective buffering (68). Other modifications consist of adding certain nonessential amino acids (77). The medium can be prepared with either a Hanks or Earle BSS base. The Appendix of this chapter describes the preparation of Eagle MEM as an example of the compounding of a synthetic cell culture medium.

Now that cell culture media are available from several reliable commercial sources, it is usually more efficient and economical for virus laboratories to purchase complex media rather than to attempt to prepare them. The media are made in large lots according to standard formulations (77, 92), and are pretested by the manufacturers for ability to support cellular growth. This ensures greater uniformity of quality than can be achieved by preparing small lots of media in individual laboratories. However, it is good practice to test all lots of new media, from any source, for suitability in cell culture by comparing growth and maintenance of cells in the new medium with that obtained in parallel cultures on a previous lot of the same type of medium known to be satisfactory.

Cell culture media are available commercially in either liquid or powdered form, and the liquid media may be obtained in completed form (1X) or as concentrated stock solutions. If powdered or concentrated media are used, careful attention should be given to the quality of water used for preparing the final medium. Water for use in cell culture media is most satisfactorily prepared by demineralization followed by distillation in an all-glass still, and it should have a minimum of 1,000,000 ohms resistance. While powdered cell culture media have generally been highly satisfactory for use in virology laboratories, there may be a few situations, such as for the growth of certain very fastidious transformed cell lines and for establishing human fibroblast cultures, in which they have been found somewhat less satisfactory than liquid media. Therefore, if unsatisfactory results are obtained with powdered media, it might be advisable to try the same media in liquid form.

Liquid and powdered cell culture media are generally stored at 4–5 C, while serum and stock solutions of vitamins, glutamine, and antibiotics are stored at −20 C. It has recently been shown that fluorescent light may be detrimental to cell culture media (124), since it causes the formation of toxic photoproducts from riboflavin and tryptophane in the media. Therefore, it is recommended that liquid media be stored in the dark.

Certain components such as $NaHCO_3$, antibiotics, and glutamine are not incorporated into the media initially, but are prepared as stock solutions and added at the time of use.

Many cell culturists recommend omitting antibiotics from cell culture media, and there are obvious advantages to this. It necessitates the use of stringent aseptic techniques, which in turn reduces the risk of contamination. If contamination does occur, it is readily recognizable, and antibiotic resistant contaminants are not induced by exposure to low levels of antibiotics. However, from a practical standpoint this approach is seldom feasible in the diagnostic virology laboratory. This is because work is usually done on a relatively large scale which entails a greater risk of contamination, and because potentially contaminated clinical specimens are inoculated into the cell cultures. A combination of penicillin and streptomycin, sometimes supplemented with amphotericin B as an anti-fungal agent, has been most widely used; however, it is recognized that these may be less adequate than some of the wider spectrum antibiotics in controlling contamination. Gentamicin has received increasing use as a cell culture antibiotic (1, 93). In addition to its broad-spectrum activity, it also possesses the advantage of being extremely stable and even resistant to autoclaving. Gentamicin generally has no toxic effect on cells at the concentrations recommended in media, and no adverse effect on virus replication. However, in our experience it seems to be slightly more toxic than penicillin and streptomycin for certain delicate lines of human fetal diploid cells. A recent review by Armstrong (1) discusses the control of bacterial and fungal contamination of cell cultures and recommends concentrations of various antibiotics for use in cell cultures.

Handling and storage of fresh tissues

Fetuses, organs, and membranes to be cultivated *in vitro* should be placed in a sterile container immediately after collection and covered with fluid. This may be a BSS if the tissue is to be processed within a short time, but if it is to be stored, nutrient medium should be employed. The holding medium should contain antibiotics to suppress bacterial contamination. Although it is preferable to culture the tissues as soon as possible after they are obtained, they can be stored satisfactorily for periods of 24–48 hr, and even longer, if certain precautions are observed. To maintain viability during storage, it is essential that nutrients diffuse throughout the tissues; therefore, large organs should be cut into smaller pieces, and organs of fetuses should be excised for storage. The temperature at which the tissues are stored is also important as metabolites are depleted more rapidly at higher temperatures. Thus, storage at refrigerator temperatures is recommended, and tissue fragments which are transported to distant points should be packed in an iced container. Prior to treatment with dispersing agents the tissues should be washed several times with a BSS.

Cell dispersing techniques
Treatment with proteolytic enzymes

Various proteolytic enzymes selectively degrade the protein matrix which binds cells in tissues and in cultures and disperse the cells before they are seriously damaged. Prolonged proteolytic treatment can, however, have a damaging effect on cells, and therefore most cell dispersal methods are designed to expose tissues and cells for the minimum length of time required to give monodispersed cell suspensions. Some procedures use a combination of a proteolytic enzyme with a chelating agent such as ethylenediaminetetraacetic acid (EDTA) or sodium citrate, and this may give better cell dispersion and higher yields of viable cells than can be obtained with enzymes alone (74, 84).

Trypsin is the enzyme most widely employed in dispersing mammalian cells for culture. However, the crude trypsin preparations used for this purpose contain other proteolytic enzymes, particularly elastase, and there is evidence that these enzymes are the most active in dissociating cells (86); crystalline trypsin is relatively ineffective in dispersing cells in certain fresh tissues and cultures.

Pronase has been found to disperse monolayer fibroblast cultures more rapidly and effectively than does trypsin, but it is less efficient for dispersing certain types of epithelial cell lines (30). Pronase is not inactivated by serum as is trypsin and must be thoroughly washed from cells before they are cultured.

For the most effective dissociation of cells, it is recommended that enzyme solutions be prepared in buffered saline free from calcium and magnesium, as the presence of these ions increases the stability of the intercellular matrix.

Trypsinization of fresh tissues. Methods for dispersing cells from kidney tissue are given as examples of this procedure. Cells can be dispersed from kidney tissues by multiple extraction methods based upon the procedure originally described by Youngner (130), by overnight trypsinization as devised by Bodian (7), or by various automatic methods based upon the technique developed by Rappaport (89). In this laboratory a modification of the high-yield trypsin-versene extraction method developed by Montes de Oca et al (74) is used for dispersal of monkey kidney cells. This method is reportedly suitable for dispersing rabbit and human kidney cells as well; the additional use of collagenase facilitates dispersal of human kidney cells (73). Kidney tissue from other species is generally dispersed by overnight trypsinization in this laboratory. All manipulations are conducted with sterile equipment under aseptic conditions.

Animals are exsanguinated and the kidneys are excised, placed in a sterile beaker, washed in 3 changes of Hanks BSS, and then transferred to a sterile Petri dish where the pelvis and capsule are removed from kidneys of larger species. The tissue is then minced in a small amount of phosphate-buffered saline (PBS), pH 7.5 (see Appendix) into pieces 2-4 mm, using paired scalpels.

The kidney-mince is put into a trypsinization flask (an Erlenmeyer flask with a side arm and 4-8 equally spaced indentations near the base) containing a magnetic stirring bar, in which it is washed by stirring for 30 min in 200 ml of PBS, pH 7.5. After the tissue has settled and the wash fluid is removed, the tissue is trypsinized by one of the following methods.

Trypsin-versene extraction method. The volumes of reagents indicated below are those used for processing one pair of monkey kidneys.

1. A trypsin-versene solution is prepared by mixing 250 ml of a 1% solution of trypsin (see Appendix), 600 ml of PBS, pH 7.5, 2 ml of 8% versene (EDTA), 8.5 ml of penicillin-streptomycin-neomycin-bacitracin solution (see Appendix), and 0.85 ml of fungizone solution (see Appendix).

2. To the washed tissue-mince in the trypsinization flask is added 100 ml of pre-warmed (37 C) trypsin-versene solution, and the suspension is stirred, at a rate just short of bubbling, at room temperature for 15 min.

3. The supernatant cell suspension is harvested, 100 ml of fresh trypsin-versene solution is added to the trypsinization flask, and the tissue is again stirred for 15 min. This is continued for about 8 changes of trypsin-versene solution or until the cortical tissue is completely digested.

4. Harvested cells are pooled into a flask containing 300 ml of growth medium and held at 4 C until extraction is completed.

5. At the end of the extraction, the pooled cell suspension is passed through a funnel lined with stainless steel wire gauze (72 mesh, wire diameter 0.0037″, Newark Wire Cloth Co, Newark, NJ or Colorado Fuel and Iron Corp, Emeryville, CA) into 250-ml centrifuge bottles.

6. The cells are sedimented by horizontal centrifugation at 800 rpm for 15 min, and the supernatant fluid is aspirated from the packed cells.

7. The cells in each 250-ml bottle are collected into 10 ml of growth medium and transferred to 15-ml conical, graduated centrifuge tubes. The cells are packed by centrifugation at 700 rpm for 10 min, and the volume of the cell pack is noted.

8. The supernatant fluid is removed and, based upon the packed cell volume or upon counting of viable cells by the trypan blue exclusion method (see below), the cells are suspended in the appropriate volume of growth medium (see below under preparation of cultures of individual cell types) and planted in culture vessels.

Overnight trypsinization method. This procedure can be used for dispersing cells from monkey, human, hamster, rabbit, porcine, bovine, and canine kidneys. The volume of reagents indicated below are those used for processing one pair of monkey kidneys.

1. To the washed tissue-mince in the trypsinization flask is added 150–200 ml of fresh 0.25% trypsin solution in Hanks BSS and the suspension is stirred at a rate just short of bubbling, at 4 C overnight.

2. The following day the suspension is passed through a funnel lined with 72-mesh stainless steel wire gauze into 250-ml centrifuge bottles, and the cells are sedimented by horizontal centrifugation at 800 rpm for 15 min.

3. The supernatant fluid is removed and the cells are washed 3 times by resuspending in 100 ml of Hanks BSS and centrifuging at 800 rpm for 15 min.

4. The cells are then resuspended in 10–15 ml of Hanks BSS and transferred to conical, graduated centrifuge tubes. The cells are packed by horizontal centrifugation at 700 rpm for 10 min, and the volume of the cell pack is noted. Alternatively, the viable cells can be enumerated using the trypan blue exclusion method (see below).

5. Based upon the packed cell volume or the count of viable cells, the cells are suspended to the appropriate concentration in growth medium (see below under preparation of cultures of individual cell types) and planted in culture vessels.

Multiple extraction trypsinization method. The procedure given below is that used by Tyrrell et al (118) for dispersing cells from human fetal kidney tissue, and the volumes of reagents given are those used for this type of kidney.

1. Minced kidney tissue is washed 3 times in Hanks BSS in a trypsinization flask. Fifty ml of a 0.25% trypsin solution in Hanks BSS (or PBS, pH 7.5) is added and the mixture is stirred for 5 min. The tissue is then allowed to settle and the supernatant fluid is discarded.

2. Fifty to 100 ml of fresh 0.25% trypsin solution is added to the tissue and stirred for 20 min at room temperature. The supernatant fluid (first extraction) is decanted into a large centrifuge bottle, and the cells are sedimented by centrifugation at 600 rpm for 20 min. The trypsin solution is removed, and the cells are washed twice by resuspending in Hanks BSS and centrifuging at 600 rpm for 2 min. The cells are then resuspended in a small volume of Hanks BSS and held in an ice-bath to await pooling with cells from subsequent extractions.

3. Fresh trypsin solution is added to the tissue, and 2–3 more extractions and washings are conducted as described in (2.) above.

4. The pooled suspensions from all of the extractions are passed through a funnel lined with 72-mesh stainless steel wire gauze into a large centrifuge tube.

5. The cells are sedimented by horizontal centrifugation at 800 rpm for 15 min, and the supernatant fluid is discarded. The cells are then resuspended in 10–15 ml of growth medium and transferred to a conical, graduated centrifuge tube. The cells are packed by horizontal centrifugation at 1000 rpm for 10 min, and the volume of the cell pack is noted.

6. Cells are diluted appropriately in growth medium (see below under preparation of cultures of individual cell types) and planted in culture vessels.

Automatic trypsinization. Rappaport (89) first described an apparatus for the continuous, automatic addition of trypsin and withdrawal of dispersed cells which could be used for processing large amounts of tissue. Devices of various complexity were subsequently described for automatic trypsinization of kidney tissue. A simple glass device developed by Shipman and Smith (111) which minimizes exposure time to trypsin and gives high yields of viable cells is available commercially (Bellco Glass Inc, Vineland, NJ)

Trypsinization of monolayer cell cultures. Cells in monolayer cultures can be dispersed for subculture using either trypsin, or a trypsin-versene (EDTA) mixture. The latter gives faster and more complete dispersion of most cell types. Either of the following two methods can be used, but the first requires fewer manipulations.

Method A

1. Growth medium is removed from the cell culture, and the monolayer is washed with PBS, pH 7.5 (see Appendix).

2. A 0.25% trypsin solution (or equal parts of 0.25% trypsin and 1:2000 versene solutions) in PBS, pH 7.5 is added to the monolayer and left in contact with the cells for 15–30 sec, after which the solution is removed.

3. The culture is held at 37 C until microscopic examination shows that the cells have pulled apart.

4. The cells are then suspended to the proper concentration in growth medium, based either upon counting the cells, or upon an arbitrary "split" of 1 culture into 2 or more. The serum in the growth medium halts the action of the trypsin.

Method B

1. Growth medium is removed from monolayer cell cultures and the cell sheets are washed with PBS, pH 7.5.

2. A 0.25% trypsin solution (or equal parts of 0.25% trypsin and 1:2000 versene solutions) in PBS, pH 7.5, is added to the monolayer in a volume sufficient to cover the cell sheet.

3. Cultures are incubated at 37 C until the cells are completely dislodged into the medium.

4. The cell suspension is centrifuged at 1000 rpm for 10 min, and the dispersing solution is removed.

5. Cells are resuspended in the desired volume of growth medium and planted in culture vessels.

Treatment with chelating agents

Certain types of cells in culture can be dispersed by treatment with chelating agents which dissociate the cells by binding the divalent cations stabilizing the intercellular bonds. The most commonly employed chelating agents are versene (EDTA) and sodium citrate. These agents will not disperse cells from fresh tissues, and they are not effective for dispersing certain types of cultured fibroblast cells. However, they can be used on cultures of epithelial cells. An advantage is the fact that these solutions can be sterilized by autoclaving, and thus avoid the risk of introducing contaminants which may be present in trypsin, such as mycoplasmas and parvoviruses, into cultured cells. The following procedure is used for dispersing cell monolayers with versene.

1. Growth medium is removed from the culture and the cell sheet is washed 3 times with PBS, pH 7.5.

2. Versene in PBS (a 1:3000 dilution for monkey or other animal kidney cells and a 1:5000 dilution for human cells) is added directly to the cell sheet, and the cultures are shaken and incubated at 37 C for 15–30 min with the versene covering the cell sheet.

3. Remaining clumps of cells are dispersed by pipetting back and forth, and the cells in suspension are counted in a hemocytometer.

4. A volume of the cell suspension containing the desired number of cells is centrifuged at 1000 rpm for 10 min, the versene is removed, and the cells are resuspended in the appropriate volume of growth medium.

Mincing of fresh tissues

Initiation of cell cultures from certain types of human tissues, such as biopsy tissues or human fetal lung or kidney, can also be accomplished by using minced or fragmented, rather than trypsinized, tissue. Mincing is done in a Petri dish using paired scalpels or scissors and a small volume of growth medium. The tissue is reduced to pieces approximately 1–4 mm. Fragmented tissue preparations are obtained by tearing the tissue apart in a small volume of medium using 2 pairs of forceps; this is continued until the fragments are too small to be grasped and further shredded. The tissue mince is placed into a culture vessel, and sufficient growth medium is added to cover the surface of the vessel.

Enumeration of cells

Packed cell volume. A rough estimate of the number of cells obtained by dispersion techniques may be derived by measuring the volume of packed cells under standard conditions of centrifugation. This measurement can be made in a graduated, conical centrifuge tube or, more accurately, in a hematocrit. Although this method does not give an estimate of viable cells, it has been found suitable for use in preparing cultures of a variety of cell types. The packed cells are simply diluted in the appropriate volume of growth medium and dispensed into suitable culture vessels.

Cell counting. More accurate determinations of cell numbers can be performed by counting the cells in a hemocytometer. It is important to disperse the cells thoroughly by pipetting back and forth and to charge the chambers immediately. The cells in 5 large squares (each corner square and the middle square) of both chambers are counted, omitting cells lying on the top and left-hand lines, but including cells lying on the bottom and right-hand lines. The *mean* count of the 10 squares is multiplied by 10,000 to give the number of cells/ml of suspension. Staining the cells with crystal violet may aid in distinguishing cells from extraneous material. One part of the cell suspension is mixed with 2 parts of 0.1% crystal violet in 0.1 M citric acid, and the cells are counted in a hemocytometer as described above. As the cell suspension is diluted 1:3 in the staining solution, the count is multiplied by 3 to give the number of cells/ml of the original suspension.

Trypan blue exclusion method for viable cell count. Certain dyes stain only dead cells, while viable cells exclude the dye and remain unstained. Trypan blue is the dye generally used for determination of viable cell counts. One volume of 1% trypan blue solution in Hanks BSS is added to 9 volumes of cell suspension, and the mixture is held at room temperature for 10 min. The suspension is then centrifuged at 1000 rpm for 10 min, the supernatant fluid is removed, and the cells are resuspended in Hanks BSS to the original volume of the cell suspension. Further dilution may be required for counting if the cell suspension is very heavy. The cells are then counted in a hemocytometer as described above, enumerating only the unstained viable cells. Both stained and unstained cells can be counted if the relative proportions of viable and nonviable cells in the preparation need to be determined.

Preparation of *in vitro* cell cultures of various types

The compositions and methods for preparing most of the media components are given in the Appendix of this chapter. Formulations of some of the complex media, which most laboratories obtain from commercial sources, are given elsewhere (77, 92). In most instances calf or bovine serum can be substituted for fetal bovine serum in the growth media, but if this is done, the cultures must be washed 2 or 3 times before they are used for virus propagation. In this laboratory the antibiotics generally employed in cell culture media are either a combination of pencillin (100–200 u/ml) and streptomycin (100–200 μg/ml); a combination of penicillin (250 u/ml), streptomycin, neomycin (250 μg each/ml), and bacitracin (2.5 u/ml); or gentamicin (50–100 μg/ml). In some instances fungizone (amphotericin B) is also used at a concentration of 0.5–1.0 μg/ml.

Human fetal kidney cell cultures, primary:

1. Kidneys from fetuses 3–5 months of gestation are rinsed in Hanks BSS, then placed in a Petri dish where the capsule and pelvis are removed and the remainder of the kidney is minced finely with paired scalpels.

2. If there is uncertainty about the quality of the tissue, it is tested for viability by preparing pilot cultures. One or 2 pieces of minced tissue are put into a tube with 4–5 ml of 0.25% trypsin and held at room temperature for 15 min. The cells are then dispersed by pipetting, sedimented by centrifugation at 600 rpm for 10 min, and the supernatant fluid is removed. The cells are suspended in 1–2 ml of growth medium, and each of 2 culture tubes is seeded with 0.5–1.0 ml of the cell suspension and incubated overnight at 36–37 C.

3. The minced tissue is transferred from the Petri dish to a trypsinizing flask containing a magnetic stirring bar, where it is washed in Hanks BSS for 5 min. After the tissue has settled, the wash fluid is removed.

4. To the trypsinization flask is added 100–150 ml of 0.25% trypsin solution in Hanks BSS, and the tissue is dispersed by overnight trypsinization.

5. If cellular growth is evident in the pilot cultures, processing of the cells is continued the following morning.

6. Based on the volume of packed cells, the cells are suspended to a 1:100 dilution in the following growth medium:

Fetal bovine serum	10.0 ml
Eagle MEM (in Hanks BSS)	86.9 ml
2.8% NaHCO$_3$	2.5 ml

Penicillin (20,000 u/ml)-streptomycin (20,000 μg/ml) . . . . 0.5 ml
Fungizone (1 mg/ml) . . . . 0.1 ml

7. Tube cultures are seeded with 0.5 ml of cell suspension, and 2-oz bottle cultures with 5 ml, and incubated at 36-37 C.

8. If the cells are to be preserved by freezing in liquid nitrogen, they are diluted 1:100 in 9 parts of growth medium and 1 part of dimethylsulfoxide, and stored in 1-ml volumes.

9. Growth medium is replaced in a volume of 1 ml on cell cultures at 2 days after initiation, and confluent monolayers are obtained 4-5 days after the cells are planted.

10. Before the cultures are inoculated with virus, the growth medium is removed and replaced with 1 ml of the following maintenance medium:

Fetal bovine serum (inactivated 56 C 30 min) . . . . 2.0 ml
Eagle MEM (in Earle BSS) . . . . 94.9 ml
8.8% NaHCO₃ . . . . 2.5 ml
Penicillin (20,000 u/ml)-streptomycin (20,000 μg/ml) . . . . 0.5 ml
Fungizone (1 mg/ml) . . . . 0.1 ml

Human fetal skin and muscle cell cultures, primary:

1. Tissue of the limbs and torsos from fetuses of 2-5 months gestation is minced and washed in 3 changes of Hanks BSS.

2. The minced tissue is dispersed by overnight trypsinization.

3. Dispersed cells are diluted 1:100 in the following growth medium:

Fetal bovine serum . . . . 10.0 ml
Eagle MEM (in Hanks BSS) . . . . 86.4 ml
2.8% NaHCO₃ . . . . 2.5 ml
Penicillin (20,000 u/ml)-streptomycin (20,000 μg/ml) . . . . 1.0 ml
Fungizone (1 mg/ml) . . . . 0.1 ml

4. Tube cultures are seeded with 0.5 ml, and 200-ml bottle cultures with 10 ml of the cell suspension and incubated at 36-37 C.

5. After 2 days, growth medium is replaced in the cultures (increasing the volume to 1 ml in tube cultures), and incubation is continued until the cultures contain continuous monolayers of cells, usually 4-5 days after planting.

6. For propagation of viruses, the growth medium is removed and replaced with the maintenance medium described above for human fetal kidney cell cultures.

7. Monolayer cultures can be dispersed with trypsin for subculture and establishment of cell lines. Growth and maintenance media used for these cultures are the same as those employed for primary cell cultures.

Human fetal diploid cell lines

Human fetal lung and kidney are the diploid cell types most widely used for propagation of viruses. Human fetal diploid lung (HFDL) cells are generally considered to be more sensitive for propagation of certain respiratory viruses, while human fetal diploid kidney (HFDK) are slightly more sensitive for growth of enteroviruses. Both types of diploid cell lines are available from commercial sources, and a new, extensively characterized HFDL line designated IMR-90 (82) is now available for use in virology. Human fetal diploid cell lines can not be subcultivated indefinitely, but tend to go into a decline phase between the thirtieth to the fiftieth passage; thus, it is important to bank cells at low passage levels in liquid nitrogen to avoid loss of the lines through excessive passage.

Initiation of human fetal diploid cell cultures (43)

1. Fetal lung or kidney tissue is minced and dispersed by the multiple extraction trypsinization procedure.

2. Cells are either diluted 1:100 in growth medium, based upon the packed cell volume, or viable cells are enumerated by the trypan blue exclusion method, and diluted in growth medium to contain approximately 100,000 viable cells per ml.

3. Growth medium used for initiation of cultures has the following composition. The pH of the medium after equilibration of the culture at 36–37 C should be less than 7.4.

Fetal bovine serum .... 10.0 ml
Eagle MEM (in Hanks BSS) .... 86.9 ml
2.8% NaHCO$_3$ .... 2.5 ml
Penicillin (20,000 u/ml)-streptomycin (20,000 μg/ml) .... 0.5 ml
Fungizone (1 mg/ml) .... 0.1 ml

4. Cells are planted in culture vessels of appropriate size for the amount of cell suspension available and incubated at 36–37 C.

5. The growth medium is replaced at 3–4 day intervals until a confluent monolayer of cells is formed, at which time the cultures are subcultivated.

Subcultivation of diploid cell lines

Cultures are placed on a strict schedule of subcultivation, preparing 2 new cultures from each one harvested (1:2 split) at 3–4 day intervals. After the line is established, 1:4 splits can be made at weekly intervals. In subpassaging diploid cells it is important that the cells be well dispersed; otherwise, cultures will contain microcolonies derived from clumps of cells, and this will lead to early senescence of the culture (44).

1. Growth medium is removed and the cells are dispersed (Method A, page 79), using a trypsin-versene solution.

2. Cells are resuspended in the growth medium described above, using 2 volumes of medium for each culture harvested. Two bottle cultures are prepared for each one harvested. Tube cultures are prepared by seeding each tube with 1 ml of the suspension from the 1:2 split, or by counting the cells, adjusting the suspension to contain 100,000 cells in a volume of 1.5 ml, and seeding each tube with 1.5 ml of the suspension.

3. After 2 days incubation at 36–37 C the growth medium is changed, and the cultures should contain confluent monolayers at 3–4 days after initiation.

4. For propagation of viruses, the growth medium is removed from the cultures and replaced with either of the following maintenance media:

Fetal bovine serum (inactivated 56 C 30 min) .... 2.0 ml
Eagle MEM (in Earle BSS) .... 94.9 ml
8.8% NaHCO .... 2.5 ml
Penicillin (20,000 u/ml)-streptomycin (20,000 μg/ml) .... 0.5 ml
Fungizone (1 mg/ml) .... 0.1 ml
or
Fetal bovine serum (inactivated 56 C 30 min) .... 2.0 ml
Leibovitz Medium No. 15 (L-15) .... 97.4 ml
Penicillin (20,000 u/ml)-streptomycin (20,000 μg/ml) .... 0.5 ml
Fungizone (1 mg/ml) .... 0.1 ml

Preservation of human fetal diploid cell lines in the frozen state

1. Cell monolayers which have just reached confluency are dispersed with trypsin-versene (Method A, page 79), suspended in growth medium, centrifuged at 800 rpm for 10 min, and the supernatant fluid is removed.

2. The cells are then suspended in 9 parts of growth medium and 1 part of dimethylsulfoxide to a concentration of approximately 2×10^7 cells per ml.

3. The suspension is dispensed into ampules in 1-ml volumes and stored in liquid nitrogen.

4. To revive the cultures, the frozen suspension is thawed rapidly by placing the ampule in a 37 C water bath, and the contents of the 1-ml ampule are distributed into 2 or 3, 32-oz prescription bottles each containing 40 ml of growth medium. The freezing and

reviving of ampules containing high concentrations of cells permits rapid recovery of large numbers of cells and eliminates the need to "build up" the line through several subpassages. Alternatively, cells can be frozen at a concentration of 2×10^6 cells per ml, and these can be planted in 10 ml of growth medium in an 8-oz prescription bottle.

5. After 2 days incubation at 36-37 C the medium is replaced, and incubation is continued until the cells become confluent.

Human amnion cell cultures

Human amnion cells in culture (19) support the replication of a variety of human viruses, and the tissue is relatively easy to obtain. However, in recent years this cell type has been supplanted to some extent by human fetal diploid cell lines and certain established cell lines which are more readily available, and less subject to variation in virus susceptibility. The following procedure is used in this laboratory for preparing cell cultures.

1. Placentas collected from cesarean sections are placed in 300-500 ml of Hanks BSS and held at refrigerator temperature no longer than 10-12 hr before processing.

2. The membranes are spread out in a large, sterile pan with the cord side up and, with forceps and scissors, the amnion is stripped away from the chorion starting at the edge of the tear and working toward the cord. An area of membrane 1-2 inches wide adjacent to the cord is discarded because of the high hyaluronic acid content of the cord.

3. The amniotic membrane is placed in a beaker containing 200-300 ml of Hanks BSS and rinsed free of blood and debris in 3 changes of Hanks BSS. The membrane is allowed to stand in the fluid for 5 min for each rinsing.

4. To determine the suitability of the membrane for culture, 1 or 2 small pieces of tissue are placed in a tube containing 1 ml of Hanks BSS and 1 drop of 1% trypan blue and held at room temperature for 2 min. The tissue is then spread out on a microscope slide and examined under low power magnification. Microscopic examination should reveal a layer of cells of uniform appearance, tightly packed together on an almost transparent basement membrane. Dead cells stain dark blue. Membranes with many dead cells or with large areas of abnormal appearing cells are unsuitable for culture.

5. Membranes with a satisfactory microscopic appearance are placed into a beaker containing 300 ml of 0.01% trypsin in Hanks BSS and held in this solution for 2 hr at room temperature.

6. The membrane is then placed in a flask containing 300 ml of 0.25% trypsin in PBS, pH 7.5, and held at room temperature overnight.

7. The following day the flask is shaken several times and then held at 37 C for 2-4 hr.

8. The cell suspension is then passed through a funnel lined with stainless steel wire gauze (72 mesh, wire, diameter 0.0037″, Newark Wire Cloth Co, Newark, NJ or Colorado Fuel and Iron Corp, Emeryville, CA) into 250-ml centrifuge bottles, and the cells are sedimented by horizontal centrifugation at 800 rpm for 10 min.

9. The cells are washed 3 times in 100 ml of Hanks BSS by centrifugation at 800 rpm for 10 min. Cells suspended in the third wash fluid are counted in a hemocytometer, and after sedimentation and removal of the wash fluid, the cells are suspended in the following growth medium to give a concentration of 450,000 cells per ml.

Fetal bovine serum . . . . 20.0 ml
Medium No. 199 (in Earle BSS) . . . . 77.9 ml
8.8% NaHCO$_3$ . . . . 1.0 ml
Penicillin (20,000 u/ml)-streptomycin (20,000 μg/ml) . . . . 1.0 ml
Fungizone (1 mg/ml) . . . . 0.1 ml

10. Tube cultures are seeded with 1 ml of cell suspension, 16-oz prescription bottles with 20 ml, and 32-oz prescription bottles with 30 ml.

11. After 72-hr incubation at 36-37 C, the medium is replaced with growth medium in which the concentration of fetal bovine serum is reduced to 10%. Cultures usually contain confluent monolayers by 5-7 days after initiation.

12. For virus propagation, the growth medium is removed and replaced with the following maintenance medium in a volume of 2 ml for tube cultures or appropriate volumes for bottle cultures.

Fetal bovine serum (inactivated 56 C 30 min)	2.0 ml
Medium No. 199 (in Earle BSS)	94.4 ml
8.8% NaHCO$_3$ . . . . :	2.5 ml
Penicillin (20,000 u/ml)-streptomycin (20,000 μg/ml)	1.0 ml
Fungizone (1 mg/ml)	0.1 ml

13. "Secondary" human amnion cell cultures can be prepared by one subpassage of primary cultures.

a. Cells in primary cultures are dispersed with trypsin.

b. The cell suspension is counted in a hemocytometer, suspended in growth medium (with 20% fetal bovine serum) to a concentration of 120,000 cells per ml, and planted in appropriate volumes.

c. After 2-3 days incubation at 36-37 C, the medium is replaced with growth medium containing 10% fetal bovine serum, and incubation is continued until confluent monolayers are formed.

d. The maintenance medium described above is used when cultures are inoculated with virus.

Established cell lines of human origin

A variety of human cells of both malignant and nonmalignant origin have been carried in continuous passage for many years and some have found widespread use in virus laboratories. Most of these established lines have a narrower range of virus susceptibilities than do primary or diploid cell cultures, but they are suitable for isolating many of the viruses infecting humans. Many viruses which cannot be isolated directly in these cell lines can nevertheless be adapted to growth in them for use in Nt tests or for preparation of serologic antigens. Established cell lines generally multiply rapidly, making it possible to obtain large populations of cells in culture and thus, in many instances, to produce more potent serologic antigens than those derived from primary or diploid cultures containing fewer host cells.

The HeLa line of continuous passage cells, established in 1951 by Gey et al (34) from a cervical carcinoma, has been the one most commonly employed for virus propagation. Others include the KB line established by Eagle et al (22) from a carcinoma of the nasopharynx, the HEp-2 human epithelial line of Toolan (117), and the FL line of human amnion established by Fogh and Lund (29). For the most part these lines are similar in their susceptibility to human viruses, although some are more suitable than others for demonstrating the CPE of particular viruses. The RD cell line, established by McAllister et al (64) from a human rhabdomyosarcoma, has been found to be more sensitive than other cell types for isolation and propagation of certain group A coxsackieviruses, some of which could previously be propagated only in suckling mice (97).

The following procedure can be used for propagation of all of the established human cell lines mentioned above.

1. Cells in monolayer cultures are dispersed with versene or trypsin-versene solution and counted in a hemocytometer.

2. Either of the following growth media may be used; the second one gives larger cell populations and is used for cultures intended for the production of serologic antigens.

Fetal bovine serum	10.0 ml
Eagle MEM (in Hanks BSS)	86.5 ml
2.8% NaHCO$_3$	2.5 ml
Penicillin-streptomycin-neomycin-bacitracin soln	1.0 ml

or

Fetal bovine serum	10.0 ml
Lactalbumin hydrolysate-yeast extract medium	89.0 ml
Penicillin-streptomycin-neomycin-bacitracin soln	1.0 ml

3. Cells are diluted in growth medium to contain 50,000–100,000 cells per ml, and planted in appropriate volumes in culture vessels.

4. Cultures are incubated at 36-37 C, and the medium is replaced 1 or 2 times during the 5-7 day period required for confluent monolayers to form.

5. Before the cultures are used for virus propagation, the growth medium is removed and replaced with either of the following maintenance media.

Fetal bovine serum (inactivated 56 C 30 min)	5.0 ml
Eagle MEM (in Earle BSS)	91.5 ml
8.8% NaHCO$_3$	2.5 ml
Penicillin-streptomycin-neomycin-bacitracin soln	1.0 ml

or

Fetal bovine serum (inactivated 56 C 30 min)	5.0 ml
Leibovitz medium No. 15 (L-15)	94.0 ml
Penicillin-streptomycin-neomycin-bacitracin soln	1.0 ml

Organ cultures of human embryonic tracheal or nasal ciliated epithelium (47)

1. Tissues excised from fetuses 5-9 months of gestation are placed in holding medium consisting of Hanks BSS with 10% fetal bovine serum. They should be prepared for culture within 24 hr.

2. The tissues are trimmed, washed in several changes of Hanks BSS, and then the mucuous membrane and underlying bone or cartilage are cut into pieces 2-3 mm square. Very sharp instruments should be used to avoid damaging the ciliated cells by pressure.

3. In the bottom of a 60-mm Petri dish, 4-6 small areas (5-6 mm across) are lightly scratched with a scalpel blade (parallel scratches at right angles to each other).

4. A piece of tissue is placed, ciliated side upward, on each scratched area, care being taken to avoid touching the ciliated membrane with the blade of the scalpel. The tissue fragments adhere strongly to the scratched area.

5. Nutrient medium may be either medium No. 199, Eagle MEM, or Leibovitz medium No. 15, supplemented wtih 0.2% bovine albumin. Media should contain 100-200 u penicillin/ml and 100-200 μg streptomycin/ml. Medium should be added until it is just level with the top of the tissue fragments.

6. Ciliary activity is observed using a dissecting microscope with reflected light, and only cultures showing strong ciliary beating are used for virus propagation. Virus may be inoculated into the cultures immediately after initiation or after 2 days incubation at 33 C with 2 medium changes.

7. After inoculation with virus or clinical materials the cultures are incubated at 33 C, and the fluids are harvested daily and stored at -70 C to await examination for virus content. Ciliary activity is also observed over the course of the incubation period.

Primary monkey kidney cell cultures

1. Cells from excised kidneys are dispersed by the trypsin-versene method.

2. After the cells are washed and packed by low-speed centrifugation they are diluted 1:300 in growth medium (see below), or the viable cells can be counted by the trypan blue exclusion method and diluted in growth medium to give 100,000– 300,000 cells/ml.

3. The following growth medium is used for initiation of monkey kidney cell cultures.

Fetal bovine serum .... 5.0 ml
Lactalbumin hydrolysate, 5% .... 10.0 ml
Hanks BSS .... 82.9 ml
2.8% NaHCO$_3$ .... 1.0 ml
Penicillin-streptomycin-neomycin-bacitracin soln .... 1.0 ml
Fungizone (1 mg/ml) .... 0.1 ml

4. Tube cultures are seeded with 0.5 ml of a 1:300 cell suspension, or 1 ml of a suspension containing 100,000–300,000 cells per ml. Four-oz prescription bottles are seeded with 8 ml of cell suspension, 8-oz bottles with 10 ml, and 16-oz bottles with 20 ml.

5. The dispersed monkey kidney cells can also be stored in liquid nitrogen for planting at a later time. One volume of packed cells is suspended in 5 volumes of freezing medium which consists of 1 part of dimethylsulfoxide and 9 volumes of growth medium (with the concentration of fetal bovine serum increased to 10%). This suspension is dispensed in 1-ml volumes for freezing. When the cells are revived, the contents of each 1-ml ampule are diluted in 40 ml of growth medium and planted in the volumes indicated above.

6. Cultures are incubated at 36–37 C for 24–72 hr, and the growth medium is replaced with growth medium in which the concentration of fetal bovine serum is reduced to 2%, and the concentration of 2.8% NaHCO$_3$ is increased to 2%. Tube cultures receive 2 ml of this medium. Cell sheets should be confluent 5–7 days after initiation of the cultures.

7. For virus propagation the cells can be maintained on a serum-free medium consisting of Eagle MEM (in Earle BSS) containing 2.5 ml of 8.8% NaHCO$_3$ solution and 1 ml of penicillin (20,000 u/ml)-streptomycin (20,000 μg/ml) solution per 100 ml of medium, or this medium can be supplemented wtih 2% inactivated fetal bovine serum. The most satisfactory maintenance medium for isolation and propagation of certain respiratory viruses, which are inhibited by high concentrations of NaHCO$_3$, is Leibovitz medium No. 15 containing 2% inactivated serum and 1% of the penicillin (20,000 u/ml)-streptomycin (20,000 μg/ml) solution.

8. The yield of cell cultures from monkey kidneys may be increased through the use of "secondary" cultures prepared by dispersing and subculturing cells from primary cultures. However, contaminating simian foamy viruses may become more apparent in secondary cultures than in primary cultures.

a. Primary cultures are dispersed with trypsin-versene solution in PBS, pH 7.5 (Method A, page 79) or with a 1:3000 dilution of versene.

b. The cells are counted in a hemocytometer and suspended in growth medium to a concentration of 120,000 cells/ml.

c. The suspension is planted in culture vessels in the volumes indicated above, and incubated at 36–37 C, with a medium change after 24 hr.

Fetal monkey cell lines

A variety of cell lines has been established from fetal monkey tissues, primarily lung and kidney (31, 120, 121). In some cases the lines remained in the diploid state and had a finite life span (31, 120), while in others the cells became heteroploid at an early passage level, and appeared to have the properties of established cell lines (121). The range of virus susceptibilities of most of these cell lines has been almost as broad as that of primary monkey kidney cells, but they are less satisfactory for isolation and propagation of some of the ortho- and paramyxoviruses.

In addition to conserving primary monkey kidney cells, which are becoming increasingly difficult and expensive to obtain, the use of fetal monkey kidney cell lines has other advantages in virology laboratories. The lines have been well characterized and shown to be free from adventitious agents such as simian viruses and mycoplasmas. The lines can be stored in the frozen state to provide large supplies of readily available cells.

Cell lines are established from fetal monkey tissues by essentially the same procedures used for establishing human fetal diploid cell lines. Rhesus or African green monkeys are usually employed.

1. Fetuses of approximately 150–160 days gestation are taken by cesarean section, and the kidneys, lungs, and other selected tissues are removed.

2. Cells are dispersed in 0.25% trypsin by the multiple extraction method.

3. Using the same growth medium employed for initiation of human fetal diploid cell lines, the cells are either diluted 1:100 based upon the packed cell volume, or counted and diluted to contain approximately 3×10^5 cells/ml.

4. Cells are planted in culture vessels of appropriate size for the amount of cell suspension available and incubated at 36–37 C.

5. The growth medium is replaced at 3–4 day intervals until a confluent monolayer of cells is formed, at which time the cultures are subcultivated, preparing 2 new cultures from each one harvested (1:2 split).

6. For preparation of tube cultures and bottle cultures for virus propagation, the cells are diluted in growth medium at a 1:3 split, or to contain approximately 100,000 cells/ml.

7. Maintenance media employed during virus propagation are the same as those used for human fetal diploid cell culture.

8. Cells are preserved in the frozen state in the same manner as human fetal diploid cells.

Established monkey kidney cell lines

Certain established cell lines derived from adult monkey kidney tissue are widely used for virus propagation. These lines have the property of indefinite subcultivation, and some have been carried for more than 100 passages. However, it is recognized that decreased virus susceptibility may result with continuous passage, and it is desirable to use the cells at as low a passage as is available and to bank low passage cells in the frozen state to avoid excessive subcultivation. These cell lines have a narrower range of virus susceptibilities than do primary or diploid simian cells, but they are useful for isolation and propagation of many enteroviruses, rubella virus, and certain arboviruses.

Hull et al (54) established several continuous lines of rhesus monkey kidney cells, and the LLC-MK₂ line is the one which has been used most extensively. Two lines of African green monkey kidney cells, the BS-C-1 line established by Hopps et al (48), and the Vero line developed by Yasumura and Kawakita (129) are also widely used in virus laboratories. The following procedure can be used for preparing cultures of these cell lines.

1. The cells in monolayer cultures are dispersed with a trypsin-versene solution (Method A, page 79).

2. The following growth medium is used to dilute the cells to contain 100,000 cells/ml, or cells can be diluted in 5 volumes of medium for each culture harvested (1:5 split).

Fetal bovine serum . . . . 10.0 ml
Eagle MEM (in Hanks BSS) . . . . 86.4 ml
2.8% NaHCO₃ . . . . 2.5 ml
Penicillin-streptomycin-neomycin-bacitracin soln . . . . 1.0 ml
Fungizone (1 mg/ml) . . . . 0.1 ml

3. Culture vessels are seeded with appropriate volumes of the suspension (0.5 ml for tube cultures and 20 ml for 16-oz bottle cultures) and incubated at 36–37 C.

4. The growth medium is replaced after 2 days incubation, increasing the volume on tube cultures to 2 ml, and incubation is continued until the cell sheets are confluent.

5. For virus propagation the growth medium is replaced with the following maintenance medium.

Fetal bovine serum (inactivated 56 C 30 min)	2.0 ml
Eagle MEM (in Earle BSS)	86.4 ml
8.8% NaHCO$_3$	2.5 ml
Penicillin-streptomycin-neomycin-bacitracin soln	1.0 ml
Fungizone (1 mg/ml)	0.1 ml

Rabbit kidney, primary cultures

Primary rabbit kidney cell cultures are suitable for propagation of herpes simplex, vaccinia, and rubella viruses, and they are also used for propagation of the simian foamy viruses which frequently occur as contaminants of monkey kidney cell cultures.

1. Kidneys from 3-week-old albino rabbits are decapsulated and minced, and the cells are dispersed by the overnight trypsinization method.

2. The dispersed cells are diluted 1:300 in the following growth medium:

Fetal bovine serum	10.0 ml
Eagle MEM (in Hanks BSS)	87.0 ml
2.8% NaHCO$_3$	2.5 ml
Penicillin-streptomycin-neomycin-bacitracin soln	0.5 ml

3. Tube cultures are seeded with 0.5 ml of cell suspension, and 8-oz prescription bottles with 10 ml. After 2–3 days incubation at 36–37 C the medium is replaced, increasing the volume in tube cultures to 2 ml. Incubation is continued until monolayers are confluent.

4. For virus propagation the growth medium is replaced with the following maintenance medium:

Fetal bovine serum (inactivated 56 C 30 min)	2.0 ml
Eagle MEM (in Earle BSS)	95.0 ml
8.8% NaHCO$_3$	2.5 ml
Penicillin-streptomycin-neomycin-bacitracin soln	0.5 ml

Established rabbit cell lines

The RK-13 (6) and LLC-RK$_1$ (55) lines of rabbit kidney cells, and the SIRC line of rabbit cornea cells (60) are used principally for propagation of rubella virus. The procedure given below can be used for cultivation of all three lines.

1. Cells in monolayer cultures are dispersed with a trypsin-versene solution (Method A, page 79).

2. Cells are diluted in 5 times the original culture volume (1:5 split) of the following growth medium.

Fetal bovine serum	10.0 ml
Eagle MEM (in Hanks BSS)	86.5 ml
2.8% NaHCO$_3$	2.5 ml
Penicillin-streptomycin-neomycin-bacitracin soln	1.0 ml

3. Tube cultures are seeded with 1 ml of the cell suspension, and 8-oz prescription bottles with 10 ml. After 2 days incubation at 36–37 C, the medium is replaced with fresh growth medium. The cultures should contain confluent monolayers of cells at 5–7 days after initiation.

4. For virus propagation, the growth medium is removed and replaced with the following maintenance medium:

Fetal bovine serum (inactivated 56 C 30 min)	2.0 ml
Eagle MEM (in Earle BSS)	94.5 ml
8.8% NaHCO$_3$	2.5 ml
Penicillin-streptomycin-neomycin-bacitracin soln	1.0 ml

Hamster kidney, primary cultures

Kissling (58) first described the replication of certain arboviruses in primary hamster kidney cells, and this host system has subsequently been used for isolation and propagation of a variety of arboviruses. Cultures are prepared by the following procedure.

   1. Kidneys from hamsters 4–8 weeks of age are trypsinized by the overnight procedure.
   2. Dispersed cells are either diluted 1:300 in growth medium or counted in a hemocytometer and diluted in growth medium to give a suspension containing 600,000 cells/ml. The following growth medium may be used.

Fetal bovine serum	10.0 ml
Eagle MEM (in Hanks BSS)	86.5 ml
2.8% NaHCO$_3$	2.5 ml
Penicillin-streptomycin-neomycin-bacitracin soln	1.0 ml

   3. Tube cultures are planted with 1 ml of the suspension, and 8-oz prescription bottles with 10 ml. After 2–3 days incubation at 36–37 C, the growth medium is replaced. Confluent monolayers should be formed at 5–6 days after initiation of the cultures.
   4. The following maintenance medium is used for virus propagation:

Fetal bovine serum (inactivated 56 C 30 min)	2.0 ml
Eagle MEM (in Earle BSS)	94.5 ml
8.8% NaHCO$_3$	2.5 ml
Penicillin-streptomycin-neomycin-bacitracin soln	1.0 ml

BHK-21 established hamster kidney cell line

The BHK-21 (Clone-13) line of baby hamster kidney cells established by Macpherson and Stoker (69) is useful for propagation of rubella virus, many of the arboviruses, and various other human and animal viruses.

   1. Monolayer cell cultures are dispersed with trypsin-versene solution (Method A, page 79).
   2. Cells are counted in a hemocytometer and diluted in growth medium to contain 50,000 cells/ml. Alternatively, the cells may be diluted in 40 times the original culture volume of growth medium (1:40 split). Growth medium has the following composition:

Fetal bovine serum	10.0 ml
Eagle MEM (in Hanks BSS)	86.5 ml
2.8% NaHCO$_3$	2.5 ml
Penicillin (20,000 u/ml)-streptomycin (20,000 μg/ml)	1.0 ml

   3. Tube cultures are planted with 0.5 ml of the cell suspension, 8-oz bottle cultures with 10 ml, and 32-oz bottle cultures with 40 ml. Cell sheets should become confluent after 2–4 days incubation at 36–37 C.
   4. The following maintenance medium is used for virus propagation:

Fetal bovine serum (inactivated 56 C 30 min)	2.0 ml
Eagle MEM (in Earle BSS)	94.5 ml
8.8% NaHCO$_3$	2.5 ml
Penicillin (20,000 u/ml)-streptomycin (20,000 μg/ml)	1.0 ml

Chick embryo cell cultures

In vitro cultures of chick embryo fibroblasts may be used for propagation of some of the arboviruses, herpes simplex viruses, and certain pox viruses. The following procedure can be employed for preparation of cultures.

   1. Nine-day-old chick embryos are harvested and placed in a sterile Petri dish where the eyes, beaks, legs and wings are removed and discarded. The torsos are then washed in 3 changes of Hanks BSS and minced into pieces approximately 3 mm in diameter.

2. The tissue-mince is washed in 3 changes of Hanks BSS and then passed through a 50-ml syringe (without a needle) into a flask where it is washed twice with Hanks BSS.

3. An appropriate volume of 0.25% trypsin in Hanks BSS is added (200 ml for 5-10 embryos, 300 ml for 11-20 embryos), and a magnetic stirring bar is added to the flask.

4. The suspension is stirred for 1 hr at room temperature, and then passed through a funnel lined with stainless steel wire gauze (72 mesh, wire, diameter 0.0037″, Newark Wire Cloth Co., Newark, N.J., or Colorado Fuel and Iron Corp., Emeryville, Ca.) into 250-ml centrifuge bottles.

5. The cells are sedimented by horizontal centrifugation at 600 rpm for 10 min, washed once in Hanks BSS by centrifugation at 600 rpm for 10 min, and then suspended in 15-30 ml of Hanks BSS in graduated, conical centrifuge tubes and packed by centrifugation at 600 rpm for 10 min.

6. The volume of the cell pack is noted, and the cells are diluted 1:200 in the following growth medium.

Fetal bovine serum	5.0 ml
Eagle MEM (in Hanks BSS)	91.5 ml
2.8% NaHCO$_3$	2.5 ml
Penicillin-streptomycin-neomycin-bacitracin soln	1.0 ml

7. Tube cultures are planted with 1 ml of the suspension, and 8-oz prescription bottle cultures with 10 ml. After incubation at 36-37 C for 1-2 days, complete monolayers of cells are formed, and the cultures are ready for inoculation with virus.

8. The growth medium on the cultures is replaced with the following maintenance medium.

Eagle MEM (in Hanks BSS)	96.5 ml
2.8% NaHCO$_3$	2.5 ml
Penicillin-streptomycin-neomycin-bacitracin soln	1.0 ml

Storage, Preservation, and Transport of Cell Cultures

Over the past years advances have been made in techniques for storage and preservation of cells in culture which have greatly facilitated the use of cell culture host systems in virus laboratories. Cell harvests from freshly dispersed tissues can be stored in the frozen state for future preparation of primary cultures. In addition to extending the use of the cells, this permits examination of pilot cultures for growth properties and possible contamination with adventitious agents before the entire lot is processed. Diploid cell lines can be maintained in the frozen state at low passage levels to prevent loss of the lines through excessive passage. Stocks of cells can be maintained to serve as a back-up in the event that the line is lost through contamination or adverse culture conditions. Cell lines used infrequently can be maintained frozen to avoid the need for continuous subcultivation. In addition, simple procedures have been devised to prolong the utility of cell cultures and to reduce the amount of subculturing required for maintaining established cell lines.

Storage of cells in the frozen state

The viability of mammalian cells can be maintained for months at dry-ice temperatures, and for years at liquid-nitrogen temperatures. Four factors are important in preserving cells in the frozen state. First, cryoprotective agents such as glycerol or dimethylsulfoxide (DMSO) must be used (71).

These presumably protect the cells during freezing and thawing by binding water, thus reducing the build-up of intracellular electrolytes, and also reducing the amount of water available to form ice crystals. Requirements for effective cryoprotective agents are that they must penetrate the cells rapidly, they must prevent a significant amount of water from freezing, and they must be nontoxic in useful concentrations. They are usually employed in freezing media at concentrations of 5–10%. Although many cell types have been preserved satisfactorily for years in glycerol, DMSO is more widely used now, particularly for preservation of primary cells.

The second important factor is slow freezing of the cell suspension. This causes ice crystals to form extracellularly rather than intracellularly, and thus they do not disrupt the cells (71). Cooling rates of 1–3 C per min are recommended. This can be accomplished through the use of a mechanical programmed slow-freeze apparatus (Linde Division, Union Carbide Corp., New York, NY), by using a polystyrene plug (also from Linde) which fits into the opening of a liquid nitrogen freezer and can be positioned to control the rate of cooling, or simply by placing the cells in a −70 C freezer for 2–3 hr.

Third, frozen cell suspensions must be maintained at temperatures of −70 C or lower. At dry-ice temperatures, cells maintain 80–90% viability for 6 months, and then viability rapidly decreases to 2–3% by 1–2 years. In liquid-nitrogen temperatures of −196 C, all chemical and physical activity is reduced to a negligible level, and cell suspensions maintain high levels of viability for years (109).

Fourth, rapid thawing is required to prevent damage to the cells; ampules of frozen cells are removed from the freezer and immediately immersed in a waterbath at 37 C.

The following procedure can be employed for liquid-nitrogen storage of cells freshly dispersed from original tissue, as well as for diploid and established cell lines. Cell cultures which have just become confluent, and which were fed with growth medium 24 hr previously should be used. The preceding section on preparation of various types of cell cultures describes the growth media and cell concentrations used for storage of cells in the frozen state. In general it is recommended that 2–6 million viable cells be stored in 1-ml volumes of freezing medium.

1. Cells dispersed with trypsin or trypsin-versene solution are suspended in freezing medium to a concentration of approximately 2–6 million viable cells/ml. Freezing medium is the growth medium used for the particular cell type, containing 10% fetal bovine serum and supplemented with 10% DMSO. This should be freshly prepared. It is important to recognize that *DMSO is rapidly absorbed through the lungs, and readily penetrates the skin, and therefore appropriate precautions should be taken in handling this reagent.* Also, DMSO produces an exothermic reaction when mixed with growth medium, and the freezing medium should be cooled before it is added to cells.

2. The cell suspension is dispensed in 1-ml volumes into Cryule (Wheaton Scientific Co., Millville, NJ) glass ampules. Small volumes should be frozen to ensure good penetration of the cryoprotective agent and uniform freezing rates. Plastic ampules (Corning Glass Works, Corning, NY) can be used if they are stored in the vapor, rather than the liquid phase of the liquid nitrogen freezer.

3. Proper sealing of the glass ampule is very important; if it is improperly sealed and liquid nitrogen penetrates, the pressure built up inside the ampule upon warming is likely to cause it to explode. A semi-automatic ampule sealer is available commercially (Kahl-

enberg-Globe Equipment Co., Sarasota, FL) which seals ampules by the pull-seal method, and minimizes the risk of small leaks in the seal. Proper sealing of the ampules can be confirmed by immersing them in a 0.05% methylene blue solution for 30–45 min at refrigerator temperature; dye will seep into improperly sealed ampules (109). Ampules to be immersed in the liquid phase of the liquid nitrogen freezer should always be checked for leaks before storage.

4. Ampules are racked on appropriately labeled canes and placed in a −70 C freezer for 2–3 hr, which provides an appropriately slow cooling rate.

5. The canes are then transferred rapidly to a liquid nitrogen freezer. *A protective face mask and gloves should always be worn when opening a liquid nitrogen freezer* as a precaution against the possibility of an ampule explosion.

6. To revive the frozen cells, ampules are removed from the liquid nitrogen freezer and quickly placed in a stainless steel pan fitted with a cover and containing warm water at 37–39 C. *A protective face mask and gloves must be used for this manipulation.*

7. When the contents of the ampule have thawed, the ampule is immersed in 70% ethanol at room temperature, and then removed and opened.

8. The cells are suspended in the appropriate volume of growth medium (see section above), planted in culture vessels and incubated at 36–37 C. After 24 hr the growth medium is replaced, and incubation is continued until a confluent monolayer is formed.

Preservation of cell cultures at reduced temperatures

In many instances it is not possible to utilize at once all of the primary cell cultures derived from a processed tissue, and it may be desired to preserve them for use in the near future. Short-term preservation of cell cultures can be accomplished by reducing the metabolic activity of the cells through lower incubation temperatures. The cells are permitted to grow into almost confluent monolayers before the incubation temperature is reduced.

Primary cell cultures such as monkey kidney can be maintained at ambient room temperatures (or preferably at a more constant incubator temperature of 23–24 C) for 2 weeks without a medium change. Maintenance medium is added and they are used for virus propagation. Cells can actually be maintained under these conditions for longer than 2 weeks, but those kept for longer periods sometimes appear to be slightly less sensitive than younger cultures for propagation of certain viruses.

Primary cell cultures can also be maintained for up to 2 weeks at 4 C. The cells tend to pull apart and round up, but when the cultures are returned to an incubator at 36–37 C for 24 hr, the cells form a confluent monolayer. Cultures are then placed on maintenance medium for propagation of viruses.

Bead-in-tube cultures

A simple device called a bead-in-tube culture (62) may be employed to reduce the amount of subculturing necessary for maintaining established cell lines. This may be useful in laboratories that require the cells from time to time, but do not have good facilities for storage in the frozen state.

A cell suspension in 2 ml of growth medium is placed in a culture tube containing a 6-mm glass bead. The tube is capped tightly and incubated at 36–37 C in an upright position in a conventional test tube rack. Cells grow on the bottom of the tube and at approximately weekly intervals the tube is agitated vigorously to dislodge excess cells with the glass bead. The cells in suspension can then be used for initiation of subcultures, or discarded if the line is not in current use. Fresh growth medium is added and the cells left adhering to the tube continue to proliferate.

Transport of cell cultures and cell suspensions

Cultures of most cell types can be transported without refrigeration, and they will remain viable for the length of time required to ship them by air to practically any location. The main hazard is that of exposure to extremes of temperature, and the cultures should be packed in an insulated container for air shipment.

Cells may be shipped in suspension at a concentration of approximately 1×10^6 cells/ml of growth medium or as monolayer cultures. In monolayer cultures the cells are protected from being dislodged by agitation of the fluid either by completely filling the culture vessel with medium, or by removing most of the medium, leaving only a small amount to cover the monolayer and prevent it from drying.

Virus Isolation Attempts in Cell Cultures

Preparation of inocula

Stool suspensions. Stool suspensions for virus isolation attempts are prepared in 30-ml polycarbonate centrifuge tubes with screw caps containing glass beads and 15 ml of Hanks BSS. Approximately 1.5–2.0 g of the stool specimen is placed in the tube, and a portion of the specimen is stored at −20 C for retesting if necessary. The tubes are balanced for centrifugation by the addition of sterile glass beads. Tubes are then tightly capped and shaken vigorously to emulsify the specimen with the glass beads. After centrifugation at 10,000 rpm for 30 min at 4 C, the supernatant fluid is removed for testing. A portion of the clarified suspension is treated with antibiotics for inoculation into cell cultures. To each ml of the suspension is added 0.1 ml of a solution containing 1,000 μg gentamicin/ml or, to each ml of suspension is added 0.1 ml of a solution containing 10,000 u of penicillin and 50,000 μg of streptomycin per ml. The remainder of the suspension is held at −20 C until testing is completed.

The antibiotic-treated suspension is held at 4 C until it is inoculated in 0.25 ml amounts into 2 tube cultures of monkey kidney cells and 2 tube cultures of human fetal diploid kidney cells. Inoculated cell cultures are incubated at 36–37 C (preferably in a roller drum) and observed microscopically for evidence of a viral CPE. If the inoculum is so toxic that the cells degenerate nonspecifically, the cultures should be subpassaged as soon as possible.

Rectal swabs. Rectal swabs are less satisfactory than stool specimens for virus isolation and should be tested only if it is not feasible to obtain sufficient fecal material. The swab should be placed in approximately 3.5 ml of nutrient broth or Hanks BSS with 0.5% gelatin for transport to the laboratory where the specimen is stored at −20 C to await testing. After thawing, the fluid is expressed and the swab is discarded. The fluid is clarified by centrifugation at 2,500 rpm for 15 min at 4 C, and the supernatant fluid is removed, treated with antibiotics and inoculated into cell cultures as described above for stool specimens.

Urine specimens. Urine specimens are most often used for cytomegalovirus isolation attempts, but other viruses such as rubella, enteroviruses, or adenoviruses may also be recovered. Because of the instability of cytomegalovirus (CMV) upon freezing, specimens should be processed and inoculated as soon as possible after collection. They should be held at 4 C if they can be inoculated with 24 hr after collection; if there is to be a longer delay, the specimen should be mixed with an equal volume of 70% sorbitol and stored at −70 C. The pH of the specimen should be tested, and adjusted to 7.0–7.4 with 8.8% $NaHCO_3$ if necessary. Concentration of the urine specimen may enhance chances for virus recovery, but concentrates may be toxic for cell cultures. Therefore it is desirable to inoculate both unconcentrated and concentrated samples of each urine specimen for virus isolation attempts.

To each milliliter of unconcentrated urine is added 0.1 ml of a solution containing 10,000 u penicillin and 50,000 μg streptomycin/ml, or 0.1 ml of a solution containing 1,000 μg gentamicin/ml. Fungizone is also added to a final concentration of 10 μg/ml of specimen. The antibiotic-treated specimen is held at 4 C until it is inoculated into appropriate cell cultures in a volume of 0.25 ml per tube.

Urine is concentrated by centrifuging at 2,500 rpm for 20 min at 4 C, and resuspending the sediment in one-tenth or less of the original volume of supernatant urine. A portion of this concentrate is treated with antibiotics and inoculated into cell cultures as indicated above for unconcentrated urine. A portion of the concentrate is mixed with an equal volume of 70% sorbitol and stored at −70 C. If the specimen was originally received in sorbitol, it is not necessary to add more for storage in the frozen state.

Throat and nasopharyngeal specimens. Washings are collected in a buffered broth containing 0.5–1.0% protein, and swabs should be placed into 5 ml of similar holding medium. Hanks BSS with 0.5% gelatin can be used for this purpose. Virus isolation rates are highest when freshly collected specimens are inoculated directly into cell cultures without freezing. Specimens should be held at 4 C if they can be inoculated within 24 hr; otherwise they should be stored at −70 C. Fluid is expressed from swab specimens, and the swabs are discarded. A portion of the specimen is treated with antibiotics for inoculation. To each milliliter of specimen is added 0.1 ml of a solution containing 10,000 u penicillin and 50,000 μg streptomycin/ml, or 0.1 ml of a solution containing 1,000 μg gentamicin/ml. Fungizone is also added to a final concentration of 10 μg/ml of specimen.

The antibiotic-treated specimen is held at 4 C until it is inoculated in 0.25-ml volumes into appropriate cell culture tubes. A portion of the untreated specimen is stored at −70 C.

Vesicular lesion specimens. Vesicular fluids and lesion material collected on swabs or with a scalpel are placed into 2–3 ml of holding medium containing 0.5–1.0% protein. If dry swabs are received in the laboratory they are eluted into 2.5 ml of Hanks BSS with 0.5% gelatin. A portion of the specimen is treated with antibiotics, using 0.1 ml of a solution containing 10,000 u penicillin/ml and 50,000 μg streptomycin/ml or 0.1 ml of a solution containing 1,000 μg gentamicin/ml for each 1 ml of specimen. Fungizone is also added to a final concentration of 10 μg/ml of specimen. The antibiotic-treated specimen is held at 4 C until it is inoculated in 0.25-ml volumes into cell culture tubes. A portion of the untreated specimen is stored at −70 C.

Cerebrospinal fluid. Cerebrospinal fluid should be inoculated into cell cultures as soon as possible after collection or held at −70 C, since viruses are very labile in this medium. The fluid is inoculated directly into cell cultures without antibiotic treatment.

Tissue suspensions. Tissues taken at autopsy and biopsy can be homogenized into a suspension for inoculation into cell cultures or, preferably, they can be cultivated *in vitro* to provide a more sensitive system for virus recovery. If cultivation is to be attempted, the specimen should be held at 4 C and processed as soon as possible. If only suspensions are to be prepared, the tissue can be frozen at −70 C until it is processed.

A representative sample of the tissue is weighed in a sterile Petri dish and then transferred to a mortar and ground into a 20% suspension with the appropriate volume of 0.75% bovine albumin buffered saline, or Hanks BSS containing 0.5–1.0% protein. If the specimen contains a great deal of connective tissue, alundum is used for grinding. The suspension is then centrifuged at 2,500 rpm for 10 min at 4 C. The supernatant fluid is removed, and a sample of sufficient volume is treated with antibiotics. To each milliliter of clarified tissue suspension is added 0.1 ml of a solution containing 10,000 u penicillin/ml and 50,000 μg streptomycin/ml, or 0.1 ml of a solution containing 1,000 μg gentamicin/ml. For lung tissue, fungizone is also used at a concentration of 10 μg/ml of suspension. Both the original specimen and the remainder of the untreated suspension are stored at −70 C for retesting if necessary.

The antibiotic-treated specimen is held at 4 C until it is inoculated in 0.25-ml volumes into appropriate cell culture tubes.

Inoculation and incubation of cell cultures for virus isolation attempts

Certain measures should be taken to ensure sensitivity and reliability of virus isolation attempts performed in cell cultures.

Different cell types should be handled separately and inoculated with clinical materials as separate runs to prevent cross-contamination of human cells with simian viruses and to prevent cross-contamination of cell types. Contamination of fibroblast cells with epithelial cells may sometimes be mistaken for a viral CPE.

The same pipette should never be used for inoculating a clinical specimen into different cell types such as monkey kidney cells and then human cells. This may cross-contaminate cell types or, more importantly, may introduce simian viruses into human cell cultures and lead to erroneous assumptions that the viruses were isolated from human clinical specimens.

For recovery of most human viruses, incubation temperatures within the range of 35-37 C are optimal. However, the rhinoviruses grow optimally at 33 C, and thus, for isolation of respiratory viruses a reduced temperature may be employed to facilitate recovery of these fastidious agents; this temperature is also satisfactory for recovery of other respiratory viruses.

It is well-recognized that most viruses reach higher titers and produce a more marked CPE in cultures which are rotated or rocked to provide an exchange of the fluid and gas phase on the cell sheet. Therefore, roller drums are usually employed for virus isolation attempts wherever possible, while stationary cultures, which require less incubator space, are used for propagation of established virus strains.

If at all feasible, medium should not be changed on cell cultures after they have been inoculated with clinical materials, since this increases the risk of cross-contamination. If long-term maintenance is necessary, as for isolation of cytomegalovirus, the fluids should be carefully removed from the tubes using a separate pipette for each set of cultures; medium should never be decanted from inoculated tubes. Refeeding should also be done using a separate pipette for each set of cultures.

Although the use of cell cultures in microtiter plates for virus identification and antibody assays has contributed to greater economy and efficiency in virus diagnosis, the use of microcell cultures for virus isolation is to be discouraged. This is primarily because of the increased risk of cross-contamination between specimens. Also, the amount of infected material derived from such cultures may not be adequate for subsequent testing, and the need for subpassage of the isolate delays its identification. Further, clinical specimens show greater toxicity in micro cultures than in tube cultures, and the destruction of viable cells may hinder viral replication.

Problems encountered in isolating viruses in cell cultures

Certain inocula, notably tissue specimens and some fecal specimens, may be toxic to the cells and cause them to degenerate before a specific viral CPE can be manifested. Cell cultures showing marked degeneration within the first 24-48 hr after inoculation should be subpassaged to dilute out toxic effects of the inoculum and to provide viable cells for virus which may be present. In rare cases, toxicity of specimens may be so great that 3 cell culture passages are required to dilute it out. One useful way to distinguish between toxicity and a viral CPE is to make a reading 3-4 hr after inoculation, which is too early for viral CPE to occur, but sufficient time for a toxic effect to be exerted.

Also, cultures may undergo spontaneous degeneration before the desired incubation period is reached. This is indicated by degeneration of uninoculated control cultures incubated with the test series and, again, the cell cultures on each specimen should be harvested, pooled and subpassaged into a second set of cultures.

The presence of indigenous simian viruses in monkey kidney cell cultures presents serious problems in virus isolation attempts. These agents may produce a CPE or HAd reaction which can be mistaken for that of human viruses. The CPE of simian foamy viruses may mask that of the test viruses, or may prevent long maintenance and observation of the cells. There are no completely satisfactory methods for overcoming the problems of contaminating simian viruses, and other cell types should be substituted for primary and secondary monkey kidney wherever possible. The inclusion of SV-5 or SV-40 antiserum in cell culture media is not a reliable method for suppressing these viruses. Quarantine of rhesus monkeys for at least 6 weeks before using their tissues for cell cultures has been relatively effective in controlling contamination with SV-5 virus, but spotty contamination with this hemadsorbing virus still occurs in monkey kidney cells from commercial sources. Cell culture isolates showing hemadsorption, but which are not identifiable with antisera to the human ortho- and paramyxoviruses, should be tested against antisera to SV-5 and SV-41 viruses. SV-40 contaminants can be identified by immunofluorescent staining, and simian CMV can be distinguished from human CMV by its ability to produce a CPE in monkey kidney cells.

Culturing tissue specimens for virus recovery

Various comparative studies have established that culturing viable cells from biopsy or autopsy tissues is a more sensitive method for virus recovery than is inoculating tissue homogenates into cell cultures; this approach should be considered whenever unfrozen tissue is available in sufficient quantity. Three different cell culture methods can be used. First, the minced or trypsinized tissue can simply be placed in nutrient medium and cultured; secondly, dispersed cells from the test tissue can be co-cultivated with cell lines or primary cells; third, after cells from the tissue are established in culture, they can be fused with other cell types using one of several cell fusing agents such as inactivated Sendai virus (80), lysolecithin (15, 116) or polyethylene glycol (87). Co-cultivation or cell fusion have yielded viruses in some instances where cultivation of the tissue alone failed to do so (13, 50, 51, 85, 116).

The greater success of virus isolation using cultured cells may be related to the low levels of virus in the tissue or to the need for cell-to-cell transfer of virus from viable cells in some instances. In co-cultivation the helper cells apparently contribute some factor essential to the production of complete infectious virus which is lacking or ineffective in cells from the original tissue, and in the case of cell fusion, it appears that barriers to infection are somehow eliminated in the formation of heterokaryons. Also, homogenization of organs or tissues may release virus-inhibiting substances (9, 79), and these may interfere with virus recovery from tissue homogenates.

The following procedures are used in this laboratory for culturing cells from tissue specimens for virus isolation attempts (13; Cremer NE, personal communication).

With some tissue specimens, success in establishing cell cultures may differ using minced tissue and using trypsin-dispersed cells; therefore, it is advisable to use both approaches in culturing the cells. If insufficient tissue is available to do this, minced tissue should be employed.

Finely minced tissue is washed once with Hanks BSS and then planted in a 25-cm² Falcon flask in medium consisting of 20% fetal bovine serum and 80% fortified Eagle MEM (2X the standard concentration of vitamins and amino acids). The culture flask is incubated with a loose cap at 35–36 C in a CO_2 incubator, and one-half of the medium is replaced with fresh medium after 10 days. As long as 2–3 weeks may be required before cellular proliferation can be seen microscopically. Medium is changed at weekly intervals, and the cells are subpassaged by trypsinization when large colonies of cells have formed. The first subpassage is at a 1:1 split, i.e., the cells from 1 culture are planted into a new culture of the same size. Thereafter cultures are subpassaged at a 1:2 split when the cells become confluent, and the concentration of fetal bovine serum in the growth medium is reduced to 10%. When cell lines are well established, the cultures can be incubated in sealed flasks in a dry incubator.

Trypsin dispersed cells are prepared by extracting the tissue mince twice with 0.25% trypsin in PBS, pH 7.5, for 15 min at room temperature. The cell suspensions from the 2 extractions are filtered through a No. 72 stainless steel wire mesh and centrifuged at 700 rpm for 10 min. The cells are then suspended in the growth medium described above and approximately 1×10^6 cells are planted in a 25-cm² Falcon flask, incubated, fed, and subcultivated as described above.

For co-cultivation, trypsin-dispersed cells from the tissue specimen are cultured with roughly equal numbers of helper cells in a 25-cm² Falcon flask using the growth medium of choice for the helper cells (see above). Cultures are incubated in a CO_2 incubator, fed, and subpassaged as described above for cultures derived from tissue minces. Helper cells most commonly employed for recovery of viruses from human tissues are HFDL and established lines of monkey kidney cells, although other cell lines or primary cells may be used.

When cell lines have been established from minced or trypsinized samples of the test tissue, cell fusion may be used in efforts to recover virus. These procedures using inactivated Sendai virus (80), lysolecithin (15, 116) or polyethylene glycol (87) are given in detail elsewhere. Disadvantages to the use of inactivated Sendai virus are difficulties which may be encountered in producing material with high fusing activity, instability of the fusing factor on storage and the risk that the virus is not completely inactivated and may infect the cultures. Use of lysolecithin circumvents these disadvantages, but this agent may be toxic for cells in culture. Polyethylene glycol has only recently come into use as a cell fusing agent; it is less toxic than lysolecithin and may prove to be the fusing agent of choice.

Cells cultured from tissue samples are generally carried for at least 10 subpassages or, if time and facilities permit, for as long as the cultures maintain their viability. At regular intervals the cells are observed for viral CPE, examined by EM, stained with fluorescein-labeled antisera to the most appropriate viruses, and also examined by indirect FA against serum from the patient from whom the tissue was derived. Cultures can also be examined for hemadsorption or interference. Fluids from the cultures are inoculated into cell cultures or animals in which human viruses may be recovered. In some instances the cultures may be treated with agents such as iododeo-xyuridine (IUDR) or bromodeoxyuridine (BUDR) which may activate production of complete virus from latently infected cells (32, 36, 40).

Titration of Virus in Monolayer Cell Cultures, TCID$_{50}$ Endpoints

The amount of infectious virus present in a cell culture fluid can be titrated by determining the highest dilution of the fluid which produces degeneration (or hemadsorption or interference) in 50% of the cell cultures inoculated; this dilution is the 50% tissue culture infectious dose endpoint (TCID$_{50}$).

To determine the TCID$_{50}$ of a virus suspension, logarithmic or half-logarithmic dilutions are prepared in BSS or maintenance medium. In preparing virus dilutions it is necessary to discard pipettes between each dilution to avoid carrying virus particles on the pipette to the next dilution; failure to do so gives misleading high infectivity endpoints. Each dilution is added in a volume of 0.1 ml to 4 or more culture tubes. The inoculated cultures are incubated under optimal conditions and observed microscopically at intervals over a 7-day period, or longer for slower-growing viruses. If the cells in the inoculated culture show a specific viral CPE (or if the culture shows hemadsorption or interference), it is considered positive (or infected), and the TCID$_{50}$ endpoint is calculated by the method of Reed and Muench or Karber (see Chapter I).

For most Nt tests 100 TCID$_{50}$ of virus are tested against dilutions of serum. To calculate the dilution of virus suspension containing 100 TCID$_{50}$ the following procedure is used:

Log of TCID$_{50}$ titer + 2 = Log of virus suspension containing 100 TCID$_{50}$

Example: TCID$_{50}$ titer = $10^{-6.5}$ per 0.1 ml of suspension

$$\begin{array}{r} -6.5 \\ +2.0 \\ \hline -4.5 \end{array}$$ = Log of dilution of virus suspension containing 100 TCID$_{50}$ in a volume of 0.1 ml.

Viral Plaque Assays

A measurement of viral infectivity more precise than the TCID$_{50}$ endpoint can be obtained by plaquing viruses in monolayer cell cultures. A plaque is a localized focus of virus-infected cells, which under optimal conditions originates from a single infectious virus particle. Enumeration of these foci is a highly quantitative method for assay of viral infectivity, and demonstrating reduction in virus plaque counts provides a very sensitive means for measuring virus neutralizing capacity of antibody and antiviral substances.

Plaques of virus-infected cells can be demonstrated in a variety of ways. The method most commonly used for cytopathic viruses is to stain the cell monolayer with the vital stain, neutral red; the foci of dead, virus-infected cells appear as clear, unstained areas against a background of stained, viable

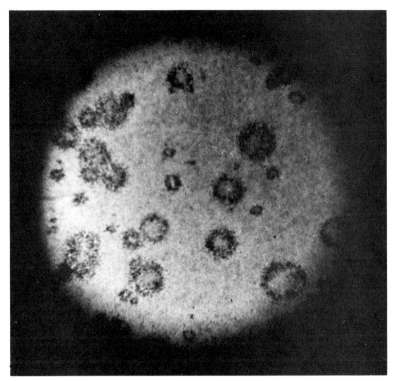

Figure 3.5—Foci of CMV-infected human fetal diploid lung cells showing enhanced uptake of neutral red.

cells (Fig 3.2). Dilutions of virus suspension are added to cell monolayers in Petri dish or bottle cultures, and after adequate time is allowed for adsorption of virus particles to the host cells, the monolayer is overlaid with a nutrient medium containing a solidifying agent such as purified agar, agarose or starch. Virus particles infecting and replicating in the cells are localized by the solid overlay and virus spreads from the initially infected cell to adjacent cells, producing circumscribed foci of cellular degeneration. In some instances neutral red is incorporated into the initial nutrient overlay, but if prolonged incubation is necessary for plaque demonstration, it is added in a second overlay toward the end of the incubation period. Neutral red stain may, through its photodynamic action, destroy host cells and inhibit virus plaque formation. Thus, it is important that cultures with neutral red overlays be incubated in the dark.

Cells infected with certain viruses which do not produce a rapid CPE may acquire a greater affinity for neutral red than that of uninfected cells, and "red" plaques may be demonstrated by enhanced staining of cells in infected foci (Fig 3.5).

Plaques produced by cytopathic viruses can also be demonstrated using stains other than neutral red. Since these stains kill the cells it is not possible to isolate viruses from the plaques, and the methods are useful only for enumerating infectious virus particles. These methods employ an overlay which can be removed from the cell sheets before they are stained. The overlays are solidified with either a low concentration of agar or agarose (126), methyl cellulose (51), or with tragacanth gum (72). Cells destroyed by virus are removed along with the overlay, and plaques appear as clear areas against a background of stained cells. Stains used for these procedures include crystal violet, Giemsa stain, tetrazolium salt, and carbolfuchsin. An advantage of these plaquing techniques is the fact that cultures can be stained and preserved for plaque counting at a later time.

Plaques produced by ortho- and paramyxoviruses, and by rubella virus, can be detected by the HAd technique. Infected cultures are overlaid with a nutrient medium sufficiently fluid to be aspirated by suction and, after a suitable incubation period, the overlay is removed and a suspension of appropriate RBC is added. The RBC adsorb to foci of infected cells, and plaques can be counted macroscopically.

Viruses such as rubella which render infected cells resistant to a challenge virus can be plaque assayed by interference tests. Virus suspensions are inoculated onto cell sheets, and after a suitable incubation period the cultures are superinfected with a large dose of challenge virus which produces HAd or CPE in the cell type. Foci of cells infected with the first virus are resistant to this challenge, and they appear as "negative" areas, which fail to show HAd or CPE, against a background of cells which hemadsorb RBC or show the CPE of the challenge virus. The delicate balance between interfering and challenge viruses in this test system necessitates very concise standardization of test conditions.

Sensitive and rapid virus plaque assays have been developed based upon FA or IP staining. In most instances single infected cells are enumerated microscopically after the first cycle of infection before secondary foci are evident. If a solidifying agent is used which can be removed for staining, or if the virus is one such as varicella-zoster virus which spreads in discrete foci by cell-to-cell transfer, incubation can be continued until larger foci of infected cells are developed, and IP staining can then be used to detect plaques which can be seen macroscopically (33).

Viruses may be "plaque-purified", i.e., pure lines may be isolated by subpassaging the progeny of a single plaque (which is presumed to have originated from a single viral particle). For effective purification the monolayer should be washed free from unadsorbed virus prior to addition of the overlay, plaques should be picked from cultures having fewer than 10 plaques, and they should be at least 10 mm from adjacent plaques. Also, two or more serial passages should be made (18). Virus may diffuse from plaques to the surface of the overlay (78), and the addition of a second neutral red overlay or the accumulation of water of condensation on the overlay surface may serve to cross-contaminate plaques. Thus, if cultures requiring a second overlay or those which are not inverted during incubation are used for plaque purification, it is important to select plaques from cultures having few, or preferably single, plaques.

If plaque assays are used for quantitation of viruses directly from clinical specimens, particularly in sewage or wastewater samples, it must be recognized that the specimens may contain toxic materials which become immobilized on the monolayer and produce foci of necrotic cells which may be mistaken for virus plaques. Thus, it is important to confirm that plaques are virus-induced by subculturing virus from the plaque.

The following two procedures are given as examples of plaquing techniques which are applicable to a wide variety of viruses. The first is performed in bottle cultures, and the second is conducted in Petri dish cultures which are incubated in a CO_2 atmosphere.

Plaquing enteroviruses in bottle cultures of monkey kidney cells

The following procedure is a minor modification of the technique originally described by Hsiung and Melnick (53). Additives such as 25 mM $MgCl_2$ or 100-400 μg/ml of DEAE-dextran may be used in the overlay to enhance plaque formation by certain enteroviruses (122, 123). The procedure can be used either with primary monkey kidney cells or with lines of monkey kidney cells.

1. Growth medium is removed from monolayer cell cultures in 3-oz prescription bottles.

2. Dilutions of the virus suspension are inoculated onto the monolayers in a volume of 0.2 ml, using at least 2 cultures for each virus dilution. The inoculum is distributed over the monolayer and the cultures are incubated at 36-37 C for 1.5 hr to permit virus adsorption. When plaque-purifying viruses, the cell sheets are washed once with 8 ml of Hanks BSS to remove unadsorbed virus prior to overlaying.

3. A 2X nutrient overlay solution prepared as follows is brought to a temperature of 46-47 C and mixed with an equal volume of melted 2% Difco purified agar (at 46-47 C).

2X Nutrient Overlay Solution

10X Eagle MEM (in Earle BSS)	20.0 ml
Glutamine, 3%	2.0 ml
Fetal bovine serum (inactivated 56 C 30 min)	4.0 ml
8.8% $NaHCO_3$	5.0 ml
Neutral red, 1:1000 dilution	3.0 ml
Penicillin-streptomycin-neomycin-bacitracin soln	2.0 ml
Sterile, double distilled water	64.0 ml

4. The nutrient agar overlay (equal parts of 2% agar solution and the 2X nutrient overlay solution) is held at 46-47 C during addition to the cultures with a Cornwall automatic pipette. Each culture receives 10 ml of the overlay, which is spread carefully over the monolayer.

5. The bottles are placed on a flat surface for 1 hr to permit the agar to harden, after which they are inverted and incubated in the dark at 36-37 C. Poliovirus plaques should appear in 2-4 days, but some of the echoviruses may require 7-10 days to produce plaques.

Plaquing viruses in Petri dish cultures of human fetal diploid cells

The following procedure can be used to plaque a variety of viruses which are cytopathic in HFDL cells, including herpes simplex viruses (104), varicella-zoster virus (104) and certain enteroviruses (99). The method can also be used with established monkey kidney cell lines such as Vero or BS-C-1 if the concentration of neutral red used in the second overlay is doubled. Tests are conducted in 30-mm plastic Petri dishes, or more conveniently in 30-mm wells in plastic trays.

1. Monolayer cultures are prepared by seeding with 300,000 HFDL cells in 3 ml of the following growth medium.

Fetal bovine serum . . . . 10.0 ml
Eagle MEM (in Hanks BSS) . . . . 86.5 ml
2.8% $NaHCO_3$ . . . . 2.5 ml
Penicillin (20,000 u/ml-)-streptomycin (20,000 μ g/ml) . . . . 1.0 ml

2. Cultures are incubated at 36–37 C in a humidified 5% CO_2 atmosphere until confluent monolayers are formed (2–3 days).

3. Growth medium is removed and dilutions of the virus suspension are inoculated onto the monolayers in a volume of 0.1 ml, using at least 2 cultures for each dilution, and distributed over the cell sheet. Cultures are incubated in a CO_2 incubator at 36–37 C for 1.5 hr to permit virus adsorption.

4. A 2X nutrient overlay solution prepared as follows is brought to a temperature of 46–47 C and mixed with an equal volume of melted 1% agarose or Oxoid purified agar (at 46–47 C).

2X Nutrient Overlay Solution

10X Eagle MEM (in Earle BSS) . . . . 20.0 ml
Glutamine, 3% . . . . 2.0 ml
Fetal bovine serum (inactivated 56 C 30 min) . . . . 10.0 ml
8.8% $NaHCO_3$ . . . . 5.0 ml
Penicillin (20,000 u/ml)-streptomycin (20,000 μg/ml) . . . . 2.0 ml
Sterile, double distilled water . . . . 61.0 ml

5. The nutrient agar overlay (equal parts of 1% agar or agarose solution and the 2X nutrient overlay solution) is held at 46–47 C during addition to the cultures with a Cornwall automatic pipette. Each culture receives 3 ml of the overlay.

6. After the overlay has hardened, cultures are placed in a CO_2 incubator at 36–37 C.

7. The time at which the second overlay is added depends upon the virus being plaqued. Herpes simplex viruses require 3 days of incubation, varicella-zoster virus requires 7–8 days, and enteroviruses require 5 or 6 days.

8. The second overlay has the same composition as the first, with the exception that it also contains 5% of a 1:1000 solution of neutral red. (Ten percent of the solution is used if Vero or BS-C-1 monkey kidney cells are used for the assay.) Each culture receives 2 ml of this second overlay.

9. Incubation is continued in a CO_2 incubator at 36–37 C (in the dark), and plaques are enumerated after 24–48 hr.

Neutralization Tests in Cell Culture Systems

Neutralization tests conducted in cell cultures may be applied in two ways to the laboratory diagnosis of viral infections. First, virus strains isolated from the patient may be identified by demonstrating the ability of known, specific immune serum to neutralize the infective capacity of the virus, i.e., to prevent a CPE, HAd, plaque formation, or other manifestations of infection in cell cultures. Secondly, infections may be diagnosed by demonstrating a significant increase in Nt antibody for a given virus between acute- and convalescent-phase serum specimens collected from the patient.

In cell culture systems, serum specimens are generally assayed for Nt-antibody content by testing serial dilutions of the serum against a standard dose (usually 100 $TCID_{50}$) of the virus. This is referred to as the constant virus-varying serum technique, and it is more useful for demonstrating significant increases in Nt antibody than is the constant serum-varying virus procedure in which undiluted serum is tested against serial dilutions of virus.

In the constant virus-varying serum system the antibody titer is expressed as the highest serum dilution which neutralizes the test dose of virus.

Neutralizing-antibody assays in monolayer tube cultures

1. The serum specimen (either known immune serum or unknown serum to be assayed for Nt antibody) is inactivated at 56 C for 30 min to destroy heat-labile, nonspecific viral inhibitory substances.

2. Appropriate serum dilutions are prepared in either BSS or the maintenance medium to be used on the cell cultures.

3. Virus is diluted to contain 100 $TCID_{50}$ in a volume of 0.1 ml (as determined by previous titration of the virus). Virus dilutions are prepared in the same diluent used for serum dilutions.

4. Equal volumes of the serum dilutions and the test virus dilution are mixed. The volume of serum-virus prepared is dependent upon the number of cell cultures to be inoculated. For a "virus control" the test virus dilution is mixed with an equal volume of diluent, or known "normal" serum of the same species as the test serum and incubated under the same conditions as the serum-virus mixtures. For Nt antibody assay runs it is necessary to perform a concurrent titration of the virus to establish that the test dose actually contained approximately 100 $TCID_{50}$.

5. The conditions recommended for incubation of serum-virus mixtures vary widely. For certain viruses it has been demonstrated that preliminary incubation does increase the neutralizing capacity of the serum. However, it is important to avoid incubation conditions under which the virus might be labile, e.g., prolonged periods at -37 C. For most Nt tests, serum-virus mixtures are incubated for 0.5–1 hr at 37 C.

6. After the incubation period the serum-virus mixtures and virus controls are inoculated in a volume of 0.2 ml into monolayer tube cultures. At least 2 cultures are employed for each serum-virus mixture.

7. The inoculated cultures are incubated under conditions most suitable for optimal growth of the virus and examined microscopically for ability of the serum to inhibit the CPE of the virus. Final readings are usually made when the virus control shows that 100 $TCID_{50}$ are present in the test. In the case of non-cytopathic ortho- or paramyxoviruses, the cultures are tested for hemadsorption after a suitable incubation period, and neutralization of the virus is evidenced by failure of the cultures inoculated with serum-virus mixtures to hemadsorb the RBC.

Neutralization tests for identification of viral isolates employing immune serum pools

Neutralization tests for identification of viruses belonging to large groups consisting of a multiplicity of distinct immunotypes can be greatly facilitated through the use of immune serum pool schemes. A procedure developed in our laboratory for identification of enteroviruses is called the "intersecting serum" scheme (96). Each type-specific immune serum is incorporated into 2 different serum pools, and identification is made by demonstrating neutralization of an isolate by 2 pools sharing a common type-specific immune serum. Figure 3.6 shows how the pools are composed. The same pool scheme can also be used for the identification of rhinoviruses and adenoviruses.

The serum pools are prepared, their reactivity tested against all of the viral types for which sera are included, and then stored in the frozen state in convenient working volumes. This eliminates the need to prepare pools each time Nt tests are performed and assures the proper composition of pools used in each run.

COMPOSITION OF SERUM POOLS

Serum pool numbers	8 ↓	9 ↓	10 ↓	11 ↓	12 ↓	13 ↓	14 ↓
1 →	P1*	P2	P3	CA7	CA9	CA16	CB1
2 →	CB2	CB3	CB4	CB5	CB6	E1	E2
3 →	E3	E4	E5	E6	E7	E8	E9
4 →	Reo1	E11	E12	E13	E14	E15	E16
5 →	E17	E18	E19	E20	E21	E22	E23
6 →	E24	E25	E26	E27	E29	E30	E31
7 →	E32	E33	En68	En69	En70	En71	++

*P = poliovirus immune serum; CA = group A coxsackievirus; CB = group B coxsackievirus; E = echovirus; En = enterovirus immune serum type

++ Immune serum to enterovirus candidate strain

IDENTIFICATION OF ISOLATES

Serum pool numbers	8 ↓	9 ↓ (Neutralization)	10 ↓	11 ↓	12 ↓	13 ↓	14 ↓
1 →							
2 →							
Neutralization 3 →		X	Identified as echovirus type 4				
4 →							
5 →							
6 →							
7 →							

Figure 3.6—Fourteen-pool intersecting serum scheme for identification of enteroviruses

For screening isolates each serum pool-virus mixture is inoculated into a single culture tube. The isolate is then tested against the individual immune serum showing neutralization in the pool scheme.

The success of the scheme depends upon the use of *well-standardized* antiserum known to possess little or no Nt activity for heterologous virus types and with high enough homotypic Nt titers that they can be diluted sufficiently to obviate any heterologous Nt activity which may be contributed by pooling sera containing low levels of heterotypic activity. No more than 7 antisera are included in each pool, as pooling larger numbers of sera tends to increase heterotypic activity.

1. Immune serum is inactivated at 56 C for 30 min and then dispensed into appropriate pools. Hanks BSS is added to give a final dilution of *each serum* of 1:50. High-titer immune serum can be used more dilute, but for identification of viral isolates it is generally desirable to use high concentrations of immune serum to permit identification of possible antigenic variants. Rather than using an arbitrary single dilution for each antiserum, each serum may be diluted to contain 50 antibody units in the pool (106). The pools are dispensed in volumes conveniently employed for a single day's test and stored at -20 C.

2. The serum pools are then checked by testing against 100 $TCID_{50}$ of each virus type for which immune serum is included in the scheme. This gives a complete picture of the homotypic and possible heterotypic Nt activity of the pools for every virus type in the scheme.

3. Virus isolates are arbitrarily tested at a dilution of 1×10^2 (or 1×10^{-1} if they are weakly cytopathic) against the immune serum pools. The virus dilution is prepared in Hanks BSS.

4. An 0.15 ml volume of the viral isolate is added to 0.15 ml of each serum pool and, after an incubation period of 1 hr at room temperature or 4 C, each serum pool-virus mixture is inoculated in a volume of 0.2 ml into a single cell culture tube. The virus dilution, in a volume of 0.1 ml, is inoculated into a culture tube as a "virus control" to determine that it contains a sufficiently cytopathic virus dose. Preferably, successive log_{10} dilutions made from the test virus dilution are inoculated into 2–4 cell cultures to give a more accurate determination of the virus dose present in the test.

5. Inoculated cultures are incubated under appropriate conditions and examined microscopically at intervals over a 7-day period (or longer for some of the slower-growing rhinoviruses). The tests are considered satisfactory if the cultures inoculated with virus alone show complete or almost complete viral degeneration at the end of the incubation period.

6. If neutralization of the isolate is seen in 2 of the pools, definitive identification is made by testing the isolate against the individual immune serum shared by these 2 pools.

Plaque reduction neutralization tests

Plaque reduction Nt tests provide a very sensitive assay for virus Nt antibodies. After an appropriate incubation period, serum-virus mixtures are inoculated onto monolayers in bottles or Petri dishes, and the cultures are incubated for 1.5 hours at 36–37 C to permit virus adsorption. The monolayers are then washed with Hanks BSS, and covered with an appropriate nutrient overlay containing a solidifying agent. After a suitable incubation period at 36–37 C, plaques are demonstrated using a neutral red stain or by removing the overlay and staining with one of the stains indicated above. FA and ID systems can also be used.

The Nt activity of a test serum is determined by its ability to reduce the number of virus plaques as compared to the number seen in control cultures inoculated with the virus and diluent. In some systems a reduction in plaque count of 80% is considered significant, and in others 50% plaque reduction is taken as the Nt antibody endpoint.

For antigenic analysis of certain viruses, e.g., poliovirus strains, antiserum may be incorporated into the overlay at various concentrations and virus can either be inoculated onto the monolayer prior to overlaying (125), or discs impregnated with 1,000 plaque-forming units (pfu) of virus are placed on the agar surface (70); heterologous strains break through at higher serum concentrations and produce plaques.

Microneutralization tests in cell cultures

Microneutralization tests conducted in cell cultures in wells in disposable plastic microtiter plates are more economical than tube Nt tests in terms of cell cultures and reagents. They also require less incubator space and are easier to perform and read than tests in tube cultures. It is advisable to use plates specified by the manufacturer to be processed for tissue culture; other plates may vary in their suitability for growth of cell cultures.

Cell monolayers may be prepared before they are inoculated with virus and serum-virus mixtures or, more conveniently, the cells, serum, and virus may be added at the same time. In the latter system un-neutralized virus degenerates the cells and monolayers are not formed, while in cultures containing neutralized virus, the cells proliferate into a confluent monolayer. Endpoints may be based upon microscopic observation of viral CPE or HAd, or tests may be based upon metabolic inhibition, in which case the results are read colorimetrically.

Tests in preformed monolayer cultures

Although microneutralization tests conducted in preformed cell monolayers are more cumbersome than those in which cells in suspension are added to serum-virus mixtures, these procedures may be required in certain instances. Some hyperimmune animal sera contain antibodies to host cells or toxic substances which inhibit outgrowth of cells into monolayers. However, such sera can generally be used in microneutralization tests in preformed monolayer cultures. This method is used in identifying viral isolates with "intersecting serum" pools by microneutralization tests, or for testing other sera which can not be assayed satisfactorily by microneutralization procedures based upon the growth of cells in the presence of test serum.

Simple, inexpensive plastic templates have been devised in this laboratory to aid in proper identification of cell cultures in microtiter plates during inoculation and microscopic observation (16). These increase accuracy in performing and reading the tests, and also reduce the time required to conduct the tests.

1. Tests are conducted in flat-bottom cups in sterile microtiter plates processed for cell culture and fitted with sterile covers.

2. Either HFDL cells or the BS-C-1 line of monkey kidney cells are used for the tests. Cells are dispersed with trypsin-versene solution. HFDL cells or BS-C-1 cells are suspended to a concentration of 150,000–200,000 cells/ml in the following growth medium.

Fetal bovine serum . . . .   10.0 ml
Eagle MEM (in Hanks BSS) . . . .   86.9 ml
2.8% NaHCO$_3$ . . . .   2.5 ml
Penicillin (20,000 u/ml)-streptomycin (20,000 μg/ml) . . . .   0.5 ml
Fungizone (1 mg/ml) . . . .   0.1 ml

3. Cell suspensions are dispensed into cups in a volume of 0.2 ml, and the cultures are incubated at 36 C in a CO_2 incubator until confluent monolayers have formed (2–3 days).

4. Growth medium is aspirated from each well, and replaced with 0.1 ml of the following maintenance medium.

Fetal bovine serum (inactivated 56 C 30 min) . . . .   2.0 ml
Eagle MEM (in Earle BSS) . . . .   94.9 ml
8.8% NaHCO$_3$ . . . .   2.5 ml
Penicillin (20,000 u/ml)-streptomycin (20,000 μ/ml) . . . .   0.5 ml
Fungizone (1 mg/ml) . . . .   0.1 ml

5. Serum (inactivated at 56 C for 30 min) and virus dilutions are prepared in maintenance medium, and equal volumes are mixed and held at 4 C for 1 hr. Controls consist of a virus titration for which $\log_{10}$ dilutions of virus, starting with the test dose, are mixed with an equal volume of diluent, and serum controls to detect possible toxicity in which the lowest serum dilution tested is mixed with an equal volume of diluent; these are held at 4 C with the test specimens.

6. Serum-virus mixtures and control mixtures are inoculated into micro cell cultures in a volume of 0.1 ml. Each dilution in the virus titration is inoculated into 4 cultures. Cell control cultures consisting of monolayers with 0.2 ml of maintenance medium should be included in each plate as controls on nonspecific cellular degeneration. An inoculating template (16) is used to aid in identifying the appropriate cultures to be inoculated.

7. To each culture is added 0.1 ml of sterile mineral oil, viscosity 350, and after blotting with a sterile blotter, the plates are sealed with 3 ¼" Paklon tape (Minnesota Mining and Manufacturing Co., St. Paul, Minn.). Other laboratories have used medium with a HEPES buffer and incubation in a humidified chamber to circumvent the need for sealing micro-cell-culture plates (39).

8. Plates are incubated at 36 C in a dry incubator until the virus control indicates that the desired dose of virus is present in the test system.

9. With the aid of a reading template (16), the cultures are examined for viral CPE using an inverted microscope.

Microneutralization test for paramyxoviruses

The following procedure is given as an example of a microneutralization test in which cells in suspension are added to serum-virus mixtures in microtiter plates, and then grow into monolayers. It was developed in our laboratory for assay of antibodies to human and animal parainfluenza viruses (102), and it is also applicable to the influenza viruses. In this test system virus is detected by hemadsorption.

1. Tests are conducted in sterile microtiter plates with "U" cups which have been processed for cell culture.

2. Serum dilutions, virus dilutions and the cell suspension are all prepared in a medium consisting of 10% fetal bovine serum (inactivated at 56 C for 30 min) and 90% Leibovitz medium No. 15.

3. Serum is inactivated at 56 C for 30 min and 2-fold dilutions (from 1:8 through 1:1024) are prepared in the medium described above, using 0.025-ml diluters. A set of serum dilutions is prepared for each test virus, and dilutions of 1:8 through 1:32 are prepared for a "serum control" to test for possible toxicity of the serum for the cells.

4. To each set of serum dilutions is added 0.025 ml of virus diluted to contain 100 TCID$_{50}$ as determined by a previous titration. To the "serum control" dilutions is added

0.025 ml of medium instead of virus. Serum-virus mixtures are incubated at room temperature for 1 hr.

5. Monkey kidney cells (dispersed from primary cultures) are diluted in medium to contain 200,000 cells/ml, and 0.025 ml of the suspension is added to each cup.

6. A titration of the test virus is performed in each run, adding 0.025 ml of $\log_{10}$ virus dilutions to 0.025 ml of medium, and using 4 cups per dilution, to establish that the test dose contained approximately 100 $TCID_{50}$.

7. The plates are sealed with 3 ¼″ Paklon tape and set to incubate at 36 C for 6 days.

8. The tape seal is removed and the medium in each cup is aspirated carefully using a blunt 23-gauge needle. In order to remove nonspecific inhibitors which might be present in the test serum or growth serum, each cup is rinsed by the addition of 0.05 ml of physiological saline which is then aspirated.

9. To each cup is added 0.05 ml of a 0.5% suspension of guinea pig RBC prepared in physiological saline. The plates are sealed with tape and incubated at 4 C for 30 min.

10. The tape is checked to make certain that all cups are sealed and the plates are inverted, permitting unadsorbed RBC to flow from the cell sheet while RBC adsorbed to virus-infected cells remain attached. Hemadsorption is detected microscopically with the plates inverted, using a standard light microscope. Viral neutralization is evidenced by inhibition of hemadsorption.

Colorimetric (metabolic inhibition) microneutralization tests

The principle upon which metabolic inhibition tests are based is discussed above. Colorimetric techniques have been utilized for assay of Nt antibodies to a variety of viruses, and they possess several advantages over Nt tests conducted in monolayer cultures. Reading the tests colorimetrically eliminates the need for time-consuming microscopic observation, and the cell suspension, virus, and test serum are all added on the same day. Also, the cells need not form a smooth monolayer which holds up over a long observation period, but must merely produce sufficient acid to shift the color of the indicator by the end of the incubation period. Metabolic inhibition tests are sometimes more sensitive than monolayer Nt tests for detecting viral antibody. This is probably a reflection of the fact that antibody need only delay the viral CPE until the cells have produced sufficient acid to convert the indicator; late "breakthrough" of un-neutralized virus is not so likely to be detected in the metabolic inhibition system as in monolayer Nt tests in which the CPE of un-neutralized virus is detected microscopically.

The procedure given below is used in our laboratory for Nt-antibody assays for the enteroviruses and for identification of certain enterovirus isolates. Metabolic inhibition tests can also be performed with some of the slower-growing viruses such as reoviruses if a "two-phase" system (103) is used. In this case the test is initiated in a medium in which cellular metabolism produces little change in pH, and after the virus has had an opportunity to exert a CPE, a second "indicator" medium is added which contains a CO_2-bicarbonate buffering system and a high level of glucose; this permits cultures in which virus is neutralized to convert the phenol red indicator.

1. Tests are conducted in sterile microtiter plates with "U" cups which have been processed for cell culture.

2. BS-C-1 grivet monkey kidney cells are used for the test. Cells in monolayer cultures are dispersed with a trypsin-versene solution, and counted using the trypan blue exclusion method. Cells are suspended to a concentration of 30,000 viable cells/ml in the following medium.

Fetal bovine serum (inactivated 56 C 30 min) . . . .   5.0 ml
Medium No. 199 in Earle BSS (containing 2.75 mg/dl alcohol-soluble
   phenol red) . . . .   88.9 ml
Glucose, 20% solution . . . .   1.5 ml
8.8% NaHCO$_3$ . . . .   2.5 ml
Penicillin-streptomycin-neomycin-bacitracin soln . . . .   1.0 ml
Fungizone (1 mg/ml) . . . .   0.1 ml

    3. Serum to be assayed for Nt antibodies is inactivated at 56 C for 30 min, and 2-fold dilutions (from 1:8 through 1:1024) are prepared in the above medium using 0.05 ml diluters. A set of serum dilutions is prepared for each test virus, and dilutions of 1:8 through 1:32 are prepared for a "serum control" to test for possible toxicity of the serum for the cells.

    4. To each set of serum dilutions for the test proper is added 0.05 ml of a dilution of test virus containing 100 to 320 TCID$_{50}$, as determined by a previous titration. Virus dilutions are also prepared in the above medium. To the "serum control" dilutions is added 0.05 ml of medium instead of virus.

    5. Positive- and negative-control sera are included for each virus type in the test.

    6. A concurrent titration of each test virus must be included in every run to establish that the test dose actually contained 100–320 TCID$_{50}$. The test virus dilution is further diluted in half-log steps past the expected endpoint, and each dilution is dispensed in a volume of 0.05 ml into 4 cups containing 0.05 ml of medium.

    7. Tests are held for 30-60 min at room temperature before addition of the cell suspension.

    8. The cell suspension is added in a volume of 0.05 ml to all serum-virus mixtures, the "serum controls" and the virus titration.

    9. A cell control, included in each run, is prepared as follows. To each of 4 cups containing 0.05 ml of medium is added 0.1 ml of the cell suspension; to 4 cups containing 0.1 ml of medium is added 0.05 ml of the cell suspension; to 4 cups containing 0.1 ml of medium is added 0.05 ml of a 1:2 dilution of the suspension; and to 4 cups containing 0.1 ml of medium is added 0.05 ml of a 1:4 dilution of the cell suspension. Thus, the cups contain 2X, 1X, ½X and ¼X the concentration of cells used in the test proper.

    At the time the test is read the medium in cups containing 2X and 1X concentrations of cells should have a pH of 6.8-7.0, the medium in cups with cells at half the concentration used in the test should have a pH of 7.2-7.6, and that in cups with cells at one-fourth the test concentration should have a pH of 8. If the pH values in the respective sets of cups are higher than this, it is an indication that too few cells were used, or that the cells metabolized too slowly; if the pH values are lower, it indicates that the suspension contained too many cells.

    11. Moisture is removed from the surface of each plate with a sterile blotter, and 0.1 ml of sterile mineral oil, viscosity 350, is added to each cup. The plates are then sealed with 3¼" Paklon tape, using a roller to ensure a tight seal.

    12. Tests are incubated at 36-37 C for 6-8 days.

    13. At the end of the incubation period, the tests are read colorimetrically. A pH of 7.4 or higher indicates virus replication and CPE, while a pH of 7.2 or lower is indicative of lack of viral infectivity (in the virus titration) or specific neutralization of the virus (in the antibody assay). The cell controls should show the pH values indicated above.

Preparation of Viral Serologic Antigens in Cell Cultures

    Many of the antigens employed for serologic diagnosis of viral infections are derived from infected cell cultures. Procedures for antigen preparation vary with the agent and the intended use of the antigen, and optimal conditions must be individually defined for each group of viruses and type of antigen.

Antigens for use in Nt tests need not have a high degree of purity, but they should contain a high proportion of infectious virus as compared to the content of noninfectious virus, which is also capable of binding antibody. Infectivity titers should be high enough to permit dilution to eliminate much of the host material and noninfectious virus. Thus, virus should be propagated under conditions giving maximum infectivity titers and should be handled and stored so as to prevent loss of infectivity.

Hemagglutinating (HA) antigens must possess sufficiently high titers to permit their use at dilutions containing 4 or 8 antigenic units; they must be free of serum, host tissue, or microbial contaminants which might agglutinate the test RBC; and they must also be free from nonspecific inhibitors of viral hemagglutinins. The use of kaolin-treated serum in the maintenance medium (114) or serum-free maintenance medium avoids the problem of nonspecific inhibitors. In some instances hemagglutinins in infected cell culture fluids can be "unmasked" by treatment with fluorocarbon (35, 95). The HA titers of certain antigens can be increased by alternate cycles of freezing and thawing, by sonication, or by treatment with Tween 80 and ether (83, 114).

Important qualities of viral complement-fixing (CF) antigens are high potency, freedom from host materials which might fix complement with the test sera, and freedom from anticomplementary activity.

Viral antigens for use in immunodiffusion or counterimmunoelectrophoresis procedures must be highly concentrated in order to form visible immunoprecipitates. In most instances physical or chemical concentration procedures are employed, but it is essential to have high-titer starting materials for these preparations.

In using purification and concentration procedures for preparation of viral antigens, it is important to avoid chemical or physical treatments which denature viral proteins, producing changes in antigenic properties.

Various studies on optimal conditions for producing viral serologic antigens have helped to define some of the most important factors in obtaining high-titer and specific antigens.

As would be expected, cell cultures with large populations of host cells give rise to higher titered antigens than do cultures with lower cell populations. Established cell lines generally attain higher cell numbers in culture than do diploid or primary cells, and thus are more suitable for antigen production, if the virus replicates well in the line. Some concentration of viral antigens is achieved simply by infecting a large population of host cells in a small volume of maintenance medium; antigens are concentrated by virtue of being released into a small volume of fluid. Roller bottle cultures and suspension cell cultures are particularly useful for viral antigen production.

Higher-titer viral serologic antigens are generally produced in cell cultures maintained on medium containing serum than in serum-free medium. It should be determined that the serum to be used in maintenance medium is free from anticomplementary activity. For preparation of HA antigens it must also be free from nonspecific inhibitors and agglutinins for the indicator RBC.

One of the most important factors in producing high-titer CF and HA antigens is that of infecting cell cultures at a high multiplicity of from 1 to 10 infectious doses of virus per cell (95, 100, 114). In heavily infected cell cultures which show rapid cellular degeneration there is decreased production by host cells of anticomplementary substances and of inhibitors which may mask viral hemagglutinins.

In developing methods for preparing viral serologic antigens, it is important to determine whether the antigens remain associated with the cellular phase of the culture or are released into the culture fluids (100). Much of the viral antigen produced in cell cultures is cell-associated at the time the cultures first show an extensive viral CPE, and disrupting the virus-infected cells in a small volume of medium by freezing and thawing or by sonication is a useful method for producing high-titer antigens for a variety of viruses (94, 100, 105). However, harvesting only cell-associated virus is not an optimal procedure for producing antigens for all viruses. Some viruses, e.g., respiratory syncytial and adenoviruses, release additional CF antigens into the culture fluids, and higher antibody titers are demonstrable by using the whole culture material (cells and fluids) as antigen than by using antigen derived from the infected cells alone (100). It is also important to establish the optimal method for releasing viral antigens from infected host cells. Highly reactive CF antigens for certain viruses can be obtained by extracting the host cells with alkaline buffers (14, 98, 100), but for some viruses sonic treatment or freezing and thawing is more effective.

The following three procedures are given as examples of methods for producing viral serologic antigens in cell cultures. In the first procedure antigen is prepared from the whole infected culture, in the second it is derived from infected cells disrupted by sonication, and in the third it is prepared by extraction of infected cells with an alkaline buffer. Control antigens are prepared in the same manner from uninfected cell cultures of the same lot used for preparation of the viral antigen.

Preparation of adenovirus or respiratory syncytial virus CF antigen in HeLa cells

    1. Sterile 16-oz prescription bottles are seeded with 2×10^6 HeLa cells in 20 ml of growth medium consisting of 10% fetal bovine serum and 90% lactalbumin hydrolysate-yeast extract medium buffered with 1.25 ml of 8.8% $NaHCO_3$/100 ml of medium.

    2. Cultures are incubated at 35–36 C for 4 days, and the medium is replaced with fresh growth medium containing 5 ml of 8.8% $NaHCO_3$/100 ml of medium. Incubation is continued for 1–2 days.

    3. The growth medium is removed from a representative culture, and the cells are dispersed with a mixture of equal parts of 0.25% trypsin and 1:2000 versene and then counted in a hemocytometer.

    4. Growth medium is removed from the remaining cultures, and they are infected with seed virus at a ratio of 1-10 infectious doses of virus per cell. The total volume of fluid in each culture is brought up to 6 ml with Hanks BSS if the volume of seed virus is less than that. Cultures are incubated at 35–36 C for 1.5 hr.

    5. Inocula are removed from the cultures and 20 ml of maintenance medium is added, consisting of 2% inactivated fetal bovine serum and 98% Leibovitz medium No. 15. Cultures are incubated at 35–36 C until they show a 4-plus viral CPE.

    6. Cells are dislodged into the culture fluids by shaking with sterile glass beads, and materials from each culture are pooled.

    7. The pooled cells and fluids are then sonically treated at 20 Kc/sec for 2 min.

    8. The sonicated material is clarified by centrifugation at 2000 rpm for 20 min at 4 C, and the supernatant fluid, which contitutes the antigen, is distributed into appropriate working volumes and stored at −70 C.

Preparation of measles virus CF and HA antigens in HeLa cells

1. Cultures of HeLa cells are prepared and the cells enumerated as described in steps 1 through 3 of the above procedure.

2. Growth medium is removed from the cultures, and they are infected with measles seed virus at a multiplicity of 1 to 10 infectious virus doses per cell. The total volume of fluid in each culture is brought up to 6 ml with Hanks BSS if the volume of seed virus is less than that. Cultures are incubated at 35–36 C for 1.5 hr.

3. Inocula are removed from the cultures and 20 ml of maintenance medium consisting of 5% inactivated fetal bovine serum and 95% Leibovitz medium No. 15 is added. Cultures are incubated at 35–36 C until they show a 4-plus viral CPE.

4. Cells are dislodged into the culture fluid by shaking with sterile glass beads, and materials from each culture are pooled.

5. The cells and fluids are separated by centrifugation at 2000 rpm for 20 min at 4 C. The supernatant fluid is discarded.

6. The cells are resuspended to one-tenth of the original volume in Hanks BSS, and the suspension is sonicated at 20 Kc/sec for 2 min.

7. The sonicated material is clarified by centrifugation at 2000 rpm for 20 min at 4 C, and the supernatant fluid, which constitutes the CF antigen, is distributed into appropriate working volumes and stored at −70 C.

8. The clarified antigen obtained in the previous step is treated with Tween 80 and ether for use as a HA antigen.

   a. To 9 parts of antigen is added 1 part of a 1.25% solution of Tween 80, and the mixture is shaken at 4 C for 5 min.

   b. One-half volume of anesthetic ether is added, and the preparation is shaken at 4 C for 15 min.

   c. After centrifugation at 1500 rpm for 15 min, the aqueous phase is removed for use as antigen.

   d. Residual ether is removed by bubbling with nitrogen.

9. The HA antigen is also stored at −70 C.

Preparation of rubella virus CF and HA antigen by alkaline buffer extraction of infected BHK-21 cells (98, 101)

1. Cells from monolayer cultures of the BHK-21 line of baby hamster kidney are dispersed with trypsin-versene solution and counted. Sufficient cultures are dispersed to give $3-4 \times 10^8$ cells.

2. The dispersed cell suspensions are divided between two 200-ml centrifuge bottles and the cells are sedimented by centrifugation at 1000 rpm for 10 min. The supernatant fluid is removed.

3. To each cell pack is added rubella seed virus in a volume sufficient to infect the cells at a ratio of at least 1 infectious dose of virus per cell. The cells are carefully suspended in the seed virus preparation, and the mixture is incubated at 35–36 C for 1.5 hr with occasional shaking.

4. The cells are then sedimented by centrifugation at 1000 rpm for 10 min, and the seed virus is removed.

5. The infected cells are resuspended in 40 ml of growth medium consisting of 10% fetal bovine serum and 90% Eagle MEM in Hanks BSS (buffered with 1.25 ml of 8.8% $NaHCO_3$/100 ml of medium).

6. Each of 4 roller bottles is seeded with 10 ml of infected cell suspension and an additional 90 ml of growth medium is added.

7. Cultures are incubated at 35–36 C for 18–24 hr on a roller apparatus.

8. The growth medium is removed, the cultures are washed once with 100 ml of Hanks BSS, and 100 ml of serum-free maintenance medium is added, consisting of Eagle MEM prepared in Earle BSS and buffered with 2 ml of 8.8% $NaHCO_3$/100 ml of medium.

9. Cultures are incubated at 35–36 C for an additional 2–3 days.

10. Cells are then dislodged into the culture fluid by shaking with glass beads, and the cells and fluids are separated by centrifugation at 1500 rpm for 15 min.

11. After removal of the culture fluid, the cells are resuspended in 10 ml of physiological saline; they can be stored at -20 C until it is convenient to extract with alkaline buffer, or they can be extracted immediately.

12. The cells suspended in saline are centrifuged at 1500 rpm for 15 min, and the supernatant fluid is removed. The cells are then resuspended in 7 ml of 0.1 M glycine buffer, pH 9.5, and incubated in a 37 C water bath for 6 hr with occasional shaking. After centrifugation at 2000 rpm for 20 min, the supernatant fluid (alkaline buffer extract) is removed for use as antigen. This preparation is suitable for use as both a CF and HA antigen.

13. Antigen is dispensed into convenient working volumes and stored at -70 C.

Mycoplasma Contamination of Cell Cultures

Effects

Mycoplasma contamination is one of the most serious and widespread problems encountered by workers utilizing cell cultures for virus propagation. Effects of these contaminants on cultured cells are numerous and varied. They alter various metabolic activities of the culture so that valid biochemical studies cannot be conducted in the cells; they can reduce cellular growth rate, force diploid cell lines into early senescence, produce chromosomal aberrations, and cause permanent changes in cellular morphology (3, 56, 113). Mycoplasma contamination has been shown to decrease the synthesis of many different viruses in cell cultures, but in some cases increased virus yields have been obtained in contaminated cultures, possibly due to inhibition of interferon production by the mycoplasmas (3, 113).

In some instances mycoplasma contaminants produce an extensive CPE in cell cultures, but in many cases they produce few or no observable changes, and they may go unrecognized unless special efforts are made to detect them. Virus preparations produced in contaminated cells contain mycoplasma antigens as well as viral antigens, and this may create problems in the production of serologic antigens or immune sera. Mycoplasmas are not infrequently confused with viruses because of their CPE, HAd, or HA activity, small size and filterability, and resistance to certain antibiotics. When problem isolates are recovered or when an agent is suspected to represent a new virus, the possibility that it is actually a mycoplasma should always be excluded.

Sources

Various studies (3) on the incidence of mycoplasma contamination in cell cultures have shown that primary cultures are rarely contaminated (approximately 1%), whereas continuous cell lines frequently are (50-90%). This suggests that the contaminants are not generally derived from the original tissues, but are introduced in the laboratory. The major mycoplasma contaminants are strains of human, bovine, and swine origin (3). The mode by which human strains are introduced into cell cultures is generally considered to be through mouth pipetting and by failure to use adequate aseptic techniques. Bovine strains are probably introduced through commercial bovine serum used in cell culture media, since it was shown, through the use of a large-specimen broth culture technique, that a high proportion of bovine sera from commercial sources contained low levels of contaminating mycoplasmas (5). The origin of swine strains is more obscure; it was long thought to be from trypsin, which is produced from swine tissues and is widely used for preparation of cell cultures. However, efforts to isolate mycoplasma contaminants from this source have not been successful (3). It is now felt that since swine and cattle are often processed through the same slaughterhouses, the opportunity exists for swine mycoplasma strains to contaminate bovine serum; in fact a swine strain has been isolated from commercial bovine serum (3).

However, contaminated cell cultures are the vehicle usually responsible for introducing mycoplasma contaminants into the virology laboratory. Therefore, it is extremely important that cells from commercial sources and from other laboratories be examined for mycoplasma contamination upon receipt, and that contaminated cells be discarded as soon as is feasible. Mycoplasma-contaminated virus preparations and antisera from outside laboratories can also serve to contaminate cell cultures.

Detection of Mycoplasma Contaminants

Culture procedures

Standard culture procedures (3, 42, 56) for which cell culture materials are inoculated into tubes of mycoplasma broth and onto plates of mycoplasma agar usually suffice for isolation of cultivable mycoplasmas from cell cultures, since the contaminants are present in relatively high concentrations. The sensitivity of culture procedures for detecting small numbers of contaminating organisms, e.g., from bovine serum, can be markedly increased by using a so-called large-specimen broth culture method (5) for which at least 25 ml of the sample is inoculated into 100 ml or more of broth. A semi-solid broth medium (3) which provides an oxygen gradient is suitable for isolation of bacteria and fungi, as well as mycoplasma contaminants, if antibiotics are omitted. Inoculated cultures should be incubated both aerobically and anerobically in a 5% CO_2-95% N_2 atmosphere (3).

Media

Mycoplasma culture media consist of a basic broth supplemented with yeast extract and horse serum, and with agar for solid or semi-solid media. Various formulas have been used for the broth base (3, 42, 56), and none would appear to have any marked advantage in terms of sensitivity for mycoplasma isolation. Some workers add additional supplements such as dextrose, arginine, DNA, and phenol red (3, 65). Mycoplasma broth and agar, supplements, and even complete media are available from several commercial sources, and most of these have been pretested for ability to support the growth of mycoplasmas. However, it is advisable to check the sensitivity of any new lot of medium by testing its ability to support the growth of a low-passage preparation of *Mycoplasma pneumoniae*.

The following media are used routinely in our laboratory for monitoring cell cultures and bovine serum for mycoplasma contamination:

1. Mycoplasma broth base (1 liter)
Difco-Bacto PPLO broth (without crystal violet) . . . .   35 g
Distilled water to . . . . 1,000 ml
The powdered broth is dissolved by gentle heating, and while still hot, the broth is dispensed into screw-cap tubes or bottles in the desired volumes and then autoclaved at 15 lb for 15 min. When cool, the caps are tightened, and the broth is stored at 4 C.

2. Mycoplasma agar base (1 liter)
Difco-Bacto PPLO agar base . . . .   35 g
Distilled water to . . . . 1,000 ml
The medium is prepared and sterilized in the same manner as the broth base.

3. Yeast extract, 25%
Fleischmann's dry yeast (type 20-40) . . . .   250 g
Distilled water to . . . . 1,000 ml
The solution is carefully heated to boiling and filtered through 2 sheets of Whatman No. 12 filter paper, using a number of filtration set-ups since the process is slow. The pH is adjusted to 8 with NaOH, and the solution is dispensed into convenient working volumes and autoclaved at 15 lb for 15 min. The yeast extract is stored at −20 C and is stable for about 2 months.

Sterile yeast extract for mycoplasma culture media is also available from commercial sources.

4. Horse serum

Horse sera employed for cell culture procedures are also suitable for cultivation of mycoplasmas. Some commercial firms market horse serum specifically for mycoplasma media.

The fact that mycoplasma contamination has been demonstrated in commercial horse serum (45) stresses the importance of using horse serum shown to be negative by the large-specimen broth culture procedure as a supplement in mycoplasma isolation media to avoid false-positive results.

Use of agamma horse serum eliminates the appearance of pseudo-colonies, artifacts which may resemble mycoplasma colonies (42, 45), but some workers have noted that fewer mycoplasma isolations were made with agamma serum than with whole serum (GE Kenny, personal communication).

Since fresh horse serum may occasionally be toxic for certain mycoplasmas, it has been recommended that the serum be heated at 56 C (3). However, this may destroy some of the nutritive value of the serum. Horse serum used in this laboratory for mycoplasma cultivation is not inactivated.

5. Penicillin G (Crystalline Sodium) stock solution
Penicillin G . . . . 1,000,000 u vial
Sterile distilled water . . . .   2.0 ml

6. *Complete* mycoplasma broth
Mycoplasma broth base . . . . 70.0 ml
Yeast extract, 25% . . . . 10.0 ml
Horse serum . . . . 20.0 ml
Penicillin stock solution . . . .   0.2 ml
The complete broth is added in a volume of 3 ml for tubes of diphasic medium (see below), or dispensed in 50-ml volumes in 4-oz prescription bottles for large-specimen broth culture testing.

7. *Complete* mycoplasma agar
Mycoplasma agar base, melted and cooled to approximately 56 C . . 70.0 ml
Yeast extract, 25% . . . . 10.0 ml
Horse serum . . . . 20.0 ml
Penicillin stock solution . . . .   0.2 ml
The complete agar is dispensed in a volume of 2 ml for tubes of diphasic medium, and slanted to harden. It is dispensed into 60-mm Petri dishes in a volume of 6 ml. After the plates are poured and before the agar hardens, the agar surface should be stroked with a Bunsen burner flame to prevent formation of bubbles which might be mistaken for mycoplasma colonies.

8. Diphasic tube cultures
To 2 ml of slanted solidified *complete* mycoplasma agar in a screw-cap tube is added 3 ml of *complete* mycoplasma broth.

Isolation procedures

Culturing for mycoplasmas should be done in a room separate from those used for cell culture preparation in order to prevent contamination of cells. Cell cultures to be examined for the presence of mycoplasmas should be incubated with the same medium on the cells for 5 days before testing. To increase the likelihood of detecting contaminants the cells should be cultured for 3 or more passages in the absence of antibiotics. Both culture fluid and cells should be examined, since mycoplasmas exist in close association with the cell membranes; however, the cells should not be disrupted by homogenization, freezing, or sonication, since cell extracts may possess mycoplasmicidal activity (113).

The cells are scraped into the culture medium, and 0.3 ml of the suspension is inoculated into each of 2 diphasic tube cultures, and 0.1 ml is added to each of 2 complete mycoplasma agar plates and streaked across the surface with the tip of the pipette. One tube and 1 plate are incubated aerobically at 37 C; the plate is sealed with masking tape and the tube is capped tightly. One tube and 1 plate are incubated at 37 C in a Gaspak (BioQuest, Inc, Cockeysville, MD) anaerobic system; the plate lid is secured with a small strip of tape, but not sealed, and the tube culture is incubated with a loose cap.

After 1 week, the plates are examined for mycoplasma colonies using a dissecting microscope and transmitted light. If no colonies are seen, each of the diphasic cultures is subpassaged by inoculating 0.1 ml of the broth onto a complete mycoplasma agar plate. The plate inoculated with the aerobic culture is incubated aerobically, and the one inoculated with the anaerobic culture is incubated anaerobically. Original plates are incubated for 3 weeks, and the subpassage plates for 2 weeks before they are considered negative.

For testing serum or other materials by the large-specimen broth culture procedure, 5-ml volumes of the sample are inoculated into each of 10 4-oz prescription bottles containing 50 ml of complete mycoplasma broth medium. Five of the bottles are incubated aerobically, and 5 anaerobically. After 1 week, 0.1 ml of broth from each bottle is cultured onto a complete mycoplasma agar plate, and these are incubated under the same conditions as the original broth cultures. Agar cultures are examined for 3 weeks before they are considered negative.

Identification of mycoplasma colonies

Mycoplasma colonies on agar plates can usually be demonstrated only by microscopic observation. A 10X objective and 10X–15X oculars are employed. The plates are inverted, without removing the cover, on the microscope stage, and the plane of focus is oriented to the agar surface by focusing through the agar onto the lines created when the inoculum was streaked over the surface.

Mycoplasma colonies vary from 10–500 μ in diameter, and they generally consist of an opaque center with a translucent periphery, giving them a "fried egg" appearance; however, on primary isolation mycoplasma colonies may not have this typical appearance. Instead, they are small and dense with a granular core, and lack a well-developed periphery. Characteristically mycoplasma colonies grow downward into the agar, and the center or the whole colony is embedded, making them difficult to dislodge.

Certain artifacts can be confused with mycoplasma colonies. These include small air bubbles which may form on the agar surface when plates are poured, microdroplets of water condensate on the agar surface, cells from the original inoculum, and so-called pseudocolonies (42, 45) which are crystalline aggregates of calcium and magnesium soaps present in serum used in the medium. Pseudocolonies are particularly misleading, as they increase in size on incubation, and may even be "subcultivated" on agar. The use of agamma rather than regular horse serum reportedly prevents the formation of these crystalline structures.

Mycoplasma colonies can be identified as such and distinguished from colonies of bacterial L-forms by staining with Dienes stain (17). The staining solution consists of 2.5 g methylene blue, 1.25 g azur II, 10 g maltose, and 0.25 g Na_2CO_3 dissolved in 100 ml of distilled water. A cotton swab is moistened with the stain and then stroked over an area of agar just adjacent to the suspected colony. The stain diffuses to the colony, which is then examined microscopically. Mycoplasma colonies stain with a dense blue center and light blue periphery. Bacterial colonies, which also stain, are distinguished from mycoplasma colonies by the fact that they decolorize the stain after 30 min, while mycoplasma colonies fail to do so.

If warranted, species identification of mycoplasma contaminants can be accomplished by FA staining of colonies (4) or by growth inhibition tests (12).

Subcultivation of mycoplasmas

Colonies are subcultured by cutting an agar block containing the colony out of the agar with a sterile scalpel, placing the block face downward on a fresh agar plate, and rubbing it across the surface of the agar. The block is then left in contact with the agar, as in some instances growth may occur only under the agar block. Also, agar blocks containing colonies can be placed directly into broth, or broth-to-broth transfers can be made.

Use of cell culture systems for isolation of mycoplasmas

Several investigators have reported that cell cultures may provide a more sensitive host system than artificial media for isolation of certain mycoplasma contaminants (49, 52, 131). The organisms were grown in various types of cultured cells together with mycoplasma agar or broth media. In some instances the agents were cultivable on artificial media after one or more passages in the cell culture-supplemented media (49, 131). One group of workers (131) used a BHK-21 cell culture-agarose medium for separating virus from contaminating mycoplasmas; each agent produced distinguishable plaques in the system, and those produced by the virus could be selected and subpassaged.

Detection of noncultivable mycoplasma contaminants

Over the past years it has become increasingly apparent that certain mycoplasma contaminants of cell cultures cannot be isolated in any of the media currently available, despite the fact that the organisms may be present in the cultures in high concentrations. Therefore, a variety of indirect methods has been recommended for detection of these agents. Although none is able to detect all mycoplasma contaminants, the procedures are very useful adjuncts to mycoplasma culturing, and wherever feasible, it is desirable to add one, particularly a biochemical procedure, to mycoplasma screening programs (107).

Microscopic methods

Orcein staining. Fogh and Fogh (28) developed a method for microscopic detection of mycoplasmas in cell cultures which is based upon hypotonic treatment followed by orcein staining. Examination by phase microscopy reveals the organisms primarily at the cell borders associated with the plasma membrane and in the intercellular spaces. The specimen is inoculated into an uncontaminated FL cell line for an indicator host system, since these cells have a uniform morphology and are free from other structures which might be mistaken for mycoplasma bodies. Relatively high levels ($\geq 3 \times 10^5$ cfu/ml) of organisms must be present to permit detection by this method.

Fluorescent staining of mycoplasma DNA. A microscopic method utilizing a fluorescent stain which binds specifically to DNA has recently been described for detection of mycoplasma contaminants in cell cultures (11). It is a rapid and simple procedure which might be useful in laboratories which are unable to perform some of the more sophisticated biochemical methods for detection of noncultivable mycoplasmas. Uncontaminated cells stained with the so-called H-stain show fluorescence only in the nuclei, whereas in contaminated cultures the stain binds to the DNA of the mycoplasmas, and fluorescence of spherical, uniform-sized mycoplasma bodies 0.1 to 0.3 μ in diameter is seen over the cell surfaces and between the cells. It is probable that this method may fail to detect very low levels of contamination.

Autoradiography. Autoradiographic detection of mycoplasmas in infected cell cultures is based upon the fact that when uninfected cells are labeled with tritiated thymidine, it is incorporated primarily into the nucleus, whereas in cells contaminated with mycoplasmas it is incorporated preferentially into extranuclear acid-insoluble material, especially along the cell margins (115), and autoradiograms show grains over the cell cytoplasm in greater amounts than in the background. The test is relatively simple but requires 3 days for completion, and it may lack sensitivity for detecting low levels of contamination.

Biochemical methods

Uracil incorporation. Mycoplasmas readily take up exogenous uracil into their RNA, whereas animal cell cultures take up very little, and this provides the basis for detection of mycoplasma contamination in cell cultures by demonstrating high uptake of tritiated uracil (57). This is a relatively simple biochemical method which can be performed rapidly. Drawbacks are the fact that some mycoplasma species do not show high uracil incorporation and that the method is not specific for mycoplasma contaminants, since many bacteria also incorporate uracil.

Nucleoside phosphorylase activity. Mycoplasma-contaminated cell cultures show high levels of nucleoside phosphorylase activity, while uncontaminated cultures show low levels of this activity. Thus, measurement of nucleoside phosphorylase activity by incubation of radioactive uridine with culture lysates, and subsequent chromatographic separation of uridine from the reaction product, uracil, can be used as an indirect method for detecting mycoplasma contamination of cell cultures (63). Results can be obtained within 4 hours, and the method has detected infected cultures which were negative by culture methods. However, a few uncontaminated cell lines were shown to have relatively high levels of uridine phosphorylase activity.

Uridine/uracil uptake ratios. The nucleoside phosphorylase activity of mycoplasma-infected cell cultures greatly reduces the uptake of exogenous uridine; however, as indicated above, there is an increase in the uptake of exogenous uracil in the culture. Schneider et al (108) have taken advantage of this difference in the uptake of uridine and uracil to devise a technique for detection of mycoplasma contamination. Parallel cell cultures are incubated with either tritiated uridine or tritiated uracil, and the ratio of tritiated uridine to tritiated uracil in the RNA is determined. Low ratios are observed in contaminated cultures, while high ratios are seen in uncontaminated ones. Results obtained by this procedure agreed with those obtained by a polyacrylamide gel electrophoresis method for detection of mycoplasma RNA, and the test revealed mycoplasmas in cells that were negative by culture methods (108). This method is now available in commercial mycoplasma monitoring services.

Prevention of mycoplasma contamination in cell cultures

It is apparent that mycoplasma contaminated cell cultures are the most important source of further contamination in the laboratory. An excellent study by McGarrity (66) has illustrated how readily and extensively mycoplasma infected cultures can contaminate the exterior of laboratory glassware, workers' hands, and working surfaces, and it also demonstrated prolonged viability of the organisms in droplets on working surfaces, including the interior of laminar flow hoods.

Cell cultures should be obtained only from commercial companies which guarantee them to be free from mycoplasmas, but even so, they should be tested when they are received in the laboratory, as should cell cultures from other outside sources. Cell lines carried in the laboratory should be monitored on a regular and frequent basis for mycoplasma contamination. As soon as a contaminated cell line is detected, it should be discarded. It is much better practice to maintain stocks of uncontaminated cells in liquid nitrogen to be used as a back-up in the event that the line becomes contaminated, rather than to attempt to eradicate mycoplasma contaminants. Known contaminated lines should never be handled in a work area used for uncontaminated cells.

Sera used in cell culture media are also a potential source of mycoplasma contamination and should be obtained from firms which use the large-specimen broth culture method in pretesting for mycoplasma contaminants, or sera should be tested by this method in the user's laboratory. Inactivation at 56 C for 20 min, or double filtration through 0.22 μ membranes have also been recommended as aids in preventing mycoplasma contamination from serum, but it is recognized that these procedures may reduce the nutritional properties of the serum.

In handling cell cultures, strict aseptic techniques should be observed. Mouth pipetting should be prohibited, there should be no eating or smoking in the laboratory, and traffic and talking in the work area should be kept to a minimum. Work surfaces should be disinfected between handling of different cell cultures, and wherever feasible, cell cultures should be prepared in laminar flow hoods or in cubicles with high efficiency particulate air (HEPA) filters. Cell culture laboratories should adopt suitable quality control procedures to assure the efficiency of sterilization methods for media, glassware and other apparatus (65, 67).

It has been noted that mycoplasma contamination was virtually absent in cell cultures carried in laboratories using antibiotic-free media (3, 45), and this approach has been suggested as a means of preventing mycoplasma contamination. Obviously, the exclusion of antibiotics does not in itself prevent contamination, but rather it fosters greater care and skill in handling cell cultures, and this reduces the risk of mycoplasma contamination. Also, work with antibiotic-free media is usually done on a relatively small scale, for which very stringent aseptic techniques can be employed.

Cultivation of cells in the presence of antibiotics known to be effective against mycoplasmas is another approach to preventing contamination, and chlortetracycline has been recommended, since few resistant mycoplasma strains have been encountered (42, 45). The antibiotic (Aureomycin·HCl, crystalline intravenous, Lederle product No. 4691-96, 500-mg vial) is used at a concentration of 50 μg/ml of medium. It is reconstituted in 50 ml of warm (37 C) sterile distilled water and stored in convenient working volumes at -20 C.

Eradication of mycoplasma contaminants in cell cultures

Although there have been reports of the successful elimination of mycoplasma contaminants from cell cultures, it is now well recognized that permanent eradication of the contaminants is extremely difficult to achieve. In most instances the infection is merely suppressed rather than eliminated, and mycoplasma resistance to all of the commonly employed antibiotics has been encountered (3, 113). Physical or chemical treatment of contaminated cells is undesirable, since most methods are toxic to the cells and may serve to select out a population with altered characteristics. Rather than attempting to decontaminate cultures, they should be replaced, either from frozen stocks or outside sources.

If efforts must be made to eliminate mycoplasma contaminants from cell cultures, treatment with a combination of a high-titer Nt antiserum and an antibiotic is recommended (3). This is a difficult and lengthy procedure which should be considered only as a last resort.

Elimination of mycoplasma contaminants from virus stocks

Mycoplasma contaminated virus preparations may be a source of contamination for cell cultures and other reagents, and the contaminants may also interfere with virus replication or give misleading results in virus assays.

Viruses without an essential lipid can simply be treated with an organic solvent such as chloroform or ether to free them from contaminants (3). One milliliter of ether is mixed with 1 ml of the virus preparation, incubated at 22–25 C overnight, and the ether is removed by evaporation at 37 C.

A method for freeing enveloped viruses from mycoplasma contaminants is based upon the fact that phenethyl alcohol (PEA) readily inactivates mycoplasmas while affecting enveloped viruses little or not at all (112). A 2% solution of PEA in PBS, pH 7.4, is added to an equal volume of virus preparation to give a final PEA concentration of 1%; the mixture is held at room temperature for 20 min with stirring, and then serially diluted and assayed. Subpassages are made from the highest dilution of the treated material which shows a specific viral effect.

An alternative method for inactivating mycoplasma contaminants of enveloped viruses is to treat the preparation with a high concentration of pretested antibiotic at 22–25 C overnight followed by filtration through a 100-nm filter once or a 220-nm filter twice (3).

Cell Culture Apparatus

Culture vessels

Cell culture tubes or bottles with screw caps which cover the lip of the container are preferred to containers closed with rubber stoppers. They reduce the risk of contaminating the cultures and also the risk of contaminating the outside of the culture with infectious material.

Disposable. Cell culture vessels ranging in size from microtiter cups to roller bottles are available in disposable plastic or glass, and these are much more convenient and usually more economical to employ than are reusable glass containers. The plastic items are received sterile, ready for use. It has been noted that certain types of fastidious cells may grow somewhat better in disposable plastic containers than in disposable glass ones. A disadvantage to the use of plastic vessels is the fact that the openings cannot be flamed during aseptic handling of cell cultures.

Glass prescription bottles have been employed for many years for growth of cell cultures and for storage of cell culture media, and they are inexpensive enough to permit their discard after a single use. Disposable glass tubes are also widely used for cell culture. The high temperature at which glass vessels are molded incinerates dirt which may be present, and if the containers are covered after molding to prevent dirt from entering, they are usually clean enough to provide a satisfactory surface for cell growth without preliminary washing or after a single distilled water rinse. Most disposable glass culture vessels are not sterile upon receipt and must be sterilized by the user.

Cleaning nondisposable glassware. Although most laboratories employ disposable items for cell culture, this may not be feasible in some instances, and some nondisposable glassware is used in most laboratories. Certain basic procedures are essential to the proper cleaning of cell culture glassware. The first is the *immediate* soaking of the glassware in a cleaning agent. This is essential to prevent drying of materials in the glass vessels, and is particularly important for materials which have been decontaminated in the autoclave, as the heat causes protein material to dry rapidly and become difficult to remove, even with good washing procedures.

Several detergents (7X, Linbro Chemical Co, New Haven, CT; Micro-Solv, Microbiological Associates, Inc, Bethesda, MD; Lennox, Magic Soap and Chemicals Co, Oakland, CA; Alconox, Alconox, Inc, New York, NY), most of which contain a wetting agent, are recommended for cleaning cell culture glassware. The effectiveness of any detergent is dependent upon the qualities of the water supply, and the most satisfactory detergent for a given laboratory is usually determined by experimentation.

After soaking, the glassware is usually boiled in a fresh detergent solution for at least 10 min. It is generally necessary to brush culture vessels individually to provide adequately clean surfaces for growth of cells, but the use of ultrasonic equipment may eliminate the need for hand brushing. Automatic washers are generally satisfactory for cleaning pipettes.

After soaking, boiling, and brushing in detergent, it is essential to rinse the glassware adequately. A minimum of 8-10 rinses in tap water followed by 2 rinses in distilled or deionized water is generally recommended. For certain purposes a final rinse in glass-distilled water may be necessary.

Clean glassware should not be touched with bare hands while it is wet, as it will become contaminated by oils from the skin. Stainless steel wire baskets should be used for handling tubes and small bottles in bulk, and larger items should be handled with clean rubber gloves.

The cleanliness of the washed glassware can be ascertained by its wettability—fluid should wet the surface evenly rather than clinging in droplets.

Rubber items

Stoppers and tubing used for cell culture procedures should be of nontoxic silicone rubber. Ordinary rubber stoppers and rubber tubing can be prepared for use in cell culture (if prolonged contact with the medium is to be avoided) by boiling in a 5% sodium carbonate solution and rinsing repeatedly in distilled water.

Sterilization of cell culture apparatus

In sterilizing glassware it is important to recognize that cotton stoppers may contain oily substances which vaporize when heated, coating the interior of the vessels and making the surfaces unsuitable for adherence and growth of cells. The use of stainless steel or plastic closures obviates this problem. Unclosed tubes or bottles can be placed in stainless steel boxes with lids for sterilization in dry air and then closed with sterile screw caps at the time of use. Certain types of wrapping paper may also release volatile toxic substances when charred, and thus proper regulation of the temperature employed for dry-heat sterilization is important. If it is necessary to employ cotton stoppers during sterilization, they may be wrapped in heavy foil to prevent contamination of the interior surfaces of the container with vaporized oils from the cotton.

When employing moist heat for sterilization it is essential that the steam be free from impurities which might contaminate the glassware; these can be introduced by compounds used to prevent oxidation of steam pipes. Steam may be cleaned by filters (Selas Corp of America, Dresher, PA) placed in the line near the point of entry into the autoclave. Ideally, autoclaves used for sterilization of cell culture apparatus should be equipped with an indirect distilled water steam generator (90), and the interior, pipes, valves, fittings and connections should all be of stainless steel (American Sterilizer Co, Erie, PA).

To ensure adequate sterilization, temperature monitoring devices such as diacks, indicator tapes, and temperature recording charts should be used. The date of sterilization should be stamped on items *after* they are removed from the sterilizer.

Sterilization of plastics with ethylene oxide leaves a toxic residue which requires relatively long periods of aeration for its removal (91). Manufacturers of plastic cell culture vessels generally sterilize them by radiation to avoid this problem.

Method for testing cell culture apparatus for toxicity

A useful method for testing possible toxicity of certain items which contact cell cultures or culture media is to place them in double distilled water, sterilize by autoclaving, and then use the water for preparing cell culture maintenance medium. The maintenance of cells on this medium is compared with that of cells in identical medium prepared in the same water which was not exposed to the test item. This procedure has permitted us to detect toxicity of certain rubber tubing, linings for cell culture tube caps, membrane filters, and plastic film used for sealing cell cultures. It is a stringent test, but one which gives clear-cut results in that media prepared with water exposed to toxic items produce rapid and extensive destruction of the cell cultures, while those prepared with water exposed to nontoxic items maintain the cultures for as long as the control medium.

Miscellaneous equipment for cell culture procedures

Racks for stationary tube cultures. Racks designed for incubating stationary tube cultures are available from numerous commercial sources. The tubes are held in position by metal clips which prevent the tubes from turning during handling, with a resultant drying of the monolayer. This also permits decanting of used medium or rinsing fluid from an entire rack of tubes in a single operation. The racks are constructed so that the tubes are held in a slightly inclined position, which permits attachment and growth of cells toward the bottom of the tubes and ensures covering of the monolayers with the nutrient medium.

Sealing devices for tube cultures. During the outgrowth of cell cultures all of the tubes in a rack may be sealed with a press device rather than with individual closures. This greatly facilitates feeding and preparation of the cultures for use. (After inoculation with virus, however, the tubes must be individually sealed with caps to prevent cross contamination.) These sealing devices are based upon the use of a plastic film (Saran Wrap, Dow Chemical Co, Midland, MI) to cover the tops of the tubes and then sealing through the use of a ¾" sponge-rubber pad which is pressed against the tops of the tubes to provide an airtight seal. Racks with these sealing devices are available from commercial sources; they have a metal cover which fits over the foam rubber pad and snaps onto the rack so as to exert pressure on the pad and seal the tubes. Alternatively, a simple "sandwich" press can be fashioned from 2 plywood boards placed at the top and bottom of the rack with edges which extend beyond the rack; the boards are bolted together at the 4 corners, and pressure is exerted through the use of wing nuts. It must be cautioned that certain plastic films other than Saran Wrap have been shown to be toxic to cell cultures (2), and their used should be avoided. Possible toxicity of plastic films can be detected by the method described above.

Tube cultures can also be sealed with pressure tape before tubes are inoculated with virus. The tops of the tubes are warmed by flaming before they are sealed. Pressure sensitive tape is satisfactory for this purpose (Minnesota Mining and Manufacturing Company No. 471 in yellow, white, or red).

Roller devices for cell cultures. Rotation of virus-infected cell cultures during incubation provides an exchange of fluid and gas phases and may enhance virus replication, as evidenced by more extensive and earlier CPE effects and higher titers. This is advantageous in primary isolation attempts on clinical materials and in the production of high-titer virus preparations for use as serologic antigens or vaccines. Roller drums for rotating tube cultures may be moved by a motor-driven shaft or on parallel, motor-driven rollers; in either case the drums can be removed for loading or for observation of the cultures. Roller devices for large bottle cultures are also available in a variety of sizes. Monolayers are grown on the entire horizontal bottle surface, and the cultures reach high population densities.

Apparatus for large-scale cell culture. In addition to roller bottle apparatus, several other devices are commercially available which permit large-scale cultivation of host cells, and production of high-titer virus preparations. These include spinner flasks for propagation of cells in suspension (Bellco Glass, Inc, Vineland, NJ), a cartridge device containing a series of discs which provide a large surface for cell attachment (Linbro Chemical Co, New Haven, CT), and a cartridge device in which spirally-wound plastic film provides a large surface area for cellular growth (Dyna-Cell, Costar, Cambridge, MA).

Appendix

Composition and preparation of cell culture media and reagents

Water used for preparation of cell culture media and reagents should be deionized and then distilled in an all-glass still. Chemicals should be of analytical reagent grade. Spatulas should be rinsed in double-distilled water between each weighing to prevent cross-contamination of reagents, and reagents should not be transferred from their original containers, because of errors which may occur in labeling or distribution. As each batch of medium is prepared, the lot number of each reagent should be recorded as it is weighed out.

Antibiotic and antimycotic solutions

Gentamicin solution

Vials of Gentamicin Reagent Solution (Schering Corp, Kenilworth, NY) are reconstituted in Hanks BSS to contain either 10 or 50 mg/ml, depending upon the size of the vial. These are stored at 4 C, and further diluted to appropriate concentrations in Hanks BSS for inclusion in cell culture media or for treatment of clinical materials.

Penicillin-streptomycin-neomycin-bacitracin solution

This antibiotic solution is incorporated into media for the cultivation of a variety of cell types, and it may also be employed for treating certain clinical specimens. It contains 25,000 u of penicillin, 25,000 μg each of streptomycin and neomycin, and 250 u of bacitracin per ml and is prepared by diluting lyophilized materials (Obtainable in bulk, Chas. Pfizer and Co, Brooklyn, NY) in Hanks BSS as follows:

Penicillin (potassium)	5,000,000 u
Dihydrostreptomycin	5,000,000 μg
Neomycin sulfate	5,000,000 μg
Bacitracin	50,000 u

The antibiotics are dissolved in a total of 200 ml of Hanks BSS.

Penicillin, 20,000 u and streptomycin, 20,000 μg/ml

This antibiotic solution may be incorporated into cell culture media or used for treating clinical specimens. It is prepared by dissolving 1,000,000 u penicillin and 1,000,000 μg streptomycin in 50 ml of Hanks BSS.

Penicillin, 10,000 u and streptomycin, 50,000 μg/ml

This antibiotic solution is used for treating clinical specimens before inoculating them into cell cultures. It is prepared by dissolving 500,000 u penicillin and 2,500,000 μg streptomycin in 50 ml of Hanks BSS.

Fungizone (amphotericin B, ER Squibb and Sons, New York, NY) solution

This antimycotic solution can be incorporated into cell culture media, or used for treating clinical specimens. A stock solution containing 1 mg/ml is prepared by dissolving 50 mg in 50 ml of distilled water.

With the exception of the gentamicin, all of the above antibiotic or antimycotic solutions are sterilized by Millipore filtration, stored at −20 C, and added to the media at time of use.

Balanced salt and buffered saline solutions

Earle balanced salt solution, 10X concentrated

	Per liter of 10X solution
NaCl	68.0 g
KCl	4.0 g
$CaCl_2$	2.0 g
$MgSO_4 \cdot 7H_2O$	2.0 g
$NaH_2PO_4 \cdot H_2O$	1.4 g
Glucose	10.0 g
Phenol red, 1%	20.0 ml

The $CaCl_2$ should be dissolved separately in 100 ml of double distilled water and added to the other dissolved reagents just before the solution is brought to a final volume of 1,000 ml with double distilled water.

The 10X solution is sterilized by Millipore filtration. For use the 10X solution is diluted to 1X with sterile double distilled water and *buffered by the addition of 2.5% of an 8.8% NaHCO₃ solution.*

Hanks balanced salt solution, 10X concentrated

	Solution 1	Per liter of 10X solution
NaCl		80.0 g
KCl		4.0 g
$CaCl_2$		1.4 g
$MgSO_4 \cdot 7H_2O$		2.0 g

	Solution 2	Per liter of 10X solution
$Na_2HPO_4 \cdot 12H_2O$		1.2 g
KH_2PO_4		0.6 g
Glucose		10.0 g
Phenol red, 1%		16.0 ml

The reagents for each solution are dissolved in slightly less than 500 ml of double distilled water, and Solution 2 is added to Solution 1 with stirring. The 10X solution is then brought to a final volume of 1,000 ml with double distilled water.

The 10X solution is sterilized by Millipore filtration, or it may be diluted to IX with double distilled water and sterilized by autoclaving at 10 lbs pressure for 10 min.

For use the 10X solution is diluted to 1X with sterile double distilled water and *buffered by the addition of 1.25% of a 2.8% NaHCO₃ solution.*

Phosphate-buffered saline, pH 7.5

This solution is used for diluting cell dispersing agents, and for washing cells before dispersion.

Per liter IX

NaCl	8.00 g
KCl	0.20 g
KH_2PO_4	0.12 g
Na_2HPO_4 (anhydrous)	0.91 g
Double distilled water to	1,000 ml

The solution may be sterilized by autoclaving at 18 lb pressure for 35 min.

Buffering solutions

Sodium bicarbonate

There are added, *at the time of use,* to balanced salt solutions or media containing Earle BSS or Hanks BSS bases to provide the proper buffering capacity.

2.8% NaHCO₃

$NaHCO_3$	2.8 g
Double distilled water	100.0 ml

8.8% NaHCO₃

$NaHCO_3$	8.8 g
Double distilled water	100.0 ml

These solutions are sterilized by Millipore filtration.

HEPES buffer, 1 M stock solution, pH 7.3

HEPES (N-2-hydroxyethylpiperazine-N'-2-ethanesulfonic acid)	235.3 g

This reagent is dissolved in 900 ml of double distilled water, and the pH is adjusted to 7.3 with 5N NaOH. The volume is adjusted to 1,000 ml with double distilled water. The solution is sterilized by Millipore filtration and stored at 4 C. HEPES buffer is usually employed in cell culture media at concentrations of 20–25 mM.

Cell dispersing agents

Trypsin solution, 1%

One gram of powdered trypsin (Trypsin, 1:300, Nutritional Biochemicals Corp., Cleveland, OH) is dissolved in 100 ml of PBS, pH 7.5, and the solution is passed through ash-free filter paper (Schleicher and Schull No. 589).

The solution is then sterilized by Millipore filtration and stored at −20 C.

Versene (Tetrasodium salt of ethylenediaminetetraacetic acid [EDTA], Versenes Inc, Framingham, MA) solutions

1:2000 dilution

Versene	0.5 g
PBS, pH 7.5	1,000 ml

1:3000 dilution

Versene .... 1.0 g
PBS, pH 7.5 .... 3,000 ml

1:5000 dilution

Versene .... 0.5 g
PBS, pH 7.5 .... 2,500 ml

The solutions are dispensed into *hard glass* containers and sterilized by autoclaving at 18 lb pressure for 35 min.

Cryoprotective agents

Dimethylsulfoxide (Mallinckrodt Chemical Co, St. Louis, MO)

Care should be used in handling this reagent because of its unusual ability to penetrate the skin and to be absorbed through the lungs.

Dimethylsulfoxide is sterilized for use as a cell protective agent by filtering through a polytetrafluoroethylene Millipore FGLP 047 00 filter using a stainless steel holder. The reagent will dissolve an ordinary Millipore filter. It is stored at 4 C.

Glycerol

This cryoprotective agent is sterilized by autoclaving for 15 min at low exhaust, and stored at 4 C.

Sorbitol, 70% solution

To 350 g of sorbitol is added 150 ml of double distilled water and the mixture is stirred until the sorbitol is dissolved; this can be aided by warming at 37 C. The volume is brought to 500 ml with double distilled water, and the solution is sterilized by Millipore filtration. It is stored at 4 C.

Indicator and staining solutions

Phenol red, 1%

1. A 1 N NaOH solution is prepared by mixing 10 ml of saturated, concentrated NaOH with 90 ml of double distilled water.
2. Ten grams of alcohol-soluble phenol red (USP) is placed in a 100-ml beaker, and approximately 20 ml of the NaOH solution is added, mixed, and allowed to stand for a few minutes.
3. The dissolved dye is transferred to a 1,000-ml volumetric flask.
4. Additional 10-ml volumes of the NaOH solution are added to the beaker and the dissolved material is added to the volumetric flask. *No more than a total of 70 ml of the NaOH solution should be used.*
5. The solution is brought to a final volume of 1,000 ml with double distilled water, and stored at room temperature.

Neutral red, 1:1000 dilution

One gram of neutral red is dissolved in 1,000 ml of double distilled water and the solution is sterilized by Millipore filtration.

Nutrient media

Eagle Minimum Essential Medium (MEM)

The following is given as an example of a procedure for the preparation of a complex cell culture medium. Most laboratories will obtain complex media from commercial sources. Formulations for preparations of other media such as medium No. 199 and Leibovitz medium No. 15 are given in other sources (77, 92). As indicated below, Eagle MEM can be prepared with either an Earle BSS or Hanks BSS base. The concentrations of amino acids and vitamins may be doubled to give "fortified" MEM. The medium is prepared 10X concentrated and stored in the refrigerator. At the time of use glutamine and antibiotics (stored at -20 C) and $NaHCO_3$ are added to the 1X solution.

Solution A

	Per liter 10X medium
l-Arginine · HCl	1.05 g
l-Histidine · HCl	0.31 g
l-Lysine · HCl	0.58 g
l-Tryptophane	0.10 g
l-Phenylalanine	0.32 g
l-Threonine	0.48 g
l-Leucine	0.52 g
l-Valine	0.46 g
l-Isoleucine	0.52 g
l-Methionine	0.15 g

Solution B

	Per liter 10X medium
l-Tyrosine	0.36 g
l-Cystine	0.24 g

These 2 amino acids are dissolved in 200 ml of 0.075 N HCl (1 ml of commercial CP HCl [11.9 N] + 157.7 ml double distilled water = 158.7 ml of 0.075 N HCl) with gentle heating (80 C).

Solution C

Nicotinamide	200	mg
Pyridoxal	200	mg
Thiamine	200	mg
Pantothenic acid	200	mg
Choline	200	mg
i-Inositol	400	mg
Riboflavin	20	mg

These are dissolved in approximately 175 ml of double distilled water then brought to a final volume of 200 ml with double distilled water. The solution is dispensed in 10-ml volumes and stored at -20 C. Ten milliliters of Solution C is added to each liter of 10X medium.

Solution D

Dissolve 200 mg of biotin in 150 ml of double distilled water. To increase stability upon storage, 1 ml of 1 N HCl (10 ml of commercial CP HCl [11.9 N]+ 90 ml double distilled water = 100 ml of 1 N HCl) is added.

The total volume is brought to 200 ml with double distilled water and the solution is dispensed in 10-ml amounts and stored at $-$ 20 C. Ten milliliters of solution D is added to each liter of 10X medium.

Solution E

Dissolve 200 mg folic acid (crystalline) in 200 ml of 1X Hanks BSS, pH 7.8. The solution is dispensed in 10-ml amounts and stored at − 20 C. Ten milliliters of Solution E is added to each liter of 10X medium.

Glutamine solution, 3%

(To be added at the time of use, *not added to the 10X medium*). Dissolve 12 g 1-glutamine in 400 ml double distilled water and sterilize by filtration through a Millipore pad. The solution is stored at − 20 C, and 1 ml is added to each 100 ml of 1X MEM.

Preparation of the final mixture of 10X *Eagle MEM in Earle BSS.*

1. The following are dissolved in Solution B:

NaCl . . . . 68.0 g
KCl . . . . 4.0 g
$MgSO_4 \cdot 7H_2O$ . . . . 2.0 g

2. 1.4 g $NaH_2PO_4 \cdot H_2O$ is dissolved in 55 ml of double distilled water and added to the above pool.

3. Dissolve 10 g glucose in 50 ml double distilled water and add 20 ml of a 1% phenol red solution to the pool.

4. The volume of the pool is brought to 600 ml with double distilled water and the following solutions are added:

Solution	Per liter of 10X medium
C	10 ml
D	10 ml
E	10 ml

5. In a separate flask containing 160 ml of double distilled water, 2 g anhydrous $CaCl_2$ is dissolved and then added to the pool slowly with vigorous shaking.

6. The amino acids of Solution A are added to the pool and the volume is brought to approximately 950 ml with double distilled water; the mixture is held in the refrigerator overnight.

7. The total volume is brought to exactly 1,000 ml with double distilled water and the solution is sterilized by Millipore filtration. The 10X medium is stored at 4 C.

8. For use, the 10X medium is diluted to 1X with sterile double distilled water, and 1% of the *3% glutamine solution* and 2.5% of an *8.8% NaHCO₃ solution* are added.

Preparation of the final mixture of 10X *Eagle MEM in Hanks BSS.*

1. The following are dissolved in Solution B:

NaCl . . . . 80.0 g
KCl . . . . 4.0 g
$MgSO_4 \cdot 7H_2O$ . . . . 2.0 g

2. The following are dissolved in 50 ml of double distilled water and added to the pool:

$Na_2HPO_4 \cdot 12H_2O$ . . . . 1.2 g
KH_2PO_4 . . . . 0.6 g

3. Dissolve 10 g glucose in 50 ml double distilled water and add 20 ml of a 1% phenol red solution to the pool.

4. The volume of the pool is brought to 600 ml with double distilled water and the following solutions are added:

Solution	Per 1 liter of 10X medium
C	10 ml
D	10 ml
E	10 ml

5. In a separate flask containing 160 ml double distilled water, 1.4 g anhydrous $CaCl_2$ is dissolved and then added to the pool slowly with vigorous shaking.

6. The amino acids of Solution A are added to the pool and the volume is brought to approximately 950 ml with double distilled water; the mixture is held in the refrigerator overnight.

7. The total volume is brought to exactly 1,000 ml with double distilled water and the solution is sterilized by Millipore filtration. The 10X medium is stored at 4 C.

8. For use the 10X medium is diluted to 1X with sterile double distilled water, and 1% of the 3% *glutamine solution* and 2.5% of a *2.8% NaHCO₃ solution* are added.

Lactalbumin hydrolysate-yeast extract medium

This simple medium is employed, in combination with 10% fetal bovine serum, for propagation of a variety of established cell lines. It is prepared 5X concentrated and diluted 1 in 5 with sterile double distilled water for use.

	Per liter 5X medium
Lactalbumin hydrolysate	25.0 g
Glucose	22.5 g
Yeast extract	5.0 g
NaHCO₃	5.5 g
Phenol red, 1% solution	8.0 ml

These ingredients are dissolved in 5X Earle BSS as follows. All of the ingredients *except the NaHCO₃* are added to 1,000 ml of 5X Earle BSS and held at 4 C overnight. The following day the mixture is heated to approximately 80 C under a hot water tap to dissolve the components completely. The solution is then allowed to cool, the NaHCO₃ is added and dissolved, and the solution is sterilized by Millipore filtration.

Nutrient solutions

Glucose, 20%

Glucose (dextrose)	20.0 g
Double distilled water to	100.0 g

Sterilized by Millipore filtration.

Lactalbumin hydrolysate, 5% in physiological saline

Lactalbumin hydrolysate	5.00 g
NaCl	0.85 g
Double distilled water to	100.00 ml

Sterilized by Millipore filtration or by autoclaving at 120 C for 15 min.

Sera

All sera are sterilized by Millipore filtration and stored at − 20 C.

Sterilization of cell culture media by filtration

At this time cell culture media are usually sterilized by membrane filtration, and this type of filter possesses several advantages over the asbestos pad filters which were often used in the past. They are more effective for sterilization, since they are sieves, and all particles with dimensions exceeding the pore size are retained; this is in contrast to asbestos pads which are "gradient" type filters and retain particles but do not act as an absolute barrier. No appreciable volume of fluid is retained on membrane filters, and filtration rates are rapid. However, the filters tend to clog, due to the efficient retention of particles on the membrane, and it is generally necessary to use prefilters for clarification, and in some cases to filter the material through successively finer filters prior to passing it through a 0.22 μ sterilizing pad.

In this laboratory, Millipore membrane filters are used for sterilizing cell culture media; although other types of membranes may be satisfactory, we have found those from some sources to be toxic to cell cultures when tested by the procedure described above. If membranes other than Millipore filters are to be used for media sterilization, it would be advisable to check them for toxicity by the method described.

It has been recognized for some years that membrane filters may contain detergents which are toxic for cells in culture (10). Washing the membranes and discarding the first 100 ml of medium filtered can reduce, but not entirely eliminate, this problem; therefore, it is recommended that detergent-free filters (Triton-free filters, Millipore Corp, Bedford, MA) rather than regular filters be used for sterilizing cell culture media.

Pressure rather than suction is used for filtering cell culture media, as suction removes carbon dioxide from the solution, causing changes in pH. Also, protein components of cell culture media do not foam when filtered with pressure. Compressed nitrogen is usually employed for this purpose.

Filtered media should be checked for sterility at frequent intervals during the filtration procedure. At least 1%, and ideally 10%, of each lot of medium should be sampled for sterility. One should use culture media and incubation conditions which are optimal for growth of yeasts and molds as well as those optimal for growth of bacteria.

References

1. ARMSTRONG D: Contamination of tissue culture by bacteria and fungi. *In* Contamination in Tissue Culture, Fogh J (ed), Academic Press Inc, New York, 1973, pp 51–64
2. BANDO BM and ROSENBAUM MJ: Toxicity in HeLa cells mediated by plastic wraps. Lab Pract, January, p 26, 1973
3. BARILE MF:Mycoplasmal contamination of cell cultures: mycoplasma-virus-cell culture interactions. *In* Contamination in Tissue Culture, Fogh J (ed), Academic Press Inc, New York, 1973, pp 131–172
4. BARILE MF and DELGIUDICE RA: Isolations of mycoplasmas and their rapid identification by plate epi-immunofluorescence. *In* Pathogenic Mycoplasmas, Ciba Foundation Symposium, Elsevier, Amsterdam, 1972, pp 165–185
5. BARILE MF and KERN J: Isolation of *Mycoplasma arginini* from commercial bovine sera and its implication in contaminated cell cultures. Proc Soc Exp Biol Med 138:432–437, 1971
6. BEALE AJ, CHRISTOFINIS GC, and FURMINGER IGS: Rabbit cells susceptible to rubella virus. Lancet 2:640–641, 1963
7. BODIAN D: Simplified method of dispersion of monkey kidney cells with trypsin. Virology 4:575–577, 1956
8. BOONE CW: A surveillance procedure applied to sera. *In* Tissue Culture Methods and Applications, Kruse PF Jr and Patterson MK Jr (eds), Academic Press Inc., New York, 1973, pp 677–682
9. BURNSTEIN T and BYINGTON DP: On the isolation of measles virus from infected brain tissue. Neurology 18:162–164, 1968
10. CAHN RD: Detergents in membrane filters. Science 155:195–196, 1967
11. CHEN TR: Microscopic demonstration of mycoplasma contamination in cell cultures and cell culture media. Procedure 75361. Tissue Culture Association Manual 1:229–232, 1975

12. CLYDE WA JR: Mycoplasma species identification based upon growth inhibition by specific antisera. J Immunol 92:958-965, 1964

13. CREMER NE, OSHIRO LS, WEIL ML, LENNETTE EH, ITABASHI HH, and CARNAY L: Isolation of rubella virus from brain in chronic progressive panencephalitis. J Gen Virol 29:143-153, 1975

14. CREMER NE, SCHMIDT NJ, JENSEN F, HOFFMAN M, OSHIRO LS, and LENNETTE EH: Complement-fixing antibody in human sera reactive with viral and soluble antigens of cytomegalovirus. J Clin Microbiol 1:262-267, 1975

15. CROCE CM, SAWICKI W, KRITCHEVSKY D, and KOPROWSKI H: Induction of homo-karyocyte, heterokaryocyte and hybrid formation by lysolecithin. Exp Cell Res 67:427-435, 1971

16. DENNIS J, DUPUIS KW, and CRAWFORD LK. Templates for inoculation and microscopic observation of micro cell cultures. Am J Clin Pathol 63:281-283, 1975

17. DIENES L: L organisms of Klieneberger and *Streptobacillus monoliformis*. J Infect Dis 65:24-42, 1939

18. DULBECCO R and VOGT M: Plaque formation and isolation of pure lines with poliomyelitis viruses. J Exp Med 99:167-182, 1954

19. DUNNEBACKE TH and ZITCER EM: Preparation and cultivation of primary human amnion cells. Cancer Res 17:1043-1046, 1957

20. EAGLE H: Nutrition needs of mammalian cells in tissue culture. Science 122:501-504, 1955

21. EAGLE H: Amino acid metabolism in mammalian cell cultures. Science 130:432-437, 1959

22. EAGLE H, HABEL K, ROWE WP, and HUEBNER RJ: Viral susceptibility of a human carcinoma cell (strain KB). Proc Soc Exp Biol Med 91:361-364, 1956

23. EARLE WR: Production of malignancy *in vitro*. IV. The mouse fibroblast cultures and changes seen in the living cells. J Nat Cancer Inst 4:165-212, 1943

24. ENDERS JF, WELLER TH, and ROBBINS FC. Cultivation of the Lansing strain of poliomyelitis virus in cultures of various human embryonic tissues. Science 109:85-87, 1949

25. ESPMARK JÅ: Rapid serologic typing of herpes simplex virus and titration of herpes simplex antibody by the use of mixed hemadsorption—a mixed antiglobulin reaction applied to virus infected tissue cultures. Arch Gesamte Virusforsch 17:89-97, 1965

26. FAGRAEUS A and ESPMARK Å: Use of a "mixed hemadsorption" method in virus-infected tissue cultures. Nature 190:370-371, 1961

27. FEDOROFF S: Proposed usage of animal tissue culture terms. Procedure 81169. Tissue Culture Association Manual 1:53-57, 1975

28. FOGH J: Contaminants by microscopy. *In* Contamination in Tissue Culture, Fogh J (ed), Academic Press Inc., New York, 1973, pp 66-106

29. FOGH J and LUND RO: Continuous cultivation of epithelial cell strain (FL) from human amniotic membrane. Proc Soc Exp Biol Med 94:532-537, 1957

30. FOLEY JF and AFTONOMOS BT: Pronase. *In* Tissue Culture Methods and Applications. Kruse PF Jr and Patterson MK Jr (eds), Academic Press Inc, New York, 1973, pp 185-188

31. FORMAN ML, INHORN SL, SHEAFF E, and CHERRY JD: Biological characteristics and viral spectrum of serially cultivated fetal rhesus monkey kidney cells. Proc Soc Exp Biol Med 131:1060-1067, 1969

32. GERBER P: Activation of Epstein-Barr virus by 5-bromodeoxyuridine in "virus-free" human cells. Proc Nat Acad Sci USA 69:83-85, 1972

33. GERNA G and CHAMBERS RW. Varicella-zoster plaque assay and plaque reduction neutralization test by the immunoperoxidase technique. J Clin Microbiol 4:437-442, 1976

34. GEY GO, COFFMAN WD, and KUBICEK MT: Tissue culture studies of proliferative capacity of cervical carcinoma and normal epithelium. Cancer Res 12:264-265, 1952

35. GIRARDI AJ: The use of fluorocarbon for "unmasking" polyoma virus hemagglutinin. Virology 9:488-489, 1959

36. GLASER R and RAPP F: Rescue of Epstein-Barr virus from somatic cell hybrids of Burkitt lymphoblastoid cells. J Virol 10:288-296, 1972

37. GOOD NE, WINGET GD, WINTER W, CONNOLLY TN, IZAWA S, and SINGH RMM: Hydrogen ion buffers for biological research. Biochemistry 5:467-477, 1966

38. GOODHEART CR, CASTRO BC, ZWIERS A, and REGNIER PR: Plating efficiency for primary hamster embryo cells as an index of efficacy of fetal bovine serum for cell culture. Appl Microbiol 26:525-528, 1973

39. HALLIBURTON G and BECKER ME: The use of HEPES buffer in microtissue culture plates for routine enterovirus diagnosis. Health Lab Sci 8:155–159, 1971

40. HAMPAR B, DERGE JG, MARTOS LM, and WALKER JL: Synthesis of Epstein-Barr virus after activation of the viral genome in a "virus-negative" human lymphoblastoid cell (Raji) made resistant to 5-bromodeoxyuridine. Proc Natl Acad Sci 69:78–82, 1972

41. HANKS JH and WALLACE RE: Relation of oxygen and temperature in the preservation of tissues by refrigeration. Proc Soc Exp Biol Med 71:196–200, 1949

42. HAYFLICK L: Tissue cultures and mycoplasmas. Texas Rep Biol Med Suppl 1, 23:285–303, 1965

43. HAYFLICK L: Fetal human diploid cells. In Tissue Culture Methods and Applications, Kruse PF Jr and Patterson MK Jr (eds), Academic Press Inc, New York, 1973, pp 43–45

44. HAYFLICK L: Subculturing human diploid fibroblast cultures. In Tissue Culture Methods and Applications, Kruse PF Jr and Patterson MK Jr (eds), Academic Press Inc, New York, 1973, pp 220–223

45. HAYFLICK L: Screening tissue cultures for mycoplasma infections. In Tissue Culture Methods and Applications, Kruse PF Jr and Patterson MK Jr (eds), Academic Press Inc, New York, 1973, pp 722–728

46. HEALY GM, MORGAN JF, and PARKER RC: Trace metal content of some natural and synthetic media. J Biol Chem 198:305–312, 1952

47. HOORN B and TYRRELL DAJ: Organ cultures in virology. Prog Med Virol 11:408–450, 1969

48. HOPPS HE, BERNHEIM BC, NISALAK A, TJIO JH, and SMADEL JE: Biologic characteristics of a continuous kidney cell line derived from the African green monkey. J Immunol 91:416–424, 1963

49. HOPPS HE, MEYER BC, BARILE MF, and DELGIUDICE RA: Problems concerning "non-cultivable" mycoplasma contaminants in tissue cultures. Ann NY Acad Sci 225:265–276, 1973

50. HORTA-BARBOSA L, FUCCILLO DA, LONDON WT, JABBOUR JT, ZEMAN W, and SEVER JL: Isolation of measles virus from brain cell cultures of two patients with subacute sclerosing panencephalitis. Proc Soc Exp Biol Med 132:272–277, 1969

51. HOTCHIN JE: Use of methyl cellulose gel as a substitute for agar in tissue culture overlays. Nature 175:352, 1955

52. HOUSE W and WADDELL A: Detection of mycoplasma in cell cultures. J Pathol Bacteriol 93:125–132, 1967

53. HSIUNG GD and MELNICK JL: Morphologic characteristics of plaques produced on monkey kidney monolayer cultures by enteric viruses (poliomyelitis, Coxsackie, and ECHO groups). J Immunol 78:128–136, 1957

54. HULL RN, CHERRY WR, and TRITCH OJ: Growth characteristics of monkey kidney cell strains LLC-MK₁, LLC-MK₂ and LLC-MK₂ (NCTC-3196) and their utility in virus research. J Exp Med 115:903–918, 1962

55. HULL RN, DWYER AC, CHERRY WR, and TRITCH OJ: Development and characteristics of the rabbit kidney cell strain, LLC-RK₁. Proc Soc Exp Biol Med 118:1054–1059, 1965

56. KENNY GE: Contamination of mammalian cells in culture by mycoplasmata. In Contamination in Tissue Culture, Fogh J (ed), Academic Press Inc, New York, 1973, pp 107–129

57. KENNY GE: Rapid detection of mycoplasmata and nonculturable agents in animal cell cultures by uracil incorporation. In Microbiology-1975, Schlessinger D (ed), Am Soc Microbiol, Washington, DC, 1975, pp 32–36

58. KISSLING RE: Growth of several arthropod-borne viruses in tissue culture. Proc Soc Exp Biol Med 96:290–294, 1957

59. KOPROWSKI H: Cell fusion and virus rescue. Fed Proc 30:914–920, 1971

60. LEERHØY J: Cytopathic effect of rubella virus in a rabbit-cornea cell line. Science 149:633–634, 1965

61. LEIBOVITZ A: The growth and maintenance of tissue-cell cultures in free gas exchange with the atmosphere. Am J Hyg 78:173–180, 1963

62. LEIGHTON J: Economic maintenance of continuous lines of human cells with bead-in-tube cultures. Lab Invest 7:513–514, 1958

63. LEVINE EM: Mycoplasma contamination of animal cell cultures: a simple, rapid detection method. Exp Cell Res 74:99–109, 1972

64. McALLISTER RM, J MELNYK, JZ FINKLESTEIN, EC ADAMS JR, and GARDNER MB: Cultivation in vitro of cells derived from a human rhabdomyosarcoma. Cancer 24:520–526, 1969
65. McGARRITY GJ: Control of microbiological contamination. Procedure 16183. Tissue Culture Association Manual 1:181–184, 1975
66. McGARRITY GJ: Spread and control of mycoplasmal infection of cell cultures. In Vitro 12:643–648, 1976
67. McGARRITY GJ and CORIELL LL: Procedures to reduce contamination of cell cultures. In Vitro 6:257–265, 1971
68. McLIMANS WF, DAVIS EV, GLOVER FL, and RAKE GW: The submerged culture of mammalian cells: the spinner culture. J Immunol 79:428–433, 1957
69. MACPHERSON I and STOKER M: Polyoma transformation of hamster cell clones—an investigation of genetic factors affecting cell competence. Virology 16:147–151, 1962
70. MELNICK JL: Problems associated with the use of live polio-virus vaccine. Am J Public Health 50:1013–1031, 1960
71. MERYMAN HT: Preservation of living cells. Fed Proc 22:81–89, 1963
72. MIRCHAMSY H and RAPP F: A new overlay for plaquing animal viruses. Proc Soc Exp Biol Med 129:13–17, 1968
73. MONTES DE OCA H and MALININ TI: Dispersion and cultivation of renal cells after short-term storage of kidneys. J Clin Microbiol 2:243–246, 1975
74. MONTES DE OCA H, PROBST P, and GRUBBS R: High-yield method for dispersing simian kidney for cell cultures. Appl Microbiol 21:90–94, 1971
75. MOORE GE, GERNER RE, and FRANKLIN HA: Culture of normal human leukocytes. J Am Med Assoc 199:519–524, 1967
76. MORGAN JF, MORTON HJ, and PARKER RC: Nutrition of animal cells in tissue culture. I. Initial studies on a synthetic medium. Proc Soc Exp Biol Med 73:1–8, 1950
77. MORTON HJ: A survey of commercially available tissue culture media. In Vitro 6:89–108, 1970
78. Mosley JW and Enders JF: A critique of the plaque assay technique in bottle cultures. Proc Soc Exp Biol Med 108:406–408, 1961
79. NASH DR, HALSTEAD SB, STENHOUSE AC, and McCUE C: Nonspecific factors in monkey tissues and serum causing inhibition of plaque formation and hemagglutination by dengue viruses. Infect Immun 3:193–199, 1971
80. NEFF JM and ENDERS JF: Poliovirus replication and cytopathogenicity in monolayer hamster cells fused with beta propiolactone-inactivated Sendai virus. Proc Soc Exp Biol Med 127:260–267, 1968
81. NELSON-REES WA and FLANDERMEYER RR: HeLa cultures defined. Science 191:96–98, 1976
82. NICHOLS WW, MURPHY DG, CRISTOFALO VJ, TOJI LH, GREENE AE, and DWIGHT SA: Characterization of a new human diploid cell strain, IMR-90. Science 196:60–63, 1977
83. NORRBY E: Hemagglutination by measles virus. A simple procedure for production of high potency antigen for hemagglutination-inhibition (HI) tests. Proc Soc Exp Biol Med 111:814–818, 1962
84. PARISIUS W, CUCAKOVICH NB, MACMORINE HG, VAN WEZEL AL, and VAN HEMERT PA: An improved method for the cell dispersion of tissue in trypsin-citrate solution. Procedure 46182. Tissue Culture Association Manual 2:345–348, 1976
85. PAYNE FE, BAUBLIS JV, and ITABASHI HH: Isolation of measles virus from cell cultures of brain from patients with subacute sclerosing panencephalitis. N Engl J Med 281:585–589, 1969
86. PHILLIPS HJ: Dissociation of single cells from lung or kidney tissue with elastase. In Vitro 8:101–105, 1972
87. PONTECORVO G: Production of mammlian somatic cell hybrids by means of polyethylene glycol treatment. Somatic Cell Genetics 1:397–400, 1975
88. PYE D: Procedures for evaluating growth-promoting qualities of cell culture reagents. Procedure No. 75192. Tissue Culture Association Manual 1:171–176, 1975
89. RAPPAPORT C: Trypsinization of monkey kidney tissue: An automatic method for the preparation of cell suspensions. Bull WHO 14:147–166, 1956
90. ROBBINS JH and JONES GA: Autoclave which sterilizes with highly purified steam for tissue-culture laboratories. Lancet 2:1236–1237, 1971

91. RUETER A and SCHLEICHER JB: Elimination of toxicity from polyvinyl trays after sterilization with ethylene oxide. Appl Microbiol 18:1057–1059, 1969

92. RUTZKY LP and PUMPER RW: Supplement to a survey of commercially available tissue culture media (1970). In Vitro 9:468–469, 1974

93. SCHAFER TW, PASCALE A, SHIMONASKI G and CAME PE: Evaluation of gentamicin for use in virology and tissue culture. Appl Microbiol 23:565–570, 1972

94. SCHELL K, HUEBNER RJ, and TURNER HC: Concentration of complement fixing viral antigens. Proc Soc Exp Biol Med 121:41–46, 1966

95. SCHMIDT NJ, FOX VL, and LENNETTE EH: Studies on the hemagglutination of Coe (Coxsackie A21) virus. J Immunol 89:672–683, 1962

96. SCHMIDT NJ, GUENTHER RW, and LENNETTE EH: Typing of ECHO virus isolates by immune serum pools. The "intersecting serum scheme." J Immunol 87:623–626, 1961

97. SCHMIDT NJ, HO HH, and LENNETTE EH: Propagation and isolation of group A coxsackieviruses in RD cells. J Clin Microbiol 2:183–185, 1975

98. SCHMIDT NJ and LENNETTE EH: Rubella complement-fixing antigens derived from the fluid and cellular phases of infected BHK-21 cells: extraction of cell-associated antigen with alkaline buffers. J Immunol 97:815–821, 1966

99. SCHMIDT NJ and LENNETTE EH: Antigenic variants of coxsackievirus type A24. Am J Epidemiol 91:99–109, 1970

100. SCHMIDT NJ and LENNETTE EH: Comparison of various methods for preparation of viral serological antigens from infected cell cultures. Appl Microbiol 21:217–226, 1971

101. SCHMIDT NJ, LENNETTE EH, GEE PS, and DENNIS J: Physical and immunologic properties of rubella antigens. J Immunol 100:851–857, 1968

102. SCHMIDT NJ, LENNETTE EH, and HANAHOE MF: A micro method for performing parainfluenza virus neutralization tests. Proc Soc Exp Biol Med 122:1062–1067, 1966

103. SCHMIDT NJ, LENNETTE EH, and HANAHOE MF: Microneutralization test for the reoviruses. Application to detection and assay of antibodies in sera of laboratory animals. Proc Soc Exp Biol Med 121:1268–1275, 1966

104. SCHMIDT NJ, LENNETTE EH, and MAGOFFIN RL: Immunological relationship between herpes simplex and varicella-zoster viruses demonstrated by complement-fixation, neutralization and fluorescent antibody tests. J Gen Virol 4:321–328, 1969

105. SCHMIDT NJ, LENNETTE EH, SHON CW, and SHINOMOTO TT: A complement-fixing antigen for varicella-zoster derived from infected cultures of human fetal diploid cells. Proc Soc Exp Biol Med 116:144–149, 1964

106. SCHMIDT NJ, MELNICK, JL WENNER HA, HO HH, and BURKHARDT MA: Evaluation of enterovirus immune horse serum pools for identification of virus field strains. Bull WHO 45:317–330, 1971

107. SCHNEIDER EL and STANBRIDGE EJ: Comparison of methods for the detection of mycoplasmal contamination of cell cultures: a review. In Vitro 11:20–34, 1975

108. SCHNEIDER EL, STANBRIDGE EJ, and EPSTEIN CJ: Incorporation of ^{3}H-uridine and ^{3}H-uracil into RNA; a simple technique for the detection of mycoplasma contamination of cultured cells. Exp Cell Res 84:311–318, 1974

109. SHANNON JE and MACY ML: Freezing, storage, and recovery of cell stocks. In Tissue Culture Methods and Applications. Kruse PF Jr and Patterson MK Jr (eds), Academic Press Inc, New York, pp 112–718, 1973

110. SHIPMAN C JR: Evaluation of 4-(2-Hydroxyethyl)-1-piperazine-ëthanesulfonic acid (HEPES) as a tissue culture buffer. Proc Soc Exp Biol Med 130:305–310, 1969

111. SHIPMAN C JR and SMITH DF: Automatic device for the trypsinization of animal tissues. Appl Microbiol 23:188–189, 1972

112. STAAL SP and ROWE WP: Differential effect of phenethyl alcohol on mycoplasmas and enveloped viruses. J Virol 14:1620–1622, 1974

113. STANBRIDGE E: Mycoplasmas and cell cultures. Bact Rev 35:206–227, 1971

114. STEWART GL, PARKMAN PD, HOPPS HE, DOUGLAS RD, HAMILTON JP, and MEYER HM, JR: Rubella-virus hemagglutination-inhibition test. N Engl J Med 276:554–557, 1967

115. STUDZINKSKI GP, GIERTHY JF, and CHOLON JJ: An autoradiographic screening test for mycoplasmal contamination of mammalian cell cultures. In Vitro 8:466–472, 1973

116. TER MEULEN V, KOPROWSKI H, IWASAKI Y, KÄCKELL YM, and MÜLLER D: Fusion of cultured multiple sclerosis brain cells with indicator cells: presence of nucleocapsids and virions and isolation of parainfluenza type virus. Lancet 2:1–5, 1972

117. TOOLAN HW: Transplantable human neoplasms maintained in cortisone-treated laboratory animals: H.S. No. 1; H.Ep. No. 1; H.Ep. No. 2; H.Ep. No. 3 and H.Emb.Rh. No. 1. Cancer Res 14:660-666, 1954

118. TYRRELL DAJ, BYNOE ML, HITCHCOCK G, PEREIRA HG, and ANDREWES CH: Some virus isolations from common colds. I. Experiments employing human volunteers. Lancet 1:235-237, 1960

119. VAN WEZEL AL: Microcarrier cultures of animal cells. *In* Tissue Culture Methods and Applications, Kruse PF Jr and Patterson MK Jr (eds), Academic Press Inc, New York, 1973, pp 372-377

120. WALLACE RE, VASINGTON PJ, PETRICCIANI JC, HOPPS HE, LORENZ DE, and KADANKA Z: Development of a diploid cell line from fetal rhesus monkey lung for virus vaccine production. In Vitro 8:323-332, 1973

121. WALLACE RE, VASINGTON PJ, PETRICCIANI JC, HOPPS HE, LORENZE DE, and KADANKA Z: Development and characterization of cell lines from subhuman primates. In Vitro 8:333-341, 1973.

122. WALLIS C and MELNICK JL: Mechanism of enhancement of virus plaques by cationic polymers. J Virol 2:267-274, 1968

123. WALLIS C, MORALES F, POWELL J, and MELNICK JL: Plaque enhacement of enteroviruses by magnesium chloride, cysteine, and pancreatin. J Bacteriol 91:1932-1935, 1966

124. WANG RJ: Effect of room fluorescent light on the deterioration of tissue culture medium. In Vitro 12:19-22, 1976

125. WECKER E: A simple test for serodifferentiation of poliovirus strains within the same type. Virology 10:376-379, 1960

126. WENTWORTH BB and FRENCH L: Plaque assay of *Herpesvirus hominis* on human embryonic fibroblasts. Proc Soc Exp Biol Med 131:588-592, 1969

127. WILLIAMSON JD and COX P: Use of a new buffer in the culture of animal cells. J Gen Virol 2:309-312, 1968

128. WYATT RD, KAPIKIAN AZ, THORNHILL TS, SERENO MM, KIM HW, and CHANOCK RM: In vitro cultivation in human fetal intestinal organ culture of a reovirus-like agent associated with nonbacterial gastroenteritis in infants and children. J Infect Dis 130:523-528, 1974

129. YASUMURA Y and KAWAKITA Y: Studies on SV_{40} in relationship with tissue culture. Nippon Rinsho 21:1201-1209, 1963

130. YOUNGNER JS: Monolayer tissue cultures. I. Preparation and standardization of suspensions of trypsin-dispersed monkey kidney cells. Proc Soc Exp Biol Med 85:202-205, 1954

131. ZGORNIAK-NOWOSIELSKA I, SEDWICK WD, HUMMELER K, and KOPROWSKI H: New assay procedure for separation of mycoplasmas from virus pools and tissue culture systems. J Virol 1:1227-1237, 1967

CHAPTER 4

IMMUNOFLUORESCENT STAINING

John L. Riggs

Introduction

Immunofluorescence procedures, more commonly referred to as the direct fluorescent-antibody (FA) procedure and the indirect fluorescent-antibody (IFA) procedure, provide a means whereby the site of an antigen-antibody reaction can be observed by microscopic examination. Specific antibody molecules are chemically linked to a fluorescent dye, such as fluorescein isothiocyanate (FITC) or tetramethyl rhodamine isothiocyanate (TMRITC). Such "labeled" antibodies retain their specificity for their respective antigens and, after a short reaction period, the reaction site can be visually detected using a fluorescence microscope. Such attributes as specificity and the short time required to stain and observe the specimen make immunofluorescence an ideal diagnostic tool for viral diseases.

In 1941 the technique was introduced by Coons et al (3), who employed the labile isocyanate derivative of fluorescein for conjugation of fluorescein to antibodies or antigens. The conjugation procedure was later modified by Riggs et al (20), who replaced the labile isocyanate radical with stable isothiocyanate, thus permitting a wider use of the procedure. Over 500 English-language references for immunofluorescence methods, most applying this modification to diagnostic virology, have appeared in the literature since that time. Some of the earliest examples of the use of immunofluorescence for diagnosis of viral diseases were influenza by Liu (13), rabies by Goldwasser and Kissling (7) and also by McQueen et al (16), measles by Cohen et al (2), herpes simplex by Biegeleisen et al (1), varicella-zoster by Weller and Coons (23), and poliomyelitis by Kalter et al (11). The list of viral diseases to which immunofluorescence procedures have been applied since that time has been expanded by others (4) and is very extensive, although examples of the routine use of FA for viral diagnosis remain surprisingly few.

In this chapter it is the intent to present a more general treatment of the application of immunoflurescence to viral diagnosis. For a more in-depth presentation, the reader is referred to the many excellent reviews of the subject matter, such as Gardner and Mcquillin (5), Nairn (17), Goldman (6), and Kawamura (12). Application of the technique to specific viral diseases is discussed when applicable in the appropriate chapters.

Methods

Fluorescence microscopes

Until recently most fluorescence microscopes were fitted with a high-intensity light source such as the Osram HBO 200 mercury burner filtered through a system of glass filters to provide the ultraviolet light (UV) which excites the fluorescent preparation under examination. Such filter systems consist of a heat-absorbing filter (e.g., Zeiss KG-1), excitation filters (Schott BG-12, UG-2, UG-5) of different thicknesses, and a barrier filter to exclude the UV irradiation from the observer's eyes. These filter combinations are used in conjunction with a cardioid dark-field condenser in a binocular microscope with 10X oculars. A monocular microscope provides a somewhat more intense field, but the ease and convenience of a binocular microscope more than offsets this advantage.

More recently interference filters have been utilized in fluorescence microscopy and have made possible the substitution of a less expensive and more convenient filament lamp for the mercury burner to excite fluorescence (21, 22). Interference filters have been developed to produce a transmission band of up to 85% in the 400–500 nm (blue) range, and a smaller band (1% transmission at approximately 630 nm [red]). The interference filters effectively excite the typical green fluorescence of fluorescein since the absorption peak of FITC is at approximately 495 nm. The smaller red band provides a contrasting red background which helps in interpreting morphologic detail when viewing a specimen in the fluorescence microscope, but it can, however, be reduced or eliminated by using a blue, red-excluding filter (BG-38) of the appropriate thickness as part of the barrier filter system.

A tungsten light source can be used with the interference filters; however, the substitution of the Osram 12-volt 100-watt halogen lamp provides a more intense light source.

A comparatively recent introduction in fluorescence microscopy is the use of incident light or epi-illumination (18). The illumination in this system is directed to the specimen from above, thus eliminating the need for a substage condenser. Light from a source is directed horizontally to a dichroic mirror set at an angle of 45° in the microscope tube. The interference mirror reflects light of selected wavelength for excitation down the microscope tube through the objective onto the surface of the specimen. The fluorescent emission of the specimen passes back through the objective to the dichroic mirror, which transmits light of this wavelength through to the barrier filter and finally to the eyepiece and observer.

The type of microscope, light source, and filter system chosen is, of course, dictated by its intended use, i.e., routine diagnostic procedures or research and the fluorochromes employed (fluorescein, rhodamine, etc.). A simple, workable system includes a binocular microscope fitted with a quartz-halogen light source, FITC interference filters with appropriate red-suppressing and barrier filters used in conjunction with a cardioid dark-field condenser. Such a system provides an adequate instrument at moderate cost that can handle almost any FA procedure.

Preparation of reagents

Immune serum production

When producing immune serum for use in immunofluorescence procedures, one must bear in mind that the nature of the reaction itself makes it a
very sensitive immunologic technique. Antigen-antibody reactions can be
visualized by FA that cannot be easily determined in any other manner.
Thus, antibodies inadvertently produced to minute quantities of contaminating components in the viral antigen preparation, such as host cell
antigens or growth medium components, may react with their antigen in the
test system, producing unwanted staining which masks the actual viral antigen-antibody reaction and makes interpretation very difficult or impossible.

In certain instances viral antigens can be produced in animal cells of the
same species as the animal to be immunized, thus avoiding the production of
antibodies to host cell components in the viral antiserum. Viral antigens produced in cells of a species heterologous to the animal intended for immunization must be purified in some manner to eliminate or reduce the production
of antibodies to unwanted components. Often differential centrifugation or,
preferably, density-gradient centrifugation suffices to reduce such contaminating components to an acceptable level.

Convalescent-phase serum from animals infected with a virus can also
be used to avoid unwanted anti-host-cell antibodies, since the antibody in
such animals is directed only against viral components.

Most common laboratory animals such as rabbits, mice, hamsters, guinea
pigs, monkeys, or goats can be used for immune serum production. Newly
obtained animals should be conditioned for a period of time to ensure that
they are disease free, and any animals showing signs of illness should be
discarded and not used for immune serum production. Young adult animals
should be used since older animals usually have had experience with a variety of antigens and already possess unwanted antibodies which interfere in
the FA procedure.

An immunization schedule should be designed to produce a high-titer,
specific antibody response with as few injections as possible. Prolonged
schedules tend to produce antibodies that cross-react with other viruses,
thus defeating the purpose of the specificity of the reaction.

The following schedule has been employed in our laboratories and has
consistently produced immune serum suitable for use in the FA technique in
most instances.

  1. A sample of serum is obtained from the larger animals (goats, monkeys, rabbits)
before immunization, to be used as control serum.
  2. The viral antigen (1.0 ml containing 10^6 pfu) is mixed with an equal volume of
complete Freund adjuvant, and one-half is inoculated into each hamstring muscle.
  3. At 7- to 10-day intervals after the first inoculation, the viral antigen without adjuvant is inoculated into each hamstring muscle for 3 additional times.
  4. Ten to 14 days following the final injection, the animal is test bled, and the antibody titer is determined by the appropriate procedure, i.e., neutralization, hemagglutination inhibition, indirect FA, etc.
  5. Animals showing a good response to the viral antigen are exsanguinated, and the
serum is recovered by centrifugation.

Animals which fail to respond to this regimen, upon further immunization usually begin production of unwanted antibodies to minor contaminating components in the antigen preparation. There are exceptions, however, depending upon the source and purity of the virus preparation used for immunization.

Details of the immunization schedule and choice of antigen may vary, but the basic principles remain the same: If possible, do not include any antigens in the immunizing material except homologous host tissue and the desired viral antigens; keep the number of inoculations to a minimum sufficient to produce a good antibody titer. Live viruses need be inactivated only when the virus is lethal for the animal species being immunized.

Conjugation with fluorescein isothiocyanate

Overlabeled antibodies, those possessing an excess number of fluorescein molecules over the number needed for visualization in the fluorescence microscope, have a tendency to combine nonspecifically with normal cellular components, thereby producing nonspecific staining. The fluorescein to protein (F/P) ratio has been used by many investigators as an indication of the amount of nonspecific staining one may obtain with a certain conjugate. The higher the F/P ratio, the more nonspecific staining is encountered and, conversely, the lower the F/P ratio, the less nonspecific staining is encountered. The F/P ratio can be controlled to some extent by adjusting the amount of dye used in the conjugation procedure followed by fractionation of the conjugate by DEAE chromotography.

Currently, many procedures are described in the literature for the production of usable conjugates, although there is no universally accepted conjugation procedure which produces conjugates of acceptable sensitivity and specificity for all immunofluorescence work.

The following conjugation procedure is used in our laboratory and has given consistently good results.

1. Two consecutive precipitations of the immune serum with 35–45% ammonium sulfate are performed by adding 70–90% saturated ammonium sulfate to the immune serum, which has been diluted with an equal volume of distilled water.

2. The precipitates are recovered by centrifugation, and the final precipitate is dissolved in 0.1 M phosphate-buffered saline (PBS), pH 7.2, in a volume smaller than that of the starting serum.

3. The crude globulin solution is dialyzed against PBS to remove the ammonium sulfate.

4. The protein content of the crude globulin solution is determined either by the Biuret procedure (9) or by the method of Lowry (14).

5. The globulin solution containing 0.5–1.5% protein is buffered by adding 10–15% by volume of 0.5 M carbonate-bicarbonate buffer, pH 9.

6. FITC at a ratio of 1 mg dye/100 mg protein is dissolved in 0.5 ml of acetone and added dropwise to the stirred buffered globulin solution. (Should the dye fail to dissolve in the acetone, it can be added as a slurry.)

7. The mixture is transferred to a cold room (4 C) and stirred slowly overnight with a magnetic stirrer.

DEAE fractionation

Antibodies which possess the correct F/P ratio and show little or no nonspecific staining can be separated from the underlabeled or overlabeled antibodies in a conjugate on a DEAE-cellulose column in the following way.

1. DEAE-cellulose obtained from a commercial source is prepared by first washing with a solution of 0.5 M NaOH. The DEAE-cellulose is recovered by vacuum filtration on a large Buckner funnel and is then thoroughly washed with copious amounts of distilled water. To ensure removal of the NaOH, the eluate is checked on a pH meter, and washing is continued until the pH of the washing is the same as that of the added distilled water.

2. The washed DEAE-cellulose is then equilibrated with 0.0175 M phosphate-buffer by washing, and washing is continued until the eluate has a pH of 6.3. The DEAE-cellulose can then be stored as a slurry in the pH 6.3 buffer at 4 C.

3. The conjugated globulin solution is dialyzed against 0.0175 M phosphate buffer, pH 6.3, at 4 C. A fine precipitate forms in the globulin solution under these conditions and is discarded.

4. A chromatography column is prepared from the washed, buffered DEAE-cellulose. (A 2-cm diameter column packed with cellulose to a height of 15 cm is sufficient for the globulins obtained from 20 ml of whole immune serum.)

5. The column is packed with the DEAE-cellulose and washed with the 0.0175 M buffer, pH 6.3, with 3–5 lb of air pressure being applied. The dialyzed conjugate is then applied to the column, with care being taken not to let the miniscus of the fluid fall below the surface of the DEAE-cellulose. Once the conjugate is on the DEAE-cellulose bed, the column is washed with 100 ml of the starting buffer. The eluate from this wash is discarded since it contains the unwanted, unlabeled, and underlabeled globulins.

6. The column is then eluted with 0.075 M NaCl in the 0.0175 M phosphate buffer, pH 6.3. As the elutant is applied, a colored fraction can be seen to move down the column. This fraction is retained since it contains the optimally labeled globulins. The eluate is collected in small fractions (3–5 ml), and as elution continues the intensity of the color of the fractions can be seen to decrease. The most highly colored fractions are combined (usually 1.5–2 times the volume of the starting conjugate solution).

7. The combined fractions are dialyzed against PBS, pH 7.2, and are ready for use in the immunofluorescence procedure.

Storage of conjugates

The finished conjugate is divided into 1- to 2-ml portions, suitably labeled, and either lyophilized or stored frozen at −20 C. Upon reconstitution or thawing, the conjugate is diluted appropriately, filtered through a 0.45 μm Millipore filter to remove any precipitate which may have formed, and stored at 4 C for use. Conjugates stored frozen in this manner have retained their titer as long as 8 years in our laboratory.

Titration and specificity of conjugates

Each conjugate must be thoroughly characterized for specificity, sensitivity, or titer, and amount of nonspecific staining before being used as a diagnostic reagent. When antiserum has been conjugated for use in the direct technique, the conjugate from the DEAE-cellulose column after dialysis is serially diluted in PBS, and the dilutions are applied to preparations of the homologous antigens (infected cell cultures, slip smears, or impression smears from known virus, positive tissues, etc.) and allowed to react in a humid atmosphere for 45–60 min at 37 C. The preparations are then washed in 3 changes of PBS, 5 min washing per change, are mounted in Elvanol mounting medium (10), and are examined in the fluorescence microscope. The staining titer of the conjugate is determined as the last dilution giving a 1+ or 2+ reaction; however, for use, the dilution 2- to 4-fold below the last dilution showing a 3+ or 4+ reaction is the working dilution of the conjugate (usually a 1:5 or 1:10 dilution of the conjugate obtained by DEAE-cellulose fractionation). Nonspecific staining is determined in the same manner by reacting the dilutions of the conjugate with uninfected cell cultures or tissue specimens. Cross-reacting staining is also determined using cell cultures or tissues infected with heterologous viral antigens. A conjugate showing excess nonspecific staining or cross-reaction with a heterologous virus, except where the cross-reaction is expected, cannot be used as a diagnostic reagent.

Anti-species conjugates prepared for use in the indirect procedure are characterized in the same manner using a chessboard titration of dilutions of the conjugate against dilutions of the intermediate serum consisting of viral immune serum of the appropriate species. Nonspecific staining and cross-reactions to heterologous viral antigens are determined as described above using uninfected cell cultures or tissues for nonspecific staining and cell cultures or tissues infected with heterologous viruses for cross-reactions. In addition, conjugates should also be tested by utilizing normal serum on virus-infected specimens from the same species of animal against which the antiglobulin conjugate was prepared.

Staining procedures

Direct procedure

The direct staining procedure is usually the method of choice when examining material for viral antigen. It is the simplest and most reliable of the various staining methods in that fewer nonspecific reactions occur, and the results of staining are therefore less subject to misinterpretation.

The appropriately prepared and diluted conjugate is applied directly to the material being examined (infected cell culture, tissue smear, etc.) and is allowed to react for a period of time (usually 30–45 min) in a humid atmosphere at 37 C. The conjugate is then removed, and the stained preparations are washed in 3 changes of PBS, 5 min per washing. After brief rinsing in distilled water, the preparations are air dried, are mounted in Elvanol mounting medium, and are then ready for examination. Although it is necessary to prepare and maintain conjugates for each virus, the greater specificity afforded by the direct technique overcomes this one drawback.

Indirect procedure

The indirect procedure can be used for detecting and identifying viral antigens. While the technique may be slightly more sensitive than the direct method, there also can be a greater problem with specificity. It is the only method, however, which can be used to detect antibodies in a serum and to determine complement-fixing antibodies in a serum by immunofluorescence.

The material to be examined is first overlayed with an appropriate dilution of immune serum and is allowed to react for a period of time (30–45 min) in a humid atmosphere at 37 C. Washing is then carried out in PBS, as in the direct procedure (3 changes of PBS, 5 min per washing). The material is then reacted with an optimal dilution of conjugate prepared from antiserum against the species of immunoglobulin in which the viral antiserum was prepared. The reaction is again maintained for 30–45 min in a humid atmosphere at 37 C, and in this manner the primary antibody-antigen complex is detected. The preparations are washed and mounted as before and are ready for examination.

Indirect procedure for antibody. The serologic response of an individual to a specific viral antigen can be determined by use of the indirect procedure. Commercial preparations of antiserum against the different classes of human immunoglobulins are available (anti-IgG, γ chain specific; anti-IgA, α chain specific; and anti-IgM, μ chain specific). The specificity of such preparations should be thoroughly checked by the investigator. Conjugates are prepared and fractionated as described before from these sera and are used in the indirect procedure to assess the response of an individual against almost any virus that can be grown in cell culture (rubella, cytomegalovirus, rabies, etc.).

Indirect procedure for complement-fixing antibody. The determination of complement-fixing antibody in a serum by immunofluorescence is a modification of the indirect procedure and was first described by Goldwasser and Shepard in 1958 (8). Reedman and Klein (19) later modified the procedure to detect complement-fixing antigens of the Epstein-Barr virus by adding the various components sequentially. In the original description of the technique, a dilution of heat-inactivated immune serum mixed with an optimal dilution of guinea pig complement (C) is allowed to react with the virus preparation. After washing, a conjugate of anti-guinea pig C is added, which will react with the antigen-antibody C complex. After washing and mounting, the preparation is ready for examination.

For certain viruses the reagents must be added sequentially in order for staining to be obtained by the anti-C technique.

The diluted immune serum is reacted with the virus preparation for 1 hr at 37 C or for 30 min at 37 C and then at 4 C overnight. After washing, the suitably diluted C is added and allowed to react for 45 min at 37 C. After further washing, the labeled anti-C is added and allowed to react for 45 min at 37 C; the preparation is again washed, mounted, and is ready for examination. Commercial preparations of anti-human C3 complement component or anti-guinea pig C3 complement component have been used successfully in this technique.

Fluorescent focus inhibition test for neutralizing antibody

Neutralizing antibody endpoint titers can be determined for almost any virus that can be grown in cell culture by detecting the breakthrough virus by the use of the direct FA procedure, rather than by cytopathic effect (CPE), animal death, or plaque formation. This type of test has the advantages of economy and ease of adaptations to large-scale routine use and is especially helpful in cases where the virus does not produce recognizable CPE or plaques. Microscope slides suitable for cell cultures can be obtained commercially (Lab-tek or "Printed Slides," Roboz Surgical Instrument Co., Washington, D.C.), although they are relatively expensive. A more economical cell culture can be prepared as follows:

1. Arrange slides (50–100) on a paper-covered work area with 2–3 14-mm diameter coverslips on each slide.
2. Frost the slides with Fluoroglide spray (Chemplast Co., Inc., Wayne, NJ).

3. Allow slides to dry; then remove the coverslips and save for repeated use.
4. Autoclave the slides (5 slides per 150-mm filter-paper-lined Petri dish).

The appropriate cell cultures for the virus are prepared on the slides in the following manner:

1. Trypsin dispersed cells in growth medium are applied to the unfrosted areas of the slides (0.1 ml of appropriately diluted cells).
2. The filter paper in the Petri dish is soaked with sterile distilled water to maintain humidity.
3. The slide cultures are incubated in a CO_2 incubator 37 C until confluent monolayers are formed.

For the test proper, the serum is first heat-inactivated (56 C, 30 min) and dilutions are made in the maintenance medium used for the cell culture (usually 1:4 to 1:128). The virus to be neutralized is diluted in the same maintenance medium to contain 100–300 fluorescent focus-forming units per 0.1 ml of the final serum-virus mixture. The virus and serum dilutions are combined in equal volumes and are incubated at 37 C for 1 hr. The medium is removed from the cell culture on the microscope slides prepared previously, and each serum-virus mixture is inoculated (0.1 ml) onto 2 micro-culture monolayers. The cultures are then incubated for a sufficient length of time to form foci of infected cells. The maintenance medium is then removed, and each slide is fixed in acetone, air dried, stained by the usual direct FA procedure, and examined with the fluorescence microscope.

The antibody titer can be expressed as the highest dilution which reduces the number of fluorescent foci by a certain amount ($\geq$ 80% reduction or complete reduction). In each test run, controls consisting of uninoculated cells, a virus titration series, antibody-positive serum, and antibody-negative serum are included.

Controls

Controls for the direct FA procedure, which are incorporated into each test, include homologous virus preparations or the "positive" control, and uninfected cell culture or tissue preparations as the "negative" control. Each conjugate, of course, is tested previously for its specificity, sensitivity, and nonspecific staining. In addition to the above, in the indirect procedure, either omission of the intermediate immune serum or substitution of a "normal" serum of the same species for the immune serum in the reaction serves as an additional control.

The complement staining procedure requires controls in addition to the positive and negative contols mentioned above. Omission of the intermediate immune serum or substitution of a "normal" serum is included, along with the omission of the complement-containing reagent or substitution of a heat-inactivated complement reagent.

Preparation of specimens—fixation

Virus isolates from cell cultures. Cell cultures which have been prepared for routine virus isolation procedures can also be used for identification by FA staining. Example of viruses that can be identified in this manner are herpes simplex, measles, rubella, varicella-zoster, and vaccinia viruses.

Cell culture tubes showing 2+ to 3+ CPE are removed from the glass surface by scraping and pipetting vigorously to produce single cells in suspension, or cells are removed by trypsin or trypsin-versene solutions. An equal number of normal, uninfected control cells are removed from the growth surface in the same manner and are combined with the virus-infected cells to provide a negative contrast and to act as a "built in" control in the stained preparation. In addition, uninfected cells are prepared separately to serve as an uninfected cell control. The cells are sedimented by centrifugation and are resuspended in a small amount (0.05–0.1 ml) of PBS containing 1–2% fetal bovine serum or 0.05% gelatin. The cell suspension is taken up in a Pasteur pipette equipped with a bulb, and while holding the pipette vertically, 2–3 small spot drops (3–5 mm in diameter) are deposited on a microscope slide. The drops are viewed microscopically under low power to assure an adequate cell suspension has been produced, and the spots are allowed to air dry at room temperature. Uninfected control cell spots are prepared in the same manner, and after drying the slides are fixed in acetone for 5 min at room temperature. After fixation the slides can be stored at −65 C until used in the staining procedure.

Tissues. Slip smears or impression smears of infected tissues from autopsies or biopsies or for identification of viral isolates in an animal host tissue such as mouse brain (rabies, herpes, arboviruses, etc.) are suitable for examination by the FA technique. When preservation of tissue architecture is desired, frozen sections of the tissues can be prepared and stained. Swabs can be used to collect specimens from nasal or conjunctival infections and smears made for direct identification. Swabs can also be used to collect material from vesicular lesions for making smears.

Fixation. A number of fixatives have been used successfully in FA procedures, including ethanol, methanol, carbon tetrachloride, formalin, paraformaldehyde, glutaraldehyde, glyoxal, and many others. The suitability of the fixative, of course, depends upon the antigen in question. Viral antigens are notoriously unstable and lose their antigenic characteristics when treated with many of the fixatives mentioned above. The one fixative that is universally acceptable for viral antigens is acetone at room temperature for from 5 to 10 min or in acetone at −20 C overnight. Often acetone will not inactivate all infectious viruses, however, and care must be taken to autoclave or otherwise decontaminate preparations before disposing of them after examination.

Clinical Aspects

Theoretically, the FA procedure can be used to identify any viral, rickettsial, or chlamydial agent for which specific immune serum can be prepared. It can also be used to detect and titrate antibodies to any such agents which can be propagated in a cell-culture system or animal host. In this respect antibody assay by the IFA procedure is especially helpful in viral diagnosis if used as a confirmatory procedure when the complement fixation or hemagglutination inhibition tests are equivocal. There are certain viral or rickettsial diseases of clinical or public health importance where the use of FA techniques to facilitate a more rapid diagnosis can be of substantial benefit because specific therapy is available. Examples of such diseases are: Rocky Mountain spotted fever, Q fever, trachoma (specific antibiotic therapy), herpes simplex (specific antiviral drug therapy), or rabies, Lassa fever (passive immunization).

Certain other viral diseases of public health importance can be better managed clinically if the diagnosis is confirmed early, even though no specific treatment is available (e.g., influenza, cytomegalovirus, respiratory syncytial virus). In addition, FA staining of nasal smears can give probably the earliest proof of influenza virus infections in a community. In this regard an intersecting serum scheme such as described by McLure et al (15) can be utilized and can differentiate and identify many of the common upper respiratory viral agents prevalent at any one time in a community.

In most cases the identification of a viral agent can be completed the same day its presence is recognized. For some viruses (rubella, measles, lymphocytic choriomeningitis) the CPE in cell culture may be obscure and difficult to recognize, and in such cases FA staining is the best method for recognition and identification. When incorporated as routine in the diagnostic laboratory, FA staining procedures can provide great savings in time, money, and resources.

References

1. BIEGELEISEN JZ JR, SCOTT LV, and LEWIS V JR: Rapid diagnosis of herpes simplex virus infections with fluorescent antibody. Science 129:640–641, 1959
2. COHEN SM, GORDON I, RAPP F, MACAULAY JC, and BUCKLEY SM: Fluorescent antibody and complement-fixation tests of agents isolated in tissue culture from measles patients. Proc Soc Exp Biol Med 90:118–122, 1955
3. COONS AH, CREECH HJ, and JONES RN: Immunological properties of an antibody containing a fluorescent group. Proc Soc Exp Biol Med 47:200–202, 1941
4. EMMONS RW and RIGGS JL: Application of immunofluorescence to diagnosis of viral infections. In Methods in Virology, Vol VI, Maramorosch K and Koprowski H (eds), Academic Press, NY, 1977
5. GARDNER PS and McQUILLIN J: Rapid Virus Diagnosis, Application of Immunofluorescence, Butterworth and Co, London, 1974
6. GOLDMAN M: Fluorescent Antibody Methods. Academic Press, Inc, New York, 1968
7. GOLDWASSER RA and KISSLING RE: Fluorescent antibody staining of street and fixed rabies virus antigens in mouse brains. Proc Soc Exp Biol Med 98:219– 223, 1958
8. GOLDWASSER RA and SHEPARD CC: Staining of complement and modifications of fluorescent antibody procedures. J Immunol 80:122–131, 1958
9. GORNALL AG, BARDAWILL CJ, and DAVID MM: Determination of serum proteins by means of the Biuret reaction. J Biol Chem 177:751–766, 1949
10. HEIMER GV and TAYLOR CED: Improved mountant for immunofluorescence preparations. J Clin Pathol 27:254–256, 1974
11. KALTER SS, HATCH MH, and AJELLO GW: The laboratory diagnosis of poliomyelitis with fluorescent antibodies. Bacteriol Proc 89–90, 1959
12. KAWAMURA A JR (ED): Fluorescent Antibody Techniques and Their Applications, 2nd edition, University Park Press, Baltimore, 1977
13. LIU C: Rapid diagnosis of human influenza infection from nasal smears by means of fluorescein-labeled antibody. Proc Soc Exp Biol Med 92:883–887, 1956
14. LOWRY OH, ROSEBROUGH NJ, FARR AL, and RANDALL RJ: Protein measurement with the Folin phenol reagent. J Biol Chem 193:265–275, 1951

15. McLure AR, MacFarlane DE, and Sommerville RG: An intersecting anti-serum pool system for the immunofluorescent identification of respiratory viruses. Arch Gesamte Virusforsch 37:6–11, 1970

16. McQueen JL, Lewis AL, and Schneider NJ: Rabies diagnosis by fluorescent antibody. I. Its evaluation in a public health laboratory. J Public Health 50:1743–1752, 1960

17. Nairn RC: Fluorescent Protein Tracing, 4th edition, Williams and Wilkins Co., Baltimore, 1976

18. Ploem JS: The use of a vertical illuminator with interchangeable dichroic mirrors for fluorescence microscopy with incident light. Z Wiss Mikrosk 68:129–142, 1967

19. Reedman BM and Klein G: Cellular localization of an Epstein-Barr virus (EBV)-associated complement-fixing antigen in producer and nonproducer lymphoblastoid cell lines. Int J Cancer 11:499–520, 1973

20. Riggs JL, Seiwald RJ, Burckhalter JH, Downs CM, and Metcalf TG: Isothiocyanate compounds as fluorescent labeling agents for immune serum. Am J Pathol 34: 1081–1097, 1958

21. Rygaard J and Olsen W: Interference filters for improved immunofluorescence microscopy. Acta Pathol Microbiol Scand 76:146–149, 1969

22. Rygaard J and Olsen W: Determination of characteristics of interference filters. Ann NY Acad Sci 177:430–433, 1971

23. Weller TH and Coons AH: Fluorescent antibody studies with agents of varicella and herpes zoster propagated in vitro. Proc Soc Exp Biol Med 86:789–794, 1954

CHAPTER 5

IMMUNOENZYMATIC METHODS

Denis R. Benjamin

Theory of Methods

The development of immunoenzymatic methodology was a logical extension of the already successful antibody-labeling techniques with agents such as fluorescein and ferritin (5, 47). The role of these methods, both in diagnostic and investigative virology, has burgeoned recently. The replacement of fluorescein with an enzyme marker proved to have a number of distinct advantages, and its flexibility has broadened the applicability and use of enzyme-labeled antibodies.

The underlying principles of the immunoenzymatic procedures are very similar to those of immunofluorescence. An enzyme is chemically or immunologically linked to an antibody. This reagent is used to detect the antigen-antibody reaction as the presence of the enzyme-labeled antibody is revealed by incubation with the enzyme's specific chromogenic substrate.

The advantages of selecting enzyme labels over fluorescent dyes include:

1. The enzyme-substrate reaction is detected with a light microscope or even macroscopically, avoiding the problems of ultraviolet dark-field microscopy.

2. Many of the products of the enzyme-substrate reaction are electron dense, making electron microscopy possible. Peroxidase itself is electron dense.

3. Most preparations are permanent, allowing retrieval and review of old preparations, whereas fluorescent dyes rapidly fade.

4. The catalytic activity of the enzyme and the number of enzyme molecules attached to the antibody act as an amplification system. By prolonging the substrate incubation the sensitivity can be enhanced.

5. Endogenous enzyme activity (e.g., peroxidase activity in granulocytes) can be easily blocked without altering antigenic specificity. Autofluorescence of tissues and cells has proved a difficult problem to solve in many fluorescent-antibody (FA) procedures.

6. Reagents, especially the enzyme-antibody conjugates, are more readily standardized and more stable than most fluorescent conjugates.

153

7. There are reportedly fewer nonspecific reactions than with FA methods. This may be due to the fact that the conjugates are not charged and have less tendency to aggregate (31).

8. With certain procedures (e.g., the soluble peroxidase-antiperoxidase method) there is no chemical alteration of the antibody.

9. A number of immunoenzymatic procedures have performed more successfully on routinely processed tissue (e.g., paraffin embedding) than have FA methods.

For routine diagnostic virology, immunoenzymatic methods are of value in 4 major areas.

1. Direct detection of viral antigen in clinical samples (e.g., biopsy, cell scrapings, secretions)

2. Detection and identification of viral antigen in tissue culture

3. Rapid typing of viruses in tissue culture

4. Serology

The ideal application for this rapid diagnostic procedure is for the direct detection of viral antigen in patient material. This has been successfully accomplished in herpes simplex infection (10). Early detection, identification, and typing of tissue and culture isolates reduces the usual lag time in diagnosis and obviates the need for large amounts of tissue culture as well as the problems and expense of neutralization procedures. Immunoenzymatic methods offer considerable advantages for serologic measurements, including more accurate quantitation of antibody levels.

This chapter emphasizes the general technical characteristics of the various methods. The application of the methods for specific viruses and specific situations is only highlighted. More detailed descriptions can be found in the referenced literature. Recently, comprehensive reviews of the immunoenzymatic procedures have been published (3, 38, 49, 66, 72, 73).

Direct method

As in direct FA methods, an antibody is conjugated with a marker (enzyme) and then incubated directly with the appropriate preparation containing suspected antigen. Following a wash to remove unreacted antibody, the preparation is incubated with the enzyme's substrate in order to visualize the sites of antigen-antibody binding. This method is seldom employed as it lacks sensitivity and versatility; for each antigen, the specific antibody requires enzyme conjugation.

Indirect method and enzyme-linked immunosorbent assay (ELISA)

The indirect method is far more versatile and considerably more sensitive than the direct method. It can be employed for both antigen identification and antibody measurement. A suitable antigen preparation (e.g., infected tissue culture, cell scraping, frozen section of tissue) is incubated with specific antibody. After washing to rid the preparation of any unreacted antibody, the preparation is incubated with an enzyme-labeled-antigamma globulin antibody directed against the species in which the specific antibody was raised (i.e., if the initial antibody was raised in rabbits an antirabbit gamma globulin is used). This second antibody may be specifically selected to detect IgG, IgM, or IgA classes. Following the period of incubation and washing, the preparation is reacted with the enzyme's substrate, mounted routinely, and viewed with the light microscope. The procedure is diagrammatically represented in Figure 5.1.

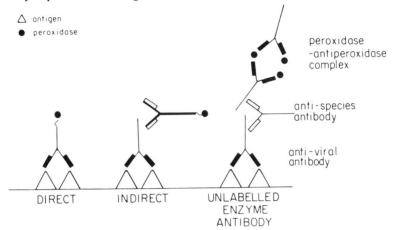

Figure 5.1—Diagrammatic representation of the direct, indirect and unlabelled enzyme antibody methods.

The ELISA is similar to the indirect immunoenzymatic procedure, but it is rendered more quantitative by absorbing the antigen (or antibody) to a solid phase (e.g., base of microtiter plate wells, agarose beads) and measuring the amount of enzyme-labeled antibody reacting with it. Once again 2 basic criteria are required to be fulfilled for the development of a satisfactory assay: 1) The antigen or antibody must be attached, usually adsorbed, onto a solid-phase support without altering immunologic activity. 2) The antibody-enzyme complex must retain both immunologic and enzymatic activity.

While the ELISA assay has been used for antigen detection and measurement, usually with a double antibody sandwich method, its major utility is for antibody quantitation. In this latter case, antigen is absorbed onto the polystyrene of microtiter wells or coupled to agarose beads, incubated with varying dilutions of serum, washed, and reincubated with enzyme-labeled gamma globulin, rinsed once again, and then reacted with the enzyme substrate. The enzyme activity is then measured spectrophotometrically. The ELISA assay is essentially similar to and has the same sensitivity as solid-phase radioimmunoassays, capable of measuring nanogram quantities of protein.

Unlabeled enzyme antibody method (soluble peroxidase-antiperoxidase, PAP)

The attractive advantages of the unlabeled enzyme antibody method are its extreme sensitivity and the fact that all reactions are immunologic (46, 58). Antibody is not altered by chemical reaction. Its drawbacks are its relative complexity and greater number of controls that are required for satisfactory interpretation.

The basic reagent is a soluble complex of the peroxidase enzyme and its antibody, usually made in rabbits or goats. This reagent is used to detect the presence of the initial antigen-antibody reaction via an intermediate or bridging antibody (either antirabbit or antigoat gamma globulin). The steps are outlined in Figure 5.1.

This second (bridging) antiserum is added in sufficient excess so that many molecules are bound to the first specific antiserum by only a single site in the Fab portion, allowing the second site to react with the PAP complex.

The initial antiviral antibody can frequently be used in a very high dilution (e.g., 1:100–1:5000) because of the sensitivity of the assay. More concentrated solutions have been demonstrated to produce false-negative reactions due to a prozone phenomenon (11). High dilutions also reduce the incidence of nonspecific staining.

An added attraction to the PAP method for electron microscopy is the ease with which the peroxidase-antiperoxidase complexes can be identified, either by their unique shape (45) or the presence of Fresnel fringes (23).

Technical Procedures

Preparation and purification of antiserum

The production of specific viral antisera is identical to that for all immunochemical methods. Presumably any specific high-titer antiserum works satisfactorily in the immunoenzymatic procedures. For laboratories that do not have the facilities or expertise to produce their own viral antiserum, commercial preparations are available that have proved very satisfactory for most uses (see Appendix). At present there is considerable variation from one lot of commercially prepared antiserum to the next, not only in terms of titer, but also in the extent of cross-reactivity and nonspecificity. Each lot of antiserum must be tested with its appropriate antigen and control preparations (see below) before it can be satisfactorily used for diagnostic purposes.

A well-prepared antiserum, made by injection of purified antigen, can be used without additional purification, but may require further handling to improve its specificity. The most frequent and convenient procedure is to absorb the antiserum with tissue powder such as rabbit or bovine liver powder. This largely empirical procedure often removes the majority of the nonspecificity of the antiserum. One simple absorption procedure is to place approximately 0.5 g of tissue powder (e.g., rabbit liver) in a conical centrifuge tube, add 2 ml of a 1:20 dilution of antiserum, mix thoroughly, and incubate at 37 C for 1 hr. Centrifuge the mixture at 800 × g for 20 min to sediment the tissue powder, and carefully pipette off the supernatant. It is usually unnecessary to use higher centrifugal forces in order to remove immune complexes. Absorption may have to be repeated a number of times before a satisfactory reagent is produced. Other absorption substrates include uninfected tissue culture from which the antigen had been made or tissue culture infected with a heterologous virus. This latter procedure should remove cross-reacting antibody.

For reasons that are not entirely understood, some antisera, although of high titer and specific as demonstrated in other immunologic assays, do not prove to be suitable in the immunoperoxidase (IP) method. This may relate to the nature of the antigen or the antigen-antibody reaction. While many viruses are easily identified, certain viruses such as the group B coxsackieviruses have defied most attempts.

The appropriate antibody dilution should be chosen after performing the assay using serial dilutions of antibody on both infected and noninfected cells. Select the greatest dilution that gives the most positive result with the infected cells and no reaction with the uninfected cells. In the example below, the 1:80 dilution should be chosen.

	Antiserum Dilution				
	1:10	1:20	1:40	1:80	1:160
Infected cells	4+	4+	4+	4+	2+
Noninfected cells	2+	1+	–	–	–

The great sensitivity of the unlabeled antibody enzyme method often necessitates high dilutions of the primary antiserum. At low dilutions a type of prozone phenomenon can cause false-negative results (11).

Once an antiserum has been found satisfactory and an optimal dilution established, it should be divided into appropriate working volumes that can be frozen. Once thawed for use it is best to discard any unused portion.

Nonspecific staining can arise in a number of ways. There may be nonimmune binding of the antiserum with the tissue or cellular substrates. This can be detected in control preparations using normal (i.e., nonimmune) serum or antiserum to unrelated antigens. A preimmunization serum from the same animal in which the antibody was prepared is the best normal control serum but is not always available. This type of nonimmune binding can usually be eliminated by diluting the antiserum as illustrated above. Another useful method is to preincubate the preparation with a normal serum protein solution. The species selected should be the same as that used to make the second antibody. If, for example, a goat anti-rabbit IgG-peroxidase is used as the second antibody in the indirect IP method, the preparation should be preincubated with a 1:10–1:20 dilution of normal goat serum. If the bridging antibody in the PAP method is a swine anti-rabbit IgG, then normal swine serum should be used.

The second frequent cause of nonspecific staining is the presence of other antibody activities in the primary antiserum in addition to its major specificity. These "contaminating" antibodies are often directed against cell components since many of the antigen preparations used to inoculate animals contain cell fragments. The presence of these antibodies cannot always be excluded by standard immunoelectrophoretic study as this procedure is less sensitive and may fail to detect antibodies which are too "weak" to result in precipitin reactions. These contaminating antibodies can form a major component of some antisera and can lead to confusing results or even a frank misdiagnosis. This was highlighted in a report of a case of encephalitis in which a brain biopsy was performed for immunodiagnosis (51). A herpes simplex antiserum was used in an indirect FA procedure, demonstrating many "positive" cells. At autopsy, tuberculous meningoencephalitis was discovered. The so-called "herpes simplex" antiserum had been made by injecting herpes-infected tissue culture and Freund complete adjuvant, the latter containing *Mycobacterium*. This sanguine lesson must always be kept in mind when working with "specific" antiserum.

Another technique, reportedly useful for reducing the amount of background staining on formalin-fixed, paraffin-embedded tissue, is to digest the tissue with pepsin. This method has been used with the PAP method, dramatically decreasing the nonspecific background staining of the connective tissue (52). The effect of pepsin digestion on various viral antigens and the ability to subsequently detect them with the IP method are variable and unpredictable and should be determined by empirical observation.

Choice of enzyme

A number of enzymes have been used successfully as markers. The ideal enzyme should be available in pure form, be simple to conjugate to an antibody without losing activity, be stable, and have a high specific activity. When used to detect antigens in cells or tissues it should have a relatively low molecular weight and be easily identifiable histochemically. When used for quantitative antibody measurement as in the ELISA method, it is more convenient to select an enzyme that can be readily measured spectrophotometrically either in a kinetic or endpoint assay. Horse-radish peroxidase (mol wt 40,000) satisfies most of the requirements for a histochemically identifiable enzyme. It is by far the most widely employed agent. A number of substrates can be used to detect its presence, a few of which yield electron-dense products ideal for electron microscopy. Conjugated to an antibody it is stable for many months and has high specific activity.

Alkaline phosphatase (mol wt 100,000) and glucose oxidase (mol wt 150,000) have been used for both histochemical identification and the ELISA assay, although they are far better suited to the latter.

Enzyme-antibody conjugation

The enzyme labeling of antiserum can be performed in most laboratories with little problem. Commercially prepared conjugates have recently become available which are entirely satisfactory for most uses (Appendix).

Three methods are commonly used, all producing similar conjugates. The 2-stage technique of Avrameas and Ternynck (4) using glutaraldehyde as the bifunctional reagent is said to result in smaller conjugates having an enhanced ability to penetrate cells, while the procedure of Nakane and Kawaoi (48) reportedly results in increased labeling efficiency. However, these conjugates tend to have a higher molecular weight. This procedure produces a Schiff base that is stabilized by borohydride reduction. We have relied on the 2-stage procedure with glutaraldehyde obtaining reproducibly satisfactory results. A number of studies have compared the various methods and characterized the conjugates (12, 13).

Two-stage procedure with glutaraldehyde (after Avrameas and Ternynck, 4)

    1. Dissolve 10 mg of horseradish peroxidase (Type IV, RZ~3.0) in 0.2 ml of 0.1 M phosphate buffer, pH 6.8, containing 1.25% glutaraldehyde.
    2. Allow to stand overnight (12-18 hr) at room temperature.
    3. Chromatograph on a Sephadex G-25 column (60 × 0.9 cm) equilibrated with 0.15 M sodium chloride.
    4. Collect the brown fractions (activated peroxidase).
    5. To this solution add 1 ml of 0.15 M sodium chloride containing 5 mg of IgG antispecies antibody.
    6. Add 0.1 ml of 1 M carbonate-bicarbonate buffer, pH 9.5.
    7. Incubate at 4 C for 24 hr.
    8. Add 0.1 of 0.2 M lysine and allow to stand for 2 hr.
    9. Dialyze at 4 C against 3 × 1 liter of phosphate-buffered saline (PBS).
    10. Precipitate conjugate with an equal volume of saturated ammonium sulphate.
    11. Wash precipitate twice with half-saturated ammonium sulphate.
    12. Dissolve final precipitate in a minimal volume of distilled water.
    13. Dialyze for 48 hr at 4 C against 6 × 1 liters PBS.

One-stage glutaraldehyde method (after Avrameas, 2)

    1. To 1 ml of 0.1 M phosphate buffer, pH 6.8, containing 5 mg of protein (antibody), add 12 mg of horseradish peroxidase (Type IV RZ~3.0).
    2. Add 0.05 ml of 1% aqueous glutaraldehyde dropwise while stirring.
    3. Allow to stand at room temperature for 2 hr.
    4. Dialyze at 4 C against 3 × 1 liters of PBS for 12-24 hr.
    5. Remove any precipitate by centrifugation at 20,000 rpm for 30 min at 4 C.

Schiff base method (after Nakane and Kawaoi, 48)

    1. Dissolve 5 mg of horseradish peroxidase (Type IV RZ~3.0) in 1 ml of freshly made 0.3 M sodium bicarbonate, pH 8.1.
    2. Add 0.1 of freshly made 1% 2, 4, dinitro-fluorobenzene in absolute ethanol.
    3. Mix gently for 1 hr at room temperature.
    4. Add 1 ml of 0.04-0.08 M NaIO$_4$ in distilled water. Mix gently for 30 min at room temperature. Solution should appear yellow-green.
    5. Add 1.0 ml of 0.16 M ethylene glycol in distilled water. Mix gently for 1 hr at room temperature.
    6. Dialyze the solution overnight against at least 3 × 1 liter of 0.01 M sodium carbonate buffer, pH 9.5, at 4 C.
    7. Add 5 mg of antispecies IgG to 3 ml of the above peroxidase-aldehyde solution, and mix gently for 2-3 hr at room temperature.
    8. Add 5 mg sodium borohydride. Leave at 4 C for 3-12 hr.
    9. Dialyze against PBS at 4 C for 48 hr.
    10. Freeze conjugate at −20 C in convenient working volumes.

Enzyme detection

Horseradish peroxidase

    Horseradish peroxidase can be detected with a variety of substrates which become oxidized, usually to an insoluble polymer, when the peroxidase catalyzes the release of oxygen from hydrogen peroxide. Commonly used substrates include benzidine (blue reaction product) 3-3'diaminobenzidine (brown), o-dianisidine (brown), α-naphthol (red). Unfortunately, most of these are potentially carcinogenic so that the use of benzidine and napthol must conform to federal safety regulations (16). An alternative reagent which produces red-brown granules at the site of peroxidase activity is 3-amino-9-ethylcarbazole (AEC). The following 3 methods are commonly employed.

AEC method (modified from Kaplow, 36)

1. Dissolve 2 mg of 3-amino-9-ethylcarbazole in 0.5 ml of diethylformamide (made fresh each time).
2. Add 9.5 ml of acetate buffer (pH 5).
3. Add 1 drop of 3% hydrogen peroxide immediately prior to use.
    Acetate buffer
    Solution A–0.68 g sodium acetate in 100 ml H₂0
    Solution B–0.3 ml acetic acid in 100 ml H_2O
    Add 70 ml Sol A to 30 ml Sol B to make 100 ml of buffer.
4. Incubate at room temperature for 10–20 min.
5. Rinse with water and mount in glycerol.

Benzidine (Kaplow, 35)

To make Kaplow medium

1. Dissolve 0.3 g benzidine dihydrochloride in 100 ml of 30% ethyl alcohol.
2. Add 1 ml of 0.132 M zinc sulphate, 1 g of sodium acetate, 0.7 ml of 3% hydrogen peroxide, and 1.5 ml of 1.0 N sodium hydroxide.
3. Dissolve 0.2 g of safranin O in the above to act as a counterstain.
4. Filter solution and adjust pH to 6.1 with 1 N hydrochloric acid. *This stock solution is stable for approximately 3 months*
5. Place 1 drop of the solution into each well for 30–60 sec.
6. Rinse with water.
7. Dehydrate through graded alcohols to xylene.
8. Mount coverslip with a permanent mounting medium (e.g., Permount).

3-3'-diaminobenzidine (Graham and Karnowsky, 29)

1. Dissolve 5 mg of 3-3'-diaminobenzidine tetrahydrochloride in 10 ml of 0.05 M Tris buffer, pH 7.6.
2. Add 0.1 ml of 1% H_2O_2.
3. Incubate for 15–30 min.
4. Wash briefly in water.
5. (May poststain in 2% OsO_4 for 5 min to stabilize reaction product.)
6. Dehydrate through graded alcohols to xylene.
7. Mount coverslip with a permanent mounting medium.

Preparation of samples for examination

For most purposes standard glass microscope slides are used. It is usually convenient to place a number of specimens on each slide, as some will serve as controls, or may receive varying dilutions of antiserum. Commercial slides are available that contain shallow wells of varying size and number allowing the performance of multiple assays on a single slide without reagents spilling from a well to an adjacent one. *Slides can be prepared in the following manner:*

1. Clean slide with 100% alcohol.
2. Place small drops of glycerol on slide with syringe or Pasteur pipette, in the desired configuration, e.g., 2 rows of 8 (up to 40 small wells can be made on a standard slide).
3. Spray with a fluorocarbon (Fluoroglide-film bonding grade, Chemplast Inc).
4. Allow to dry and then rinse off glycerol under running tap water.

The specimen preparation depends largely on the purpose of the assay. For the direct detection of viral antigen in clinical samples, the sample such as vesicular fluid, nasopharyngeal swab, or tissue imprint is placed directly onto the wells and allowed to air dry. With vesicular lesions, e.g., herpes simplex, it is important to scrape the base of the lesion in order to detach infected cells, as the vesicular fluid alone seldom contains adequate numbers of cells.

Tissue culture may be scraped off the side of roller tubes and centrifuged at $800 \times g$ for 10 min; the medium is removed and the cell button suspended in 0.1–0.2 ml of PBS. Drops of this cell suspension are placed in the wells and allowed to air dry. This method produces considerable artifact due to cell fragments but is our standard procedure for routine identification and serology. Better morphologic detail is obtained if the cell culture is grown on coverslips and the entire procedure performed on each coverslip (these may be gently broken into a number of fragments to serve as controls). Commercial slides are also available in which monolayers can be cultured for subsequent IP assays.

Frozen section is the standard procedure for identifying viral antigen in tissue fragments. However, a variety of antigens have been detected with the PAP method following routine formalin fixation and paraffin embedding.

Tissue fixation is of considerable importance in determining the success of the assay. All common fixatives alter the viral antigens in various ways, but results cannot be predicted. For most purposes, cold acetone (4 C for 10–20 min) has proved satisfactory. There is some concern that short fixation may not kill viruses, especially nonlipid-containing viruses such as adenovirus and coxsackievirus (6).

Other fixatives such as formalin, alcohol, and gluteraldehyde do appear to decrease the staining of many human pathogenic viruses. However, sufficient antigenic determinants can remain so that they can be identified with the more sensitive techniques such as PAP and electron microscopy, especially following relatively brief periods of fixation. Because of current lack of information concerning the effect of fixatives on viral antigens, a trial of various fixatives may have to be performed before the optimal fixative is selected.

Procedures to eliminate endogenous peroxidase

Endogenous peroxidase does not usually pose any problem in tissue culture preparations but may be troublesome in certain clinical samples, especially those specimens from an acute inflammatory reaction, as neutrophils and eosinophils are particularly rich sources of the enzyme. A number of procedures have been described which eliminate this endogenous peroxidase or the pseudo-peroxidase activity of cells such as erythrocytes.

For tissue sections, it has recently been reported (32) that treatment with 0.1 M periodic acid for 5 min followed by 2 min with 0.02% fresh sodium borohydride is very successful in obliterating all endogenous peroxidase activity. It is important that these concentrations and incubation times be observed, as longer periods will lift the sections off the slides. Egg albumin must be used on the slides in order to maintain adequate adherence of the sections to the glass.

A technique that has worked successfully on many clinical samples is the use of an acid-alcohol solution. A 15-min incubation of the slides in 0.074% hydrochloric acid in ethanol (0.2 ml concentrated hydrochloric acid in 100 ml of absolute ethyl alcohol) usually abolishes all endogenous peroxidase activity without significantly reducing the staining reaction of many antigens (70).

Methanol partially inhibits the activity of peroxidase and has been combined with a number of other reagents to eliminate endogenous peroxidase. Straus (59) reported the use of 1% sodium nitroferricyanide and 1% acetic acid in methanol for 15 min, while Streefkerk (60) recommends pretreatment with methanol followed by hydrogen peroxide in PBS (0.006% to 0.0125%).

The success of any of these methods is also dependent on the type of tissue or sample used, the initial fixation of and the substrate used to detect peroxidase activity. Their effect on antigenic activity cannot be predicted, so that a trial of a number of these may have to be performed before selecting the one that eliminates all endogenous peroxidase while maintaining optimal staining of the viral antigen.

Methods of procedure

Direct method

1. Prepare sample as described under Preparation of Samples for Examination.
2. Incubate with suitable dilution of peroxidase-labeled antiserum for 30–60 min at 37 C in humidified chamber.
3. Rinse with PBS for 15 min.
4. Stain.

Controls for the direct method should include:

1. Uninfected cells—must be negative (test for nonspecificity).

2. Blocking (inhibition test)—unlabeled antibody, applied for 30–60 min prior to the start of the assay, should markedly diminish or abolish the staining reaction (test for specificity). The unconjugated antiserum used for blocking should not be from the same source as the labeled antibody in order to confirm the specificity of the viral antigen-antibody reaction.

3. Heterologous conjugate should not produce any staining (test for cross-reactivity).

4. Direct incubation of infected cells with enzyme substrate should not produce any reaction (test for endogenous enzyme).

Indirect immunoperoxidase procedure

1. Prepare and fix sample.
2. Optional—block endogenous peroxidase, if appropriate.
3. Optional—incubate with 1:20 dilution of normal swine, normal goat, or normal horse serum) for 15-30 min. Rinse in PBS for 15 min.
4. Incubate with drop of suitably diluted antiserum for 30-60 min in humidified chamber at 37 C.
5. Rinse briefly in running tap water.
6. Rinse in PBS bath for 15 min.
7. Incubate with drop of peroxidase-labeled antispecies antibody (1:50 to 1:100 dilution) for 30-60 min in humidified chamber.
8. Rinse briefly in running tap water.
9. Rinse in PBS bath for 15 min.
10. Blot dry.
11. Stain and mount.

NOTE: Peroxidase-labeled antibody is stable at 4 C or -20 C for prolonged periods if undiluted. Once it is diluted to 1:50 or 1:100, any remaining should be discarded or used within 1 week.

The following controls should be performed:

1. Uninfected cells (must be negative—test for nonspecificity).

2. Heterologous unlabeled serum, nonimmune serum, or PBS should not produce any staining when used in place of the specific antiserum (i.e., in place of the first antibody or step 4 above).

3. Absorption of the specific antiserum with its homologous antigen should decrease or abolish the staining reaction.

4. The peroxidase-labeled antiglobulin conjugate alone should not produce staining of either infected or uninfected cells.

5. The enzyme substrate alone should not produce any reaction (test for endogenous peroxidase).

Soluble peroxidase antiperoxidase method

1. Prepare tissue sample as described above (note—some antigens "survive" formalin fixation and paraffin embedding).
2. Incubate with 1:20 dilution of normal swine serum for 30 min.
3. Wash in PBS for 15 min.
4. Incubate with primary antiviral antibody (made in rabbit) for 30-60 min (note—appropriate dilution must be found by trial but is generally very high, e.g., 1:100-1:5000).
5. Rinse in PBS for 15 min.
6. Incubate in 1:20 dilution of swine antirabbit IgG for 30 min.
7. Rinse in PBS for 15 min.
8. Incubate in 1:50 dilution of soluble peroxidase-antiperoxidase (rabbit) for 30 min.
9. Rinse in PBS for 15 min.
10. Stain and mount.

The following controls should be performed:

1. Uninfected cells (must be negative—test for nonspecificity).

2. Nonimmune serum or PBS in place of the primary specific antiviral antiserum should not produce any staining.

3. Absorption of specific antiserum with homologous antigen should decrease or abolish staining reaction (test for specificity).

4. The soluble peroxidase-antiperoxidase complex alone should not stain either infected or uninfected cells.

5. The enzyme substrate alone should not produce any reaction (test for endogenous peroxidase).

Diagnostic Applications

Antigen detection and identification in tissue culture

The majority of the reported uses of immunoenzymatic techniques have been for the identification of viral antigen in tissue culture systems. In certain circumstances antigen can be detected prior to the development of specific cytopathic effect (CPE) (8) or in cell lines in which the virus does not produce any microscopic changes. This reduces the usual delay in viral diagnosis and allows the positive identification of the virus without having to resort to neutralization tests. We have found it most useful for the routine identification of the myxo- and paramyxovirus groups and for the identification and typing of herpes simplex and cytomegalovirus.

Using antibodies raised against specific viral protein components, virus replication can be studied in more detail at both the light and electron-microscopic level.

Table 5.1 lists those viruses that have been successfully identified with the IP method. Specific details for each virus can be found in the references.

TABLE 5.1—VIRAL ANTIGENS DETECTED BY IMMUNOPEROXIDASE METHODS

Common Human Pathogens

Adenovirus (type 12)	66,72*	Measles	21,39
Cytomegalovirus	9,37,66	Mumps	8
Dengue	17	Parainfluenza (types 1,2,3)	8
Epstein-Barr	57	Poliovirus	30,31
Echovirus (type 11)	31	Rabies	34
Hepatitis B	15,50,62	Reovirus	65
Herpes simplex	7,66	Respiratory syncitial	8,66
Influenza A, A_2	8,19	Rubella	26
Influenza B	8	Vaccinia	44,56
Lymphocytic choriomeningitis	1	Varicella zoster	55

Miscellaneous Pathogens

Avian Leukosis	18,20,66	Myxomatosis	66
Bacteriophage P1	71	Newcastle disease	33
Densonucleosis	66	Polyoma	72
Foot & mouth disease	63	Simian virus 40	40,43,55,72
Fowlpox	64	Simian virus 5	8
Mareks disease	66	Tipula iridescent	66

*Reference numbers

Direct detection of viral antigen in clinical samples

The direct detection of viral antigen using IP methods has been reported for only a limited numbers of viruses. It has been most successful for herpes simplex, both for mucocutaneous lesions and in preparations of the central nervous system from patients with encephalitis (10, 66). Similarly, measles virus antigen has been demonstrated in the brain of patients with subacute sclerosing panencephalitis (14). Hepatitis B surface antigen has also been demonstrated in liver sections, even following formalin fixation and paraffin embedding (15, 50, 62). However, it is anticipated that it will soon be applied to a wide range of viruses, similar to the manner in which immunofluorescence has been used for rapid viral diagnosis.

Identifying viral antigen in clinical samples has a number of unique problems. Endogenous peroxidase is found in a variety of cells, but especially at sites of inflammation in which eosinophils are a particularly rich source. This should always be blocked or abolished prior to the start of the assay, using one of the methods described above.

Aside from the quality of the specific antiviral antibody which is always crucial for the development of a satisfactory assay, the method of sampling and sample preparation is critical. This has been well demonstrated in the case of the respiratory viruses with immunofluorescence procedures; only nasopharyngeal swabs taken carefully at the early phase of infection are likely to yield antigen-containing cells (24, 25).

Similarly in herpes simplex infections one is far more likely to be able to demonstrate viral antigen in cells from the early vesicular lesions rather than during the stage of ulceration or crusting. It is important in these cases to scrape the base of the vesicle in order to detach infected cells, as the fluid seldom contains sufficient numbers of cells.

Serology

Many serologic determinations can be conveniently performed using the indirect IP procedure. A standard virus should be cultured and the cells harvested when there is $2+$ to $3+$ CPE or when at least half the cells appear infected. The cell suspension, once dried and fixed in individual wells on slides, remains stable for prolonged periods. Many viral antigens have remained identifiable for at least 12 months at room temperature, although it is recommended that the slides be stored at -20 C for optimal preservation. Using serial dilutions of the patient's serum followed by antihuman IgG or IgM peroxidase conjugate, titers are read as the reciprocal of the highest dilution giving positive staining. A procedure is described for preparing and standardizing peroxidase-labeled antihuman IgG antibody which is useful in producing a reproducible plateau endpoint (69). We have used this method for herpes simplex, varicella-zoster, cytomegalovirus, and mumps. It is comparable to similar indirect immunofluorescence assays.

An alternative method is the ELISA (22). A standard quantity of antigen is attached to polystyrene tubes or wells of microtiter plates or can be chemically linked to agarose beads (61). There is a wide choice of enzymes which can be linked to the antihuman gamma globulin, with alkaline phosphatase being favored by many workers. In this case, the enzyme activity is measured spectrophotometrically rather than visually, allowing more accurate quantitation. There are a number of problems associated with ELISA that have precluded its widespread adoption. These include the variable antigen preparations, the difficulties in absorbing standard amounts of antigen to the solid phase, the leaching off of antigen during the procedure, and the variation in enzyme-antibody conjugates. Because of these it is not yet possible to compare results from one laboratory to another. However, once a standard curve has been established for a particular batch of antigen, the reproducibility of the assay is surprisingly good. Because of the relatively low interassay variation, smaller changes in antibody titer can be regarded as significant. This allows paired sera to be drawn much closer together (e.g., 5-6 days rather than the traditional 2-3 weeks) so that a serologic diagnosis can be established in a more clinically relevant time frame. This has been demonstrated by an ELISA procedure for influenza A (41). One additional advantage of this procedure is that it can be well adapted for large-scale seroepidemiologic investigations. Automation of the procedure is feasible so that large numbers of specimens may be handled.

Table 5.2 lists those viruses for which an indirect IP procedure or an ELISA assay has been reportedly useful.

TABLE 5.2—SEROLOGIC DETERMINATIONS WITH IMMUNOENZYMATIC METHODS

PATHOGEN	REFERENCE
Cytomegalovirus	27,54,68
Ebstein-Barr Virus	68
Influenza	41
Herpes simplex	42,66,68
Hog cholera	53
Measles	68
Mumps	65
Rubella	28,67,68

Appendix

Sources of antiviral antibodies and peroxidase-labeled antibodies

1. Accurate Chemical and Scientific Company   Peroxidase-labeled antibodies
   28 Tec Street, Hicksville, NY 11801
2. Antibodies Incorporated   Antibodies
   P.O. Box 442, Davis, CA 95616
3. Behring Diagnostics   Antibodies
   Route 202-206 North, Somerville, NJ 08876
4. Center for Disease Control   Antiviral antibodies
   1600 Clifton Road, Atlanta, GA 30333
5. Flow Laboratories   Antiviral antibodies
   P.O. Box 2226
   1710 Chapman Avenue
   Rockville, MD 20852

6. Hyland   Antibodies
   3300 Hyland Avenue
   P.O. Box 2214
   Costa Mesa, CA 92626
7. Microbiological Associates   Antiviral antibodies
   4733 Bethesda Avenue
   Bethesda, MD 20014
8. Miles Laboratories, Inc (Research Products)   Peroxidase-labeled antibodies
   Elkhart, IN 46514

References

1. ABELSON HT, SMITH GM, HOFFMAN HA, and ROWE WP: Use of enzyme labelled antibody for electron microscope localization of lymphocytic choriomeningitis virus antigen in infected tissue culture. J Natl Cancer Inst 42:497-515, 1969
2. AVRAMEAS S: Coupling of enzymes to proteins with gluteraldehyde. Use of the conjugates for the detection of antigens and antibodies. Immunochemistry 6:43-52, 1969
3. AVRAMEAS S: Immunoenzyme techniques: enzymes as markers for the localization of antigens and antibodies. Int Rev Cytol 27:349-385, 1970
4. AVRAMEAS S and TERNYNCK T: Peroxidase labelled antibody and Fab conjugates with enhanced intracellular penetration. Immunochemistry 8:1175-1179, 1971
5. AVRAMEAS S and URIEL J: Methode de marquage d'antigenes et d'anticorps avec des enzymes et son application en immuno diffusion. CR Acad Sci (Paris) 262:2543-2545, 1966
6. BARDELL D: A study of possible biohazards in fluorescent antibody test using adenovirus, coxsackie virus, herpesvirus and RSV as antigen. J Clin Microbiol 4:322-325, 1976
7. BENJAMIN DR: Rapid typing of herpes simplex virus strains using the indirect immunoperoxidase method. Appl Microbiol 28:568-571, 1974
8. BENJAMIN DR and RAY CG: Use of immunoperoxidase for the rapid identification of human myxoviruses and paramyxoviruses in tissue culture. Appl Microbiol 28:47-51, 1974
9. BENJAMIN DR: Use of immunoperoxidase for rapid viral diagnosis In Microbiology, 1975. Am Soc Microbiol, Washington, DC, pp 89-96
10. BENJAMIN DR and RAY CG: Use of immunoperoxidase on brain tissue for the rapid diagnosis of herpes encephalitis. Am J Clin Path 64:472-476, 1975
11. BIGBEE JW, KOSEK JC, and ENG LF: Effects of primary antiserum dilution on staining of "antigen-rich" tissue with the peroxidase-antiperoxidase technique. J Histochem Cytochem 25:443-447, 1977
12. BOORSMA DM and KALSBEEK GL: A comparative study of horse-radish peroxidase conjugates prepared with a one-step and two-step method. J Histochem Cytochem 23:200-209, 1975
13. BOORSMA DM, STREEFKERK JG, and KORS N: Peroxidase and fluorescein isothiocyanate as antibody markers. A quantitative comparison of two peroxidase conjugates prepared with gluteraldehyde or periodate and a fluorescein conjugate. J Histochem Cytochem 24:1017-1025, 1976
14. BROWN HR and THORMAR H: Immunoperoxidase staining of simple nuclear bodies in subacute sclerosing panencephalitis (SSPE) by antiserum to measles nucleocapsids. Acta Neuropathol 36:259-264, 1976
15. BURNS J: Immunoperoxidase localization of hepatitis B antigen in formalin-paraffin processed liver tissue. Histochemistry 44:133-135, 1975
16. CARCINOGENS. Federal Register, Vol 39, No 125, Part 2
17. CATANZARO PJ, BRANDT WE, HOGRAFE WR, and RUSSEL PK: Detection of dengue cell-surface antigens by peroxidase labelled antibodies and immune cytolysis. Infect Immun 10:381-388, 1974
18. DISTEFANO HS, MARUCCI AA, and DOUGHERTY RM: Immunohistochemical demonstration of avian leukosis virus antigens in paraffin embedded tissue. Proc Soc Exp Biol Med 142:1111-1116, 1973
19. DOBARDZIC R, BOUDREAULT A, and PAVILANIS V: L'identification du virus de l'influenza a' l'aide de l'immunoperoxydase. Can J Microbiol 19:146-149, 1973

20. DOUGHERTY RM, MARUCCI AA, and DiSTEFANO HS: Application of immuno-histochemistry to study of avian leukosis virus. J Gen Virol 15:149-154, 1972

21. DUBOIS-DALCQ M and BARBOSA LH: Immunoperoxidase stain of measles antigen in tissue culture. J Virol 12:909-918, 1973

22. ENGVALL E and PERLMAN P: Enzyme linked immunosorbent assay (ELISA) III. Quantitation of specific antibodies by enzyme labelled antiimmunoglobulin in antigen coated tubes. J Immunol 109:129-135, 1972

23. ERLANDSEN SL, PARSONS JA, and TAYLOR TD: Ultrastructural immunocytochemical localization of lysozyme in the Paneth cells of man. J Histochem Cytochem 22:401-413, 1974

24. FULTON RE and MIDDLETON PJ: Comparison of immunofluorescence and isolation techniques in the diagnosis of respiratory viral infections of children. Infect Immun 10:92-101, 1974

25. GARDNER PS and McQUILLIN J: Application of immunofluorescent antibody technique in rapid diagnosis of respiratory syncytial virus infection. Br Med J 3:340-343, 1968

26. GERNA G: Rubella virus identification in primary and continuous monkey kidney cell cultures by the immunoperoxidase technique. Arch Virol 46:291-295, 1975

27. GERNA G, McCLOUD CJ, and CHAMBER RW: Immunoperoxidase technique for detection of antibodies to human cytomegalovirus. J Clin Microbiol 3:364-372, 1976

28. GERNA G and CHAMBER RW: Rubella antibody assay by the immunoperoxidase technique; comparison with the hemagglutination inhibition test for determination of immune status. J Infect Dis 133:469-472, 1976

29. GRAHAM RC and KARNOVSKY MJ: The early stage of absorption of injected horse-radish peroxidase in the proximal tubule of the mouse kidney; ultrastructural cytochemistry by a new technique. J Histochem Cytochem 14:291-302, 1966

30. HERRMANN JE and MORSE SA: Coupling of peroxidase to poliovirus antibody; characteristics of the conjugates and their use in virus detection. Infect Immun 8:645-649, 1973

31. HERRMANN JE, MORSE SA, and COLLINS MF: Comparison of techniques and immunoreagents used for indirect immunofluorescence and immunoperoxidase identification of enteroviruses. Infect Immun 10:220-226, 1974

32. HEYDERMAN E and NEVILLE AM: A shorter immunoperoxidase technique for the demonstration of carcinoembryonic antigen and other cell products. J Clin Pathol 30:138-140, 1977

33. HOSHINO M and MAENO K: The usefulness of enzyme labelled antibody method of ultrastructural localization of Newcastle disease virus antigens in infected HeLa cells. J Electron Microsc 20:49-56, 1971

34. JENTZSCH KD and ZIPPER J: Light microscopic localization of rabies virus antigen by means of peroxidase-labelled immunoglobulin. Exp Pathol 9:163-168, 1974

35. KAPLOW LS: Simplified myeloperoxidase stain using benzidine hydrochloride. Blood 26:215-219, 1965

36. KAPLOW LS: Substitute for benzidine in myeloperoxidase stains. Am J Clin Pathol 63:451, 1975

37. KURSTAK E, BELLONCIK S, ONJI PA, MONTPLAISIN S, and MARTINEAU B: Localisation par l'immunopaxy-dase dos antigens du virus cytomegalique en culture cellulaire de fibroblasts humans. Arch Gesamte Virusforsch 38:67-76, 1972

38. KURSTAK E: The immunoperoxidase technique; localization of viral antigens in cells, In Methods in Virology Vol 5, Maramorsch K and Koprowski H (eds), Academic Press Inc, NY, 1971, pp 423-444

39. LAMPERT PW, JOSEPH BS, and OLDSTONE MBA: Antibody induced capping of measles virus antigens on plasma membranes studied by electron microscopy. J Virol 15:1248-1255, 1975

40. LEDUC EM, WICKER R, AVRAMEAS S, and BERNHARD W: Ultrastructural localization of SV40 T antigen with enzyme labelled antibody. J Gen Virol 7:609-614, 1969

41. LEINIKKI P and PÄSSILÄ S: Solid phase antibody assay by means of enzyme conjugated to antiimmunoglobulin. J Clin Pathol 29:1116-1120, 1976

42. MARUCCI AA and DOUGHERTY RM: Use of the unlabeled antibody immunohistochemical technique for the detection of human antibody. J Histochem Cytochem 23:618-623, 1975

43. MILLER MM, KARNOVSKY MJ, and DIAMANDOPOULOUS AT: An improved immuno-peroxidase technique for identifying SV40 V and T antigens by light microscopy. Proc Soc Exp Biol Med 146:432–437, 1974

44. MIYAMOTO H: Vaccinia virus infection in vitro studied by peroxidase labelled antibody method. Acta Histochem Cytochem 8:56–64, 1975

45. MORIARTY GC and HALMI NS: Electron microscopic study of the adreno-corticotrophin producing cell with the use of unlabelled antibody and the soluble peroxidase-anti-peroxidase complex. J Histochem Cytochem 20:590–603, 1972

46. MORIARTY GC, MORIARTY CM, and STERNBERGER LA: Ultrastructural immuno-cytochemistry with unlabelled antibodies and the peroxidase-antiperoxidase complex; a technique more sensitive than radioimmunoassay. J Histochem Cytochem 21:825–833, 1973

47. NAKANE PK and PIERCE GB: Enzyme labelled antibodies; preparation and application for the localization of antigens. J Histochem Cytochem 14:929–931, 1966

48. NAKANE PK and KAWAOI A: Peroxidase labeled antibody. A new method of conjugation. J Histochem Cytochem 22:1084–1091, 1974

49. NAKANE PK and PIERCE GB: Enzyme labelled antibodies for the light and electron micro-scopic localization of tissue antibodies. J Cell Biol 33:307–318, 1967

50. NAYAK NC and SACHDEVA R: Localization of hepatitis B surface antigen in conventional paraffin sections of liver. Comparison of immunofluorescence, immunoperoxidase and orcein staining methods with regard to their specificity and reliability as antigen mark-ers. Am J Pathol 81:479–490, 1975

51. PURDHAM DR, SALMON MV, and WILLIAMS B: False-positive immunofluorescence test for herpes simplex in tuberculous meningitis. Lancet 1:1235–1236, 1976

52. READING M: A digestion technique for the reduction of background staining in the immuno-peroxidase method. J Clin Pathol 30:88–90, 1977

53. SAUNDERS GC and WILDER ME: Disease screening with enzyme labelled antibodies. J Infect Dis 129:362–364, 1974

54. SCHMITZ H, DOERR HW, KAMPA D, and VOGT A: Solid-phase enzyme immunoassay for immunoglobulin M antibodies to cytomegalovirus. J Clin Microbiol 5:629–634, 1977

55. SHABO AL, PETRICCIANI JC, and KIRSCHSTEIN RL: Immunoperoxidase localization of her-pes zoster and simian virus 40 in cell culture. Appl Microbiol 23:1001–1009, 1972

56. SIVERD JJ and SHARON N: Immunohistochemical method for detection of vaccinia virus. Proc Soc Exp Biol Med 131:939–941, 1969

57. STEPHENS R: Comparative studies on EBV antigens by immunofluorescent and immuno-peroxidase techniques. Int J Cancer 19:305–312, 1977

58. STERNBERGER LA, HARDY PM JR, CUCULIS JT, and MEYER HG: Unlabelled antibody en-zyme method of immunochemistry. Preparation and properties of soluble antigen-anti-body complex (horse-radish peroxidase-antihorse-radish peroxidase) and its use in identification of spirochaetes. J Histochem Cytochem 18:315–333, 1970

59. STRAUS W: Inhibition of peroxidase by methanol and by methanolnitroferricyanide for use in immunoperoxidase procedures. J Histochem Cytochem 19:682–688, 1971

60. STREEFKERK JG: Inhibition of erythrocyte pseudoperoxidase activity by treatment with hydrogen peroxide following methanol. J Histochem Cytochem 20:829–831, 1972

61. STREEFKERK JG and DEELDER AM: Serodiagnostic application of immunoperoxidase reac-tions on antigen coupled agarose beads. J Immunol Methods 7:225–236, 1975

62. SUMITHRAN E: Methods for detection of hepatitis B surface antigen in paraffin sections of liver: a guideline for their use. J Clin Pathol 30:460–463, 1977

63. SUTMOLLER P and COWAN KM: The detection of foot and mouth disease virus antigens in infected cell cultures by immunoperoxidase techniques. J Gen Virol 22:287–291, 1974

64. TRIPATHY DN, HANSON LE, and KILLINGER AH: Immunoperoxidase technique for detec-tion of fowlpox antigen. Avian Dis 17:274–278, 1973

65. UBERTINI T, WILKIE BN, and NORONHA F: Use of horse-radish peroxidase labelled anti-body for light and electron microscopic localization of reovirus antigen. Appl Micro-biol 21:534–538, 1971

66. VIRAL IMMUNODIAGNOSIS, Kurstak E and Morriset R (eds), Academic Press Inc, NY, 1974

67. VOLLER A and BIDWELL DE: A simple method for detecting antibodies to rubella. Br J Exp Pathol 56:338–340, 1975

68. VOLLER A, BIDWELL DE, and BERTLETT A: Microplate enzyme immunoassays for the immunodiagnosis of virus infections *In* Manual of Clinical Immunology, Rose NR and Friedman H (eds), Am Soc Microbiol, Washington, DC, 1976, pp 506–512

69. WALWICK ER, INAMI YH, and NAKAMURA RM: Preparation and standardization of peroxidase-labelled antihuman IgG antibody for use in determination of serum antinuclear antibody levels. Am J Clin Pathol 63:219–230, 1975

70. WEIR EE, PRETLOW TG, PITTS A, and WILLIAMS EE: Destruction of endogenous peroxidase activity in order to locate cellular antigens by peroxidase labelled antibodies J Histochem Cytochem 22:51–54, 1977

71. WENDELSCHAFER-CRABB G, ERLANDSEN SL, and WALKER DH: Ultrastructural localization of viral antigens using the unlabelled enzyme-antibody method. J Histochem Cytochem 24:517–526, 1976

72. WICKER R: Comparison of immunofluorescent and immunoenzymatic techniques applied to the study of viral antigens. Ann NY Acad Sci 177:490–500, 1971

73. WICKER R and AVRAMEAS S: Localization of virus antigens by enzyme labeled antibodies. J Gen Virol 4:465–471, 1969

CHAPTER 6

RADIOIMMUNOASSAY

Bagher Forghani

Introduction

Radioimmunoassay (RIA) combines the high sensitivity of radioisotope labeling with the marked specificity of immunologic reactions, and, following the development of an RIA method by Yalow and Berson in 1960 (57) for determination of insulin levels in plasma, the procedure was widely applied in the field of clinical chemistry for assay of trace amounts of a variety of biologic substances.

RIA was first applied in virology for assay of hepatitis B surface antigen (HBsAg) and antibody (anti-HBs) (36, 39). HBsAg has unique features that contribute to the sensitivity and reliability of RIA, including its high degree of antigenic stability and the fact that it is present in high concentrations in serum, unassociated with host tissue, and thus can be readily isolated, purified, and concentrated. Since other viral antigens do not possess these characteristics, development of sensitive and specific RIA methods proceeded more slowly. Hayashi et al (25, 26) showed that ^{125}I-labeled antibody could be used to demonstrate viral antigen on the surface of infected cells, and Rosenthal et al (48, 49) first described the use of lysates of virus-infected cells, or semipurified virus, adsorbed to microtiter plates as a source of antigen for detection of viral antibodies. Subsequently, RIA procedures using virus-infected cells on glass or plastic supports (16–19, 52), viral antigens passively adsorbed to polystyrene tubes (12), polystyrene beads (1, 32, 43), imitation pearls (52), wells in polyvinyl microtiter plates (30, 35, 59), or viral antigen covalently bonded to activated bromoacetyl cellulose (4) were developed for assay of viral antigens or antibodies.

RIA for detection of viral antigens and antibodies are based upon the fact that antibodies can be labeled with a radioisotope (usually ^{125}I) without losing their immunologic specificity and can then be used as probes for detecting homologous antigen. In the case of assays for viral antigen, the labeled antibody can be a specific viral antibody, which is then used for direct detection of homologous viral antigen. More often, however, viral antigen is detected by the indirect RIA procedure in which test material is mixed with an unlabeled viral antibody preparation, and radiolabeled antibody directed against the species of the viral antiserum is then added to detect an initial

171

antigen-antibody reaction. The indirect procedure is also used for detection of viral antibodies. The sensitivity and specificity of RIA depend upon the preservation of specific antibody activity upon labeling and also to a large extent upon the initial potency and specificity of the antiserum used for labeling or as an intermediate serum.

The major advantage of RIA as compared with conventional methods for detection of viral antigen or antibody is its greater sensitivity. This permits the use of highly dilute immune reagents, which in turn reduces nonspecific reactivity, and also results in economy of reagents. Also, RIA results based upon counting isotope emissions are more quantitative and less subjective than are results based upon visual reading. Disadvantages are the fact that radiolabeled antibodies can be used for only about 3–4 months, the potential hazard of radioisotopes, the need for expensive equipment for counting, and the fact that localization of viral antigen in infected cells is not possible.

RIA for detection of viral antibody is performed either by a radioisotope precipitation (RIP) method (23) or, more commonly, by a solid-phase procedure. For the former, virus is radiolabeled, added to the test serum and, after incubation, anti-gamma globulin directed against the species of the test serum is added; this precipitates gamma globulin in the test serum, and radiolabeled virus is also present in the precipitate if the test serum contained homologous viral antibodies. The amount of radioactivity in the precipitate gives a measure of the degree of virus-antibody reaction. RIA has been used most extensively in the assay of antibodies to HBsAg and antibodies to hepatitis B core antigen (see Chapter 29).

Solid-phase RIA (5), in which viral antigen is fixed to a solid glass or plastic support, is easier to perform than RIP, and most methods for assay of viral antigens and antibodies are based upon this principle. The solid phase consists of cells or cell lysates infected with a known virus (for antibody assay) or of cells, lysates, smears or sections of tissue to be examined for a viral antigen. These are fixed, or simply dried, depending upon the method, and then treated with the primary or intermediate serum. If the test is being used to identify a virus, this is a known viral antiserum, and a preimmunization serum is also used on representative antigen preparations for control purposes. On the other hand, the primary serum can be one which is being assayed for antibodies to a known virus infecting the cells. In this case, the serum is also added to uninfected cell preparations for controls. After incubation and washing, radiolabeled immune globulins directed against the species of the primary serum are added. Labeled immunoglobulins specific for heavy chains of immunoglobulins can also be used for class-specific antibody detection. After further incubation and thorough washing, the amount of bound reactivity is counted in a gamma counter, and binding ratios are calculated by dividing the counts per minute (cpm) in the test specimens by those in the controls. Ratios of ≥ 2.1 are generally considered positive for virus or viral antibody.

Indirect solid-phase RIA procedures developed in our laboratory, which utilize fixed virus-infected cells, have been shown to be highly sensitive for detecting viral antigen in cell cultures and brain tissue and for assaying viral antibodies in serum and cerebrospinal fluid (16–18, 20, 21). These procedures are described in detail in this chapter; however, other sources for detailed descriptions of additional viral RIA procedures are available (see below).

Solid-phase Radioimmunoassay

Antigen preparations

Virus-infected cells produce a variety of antigens, including intact virions, viral subunits, and in some cases, nonstructural proteins. These have different antigenic specificities and vary in their stability to chemical and physical effects, such as those which may be encountered in purification, adsorption, or bonding to a solid surface. A major concern in the preparation of viral antigens for RIA is the maximal preservation of antigenic determinants to provide the broadest possible spectrum of antigens for reaction with antibody preparations. Based upon the sensitivity of the assays, virus-infected cells fixed with acetone appear to provide a broad spectrum of well-preserved antigens.

Infected cell monolayers.

The method described uses virus-infected cell monolayers prepared in the bottom of 1-dr glass vials as a source of antigen. The vials provide a convenient and safe vessel for initiation and infection of cell cultures, for performance of all steps of the RIA, and finally for counting radioactivity directly in the vials. The amount of infected cells required for each test is approximately the same as that for immunofluorescent staining.

Because sensitivity of the assay depends upon an extensive infection of the host cells, cultures are infected and harvested under conditions which produce infection in ≥90% of the cells in the culture, as indicated by immunofluorescent staining. Optimal conditioning for infection and harvesting must be defined for each virus system. Those for a variety of viruses are given in greater detail elsewhere (17, 18).

1. Prepare a suspension of the appropriate cell type containing approximately 50,000 cells per ml in growth medium consisting of 10% fetal bovine serum and 90% Eagle minimal essential medium (MEM) prepared in Hanks balanced salt solution (BSS). Put 1 ml of suspension into 1-dr glass vials.

2. Incubate cultures loosely covered in a CO_2 incubator 2–3 days until a confluent cell monolayer is formed. Aspirate growth medium and replace with 1 ml of maintenance medium consisting of 2% fetal bovine serum and 98% Eagle MEM.

3. Infect cells with virus of known titer, ideally at a ratio of 1 plaque-forming unit (pfu) per cell, or with a virus dose which produces infection in ≥90% of the cells in the culture in 3–5 days. The extent of virus infection is determined by immunofluorescent staining of representative cultures. For viruses which do not produce an extensive cytopathic effect (CPE), e.g., rubella or cytomegalovirus, cells can be infected in suspension and then planted in growth medium to grow into a confluent monolayer.

4. Aspirate the medium, and rinse the cells briefly with 1 ml of distilled water.

5. Without drying, fix the cells with 1 ml of acetone at room temperature for 10 min.
6. Aspirate the acetone and dry the cells at room temperature for 30 min. They can be used as a source of antigen immediately or stored at −70 C indefinitely.

Frozen tissue sections.

Sections prepared from frozen virus-infected tissue are also a suitable source of viral antigen for RIA, as demonstrated in studies on measles virus-infected human and animal brain tissue (21).

1. Freeze a small sample of tissue approximately 4–5 mm in diameter at −70 C in a tube.
2. Put a few drops of embedding medium (Tissue-Tek, Ames Co., Division of Miles Laboratories) onto a precooled (−16 to −18 C) specimen-holder plate in a microtome.
3. Before the embedding medium solidifies, place the frozen tissue into it with cold forceps. Add additional medium to cover the tissue.
4. When the preparation is completely frozen, cut sections 3–4 μ thick and carefully mount onto round coverslips 15 mm in diameter, using 4–5 sections per coverslip without overlapping. Attachment of the sections to the coverslip can be enhanced by precoating the coverslips with a 1–2% solution of bovine albumin in 0.01 M phosphate-buffered saline (PBS), pH 7.2, and then drying.
5. Air dry the preparations, fix in cold acetone for 10 min, and place the coverslips in scintillation vials for use in RIA.

Antiserum

Viral antiserum

Viral antisera for RIA have the same requirements for potency and freedom from reactivity with host cell components as those used for immunofluorescent staining (see Chapter 4). Freedom from host cell reactivity can best be achieved by immunizing animals with virus propagated in a homologous host system (see chapters on individual viruses). If this is not feasible, purification procedures can be used, as exemplified by that used for preparation of antiserum to human cytomegalovirus (19).

Antiserum to gamma globulin

Whole or partially purified antisera to various species of gamma globulin are available from a number of commercial sources, and these are generally suitable for radiolabeling and use in RIA. However, specific binding can be increased by radiolabeling only those antibodies directed against the desired immunoglobulin in the primary serum. A radiolabeled preparation of purified goat antibodies to human IgG was found by the author to give specific binding ratios with human IgG that were twice as high as those obtained with radiolabeled total IgG from the same goat antiserum. The following procedure can be used for purification of antibodies specific for human IgG. It consists of adsorbing antibodies specific for human IgG from goat antiserum to whole human gamma globulin, using insolubilized, purified human IgG as the immunoadsorbent, and subsequent elution of the isolated and purified antibodies.

Preparation of the immunoadsorbent (2).

1. Separate the IgG from 200–300 ml of pooled human sera (negative for HBsAg) by 3 precipitations with ⅓ saturated ammonium sulfate, pass through a DEAE cellulose

column (see Chapter 4), and concentrate to 5–10 ml by ultrafiltration through an Amicon membrane (Amicon Corp., Lexington, Mass.). The pH is controlled by filtering in the presence of 0.1 M phosphate buffer (PB), pH 7.0.

2. Determine the protein concentration of the concentrate by the biuret or Lowry method.

3. For each 500 mg of protein, add 2 ml of a 2.5% aqueous solution of glutaraldehyde dropwise with constant stirring. A gel forms immediately upon addition of the glutaraldehyde.

4. Keep the gel at room temperature for 2–3 hr to ensure complete insolubilization and cross-linkage.

5. After centrifugation of the gel at 3000 rpm for 15 min, discard the supernatant fluid, which should contain little or no protein.

6. Homogenize the pelleted gel into fine particles with a glass rod and then wash 3–4 times with 200 ml of 0.2 M PB, pH 7.2, by centrifugation at 3000 rpm for 15 min at 4 C.

7. Add 200 ml of 0.1 M glycine-HCl buffer, pH 2.8, to the gel to remove any soluble IgG. Repeat this step once. Wash the immunoadsorbent twice in 200 ml of 0.02 M PB, pH 7.2.

8. The immunoadsorbent can be used immediately, or it can be stored at 4 C with 0.02% sodium azide.

Purification of antibodies to human IgG.

1. Separate the IgG fraction from 10 ml of goat antiserum to human gamma globulin (Antibodies Inc., Davis, Calif.) by 3 precipitations with $^1/_3$ saturated ammonium sulfate and pass through a DEAE cellulose column.

2. Add the IgG preparation to the immunoadsorbent (insolubilized human IgG) and incubate for 30 min at 37 C with occasional shaking, then incubate overnight at 4 C with gentle shaking.

3. After centrifugation at 3000 rpm for 15 min, remove the supernatant fluid and wash the pelleted immunoadsorbent 4–5 times with 200 ml of 0.1 M PBS, pH 7.2, by centrifugation at 3000 rpm.

4. Elute the antibodies specific for human IgG from the immunoadsorbent by adding of 0.1 M glycine-HCl buffer, pH 2.8, for 30 min at room temperature, follow by centrifugation at 3000 rpm for 15 min. Repeat elution 3–4 times with small volumes of the buffer to remove all of the IgG. Generally the first elution releases little IgG because the pH is not sufficiently low.

5. Clarify pooled eluates by centrifugation at 3000 rpm, and then concentrate and adjust the pH by Amicon membrane filtration in the presence of 0.05 M PB, pH 7.0. Concentrate the purified antibodies from 10 ml of antiserum to a volume of 2–3 ml; this should contain 4–6 mg of specific antibody protein. Remove the small amount of precipitate which forms by centrifuging.

6. The method given above can also be used for purification and concentration of antibodies specific for human IgA and IgM using appropriate immunoadsorbents.

Radiolabeling of proteins

In most of the RIA procedures used for clinical chemistry, the antigen is labeled with a radioisotope. However, with the exception of hepatitis B antigens, radiolabeling of viral antigens has generally been restricted to research studies. Because of the lability of viral antigens and their close association with host cell components, it has been more feasible to use radiolabeled antibodies in RIA procedures for viral diagnosis. Also, the use of labeled antibodies against IgG provides a highly versatile reagent which is applicable to use in a variety of virus systems.

Several different radioisotopes have been used for labeling antigens or antibodies, but ^{131}I and ^{125}I have been most widely employed. ^{131}I, a beta-gamma emitter with a half-life of 8 days, is used much less frequently than ^{125}I, a low gamma emitter with a longer half-life of approximately 60 days. Additional attributes of ^{125}I are ease of preparation, accuracy of counting, and stability *in vitro* and *in vivo*. Also, it is not reincorporated into new protein, since iodine is not normally present in protein, with the exception of thyroglobulin.

Radioiodination of proteins is based upon the substitution of an iodine molecule for 1 hydrogen molecule on a tyrosyl group. However, under certain conditions iodine may react with sulfhydryl groups. It is important to limit the incorporation of iodine into proteins to prevent changes in their immunologic properties. Several methods have been described for iodinating proteins, and each uses an oxidizing agent to effect substitution. The methods most frequently used are the iodine monochloride method, the nitrous acid method, the lactoperoxidase method, and the chloramine-T method.

In 1958 McFarlane (42) introduced the use of iodine monochloride as an oxidizing agent, and this has been used primarily for radioiodination of insulin. Nitrous acid oxidizes iodide to form free iodine which reacts with tyrosyl groups. Although good results have been obtained in radiolabeling with this reagent (42), the alkaline conditions may have an adverse effect on the immunologic properties of certain proteins. It is most applicable to large scale labeling. The lactoperoxidase method is a fairly new procedure introduced by Marchalonis in 1969 (40). Lactoperoxidase catalyzes the iodination reaction in the presence of hydrogen peroxide. High efficiency of labeling has been reported, including labeling of gamma globulin (54).

The chloramine-T method, introduced by Hunter and Greenwood in 1962 (27), has been universally used for labeling micro- and milligram amounts of proteins, and it was further adapted by McConahey and Dixon (41) for labeling microgram quantities of gamma globulins. This is the procedure employed in our laboratory for efficient radiolabeling of IgG from various species, and it is described here in detail.

Chloramine-T is the sodium salt of the N-monochloro- derivative of p-toluene sulfonamide. In an aqueous solution it slowly yields hypochlorous acid, which is a mild oxidizing agent. Addition of chloramine-T to a mixture of protein and iodate results in incorporation of iodine into the protein. According to Hunter (28), the mechanism of the reaction is not fully understood, but it presumably involves the formation of cationic iodine in the presence of chloramine-T and subsequent labeling of the protein.

Chloramine-T method for labeling IgG with [125]I

The following procedure is for labeling 1 mg of purified IgG with 1 mCi of [125]I (sodium iodide, carrier-free, New England Nuclear). For labeling different quantities of protein, the amount of radioisotope is adjusted proportionately.

1. Add 1 mg of purified IgG to a clean scintillation vial containing a small polyethylene-coated magnetic stirring bar. Place the vial in a cracked-ice bath in a large Petri dish, and place the whole assembly on a magnetic stirrer.

2. Perform the labeling procedure in a well-ventilated hood. Open the vial of radioisotope (most manufacturers sell a minimum quantity of 2 mCi of the isotope) carefully

and add 0.1 ml containing approximately 2 mCi to 0.9 ml of 0.05 M PB, pH 7.0, and mix well.

3. Add to the protein solution in the scintillation vial a volume of the isotope solution containing 1 mCi, dropwise with constant stirring.

4. Rapidly add 500 μg of chloramine-T in a volume of 0.5 ml with a 1 ml syringe. Prepare the chloramine-T solution just before use by dissolving 10 mg of the reagent in 10 ml of cold 0.05 M PB, pH 7.0.

5. After 5 min of stirring on the ice bath, stop the action of the chloramine-T by the addition of 500 μg of sodium metabisulfite in a volume of 0.5 ml. Pepare the solution just before use by dissolving 10 mg of the reagent in 10 ml of cold 0.05 M PB, pH 7.0.

6. Prepare a Sephadex G25 column (0.6 × 11 cm). To increase recovery of the labeled IgG, saturate the column with 1 ml of 2% bovine serum albumin (BSA) (prepared in 0.05 M PB, pH 7.0). Then wash with 20 ml of 0.05 M PB, pH 7.0, and determine the void volume by adding blue dextran solution in PB in a volume equal to that of the labeled protein solution and wash the column with additional PB. Measure the volume eluted before the color disappears and discard that volume of eluate before collecting the labeled protein.

7. Add the labeled protein, together with 0.4–0.5 ml of fluid (3 mg KI per ml of 0.05 M PB, pH 7.0) used to rinse out the vial, to the column and elute with 0.05 M PB, pH 7.0. Discard the fluid in the void volume, and collect the labeled protein in a single fraction of approximately 4–6 ml.

8. Transfer the labeled protein to dialyzing tubing (pretreated with 2% BSA) and dialyze at 4 C against several changes of 0.05 M PB, pH 7.0, until the radioactivity count of the dialyzing fluid is negligible. For more effective removal of unbound ^{125}I, add 3 ml of 1 N KI to each liter of dialyzing fluid. However, the final dialysis should be against PB only, so that the KI is removed from the protein preparation.

9. If only a small amount of protein is labeled, column chromatography can be omitted, and the labeled protein can be dialyzed directly.

Evaluation of radiolabeling

1. Prepare a 1:200 dilution of the labeled protein by adding 5 μg to 1 ml of 0.05 M PB, pH 7.0, in a plastic tube which can be accommodated in both a gamma counter and a preparative centrifuge, and count this in a gamma counter for 1 min to obtain the total cpm.

2. Add 1 ml of 2% BSA in 0.05 M PB, pH 7.0, to the tube, followed by 2 ml of 10% trichloracetic acid.

3. Mix and let stand at room temperature for 5–10 min, then centrifuge the preparation at 3000 rpm for 5 min.

4. Remove 1 ml of supernatant fluid carefully and count the radioactivity in a gamma counter for 1 min. Multiply this by 4 to give the total unbound ^{125}I. Subtract the total unbound ^{125}I from the total protein cpm to give the cpm of ^{125}I-bound protein. The following calculations are done to determine the quality of labeling.

(Express the cpm of bound protein as disintegration per minute (dpm) corrected for ^{125}I counting efficiency of the gamma counter and for ^{125}I decay.)

a. Percent ^{125}I bound to protein =

$$\frac{\text{Total cpm} - \text{total unbound cpm}}{\text{Total cpm}} \times 100$$

b. Percent efficiency of protein labeling =

$$\frac{\text{cpm of bound protein} \times \text{final volume of labeled protein}}{\text{Total } \mu\text{Ci used for labeling (Expressed as dpm)}}$$

c. Specific activity of the labeled protein = μCi ^{125}I/μg protein.

With the above procedure, the amount of ^{125}I bound to IgG is >98%, and assuming that no protein is lost in the labeling process, a specific activity of 0.5 μCi/μg of protein is achieved.

Storage of radiolabeled protein

The radiolabeled IgG can be stored at 4 C or dispensed in convenient working volumes and stored frozen at −20 C or −70 C. We generally store the labeled IgG at 4 C with 5% BSA as a protective agent and a carrier protein, and with 0.02% sodium azide to prevent microbial contamination. The labeled IgG maintains its sensitivity for use in RIA for 3-4 months, provided the same amount of radioactivity is used in each RIA run.

Direct solid-phase radioimmunoassay

A viral antiserum to be radiolabeled for use in direct RIA for detection of viral antigens should be of high initial potency and specificity. Potency can be determined by other conventional viral antibody assays, such as neutralization, hemagglutination inhibition, or complement fixation, or even by indirect RIA. Specificity can be assessed by testing against uninfected host cell material corresponding to that in which the virus is prepared. In some cases it is possible to eliminate host cell reactivity from a viral antiserum by absorption with uninfected host cells or with insolubilized serum of the species used for growth or maintenance of the host cells. However, it is more desirable to begin with an immune serum free from anti-host reactivity.

The IgG fraction of the antiserum is purified and radiolabeled as described above. It is then tested, as described below, in varying dilutions against homologous virus-infected cells and uninfected cells to determine an optimal working dilution, that is, one which gives maximum reactivity with infected cells and shows no nonspecific reactivity with uninfected cells. A preimmunization serum from the same animal, radiolabeled in the same manner, is useful for determining the viral specificity of the labeled IgG. In some instances it is necessary to confirm the specificity of the labeled immune globulins by testing against other heterotypic viruses which are likely to be recovered from similar sources or similar syndromes, e.g., antisera to herpes simplex virus are tested against cells infected with other human herpesviruses and with vaccinia virus.

1. Dilute the radiolabeled viral antibody preparation in 0.01 M PBS, pH 7.2, containing 5% BSA and 0.05% Tween 20 to contain approximately 50,000 cpm in a volume of 0.1 ml, and apply to virus-infected and uninfected cells (at least in duplicate).

2. Incubate for 2-3 hours at room temperature, or 30 to 60 min at 37 C, aspirate the fluids, and wash the vials 3 times with PBS, pH 7.2.

3. Count the residual radioactivity in a gamma counter for 1 min. Binding ratios are expressed as the mean cpm obtained against virus-infected cells divided by the mean cpm obtained with uninfected cells, and ratios ≥2.1 are considered to indicate the presence of homologous viral antigen.

4. If the test is done to search for viral antigen in clinical materials and, thus corresponding uninfected cells are not available for controls, controls should include a radiolabeled preimmunization serum and heterotypic radiolabeled viral antibodies, and binding ratios are based on these.

The above procedure can also be applied to smears or frozen sections of tissue. The direct RIA is simple and results can be obtained within a few hours. However, the disadvantage is the fact that labeled antibodies to individual viruses must be used, and thus versatility is not as great as that of indirect RIA.

Indirect solid-phase radioimmunoassay

This procedure can be used for detecting viral antigen in infected cells or tissue, or for assaying viral antibody in serum or cerebrospinal fluid.

   1. Prepare dilutions of known viral antiserum or serum to be assayed for viral antibody in 0.01 M PBS, pH 7.2, containing 0.02% BSA.
   2. Add the serum dilutions in a volume of 0.2 ml to infected and uninfected cells, and incubate for 2 hr at 37 C or at room temperature overnight.
   3. Aspirate the contents of the vials and wash the vials twice with 3 ml of PBS.
   4. Dilute ^{125}I-labeled immune globulins directed against the species of the primary serum in PBS with 5% BSA and 0.05% Tween 20 to contain 50,000 cpm in 0.1 ml and add to the vials in a volume of 0.1 ml.
   5. Incubate at room temperature for 70-80 min, aspirate the contents of the vials, and then wash the vials twice with 3 ml of PBS.
   6. Count the residual radioactivity in the vials in a gamma counter for 1 min. If the test is used to detect viral antigen in cells or tissues, examine the test material against preimmunization serum from the same animal in which the viral antiserum was prepared, and calculate the binding ratios by dividing the cpm obtained with the immune serum by the cpm obtained with the preimmunization serum. If viral antibody is being assayed, test the serum against uninfected cells of the same lot as those used for preparation of the viral antigen, and calculate the binding ratios by dividing the cpm obtained with virus-infected cells by the cpm obtained with uninfected cells. Consider ratios ≥2.1 positive for viral antigen or antibody.

Specificity testing by inhibition of binding

The virus specificity of binding in a direct RIA can be confirmed in a blocking test for which portions of the specimen are first incubated at room temperature for 1-2 hours with a known viral antiserum and with preimmunization serum, and then tested against the ^{125}I-labeled viral antibodies. The positive viral antiserum used for blocking should be a different one from that used for radiolabeling. If binding of the ^{125}I-labeled antibodies is virus-specific, it is inhibited by the positive antiserum, which has blocked the virus determinants so that they are not available to the ^{125}I-labeled antibodies. A more convenient, but somewhat less reliable, method is the addition of unlabeled and labeled antibodies to the specimen at the same time, followed by incubation conditions for direct RIA. The amount of inhibition is calculated from the following formulae, and inhibition of ≥50% is considered to confirm the specificity of the reaction.

If the specificity test is being applied to a viral isolate propagated in cell cultures, the percent inhibition of binding ratios can be calculated as follows. The binding ratios of labeled immune and preimmunization sera are first calculated as described above by dividing the binding (cpm) obtained against infected cells by that obtained with uninfected cells, and binding ratios of these labeled sera are also calculated using infected and uninfected cells pretreated with the specific, unlabeled viral antiserum. The following calculations are then made:

a. Percent inhibition of binding ratio for immune serum =

$$1 - \frac{\text{Binding ratio for immune serum with cells pretreated with viral antiserum}}{\text{Binding ratio for immune serum with untreated cells}} \times 100$$

b. Percent inhibition of binding ratio for preimmunization serum =

$$1 - \frac{\text{Binding ratio for preimmunization serum with cells pretreated with viral antiserum}}{\text{Binding ratio for preimmunization serum with untreated cells}} \times 100$$

Specificity of the binding obtained in direct RIA is confirmed by ≥50% inhibition of the binding ratio for immune serum and negligible inhibition of the binding ratio for preimmunization serum.

If the specificity test is being applied directly to clinical material (e.g., brain tissue) suspected of containing viral antigen, there is no corresponding uninfected material, and binding ratios are determined by dividing the cpm obtained with labeled immune serum by that obtained with labeled preimmunization serum. The percent inhibition of binding is determined as follows:

Percent inhibition of binding ratio =

$$1 - \frac{\text{Binding ratio with specimen pretreated with viral antiserum}}{\text{Binding ratio with untreated specimen}} \times 100$$

To test the virus specificity of an indirect RIA reaction for antigen detection, the viral antiserum and preimmunization serum are absorbed with homologous viral antigen and with control antigen and then assayed in the indirect RIA against the test material (17). The following calculation can be applied to determine the extent of inhibition of specific viral antibody activity.

Percent inhibition of binding =

$$1 - \frac{\text{cpm of immune serum absorbed with viral antigen}}{\text{cpm of immune serum absorbed with control antigen}} \times 100$$

The inhibition technique can also be applied for indirect detection of viral antigen in a specimen. A standard dilution of viral antiserum is incubated with the test specimen and with a similar known negative control specimen, and these absorbed sera are then assayed for specific viral antibody in the indirect RIA system. Presence of viral antigen in the test specimen is indicated by a reduction in binding with serum absorbed with that material as compared to the portion of serum absorbed with known negative material (personal unpublished observations).

Nonspecific reactivity in radioimmunoassay

Increased sensitivity of an assay may also enhance the nonspecific or cross-reactivity of the reagents. We have noted that an occasional serum shows high binding with uninfected cell cultures or tissues. Also, the lower dilutions of most sera show increased binding with uninfected tissue, but with dilution the activity is reduced and specific binding ratios increase (16–18).

The exact cause of binding of IgG to uninfected cells is unknown, but several possibilities exist. The binding appears similar to that of "cytophilic antibodies" which attach to macrophages and lymphoid tissue, and it may be that nonspecific activity is due to antitissue antibodies present in certain sera. It is well recognized that antinuclear and anticytoplasmic antibodies bind to uninfected tissues, and may mask specific viral antibody reactions in immunofluorescence systems. Also, the surface charge of IgG has been suggested as a factor influencing its binding to tissues.

Cross-reactivity may also be the result of antigenic relationships existing among certain viruses and, in a highly sensitive system such as RIA, antigenic relationships may be demonstrated which are not apparent in a less sensitive test system.

Nonspecific reactivity or cross-reactivity can frequently be removed from test serum by absorption with uninfected cells or cells infected with the cross-reacting virus. Serum is added to cells or tissues at a ratio of 1 part serum to 10 of packed cells, mixed well and then incubated for 30 min at 37 C followed by gentle shaking at 4 C overnight. The preparation is then centrifuged at 30,000 rpm for 2 hr at 4 C to sediment cells and immune complexes, and the supernatant serum is removed for testing.

Applications of RIA in Diagnostic Virology

This section is intended to acquaint the reader with some of the uses to which RIA has been put in the diagnosis of viral infections, to cite detailed methods for RIA procedures other than those described in this chapter, and to indicate some of the attributes and advantages of RIA for detection of viral antigens and antibodies.

Vaccinia virus. Vaccinia virus was one of the first to which RIA was applied. Hayashi et al (25, 26) introduced the use of ^{125}I-labeled antibodies to detect specific viral antigens on the surface of vaccinia-infected cells. Rosenthal et al (48, 49) sensitized wells in polyvinyl microtiter plates with partially purified vaccinia virus and used these in RIA procedures for detection of vaccinia antigens and antibodies. For this micromethod, the wells were cut apart after performance of the test and placed in tubes for counting residual radioactivity. This approach was readily adopted for micro-RIA with other viruses. Hutchinson et al (29) used fixed vaccinia virus-infected cells on glass coverslips as a source of antigen for assay of vaccinia antibody by RIA. Ziegler et al (59) used lysates of vaccinia virus-infected cells adsorbed to microtiter cups to study antibody responses in smallpox patients and vaccinees, and found RIA titers to be slightly higher than those obtained by neutralization (Nt) tests in vaccinees and those obtained by hemagglutination inhibition (HAI) in smallpox patients. The indirect RIA method described in this chapter has been applied to detection of vaccinia virus antibodies in human serum and cerebrospinal fluid (18), and RIA antibody titers were markedly higher than those obtained by conventional serology.

Herpes simplex virus (HSV). Hayashi et al (25, 26) and Rosenthal et al (48, 49) early demonstrated the feasibility of using direct and indirect RIA to demonstrate herpes simplex virus antigens on the surface of fixed infected cells in culture, and Rosenthal et al (48, 49) reported on the use of a solid-phase micro-RIA using partially purified HSV adsorbed to polyvinyl micro-titer plates for assay of antibodies. Smith et al (52, 53) used partially purified HSV adsorbed to imitation pearls for antibody assay and obtained RIA titers which were 10 times higher than those obtained by plaque reduction neutralization. Kalimo et al (33, 34) utilized polystyrene balls coated with semi-purified HSV to test for herpes simplex virus-specific IgG and IgM anti-bodies in human sera, and more recently they extended this procedure to investigate class-specific antibody responses to the capsid, envelope, and excreted antigens of HSV (34).

Forghani et al (16, 17) used indirect solid-phase RIA with cross-absorbed HSV antisera for typing HSV isolates and for direct identification of HSV antigen in brain tissue from experimental animals and human infections. Piraino et al (47) employed a direct RIA for typing HSV isolates in unfixed, infected cell cultures, and Enlander et al (15) developed a competition RIA for detection of HSV for which purified HSV was labeled with ^{125}I and polystyrene tubes were coated with antibody.

RIA has been useful for type-specific identification of HSV antibodies in human serum and cerebrospinal fluid (CSF). In this laboratory a method was devised in which sera are cross-absorbed with HSV-1 and HSV-2 infected cells to remove cross-reacting antibodies and then tested for residual anti-bodies by indirect RIA against HSV-1 and HSV-2 infected cells (17). This method was used for studies correlating HSV antibody type specificity with the virus type(s) isolated at autopsy from human trigeminal, thoracic, and sacral ganglia (20), and in all instances virus types isolated correlated with the antibody type(s) demonstrable in the patients' sera. Patterson et al (46) recently described an RIA method for detecting HSV-1 and HSV-2 specific immune responses in human serum based upon using antigens adsorbed to crushed polystyrene as an immunoadsorbent to remove cross-reacting anti-bodies and then testing the adsorbed serum against HSV-1 and HSV-2 anti-gens adsorbed to plastic-coated beads.

RIA has been shown to be much more sensitive than complement fixation (CF) for demonstrating HSV antibodies in CSF of patients with herpes simplex encephalitis (18) and in CSF of patients with multiple sclerosis and other neurologic diseases (22).

Cytomegalovirus. In our laboratory we have demonstrated the feasibility of using direct RIA with a labeled CMV antiserum prepared in hamsters for identification of CMV isolates recovered from clinical specimens (19). Lausch et al (37) reported on the detection of virus-specific antigens on the surface of cells transformed by CMV using ^{125}I-labeled antibodies produced in rabbits. Knez et al (35) have used RIA to study the specific IgG and IgM antibody responses to CMV in human infections.

Rubella virus. The solid-phase indirect RIA described in this chapter has been found to be markedly more sensitive than HAI and CF tests for demonstration of rubella virus antibody in sera and CSF, and its greater sensitivity has been particularly useful in permitting detection of rubella virus antibody in CSF of patients with chronic rubella virus infections of the central nervous system (18) and in examining CSF of multiple sclerosis patients and control patients for rubella virus antibody (22).

Kalimo et al (32) used partially purified rubella virus adsorbed to polystyrene balls as a source of antigen for assaying specific IgG and IgM antibodies in human serum, and Meurman et al (43, 44, 45) extended this technique to study the persistence of rubella IgG and IgM antibody in postnatal infection. Compared to conventional rubella serologic tests, RIA was found to be more sensitive for detection of class-specific antibodies.

Measles virus. The indirect RIA procedure described in this chapter has also been found to be more sensitive than conventional serologic methods for detection of measles virus antibodies in serum and in CSF of patients with subacute sclerosing panencephalitis (SSPE) (18); it was also more sensitive than HAI and CF tests for detecting measles virus antibody in CSF of patients with multiple sclerosis and other neurologic diseases (22). Arstila et al (1) developed an indirect RIA technique using polystyrene balls coated with semipurified measles virus antigen for detecting measles IgG and IgM antibody in human serum and CSF, and reported high sensitivity for the procedure. Cunningham-Rundles et al (8) used ^{125}I-labeled subunit antigens from detergent-disrupted measles virus in a radioimmune precipitin test to study antibody responses to measles virus structural proteins in serum and CSF of patients with various neurologic diseases.

Joseph et al (31) used ^{125}I-labeled Fab fragments of measles virus antibody from human immune serum to study expression of specific viral antigens on the surface of HeLa cells persistently and acutely infected with measles virus, and were able to determine the amount of bound antibody required for each infected cell in order for complement dependent immune lysis to occur.

Studies performed in our laboratory demonstrated the feasibility of using the indirect RIA for demonstration of measles virus antigen directly in the brain tissue of SSPE patients and experimentally infected hamsters (21). Further, it was found that brain tissue from an SSPE patient in which measles antigen was demonstrable also contained specific measles virus antibody which could be eluted at low pH or with chaotropic ions and assayed by indirect RIA. By using highly purified radiolabeled antibodies specific for the various classes of human immunoglobulins, measles virus antibody eluted from SSPE brain tissue was shown to consist solely of immunoglobulins of the IgG class (21). Earlier Smith et al (53) had demonstrated that measles virus (and also HSV) antibody could be eluted from human arteries and assayed by RIA.

Influenza virus. Daugherty et al (10, 11) used a radioimmune precipitin test to measure the class-specific immune response to influenza virus infection. Using RIA to compare binding affinities of immune globulins for influenza virus antigens, Daugherty (13) concluded that IgG antibody had greater affinity for influenza antigens than did IgM antibody. Daugherty et al (12) also devised a solid-phase indirect RIA which utilized polystyrene tubes coated with immune globulin to bind semipurified influenza virus; this solid-phase antigen was then used to assay for influenza virus antibody in human serum by the indirect RIA procedure. RIA titers correlated well with HAI titers but not with CF titers. Braciale (4) used influenza virus covalently coupled to activated bromoacetylcellulose as a solid-phase antigen for indirect RIA of influenza virus antibodies.

Schieble and Cottam (50) applied solid-phase RIA to antigenic analysis of influenza A viruses by using virus-infected primary rhesus monkey kidney cells fixed to 1-dr glass vials as a source of antigen. In addition to the greater sensitivity of RIA over that of HAI, another advantage was the fact that both hemagglutinins and neuraminidase could be characterized in the RIA system.

Paramyxoviruses. Charlton and Blandford in 1975 (6) described an indirect micro solid-phase RIA for parainfluenza type 1 virus (Sendai strain) which utilized flexible polyvinyl microtiter plates. They reported that antibody titers obtained by RIA were 1000 times higher than those demonstrated by HAI. Yung et al (58) used a similar procedure for coating microtiter plates with parainfluenza antigen, and reported that RIA could differentiate between two parainfluenza type 1 strains. An indirect micro-RIA was developed for Newcastle disease virus (NDV) by Cleland et al (7). Virus-infected chick embryo cells grown in plastic microtiter plates and fixed with formalin were used as a source of antigen; again, RIA was found to be highly sensitive for assay of viral antibody.

Mumps virus. Daugherty et al (14) applied a solid-phase RIA to determine mumps class-specific immunoglobulins and reported a good correlation between RIA and CF results. The solid-phase RIA described in this chapter has also been applied for demonstration of mumps antibody in serum and CSF of patients with parotitis, and it was found to be more sensitive than HAI or CF (18).

Arboviruses. Dalrymple et al (9) used a radioimmune precipitation procedure for antigenic analysis of western and eastern equine encephalitis viruses and found results to be comparable to those obtained with plaque reduction neutralization tests in terms of sensitivity and specificity. Trent et al (55) developed a micro-solid-phase RIA for assay of antibodies to certain purified group B arboviruses and to envelope and nonstructural viral antigens. RIA antibody titers were 10- to 100-fold higher than those obtained by conventional serologic methods, and sharp type-specificity could be achieved through the use of appropriate antigens. Levitt et al (38) adapted the solid-phase RIA described in this chapter for rapid detection and identification of western equine encephalomyelitis virus from clinical specimens.

Other viruses. The reader is referred to the chapters on hepatitis (Chapter 29) and viral gastroenteritis (Chapter 30) for descriptions of RIA procedures which are useful in the diagnosis of infections with these agents.

Some of the other viruses capable of infecting humans to which RIA has been applied include rabies virus (56), lymphocytic choriomeningitis virus (3), and adenoviruses (51).

Conclusion

RIA procedures for detecting viral antigens and antibodies are most applicable and have the greatest potential value in diagnostic virology for large-scale studies which involve replicate testing with the same viruses, rather than for routine miscellaneous virus testing in smaller laboratories. However, the indirect procedure is very versatile since only labeled antispecies immune globulins are required, rather than individually labeled viruses or virus-specific antibodies. The sensitivity of the method makes it very useful for detecting small amounts of viral antigen directly in clinical materials and for demonstrating low levels of antigen or antibody in body fluids or exudates, and increasing use of RIA will undoubtedly be made for this purpose. Nonspecific reactivity appears to be less of a problem in RIA than in enzyme immunoassay, and this is a marked advantage of RIA in the examination of clinical materials.

RIA will undoubtedly find future application in studies aimed at identifying a possible viral etiology of certain chronic or degenerative diseases by demonstrating specific viral antibody in eluates from diseased tissue. Elution with chaotropic ions has been shown to be a very effective method for release of bound viral antibody from infected tissues (21, 53), and indirect RIA provides a very sensitive method for detecting virus-specific antibody in the eluates.

Appendix

Safety procedures for working with radioisotopes

Radiation safety and protection must be an integral part of the total safety program in an infectious disease laboratory working with radioisotopes or performing RIA. As discussed earlier, ^{125}I is a gamma emitter and its radiation is similar to x-rays in penetrating biologic substances. Several factors should be considered in avoiding or reducing exposure to ^{125}I radiation; these are proper shielding, time of exposure, and the distance from radioactive material.

Shielding. Gamma radiation exposure can be effectively reduced by keeping all radioactive material in the lead container (generally provided by the manufacturer) at all times except during pipetting.

Time. The radiation effects on biologic substances are cumulative, so the longer the exposure to ^{125}I, the higher the dose received and the greater the chances for radiation damage. Therefore, regardless of the quantity of radioactive material being used, the exposure should be no longer than absolutely necessary.

Distance. Distance is a very effective way of reducing radiation exposure. Thus, the storage of all radioactive material should be as far away as possible from the working area. Isotopes should be kept within reach only when they are used, and this is only a few minutes for RIA procedures.

Safety and protection guidelines

1. A film badge and finger ring must be worn all the time when working with radioactive materials.

2. Direct contact with radioactive material must be avoided by wearing protective laboratory coats and using disposable gloves.

3. Eating, drinking, smoking, or application of cosmetics must be prohibited in the working area or isotope storage area.

4. No mouth pipetting should be permitted for *any* reagents.

5. The workbench or hood must be covered with plastic-backed paper before starting to work.

6. All radioactive samples and containers should be clearly labeled.

7. All spills must be contained immediately and decontaminated as described below.

8. The work area should be monitored periodically for unnoticed spills.

9. The bench and the floor surfaces of the laboratory should be of non-absorbent material to facilitate decontamination of spills.

10. Disposable glassware should be used wherever possible, because effective washing of radioactivity from glassware is difficult and sometimes impossible.

11. Hands must be washed thoroughly after working with radioactive material. If hands inadvertently become contaminated, they must be monitored for radioactivity after scrubbing.

Accidents and spills of radioactive material

All necessary precautions should be taken to prevent accidents and spills; however, in the event that radioactive liquids are spilled, prompt measures should be taken to avoid spreading. The spill should be contained immediately with absorbent materials such as sponges, paper towels, gauze, etc. These items should be stored close to the working area and be easily accessible.

If the worker becomes contaminated, all contaminated clothing must be removed and contaminated skin must be washed thoroughly until the skin registers near to normal background counts with a Geiger counter.

If a workbench, floor, or hood is contaminated, the contaminated area should be marked off so that spreading can be avoided. The contaminated area should be washed with water-detergent soaked absorbent material and then wiped dry. The washing must be repeated until the monitor shows ≤4 times the background count.

Disposal of radioactive waste

Working with radioactive material inevitably produces liquid and solid radioactive waste, which must be disposed of properly without exposing the general public to either radiation or infectious materials. Therefore, all radioactive infectious material must be decontaminated before disposal either by autoclaving or by a liquid disinfectant such as Clorox or Cidex.

Solid waste is placed in autoclavable plastic bags separate from liquid waste; the latter is left in the original containers, which are closed and placed in plastic bags in such a manner as to avoid spilling. All waste containers should be marked "Radioactive Waste". Infectious material must be autoclaved before discarding. The plastic bag is placed into a second bag, placed in a covered autoclave pan, appropriately labeled with "Radioactive Waste" and used only for decontamination of radioactive material, and autoclaved. The materials are then held in an area apart from the general work and storage area until monitoring shows that radioactivity has decayed to 4 times the background level. Particularly "hot" radioactive waste, e.g., vials in which the isotope was received from the manufacturer, vials used for labeling, transfer pipettes, etc., should be shielded with lead until radioactivity has decayed. The radioactive waste should be identified as to the type of isotope, e.g., ^{125}I, ^{14}C, ^{51}Cr, ^{3}H, etc., and different isotopes should not be mixed, since they have different half-lives. Regardless of the level of radioactivity, radioactive waste should not be dumped into the general laboratory disposal system. Arrangements should be made with a licensed salvage company to pick up radioactive waste periodically.

References

1. ARSTILA P, VUORIMAA T, KALIMO K, HALONEN P, VILJANEN M, and TOIVANEN P: A solid-phase radioimmunoassay for IgG and IgM antibodies against measles virus. J Gen Virol 34:167–176, 1977

2. AVREMEAS S and TERNYNCK T: The cross-linking of proteins with glutaraldehyde and its use for the preparation of immunoadsorbent. Immunochemistry 6:53–66, 1969

3. BLECHSCHMIDT M, GERLICH W, and THOMSSEN R: Radioimmunoassay for LCM virus antigen and anti-LCM virus antibodies and its application in an epidemiologic survey of people exposed to Syrian hamsters. Med Microbiol Immunol 163:67–76, 1977

4. BRACIALE TJ, GERHARD W, and KLINMAN NR: Analysis of the humoral immune response to influenza virus in vitro. J Immunol 116:827–834, 1976

5. CATT K and TREGEAR GW: Solid-phase radioimmunoassay in antibody-coated tubes. Science 158:1570–1572, 1967

6. CHARLTON D and BLANDFORD G: A solid phase micro-radioimmunoassay to detect minute amounts of Ig class specific anti-viral antibody in a mouse model system. J Immunol Methods 8:319–330, 1975

7. CLELAND GB, PEREY DYE, and DENT PB: Micro-radioimmunoassay for antibodies to Newcastle disease virus in the chicken. J Immunol 114:422–425, 1975

8. CUNNINGHAM-RUNDLES C, JERSILD C, DUPONT B, POSNER JB, and GOOD RA: Detection of measles antibodies in cerebrospinal fluid and serum by a radioimmunoassay. Scand J Immunol 4:785–790, 1975

9. DALRYMPLE JM, TERAMOTO AY, CARDIFF RD, and RUSSELL PK: Radioimmune precipitation of group A arboviruses. J Immunol 109:426–433, 1972

10. DAUGHERTY H: Immunoprecipitin reaction of influenza virus-antibody complex with anti-IgG. J Immunol 107:802–809, 1971

11. DAUGHERTY H, DAVIS ML, and KAYE HS: Immunoglobulin class of influenza antibodies investigated by radioimmunoassay (RIA). J Immunol 109:849–856, 1972

12. DAUGHERTY H, WARFIELD DT, and DAVIS ML: Solid-phase radioimmunoassay of total and influenza specific immunoglobulin G. Appl Microbiol 23:360–367, 1972

13. DAUGHERTY H: Preferential radioassay of influenza-specific 7S (IgG) over 19S (IgM) class of antibodies. J Immunol 111:404–409, 1973

14. DAUGHERTY H, WARFIELD DT, HEMINGWAY WD, and CASEY HL: Mumps class-specific immunoglobulins in radioimmunoassay and conventional serology. Infect Immun 7:380–385, 1973

15. ENLANDER D, DOS REMEDIOS LV, WEBER PM, and DREW L: Radioimmunoassay for herpes simplex virus. J Immunol Methods 10:357–362, 1976

16. FORGHANI B, SCHMIDT NJ, and LENNETTE EH: Solid-phase radioimmunoassay for identification of herpesvirus hominis types 1 and 2 from clinical materials. Appl Microbiol 28:661–667, 1974

17. FORGHANI B, SCHMIDT NJ, and LENNETTE EH: Solid-phase radioimmunoassay for typing herpes simplex viral antibodies in human sera. J Clin Microbiol 2:410–418, 1975

18. FORGHANI B, SCHMIDT NJ, and LENNETTE EH: Sensitivity of a radioimmunoassay method for detection of certain viral antibodies in sera and cerebrospinal fluids. J Clin Microbiol 4:470–478, 1976

19. FORGHANI B, SCHMIDT NJ, and LENNETTE EH: Antisera to human cytomegalovirus produced in hamsters: reactivity in radioimmunoassay and other antibody assay systems. Infect Immun 14:1184–1190, 1976

20. FORGHANI B, KLASSEN T, and BARINGER JR: Radioimmunoassay of herpes simplex virus antibody: correlation with ganglionic infection. J Gen Virol 36:371–375, 1977

21. FORGHANI B, SCHMIDT NJ, and LENNETTE EH: Radioimmunoassay of measles virus antigen and antibody in SSPE brain tissue. Proc Soc Exp Biol Med 157:268–272, 1978

22. FORGHANI B, CREMER NE, JOHNSON KP, GINSBERG AH, and LIKOSKY WH: Viral antibody in cerebrospinal fluid of multiple sclerosis and control patients: comparison between radioimmunoassay and conventional techniques. J Clin Microbiol 7:63–69, 1978

23. GERLOFF RK, HOYER BH, and McLAREN LC: Precipitation of radio-labeled poliovirus with specific antibody and antiglobulin. J Immunol 89:559–570, 1962

24. GLOVER JS, SALTER DN, and SHEPHERD BP: A study of some factors that influence the iodination of OX insulin. Biochem J 103:120–128, 1967

25. HAYASHI K, ROSENTHAL J, and NOTKINS AL: Iodine-125-labeled antibody to viral antigens binding to the surface of virus-infected cells. Science 176:516–518, 1972

26. HAYASHI K, LODMELL D, ROSENTHAL J, and NOTKINS AL: Binding of ^{125}I-labeled anti-IgG, rheumatoid factor and anti-C3 to immune complexes on the surface of virus-infected cells. J Immunol 110:316–319, 1973

27. HUNTER WM and GREENWOOD FC: Preparation of iodine-131 labeled human growth hormone of high specific activity. Nature (London) 194:495–496, 1962

28. HUNTER WM: Radioimmunoassay In Handbook of Experimental Immunology, 2nd edition, Weir DM (ed), Blackwell Scientific Publications, Chapter 17, 1973

29. HUTCHINSON HD and ZIEGLER DW: Simplified radioimmunoassay for diagnostic serology. Appl Microbiol 24:742–749, 1972

30. HUTCHINSON HD, ZIEGLER DW, and FEORINO PM: Radioimmunoassay for detection of antibodies to Epstein-Barr virus in human infectious mononucleosis serum specimens. J Clin Microbiol 1:429–433, 1975

31. JOSEPH BS, PERRIN LH, and OLDSTONE MBA: Measurement of virus antigens on the surface of HeLa cells persistently infected with wild type and vaccine strains of measles virus by radioimmune assay. J Gen Virol 30:329–337, 1976

32. KALIMO KOK, MEURMAN OH, HALONEN PE, ZIOLA BR, VILJANEN MK, GRANFORS K, and TOIVANEN P: Solid-phase radioimmunoassay of rubella virus immunoglobulin G and immunoglobulin M antibodies. J Clin Microbiol 4:117–123, 1976

33. KALIMO KOK, ZIOLA BR, VILJANEN MK, GRANFORS K, and TOIVANEN P: Solid-phase radioimmunoassay of herpes simplex virus IgG and IgM antibodies. J Immunol Methods 14:183–195, 1977

34. KALIMO KOK, MARTTILA BJ, GRANFORS K, and VILJANEN MK: Solid-phase radioimmunoassay of human immunoglobulin M and immunoglobulin G antibodies against herpes simplex type 1 capsid, envelope, and excreted antigen. Infect Immun 15:883–889, 1977

35. KNEZ V, STEWART JA, and ZIEGLER DW: Cytomegalovirus specific IgM and IgG response in humans studied by radioimmunoassay. J Immunol 117:2006–2013, 1976

36. LANDER JJ, ALTER HJ, and PURCELL RH: Frequency of antibody to hepatitis-associated antigen as measured by a new radioimmunoassay technique. J Immunol 106:1166–1171, 1971

37. LAUSH RN, MURASKO DM, ALBRECHT T, and RAPP F: Detection of specific surface antigen on cells transformed by cytomegalovirus with the techniques of mixed hemagglutination and ^{125}I-labeled antiglobulin. J Immunol 112:1680–1684, 1974

38. LEWITT NH, MILLER HV, and EDDY GA: Solid-phase radioimmunoassay for rapid detection and identification of western equine encephalomyelitis virus. J Clin Microbiol 4:382–383, 1976

39. LING CM and OVERBY LR: Prevalence of hepatitis B virus antigen as revealed by direct radioimmune assay with ^{125}I-antibody. J Immunol 109:834–841, 1972

40. MARCHALONIS JJ: An enzymic method for trace iodination of immunoglobulins and other proteins. Biochem J 113:299–305, 1969

41. McCONAHEY PJ and DIXON FJ: A method of trace iodination of proteins for immunologic studies. Int Arch Allergy Appl Immunol 29:185–189, 1966

42. McFARLANE AS: Efficient trace-labeling of proteins with iodine. Nature (London) 182:53, 1958

43. MEURMAN OH, VALJANEN MK, and GRANFORS K: Solid-phase radioimmunoassay of rubella virus immunoglobulin M antibodies: comparison with sucrose density gradient centrifugation test. J Clin Microbiol 5:257–262, 1977

44. MEURMAN OH: Persistence of immunoglobulin G and immunoglobulin M antibodies after postnatal rubella infection determined by solid-phase radioimmunoassay. J Clin Microbiol 7:34–38, 1978

45. MEURMAN OH: Antibody responses in patients with rubella infection determined by passive hemagglutination, hemagglutination inhibition, complement fixation and solid-phase radioimmunoassay tests. Infect Immun 19:369–372, 1978

46. PATTERSON WR, RAWLS WE, and SMITH KO: Differentiation of serum antibodies to herpesvirus types 1 and 2 by radioimmunoassay. Proc Soc Exp Biol Med 157:273–277, 1978

47. PIRAINO FF, SEDMACK G, ALTSHULER C, and PIERCE R: Rapid antigenic typing of herpes hominis isolates on the surface of infected cells by kinetic binding of ^{125}I-labeled HVI antibodies. Am J Clin Pathol 62:581–590, 1974

48. ROSENTHAL JD, HAYASHI K, and NOTKINS AL: Rapid microradioimmunoassay for the measurement of antiviral antibody. J Immunol 109:171–173, 1972

49. ROSENTHAL JD, HAYASHI K, and NOTKINS AL: Comparison of direct and indirect solid-phase radioimmunoassay for detection of viral antigens and antiviral antibody. Appl Microbiol 25:567–573, 1973

50. SCHIEBLE JH and COTTAM D: Solid-phase radioimmunoassay as a method for evaluating antigenic differences in type A influenza viruses. Infect Immun 15:66–71, 1977

51. SCOTT JV, DREESMAN GR, SPIRA G, and KASEL JA: Radioimmunoassay of human serum antibody specific for adenovirus type 5-purified fiber. J Immunol 115:124–128, 1975

52. SMITH KO, GEHLE WD, and McCRACKEN AW: Radioimmunoassay techniques for detecting naturally occurring viral antibody in human sera. J Immunol Methods 5:337–344, 1974

53. SMITH KO, GEHLE WD, and SANFORD BA: Evidence for chronic viral infections in human arteries. Proc Soc Exp Biol Med 147:357–360, 1974

54. THORELL JI and JOHANSSON BG: Enzymatic iodination of polypeptides with ^{125}I to high specific activity. Biochim Biophys Acta 521:363–369, 1971

55. TRENT DW, HARVEY CL, QUIESHI A, and LeSTOURGEON D: Solid-phase radioimmunoassay for antibodies to flavivirus structural and nonstructural proteins. Infect Immun 13:1325–1333, 1976

56. WIKTOR RJ, KOPROWSKI H, and DIXON F: Radioimmunoassay procedures for rabies binding antibodies. J Immunol 109:464–470, 1972

57. YALOW RW and BERSON SA: Immunoassay of endogenous plasma insulin in man. J Clin Invest 39:1157–1175, 1960

58. YUNG LLL, LOH W, and TER MEULEN V: Solid-phase indirect radioimmunoassay: standardization and application in viral serology. Med Microbiol Immunol 163:111–123, 1977

59. ZIEGLER DW, HUTCHINSON HD, KOPLAN JP, and NAKANO JH: Detection by radioimmunoassay of antibodies in human smallpox patients and vaccinees. J Clin Microbiol 1:311–317, 1975

CHAPTER 7

IMMUNOGLOBULIN CLASSES AND VIRAL DIAGNOSIS

Natalie E. Cremer and John L. Riggs

Introduction

It is at times desirable to know the immunoglobulin class of a viral antibody when evaluating the presence of viral infection by serologic techniques. Usually, a current infection can be determined by a significant rise in antibody titer between an acute-phase and a convalescent-phase serum specimen. In a test employing doubling dilutions of the serum, a 4-fold or greater rise in antibody titer is considered of significance, whereas a 2-fold difference is considered to be within the technical error of the test. If there is a delay in the collection of the acute-phase serum, the antibody titer in such a specimen may already be elevated, and no difference in antibody titer between the 2 sera may be demonstrable. In other cases, although the acute-phase serum was collected at an optimal time, the concentration of IgM antibody may be elevated, and it will mask an increase in the IgG antibody concentration when the antibody titers of the acute- and convalescent-phase sera are compared. Such a situation, of course, can only occur if the assay used for antibody determination detects both classes of antibodies. It is more likely to occur in an assay method which is more reactive with IgM than IgG antibody, as for example in the passive (indirect) hemagglutination test (PHA) (22, 23). Upon removal of the IgM fraction from the serum, the rise in titer of the IgG class of antibodies becomes apparent.

The IgM class of viral antibodies is the first to appear in an immune response and is followed by IgG antibodies, usually within a few days (22), although the latter have also been detected in serum simultaneously with the appearance of IgM antibodies (15, 22, 23, 51). IgM antibodies usually are the first to disappear after infection, and their presence in the serum suggests a recent or current infection. This does not invariably hold, however, as there are reports of persistence of IgM antibody for several months and longer (12, 22, 43, 49, 51, 53). Conversely, the absence of IgM antibody in a serum sample containing IgG antibody suggests a past exposure to the virus in question. Reinfection or revaccination can result in reappearance of IgM antibody, and so the mere presence of IgM antibody does not necessarily distinguish between a primary and a secondary infection (50, 52).

The determination of antibody class is of particular importance in the diagnosis of possible maternal infection after exposure to teratogenic viruses such as rubella or cytomegaloviruses (CMV) during pregnancy. If the maternal antibody is of the IgM class, the possibility of a current viral infection exists, with its attendant danger of infection to the fetus. Antibody of fetal origin produced in response to fetal infection is also of the IgM class. Since IgG but not IgM antibody passes the placental barrier, assay of neonatal serum for these classes of viral antibodies distinguishes between IgM antibody synthesized by the infant in response to viral infection *in utero* and maternal IgG antibody passively received by placental passage.

Fewer studies have been directed at the sequential appearance of viral antibodies of the IgA class of immunoglobulins. Demonstration of serum IgA antibody as evidence of recent infection is a controversial issue, as not all investigators are in agreement as to the time of its appearance and disappearance in the blood stream in viral infection. Thus Bürgin-Wolff et al (15) reported an early appearance and disappearance of IgA antibody during infection with rubella virus. Cradock-Watson et al (23) considered the presence of IgA antibody as indicative of recent rubella infection in adults, but they were unable to detect IgA antibody in infants congenitally infected with rubella virus (24). On the other hand, Al-Nakib et al (3) reported the persistence, for at least 1 year, of serum IgA antibodies to rubella virus detected by the hemagglutination-inhibition test (HAI). Hornsleth et al (42), using the indirect fluorescent-antibody test (IFA), noted the presence of serum IgA antibodies within a day or more of onset of rubella and their disappearance after 2 weeks to several years. They and Al-Nakib et al concluded that the presence of IgA antibodies in the serum cannot be interpreted as evidence of recent infection. Ogra et al (52, 53), using a radioimmunodiffusion test, also demonstrated the persistence of IgA antibody in rubella and poliovirus infections for a year or more.

The sequence of appearance and disappearance of antibodies reported for the various classes naturally depends on how early in the disease and how often the serum samples were taken and on the sensitivity and accuracy of the assay procedure(s) for the various classes of antibody. Table 7.1 lists some representative studies, selected because serum samples were collected and evaluated at fairly frequent intervals over an extended period.

Pitfalls in Detection of IgM Antibody

A potential source of error in the identification of viral IgM antibody is the presence in the serum of rheumatoid factor (RF) (32, 64), an anti-IgG antibody often of the IgM class but also at times of the IgG class. RF of the IgA class has also been reported (1, 39). It is present in serum of individuals with rheumatoid disease, as well as in some individuals with nonrheumatoid disease and even in some apparently healthy individuals. In a study on the presence of RF in nonrheumatoid conditions, 14–17% of patients with viral diseases that included viral pneumonia, influenza, and herpes zoster had IgM RF in their serum (9). Production of IgM RF is also reported in infec-

TABLE 7.1—SEQUENCE OF APPEARANCE OF CLASSES OF VIRAL ANTIBODY IN PATIENTS AFTER ONSET OF NATURALLY ACQUIRED DISEASE

VIRUS	ASSAY	IgM			IgG			IgA			CHECK FOR RF	IgG ABSORPTION	CITATION
		EARLY	PEAK	DURATION	EARLY	PEAK	DURATION	EARLY	PEAK	DURATION			
Epstein-Barr 23 patients	IFA	3-4d	1-2w*	8-10w	3-4d	1w*	>80w*	ND	ND	ND	yes	no	51
Rotavirus 24 patients	IFA	≤7d	2w*	5w	≤7d	3w*	>40w*	ND	ND	ND	yes	yes	54
Japanese encephalitis 6 patients	GF + HAI	3d	<10d*	≥6m	8-30d	>30*	>6m*	ND	ND	ND	no	no	43
Mumps 72 patients	IFA	≥1d	1-3w	≥6-9m	ND	ND	ND	≥5d	1-3w	≥6-9m	no	no	12
Measles 10 patients	IFA	3-5d	5-10d*	6-7w	3-5d	5-10d*	>4y*	ND	ND	ND	no	no	19
Rubella 11 patients	SG + IFA	2d	~2w*	3w	1-3d	7d*	>3m*	1-3d	~2w*	1m	yes	no	23
Rubella 8 patients	IFA	≤5d	5d*	7w	≤5d	7d*	>6m*	ND	ND	ND	no	no	36
Rubella 7 patients	IFA + HAI	≥1d	1-3w*	4-5w	ND	ND	ND	≥1d	10d*	3w to >1y	no	yes	42
Rubella 25 patients	RID	≥1d	2w*	2m	≥1d	2w*	>12m*	1m	>2m	>12m	no	no	53

Early = Day(s) antibody was first detected in some patients.
Peak = Day(s) antibody was detected in all or most of the patients.
Duration = Length of time antibody was detected in some patients.
d = day; w = week; m = month; y = year; IFA = indirect fluorescent antibody; GF = gel filtration: SG = sucrose gradient; HAI = hemagglutination inhibition; RID = radioimmunodiffusion; RF = rheumatoid factor; ND = not done
* = Antibody was detected in all patients at indicated time.

tions with CMV (44), measles, rubella, and herpes simplex viruses (64). IgM RF has been found in neonates congenitally infected with *Treponema pallidum*, CMV, rubella virus, and toxoplasma. The IgM antibody was presumably elicited by the allotypic antigens (Gm antigens) of the maternal IgG (56). In this study, 44 of 50 (88%) infected infants and 6 of 42 (16%) normal infants had IgM anti-IgG antibody titers. Formation of RF to maternal IgG allotypes in normal infants and young children is not uncommon (35, 65, 66). Titers of IgM antibody to IgG begin to rise in the infant at approximately 4 months of age, at the time of decline of circulating maternal antibody which has a half-life of about 23 days. During this period the infant is exposed to and can become infected with a variety of infectious agents. It is speculated that as the infant matures the immunologic tolerance of the infant to maternal IgG is broken because of the declining concentration in maternal IgG. Antibody production to maternal allotypes may then be stimulated by immunogenic complexes formed between residual maternal IgG antibody and infectious agents contracted by the infant (56). IgM anti-IgG production reaches a maximum between 12 and 18 months of age and then declines (35, 65, 66).

If specific viral antibody of the IgG class is present in serum also containing IgM RF, the RF will complex with the viral IgG antibody in the same manner as with any other IgG molecules. Upon density gradient centrifugation or gel filtration, the IgG viral antibody in the complex will not appear in the IgG fractions but in those containing IgM immunoglobulin, and the erroneous conclusion can be made that IgM viral antibody is present in the serum sample (57). The same problem exists with assays employing fixed infected cells or antigens, treated sequentially with patient's serum and labeled antibody specific for the μ chain, such as in IFA (20, 58), enzyme-linked immunosorbent tests (ELISA) (27, 28), or solid-phase radioimmunoassay (RIA) (30). The labeled anti-μ antibody will react with the IgM RF-IgG viral antibody complex, and the test will be erroneously scored positive for IgM viral antibody. To avoid this pitfall, serum can be tested for RF prior to assay for class of viral antibody. A useful test is the latex globulin test performed either on slides or in tubes. The reagent is available commercially from a number of sources.

More difficult to assess are those sera which do not react in tests for RF, but nevertheless contain the factor (51, 64). A prudent course, therefore, is to consider all sera as possibly RF-positive and treat them for removal of RF prior to testing for class of antibody.

If RF is present in a serum, it can be removed by absorption of the serum with IgG that has been insolubilized by heating to 73 C for 10 min (64) or by reaction with a cross-linking reagent such as glutaraldehyde (6, 7). When IgG insolubilized by glutaraldehyde is used for serum absorption, in addition to removal of RF activity there can be a loss in IgG, IgA, and non-RF IgM because of nonspecific absorption, probably due in part to binding with unreacted glutaraldehyde bonds. Such bonds can be blocked by treatment of the insolubilized IgG with 0.3 M glycine at pH 7.2 (56). Such treatment reduces, but does not eliminate, nonspecific loss of the various immunoglobulins.

A second potential problem in the detection of IgM viral antibody is the inhibitory effect of IgG viral antibody when both classes of antibody are simultaneously present in the serum sample (4, 62). The inhibitory effect can be noted in assays such as IFA, ELISA, or solid-phase RIA, but not in assays where immunoglobulin classes are physically separated, as in gel filtration or gradient centrifugation. It is also not a problem if the concentration of IgG antibody is very low and the IgM antibody concentration is high, as sometimes occurs early in infection. The inhibitory effect of IgG antibody can be reduced somewhat by prolonging the incubation period of the patient's serum and the fixed virus preparation from 1 hr to 3 hr and by allowing the reaction to occur at 37 C rather than at room temperature. Such conditions permit the larger and slower-diffusing IgM molecule to compete more successfully with the smaller, faster-diffusing IgG molecule for antigen binding sites.

In addition to altering the incubation conditions to favor IgM reaction, it is often necessary to remove physically the IgG antibody. At present the most used method is absorption with a *Staphylococcus aureus* strain (Cowan I strain) that produces a cell-wall substance designated protein A (4, 31). Protein A binds to the Fc portion of the IgG molecule, causing the IgG to adhere to the bacteria. The complex is then removed by centrifugation. In this manner IgG in a serum sample is reduced by 92–98% (31). Protein A binds to IgG subclasses IgG1, IgG2, and IgG4. IgG3, which accounts for approximately 5% of the total serum IgG, is not removed (46).

Although reported in the literature as a simple method for detection of IgM and IgA antibody (4), mere treatment of a serum with protein A is not sufficient to warrant the conclusion that the residual antibodies are of these classes. Viral antibody of the IgG3 subclass can also be present. Early reports on the removal of IgG by protein A indicated that the concentration of other serum immunoglobulins was not substantially affected (4). Later studies show, however, that IgM concentrations can be reduced by 30–60% (18, 38, 47, 59) and IgA similarly. This discrepancy in results may reflect differences in the antigenic composition of the various populations of IgM molecules studies (34, 38, 47).

Another absorption method successfully used for removal of IgG was absorption with DEAE Sephadex 50, which reduced the IgG concentration by 95% (41). IgM and IgA were reduced by 50–80%. The ratio of IgM to IgG, however, increased from 1:10 to 1:2 and allowed the detection of IgM antibody to rubella virus in serum samples taken during natural infection.

Although IgM antibody is more easily reduced by 2-mercaptoethanol (2-ME) than is IgG antibody, the use of 2-ME to distinguish between these classes in whole serum has serious drawbacks (8, 21, 29, 69). In order to demonstrate IgM antibody, a 4-fold or greater reduction in serum antibody titer after treatment with 2-ME is required. IgG antibody may represent the major portion of the antibody, even in an early immune response and certainly later in the infection. If its concentration is sufficiently greater than that of the IgM antibody, any reduction in IgM antibody titer due to the treatment with 2-ME will be masked. Also, certain populations of IgG antibody are reported sensitive to 2-ME, in the concentration used for reduction of IgM antibody (22). Neutralizing activity of IgG antibody to influenza virus was reported reduced by 2-ME, as was the precipitating ability of IgG antibody to foot-and-mouth disease (2). A satisfactory use of 2-ME is for characterization of IgM fractions after separation of serum by gradient centrifugation or gel filtration (16).

Assay of Serum for Class of Antibody

The usual methods for identification of viral antibodies by immunoglobulin class are sucrose gradient centrifugation, gel filtration, and IFA (29, 36), or some of the more recent modifications of the technique using different labels, such as in RIA (30, 45) and ELISA (27, 28). Sucrose gradients and gel filtration are useful for separation of IgM and IgG, but not of IgG and IgA, because of their similar molecular size and density. In addition these techniques are time consuming in their performance, and fractions from gel filtration require concentration prior to assay because of dilution during elution. On the other hand, because there is an actual separation of IgM and IgG, a variety of techniques can be used for the antibody assay of the separated fractions, a definite advantage in studying the different functions of viral antibodies.

The use of labeled antibodies to heavy chains, as in IFA, RIA, and ELISA, also has advantages and disadvantages. Highly specific labeled antibodies are required, and nonspecificity may be a problem. The interference between IgG antibodies and IgM antibodies has already been discussed. Although the IgG can be removed by absorption with *S. aureus* protein A, there is also a 30–60% loss of IgM. If the antibody titer of the latter is sufficiently high, the loss is not a problem. If the concentration is minimal, the titer of antibody might drop below the detectable level. On the positive side, the technique does afford the possibility of identifying any of the immunoglobulin classes, including IgD and IgE, as long as specific antiserum can be obtained.

Methods for preparation of serum
Preparation of insolubilized IgG (6, 7)

  1. Prepare an aqueous solution of 2.5% glutaraldehyde.
  2. Solubilize 500 mg of human IgG or Cohn fraction II from human serum in 10 ml of 0.1 M phosphate buffer, pH 7.
  Buffer formulation:
      Solution A: 13.8 g $NaH_2PO_4 \cdot H_2O$/1 liter H_2O
      Solution B: 21.3 g Na_2HPO_4/1.5 liter H_2O
  Mix 780 ml of solution A with 1220 ml of solution B. Add NaN_2 to a final concentration of 0.1%.
  3. With stirring, add by the drop 2 ml of 2.5% glutaraldehyde to the IgG sample. A gel will form quickly.
  4. Allow the gel to react for 3 hr at room temperature.
  5. Disperse the gel in 200 ml of 0.01 M phosphate buffered saline (PBS), pH 7.2.

Buffer formulation:

Solution A: $NaH_2PO_4 \cdot H_2O$, 0.69 g; NaCl, 4.25 g; to 500 ml with distilled H_2O

Solution B: Na_2HPO_4, 1.42 g; NaCl, 8.50 g; to 1 liter with distilled H_2O

Mix 280 ml of solution A with 720 ml of solution B. Check pH; adjust if necessary. Add NaN_2 to a final concentration of 0.1%.

6. Homogenize the gel in small increments with a mortar and pestle until a smooth suspension is achieved. Collect the insolubilized IgG by centrifugation at 1570 × g (3000 rpm with a rotating radius of 15.6 cm) for 15 min at 5 C.

7. Wash the suspension with PBS 2 times.

8. Suspend the packed, insolubilized IgG in 50 ml of 0.3 M glycine buffer, pH 7.2–7.4 (3.65 g glycine/100 ml H_2O + 1 ml 0.3 M NaOH). Allow it to react with stirring for 3 hr at room temperature.

9. Collect the insolubilized IgG by centrifugation and resuspend it in PBS. Wash the material with PBS until the optical density of the supernatant fluid at 280 nm is background.

10. Resuspend the packed insolubilized IgG in PBS to make a 50% slurry. Store the slurry at 5 C. Prior to use each time, wash it once with PBS.

11. Determine the optimal concentration of the insolubilized IgG necessary to remove the RF in a strongly reactive serum of known titer. Add 0.1 ml of serum and 0.3 ml of PBS to the packed sediment from 0.1, 0.2, 0.4 and 0.6 ml of the IgG slurry.

12. Thoroughly resuspend the sediment. Incubate the mixture for 1 hr at 37 C with intermittent mixing.

13. Collect the supernatant fluid by centrifugation. Check it for RF. Determine the amount of insolubilized IgG which completely removed the RF or which reduced it below the dilution to be used in the antibody assay.

Absorption of serum for rheumatoid factor

1. Thoroughly mix 0.2 ml serum and 0.6 ml PBS with the packed sediment from the optimal amount of the 50% IgG slurry as previously determined. Incubate the mixture with intermittent stirring for 1 hr at 37 C.

2. Collect the supernatant fluid by centrifugation at 1570 × g for 15 min at 5 C.

3. Check the fluid for RF. If negative, proceed with IgM assay. If positive, repeat the absorption.

Preparation of S. aureus, protein A (4, 48)

As previously discussed, in addition to removal of RF from serum prior to assay for IgM antibody by IFA, it is advisable to remove also IgG antibody, particularly if it is present in high concentration.

1. Prepare CCY medium (5) for cultivation of *S. aureus,* Cowan strain I (available from American Type Culture Collection, 12301 Parklawn Drive, Rockville, MD 20852).

a. CCY broth:

Casein hydrolysate	40	g
Yeast extract	10	g
Sodium lactate (50%)	10	ml
$Na_2HPO_4 \cdot 2H_2O$	1	g
KH_2PO_4	0.4	g
$(NH_4)_2SO_4$	1	g
dl-trytophane	80	mg
L-cystine	100	mg
Agar	20	g
Distilled water	900	ml

Sterilize the medium at 120 C for 15 min, at 15 lb pressure.

b. Sodium β-glycerophosphate	20	g
Distilled water	100	ml

c. Vitamin stock solution:

Thiamine   20   mg
Nicotinic acid   40   mg
Distilled water   100   ml

d. Trace elements stock solution:

$MgSO_4 \cdot 7H_2O$ . . . .   0.2   g
$MnSO_4 \cdot 4H_2O$ . . . .   0.1   g
$FeSO_4 \cdot 7H_2O$ . . . .   0.06   g
Citric acid . . . .   0.06   g
Distilled water . . . .   100.0 ml

Sterilize solution b, c, and d by filtration through a Millipore filter, 0.45 μ.

After the broth-agar medium has cooled to about 50 C, add 100 ml of solution b (sodium β-glycerophosphate) and 10 ml each of the vitamin and trace element solutions. Dispense the medium into Roux bottles or similar vessel. (For preparation of starter cultures, prepare CCY broth without agar, but adding the other solutions. Trypticase soy agar and trypticase soy broth have been also used in place of CCY medium (45).)

2. Cultivate a log-phase broth culture of S. *aureus* by incubation of inoculated broth at 37 C for 6 hr.

3. Inoculate the log-phase broth culture onto the agar medium using a volume sufficient to just cover the agar surface.

4. Incubate the cultures for 18 hr at 37 C.

5. Collect the bacteria by gentle washing of the agar surface with PBS, pH 7.2. (For formulation of the buffer, see preparation of insolubilized IgG.)

6. Wash the bacteria 3 times with PBS, collecting the bacteria each time by centrifugation at 2791 × g (4000 rpm with rotating radius of 15.6 cm) for 10 min at 5 C.

7. Suspend the bacteria in 100 ml of 0.5% formaldehyde in PBS, and allow the suspension to mix at room temperature for 3 hr.

8. Collect the bacteria by centrifugation, and wash them 2 times with PBS.

9. Resuspend the bacteria to a 10% suspension in PBS. Heat the suspension at 65 C for 30 min with intermittent mixing.

10. Wash the bacteria 2 times with PBS. Resuspend the bacteria to a 10% suspension in PBS.

11. Store the bacterial suspension at 5 C. Each time prior to use wash the bacteria once with PBS.

Absorption of serum with S. aureus, protein A

1. Mix 0.2 ml of serum with the packed bacteria from 2 ml of 10% suspension of S. *aureus*. (One ml of 10% suspension will remove 1.34 ± 0.49 mg IgG.) (4, 18).

2. Incubate the mixture at room temperature for 30 min.

3. Add 0.6 ml of PBS. Mix the suspension and centrifuge it at 2275 × g for 10 min.

4. Collect the supernatant fluid. Check the fluid for removal of IgG and for loss of IgM by radial immunodiffusion. Plates for radial immunodiffusion are available from a number of commercial sources.

Methods of distinguishing classes

Sucrose gradient centrifugation for assay of IgM antibody

1. Prepare in the cold a 10–40% linear sucrose gradient in a sterile 5-ml cellulose nitrate tube, either by using a gradient maker or by layering sequentially 1.5 ml of 40%, 25%, and 10% concentrations of sucrose (26). The sucrose solutions are prepared in PBS, pH 7.2 (see preparation of insolubilized IgG for formulation).

2. If the gradient is prepared manually by layering the various concentrations, allow the gradient to equilibrate by diffusion in the cold a minimum of 6 hr or, if more convenient, overnight. If the gradient is prepared with a gradient maker, it can be used immediately.

3. Prepare the serum sample for the particular antibody assay to be used. For example, if gradient fractions will be assayed by HAI, absorb the serum with the appropriate red blood cells. If serum inhibitors are present that have similar density as the immunoglobulin under test, remove them by appropriate treatment of the serum.

Nonspecific inhibitors of influenza hemagglutination in some sera are reported to disperse throughout the whole gradient (14), while in others they are found in the denser fractions of the gradient. In the assay of serum for antibody to rubella virus, removal of the lipoprotein inhibitor is not necessary for evaluation of IgM antibody, since the inhibitor is present at the top of the gradient. However, its removal is required if a clean separation between inhibitor and IgG antibody is desired. It should also be removed if IgM is evaluated by gel filtration rather than sucrose gradient. Lipemic inhibitory material resistant to 2-ME was reported to elute with the IgM fraction (55), even with serum treated with heparin $MnCl_2$ but stored at -20 C for a month or more. Such false-positive reactions were not seen with freshly drawn serum recently treated with heparin $MnCl_2$ for removal of nonspecific inhibitors (55). It was suggested that heparin $MnCl_2$ failed to remove lipoproteins that are altered by storage. Another source of error in determination of IgM antibody to rubella virus by HAI is the presence of inhibitory material in serum contaminated with bacteria which elutes with the IgM fraction (55).

If the serum is treated for nonspecific inhibitors by the heparin $MnCl_2$ method (17), prepare the sucrose solutions in HEPES buffered saline (N-2-hydroxyethylpiperazine-N-2-ethanesulfonic acid, 5.96 g; NaCl, 8.19 g; $CaCl_2 \cdot 2H_2O$, 0.148 g; distilled H_2O to 1 liter) instead of PBS. The phosphate ions in the PBS cause precipitation of any residual heparin $MnCl_2$ in the serum, making it unusable for gradient centrifugation. As already discussed, if RF is present, absorb the serum appropriately.

The serum *should not be heated* prior to centrifugation or gel filtration, as aggregation of the serum proteins will occur and a clean separation of immunoglobulin classes will not be achieved.

The serum should be clear and free of particulate matter. If the serum is lipemic, the lipids can be removed by centrifuging the chilled specimen for 30 min at about 25,000 $\times$ g at 0 C. The lipids will form a solid layer at the top of the specimen. The clear serum can then be withdrawn with a syringe by insertion of the needle below the lipid layer.

4. Layer onto the top of the gradient 0.5 ml of a 1:4 dilution of the serum in PBS or other appropriately buffered saline solution. Gently mix the interface between the gradient and the serum, being careful not to mix the rest of the gradient.

5. Centrifuge the gradient in the cold for 18 hr at 100,000 $\times$ g in a swinging bucket rotor capable of accommodating the 5-ml tube. A number of such rotors are available, i.e., the SW39, SW50, SW50.1, and others. At the termination of centrifugation allow the rotor to decelerate without the brake.

6. Collect 0.5-ml samples *from the bottom* of the gradient, either automatically with a fraction collector or manually by puncturing the bottom of the tube with a needle and allowing the gradient to drip into calibrated and marked tubes. Collection of the fractions from the top of the gradient is not recommended as IgM fractions may become contaminated by the prior passage of IgG through the collection outlet. There are a number of simple and useful gadgets for manual collection of gradients. One of the simplest types is depicted in Figure 7.1. The flow rate is controlled by the slow release of air from the

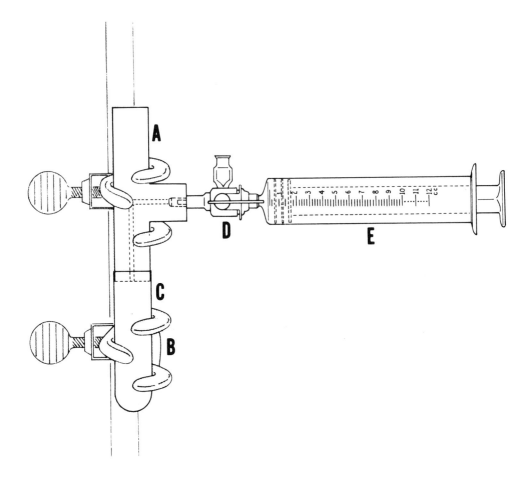

Figure 7.1—Simple arrangement for collection of gradient fractions.
       A. Lucite plug (1.2 cm in diameter at bottom for insertion into the gradient tube) with inlet 4 mm in diameter to accommodate a 3-way metal stopcock and a bore 1–2 mm in diameter for passage of air to the top of the gradient.
       B. Clamps to secure apparatus to a ring stand.
       C. Tube containing the gradient.
       D. 3-way metal stopcock.
       E. Syringe to be filled with air for displacement of the gradient through a hole pierced in the bottom of the gradient tube.

displacement syringe into the gradient tube. Another very useful and more versatile model can be constructed relatively inexpensively in a laboratory workshop (25).

    7. Check 10 μl of each fraction by Ouchterlony analysis for presence of immunoglobulins using anti-heavy chain specific antisera to γ, μ, and α chains.

    8. Depending upon the information desired, either assay for antibody those fractions containing IgM only or assay all of the fractions.

If the virus agglutinates red blood cells, HAI may be used. If the virus does not hemagglutinate, passive (indirect) hemagglutination is a useful test, particularly for IgM antibody (22, 33). If an assay employing complement is used, such as complement fixation or immune adherence, it is advisable to treat the fractions for removal of anticomplementary components prior to antibody assay. Incubate each fraction with an equal volume of a 1:4 dilution of complement at 37 C for 30 min, followed by incubation at 56 C for 30 min to inactivate the added complement. Complement-fixation assay, however, would not be a method of choice, since IgM antibody is reported not to fix complement with a number of viral antigens (10, 11, 22, 37, 60, 61, 63, 67). The reason for this is not clear and may not be true for all viruses (62, 68). IgM in some systems is very efficient in fixing complement and is more active on a molecular basis than is IgG (13).

> 9. If antibody is found in an IgM fraction, confirm the purity of the fraction by radial immunodiffusion, a more sensitive technique for detection of minor contaminants than the Ouchterlony test. The isolated IgM fractions containing antibody can also be checked for sensitivity to 2-ME (16).

Figures 7.2, 7.3 and 7.4 show patterns that can occur with sera containing IgM antibody. Figures 7.2 and 7.3 are the acute- and convalescent-phase sera from a patient with CMV infection. The sera were RF negative. The acute-phase serum had only IgM antibody, while the convalescent-phase serum showed a biphasic distribution of antibody with good separation between IgM and IgG antibody. Figure 7.4 shows the problems that can be encountered with some sera. This was an RF-positive serum from a patient with CMV infection. There was no clear separation between the IgM and IgG classes of antibody. IFA on a sample of the serum absorbed with insolubilized IgG indicated that anti-CMV antibodies were present in all 3 classes, IgM, IgG, and IgA.

Indirect fluorescent-antibody test for assay of antibody class

The IFA test has been discussed in detail in Chapter 4, and reference should be made to that chapter for the preparation of conjugates, titration of the conjugates, the light source for viewing the reaction, and other details of that nature.

In the test, immobilized antigen is reacted first with the patient's serum and then with fluorescein-labeled anti-heavy chain gamma globulin, specific for the various immunoglobulin classes. The fluorescein-labeled conjugates should be previously titrated to determine the extent to which they can be diluted to still give a 3+ to 4+ reaction with the system under test. For study of viral antibodies, infected cultures prepared either on coverslips or as spots on microscope slides are suitable. Better morphologic detail can be seen with cells growing as a monolayer on coverslips, but spots on slides can be prepared more quickly, and the slides are more easily handled during the staining and washing processes than are coverslips. The source of cells, the multiplicity of infection, and temperature and period of incubation depend upon the virus under study. Therefore only generalities can be given. Various antigens can appear at different times during virus replication, not all of which necessarily elicit antibodies of all classes in the infected individual.

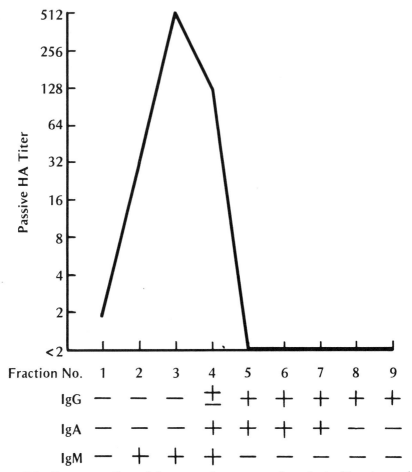

Figure 7.2—Sucrose gradient of the acute-phase serum of a patient with cytomegalovirus infection. Only antibody of the IgM class was detected by passive
(indirect) hemagglutination.

Therefore, to insure a virus preparation containing antigens reactive with the
class of antibody under test, the virus preparations (spots or coverslips) must
be checked prior to harvest with a known serum having viral antibodies of
the desired classes.

   1. Mix in suspension infected cells and noninfected cells at a ratio of 1:4. Collect the
cells by centrifugation and resuspend the cell mixture at a final concentration of approximately 6×10^6 cells/ml in PBS, pH 7.2, and containing 2% fetal bovine serum. (For
formulation of the buffered saline, see section on insolubilized IgG.) Prepare a suspension of noninfected cells similarly.
   2. Place drops of the mixture on microscope slides with frosted edge, making 2–3
spots per slide, each approximately 10 mm in diameter. Prepare similar preparations with
the noninfected cells. (Microscope slides with prepared rings for placement of drops or
for culture of monolayers are available commercially from Roboz Surgical Instrument
Co, Inc, 810 18th St NW, Washington, DC 20006. They can also be prepared by placing 2

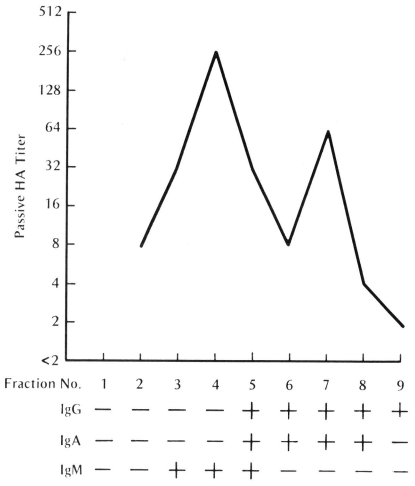

Figure 7.3—Sucrose gradient of the convalescent-phase serum of the same patient as shown in Figure 7.2. The antibody pattern separated into a
biphasic curve of IgM and IgG antibodies.

or 3, 16-mm round coverslips on a microscope slide. The slide is then sprayed with
Fluoroglide [see Chapter 4]. Upon removal of the coverslips a clear, unsprayed area is
exposed at their former site on the slide.)

3. Allow the preparations to dry at room temperature; then place the slides in acetone at room temperature for 5 min for fixation of the spots.

4. Allow the preparations to dry at room temperature for about 30 min and then
store them at −20 C. They can be kept at this temperature for several months or longer,
depending upon the virus. Better shelf-life is achieved by storage at −60 C.

5. At the time of staining allow them to defrost and dry at room temperature.

6. If slides with prepared rings are not used, ring each spot with embroidery ink (Tri
Chem Liquid Embroidery, Tri Chem, Inc, Belleville, NJ, or Roll On Decorator Paint
Tube, Artex Hobby Products, Inc, Lima, OH).

7. Prepare in PBS, pH 7.2, dilutions of the patient's serum, starting with a 1:8 or 1:4
dilution.

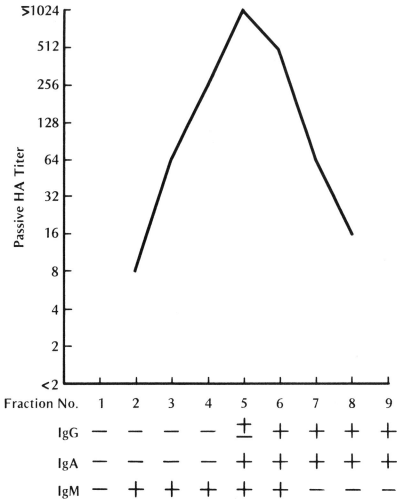

Figure 7.4—Sucrose gradient of a serum collected 19 days after onset of cytomegalovirus infection. A clear separation of immunoglobulins was
not obtained. By indirect immunofluorescence the patient had
IgM, IgA, and IgG antibodies to cytomegalovirus. The serum also
contained rheumatoid factor, which was removed by absorption
with insolubilized IgG prior to IFA assay.

8. Add the diluted serum samples to control (noninfected) and mixed infected-non-
infected cell preparations. Include in each run a known positive serum containing antibodies of the class(es) under study.

9. Incubate the preparations in a moist chamber at 37 C for 3 hr if IgM is under
study, or 1 hr if IgG or IgA is under study.

10. At the end of the incubation period, wash the slides in 3 changes of PBS, each
for 5 min with slight agitation.

11. Drain the slides of excess buffer, and add the appropriate fluorescein-labeled
anti-heavy chain antibody to each slide and to an additional preparation of infected and

noninfected cells to which no patient's serum was added. Incubate the preparations for 1 hr at 37 C.

12. Wash the slides as in step 10, ending with a *quick* dip of the slides in distilled water to remove salts. Let the slides dry at room temperature in an upright position.

13. Place a coverslip over the stained spots, using as mounting fluid Elvanol. Glycerin-PBS in a ratio of 9:1 can also be used, but less drying occurs with Elvanol and the preparations can be maintained longer for viewing.

Elvanol mounting fluid (40):

Elvanol (polyvinyl alcohol) grade 51-05	1.2 g
(E. I. Dupont De Nemours and Co., Inc., Industrial Chemicals Department, Wilmington, DE)	
Glycerol (analytical quality)	3.0 g
H_2O, distilled	3.0 ml
Tris buffer, 0.1 M, pH 8.5	6.0 ml
(1.2 g Tris base in 95.0 ml distilled H_2O, plus 3 ml 1 N HCl. Adjust if necessary to pH 8.5.)	

Place the glycerol in a centrifuge tube with a conical bottom. Add the Elvanol; stir the mixture well without getting the Elvanol onto the sides of the tube. Add the H_2O. (To avoid clumping of the Elvanol, the glycerol and Elvanol must be completely mixed before adding the water.) Stir the mixture well and leave it for 4 hr at room temperature with intermittent mixing. Add Tris buffer and place the tube in a water bath at 50 C for 10 min with intermittent stirring to dissolve the Elvanol. Clear the reagent by centrifugation at $1500 \times g$ for 15 min.

14. Examine the stained preparations with an appropriate light source and filters (see Chapter 4). Grade the intensity of the reaction on a scale of 1+ to 4+. A 1+ to 2+ reaction is usually taken as endpoint in the determination of the antibody titer of a serum. For the reaction to be valid the uninfected cells treated with the patient's serum and conjugate should show no or negligible staining. Similarly, the infected cells stained with the conjugate only should be negative.

References

1. ABRAHAM GN, CLARK RA and VAUGHAN JH. Characterization of an IgA rheumatoid factor: binding properties and reactivity with the subclasses of human γ G globulin. Immunochemistry 9:301–315, 1972
2. AL-NAKIB W, BEST JM, and BANATVALA JE. Rubella-specific serum and nasopharyngeal immunoglobulin responses following naturally acquired and vaccine induced infection. Prolonged persistence of virus-specific IgM. Lancet 1:182–185, 1975
3. AL-NAKIB W, BEST JM, and BANATVALA JE: Detection of rubella-specific serum IgG and IgA and nasopharyngeal IgA responses using a radioactive single radial immunodiffusion technique. Clin Exp Immunol 22:293–301, 1975
4. ANKERST J, CHRISTENSEN P, KJELLEN L, and KRONVALL G: A routine diagnostic test for IgA and IgM antibodies to rubella virus: absorption of IgG with *Staphylococcus aureus*. J Infect Dis 130:268–273, 1974
5. ARVIDSON S, HOLME, T, and WADSTROM, T: Influence of cultivation conditions on the production of extracellular proteins by *Staphylococcus aureus*. Acta Pathol Microbiol Scand, Section B, 79:399–405, 1971
6. AVRAMEAS S: Coupling of enzymes to proteins with glutaraldehyde. Use of the conjugates for the detection of antigens and antibodies. Immunochemistry 6:43–52, 1969
7. AVRAMEAS S: The cross-linking of proteins with glutaraldehyde and its use for the preparation of immunoadsorbents. Immunochemistry 6:53–66, 1969
8. BANATVALA JE, BEST JM, KENNEDY EA, SMITH EE, and SPENCE ME: A serological method for demonstrating recent infection by rubella virus. Br Med J 3:285–287, 1967
9. BARTFELD H: Distribution of rheumatoid factor activity in nonrheumatoid states. Ann NY Acad Sci 168:30–40, 1969
10. BELLANTI JA, RUSS SB, HOLMES GE, and BUESCHER EL: The nature of antibodies following experimental arbovirus infection in guinea pigs. J Immunol 94:1–11, 1965

11. BEST JM, BANATVALA JE, and WATSON D: Serum IgG and IgM responses in postnatally acquired rubella. Lancet 2:65–68, 1969
12. BJORVATN B: Incidence and persistence of mumps-specific IgM and IgA in the sera of mumps patients. Scand J Infect Dis 6:125–129, 1974
13. BORSOS T and RAPP HJ: Complement fixation on cell surfaces by 19S and 7S antibodies. Science 150:505–506, 1965
14. BUCHNER YI, HEATH RB, COLLINS JV, and PATTISON JR: Detection of antibodies of the IgM class in sera of patients recently infected with influenza viruses. J Clin Pathol 29:423–427, 1976
15. BÜRGIN-WOLFF A, HERNANDEZ R, and JUST M: Separation of rubella IgM, IgA and IgG antibodies by gel filtration on agarose. Lancet 2:1278–1280, 1971
16. CAUL EO, SMYTH GW, and CLARKE SKR: A simplified method for the detection of rubella-specific IgM employing sucrose density fractionation and 2-mercaptoethanol. J Hyg (Camb.) 73:329–340, 1974
17. CENTER FOR DISEASE CONTROL, Standard rubella hemagglutination-inhibition test, Public Health Service, U.S. Dept. Health, Education and Welfare, 1970
18. CHANTLER S, DEVRIES E, ALLEN PR, and HURN BAL: A rapid immunofluorescent procedure for the detection of specific IgG and IgM antibody in sera using Staphylococcus aureus and latex-IgG as absorbents. J Immunol Methods 13:367–380, 1976
19. CONNOLLY JH, HAIRE M, and HADDEN DS: Measles immunoglobulins in subacute sclerosing panencephalitis. Br Med J 1:23–25, 1971
20. COONS AH, LEDUC EH, and CONNOLLY JM: Studies on antibody production method for histochemical demonstration of specific antibody and its application to study of hyperimmune rabbits. J Exp Med 102:49–60, 1955
21. COOPER LZ, MATTERS B, ROSENBLUM JK, and KRUGMAN S: Experience with a modified rubella hemagglutination inhibition antibody test. J Am Med Assoc 207:89–93, 1969
22. COWAN KM: Antibody response to viral antigens. Adv Immunol 17:195–253, 1973
23. CRADOCK-WATSON JE, BOURNE MS, and VANDERVELDE EM: IgG, IgA and IgM responses in acute rubella determined by the immunofluorescent technique. J Hyg (Camb.) 70:473–485, 1972
24. CRADOCK-WATSON JE AND RIDEHALGH MKS: Specific immunoglobulins in infants with the congenital rubella syndrome. J Hyg (Camb.) 76:109–123, 1976
25. DENNIS J: Density gradient centrifugation: an apparatus for manual fraction collection. Lab Pract 25:696–697, 1976
26. DESMYTER J, SOUTH MA, and RAWLS WE: The IgM antibody response in rubella during pregnancy. J Med Microbiol 4:107–114, 1971
27. ENGVALL E and PERLMANN P: Enzyme-linked immunosorbent assay (ELISA). Quantitative assay of IgG. Immunochemistry 8:871–874, 1971
28. ENGVALL E and PERLMANN P: Enzyme-linked immunosorbent asay ELISA. III. Quantitation of specific antibodies by enzyme labelled antiimmunoglobulin in antigen coated tubes. J Immunol 109:129–135, 1972
29. FORGHANI B, SCHMIDT NJ, and LENNETTE EH: Demonstration of rubella IgM antibody by indirect fluorescent antibody staining, sucrose density gradient centrifugation and mercaptoethanol reduction. Intervirology 1:48–59, 1973
30. FORGHANI B, SCHMIDT NJ, and LENNETTE EH: Solid phase radioimmunoassay for typing herpes simplex viral antibodies in human sera. J Clin Microbiol 2:410–418, 1975
31. FORSGREN A and SJÖQUIST J: Protein A from S. aureus. I. Pseudoimmune reaction with human γ-globulin. J Immunol 97:822–827, 1966
32. FRASER KB, SHIRODARIA PV, and STANFORD CF: Fluorescent staining and human IgM. Br Med J 3:707, 1971
33. FREEMAN MJ and STAVITSKY AB: Radioimmunoelectrophoretic study of rabbit anti-protein antibodies during the primary response. J Immunol 95:981–990, 1965
34. GROV A: Antigenicity of human IgM in relation to interaction with staphylococcal protein A. Acta Pathol Microbiol Scand, Sect. C, 83:325–327, 1975
35. GRUBB R: The genetic markers of human immunoglobulins. Springer-Verlag, New York, Heidelberg, Berlin, 1970
36. HAIRE M and HADDEN DSM: Rapid diagnosis of rubella by demonstrating rubella-specific IgM antibodies in the serum by indirect immunofluorescence. J Med Microbiol 5:237–242, 1971

37. HANSHAW JB, HARVEY J, STEINFELD HJ, and WHITE CJ: Fluorescent-antibody test for cytomegalovirus macroglobulin. N Engl J Med 279:566–570, 1968

38. HARBOE M and FOLLING I: Recognition of two distinct groups of human IgM and IgA based on different binding to staphylococci. Scand J Immunol 3:471–482, 1974

39. HEIMER R and LEVIN FM: On the distribution of rheumatoid factors among the immunoglobulins. Immunochemistry 3:1–10, 1966

40. HEIMER G Vand TAYLOR CED: Improved mountant for immunofluorescence preparations. J Clin Pathol 27:254–256, 1974

41. HORNSLETH A, LEERHØY J, GRAUBALLE P, and SPANGGAARD H: Rubella-virus-specific IgM and IgA-antibodies. The indirect immunofluorescence (IF)-technique applied to sera with reduced IgG concentration. Acta Pathol Microbiol Scand, Sect B, 82:742–744, 1974

42. HORNSLETH A, LEERHØY J, GRAUBALLE P, and SPANGGAARD H: Persistence of rubella-virus-specific immunoglobulin M and immunoglobulin A antibodies: investigation of successive serum samples with lowered immunoglobulin G concentration. Infect Immun 11:804–808, 1975

43. ISHI K, MATSUNAGA Y, and KONO R: Immunoglobulins produced in response to Japanese encephalitis virus infections in man. J Immunol 101:770–775, 1968

44. KANTOR GL, GOLDBERG LS, JOHNSON BL, DERECHIN MM, and BARNETT EV: Immunologic abnormalities induced by post-perfusion cytomegalovirus infection. Ann Int Med 73:553–558, 1970

45. KNEZ V, STEWART JA, and ZIEGLER DW: Cytomegalovirus specific IgM and IgG response in humans studied by radioimmunoassay. J Immunol 117:2006–2013, 1976

46. KRONVALL G and WILLIAMS RC, JR: Differences in anti-protein A activity among IgG subgroups. J Immunol 103:828–833, 1969

47. LIND I, HARBOE M, and FOLLING I: A reactivity of two distinct groups of human monoclonal IgM. Scand J Immunol 4:843–848, 1975

48. MALLINSON H, ROBERTS C, and BRUCE-WHITE GB: Staphylococcal protein A; its preparation and an application to rubella serology. J Clin Pathol 29:999–1002, 1976

49. MONATH TPC: Neutralizing antibody responses in the major immunoglobulin classes to yellow fever 17D vaccination of humans. Am J Epidemiol 93:122–129, 1971

50. NAGINGTON J: Cytomegalovirus antibody production in renal transplant patients. J Hyg (Camb) 69:645–660, 1971

51. NIKOSKELAINEN J and HÄNNINEN P: Antibody response to Epstein-Barr virus in infectious mononucleosis. Infect Immun 11:42–50, 1975

52. OGRA PL, KARZON DT, RIGHTHAND F, and MacGILLIVRAY M: Immunoglobulin response in serum and secretions after immunization with live and inactivated polio vaccine and natural infection. N Engl J Med 279:893–900, 1968

53. OGRA PL, KERR-GRANT D, UMANA G, DZIERBA J, and WEINTRAUB D: Antibody response in serum and nasopharynx after natually acquired and vaccine-induced infection with rubella virus. N Engl J Med 285:1333–1339, 1971

54. ØRSTAVIK I and HAUG KW: Virus-specific IgM antibodies in acute gastroenteritis due to a reovirus-like agent (Rotavirus). Scand J Infect Dis 8:237–240, 1976

55. PATTISON JR, MACE JE, and DANE DS: The detection and avoidance of false-positive reactions in tests for rubella-specific IgM. J Med Microbiol 9:355–357, 1976

56. REIMER CB, BLACK CM, PHILLIPS DJ, LOGAN LC, HUNTER EF, PENDER BJ, and McGREW BE: The specificity of fetal IgM: antibody or anti-antibody? Ann NY Acad Sci 254:77–93, 1975

57. RIERA CM, RISEMBERG A, STRUSBERG A, and YANTORNO C: A simple method for detection of IgG rheumatoid factor. J Immunol Methods 15:223–228, 1977

58. RIGGS JL, SEIWALD RJ, BURCKHALTER JH, DOWNS CM, and METCALF TG: Isothiocyanate compounds as fluorescent labeling agents for immune serum. Am J Pathol 34:1081–1097, 1958

59. ROGGENDORF J, SCHNEWEIS KE, and WOLFF MH: Zum Nachweis Rötelnspezifischer IgM in Hämagglutinationshemmungtest. Vergleichende Untersuchungen mit der Absorption von IgG durch Protein-A-haltige Staphylokokken und der Dichtegradientenultrazentrifugation. Zentral Bakteriol Hyg Abt I. Orig A, 235:363–372, 1976

60. SCHMIDT NJ, LENNETTE EH, and DENNIS J: Characterization of antibodies produced in natural and experimental coxsackievirus infections. J Immunol 100:99–106, 1968

61. SCHMIDT NJ and LENNETTE EH: Neutralizing antibody responses to varicella-zoster virus. Infect Immun 12:606–613, 1975

62. SCHMITZ H and HAAS R: Determination of different cytomegalovirus immunoglobulins (IgG, IgA, IgM) by immunofluorescence. Arch Gesamte Virusforsch 37:131–140, 1972

63. SCHNEWEIS KE, WOLFF MH, MARKLEIN G, and STIFTER G: Untersuchungen mit der IgM-Fraktion von Patienten-seren bei Verschiedenen Viruserkrankungen. Z Immun Allergieforsch 147:S.236–249, 1974

64. SHIRODARIA PV, FRASER KB, and STANFORD F: Secondary fluorescent staining of viral antigens by rheumatoid factor and fluorescein-conjugated anti-IgM. Ann Rheum Dis 32:53–57, 1973

65. SPEISER P: New aspects of immunogenetic relationships between child and mother. 1. Children produce antibodies against their mother's antigen. Ann Paediatr 207:20–35, 1966

66. STEINBERG AG and WILSON JA: Hereditary globulin factors and immune tolerance in man. Science 140:303–304, 1963

67. STIEHM ER, HAMMANN HJ, and CHERRY JD: Elevated cord macroglobulins in diagnosis of intrauterine infections. N Engl J Med 275:971–977, 1966

68. TOKUMARU T: A possible role of IgA-immunoglobulin in herpes simplex virus infection in man. J Immunol 97:248–259, 1966

69. VESIKARI T and VAHERI A: Rubella: a method for rapid diagnosis of a recent infection by demonstration of the IgM antibodies. Br Med J 1:221–223, 1968

CHAPTER 8

ASSAY OF CELL-MEDIATED IMMUNITY AND IMMUNE COMPLEXES IN VIRAL INFECTIONS

Michael B.A. Oldstone and Luc H. Perrin

The host immune system can respond to an infecting agent in not just one but a variety of unique ways. Finding such diversity of immune responses to viral infections has led investigators to develop new laboratory diagnostic methods with which viruses or their specific effects can be distinguished with certainty. Moreover, by using these methods, the clinician can now recognize an infecting agent during the acute phase of a patient's illness. Further, in laboratory studies of the ability of immune reagents to affect directly virions and/or target cells infected with viruses, one may reflect with increasing accuracy as to how a similar event is likely to proceed *in vivo*. These new immunovirologic approaches coupled with epidemiologic and conventional virologic and immunologic studies should allow for a relatively more precise study of disease. In addition, results from such assays should contribute important knowledge as to the expected efficiency of vaccines, both attenuated and inactivated, in controlling or limiting primary infection and/or calling forth of immune lymphoid cells and secondary antibody response to limit secondary infection. Predictably, these extremely specific and sensitive assays should help in further classifying infectious agents. Besides their usefulness in experimental virology, many of these assays are now available for the diagnostic or clinical laboratories. However, some inherent disadvantages are that specialized techniques and equipment are required and that a given assay may be worked out for only several virus agents. Nevertheless, there is no reason to assume that these techniques cannot be extended for use with other agents as well.

Procedures Applicable and Useful to the Clinic and Laboratory

The virus as a replicating agent provides a supply of macromolecular antigens and, in most if not all instances, elicits host humoral and cellular immune responses. Lymphocytes respond to the viral antigens by transforming into blast-like cells and proliferating clonally. As a result, antiviral antibodies and/or lymphoid cells specifically sensitized to the virus arise. The fact that these immune products can injure or kill cells with specific viral antigens on their plasma membranes and that during infection virions or viral antigens present in the serum or at the surface of infected cells may react with antiviral antibodies and form virus antigen-antiviral antibody complexes, are the bases of several diagnostic tests. This chapter characterizes several sensitive and specific techniques to detect and measure immune reactions elicited during viral infection. No attempt is made to review or list all the various assays available (3).

Cell-mediated Immune Responses

The majority of cell-mediated immune assays used can generally be placed into 2 categories: recognition tests and recognition and effector tests. Basically, recognition tests involve using immunologically competent cells obtained from the infected host and incubating them with a known viral antigen(s). Under appropriate conditions, such cells proliferate and release specific products. The basis of recognition tests is to measure proliferation, usually by counting the amount of radiolabeled thymidine which is incorporated into cells and precipitated with trichloracetic acid (TCA) or to assay the release of a variety of cell products such as lymphokines, macrophage stimulating or inhibiting factors, chemotactic factors, interferon, etc. (3). Similarly, specific antibodies can be detected as a released product or as antibody forming cells (3, 7). In contrast, recognition and effector tests require at least 2 distinct events: first, immune-specific cells recognize infected cells and, second, immune-specific cells and/or their products alter or kill virus infected cells. The recognition-effector test systems have the disadvantage that recognition could occur without execution, thus giving a negative result. For example, tests that measure lysis of virus-infected target cells by immune lymphocytes, require immunologically specific recognition between the effector and target cell, a sufficiently dense accumulation of viral antigens on the target-cell surface and the appropriate fragility of the target's plasma membrane. Nevertheless, the recognition-effector tests show high sensitivity (18, 23) and, in terms of immunity, provide the laboratory analyst and clinician with information as to whether the cells that respond are capable of limiting the spread of virus and/or lysing virus infected cells. Thus, this assay is closer than most to the patient's response in controlling his infection and in giving insight to the resultant tissue injury.

Lymphocyte-mediated cytotoxicity assay

The object is to determine whether lymphocytes generated during a viral infection can specifically kill target cells infected with known viruses. Peripheral blood lymphocytes (PBL) stimulated *in vivo* during viral infection are obtained and mixed with cultured cells that have been infected with and are expressing viral antigens. These lymphocytes are added at different ratios to the target cells. After incubation, usually at 6 hr and again at 15–18 hr, the viability of the target cells is tested. For simplicity, reproducibility, and quantitation, target cells can be labeled with ^{51}Cr, and the amount of radio-

labeled ^{51}Cr released in the supernatant fluid measured. Ratios of lymphocytes to target cells used are usually 100, 50, 20, and 10 to 1. High lympho-
cyte-to-target ratios may result in a prozone effect in which less lysis is seen
with higher numbers of lymphocytes, and, in general, adding more than 100
lymphocytes to 1 target cell frequently results in toxic culture conditions. In
some reports, up to 200 lymphocytes to 1 target cell have been used. Fig 8.1
exemplifies the kinetics with which cytotoxic lymphocytes specific for vac-

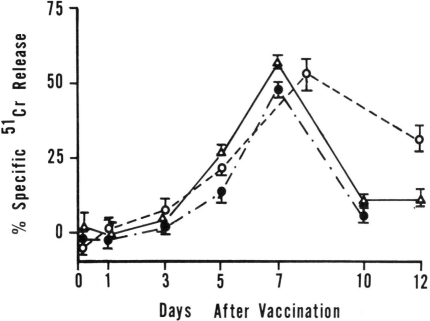

Figure 8.1—Time course of raising specific immune PBL after vaccination with vaccinia virus. Three donors' total PBL harvested at different days after
vaccination were tested against fibroblasts infected or not with vaccinia
virus at an effector to target ratio of 25:1. The amount of specific ^{51}Cr
released was calculated as described in the text. Each point represents
the mean of triplicate determinations, the vertical bar denotes 2 SEM.

cinia virus-infected target cells are generated after vaccination with standard
vaccinia virus, and Table 8.1 shows the specificity of cytotoxic lymphocytes
generated after vaccination with either measles virus or vaccinia virus vaccines.

   Tissue culture target cells. A variety of cells may be selected for the
cytotoxic assay. Requirements include that the cells be permissive for the
infecting virus, express viral antigens on their plasma membranes, demonstrate low levels of spontaneous ^{51}Cr leakiness over the assay time, and have
a membrane that is fragile to immune assault. In humans, easily detectable
killing of virus infected target cells by immune PBL can occur even though
the major histocompatibility (HLA) antigens of the target cell differ from

TABLE 8.1—DEVELOPMENT AND SPECIFICITY OF LYSIS OF VIRUS-INFECTED TARGET CELLS BY IMMUNE PERIPHERAL BLOOD LYMPHOCYTES (PBL)

| | | % SPECIFIC ^{51}CR RELEASE FROM TARGET CELLS INFECTED WITH | | | |
| | | VACCINIA VIRUS | | MEASLES VIRUS | |
VACCINE	PERSON	DAY 0	DAY 7	DAY 0	DAY 7
Vaccinia	RZ	2 ± 3	55 ± 6	10 ± 3	12 ± 3
Vaccinia	TT	6 ± 2	26 ± 3	5 ± 2	4 ± 2
Vaccinia	MB	1 ± 3	41 ± 4	23 ± 5	26 ± 5
Measles	D	ND	<1 ± 2	10 ± 2	38 ± 3
Measles	G	ND	3 ± 2	11 ± 3	46 ± 4
Measles	W	ND	1 ± 2	13 ± 2	54 ± 3
Spontaneous Release		16–21	16–20	17–23	19–23

Peripheral blood lymphocytes (PBL), harvested just before vaccination (day 0) and 7 days after vaccination, were added either to vaccinia or measles virus-infected or uninfected target cells at a ratio of 25:1. Assay was run for 18 hr and numbers represent the mean specific ^{51}Cr release ± 1 SEM of triplicate samples. The 3 PBL-target systems were autologous for the vaccinia virus study and homologous for the measles virus study.

those of the donor immune lymphocytes. This immunologically specific lysis not governed by HLA restriction has been reported by a number of laboratories after testing vaccinia virus, herpes simplex virus, measles virus, and mumps virus infections and most likely represents K or NK cell lysis (1, 15, 17). In contrast, killing of virus infected targets by murine PBL, spleen or lymph node cells often requires histocompatibility of the cell types, i.e., lysis occurs only when the *D* or *K* portions of the H-2 complex (major histocompatibility antigens of the mice) are compatible in the donor immune lymphocyte and the target cell (6). These differences between humans and mice are likely to be sorted out in the future and may be related to the fact that thymus derived (T) lymphocytes are clearly the effector cells in mice, whereas antibody-dependent lymphocytes (K cells), and perhaps other cells (NK), are easily detected in humans. Until the basis for these differences is clarified, investigators testing humans should use homologous assay systems, be aware of the H-2 restriction data in rodents, and consider the use of HLA-restricted targets with other virus systems. Table 8.2 lists a variety of target tissues used in this laboratory that have been appropriate for lymphocyte-mediated cytotoxicity assays. Target cells are generally acutely infected at a multiplicity of 2 to 4 before the assay. To simplify handling, when feasible, cells persistently (instead of acutely) infected with viruses can be used as targets (15). Such lines are established by reculturing the few cells that survive acute infection and are easily carried in culture in the laboratory. These cells are appropriate for use as targets only if the vast majority of infected cells express viral antigen on their surface.

Collection and purification of human PBL. Ten to 30 ml of blood obtained from the antecubital vein is transferred aseptically to 50-ml plastic tubes containing heparin (20 units of heparin with no preservative/ml blood). All the following manipulations are done at room temperature except when oth-

TABLE 8.2—TISSUE CULTURE LINES; HLA TYPE AND SPONTANEOUS ^{51}CR RELEASE

		SPONTANEOUS RELEASE ^{51}CR AT	
CELL LINE	HLA TYPE	6 HR	18 HR
HeLa	2,28/	10–15	20–30
HeLa PI*	2,28/	10–15	20–30
Wil-2	1,2/17,5	10–15	20–35
Daudi	No HLA	5–15	20–30
Human fibroblasts	Individually typed	10–15	20–40

HLA typing for HLA-A and HLA-B determinants were kindly done by Michele Pellegrino at Scripps Clinic and Research Foundation and Paul Terasaki, UCLA Medical School.

*HeLa cells persistently infected with measles virus (Perrin, Tishon and Oldstone, J Immunol 118:282, 1977).

erwise specified. The venous blood in heparin is diluted 1 part to 2 parts of phosphate-buffered saline (PBS) and layered on top of Ficoll-Paque sterile solution (Pharmacia Fine Chemicals, Piscataway, NJ). To a 50-ml glass or plastic tube, 15 ml of Ficoll-Paque is added over which 30 ml of diluted blood is carefully layered. The mixture is centrifuged at $800 \times g$ for 25 minutes or $400 \times g$ for 30–40 minutes, after which the interface layer is carefully collected by using a Pasteur pipette and transferred to a sterile test tube. The cells in the interface, usually 94% or more mononuclear cells, are washed twice in a balanced salt solution (MEM) and centrifuged at $700 \times g$ for 10 min. After the final wash, the mononuclear pellet is resuspended in RPMI 1640 medium containing 20% fetal calf serum (FCS). Earlier studies in our laboratory indicated little differences between using human AB-type serum or FCS in the cytotoxic assay, as long as the serum source does not contain antibodies to the virus being assayed. Mononuclear cells are counted; their viability is checked by the addition of trypan blue or eosin, and their concentration is adjusted to 5×10^6 mononuclear cells/ml of RPMI 1640 medium plus 20% FCS. The majority of monocytes can be removed by culturing mononuclear cells on glass or plastic surfaces and collecting the non-adherent cells after 1 hr at 37 C in 5% CO_2. For special studies, the PBL can be divided into subpopulations based on the presence or absence of Fc receptors, complement receptors, surface immunoglobulin, or binding to sheep erythrocytes (RBC) (3, 12, 15).

Assay method. The medium (usually MEM with 10% FCS) in which the target cells were cultured can be used to suspend the donor PBL just before their addition to the target cells. Target cells, both uninfected and virus-infected, are used at a concentration of 2×10^5 cells/ml. One hundred λ samples (containing 2×10^4 target cells) and 2 μCi ^{51}Cr (sodium chromate, New England Nuclear, Boston, MA, S. A. of 350 mCi/mg) are added to each well of a 6-mm flat-bottomed Falcon TC3040 microtest plate. After incubation for 10 hr at 37 C in a 5% CO_2 incubator, a confluent monolayer forms. The monolayers are then washed twice with medium (using gentle suction to remove the medium). In those virus systems in which one wishes to detect early antigen, infectious virus in 50 λ of growth medium or 50 λ of growth medium alone is added for 2 hr. The cells are washed once, the medium is removed, and 1 drop (30 λ) of growth medium is added to each well, followed by the addition of immune reagents. Time from infection of a cell until its use as a target varies with different viral infections and should be monitored in preliminary experiments. For example, using immunofluorescence to detect viral antigens on the surfaces of infected cells, 30 min after vaccinia-virus infection antigen can be detected, and such infected cells are used as targets 4 hr after initiating infection. In contrast, measles virus antigens appear later, and cells acutely infected with measles virus are generally used 15-24 hr after initiation of infection. Appropriate concentrations of PBL per target cells are added to each well, and the final volume of 350 λ is reached by adding growth medium. Alternately, or when target cells are nonadherent, cells are labeled with ^{51}Cr (200 μCi/2 × 10^6 lymphocytes) for 45 min at 37 C at 5% CO_2 and washed 3 times. Then 1-2 × 10^4 target cells are dispensed into each well. These various labeling procedures have been used in our laboratory with equivalent results.

The test should be performed at least in triplicate and usually in quadruplicate. Variability between triplicate samples rarely exceeds 10% and averages 4% of the total sample count. Controls recording both spontaneous ^{51}Cr release and maximal experimental release should be included in each experimental run. Maximal release is determined by the addition of 150 λ of 1% Non-idet (NP 40) at the end of the incubation period; this usually releases 80-90% of the total radioactivity. Reactants are incubated at 37 C in a 5% CO_2 incubator. At the end of 4-6 and 12-18 hr, 100 λ cell-free samples (cell debris removed by centrifugation at 400 × g for 10 min using a microtiter holder attachment) are removed and placed into tubes, and the remaining radioactivity is counted in a gamma counter.

Calculation and interpretation. The percentage of ^{51}Cr released is calculated according to the following formula:

$$\frac{E - S}{Max - S} \times 100$$

where E = ^{51}Cr released from infected target cells in the presence of PBL, S = ^{51}Cr released from infected target cells in the presence of medium alone, and Max = ^{51}Cr released upon addition of water and NP 40. ^{51}Cr released is calculated separately in each condition for both infected and uninfected cells, the specific release induced by PBL or lymphocyte subpopulations is subtracted from the values obtained with noninfected target cells. Caution in interpreting results should be used when the spontaneous release exceeds 35%. The assay should be run under conditions (MOI, length of test) where the spontaneous release of ^{51}Cr from uninfected and virus-infected cells are approximately the same. There are reports that normal (nonsensitized, nonimmune) PBL have some lytic activity against cultured cell lines (natural killer cell lysis). In our experience, lysis is on occasion greater against uninfected than infected targets and usually close to the values for spontaneous release of ^{51}Cr from target cells in the absence of PBL and hence does not interfere with the above assay.

Kinetic studies indicate a sharp rise of cytotoxic activity that peaks from the fifth to eighth day following virus inoculation and returns to baseline values by the fifteenth day after infection (Fig 8.1). In terms of assay sensitivity, studies involving vaccinia or measles virus exposure of humans indicate that the lymphocyte-mediated cytotoxic assay is about 10-fold more sensitive than cytotoxic antibody-dependent complement reactions. Similarly, in experiments with several mouse virus systems, T-lymphocyte-mediated killing is more sensitive than that by antibody and complement (18, 23). Whether different viral determinants are being recognized is not known at present.

In humans, killing of measles and vaccinia virus-infected targets suggest the participation of 2 subpopulations of PBLs: plasma cells that secrete specific antibody which is responsible for the temporal relationship of the killing and the specificity of the reaction, and Fc-positive lymphocytes which are the effector or killer cells (15). In contrast, antibody plays no known role in the H-2 restricted T-lymphocyte killing of virus-infected murine cells, instead a direct T-lymphocyte target-cell interaction produces lysis. In the human assay system, if the investigator wishes to determine whether or not killing is by an antibody-dependent lymphocyte mechanism, a Fab'2 or Fab fragment of antihuman IgG is added first and allowed to react with target cells for 5–30 min before the addition of lymphocytes. At appropriate concentrations (do dose-response curve) this will nearly totally abrogate antibody-dependent lymphocyte killing but should not alter T-lymphocyte-mediated killing (15).

Adaptation of the assay to detect antibody made early in viral infections. The ^{51}Cr release assay can be adapted to detect specific antiviral antibody production. Here the FAB parts of the antibody molecule bind specifically to the viral antigens expressed on the cells' surface, leaving the Fc piece to react with any lytic cell bearing an Fc receptor (that cross-reacts with human Fc). Various dilutions of serum (1/5 to 1/1000), previously heated at 56 C for 30 min, are added to virus-infected target cells and allowed to incubate for 5–10 min. Thereafter, PBL harvested from normal nonimmune donors or from a variety of other animals are added, and the release of ^{51}Cr at the end of 6 hr is monitored. Controls consist of using a serum source devoid of antibodies. Handling of cultures and calculations are similar to that described above. The advantage of this assay is its great sensitivity with the ability to detect, in some systems, antibody activity in serum diluted 1×10^{-5} (17). In our laboratory this assay is 20- to 50-fold more sensitive in detecting antibodies to measles or vaccinia virus than conventional immunofluorescent or complement-associated tests. Further, PBL from other mammalian species can often be used in this assay.

Proliferation assay

The objective is to identify the virus involved by obtaining PBL during the acute phase of infection and reacting these cells with a variety of known viral antigens under appropriate culture conditions. If the patient's lymphocytes are already primed by exposure to specific viral antigens, upon being re-exposed to the initiating antigen(s), the cells proliferate. This proliferation can be quantitated by adding ^{3}H or ^{14}C thymidine, and either measuring the amount of radiolabeled percursor in TCA-precipitable (DNA) counts of the whole cell culture or by counting the numbers of proliferating lymphoblasts. The specificity of this kind of assay in discriminating, for example, herpes simplex virus type 1 from herpes simplex virus type 2—viruses that share less than 50% DNA homology—is shown in Table 8.3. The response of lymphocytes stimulated with antigen *in vitro* correlates best with the existence of prior exposure to that antigen in the host. However, owing to the variability in cells' responses, it is important that determinations are at least triplicate to quadruplicate and that the given experiment includes all controls (see below). The toxicity of each new preparation of antigen should be ascertained at several doses, and nonspecific depressants or stimulants (unwanted bacterial products, tissue antigens) should be removed. Some cells (macrophages) can release thymidine into the medium and thus inhibit incorporation of radiolabeled thymidine.

Viral antigen preparation. The most reliable procedure is to obtain highly purified, characterized virus or viral antigen(s) by established techniques for the system being studied. Virus infectivity should be destroyed. For example, in our laboratory vaccinia virus is obtained from infected cell-culture fluids by centrifugation. After pelleting, virus is banded in sucrose, harvested, the sucrose removed by dialysis, and the virus is inactivated by ultraviolet (UV) treatment. An optimal amount of virus for use in the assay is that equivalent to 5 pfu before inactivation. Supernatant fluids, harvested from uninfected cells or from other virus-infected cells, are handled in the same way serve as control antigen. A variety of viruses can be prepared, titrated against known responder lymphocytes, stored, and used in subsequent tests. Alternatively, virus-infected and uninfected cells, treated with 1% paraformaldehyde or 0.5% gluteraldehyde or frozen and thawed cells in which virus infectivity is inactivated with UV light or heat, can be used. A dose-response curve, titrating varying amounts of antigen against fixed numbers of known responder PBLs, is used to arrive at optimal concentrations.

TABLE 8.3—*IN VITRO* STIMULATION OF IMMUNE LYMPHOCYTES BY TYPE 1 AND TYPE 2 HSV

	^{3}H THYMIDINE UPTAKE—CPM		
TEST MATERIAL*	LYMPHOCYTES FROM RABBITS IMMUNIZED WITH HSV-1†	LYMPHOCYTES FROM RABBITS IMMUNIZED WITH HSV-2†	LYMPHOCYTES FROM UN-IMMUNIZED RABBITS
HSV-1	41,611	12,863	3,998
HSV-2	7,566	27,232	4,151
PBS	4,066	3,226	4,207

*Materials used to stimulate lymphocytes *in vitro.*

†Lymphocytes were obtained from rabbits 7 days after immunization with HSV-1 or HSV-2. Data obtained from Rosenberg et al, J Immunol 109:413, 1972

Collection and purification of human PBL. See Lymphocyte-mediated toxicity assay.

Assay method. The procedure used is that reported by Rosenberg et al (16) and Møller-Larson et al (11). Peripheral blood mononuclear cells are suspended in RPMI-1640 medium containing antibiotics, glutamine, and 15% FCS to a concentration of 1×10^6 lymphoid cells/ml. Two hundred λ of the cell suspension are added to wells of a Linbro microplate (No. IS-MRC-96) followed by 10 λ of various test antigens; the mixtures are incubated for 72–96 hr at 37 C in 5% CO_2. During the final 4 hr of incubation, 5 λ of ^3H or ^{14}C thymidine from a thymidine solution containing 0.02 μCi/λ (SA 18 Ci/mmol) is added to each well. The amount of radioactivity depends on the test conditions used and should be diluted accordingly. Cells are precipitated by TCA and collected on glass-fiber paper or millipore filters. Filters are placed in scintillation vials, scintillation fluid is added, and radioactive counts determined. Positive control for lymphocyte stimulation consists of treatment with phytohemagglutinin (0.1 μg/ml), while a negative control is the addition of medium to test lymphocytes. The possibility of interferon induction and its effects on the system under study should be ascertained.

Immune-complex Assays

Experience with a large number of viral infections in animals (13) and in several human infections (13, 14, 19, 22) (chronic measles—subacute sclerosing panencephalitis, hepatitis B virus, cytomegalovirus, Epstein-Barr virus) indicates that immune complexes form and can be detected both in the circulation, as well as in target tissues, where they localize. Presumably, the interaction of viral antibody with virus or viral antigens in the circulation during acute and chronic virus infection not only serves as a marker of the presence of virus but also produces immune complexes that commonly cause nephritis and arteritis. Immune-complex deposits are the source of tissue damage that is immunopathologically similar in humans and animals and is likely responsible for several of the signs and symptoms that accompany acute viral infections.

Evidence for the presence of immune complexes lies in demonstrating circulating complexes and in showing localization of antigen, host immunoglobulin, and complement components at the site of tissue injury. Usually, nonantigen specific tests are performed to determine the presence of such complexes initially. Of the many techniques developed to demonstrate and quantitate circulating immune complexes, a collaborative study sponsored by the World Health Organization has indicated the general usefulness of 2 assays, in particular, the Clq-binding test and the Raji cell test (9). Both of these assays are based mainly on the interaction of immune complexes with complement components or complement receptors. Although both assays frequently give comparable results, a recent report suggests that the Clq test may be more sensitive in detecting complexes formed in antigen excess, whereas the Raji test has enhanced sensitivity for detecting immune complexes formed in antibody excess (5). Hence, the tests likely complement one another. The disadvantages of these tests are that they only measure complement-bound immune complexes and, although they measure activity occurring during viral infections, they are in themselves not virus or antigen specific. Techniques to measure antigen specificity in the circulating complex are now being developed and used in several research laboratories. Such assays in which the reactants in the complex are isolated and segregated can allow for identification of the specific antigen by standard serologic means (13). Once circulating complexes deposit, they can be recognized on the basis of their immunopathologic patterns; they form a discontinuous granular deposit of host immunoglobulin, specific viral antigen(s), and complement components in the absence of deposits of other (trapped) serum proteins in the lesion (Fig. 8.2). The methods for detecting these complexes, defining the antigenic component, and eluting and quantitating the antibody have been reviewed recently and need not be detailed here (13). With the exception of obtaining biopsies of affected skin or injured vessels from individuals with viral infection, these techniques are limited to specialized and/ or experimental studies.

Clq-binding assay

The objective is to obtain a rapid quantitation of soluble immune complexes in human serum or other body fluids. The principle of the test is to measure the amount of radiolabeled Clq that binds to macromolecular substances in a sample of fluid from the subject to be tested. Unbound Clq is separated from Clq bound to complexes by precipitation with polyethylene glycol (PEG). Disadvantages of this technique are that complexes that do not bind complement are not detected and biologic substances other than immune complexes sometimes bind to Clq and produce false-positive results. The Clq-binding test described is one used in our laboratory and follows in large part the original assay described by Lambert and his colleagues (25).

Purification and radiolabeling of human Clq. Clq is purified using a modification of the method of Youemasu and Stroud (24). Serum obtained 2 hr after clot formation is centrifuged at 30,000 $\times$ g for 30 min at 4 C so that

Figure 8.2—Fluorescent photomicrograph of an artery from a patient with chronic persistent hepatitis associated with hepatitis B antigen infection. (A) Section stained with fluoresceinated antiserum to human IgG. Note the granular discontinuous deposits of IgG. Similar results obtained with fluoresceinated antiserum to human and complement component. (B) Adjacent section stained with rhodamine-conjugated antiserum to hepatitis B antigen. (Pictures kindly supplied by A. Nowaslawski, Department of Immunopathology, State University of Warsaw, Poland.) Four-micron sections of snap-frozen tissues are placed on clean glass slides, fixed with ether-alcohol (vol. 1:1, 10 min) and 95% ethanol (20 min), washed in PBS (5 min), stained with appropriate fluorescence-conjugated reagent (30 min), and washed 3 times in PBS (5 min each wash). A drop of glycerol-PBS (1 part PBS: 9 parts glycerol) is added to the tissue which is then covered with a coverslip (13, 14).

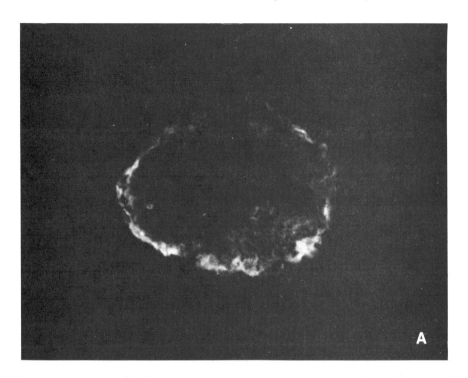

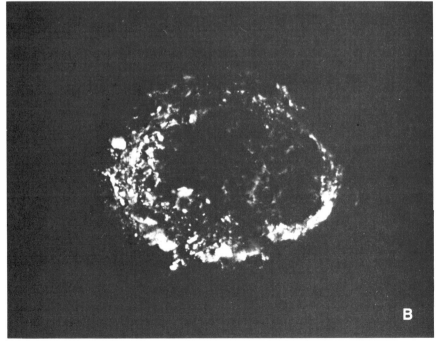

any lipid layer formed at the top of the tube can be removed. Forty milliliters of serum is then mixed with 10 ml of 0.1 M EDTA, pH 7.5, for 10 min at 37 C, and the mixture is immediately placed in an ice bath and the pH adjusted to 7.5. All subsequent steps are done with ice-cold reagents and in an ice bath. Two hundred milliliters of 0.005 M EDTA, pH 7.5, is added slowly to the serum-EDTA mixture while it is gently stirred with a glass rod. The final mixture is left in the ice bath for 1 hr and gently stirred every 15 min. The precipitate formed after centrifugation at $12,000 \times g$ for 30 min at 4 C is recovered and gently resuspended in 80 ml of 0.022 M EDTA. It is important that the conductivity of the 0.022 M EDTA corresponds to that of 0.04 M NaCl. The precipitate formed by recentrifugation is then resuspended in 0.022 M EDTA. After a repeat centrifugation, the precipitate is collected and dissolved in approximately 10 ml of 0.75 M NaCl, 0.01 M EDTA, pH 5. The solution is held at 4 C overnight then centrifuged at $30,000 \times g$ for 30 min at 4 C, and the supernatant fluid collected and dialyzed for 4 hr against 0.067 M EDTA, pH 5 (the conductivity of this solution should correspond to that of 0.078 NaCl). A precipitate forms and is recovered after centrifugation at $12,000 \times g$ for 30 min at 4 C. This precipitate is washed twice in 0.067 M EDTA, pH 5, and gently dissolved in 3 ml of 0.3 M NaCl, 0.01 M EDTA, pH 7.5, for 2 hr at 4 C. After the solution is centrifuged at $30,000 \times g$ for 30 min at 4 C to remove aggregates, the supernatant fluid contains purified non-aggregated Clq. A yield of 1-2 mg from 40 ml of serum is expected. The purity is checked immunoelectrophoretically using 1% agarose in buffer containing 10 mM EDTA and tested against antiserum to total human serum and antiserum to Clq. The purified Clq is divided into portions containing approximately 250 μg of Clq each and stored at -70 C until used. These preparations can be used as long as 6-12 months after purification.

Purified Clq is labeled with I^{125} (New England Nuclear SA ~ 350 mCi/ml) by using lactoperoxidase iodination. Two hundred fifty μg of Clq is dissolved in 500 λ of 0.3 M NaCl and 0.01 M EDTA, pH 7.5. To this mixture are added 5 λ of I^{125} (~ 500 μCi in NaOH); 5 λ of NaI [0.006 mg/ml in Veronal-buffered saline (VBS) (0.01 M sodium barbital, 0.5 M NaCl, 1mM $CaCl_2$ 1mM $MnCl_2$, pH 8]; 5 λ of lactoperoxidase (1 mg/ml in VBS); 5 λ of H_2O_2 3×10^{-3}% in VBS. The mixed reagents are gently agitated and then incubated for 15 min in an ice bath. The reaction is then stopped by the addition of 10 λ of NaI in VBS, 6 mg/ml; 10 λ of NaN_3 in VBS, 0.03 mg/ml; 2 ml of VBS with gelatin 0.1% or bovine serum albumin (BSA) carrier. The radioactive uptake is generally between 50-80%, and the ^{125}I Clq has a specific activity of more than 1 μCi/μg (range 1-1.6 μCi/μg).

Radiolabeled Clq is added to Con-A Sepharose column 1×14 cm. One-milliliter volumes of 0.5 M NaCl in VBS are added; the eluted fractions are collected, and radioactive counts are determined. This procedure removes fragments of Clq or possible immunoglobulin contamination in the Clq preparation. After radioactive counts have fallen to baseline levels, the labeled Clq is eluted from the Con-A Sepharose column by adding 1-ml volumes of 0.5 M NaCl in VBS containing 10% alpha-methyl-D mannoside. Individual fractions are monitored in a gamma counter, and material at the peak is pooled and stabilized by the addition of BSA to give a final concentration of 0.1% BSA in 0.15 M NaCl in VBS buffer. After dialysis against VBS buffer in the cold, the [125]I Clq can be stored at −75 C. Usually > 96% of [125]I Clq is precipitated by TCA. Once iodinated, the radiolabeled Clq is generally not used for more than 14 days.

Assay method. [125]Clq is centrifuged at 10,000 rpm for 40 min before use in order to remove aggregates. The deaggregated [125]I Clq is diluted in 1% BSA in 0.5 M NaCl in VBS so that approximately 4,000,000 counts of [125]I Clq are present in 1 ml. Plastic test tubes, 12- × 75-mm, are coated with 0.1% gelatin in VBS, inverted and allowed to dry overnight.

Twenty-five λ of the serum sample to be tested is placed in labeled test tubes with 50 λ of 0.2 M EDTA, pH 7.5. For the standard curve, 25 λ of aggregated human gamma globulin (see below) is placed in labeled test tubes with 25 λ from a control pool of serum (negative for Clq-binding activity, heated at 56 C for 30 min) and 25 λ of 0.2 M EDTA, pH 7.5. After 30 min incubation at 37 C, the tubes are immediately transferred to an ice bath where 25 λ of [125]I Clq (approximately 100,000 cpm) are added. Immediately thereafter, 1 ml of PEG, 3% in borate buffer (0.1 M boric acid, 0.025 M sodium tetraborate, 0.075 M NaCl, pH 8.2–8.4), is gently added to each tube. Tubes are not agitated but are left to stand in the ice bath. After 1 hr of incubation, tubes are centrifuged for 40 min at 2,200 rpm; the supernatant fluid is completely drained, and the radioactivity in the precipitates is measured. Samples are always run in triplicate, and concurrent controls are a known negative control (pooled human serum without Clq-binding activity), 25 λ of [125]I Clq mixed with 75 λ of FCS and 1 ml of 20% TCA, and standard amounts of aggregated human gamma globulin. The soluble heat aggregated human gamma globulin is formed from a solution of 10 mg Cohn fraction II per ml, NaCl 0.9%, heated at 63 C for 20 min, and centrifuged at 10,000 rpm for 10 min. Standard mixtures of aggregated human gamma globulin are used which contain 10-fold dilutions from 10 mg/ml down to 1 μg/ml.

Calculation and interpretation. The results are expressed as the percentage of TCA-precipitable Clq radioactive counts precipitated by PEG. In our experience, control human serum precipitates 5% ± 2 (mean ± 1 standard deviation) of added TCA-precipitable [125]I Clq. In comparison, the various standard solutions of aggregated human gamma globulin mixed with heat inactivated serum at concentrations of 10 mg, 1 mg, 100 μg, 10 μg, and 1 μg bind approximately 100%, 67%, 28%, 18%, and 10% of the TCA-precipitable, radiolabeled Clq counts that are offered. These data are most meaningfully expressed as the percentage of TCA-precipitable Clq bound, rather than as equivalents of aggregated human gamma globulin, since the aggregates vary among different preparations and may not reflect the size and nature of the immune complexes detected. When the presence of immune complexes is tested in mouse serum, 100 λ (instead of 50 λ) of 0.2 M EDTA, pH 7.5, is used. Experience in several laboratories has indicated that freezing and thawing the serum sample 3–5 times usually does not alter the Clq-binding efficiency. However, it is best to disperse serum being tested in small volumes to avoid repeated freezing and thawing.

As drawbacks, complexes containing only IgA have been reported as not binding Clq (2). Various polyanionic biologic substances may bind to Clq, raising the possibility of nonspecific binding in this test (9, 25).

Raji cell assay

Quantitation of immune complexes in human serum and other body fluids by the Raji cell assay is based on the observation that immune complexes containing complement attach to the large numbers of binding sites for C3–C3b, C3d, and C1 (see addendum) found on the surfaces of these cells. Since Raji cells are devoid of membrane-bound immunoglobulin, the technique quantitates immune complexes bound to the cells by measuring uptake of radioactive antibody by IgG in the immune complexes. Although the Raji cells contain IgG Fc receptors, these are of low avidity and do not interfere with the test per se. The disadvantages of this technique are similar to several of those of the Clq-binding assay; it does not detect immune complexes without complement and it is antigenically nonspecific. However, the nonspecificity allows for the detection of complexes due to multiple sources. A theoretical disadvantage is that the serum being tested can contain antibodies to the Raji cell surface and produce a false-positive result. However, even if such antibodies are present, they are generally of the IgM class and would not be detected by the radioactive anti-IgG used in the assay. The Raji cell assay described was developed by Theofilopoulos and Dixon and is used extensively in their laboratories (20–22).

Handling the Raji cell line and assaying for C3-C3b and C3d receptors. Raji cells are cultured in Eagle minimal essential medium with 1% glutamine, antibiotics and 10% FCS. The cells are seeded at 2×10^5 cells/ml in an Erlenmeyer flask, which is stoppered and agitated on a G-10 gyrorotator shaker (New Brunswick Scientific, New Brunswick, NJ) at 80 rpm per minute in a 37 C warm room. The cell cultures carried in this manner are passaged twice a week.

C3 receptors are detected by the use of an EAC rosetting technique (8). Indicator cells are prepared by exposing sheep erythrocytes (RBC) to 19S rabbit anti-erythrocyte antibody (EA) and incubating them with fresh C6-deficient rabbit serum or C5-deficient mouse serum which forms EAC3b and EAC3d cells, respectively. C6-deficient rabbits are commercially available from Rancho Conejo, Vista, CA, while several C5-deficient mouse strains are available from Jackson Laboratory, Bar Harbor, ME. To test for EAC3b and C3d-receptors, 2×10^6 Raji cells in 200 λ are placed into a 1.5-ml plastic Eppendorf conical tube (Beckman Inst., Los Angeles, CA), gently pelleted, and 20 λ of appropriate EAC cells (5×10^9 cells/ml of VBS) are added. This mixture is agitated and incubated for 30 min at 37 C. The cells are gently suspended in 900 λ of VBS and the number of Raji cells with ≥ 3 EAC attached is ascertained. More than 70% of Raji cells should possess C3b- and C3d-receptors as determined by rosetting of indicator EAC cells.

Assay method. The IgG fraction of rabbit antibody to human IgG is iodinated with ^{125}I as described above or by the procedure of McConahey and Dixon (10). The protein concentration is adjusted to 1 mg/ml of PBS with a specific activity of approximately 0.3 μCi/μg of protein.

Raji cells are harvested after 72 hr of culture. The 2×10^6 Raji cells required for each test are added to 1.5-ml plastic Eppendorf conical tube. One ml of Spinner medium is added to each tube, and the cells are centrifuged at 1800 rpm for 10 min. Supernatant fluids are aspirated, and the pellets are resuspended in 50 λ of Spinner medium. The serum to be tested is diluted 1:4 in 0.15 M NaCl, and 25 λ is added to the Raji cells. The mixture is incubated for 45 min at 37 C and gently agitated by hand every 10 min, after which the cells are washed 3 times with Spinner medium. For the first wash, 1 ml of Spinner medium is added, and the cells are centrifuged at 1800 rpm for 10 min. Supernatant fluids are aspirated and discarded. The second and the third washes are identical: 200 λ of Spinner medium is added to the cell pellet, the pellet is carefully dispersed with a pipette, and then an additional 1 ml of Spinner medium is added. Cells are centrifuged as above, and supernatant fluids are removed. Sufficient radiolabeled antibody to be in excess is added. Usually 15 μg of the radioactive antibody described above diluted with Spinner medium containing 1% human serum albumin is added to the cells and left for 30 min at 4 C, and the tube gently agitated every 5–10 min. The cells are washed 3 times in Spinner medium as before; the supernatant fluids are decanted completely, and the radioactivity in the pellet is determined in a gamma counter. All assays are done in triplicate and include a negative control consisting of normal human serum and a positive control containing various amounts of aggregated human gamma globulin diluted in normal serum. The preparation of aggregated gamma globulin is described above in the Clq assay. Test tubes with 50 λ of aggregated gamma globulin containing 40 μg of protein are each serially diluted 1- to 2-fold with saline. To each dilution of aggregated human gamma globulin in 50 λ of a 1:2 dilution, the control human serum is added, mixed, and incubated at 37 C for 30 min. Thereafter, 25 λ of each mixture is added to 2×10^6 Raji cells, incubated, washed, and handled as the test sample.

Calculation and interpretation. As reported by Theofilopoulos et al, Raji cells efficiently bind aggregated human gamma globulin that has been allowed to react with serum (21). Uptake of radioactive IgG is determined and referred to a standard curve of radioactive antibody bound by cells previously incubated with various amounts of aggregated human gamma globulin in serum. The amount of immune complexes present in serum is equated with the amount of aggregated human gamma globulin present after correcting for dilution. The estimated amount of immune complexes in each serum tested is expressed as μg of aggregated human gamma globulin equivalent per ml of serum.

Serum to be tested in the Raji cell assay should be used fresh or stored at -70 C and not frozen and thawed more than 3–4 times. The limit of detection is about 12 μg of aggregated human gamma globulin equivalents with a range of 12–30 μg. This assay has detected circulating immune complexes in patients with infections due to hepatitis B virus, measles virus, dengue hemorrhagic fever virus, and Epstein-Barr virus (Table 8.4).

TABLE 8.4—RAJI CELL RADIOIMMUNE ASSAY FOR IMMUNE COMPLEXES IN HUMAN SERUM

				μg OF AHG EQUIVALENT/ML	
DIAGNOSIS	NO. OF CASES	NO. POSITIVE	PERCENT POSITIVE	MEAN	RANGE
Serum hepatitis (with or without HB-Ag)	34	18	53	65	24–212
Systemic lupus erythematosus	13	13	100	327	24–1,100
Vasculitis*	25	14	56	155	25–1,000
Subacute sclerosing panencephalitis	6	3	50	58	24–100
Dengue hemorrhagic fever	24	15	62	62	25–225
African Burkitt lymphoma	15	9	60	256	30–1,200
Malignancies†	104	43	41	68	20–383
Hospitalized patients‡	60	5	8	39	20–100
Normal subjects	120	4	3	21	12–30

Data represent the experience of Dr. A. Theofilopoulos and F. Dixon with the Raji cell assay in several selected diseases. Reprinted with their permission.

*Eight serum samples from patients with idiopathic vasculitis, 7 from rheumatoid vasculitis, and 10 from Sjogren syndrome-cryoglobulinemia-vasculitis.

†Fifty-five serum samples from patients with solid tumors and 49 from patients with lymphoid tumors.

‡Patients with no suspected immune complex disease (hypertension, heart failure, diabetes, obstructive pulmonary disease).

Addendum

Recently Gupt et al published data suggesting that the Raji cell may also bind immune complexes via C1 receptors. (Gupta et al, Arthritis Rheum 20:119, 1977; Sauter et al, Fed Proc 37:1362, 1978)

References

1. ANDERSSON T, STEJSKAL V, and HÄRFAST B: An in vitro method for study of human lymphocyte cytotoxicity against mumps-virus-infected target cells. J Immunol 114:237–243, 1975
2. AUGENER W, GREY HM, COOPER NR, and MÜLLER-EBERHARD HJ: The reaction of monomeric and aggregated immunoglobulins with C1. Immunochemistry 8:1011–1020, 1971
3. BLOOM BR and DAVID JR (EDS): In Vitro Methods in Cell Mediated and Tumor Immunology. Academic Press, Inc, New York 1976
4. BRUNNER KT, MAUEL J, CEROTTINI JC, and CHAPUIS B: Quantitative assay of the lytic action of immune lymphoid cells on ^{51}Cr labeled allogeneic target cells in vitro; inhibition by isoantibody and by drugs. Immunology 14:181–196, 1968
5. CASALI P, BOSSUS A, CARPENTIER NA, and LAMBERT PH: Solid-phase enzyme immunoassay or radioimmunoassay for the detection of immune complexes based on their recognition by conglutinin: conglutinin-binding test. A comparative study with ^{125}I-labelled C1q binding and Raji-cell RIA tests. Clin Exp Immunol, 29:342–354, 1977
6. DOHERTY PC, BLANDEN RV, and ZINKERNAGEL RM: Specificity of virus-immune effector T cells for H-2K or H-2D compatible interactions: Implications for H-antigen diversity. Transplant Rev 29:89–124, 1976
7. JOHNSON RA, HOOFNAGLE JH, GERETY RJ, BARKER LF, and MERCHANT B: Detection of cells producing antibody to hepatitis B surface antigen by an indirect hemolytic plaque assay. Intervirology 4:287–291, 1974

8. JONDAL M, KLEIN G, OLDSTONE MBA, BOKISCH V, and YEFENOF E: Surface markers on human B and T lymphocytes. VIII. Association between complement and Epstein-Barr virus (EBV) receptors on human lymphoid cells. Scand J Immunol 5:401–410, 1976

9. LAMBERT PH, DIXON FJ, ZUBLER RH, ET AL: A WHO collaborative study for the evaluation of eighteen methods for detecting immune complexes in serum. J Clin Lab Immunol, 1:1–15, 1978

10. MCCONAHEY PJ and DIXON FJ: A method of trace iodination of proteins for immunologic studies. Int Arch Allergy Appl Immunol 29:185–189, 1966

11. MØLLER-LARSEN A, ANDERSEN HK, HERON I, and SAROV I: In vitro stimulation of human lymphocytes by purified cytomegalovirus. Intervirology 6:249–257, 1975/76

12. MORETTA L, WEBB SR, GROSSI CE, LYDYARD PM, and COOPER MD: Functional analysis of two human T-cell subpopulations: Help and suppression of B cell responses by T cells bearing receptors for IgM or IgG. J Exp Med 146:184–200, 1977

13. Oldstone MBA: Virus neutralization and virus induced immune complex disease: virus-antibody union resulting in immunoprotection or immunologic injury—two different sides of the same coin, In Progress in Medical Virology. Vol 19, Karger, Basel, 1975, pp 84–119

14. OLDSTONE MBA, THEOFILOPOULOS AN, GUNVEN P, and KLEIN G: Immune complexes associated with neoplasia: presence of Epstein-Barr virus antigen-antibody complexes in Burkitt's lymphoma. Intervirology 4:292–302, 1974

15. PERRIN LH, ZINKERNAGEL RM, and OLDSTONE MBA: Immune response in humans after vaccination with vaccinia virus: generation of a virus specific cytotoxic activity by human peripheral lymphocytes. J Exp Med 146:949–969, 1977

16. ROSENBERG GL, WOHLENBERG C, NAHMIAS AJ, and NOTKINS AL: Differentiation of type 1 and type 2 herpes simplex virus by in vitro stimulation of immune lymphocytes. J Immunol 109:413–414, 1972

17. SHORE SL, BLACK CM, MELEWICZ FM, WOOD PA, and NAHMIAS AJ; Antibody-dependent cell-mediated cytotoxicity to target cells infected with type 1 and type 2 herpes simplex virus. J Immunol 116:194–201, 1976

18. SHORE SL, CROMEANS TL, and ROMANO TJ: Immune destruction of virus infected cells early in the infectious cycle. Nature 262:695–696, 1962

19. STAGNO S, VOLANAKIS J, REYNOLDS DW, STROUD R, and ALFORD CA: Virus-host interactions in perinatally acquired cytomegalovirus infections of man: Comparative studies on antigenic load and immune complex formation, In Development of Host Defenses, Cooper MD and Dayton DH (eds) Raven Press, New York, 1977, pp 237–250

20. THEOFILOPOULOS AN and DIXON FJ: Immune complexes in human sera detected by the Raji cell radioimmune assay, In In Vitro Methods in Cell-Mediated and Tumor Immunity. Academic Press, Inc., New York, 1976, pp 555–563

21. THEOFILOPOULOS AN, DIXON FJ, and BOKISCH VA: Binding of soluble immune complexes to human lymphoblastoid cells. I. Characterization of receptors for IgG Fc and complement and description of the binding mechanism. J Exp Med 140:877–894, 1974

22. THEOFILOPOULOS AN, WILSON CB, and DIXON FJ: The Raji Cell radioimmune assay for detecting immune complexes in human sera. J Clin Invest 57:169–182, 1976

23. WELSH RM and OLDSTONE MBA: Inhibition of immunologic injury of cultured cells infected with lymphocytic choriomeningitis virus: role of defective interfering virus in regulating viral antigenic expression. J Exp Med 145:1449–1468, 1977

24. YONEMASU K and STROUD RM: Clq: Rapid purification method for preparation of monospecific antisera for biochemical studies. J Immunol 106:304–313, 1971

25. ZUBLER RH and LAMBERT PH: The ^{125}I-Clq binding test for the detection of soluble immune complexes In In Vitro Methods in Cell-Mediated and Tumor Immunity, Academic Press, Inc, New York, 1976, pp 565–572

Part Two

CHAPTER 9

ADENOVIRUSES

Julius A. Kasel

Introduction

Adenoviruses were first isolated from spontaneously degenerating cell cultures of human adenoids (134). Shortly afterward, the role of antigenically related agents in causing a major porportion of noninfluenzal acute respiratory disease in military personnel was documented (64). Progressively and rather rapidly thereafter, clinical and epidemiologic reports described the recovery of new immunotypes in association with other forms of clinical disease (70). Other studies which focused principally upon biologic, immunologic, serologic, and biochemical characteristics of the viruses led to the identification of relatively well-defined subgroupings of human adenoviruses (119, 128). These developments greatly simplified the diagnosis of adenovirus infections by virologic and serologic methodologies. Agents with similar properties were also recovered from other host species (107); none, however, have been shown to be sources of any human infections.

Clinical aspects

Adenoviruses have been recovered from virtually every organ system of man. Most of the 33 antigenically distinct adenoviruses isolated from man are rarely encountered as pathogens in recognizable disease. Indeed, only 12 types of adenoviruses so far have been associated with illnesses which are primarily manifested as respiratory and ocular infections. Pediatric and military populations bear the brunt of symptomatic infections with these agents. The illnesses caused by adenoviruses are mostly self-limited, rarely fatal, and recovery is followed by type-specific immunity. The clinical syndromes caused by adenoviruses and the types most frequently associated with the disease entities are shown in Table 9.1.

Acute febrile pharyngitis. This is an endemic disease which occurs chiefly in infants and young children and is associated with type 1, 2, and 5 infections, and less commonly with other types. Exudate on the pharyngeal walls, a granular appearance of the mucosa, and moderately tender, enlarged cervical lymph nodes are commonly seen; cough and coryza are also frequently present. Such symptomatic infections in individual cases are not clinically distinguishable from those caused by other microbial agents.

Notable features of respiratory tract infections caused mainly by types 1, 2, 5, and 6 are the persistence of virus in a "latent" state in adenoidal and tonsillar tissues in approximately 50% of infected young children (39, 70, 143, 159), and the excretion of virus rectally at intermittent intervals for many months without any recurrences of the same or different clinical manifestations (42, 66). These asymptomatic shedders of virus probably account for the endemic presence of viruses in the young pediatric age children, and they represent sources of infections transmitted to susceptibles by the fecal-oral route (42). Prior to reaching school age, a majority of

TABLE 9.1—ILLNESSES MOST COMMONLY ASSOCIATED WITH INFECTIONS BY ADENOVIRUSES

DISEASE	INDIVIDUALS MOST AT RISK	PRINCIPAL IMMUNOTYPE	REFERENCE
Acute febrile pharyngitis	Infants, young children	1,2,3,5,6,7	7,17,18,19,94, 159,168,170
Pharyngoconjunctival fever	School age children	3,7,14	8,23,63,65,70, 80,92,157
Acute respiratory disease	Military recruits	3,4,7,14,21	14,51,64,65, 88,126,152, 154
Pneumonia	Infants, young children	1,2,3,7	6,10,25,43,46, 54,83,84, 91,93,95, 99,120,121, 137,165,169
Pneumonia	Military recruits	4,7	34,89
Epidemic keratoconjunctivitis	Any age group	8,11,19	22,31,32,50, 73,160,166
Pertussis-like syndrome	Infants, young children	5	27,28,103
Acute hemorrhagic cystitis	Infants, young children	11	96,109

children have experienced at least 1 or 2 infections with the lower-numbered types of adenoviruses (70).

Pharyngoconjunctival fever. This pathologic entity is characterized clinically by fever, conjunctivitis, pharyngitis, malaise, and cervical lymphadenopathy. Typical illness with conjunctivitis is generally evident 5–6 days after exposure, and infected individuals shed virus for approximately a 10-day period (8). Pharyngoconjunctival fever is usually seen in school-age children and young adults in discrete outbreaks, but sporadic cases also occur in all age groups. Adenovirus types 1, 2, 3, 4, 6, and 7 have also been incriminated in these infections (8, 36, 38, 70, 80).

Acute respiratory disease. Epidemics of acute diffuse respiratory disease due to adenoviruses occur predominantly in military recruits, and the illnesses observed in these populations are of variable severity. Fever, pharyngitis, nonproductive cough, malaise, chills, myalgia, and headache are common signs and symptoms. Transmission of virus to susceptible individuals can occur by inhalation of infectious small-particle aerosols created by coughing and sneezing of ill persons, and the incubation period is 5–6 days. Adenovirus types 4 and 7 are most frequently involved. In recent years, immunization with live virus vaccines has markedly reduced the acute respiratory disease problem caused by adenoviruses in military populations (150, 151).

Pneumonia. Severe adenovirus pneumonias, occasionally fatal, occur in young infants and children, and are mostly associated with types 3, 7, and 21; types 1, 3, 4, 5, 7, 7a, 18, and 21 have also been isolated from fatal cases. Extrapulmonary manifestations such as encephalomeningitis, myocarditis, renal involvement, hepatomegally, hemorrhagic tendency, peripheral edema, gastroenteritis, and exanthema can be seen, especially in infants (141). Children who recover from pneumonia sometimes have residual lung disease (6, 84, 161).

Pneumonia is also a fairly frequent complication of acute respiratory disease in military recruits, and pulmonary involvement can be prolonged and extensive. Very few fatal cases have been documented, however, and these occurred in association with type 4 and 7 infections.

Epidemic keratoconjunctivitis. Recognizable illness is apparent after an 8- to 10-day silent incubation period. The initial onset of follicular conjunctivitis with preauricular lymphadenopathy can be accompanied by mild upper respiratory illness. After a 7- to 10-day delay, subepithelial corneal keratitis develops which may persist for an extended period of time. Contaminated eye instruments, ophthalmic wash solutions, hands of medical personnel, and towels are the vehicles by which ocular infections are spread to susceptible individuals.

Pertussis-like syndrome. Infrequently, whooping cough indistinguishable from that caused by the bacterial agent, *Bordetella pertussis,* can occur following type 5 infection in childhood.

Acute hemorrhagic cystitis. When caused by adenoviruses, this disease entity appears primarily in the pediatric age group, but it is sometimes also seen in adults. It is characterized by the sudden onset of gross hematuria, dysuria, and increased frequency and the urgency of urination. Adenovirus type 11 and occasionally type 21 are the incriminating immunotypes. It occurs more frequently in males than females, and viruria persists as long or longer than the hematuria and symptoms of cystitis (96).

Other syndromes. Adenoviruses have been associated with a spectrum of other illness syndromes. The evidence, however, is not sufficiently conclusive to establish a proven causal relationship. Intussusception in infants and children (81, 90, 110, 121, 171), exanthems of different types (136, 147, 171), acute mesenteric lymphadenitis (79), appendicitis (15), gastroenteritis (162), meningitis (102), encephalitis (71, 142), juvenile rheumatoid arthritis (125), orchitis (101), thyroditis (148), neonatal sepsis (3), Reye syndrome (20), and gynecologic disorders (82, 86) are among the many clinical manifestations that have been described.

Description and Nature of the Agents

Common characteristics

Both human and nonhuman adenoviruses exhibit a single type of morphology, a similar chemical composition, replicate in the cell nucleus, and have a tendency toward species specificity. These viruses produce unique and characteristic cytopathic effects (CPE) which are accompanied by the accumulation of organic acids in the host cell cultures. None of the adenoviruses hemadsorb erythrocytes, replicate in embryonated chicken eggs, and with the exception of avian adenoviruses, all possess at least 1 family-reactive antigenic determinant (119).

Size and shape

The adenoviruses are nonenveloped viruses and are 70–90 nm in diameter. They have a buoyant density in cesium chloride of 1.33–1.35 g/cm^3 and the molecular weight estimated from sedimentation coefficients is about 170–175 $\times$ 10^6. The capsid proteins of adenoviruses are arranged in an icosahedron having 20 triangular faces and 12 vertices (45). In each virion, there are 240 hexons and 12 pentons. The hexons are dispersed on the triangular faces and edges, and the 12 pentons are located in the vertices of the icosahedron. Each penton consists of a base and a fiber which is a rod-like outward projection with a terminal knob (Fig. 9.1).

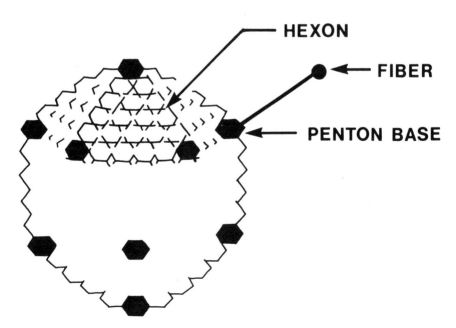

HEXON

FIBER

PENTON BASE

Figure 9.1—Schematic representation of an adenovirus.

Chemical composition

The virion contains a single molecule of double-stranded DNA in a linear form. The molecular weight and the G+C base composition of the genome for the different immunotypes ranges from 20–30 × 10⁶ and 48–61%, respectively.

Stability

Crude suspensions of most adenoviruses retain infectivity for prolonged periods of time when kept stored at −20 to −60 C in a pH environment of 6–9. Infectious virus is rapidly inactivated at 56 C and by exposure to 0.25% sodium dodecylsulfate, low concentrations of chlorine, ultraviolet irradiation, or 1:400–1:4000 concentrations of formalin. The agents are not affected by treatment with ether or chloroform, and they can be lyophilized without any appreciable loss of infectivity.

Classification

In 1976, the plenary session of the International Committee on Taxonomy of Viruses accepted proposals submitted by the Study Group on Adenoviruses, Vertebrate Virus Subcommittee, to elevate these viruses to a family named *Adenoviridae*. Presently, the family includes 2 genera and these are named *Mastadenovirus* and *Aviadenovirus* (Table 9.2). The principal criterion for the separation of adenoviruses into 2 genera is the absence of any immunologic cross-reactive antigens in mammalian and avian adenoviruses (107). For further descriptions of nonhuman adenoviruses see references 2, 49, 67 and 167.

TABLE 9.2—ADENOVIRIDAE FAMILY

GENERA	HOST SPECIES	CRYPTOGRAM
Mastadenovirus	Human, Simian, Bovine, Canine, Equine, Porcine, Ovine, Opossum, Murine, Amphibian (frog)	(D/2:20–30/12–17:55:V/I,O,R)
Aviadenovirus	Avian (turkey, fowl, goose)	(D/2:30/17:S/S:V/I,R)

A classification scheme based on the hemagglutination (HA) properties allows the separation of the human adenoviruses into 4 major subgroups (58, 128). These subgroups are identified by the interaction of adenoviruses with erythrocytes (Table 9.3 and Fig. 9.2). The HA classification is based on: the pattern of agglutination of rat erythrocytes with adenoviruses (the reaction is either complete, partial or absent); immunotypes which fail to react with rat erythrocytes but completely agglutinate rhesus erythrocytes; and the absence of hemagglutinins for either species of erythrocytes. Other viral properties such as antigenic relationships (75), oncogenicity (48), and G+C content of the human adenoviruses tend to coincide with this classification.

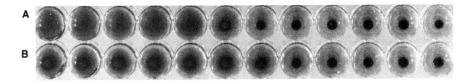

Figure 9.2—Agglutination pattern of (A) subgroup I and II and (B) subgroup III adenoviruses. (Courtesy of S. Drake).

Antigenic Composition

Number of immunotypes. Thirty-three antigenically distinct viruses of human origin have been accepted as members into the adenovirus family; 2 candidate viruses, types 34 and 35 are under consideration as additional immunotypes (Table 9.4). Naturally occurring intermediate strains which possess hexons of 1 prototype virus and fiber antigens related to another type have been recognized in human infections; however, as yet, no classification status has been assigned to these strains (30, 53, 60, 128, 164).

Viral and soluble antigens. Replication of human adenoviruses is accompanied by the excess formation of soluble antigens in addition to infectious virus (69). The adenoviral proteins are complex structures and carry many antigenic determinants. Hexons and fibers are the carriers of the major antigens and the immunologic specificities expressed by these proteins in the intact virion are also recognizable on soluble forms which accumulate in infected cells (105, 106).

Hexons and fibers of adenoviruses possess distinct type-specific and cross-reactive antigens. The type-specific determinant of the hexon, ϵ, and that of the fiber, γ, are immunologically specific for each type of adenovirus, are exposed on the surface of the intact particle, and give rise to neutralizing antibodies. The γ antigen also produces hemagglutination-inhibition (HAI)

TABLE 9.3—CLASSIFICATION OF HUMAN ADENOVIRUSES ACCORDING TO AGGLUTINATION OF ERYTHROCYTES (RBC)

SUBGROUP	IMMUNOTYPES	RBC AGGLUTINATION PATTERN	
		RAT	RHESUS
I	3,7,11,14,16,21,34,35	Absent	Complete
II	8,9,10,13,15,17,19,20,22, 23,24,25,26,27,28,29,30, 32,33	Complete	Complete or absent*
III	1,2,4,5,6,12	Partial	Absent†
IV	18,31	Absent	Absent

*Some immunotypes agglutinate these erythrocytes but to a lower titer than rat red blood cells.

†Group III immunotypes in the presence of a heterotypic antiserum produce a complete hemagglutination pattern.

TABLE 9.4—ADENOVIRUS IMMUNOTYPES

Type	Prototype Strain	Source	Diagnosis	References
1	Ad. 71	Adenoid	Hypertrophied tonsils and adenoids	135
2	Ad. 6	Adenoid	Hypertrophied tonsils and adenoids	135
3	G.B.	Nasal washing	Common cold (volunteer)	135
4	RI67	Throat washing	Primary atypical pneumonia	64
5	Ad. 75	Adenoid	Hypertrophied tonsils and adenoids	135
6	Ton. 99	Tonsil	Hypertrophied tonsils and adenoids	135
7	Gomen	Throat washing	Pharyngitis	11
7a	S-1058	Throat swab	Undifferentiated respiratory infection	132
8	Trim.	Eye swab	Epidemic keratoconjunctivitis	72
9	Hicks	Stool	Rheumatoid arthritis?	77
10	J.J.	Eye swab	Conjunctivitis	131
11	Slobitski	Stool	Paralytic polio (type 1 poliovirus also recovered)	77
12	Huie	Stool	Nonparalytic polio?	77
13	A.A.	Stool	Healthy child	131
14	DeWit	Throat swab	Acute respiratory disease	155
15	Ch. 38	Eye swab	Conjunctivitis (early trachoma?)	97
16	Ch. 79	Eye swab	Conjunctivitis (early trachoma?)	97
17	Ch. 22	Eye swab	Conjunctivitis (early trachoma?)	97
18	D.C.	Anal swab	Niemann-Pick disease?	131
19	587	Conjunctival scraping	Trachoma	9
20	931	Conjunctival scraping	Early trachoma?	9
21	1645	Conjunctival scraping	Trachoma	9
22	2711	Conjunctival scraping	Trachoma	9
23	2732	Conjunctival scraping	Trachoma	9
24	3153	Conjunctival scraping	Trachoma	9
25	BP-1	Anal swab	No specific illness	129
26	BP-2	Anal swab	No specific illness	129
27	BP-4	Anal swab	No specific illness	129
28	BP-5	Anal swab	No specific illness	129
29	BP-6	Anal swab	No specific illness	130
30	BP-7	Anal swab	No specific illness	130
31	1315/63	Stool	Healthy child	118
32	H.H.	Anal swab	Healthy child	13
33	D.J.	Anal swab	Healthy child	13
34	Compton	Urine	Renal transplant recipient	56
35	Holden	Lung and Kidney	Renal transplant recipient	98

antibodies. The family-reactive antigen, α, which is not associated with immunity, is also carried by the hexon but on an unexposed site in the intact virus. Additional specificities are also present on hexons and fibers which can evoke heterotypic HAI and neutralization (Nt) antibody responses. These determinants are shared primarily between immunotypes within the same subgroup, although intersubgroup relationships exist (105, 106, 119). The importance of penton bases in diagnostic procedures is because of their biologic rather than antigenic properties. In monomeric forms, penton bases and those with fiber attached produce CPE in cell cultures similar to that caused by infectious virus (40, 69, 112, 133).

Hemagglutinating antigens. The complete agglutination of rhesus and rat erythrocytes by adenoviruses belonging in subgroups I and II is associated with intact virus particles and 3 forms of soluble hemagglutinins (106, 119). The complete soluble forms consist of dodecons (groups of 12 pentons) and dimers of pentons and fibers. The partial agglutination of rat erythrocytes seen with adenoviruses in subgroup III is attributable to the relative excess of free pentons and fibers in crude virus cell culture suspensions. However, these soluble antigens in the presence of heterotypic adenovirus antiserum in a test diluent produce complete agglutination of rat erythrocytes (128).

For a more detailed description of soluble antigens, hemagglutinins, and other properties of the adenoviruses, several excellent reviews on these subjects are available (44, 85, 104–107, 116, 119, 144).

Pathogenicity for animals

Most human adenoviruses do not induce acute clinically apparent disease in common laboratory animals. Intravenous inoculation of adult mice with adenovirus type 5 results in the death of animals within 3–4 days (122), and subcutaneous inoculation of newborn hamsters with the same immunotype causes fatal infections mainly between 4 and 10 days (113). Intravenous and intracardiac inoculations of type 5 virus in adult rabbits and young adult guinea pigs causes asymptomatic infections, and virus can be recovered from the spleen for a prolonged period after administration of virus (41, 114). Respiratory tract inoculations of types 1, 2, 5, and 6 in piglets (12) and type 4 in dogs (24) also produce inapparent infections. However, in these instances persistence of virus is not observed. Subcutaneous inoculation of newborn hamsters, rats, and mice with types 3, 7, 11, 12, 13, 16, 18, 21, and 31 results in the formation of tumors at the site of injection after a prolonged incubation period (119).

Although common laboratory animals are not employed in the virologic diagnosis of adenovirus infections, they are excellent models for study of the different biologic and immunologic properties associated with this family of viruses.

Growth in tissue cultures

All of the human adenoviruses replicate and produce CPE in continuous human cell lines of epithelial origin such as HeLa, KB, HEp-2, and in primary human embryonic kidney (HEK) and fetal diploid (HFDL) cell cultures as

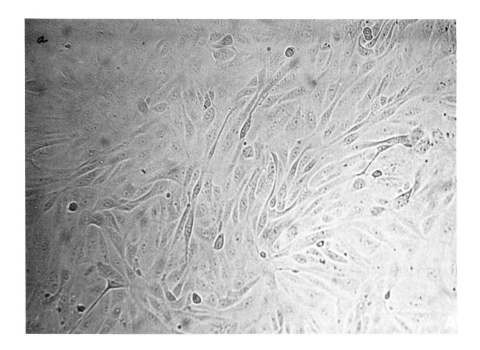

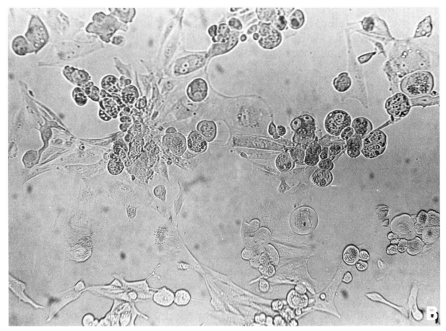

Figure 9.3—Uninoculated (A) and adenovirus infected (B) primary human embryonic kidney cell cultures. (Courtesy of S. Drake and W. Hollis).

well. In nonhuman tissue culture systems the response to adenovirus infections are variable and usually result in low yields of infectious virus.

For the isolation and propagation of adenoviruses, Eagle minimal essential medium (MEM) supplemented with 2% heat inactivated fetal calf serum and containing 100 units of penicillin, 100 μg of streptomycin, and 5 μg of amphotericin B/ml is a satisfactory cell culture maintenance medium.

Cell cultures infected with adenoviruses undergo characteristic cellular changes and these are associated with increased acidity of the medium (135). The cells become enlarged, rounded, and highly refractile, and they aggregate into irregular clusters (Fig 9.3). During the late stages of virus replication the cells may become granular in appearance (2). With adenoviruses belonging in subgroup II, cellular aggregation of infected cells is not always a constant feature. The "toxic" or pseudo-virus CPE which is induced by the penton base usually occurs within a matter of hours after inoculation of cell cultures and also lacks the granulation characteristics seen in infected cells during the late phase of the replication cycle. This effect generally occurs after inoculation of cell cultures with low dilutions of crude virus suspensions, and adenoviruses which replicate poorly in cell cultures do not produce sufficient quantities of excess penton materials to induce this early CPE.

In stained preparations of cells infected with adenoviruses, 2 types of cytologic changes can be observed (16, 127). The earliest changes are associated with the appearance of small eosinophilic, Feulgen-negative bodies surrounded by a clear halo in the nucleus, and these represent early viral products. In the later stages of infection, the inclusion bodies become larger, more basophilic, and form a Feulgen-positive mass which represents infectious virus and other viral materials.

The process of adenovirus replication is relatively inefficient; only approximately 10% of newly synthesized viral DNA and viral proteins become assembled into mature virions. Another characteristic aspect of the virus replication cycle in cell cultures is that the bulk of newly synthesized viral products is not continuously released into the medium but remains cell associated.

Preparation of Immune Serum

Although immune serum can be raised in a variety of animals, adult rabbits and young adult guinea pigs are generally used for this purpose. Crude suspensions which contain whole virus and soluble antigens are generally satisfactory immunogen preparations to produce antiserum in seronegative animals for use in HAI and Nt tests. Purified preparations of hexon are desirable to produce serum for complement-fixation (CF) and immunofluorescence tests.

One milliliter of undiluted antigen preparation is mixed with an equal volume of complete Freund adjuvant and inoculated into the animals by the intramuscular route. Thirty days later the animals are given a booster dose of antigen intramuscularly in either incomplete adjuvant or in the aqueous form. Blood is collected by cardiac puncture under light anesthesia before immunization and 3–4 weeks after the booster dose. Heterotypic Nt and HAI antibody responses occur, but these are of a lower titer than the homotypic level, and are generally restricted to adenoviruses belonging to the same subgroup as the type used for immunization (59, 146).

Collection and Preparation of Specimens for Laboratory Diagnosis

Precautions

Laboratory infections with adenoviruses can be avoided by strict adherence to safety practices described in Chapter 2. Because of the affinity of adenoviruses for the ocular area, hand-to-eye contact should be carefully avoided during processing of specimens or performance of diagnostic tests.

Virus isolation

Isolation rates are greatly enhanced by proper collection of specimens early in the disease course and by prompt shipment to the diagnostic facility. In the event of delayed transport, specimens should be stored at 4 C, or preferably frozen. The type of specimen collected is usually dictated by the clinical illness syndrome presented by the patient.

Throat swab. A sterile cotton applicator is used to swab the tonsillar fauces and posterior area of the pharynx. Immediately after collection, the swab is swirled in a virus transport medium and the fluid is expressed from the swab prior to discarding it. Several types of transport media are satisfactory for this purpose and include veal infusion broth with 0.5% bovine serum albumin or 0.5% gelatin, Hanks BSS with 0.5% gelatin, and Liebovitz medium. In addition, the media should contain 100–250 units of penicillin, 100–250 μg of streptomycin, and 5 μg of amphotericin B/ml, respectively.

Nasal wash. To collect this specimen, the head of the patient is tilted in a backward position. Sterile physiologic saline in 5-ml volumes is placed in each nostril while the subject is cautioned not to swallow. After instillation, the head is tilted forward and the patient is asked to forcibly expel the contents into a sterile container. Antibiotics are then added to the specimens. For children, specimens of nasal secretions may be obtained by direct aspiration using a small caliber dispensible plastic feeding tube with a mucous trap or by a nasal washing with cool buffered saline. The nasal washing can be performed with the child lying on a side, infusing the saline in 5-ml volumes into the upper nostril and capturing secretions in a sterile beaker, or by holding the child at a 70 angle and obtaining a 5-7 ml washing with a 1-oz soft rubber bulb syringe.

Conjunctival swab. This is collected by stroking the lower conjunctival sac of the eye approximately 5 times with a premoistened cotton swab. The swab is handled as described above.

Conjunctival scrapings. Suspect corneal epithelial cells are removed with a flattened aluminum spatula and placed in a transport medium.

Anal swab. A premoistened cotton-tipped applicator is inserted into the rectum and gently rotated. After withdrawal, the swab soiled with fecal material is handled as described above.

Urine. Clean voided midstream samples (10–20 ml) are collected in sterile containers. Freshly obtained specimens are centrifuged in the cold at 2000 × *g* for 5 min, and the sediment is resuspended in either MEM with 2% heat-inactivated bovine serum or veal infusion broth with 0.5% bovine serum albumin. Before inoculation, the cell sediment and supernatant fractions are treated with bacterial and fungal antibiotics.

Spinal fluid. Specimens are collected aseptically and used without further treatment.

Biopsy and autopsy tissues. Fresh specimens collected under sterile conditions are immersed in a transport medium. Tissues are minced into small fragments using sterile surgical scissors and then homogenized in a glass tissue grinder or in a sterile mortar with an abrasive and 5 ml of veal infusion broth which contains 0.5% bovine serum albumin. Insoluble material is removed by low-speed centrifugation.

Blood monocytes. Mononuclear cell fractions are prepared by applying 3 ml of heparinized blood cells on a Ficoll-Hypaque gradient (1). Washed cells are resuspended in RPMI medium which contains 20% fetal calf serum in a final concentration of 1.5 × 10^6 cells/ml. Portions (0.5 ml) of the suspensions are placed on human embryonic fibroblast feeder monolayers.

Serologic diagnosis

Paired blood samples are needed to establish a diagnosis by serologic methods. The first specimen should be collected as soon as possible after the onset of symptoms, and the second approximately 2–3 weeks later. After clotting, the serum is separated under sterile conditions and stored at −10 to −20 C. Serum for long-distance shipment can be conveniently stored on filter paper disks and used for antibody assay by the CF test (36). One-tenth milliliter of serum is pipetted on a disk with a diameter of 1.27 cm (Carl Schleicher & Schuell Co, Keene, NH, #740-L), dried at 37 C for 1 hr, placed in a vial, and stored at −10 or −20 C. The specimen is reconstituted by the addition of 0.4 ml of 0.15 M saline, stirred briefly by a Vortex mixer, held at 6 C overnight, and heated at 56 C for 30 min before use in the test.

Microscopy

For immunofluorescence examination, unfrozen specimens such as conjunctival scrapings and cellular sediments of urine, respiratory secretions, and infected cell cultures are placed in 0.05-ml volumes with a capillary pipette on 3–5 separately spaced areas on glass slides. After air drying, the preparations are fixed in acetone at room temperature for 5–10 min. Preparations can be frozen at either −20 or −70 C until examined. If frozen, allow slide preparations to prewarm to 25 C before staining.

Laboratory Diagnosis

Direct examination of clinical material

Electron microscopy. Two basic types of electron microscopic methods for the identification of adenoviruses in clinical specimens have been described (37, 98, 99, 153). In one procedure, fixed and stained tissue sections are examined for arrays of mature virions in the cell nucleus, and in the other method, concentrated throat-wash specimens incubated with immune serum are observed for aggregates of virus particles. Since both methods are of limited application, they are not employed routinely as a diagnostic tool.

Immunofluorescence microscopy. In recent years, the indirect fluorescent-antibody (IFA) technique has gained wide acceptance as a highly sensitive and rapid diagnostic procedure for the detection of viral antigen in clinical materials and infected tissue cultures (78, 138, 145). Since a detailed description of FA techniques is presented in Chapter 4, only the essential aspects of a suitable method as it relates to adenoviruses is described here (138).

Rabbit or guinea pig antihexon serum is usually used for the detection of antigen by the FA test. One or 2 drops of an immune serum dilution with the capacity to detect different types of adenoviruses are dropped on the test slide. Following incubation at 35–37 C for 30 min, the slides are washed for 10–15 min in each of 2 changes of PBS (0.01 M phosphate-buffered saline, pH 7.2), rinsed in distilled water, and air dried. One or 2 drops of a predetermined dilution of antiglobulin conjugate are added to the slide, and they are again incubated at 35–37 C for a period of 30 min. The washing cycle is repeated, with a final rinse in distilled water. Slide preparations of infected and uninfected cell cultures to which a negative serum and immune serum have been added are usually included as controls in the test procedure. The slides are then mounted in glycerol medium. The fluorescent staining observed is mainly localized in the cytoplasm of the cell, and a positive test shows yellow-green fluorescence.

Virus isolation

In tissue cultures. Only cell cultures of human origin should be used for the recovery of adenoviruses from clinical specimens. Although primary HEK cells provide optimal isolation of these viruses, they are not readily available in most laboratories. Infrequently, the cultures contain adeno-associated viruses which can interfere with the replication of adenoviruses (68). The continuous cell lines, HEp-2, HeLa, and KB are highly sensitive to adenoviruses. However, it is difficult to maintain the integrity of cell monolayers in a satisfactory condition for prolonged observation periods, and the cells are often contaminated with mycoplasma. HFDL cell culture, such as WI-38, is another tissue system commonly employed to isolate adenoviruses. While this type of cell line is generally less sensitive than either primary or continuous cultures, it offers the advantage of being easily maintained for long intervals with infrequent changes in maintenance medium. This latter consideration reduces the risk of cross-contamination which can occur during refeeding of cell cultures. Regardless of the cell system employed for isolation purposes, it should be recognized that different production lots may vary in their sensitivity to adenoviruses.

Specimens are inoculated into cell cultures, preferably on the same day as they are received in the laboratory. Undiluted test material (0.4 ml) is inoculated into at least 2 cell-culture tubes containing 1.5 ml of maintenance medium, and then incubated at 34–37 C either in a horizontal position or rotated on a roller drum. Additional tubes (usually 1) are inoculated with the test specimen when an immunofluorescence test is to be performed. At least 2 uninoculated tubes of each cell type should also be incubated and observed for evidence of nonspecific cellular degeneration for eventual use as negative controls in identity tests. Sometimes, inoculation of a clinical specimen, particularly anal swabs, blood, and urine, leads to transient or irreparable toxic effects on cell culture. Such toxicity is usually apparent within 24 hr, and generally can be avoided or minimized by inoculation of a 10-fold dilution of the specimen and/or washing the cell cultures and changing the medium after 60–90 min incubation with the specimen. If significant cell destruction occurs in 10–14 days in the absence of characteristic adenoviral CPE, the isolation attempt is either repeated or a subpassage is performed. After the initial examination, cell cultures are observed for the manifestation of characteristic CPE every 2–3 days for at least 28 days. If necessary, primary and diploid cells can be refed with maintenance medium once every 7–10 days and continuous lines every 2–3 days or as needed.

The rapidity with which recognizable CPE appears is dependent on the type of adenovirus and concentration of infectious virus in the specimen, in addition to the host tissue. Typical CPE generally occurs within 2–7 days with types 1, 2, 3, 5, 6, and 7 viruses. With other adenoviruses, particularly those in subgroup II, the incubation period for the expression of cellular changes can be delayed for as long as 28 days or may be demonstrable only after a blind passage of frozen and thawed cell suspensions. In diploid cell lines, the development and progression of CPE is generally slower than in primary and continuous cell cultures, and sometimes isolations may be missed with diploid cell lines. Following the appearance of CPE, degeneration should progress until 75–100% (3+ to 4+) of the cells are affected to obtain sufficient yields of soluble antigens, hemagglutinins, and infectious virus for identification of the isolate. For identification of an isolate by the FA test, CPE needs only to progress until 25–50% (1+ to 2+) are affected.

Identification of isolates. FA, CF, HAI, and Nt tests are the most commonly used methods for identifying an adenovirus isolate. The procedure selected is determined by the level of typing desired. (See Flow Chart). Indirect FA and CF methods are employed to classify an isolate as a member of the adenovirus family, agglutination with rat and rhesus erythrocytes classify the virus into a subgroup, and HAI and Nt procedures classify the virus as to a specific type.

Since the indirect FA and CF tests are based on the reactions of soluble hexons which are produced during the replication cycle, they only require

FLOW CHART FOR ISOLATION AND IDENTIFICATION OF ADENOVIRUSES

Clinical specimens:	Throat, conjunctival and rectal swabs; corneal scrapings; urine, blood, biopsy and autopsy tissues; others
Cell cultures: Type	Primary human embryonic kidney, human fetal diploid lung, Hep. 2, HeLa, KB
Maintenance	Change medium of cell cultures showing toxic effects of specimen materials within 24 hours after inoculation. Otherwise, change medium in primary and diploid cell cultures once every 7 to 10 days and in continuous cells every 2 to 3 days.
Observation period for CPE	Examine microscopically within 24 hours and 2 to 3 times weekly thereafter for 28 days. Freeze-thaw cell cultures exhibiting 3 to 4 + CPE three times and clarify by low-speed centrifugation. Retain supernatant fluid for identification of isolate by CF, HA, HAI, and Nt tests. Prepare slide preparations of cell cultures showing 1 to 2 + CPE for FA test.

Assay system
for identification

	Reagent(s)	Specificity
FA	Antiserum to hexon antigen	Group
CF	Antiserum to hexon antigen	Group
HA	Rhesus monkey and rat erythroytes	Subgroup
HAI	Antisera to immuno- types in subgroup classified by HA assay.	Mainly type
Nt	Antisera to immuno- types in subgroup classified by HA assay.	Type

the availability of a single antiserum. Of the 2 antigen detection systems, the indirect FA method is relatively simpler and less time consuming to perform, and in addition, offers the advantage of providing a more rapid identification of the isolate.

For type-specific identification by either the HAI or Nt test, a provisional subgroup classification is first obtained by determining the agglutination characteristics of the isolate with rhesus and rat erythrocytes (see Table 9.3 and Fig. 9.2). The isolate is then typed against antiserum of that subgroup. The primary division into immunotypes is based on results obtained in the Nt test (107), although the HAI method is more practical and convenient for typing of most of the adenoviruses. Antigenic cross-reactions among prototype adenoviruses must be taken into account for the proper interpretation of test results obtained by HAI and Nt methods (30, 59, 60, 106, 128, 146, 164). The pattern of cross-reactions reported with prototypic antiserum prepared in rabbits and horses are not always the same.

Among subgroup I viruses, the most significant reciprocal cross-reactions that can be observed in both HAI and Nt tests are between types 7a, 11, 14, and 21, and types 3 and 7a. Types 7 and 7a are indistinguishable by the HAI test, although they appear not to be so by the Nt test. A notable reciprocal intertypic cross-reaction seen only in the Nt test occurs with types 16 and 4. In each of the above instances, the individual immunotypes are discernible by the level of their reactions with serial dilutions of antiserum.

The major HAI and Nt cross-reactions in subgroup II do not always coincide, and the principal difficulties with typing adenoviruses occur in this subgroup. Neither types 8 and 9 nor types 23, 32, and 33 are distinguishable in the HAI test, but these are distinguishable in the Nt test. In addition, some adenoviruses in subgroup II appear to be serologic intermediates. Types 15, 25, and 29 are clearly identified as such by the HAI test, but are closely related by the Nt test. In the Nt test, the principal cross-reactions involving these adenoviruses are type 15 with types 25 and 29; type 25 with type 15; and type 29 with types 15 and 23. In contrast, types 13, 19, and 22 are separable by Nt but each cross-reacts with another immunotype in the HAI test. The major HAI cross-reactions involving these viruses are type 13 with type 30; type 19 with type 10; and type 22 with type 15.

In subgroups III and IV, intratypic and intertypic cross-reactions may be noted, and these are reciprocal crosses between types 1 and 5, and types 12, 18, and 31.

Sometimes naturally occurring strains are encountered which are not typable in a single test. Isolates with such Nt-HAI designations of 3-16, 11-14, 15-19, and 26-27 have been reported (30, 53, 60, 128, 164).

Complement-fixation test. Supernatant fluid collected after primary isolation is evaluated by the microtiter CF test as described in Chapter 1. In the CF test, duplicate serial 2-fold dilutions (1:2–1:128) of the isolate are tested against 4 CF units of a standard antihexon serum to determine its antigen titer. Four CF units of a standard hexon antigen, a negative control antigen, and dilutions (1:2 to 1:16) of supernatant fluid prepared from uninoculated cell cultures are also reacted with the antihexon serum. In addition, the complete test includes appropriate anticomplimentary controls for all materials. The titration endpoint of the isolate is read as the highest dilution which produces 3+ to 4+ fixation. After determining the CF titer, 4 CF units of the isolate are tested against serial dilutions of a standard serum; appropriate controls again are included in the test. A test is considered positive when the serum titer is about the same for the isolate and hexon control antigen.

Hemagglutination and hemagglutination-inhibition tests. HA and HAI tests are performed by the microtiter system with either flexible or hard plastic "U" type plates (128, 140). A moistened towel under the plates minimizes the effects of static electricity when reagents are dropped into the plate wells. To prepare erythrocytes for use in HA and HAI tests, collect 1 volume of blood from the femoral vein of rhesus monkeys and from albino rats by intracardiac puncture. The bloods are placed immediately into separate 5-fold larger volumes of Alsever solution. The erythrocytes (RBC) are then washed in dextrose-gelatin-veronal solution and stored as 1:10 dilution in this solution at 4 C. Cells must be used within 1 week, preferably less, after collection. Prior to use in HA and HAI tests, the erythrocytes are washed 3 times in 0.01 M PBS, pH 7.2, and adjusted to a cell concentration of 0.4% by a spectrophotometric method (61, 128). Troublesome problems with rat erythrocytes sometimes occur; these are generally avoided by pretesting cell suspensions for spontaneous agglutination in the absence of antigen, testing the agglutinability of the cells by an adenovirus with a known titer, and examining for the presence of crenated cells. If crenation is a problem, it may be reduced by washing the rat RBC in Hanks BSS immediately after collection. If possible, rats yielding satisfactory erythrocytes should be maintained in the laboratory as sources of cells.

Duplicate serial 2-fold dilutions (1:2 to 1:4096) of the isolate in 0.05-ml-volumes are prepared in plain PBS diluent, in PBS with 1% type 5 antiserum, and in PBS with 1% type 6 antiserum. (The type 5 and 6 animal antisera should have titers of at least 1:320 and should be absorbed with rat erythrocytes. The absorption is performed by adding 0.1 ml of RBC for every 1.0 ml of a 1:10 dilution of serum, incubating the mixture at 4 C for 1 hr, and collecting the supernatant fluid after centrifugation at $1800 \times g$ for 5 min in the cold). An equal volume of 0.4% rhesus RBC is added to 1 set of duplicate PBS diluent dilutions, and rat RBC are added to others. The same volume of each RBC suspension is added to 2 separate wells containing 0.05 ml of each type of diluent to serve as controls. The plates are then covered with a clear sheet of cellophane, shaken gently, and incubated at 37 C. The test is read when RBC control wells exhibit complete sedimentation and a tear drop pattern after plates are slightly tilted; this is usually evident within 1 hr. The agglutination pattern of the isolate with rhesus and rat RBC prepared in PBS diluent without heterotypic antiserum defines the subgroup in which it belongs. The HA titer is the reciprocal of the highest serial dilution which shows a complete agglutination pattern with either species of erythrocytes, and the dilution endpoint is considered to contain 1 HA unit per 0.05 ml. In the case of a subgroup III isolate, the titration performed in diluent with heterotypic serum is used for this determination.

In the HAI test, all typing sera in the same subgroup as the isolate are used. Before use, unheated serum is absorbed with the appropriate RBC as described above for types 5 and 6 immune sera. The serum is diluted serially in 0.025 ml of PBS diluent, and 4 HA units in a 0.025 volume (HA titer ÷ 8) is added to each well. For a subgroup III isolate, separate sets of dilutions are prepared in PBS diluent with both types 5 and 6 sera. The mixtures are agitated briefly and incubated at 37 C for 1 hr before the addition of 0.05 ml of RBC suspension. A back titration, i.e., 6 serial 2-fold dilutions of the test dose (0.05 ml in 0.05 ml PBS), and RBC controls are included in each test. The plates are incubated again at 37 C, and results are recorded when the RBC controls exhibit the tear drop sedimentation pattern; the first 4 serial dilutions of the back titration must exhibit a complete agglutination pattern at the time that the test is read. The isolate is identified by the typing serum which completely inhibits the agglutination reaction. When cross-reactions are observed, the antiserum which shows a ≥4-fold difference in antibody titer, in comparison to other antisera, provides the identification of the isolate. In cases where the isolate is not distinguishable, the isolate may be further characterized with the appropriate antiserum by the Nt test. An alternative sequence for the typing of an isolate is to first test 4 HA units of it against a single dilution of immune serum which contains 4 antibody units of each of the immunotypes in the appropriate subgroup (128). If this procedure shows that the isolate is of the immunotype for which cross-reactions are known to occur, it is then tested against serial dilutions of appropriate cross-reacting antisera.

Neutralization test. A method commonly used to type an isolate in the Nt test is the 48- to 72-hr procedure in human lines or rhesus monkey cell cultures (59, 124, 135, 146). To determine the challenge dose of isolate to be used in the Nt test, 0.1 ml of each serial 2-fold dilution (1:2–1:256) prepared in maintenance medium is inoculated into 3 cell cultures which contain 1.5 ml of cell medium. The titration is incubated at 34–37 C, and the degree of CPE is observed daily for 3 days. The highest dilution producing approximately 1+ to 2+ CPE in human or approximately 1+ in simian cells within 48–72 hr is considered to be 1 unit of infectious virus and the dose that is used in the Nt test. After heating at 56 C for 30 min, serial dilutions of the appropriate typing sera which encompass the known antibody titer of each are mixed with 1 unit of the isolate in equal volumes and held at 25 C for 30 min. Sufficient volumes are prepared to allow for the inoculation of 0.2 ml of serum-virus mixtures into each of 3 cell cultures. Following the incubation period, the mixtures are kept chilled and are inoculated into cell cultures within 1 hr. Uninoculated cultures and 3 containing 0.1 ml of the challenge dose are included in the test. The cell culture maintenance medium is not changed during the test period. The isolate control is examined daily, and when the appropriate degree of CPE is first demonstrable within a 48- to 72-hr period, the complete test is read 48 hr later. The antibody end point is defined as the reciprocal of the highest serum dilution which completely neutralizes CPE. The criteria for the identification of an isolate are the same as those described in the HAI test.

Flow chart for isolation procedures and methods of identification. Isolates which express characteristics common to adenoviruses but are not typed by the procedures outlined in the Flow Chart require additional study. New immunotypes are established by the fulfillment of accepted definitions of the adenovirus family (44, 107).

Serologic diagnosis

Clinical findings and epidemiologic considerations should direct attention to the possible serologic diagnosis of an adenoviral infection. Confirmation of a diagnosis requires the demonstration of a ≥4-fold rise in antibody titer between acute- and convalescent-phase sera. Even when this is evident, uncertainty of an illness association may remain because of the occurrence of asymptomatic persistent and nonpersistent infections. Not all infections result in a serologic response, and diagnostically significant responses are seen less frequently in infants and children than in adults (42, 137).

Nt, HAI, and CF tests are the procedures used for detecting an antibody response to infection, and the sensitivity for measuring an antibody response is in that order (42, 137). The CF test is a highly useful method to establish a serologic diagnosis. This is based on the fact that only a single antigen, the hexon, from any immunotype, needs to be employed in the performance of a test. Of the 2 procedures used to determine a type-specific serologic diagnosis, the Nt and HAI tests, practical considerations favor the selection of the latter method.

Complement-fixation test

Preparation of antigens. Crude preparations of hexon antigens are usually prepared in either HEp-2 or KB cell cultures (33). A dilution of an adenovirus which produces 4+ CPE by 5 days (usually type 2 or 4) is inoculated into monolayer flask cultures containing serum-free MEM. After an absorption period of 6 hr at 35 C, the medium is discarded and replaced with fresh MEM. Forty-eight hours after 4+ CPE has occurred, cell harvests are frozen and thawed 6 times, and the cellular debris is removed by low-speed centrifugation and discarded. Control preparations without virus are prepared under the same conditions. A high-quality CF antigen for use in diagnostic CF tests can be produced by further purification of the crude preparation using the following relatively simple procedure recommended by the Center for Disease Control, Atlanta, Georgia (33). One hundred volumes of undiluted crude harvest fluid are treated with 1 volume of 5% sodium lauryl sulfate (wt/vol), and dialyzed against several changes of 0.1 M sodium phosphate buffer, pH 7.3. Twenty-five volumes of this mixture are added to 1 volume of the brushite form of calcium phosphate (149) and stirred gently for 1 hr at room temperature. Following repeated washing of the gel with 0.1 M PBS, pH 7.3, the hexon is eluted by the addition of 6 volumes of 0.5 M phosphate buffer, pH 7.3, and eluates are collected after removal of the brushite by centrifugation at 2500 × *g* for 15 min.

Procedure and interpretation of test. The CF test described in Chapter 1 is used for the serologic diagnosis of adenoviral infections. Before use in the test, serum is inactivated at 56 C for 30 min. Duplicate serial 2-fold dilutions (1:2–1:1024) are tested against 4 CF units of standard hexon antigen. Suitable controls are included in the test proper for validation of results. A 4-fold difference between the acute- and convalescent-phase sera is of diagnostic significance.

Hemagglutination-inhibition test

Preparation of antigens. The procedure followed for the preparation of crude CF hexon antigens, particularly when HEp-2 cells are used, results in high yields of hemagglutinins of adenoviruses (55).

Procedure and interpretation of test. The serologic performance and interpretation of this test is identical to the description given for HA and HAI tests. For type 5 and 6 HAI tests, a PBS diluent containing the appropriate heterotypic antiserum is used. Although nonspecific inhibitors are not recognized as a problem in the HAI test with adenoviruses (62, 163), the serum should be absorbed with RBC to be used in the test before serial dilutions (1:10–1:1280) are prepared. Occurrence of nonspecific agglutination by a serum beyond the 1:20–1:40 dilution is considered an unacceptable test. The serum should be absorbed several times with RBC and retested.

Neutralization test

Preparation of antigens. The same preparations used in the HAI test are also used in the Nt procedure.

Procedure and interpretation of test. The procedure is described in the virus isolation section and an essentially similar method can be used for the serologic diagnosis of an infection by the Nt test (4, 29). The test is generally performed with primary HEK or HEp-2 cell cultures and differs in only the following respects: the use of a test dose of prototype virus calculated by the Reed-Muench method which results in an expression of 16-100 $TCID_{50}$ between 4–6 days after inoculation of 4 cell cultures; a 30-min increase in the incubation time of serum-virus mixtures; in tests with HEp-2, HeLa, or KB cell cultures, a clear 50% difference in the degree of CPE between virus control and serum-virus mixture is considered significant neutralization; the complete test is read when the virus titration indicates the presence of 16–100 $TCID_{50}$ in the virus control titration within a 4- to 6-day period. The sensitivity of the test for the detection of a serologic response is greatly increased when lower test doses of virus are used.

Other procedures

Numerous methods have been described for the serologic diagnosis of adenovirus infections and merit consideration as alternative approaches or adjuncts to those described in this chapter. These include colorimetric neutralization tests (74, 87), soluble antifluorescent-antibody test (5), immuno-osmophoresis (100), single radial diffusion (47, 115), hemagglutination-enhancement test (108), agar-gel double diffusion (35), counterimmunoelectrophoresis (57), and radioimmunoassays (139).

References

1. ANDIMAN WA, JACOBSON RI, and TUCKER G: Leukocyte-associated viremia with adeno-virus type 2 in an infant with lower-respiratory-tract disease. N Engl J Med 297:100–101, 1977

2. ANDREWES C and PEREIRA HG: Adenoviruses, *In* Viruses of Vertebrates, 3rd ed, Boilliere and Tindall, pp 309–328

3. ANGELLA JJ and CONNOR JD: Neonatal infection caused by adenovirus type 7. J Pediatr 72:474–478, 1968

4. BALLEW HC, FORRESTER FT, LYERLA HC, VELLACA WM, and BIRD BR: Laboratory Diagnosis of Viral Diseases. Center for Disease Control, Atlanta, Georgia, 1976

5. ARTENSTEIN MS and DANDRIDGE OW: A new serologic test for adenovirus infection. J Immunol 100:831–834, 1968

6. BECROFT DMO: Bronchiolitis obliterans, bronchiectasis, and other sequelae of adenovirus type 21 infection in young children. J Clin Path 24:72–82, 1971

7. BELL JA, HUEBNER RJ, ROSEN L, ROWE WP, COLE RM, MASTROTA FM, FLOYD TM, CHANOCK RM, SHVEDOFF RA: Illness and microbial experience of nursery children at junior village. Am J Hyg 74:267–292, 1961

8. Bell JA, Rowe WP, Engler JI, Parrott RH, and HUEBNER RJ: Pharyngoconjunctival fever. Epidemiological studies of a recently recognized disease entity. J Am Med Assoc 157:1083–1092, 1955

9. BELL SD, JR, ROTA TR and McCOMB DE: Adenoviruses isolated from Saudi Arabia. III Six new Serotypes. Am J Trop Med Hyg 9:523–526, 1960

10. BENYESH-MELNICK M, and ROSENBERG HS. The isolation of adenovirus type 7 from a fatal case of pneumonia and disseminated disease. J Pediatr 64:83–87, 1964

11. BERGE TO, ENGLAND B, MAURIS C, SHUEY HE, and LENNETTE EH: Etiology of actue respiratory disease among service personnel at Fort Ord, California. Am J Hyg 62:283–294, 1955

12. BETTS AO, JENNINGS AR, LAMONT PH, and PAZE E: Inoculation of pigs with adenovirus of man. Nature 193:45–46, 1962

13. BLACKLOW NR, HOGGAN MD, AUSTIN JB, and ROWE WP: Observations on two new adenovirus serotypes with unusual characteristics. Am J Epidemiol 90:501–504, 1969

14. BLOOM HH, FORSYTH BR, JOHNSON KM, MUFSON MA, TURNER HC, DAVIDSON MA, and CHANOCK RM: Patterns of adenovirus infections in Marine Corps Personnel. I A 42-month survey in recruit and nonrecruit populations. Am J Hyg 80:328–342, 1964

15. BONARD EC and PACCAUD MF: Abdominal adenovirosis and appendicitis. Hel Med Acta 2:164–171, 1966

16. BOYER GS, DENNY FW JR, and GINSBERG HS: Sequential cellular changes produced by types 5 and 7 adenoviruses in HeLa cells and in human amnion cells cytological stud-ies aided by fluorescein-labelled antibody. J Exp Med 110:827–844, 1959

17. BRANDT CD, KIM HW, JEFFERIES BC, PYLES G, CHRISTMAS EE, REID JL, CHANOCK RM, and PARROT RH: Infections in 18,000 infants and children in a controlled study of respiratory tract disease II Variation in adenovirus infections by year and season. Am J Epidemiol 95:218–227, 1972

18. BRANDT CD, KIM HW, VARGOSKO AJ, JEFFERIES BC, ARROBIO JO, RINDGE B, PARROTT RH, and CHANOCK RM: Infections in 18,000 infants and children in a controlled study of respiratory tract disease. I. Adenovirus pathogenicity in relation to serologic type and illness syndrome. Am J Epidemiol 90:484–500, 1969

19. BRETON A, GAUDIER B, SAMILLE J, PONTE C, and LELONG M: Infections a virus des voies respiratoires chez la nourrissen. Arch Fr Pediatr 18:859–883, 1961

20. BROWN JM: Reye's syndrome associated with adenovirus type 3 infection. Med J Aust 2:873–875, 1974

21. BROWN RS, NOGRADY MB, SPENCE L, and WIGLESWORTH FW: An outbreak of adeno-virus type 7 infection in children in Montreal Can Med Assoc J 108:434–439, 1973

22. BURNS RP and POTTER MH: Epidemic keratoconjunctivitis due to adenovirus type 19. John E Weeks Inst of Ophthalmology, Dept Ophthalmol, Portland, Oregon, 1975, pp 27–29

23. CALDWELL GG, LINDSEY NJ, WULFF H, DONNELLY DD, and BOHL FN: Epidemic of adenovirus type 7 acute conjunctivitis in swimmers. Am J Epidemiol 99:230–234, 1974

24. CARMICHAEL LE and BAKER JA. Secondary serological response to infectious canine hepatitis virus produced by adenovirus type 4. Proc Soc Exp Biol Med 109:75–79, 1961

25. CHANY C, LEPINE P, LELONG M, LE-TAN-VINH PS, and VIRAT J: Severe and fatal pneumonia in infants and young children associated with adenoviral infections. Am J Hyg 67:367–368, 1958

26. CLARKE MC, SHARPE HBA, and DERBYSHIRE JB: Some characteristics of three porcine adenoviruses. Arch Gesamte Virusforsch 21:91–97, 1967

27. COLLIER AM, CONNOR JD, and IRVING WR JR: Generalized type 5 adenovirus infection associated with pertussis syndrome. J Pediatr 69:1073–1078, 1966

28. CONNOR JD: Evidence for an etiologic role of adenoviral infection in pertussis syndrome. N Engl J Med 283:390–394, 1970

29. COUCH RB, CHANOCK RM, CATE TR, LANG DJ, KNIGHT V, and HUEBNER RJ: Immunization with types 4 and 7 adenovirus by selective infection of the intestinal tract. Conference on Newer Respiratory Disease Viruses, National Institutes of Health, 1962, pp 349–403

30. CRAMBLETT HG, KASEL JA, LANGMACK M, and WILKEN FD: Illnesses in children infected with an adenovirus antigenically related to types 9 and 15. Pediatr 25:822–828, 1960

31. DAWSON C and DARRELL R: Infections due to adenovirus type 8 in the United States. I. An outbreak of epidemic keratoconjunctivitis originating in a physician's office. N Engl J Med 268:1031–1034, 1963

32. DAWSON C, DARRELL R, HANNA L, and JAWETZ E: Infections due to adenovirus type 8 in the United States II Community-wide infection with adenovirus type 8. N Engl J Med 268:1034–1037, 1963

33. DOWDLE WR, LAMBRIEX M, and HIERHOLZER JC: Production and evaluation of a purified adenovirus group-specific (hexon) antigen for use in the diagnostic complement fixation test. Appl Microbiol 21:718–722, 1971

34. DUDDING BA, WAGNER SC, ZELLER JA, GMELICH JT, FRENCH GR, and TOP FH JR: Fatal pneumonia associated with adenovirus type 7 in three military trainees, N Engl J Med 286:1289–1292, 1971

35. DUPUY HJ, BLOUSE LE, and MARRARO RV: Evaluation of agar-gel double diffusion for the diagnosis of adenovirus infection. Appl Microbiol 25:1013–1014, 1973

36. EDWARDS EA: Use of serum stored on filter paper disks in complement fixation tests for adenovirus antibody. J Clin Microbiol 5:253–254, 1977

37. EDWARDS EA, VALTERS WA, BOEHM LG, and ROSENBAUM MJ: Visualization by immune electron microscopy of viruses associated with acute respiratory disease. J Immunol Meth 8:159–168, 1975

38. ELLIS AW, MCKINNON GT, LEWIS FA, and GUST ID: Adenovirus type 4 in Melbourne, 1969–1971. Med J Aust 1:209–211, 1974

39. EVANS AS: Latent adenovirus infections of the human respiratory tract. Am J Hyg 67:256–266, 1958

40. EVERETT SF, and GINSBERG HS: A toxin-like material separable from type 5 adenovirus particles. Virology 6:770–771, 1958

41. FAUCON N, CHARDONNET Y, and SOHIER R: Persistence of adenovirus 5 in guinea pigs. Infect Immun 10:11–15, 1974

42. FOX JP, HALL CE, and COONEY MK: The Seattle virus watch. VII. Observations of adenovirus infections. Am J Epidemiol 105:362–386, 1977

43. FREIMAN I, SUPER M, JOOSTING ACC, HARWIN RM, and GEAR JHS; An epidemic of adenovirus type-7 bronchopneumonia in Bantu children. S Afr Med J 45:107–111, 1971

44. GINSBERG HS: Identification and classificaion of adenoviruses. Virology 18:312–319, 1962

45. GINSBERG HS, PEREIRA HG, VALENTINE RC, and WILCOX WC: A proposed terminology for the adenovirus antigens and virion morphological subunits. Virology 28:782–783, 1966

46. GOLD R, WILT JC, ADHIKARI PK, and MACPHERSON RI: Adenoviral pneumonia and its complications in infancy and childhood. J Can Assoc Radiol 20:218–274, 1969

47. GRANDIEN M and NORRBY E: Characterization of adenovirus antibodies by single radial diffusion in agarose gels containing immobilized intact virus particles. J Gen Virol 27:343–353, 1975

48. GREEN M: Oncogenic viruses. Annu Rev Biochem 39:701–756, 1970
49. GRIMES TM and KING DJ: Serotyping avian adenoviruses by a microeutralization procedure. Am J Vet Res 38:317–321, 1977
50. GUYER B, O'DAY DM, HIERHOLZER JC, and SCHAFNNER W: Epidemic keratoconjunctivitis: a community outbreak of mixed adenovirus type 8 and type 19 Infection. J Infect Dis 32:142–150, 1975
51. HAMRE D, CONNELLY AP, JR, and PROCKNOW JJ: Virologic studies of acute respiratory disease in young adults. IV. Virus isolations during four years of surveillance. Am J Epidemiol 83:228–238, 1966
52. HARRIS DJ, WULFF H, RAY CG, POLAND JD, CHIN TDY, and WENNER HA: Viruses and disease: III. An outbreak of adenovirus type 7A in a children's home. Am J Epidemiol 93:399–402, 1971
53. HATCH MH and SIEM RA: Viruses isolated from children with infectious hepatitis. Am J Epidemiol 84:495–509, 1966
54. HENSON D and MUFSON MA: Myocarditis and pneumonitis with type 21 adenovirus infection. Am J Dis Child 121:334–336, 1971
55. HIERHOLZER JC: Further subgrouping of the human adenoviruses by differential hemagglutination. J Infect Dis 128:541–550, 1973
56. HIERHOLZER JC, ATUK NO, and GWALTNEY JM: New human adenovirus isolated from a renal transplant recipient: description and characterization of candidate adenovirus type 34. J Clin Microbiol 1:366–376, 1975
57. HIERHOLZER JC and BARME M: Counterimmunoelectrophoresis with adenovirus type-specific anti-hemagglutinin sera as a rapid diagnostic method. J Immunol 112:987–995, 1974
58. HIERHOLZER JC and DOWDLE WR: Hemagglutination properties of adenovirus types 20, 25, and 28. Proc Soc Exp Biol Med 134:482–488, 1970
59. HIERHOLZER JC, GAMBLE WC, and DOWDLE WR: Reference equine antisera to 33 human adenovirus types: homologous and heterologous titers. J Clin Microbiol 1:65–74, 1975
60. HIERHOLZER JC and PUMAROLA A: Antigenic characterization of intermediate adenovirus 14-11 strains associated with upper respiratory illness in a military camp. Infect Immun 13:354–359, 1976
61. HEIRHOLZER JC and SUGGS MT: Standardized viral hemagglutination and hemagglutination-inhibition tests. Appl Microbiol 18:816–823, 1969
62. HIERHOLZER JC, SUGGS MT, and HALL EC: Standardized viral hemagglutination and hemagglutination-inhibition tests. II. Description and evaluation. Appl Microbiol 18:824–833, 1969
63. HILLEMAN MR: Epidemiology of adenovirus respiratory infections in military recruit populations. Ann NY Acad Sci 67:262–272, 1957
64. HILLEMAN MR and WERNER JH: Recovery of new agent from patients with acute respiratory illness. Proc Soc Exp Biol Med 85:183–188, 1954
65. HILLEMAN MR, WERNER JH, DASCOMB HE, BUTLER RL, and STEWART MT: Epidemiology of RI(RI-67) group respiratory virus infecaiton in recruit populations. Am J Hyg 62:29–43, 1955
66. HILLIS WD, COOPER MR, and BANG FB: Adenovirus infections in West Bengal: I. Persistence of viruses in infants and young children. Indian J Med Res 61:980–988, 1973
67. HILLIS WD and GOODMAN R: Serological classificaiton of chimpanzee adenoviruses by hemagglutination and hemagglutination inhibition. J Immunol 102:1089–1095, 1969
68. HOGGAN MD, THOMAS GF, and JOHNSON FB: Continuous (carriage) of adenovirus associated virus genome in cell culture in the absence of helper adenovirus. In Proc Fourth Lepetit Colloquim, Silvestri LG (ed), North Holland Pub Co, Amsterdam, 1972, pp 243– 244
69. HUEBNER RJ, ROWE WP, and CHANOCK RM: Newly recognized respiratory tract viruses. Ann Rev Microbiol 12:49–76, 1958
70. HUEBNER RJ, ROWE WP, WARD TG, PARROTT RH, and BELL JA: Adenoidal-pharyncoconjunctival agents. A newly recognized group of common viruses of the respiratory system. N Engl J Med 251:1077–1086, 1954
71. HUTTUNEN L: Adenovirus type 7-associated encephalitis. Scand J Inf Dis 2:151–153, 1970

72. JAWETZ E, KIMURA SJ, NICHOLAS AN, THYGESON P, and HANNA L: New type of APC virus from epidemic keratoconjunctivitis. Science 122:1190–1191, 1955
73. JAWETZ E, THYGESON P, HANNA L, NICHOLAS A, and KIMURA SJ: The etiology of epidemic keratoconjunctivitis. Am J Ophthalmol 43:79–83, 1957
74. JOHNSTON PB, GRAYSTON JT, and LOOSLI CG: Adenovirus neutralizing antibody determination by colorimetric assay. Proc Soc Exp Biol Med 94:338–343, 1957
75. KASEL JA, BANKS PA, WIGAND R, KNIGHT V, and ALLING DW: An immunologic classification of heterotypic antibody responses to adenoviruses in man. Proc Soc Exp Biol Med 119:1162–1165, 1965
76. KASEL JA, KNIGHT V, and ALLING DW: Heterotypic hemagglutination-inhibition antibody responses in volunteers inoculated with adenovirus types 26 and 27. J Immunol 92:934–940, 1960
77. KIBRICK S, MELENDEZ L, and ENDERS JF: Clinical association of enteric viruses with particular reference to agents exhibiting properties of the ECHO group. Ann NY Acad Sci 67:311–325, 1957
78. KNIGHT V, BRASIER F, GREENBERG SB, and JONES DB: Immunofluorescent diagnosis of acute viral infection. South Med J 68:764–766, 1975
79. KJELLEN L: Studies on an unidentified group of cytopathic agents. Arch Gesamte Virusforsch. 6:45–59, 1955
80. KJELLEN L, STERNER G, and SVEDMYR A: On the occurrence of adenoviruses in Sweden. Acta Paediatr 46:164–176, 1957
81. KNOX EG, COURT SDM, and GARDNER PS: Aetiology of intussusception in children. Br Med J 5306:692–702, 1962
82. KULCSAR G, DOMOTORI J, DAN P, NASZ I, KESKENY S, HORVATH J, and GECK P: Virological studies on gynecological patients. Zentralb Bakteriol Parasitenk Infektionkr Hyg Abt 1:Orig A231:389–392, 1975
83. KUSANO N, KAWAI K, and AOYAMA Y: Intranuclear inclusion body in fatal infantile pneumonia due to adenovirus. Jpn J Exp Med 28:301–304, 1958
84. LANG WR, HOWDEN CW, LAWS J, and BURTON JF: Bronchopneumonia with serious sequelae in children with evidence of adenovirus type 21 infection. Br Med J 1:73–79, 1969
85. LAVER WG, PEREIRA HG, RUSSELL WC, and VALENTINE R: Isolation of an internal component from adenovirus type 5. J Mol Biol 37:379–386, 1968
86. LAVERTY CR, RUSSELL P, BLACK J, KAPPAGODA N, BENN RAV and BOOTH N: Adenovirus infection of the cervix. Acta Cytol 21:114–117, 1977
87. LENNETTE EH, NEFF BJ, and FOX VL: A colorimetric method for the typing of adenoviruses. Am J Hyg 65:94–109, 1957
88. LENNETTE EH, STALLONES RA, and HOLGUIN AH: Pattern of respiratory virus infections in army recruits. Am J Hyg 74:225–233, 1961
89. LEVIN S, DIETRICH J, and GUILLORY J: Fatal nonbacterial pneumonia associated with adenovirus type 4. Occurrence in an adult. J Am Med Assoc 201:975–977, 1967
90. LEVY J JR and LINDER LH: Etiology of "idiopathic" intussusception in infants. South Med J 63:642–646, 1970
91. LOKER EF JR, HODGES GR, and KELLY DJ: Fatal adenovirus pneumonia in a young adult associated with ADV-7 vaccine administered 15 days earlier. Chest 66:197–199, 1974
92. MERCHANT RK, ROWE WP, KASEL JA, and UTZ JP: Pharyngoconjunctival fever due to type 1 adenovirus. N Engl J Med 258:131–133, 1958
93. MILLER LF, RYTEL M, PIERCE WE, and ROSENBAUM MJ: Epidemiology of nonbacterial pneumonia among naval recruits. J Am Med Assoc 185:92–99, 1963
94. MOFFETT HL and CRAMBLETT HG: Viral isolations and illnesses in young infants attending a well-baby clinic. N Engl J Med 267:1213–1218, 1962
95. MOGABGAB WJ: *Mycoplasma pneumoniae* and adenovirus respiratory illnesses in military and university personnel, 1959–1966. Am Rev Resp Dis 97:345–358, 1968
96. MUFSON MA and BELSHE RB: A review of adenoviruses in the etiology of acute hemorrhagic cystitis. J Urol 115:191–194, 1976
97. MURRAY ES, CHANG RS, BELL SD JR, TARIZZO ML, and SNYDER JC: Agents recovered from acute conjunctivitis cases in Saudi Arabia. Am J Ophthalmol 43:32–35, 1957
98. MYEROWITZ RL, STALDER H, OXMAN MN, LEVIN MJ, MOORE M, LEITH JD, GANTZ,

NM, and PELLEGRINI J: Fatal disseminated adenovirus infection in a renal transplant recipient. Am J Med 59:591–597, 1975

99. NAHMIAS AJ, GRIFFITH D, and SNITZER J: Fatal pneumonia associated with adenovirus type 7. Am J Dis Child 114:36–41, 1967
100. NASZ I, CSVERBA I, and ROZSA K: Study of adenovirus type 5 antigens by immuno-osmophoresis. Z Immunitaetsforsch 134:225–234, 1967
101. NAVEH Y and FRIEDMAN A: Orchitis associated with adenoviral infection. Am J Dis Child 129:257–258, 1975
102. NEIMANN N, DELAVERGNE E, MANGIAUX M, WORMS AM, and OLIVE D: A propos de cas d'infections a adenovirus observees en Lorraine. Pediatrics 20:15–20, 1965
103. NELSON KE, GAVITT F, BATT MD, KALLICK CA, REDDI KT, and LEVIN S: The role of adenoviruses in the pertussis syndrome. J Pediatr 86:335–341, 1975
104. NEURATH AR and RUBIN BA: Viral structural components as immunogens of prophylactic value. *In* Monographs in Virology 4:1–87, 1971, S Karger, New York
105. NORRBY E: Capsid mosaic of intermediate strains of human adenoviruses. J Virol 4:657–662, 1969
106. NORRBY E: The structural and functional diversity of adenovirus capsid components. J Gen Virol 5:221–236, 1969
107. NORRBY E, BARTHA A, BOULANGER P, DREIZIN R, GINSBERG HS, KALTER SS, KAWAMURA H, ROWE WP, RUSSELL WC, SCHLESINGER W, and WIGAND R: Adenoviridae. Intervirology 7:117–125, 1976
108. NORRBY E, VAN DER VEEN J, and EPSMARK A: A new serological test for the identification of adenovirus infections. Proc Soc Exp Biol Med 134:889–895, 1970
109. NUMAZAKI Y, KUMASAKA T, YANO N, YAMANAKA M, MIYAZAWA T, TAKAI S, and ISHIDA N: Further study on acute hemorrhagic cystitis due to adenovirus type 11. N Engl J Med 289:344–347, 1973
110. NUMAZAKI Y, YANO N, IKEDA M, SEKIGUCHI H, TAKAI S, and ISHIDA N: Adenovirus infection in intrussusception of Japanese infants. Jpn J Microbiol 17:87–89, 1973
111. PARROTT RH, ROWE WP, HUEBNER RJ, BERNTON HW, and McCULLOUGH NM: Outbreak of febrile pharyngitis and conjunctivitis associated with type 3 adenoidal-pharyngeal-conjunctival virus infection. N Engl J Med 251:1087–1090, 1954
112. PEREIRA HG: A protein factor responsible for the early cytopathic effect of adenoviruses. Virology 9:601–611, 1958
113. PEREIRA HG, ALLISON AC, and NIVEN JSF: Fatal infection of new born hamsters by an adenovirus of human origin. Nature 196:244–245, 1962
114. PEREIRA HG and KELLEY B: Latent infections of rabbits by adenovirus type 5. Nature 180:615–616, 1957
115. PEREIRA HG, MACHADO RD, and SCHILD GC: Study of adenovirus hexon antigen-antibody reactions by single radial diffusion techniques. J Immunol Meth 2:121–128, 1972
116. PEREIRA MS: Adenovirus infections. Postgrad Med J 49:798–801, 1973
117. PEREIRA MS and MACCALLUM FO: Infection with adenovirus type 12. Lancet 1:198–199, 1964
118. PEREIRA MS, PEREIRA HG, and CLARKE SKR: Human adenovirus type 31: a new serotype with oncogenic properties. Lancet 1:21–23, 1965
119. PHILPSON L and LINDBERG U: Reproduction of adenoviruses. *In* Comprehensive Virology 3:143–227, Fraenkel-Contrat H and Wagner RR (eds), Plenum Press, New York, 1974
120. PINKERTON H and CARROLL S: Fatal adenovirus pneumonia in infants. Am J Pathol 65:543–545, 1971
121. POLLARD RB: Inappropriate secretion of antidiuretic hormone associated with adenovirus pneumonia. Chest 68:589–591, 1975
122. POSTLETHWAITE R: Liver damage induced in mice by human adenovirus type 5. Scott Med J 18:131–134, 1973
123. Potter CW, Shedden WIH, and ZACHARY RB: A comparative study of the incidence of adenovirus antibodies in children with intussusception with that in a control group. J Pediatr 63:420–427, 1963
124. RAFAKO RR: Production and standardization of adenovirus types 1 to 18 reference antisera. Am J Hyg 79:310–319, 1964
125. RAHAL JJ, MILLIAN SJ, and NOREIGA ER: Coxsackievirus and adenovirus infection. J Am Med Assoc 235:2496–2501, 1976

126. ROSE HM, LAMSON TH, and BUESCHER EL: An outbreak of respiratory infection with type 21 adenovirus in military recruits. Bacteriol Proc. 1968, p 150
127. ROSE HM and MORGAN C: Fine structure of virus infected cells. Ann Rev Microbiol 14:217–240, 1960
128. ROSEN L: A hemagglutination-inhibition technique for typing adenoviruses. Am J Hyg 71:120–128, 1960
129. ROSEN L, BARON S, and BELL JA: Four newly recognized adenoviruses. Proc Soc Exp Biol Med 107:434–437, 1961
130. ROSEN L, HOVIS JF, and BELL JA: Further observation of typing adenoviruses and a description of two possible additional serotypes. Proc Soc Exp Biol Med 110:710–713, 1962
131. ROWE WP, HARTLEY JW, and HUEBNER RJ: Additional serotypes of the APC virus group. Proc Soc Exp Biol Med 91:260–262, 1956
132. ROWE WP, HARTLEY JW, and HUEBNER RJ: Serotype composition of the adenovirus group. Proc Soc Exp Biol Med 97:465–470, 1958
133. ROWE WP, HARTLEY JW, ROIZMAN B, and LEVY HB: Characterization of a factor formed in the course of adenovirus infection of tissue cultures causing detachment of cells from glass. J Exp Med 108:713–729, 1958
134. ROWE WP, HUEBNER RJ, GILMORE LK, PARROTT RH, and WARD TG: Isolation of a cytopathogenic agent from human adenoids undergoing spontaneous degeneration in tissue culture. Proc Soc Exp Biol Med 84:570–573, 1953
135. ROWE WP, HUEBNER RJ, HARTLEY JW, WARD TG, and PARROTT RH: Studies of the adenoidal-pharyngeal-conjunctival (APC) group of viruses. Am J Hyg 61:197–218, 1955
136. SAHLER OJ and WILFERT CM: Fever and petechiae with adenovirus type 7 infection. Pediatrics 53:233–235, 1974
137. SCHMIDT NJ, LENNETTE EH, and KING CJ: Neutralizing, hemagglutination-inhibiting and group complement-fixing antibody responses in human adenovirus infections. J Immunol 97:64–74, 1966
138. SCHWARTZ HS, VASTINE DW, YAMASHIROYA H, and WEST WE: Immunofluorescent detection of adenovirus antigen in epidemic keratoconjunctivitis. Invest Ophthal 15:200–207, 1976
139. SCOTT JV, DREESMAN GR, SPIRA G, and KASEL JA: Radioimmunoassay of human serum antibody specific for adenovirus type 5-purified fiber. J Immunol 115:124–127, 1975
140. SEVER JL, HUEBNER RJ, CASTELLANO G, and BELL JA: Serologic diagnosis "en masse" with multiple antigens. In Conference on Newer Respiratory Diseases, 1962, pp 342–359
141. SIMILA S, YLIKORKALA O, and WASZ-HOCKER O: Type 7 adenovirus pneumonia. J Pediatr 79:605–611, 1971
142. SIMILA S, JOUPPILA R, SALMI A, and POHJONEN R: Encephalomeningitis in children associated with an adenovirus type 7 epidemic. Acta Paediatr Scand 59:310–316, 1970
143. SNEJDAROVA V, VONKA V, KUTINOVA L, REZACOVA D, and CHLADEK V: The nature of adenovirus persistence in human adenoid vegetations. Arch Virol 48:347–357, 1975
144. SOHIER R, CHARDONNET Y, and PRUNIERAS M: Adenoviruses: status of current knowledge. Prog Med Virol 7:253–325, 1965
145. SPENCE D, KENNEY G, MCCLURE AR, MACFARLAND DE, and SOMMERVILLE RG: The preparation of antiserum to adenovirus (group) hexon antigen, to be used for immunofluorescent detection of infection with different adenoviruses. Arch Gesamte Virusforsch 34: 340–345, 1971
146. STEVENS DA, SCHAEFFER M, FOX JP, BRANDT CD, and ROMANO M: Standardization and certification of reference antigens and antisera for 30 human adenovirus sertotypes. Am J Epidemiol 86:617–633, 1967
147. STROM J: Febrile mucocutaneous syndromes (ectodermosis erosiva pluriorificialis, Stevens-Johnson's syndrome etc.) in adenovirus infections. Acta Derm Venereol 47:281–286, 1967
148. SWANN NH: Acute thyroiditis. Five cases associated with adenovirus infection. Metabolism 13:908–910, 1964
149. TAVERNE JJ, MARSHALL H, and FULTON F: The purification and concentration of viruses and virus soluble antigens on calcium phosphate. J Gen Microbiol 19:451–461, 1958

150. Top FJ, Jr, Beuscher EL, Bancroft WH, and Russell PK: Immunization with live types 7 and 4 adenovirus vaccines. II. Antibody response and protective effect against acute respiratory disease due to adenovirus type 7. J Infect Dis 124:155–160, 1971

151. Top FH Jr, Grossman RA, Bartelloni PJ, Segal HE, Dudding BA, Russell PK, and Beuscher EL: Immunization with live types 4 and 7 vaccines. I. Safety, infectivity, antigenicity and potency of adenovirus type 7 vaccine in humans. J Infect Dis 124:148–154, 1971

152. Tyrrell DAJ, Balducci D, and Zaiman TE: Acute infections of the respiratory tract and the adenoviruses. Lancet 2:1326–1330, 1956

153. Valters WA, Boehm LG, Edwards EA, and Rosenbaum MJ: Detection of adenovirus in patient specimens by indirect immune electron microscopy. J Clin Microbiol 1:472–475, 1975

154. Van Der Veen J and Dijkman IH: Association of type 21 adenovirus with acute respiratory illness in military recruits. Am J Hyg 76:149–159, 1962

155. Van Der Veen J and Kok G: Isolation and typing of adenoviruses recovered from military recruits with acute respiratory disease in the Netherlands. Am J Hyg 65:119–129, 1957

156. Van Der Veen J and Lambriex M: Relationship of adenovirus to lymphocytes in naturally infected human tonsils and adenoids. Infect Immun 4:604–609, 1973

157. Van Der Veen J and Van Der Ploeg G: An outbreak of pharyngoconjunctival fever caused by types 3 and 4 adenovirus at Waalwyk, The Netherlands. Am J Hyg 68:95–105, 1958

158. Van Der Veen J and Van Zaane DJ: Infection with type 21 adenovirus in children with acute lower respiratory disease. Ned Tijdschr Geneesk 107:808–811, 1963

159. Vargosko AJ, Kim HW, Parrott RH, Jeffries BC, Wong D, and Chanock RM: Recovery and identificaiton of adenovirus in infections of infants and children. Bacteriol Rev 29:487–495, 1965

160. Vastine DW, West CE, Yamashiroya H, Smith R, Saxtan DD, Gieser DI, and Mufson MA: Simultaneous nosocomial and community outbreak of epidemic keratoconjunctivitis with types 8 and 19 adenovirus. Trans Am Acad Ophthalmol Otolaryn 81:826–840, 1975

161. Warner JO and Marshall WC: Crippling lung disease after measles and adenovirus infection. Br J Dis Chest 70:89–94, 1976

162. Whitelaw A, Davies H, and Parry J: Electron microscopy of fatal adenovirus gastroenteritis. Lancet 1:361, 1977

163. Wigand R: Non-specific serum inhibitors are irrelevant in adenovirus hemagglutination. Arch Gesamte Virusforsch 35:311–315, 1971

164. Wigand R and Fliedner D: Serologically intermediate adenovirus strains: a regular feature of group II adenoviruses. Arch Gesamte Virusforsch 24:245–256, 1968

165. Wigger HJ and Blanc WA: Fatal hepatic and bronchial necrosis in adenovirus infection with thymic alymphoplasia. N Engl J Med 275:870–874, 1966

166. Williamson J, Doig WM, Forrester JV, Dick WC, and Whaley K: Studies of the viral flora in keratoconjunctivitis sicca. Br J Ophthalmol 59:45–46, 1975

167. Wilner BI: A Classification of the Major Groups of Human and Other Animal Viruses. Burgess, Minneapolis, 1969, pp 120–132

168. Wolontis S, Tunevall G, and Sterner G: Adenovirus type 5 infections: an outbreak of febrile pharyngitis in a home for infants. Acta Paediatr Scand 56:57–65, 1967

169. Wright HT Jr, Beckwith JB, and Gwinn JL: A fatal case of inclusion body pneumonia in an infant infected with adenovirus type 3. J Pediatr 64:528–533, 1964

170. Yodfat Y and Nishmi M: Successive overlapping outbreaks of febrile pharyngitis and pharyngoconjunctival fever associated with adenovirus types 2 and 7, in a kibbutz. Isr J Med Sci 10:1505–1509, 1974

171. Yunis EJ, Atchison RW, Michaels RH, and Decicco FA: Adenovirus and ileocecal intussusception. Lab Invest 33:347–351, 1975

CHAPTER 10

POXVIRUSES

James H. Nakano

Introduction

In 1971 the US Public Health Service, following the United Kingdom's example earlier in the same year, recommended that routine childhood vaccination for smallpox be discontinued in the United States. By the end of 1977, routine vaccination was no longer required by 13 countries, namely Austria, Belgium, Canada, Denmark, Finland, the German Federation Republic, Japan, the Netherlands, New Zealand, Norway, Sweden, the United Kingdom, and the United States (143), and in January 1978, Chile joined the list. Other countries will certainly adopt the same policy eventually; however, according to available information, 81 countries and areas still require a smallpox vaccination certificate from all newly arriving persons, and 72 countries require a primary smallpox vaccination.

At this time, when smallpox is about to be eradicated and smallpox vaccination is being discontinued, any case of poxvirus infection of humans should be examined carefully, especially cases occurring in the countries where smallpox has only recently been eradicated. In this context Lennette's statement (75) is especially appropriate: "We need not necessarily expect that new and unknown viruses will turn up but rather that some of our long-known, garden variety viruses may play a hitherto unsuspected role." So it may be with poxviruses when routine smallpox immunization has ended; some of the "garden variety" poxviruses found in a common laboratory and in wild animals may become causes of human disease.

As is appropriate and timely, this chapter includes the laboratory diagnosis of human infection caused by variola, vaccinia, monkeypox, cowpox, and whitepox viruses of the orthopoxvirus group; orf and milker's nodule viruses of the parapoxvirus group; Tanapox virus of the Tanapox-Yabapox virus group, and molluscum contagiosum of the unclassified group (96).

History

Smallpox. Although the terms *variola* and *smallpox* had different origins, they are presently used synonymously. The term *variola* was used originally in the year 570 A.D. in France. It is derived either from the Latin *varius*, meaning spotted, or from *varus*, meaning small button (129). *Small-*

pox was used in a descriptive sense to differentiate the disease from syphilis, introduced into Europe in 1494 and commonly known as "large pox" (27).

The origin of smallpox as a disease is unknown (27), but ancient writings suggest that it may have started in eastern Asia (67). Although no clinical descriptions were given, it is thought to have been first recorded in Ireland in 675 A.D. and to have been introduced into France by the Moors in 731 (27). It was first recorded in England during the early 16th century and shortly thereafter was introduced by the Spaniards into the New World, where it caused epidemics in the West Indies in 1507, Mexico in 1520, and Brazil in 1563 (67). In colonial America, Winslow (138) mentions smallpox epidemics in Boston in 1628, 1634, 1677, 1689, and 1702. Bardell (8) states that in 1775, after the fighting at Lexington and Concord and the Battle of Bunker Hill, the British force under the command of General William Howe and the American force under the command of General George Washington faced each other for 9 months without any serious action because of smallpox among the troops. Smallpox also had a profound effect on the Canadian campaign, and it further hampered recruitment of soldiers for the Colonial Army in 1776.

The last outbreaks of smallpox in the United States occurred in 1946, 1947, and 1949. The 1946 outbreak was in Seattle and King County, Washington, where 16 of 51 patients died, for a case fatality rate of 32% (111). The index case, diagnosed in a soldier returning from Kyushu, Japan, was acquired in Asia and probably was variola major. The 1947 outbreak involved New York City and Milbrook, New York, where 3 of 12 patients (25%) died (134). Here, the index case was from Mexico. The last laboratory-verified smallpox outbreak in the United States occurred in Texas in 1949; 1 of the 8 patients (12%) died, and the index case was assumed to have come from Mexico (63). From 1949 to 1954, several imported suspected smallpox cases were recorded but not laboratory verified.

Vaccinia. As a prophylactic measure vaccinia virus was predominantly used in the late 1800s, after it replaced the variola and cowpox viruses formerly used to immunize humans against smallpox. The origin of vaccinia virus is obscure. According to Downie and Kempe (33), it evolved from the serial propagation of cowpox virus on the skin of calves, a method used throughout Europe in the 1860s to produce cowpox virus vaccine. Some writers, however, claim that vaccinia virus evolved from serial passaging of variola virus on calf skin during generally the same time period.

Monkeypox. Monkeypox, an exanthematous disease similar in clinical appearance to smallpox, was first noticed in 1958 as the cause of an epidemic in captured cynomolgus monkeys from Singapore and was reported by von Magnus (131). The first natural infection in humans by monkeypox virus was discovered in September 1970 in Zaire (71). Five additional cases were reported in Liberia and Sierra Leone in 1970 (49), a few months after the eradication of smallpox in the west and central African countries. Since then, 35 cases in all have been identified in 5 African countries: Liberia, Sierra Leone, Ivory Coast, Nigeria, and Zaire. Most of these were in Zaire. Information has been published on 20 of the 35 cases (6).

Whitepox. At present, 6 different strains of whitepox virus have been recovered (6). Two, designated 64-7255 and 64-7275, were isolated in 1964 from kidney cell cultures derived from 2 apparently healthy cynomolgus monkeys (52). The other 4 were isolated from the kidney tissue of apparently healthy wild animals captured in Zaire: Chimp-9 from a chimpanzee in 1971 (82), MK-7-73 from a sala monkey in 1973 (124), RZ-10-74 from a rodent (*Mastomys coucha*) in 1974 (83), and RZ-38-75 from a rodent (*Helioscorus rufobrachium*) in 1975 (83).

The strains isolated from subhuman primates or rodents cannot be differentiated either by the biologic genetic marker tests or by antigenic tests from variola virus believed to cause natural infection only in humans. Recently, the whitepox virus strains Chimp-9, MK-7-73, 64-7255, and 64-7275 were characterized by electrophoresis of their virion deoxyribonucleic acids (DNAs), fragmented by 3 restriction endonucleases. All these strains were found to group within the species *variola* of the genus *Orthopoxvirus* (46). It is important, therefore, to include whitepox virus in this chapter to alert laboratory investigators working with subhuman primates and other animals to the potential existence of this variola-like agent in their experimental animals.

Cowpox. Cowpox was reported by Jenner in 1798 (64) to be the cause of a disease in horses called "grease," which could be transmitted to cows. In cows it caused irregular pustules on nipples and was transmissible to humans, in whom it produced enlarged axillary nodes, headache, and lesions on the hands, wrists, and finger joints. As a disease in cattle it was apparently prevalent in Europe through the first half of the 20th century, but Baxby (9) states that now only a low-grade endemic form exists in the United Kingdom and the Netherlands. Recent findings support the belief that cowpox virus may have its reservoir in rodents. Since 1966, when the Center for Disease Control (CDC) began working actively to eradicate poxvirus infections, no human infection with cowpox virus has been reported in the United States.

Orf. Orf virus normally infects sheep, producing a disease known variously as contagious ecthyma of sheep, contagious pustular dermatitis, contagious pustular stomatitis, and sore mouth. It was reported by Hansen to infect humans as early as 1879, but not until 1937 was it reported in Great Britain (Peterkin as cited by Nagington and Whittle [95]); it was first reported in the United States by Schoch in 1939 (123).

Milker's nodule. Jenner's observation that "spurious cowpox" did not provide immunity against cowpox or smallpox but "classical cowpox" did (65) suggests that milker's nodule was probably known in 1799. This disease, transmitted from cattle to humans, has since been reported in Europe but was not noted in the United States until 1940 (11).

Tanapox. Two epidemics of this exanthematous disease, which occurred in 1957 and 1962 among the Wapakomo tribe along the Tana River in Kenya, were reported by Downie et al (36). Epizootics caused by a similar poxvirus occurred in the United States in 1965–1966, in a primate-importing establishment in California and in 3 primate centers (California, Oregon, and Texas) 20, 26, 42, 55).

Molluscum contagiosum. This disease has been recognized as a clinical entity since 1817 (132).

Clinical aspects

Smallpox (variola). Two distinct types of smallpox, clinically identifiable only during variola outbreaks because of relative differences in severity and the proportion of fatal cases noted, are variola major and variola minor. Variola major, which has prevailed in the Asiatic subcontinent, is severe, with case fatality rates ranging from 15% to 40%. Variola minor, formerly prevalent in South America, South Africa, and Botswana and more recently in Ethiopia and Somalia, has a case fatality rate of less than 1%.

In 1963 Bedson et al (13) reported that they had tested 23 variola strains isolated in 1961, 1962, and 1963 from Tanzania (Tanganyika) by propagating them at temperatures higher than the conventional incubation temperature range of 35–36.5 C. The reproductive capacity of these strains at 38.3 C was 1+ to 2+, that of variola major virus strains was 2+ and that of variola minor virus strains was 0. Thus, the relative reproductive capacity of these Tanzania strains at 38.3 C was designated as "intermediate." (The term "intermediate" as used by Bedson and his co-workers applied only to the reproductive capacity of the strains at the supraoptimal temperature and not to severity of disease produced in man.) Subsequently, the World Health Organization (WHO) reported case fatality rates ranging from 5.6% in Tanzania (Tanganyika) (13) to 11.1% in Sierra Leone (West Africa) to 15.4% in Indonesia (142), which implied an intermediate form of clinical smallpox. (In Indonesia the illness was originally severe, but later became less severe as the Smallpox Eradication Program progressed [personal communication, D.A. Henderson, M.D., formerly, Chief, Smallpox Eradication Unit, WHO, Geneva]). In reality, however, the spectrum of virulence ranged from very severe to very mild.

The following clinical descriptions are quoted directly from Downie and Kempe (33):

> Smallpox is usually spread by direct contact with a clinical case although it may occur indirectly by handling of clothing, bedclothes or utensils soiled by the infectious discharges of patients. It is believed that the site of entry of the virus is in the upper respiratory tract. The incubation period is most commonly 12 or 13 days but occasionally it may be as short as 8 or as long as 17 days. The clinical illness begins with fever, headache, pains in the limbs and prostration. During this preeruptive-phase, lasting 2 to 4 days, transient erythematous or petechial rash over the groins, axillae and flanks is seen in about 10% of cases. The local eruption appears usually on the 3rd or 4th day and soon afterwards the temperature drops and the patient feels much better. The focal rash usually appears first on the oral and pharyngeal mucosa, on the face or forearms and hands and then spreads to the trunk and legs. The eruption on the skin evolves through the stages of macule, papule, vesicle and pustule over a period of 5 or 6 days. In all except the

mildest cases the temperature usually rises again as the lesions become pustular. In the fully developed pustular eruption—about the 8th to 10th day of illness—the distribution is usually characteristic, the face and extremities being more extensively involved than the trunk, the back more than the front of the trunk and the chest more than the abdomen. Flexures such as the groins, axillae, the front of the elbow and popliteal skin tend to be spared. Although the eruption on the face and arms may be a day in advance of those on the legs, the eruption on any part of the body is homogenous in that all elements are at the same stage of development. In patients who are to recover, the lesions begin to dry up about the 10th to 12th day of illness and after 3 weeks most of the scabs have been shed, with the exception of the deep brown seeds in the palms of the hands and soles of the feet.

In severe cases, the eruption on the face may be confluent and when this confluent eruption evolves slowly it feels soft and velvety, with umbilication and is associated with hemorrhages in the base of the lesions; in malignant confluent cases the prognosis is bad. In the most severe cases, the fulminant or hemorrhagic, petechiae (and frank hemorrhage in many cases) appear in the skin on the 2nd or 3rd day (having a skin with a dusky purplish hue, later developing, blotchy extravasations of blood); there may be bleeding into the conjunctiva, from the mouth, nose, bladder, rectum or vagina and the patient may die in 4 to 5 days before the focal eruption can develop. In these cases the illness may be erroneously diagnosed as purpura, acute leukemia or meningococcal septicemia. In mild cases, especially where the disease is modified by previous vaccination, the eruption may be scanty, more superficial and there may be no secondary fever. Such cases are liable to be mistaken for chickenpox. Usually a leukopenia develops early in the disease followed by leukocytosis when the eruption becomes pustular. In hemorrhagic cases normoblasts and atypical white cells of the lymphocyte or lymphoblast type may appear in the peripheral blood and suggest a diagnosis of acute leukemia. Except in the acute fulminant cases most deaths occur towards the end of the 2nd week of illness.

Patients are most infectious from about the 3rd to the 10th day of illness and infection is spread at this time chiefly from the heavily infected secretions from the mouth and upper respiratory tract. However, virus is present in the crusts and the patient cannot be regarded as free from infection until all crusts have separated. The commonest complications are abscesses in the skin or subcutaneous tissues, and variolous infection of bones. Encephalitis is a rare complication; since the introduction of antibiotics secondary bacterial bronchopneumonia, once common in severe cases, is now rarely seen.

Variola minor or alastrim shows a clinical picture similar to that of variola major with discrete eruptions. The incubation period is of the same duration, there is the same preeruptive illness, but confluent rash is relatively uncommon and hemorrhagic cases are very rare. Secondary fever during the pustular stage is often absent and the eruption tends to run its course more quickly.

Pathogenesis. The virus probably enters the body through the mucosa of the upper respiratory tract. No lesion has been observed at the site of entry, and as patients are not infectious during the incubation period, no virus is shed from the respiratory passages at this time. It seems likely, as has been demonstrated in ectromelia (119) and in rabbit pox (12), that the virus passes through the mucosa and is carried possibly by phagocytic cells to the local lymph nodes where primary multiplication occurs. From this site virus probably seeps into the bloodstream, from which it is removed by cells of the reticuloendothelial system. In these tissues—spleen, lymph nodes, liver and bone marrow—the virus undergoes further multiplication and passes to the bloodstream at, or just before the onset of clinical illness. Virus can be detected in the blood at this time and from this viremia the epithelial cells of the mucosa of the mouth, pharynx, etc., and of the skin become infected. The early histologic changes in the skin suggest that the virus infects the capillary endothelium in the corium. In hemorrhagic cases, extravasation occurs around small vessels in this area. In average cases of smallpox, virus is not found in the blood after the first 2 days of illness, but in more severe and particularly in fulminant cases, virus may be present in increasing amounts up to the time of death (34). In such cases, the infection may be so intense and widespread that virus antigen may be detected in serum by precipitation or complement-fixation tests with an immune serum. The presence of virus after the first 2 days of illness, or the demonstrable presence of virus antigen in the blood, usually portends a fatal outcome.

Neutralizing antibody usually appears in the blood about the 5th or 6th day of illness when the temperature has dropped near to normal, but in severe infections the appearance of antibody may be delayed and in acutely fatal infections may not be detectable. The appearance of antibody in the blood does not, however, prevent the evolution of the skin lesions from the vesicular to the pustular stage. Virus within cells is protected from the antibody and the destruction of infected cells leads to inflammatory infiltration of polymorphonuclear leukocytes which are responsible for the pustulation. Bacteria are not usually found in unbroken pustules although secondary bacterial infection, especially of the bronchioles and pulmonary tissue, may contribute to death in a small proportion of cases; secondary bronchopneumonia has not been a common complication since the widespread use of antibiotics. The mortality rate in variola major has not been greatly reduced since the introduction of antibiotic treatment to prevent secondary bacterial infections.

Pathology. The earliest changes in the focal lesions of the skin are dilation of the capillaries in the corium, swelling of the endothelial cells, and accumulation of lymphocytes around the vessel. By the time macules are visible in the skin the virus has infected epithelial cells, and suitably stained smears of macular and early papular scrapings will usually show enormous numbers of virus particles. There is marked thickening of the epithelial layer and, as the infected cells undergo ballooning degeneration, fluid appears between the cells and its accumulation results in vesicle formation. In the fully formed vesicle or pustule in the skin, the roof is formed by a thin layer of keratinized cells, and the base by the degenerating cells in the lower malpighian layer or by the corium. Because in the lesions of the mucosa of the mouth and pharynx there is no keratin layer the virus is discharged earlier from the surface of these lesions and it is from this source that most of the infections are spread. Postmortem studies of fatal cases show that the liver and spleen are generally enlarged, but apart from occasional small hemorrhages, gross changes are not obvious (17). Large basophilic mononuclear cells are common in liver, spleen, and bone marrow. Focal degenerative changes may be found in the kidneys and testes. In fulminant cases of smallpox hemorrhages may be found in the internal organs, especially in the mucosa of the gastrointestinal tract. It is not known whether in those patients who recover focal lesions occur in the internal organs.

Vaccinia. Infection caused by vaccinia virus in humans originates either from smallpox vaccination or from contact with a recent vaccinee; therefore, as the various countries cease mandatory smallpox vaccination, its frequency will decrease. The infection can be transposed from the vaccination site to other areas of the body (e.g., periorbital disease) or to other persons. Most serious vaccinia infections occur in individuals with abnormal skin conditions, such as eczema and burns, or in people with abnormal immune mechanisms. The complications of vaccinia infections described by Fulginiti (50) and Lane et al (72) follow:

1. Erythema multiforme, a rash, usually macular and intensely erythematous, occurring 7–14 days after vaccination. It is thought to be an allergic reaction to vaccine components and may develop to be papular, vesicular, or urticarial.

2. Congenital vaccinia, a disseminated fatal disease of the fetus that can result from primary vaccination of the pregnant woman. It may occur during any trimester of pregnancy.

3. Generalized vaccinia, evidenced by the appearance of multiple lesions (containing vaccinia virus) on the body of vaccinees following viremia resulting from vaccination. The infection occurs in normal individuals whose antibody response against the virus has been delayed but adequate. The disease is almost always benign.

4. Progressive vaccinia (vaccinia gangrenosa, vaccinia necrosum), an infection in which the site of vaccination fails to heal and

the lesion progressively enlarges, developing central necroses and thick, dark eschars. The disease apparently occurs in individuals with defective cellular immune mechanisms (not necessarily defective humoral immune mechanisms) and also in persons with lymphatic malignancies who are receiving immunosuppressive therapy.

5. Postvaccinial encephalitis, a serious aftermath which occurred in the United States at the rate of 1.9 cases/million vaccinations in 1963 (99) and 2.9 cases/million vaccinations in 1968 (73). The following symptoms occur separately or in combination: meningeal signs, ataxia, muscular weakness, paralysis, lethargy, coma, and convulsions (99).

6. Eczema vaccinatum, a local or systemic dissemination of vaccinia virus in individuals with eczema or a history of eczema. The disease may be fatal.

Monkeypox. A monkeypox outbreak in a colony of captured cynomolgus monkeys was first described by von Magnus et al (131). They observed no clinical signs of the disease until the eruptive stage, which started with a generalized petechial rash and became maculopaular. The papular lesions became thick and pus-like. The lesions, almost all in the same stage of eruption, became covered with crusts that eventually dropped off, leaving distinct scars. The general health of the animals, however, appeared unaffected.

Infections in humans by monkeypox virus is basically indistinguishable from that by variola virus. Most patients are not severely ill, although 6 deaths have been associated with the disease.

Although direct person-to-person transmission from individuals with active cases to unimmunized close contacts has been rare, on 2 occasions close family contacts of patients with monkeypox virus infection contracted the disease almost 2 weeks after onset of the index case. Epidemiologic evidence has indicated that in some cases the virus was presumably transmitted from wild monkeys to humans when monkeys were eaten and their skins were processed by people living in the area where the disease occurred. However, it may on occasion have been transmitted by other animals, such as rodents, since monkeys were not always epidemiologically associated with the patients. Poxvirus (vaccinia virus) antibodies (antibodies cannot be differentiated for all viruses in the genus *Orthopoxvirus*) have been found in rodents (multimammate rat, rusty-bellied rat, African giant squirrel), larger mammals (blue duiker), and birds ("calso," touraco) captured in the general region inhabited by humans with monkeypox virus infections (18).

Whitepox. The only isolations of whitepox virus have been from apparently healthy subhuman primates and rodents. There have been no known infections in humans; therefore, the virus has never been clinically demonstrated to be a variola virus in humans. In our studies of African green monkeys infected intraperitoneally (ip) or subcutaneously (sc) by the Chimp-9 strain, the animals usually appeared ill in 4 days, had full vesicular lesions throughout their bodies on the seventh day, and recovered in about 2 weeks. Three of 10 African green monkeys used (1 inoculated by the ip route and 2 by the sc route) became acutely ill and died in 3–4 days, apparently from an overwhelming viremia. Presently, there are 6 isolates of whitepox virus.

Cowpox. This infection, a disease of cows, is now virtually nonexistent in the United States. Occurring on the skin of the udder and teats of cows, it can be transmitted by direct contact to dairy and farm workers and becomes apparent as lesions, usually on the fingers but sometimes on the hands, forearms, and face as well. The lesions begin with reddening and swelling and develop into papules that become vesicular in 4–5 days and heal in 2–4 weeks. Downie and Kempe (33) state that during the acute stage of infection the lesions are similar in histologic appearance to those of vaccinia or variola, except that large, strongly acidophilic inclusions are more numerous.

Human infections with cowpox virus have been believed to be contracted only by direct contact with infected cows. A recent report (10) of 10 human cases of cowpox in the United Kingdom, 7 in individuals with apparently no such direct contact, casts some doubt on this belief; however, they all lived in or had visited rural areas. Only 1 of the 10 patients was reported to have been previously vaccinated. A limited serologic survey of the cattle in the vicinity failed to reveal evidence that they were reservoirs of the virus, which implies that some other kinds of animals might be involved. In this same vein, apparently healthy white rats in Moscow (80) and big gerbils and yellow suslicks trapped in Turkmenia (USSR) were found to carry a poxvirus similar to cowpox virus (Prof. S.S. Marennikova, personal communication). If human infections by cowpox virus occur in the United States in the future, we should look for the source of the infections in animals such as rodents if cattle are not clearly implicated.

Orf (contagious ecthyma, contagious pustular dermatitis, contagious pustular stomatitis, sore mouth). Orf virus primarily infects sheep and goats but can infect humans, such as sheepherders, veterinarians, laboratory animal handlers, slaughter house workers, and wool shearers, who work directly with these animals. The virus is transmitted through an abraded surface on or a break such as a bite mark in the skin. Infections in humans are usually evidenced as a circumscribed single lesion on the finger, hand, arm or, occasionally, the face (58), and a generalized infection occurs only rarely (41, 90). Leavell et al (74) described 6 clinical and corresponding pathologic stages: a) 1–7 days, maculopapular stage, with erythematous spot which becomes elevated; b) 7–14 days, target stage, the lesion showing a red center, a white ring in the middle, and a red halo; c) 14–21 days, the lesion is nodular, appearing red and weeping; d) 21–28 days, regenerative stage, the lesion has a thin yellow crust with small black dots; e) 28–35 days, papilloma over the surface of the lesion; and f) 35 days or more, regressive stage, the lesion showing reduction in elevation and formation of a dry crust and subsequent shedding of several scabs before healing.

Milker's nodule. The virus causing milker's nodule in humans is primarily a pathogen of cows. The bovine disease is called pseudocowpox or paravaccinia and is manifested by development of lesions on the skin of the udder and teats. In calves the lesions are found on the lips and nose and may spread to the head, trunk, and limbs.

The virus is transmitted to humans by direct contact with infected cattle and starts at a site of abraded skin, usually on the hands and fingers. According to Becker (11), an erythematous papule develops in about 5-7 days after contact with a diseased cow and becomes a firm, elastic, bluish-red semi-globular nodule, 1-2 cm in size, with a central depression. The surface flattens as the lesion heals. Healing is complete in 4-6 weeks without scar formation. The regional glands are sometimes enlarged, and secondary pyogenic lymphangitis may develop.

Tanapox. Details of incubation and clinical features are obscure, but Tanapox infection begins with a febrile period of 3-4 days, occasionally accompanied by backache, severe headache, and prostration. Lesions, usually 1 and never more than 2, appear on the skin of the upper arm, face, neck, or trunk during the febrile stage. The pock-like lesions start as papules similar to those of smallpox and then become circular vesicles that umbilicate without pustulation. Although the lesions are similar to those of modified smallpox in a vaccinated individual, they are different in that they are larger and firmer, develop more slowly, and lack pustulation.

A number of human infections with a poxvirus similar to Tanapox virus have been reported that were transmitted from diseased, captured monkeys in 2 epidemics (42, 87), and 1 experimental infection in a human (36) has been described. None of the infected patients showed any profound systemic symptom, however. In most patients the lesions healed in 2-4 weeks; the longest period was 7 weeks.

Molluscum contagiosum. Found in individuals of all ages throughout the world, molluscum contagiosum causes a benign tumor of the skin characterized by localized proliferation of the epidermis to form lobulated and umbilicated papules (29). The umbilicated papules vary from white to pale pink and measure 2-8 mm. A semi-solid caseous material can be expressed and used for microscopic examination (79). The disease is generally transmitted by direct contact of body surfaces, but when the lesions are found in the genital regions, it can be sexually transmitted (19). Although self-limiting, it may last several months to several years.

Description and Nature of the Agents

Common Characteristics

The International Committee on Taxonomy of Virus (62) described poxvirus as:
> large, brick-shaped or ovoid virions, 300-450 nm × 170-260 nm, with external coat containing lipid and tubular or globular protein structures, enclosing one or two lateral bodies and a core, which contains the genome. Virion contains more than 30 structural proteins and several viral enzymes, including a DNA-dependent RNA (ribonucleic acid) polymerase.

The genome consists of a single molecule of double-strand DNA of molecular weight $130-240 \times 10^6$, G + C content of vertebrate poxviruses 35–40%, of entomopoxviruses about 26%. Genetic recombination occurs within genera; non-genetic reactivation occurs both within and between genera of vertebrate poxviruses.

Multiplication occurs in cytoplasm, with type B (viral factor) and type A (cytoplasmic accumulation) inclusion bodies. Mature particles are released from microvilli or by cellular disruption. Infectivity is ether resistant in some genera and ether sensitive in others. Hemagglutinin is separate from the virion and is produced by viruses of *Orthopoxvirus* only.

Size and Shape

The poxviruses discussed in this chapter can be divided into 2 morphologically distinct groups. One group, represented by vaccinia virus, is brick shaped and includes the viruses of variola, cowpox, vaccinia, monkeypox, whitepox, Tanapox, and molluscum contagiosum (Figs 10.1-6). The sizes of the viruses in this group range from 140 to 230 × 210 to 380 nm. The second group, represented by orf virus, is ovoid and elongated and includes the viruses of orf and milker's nodule (Figs 10.7-8); sizes range from 120 to 160 × 250 to 310 nm.

Chemical Composition

The vaccinia virus (92), as a representative of the orthopoxvirus group, is composed of protein (90% of the virus dry weight); DNA (2.1-7.3%, or more definitely, 3.2%); lipid (about 5%) consisting of cholesterol, phospholipid, and neutral fat; and RNA (less than 0.1-0.2%); and trace substances.

The DNA content of molluscum contagiosum virus is similar to that of vaccinia virus (114).

Resistance

Generally, poxviruses in a dry condition remain active for many months, and freeze-dried smallpox vaccine heated at 100 C for 60 min still maintains its activity (68). That freeze-dried smallpox vaccine has such great stability was one of the factors that contributed to eradication of smallpox in the tropical countries.

In the CDC laboratory variola virus could be isolated from specimens from patients with suspected smallpox even after the specimens had been held 2-8 weeks under "field" conditions in Africa, India, and Bangladesh. Of 758 specimens from smallpox patients verified to be positive by a combination of laboratory tests, only 51 (6.7%) failed to yield viable variola virus. Of 22 specimens received from Africa from human monkeypox patients and positive for poxvirus by electron microscopy (EM), only 3 (13.6%) were negative upon inoculation of tissue cultures (TC) and chicken chorioallantoic membranes (CAM).

Generally, poxviruses of the vaccinia-variola-monkeypox group are ether resistant (1, 115, 131), susceptible to 50 C when wet, and susceptible to pH 3.0 (122). Vaccinia virus (and probably other orthopoxviruses also)

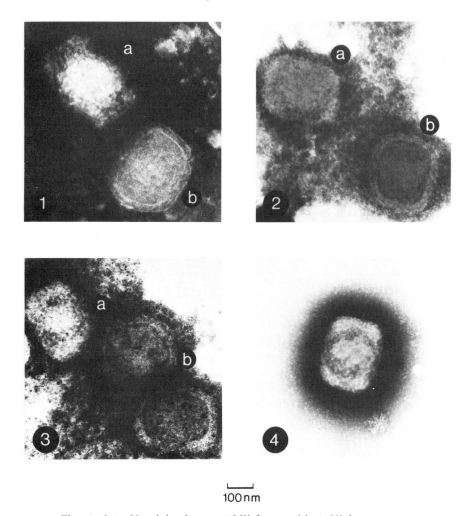

100 nm

Figure 10.1—Vaccinia virus: a. "M" form and b. "C" form.
Figure 10.2—Variola virus: a. "M" form, b. "C" form.
Figure 10.3—Monkeypox virus: a. "M" form and b. "C" form.
Figure 10.4—Whitepox virus: "M" form.

may be inactivated by alcohol, acetone (85), ultraviolet light (23), photodynamic action in the presence of methylene blue (130), formaldehyde, and
sodium hypochlorite. Orf and milker's nodule viruses are ether resistant (24, 128). The 2 viruses are inactivated by chloroform, 50 C when wet
(milker's nodule virus only), and pH 3.0 (24, 117). A half-life of Tanapox
virus at 37 C is 18 hr (102). Molluscum contagiosum virus is sensitive to
50 C and pH 3.0, but resistant to ether and chloroform (47).

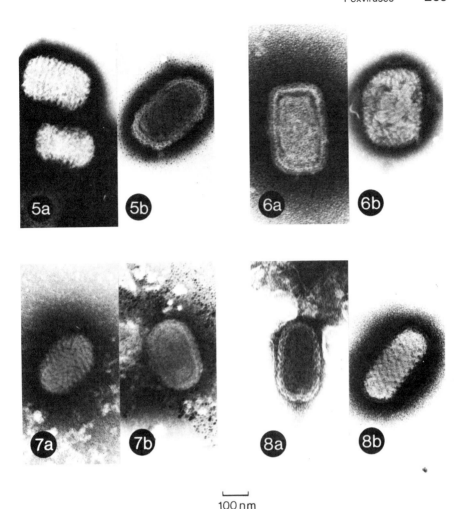

100 nm

Figure 10.5—Moluscum contagiosum virus: a. "M" form and b. "C" form.
Figure 10.6—Tanapox virus: a. "C" form and b. "M" form.
Figure 10.7—Milker's nodule virus: a. "M" form and b. "C" form.
Figure 10.8—Orf virus: a. "C" form and b. "M" form.

Classification

The names of the genera for poxviruses approved by the International Committee on Taxonomy of Viruses (62) are *Orthopoxvirus*, *Parapoxvirus*, *Avipoxvirus*, *Capripoxvirus*, *Leporipoxvirus*, *Entomopoxvirus*, and a group of viruses not yet assigned. The genus *Orthopoxvirus* includes variola, cowpox, vaccinia, monkeypox, and whitepox viruses (as well as others not considered in this chapter). The genus *Parapoxvirus* includes orf and milker's nodule viruses. Tanapox virus is not yet allocated, but Nakano (96) placed it unofficially under the Tanapoxvirus group for the sake of expediency in diagnosis; this group also contains Yabapox virus. Molluscum contagiosum is still in the unallocated group. A more extensive listing of poxviruses has been published by Nakano (96).

Antigenic composition

Virus-coded proteins are divided into 3 groups (137). They are a) the viral structural proteins, including nucleoproteins; b) the soluble antigens found in large quantity in poxvirus-infected cells; and c) the virus-induced enzymes. Only the first 2 groups will be discussed, because they are important in the routine diagnosis of poxvirus diseases and the identification of poxviruses. Furthermore, the following discussion pertains only to the poxviruses in the orthopoxvirus group.

Structural proteins. A component of the nucleoprotein antigens obtained by alkaline extraction of purified virions is apparently a group antigen common to all viruses of the family *Poxviridae* (139). Dissociated vaccinia virion proteins have been shown by polyacrylamide gel electrophoresis to contain at least 17 polypeptides (59). More recently, 31 polypeptides have been reported for vaccinia virus and 28 for fowlpox virus (107); comparison of polypeptide profiles can differentiate these 2 viruses. Polypeptides of several strains of variola virus, whitepox virus, monkeypox virus, and vaccinia virus have been observed (45) to fall into 1 of 3 basic patterns, represented by the variola, the vaccinia, and the monkeypox groups. Cowpox and rabbitpox viruses can be assigned to the vaccinia group (7) and whitepox virus to the variola group (45).

Although the poxviruses in the genus *Orthopoxvirus* produce hemagglutinin in TC, purified virions themselves do not hemagglutinate. Thus, hemagglutinin was believed not to be an integral part of the virion (66). However, when purified vaccinia virions were digested with 10–1000 μg of pepsin, hemagglutination (HA) activity was observed (84, 125). HA activity was also observed when purified variola virions were disrupted with a reducing agent (2). Furthermore, purified vaccinia virions that had been inactivated with β-propiolactone and ethyl alcohol induced the production of hemagglutination-inhibiting (HAI) antibody when inoculated into guinea pigs (57). These findings suggest that hemagglutinin or hemagglutinin-like material is present in purified vaccinia virions, although it cannot be demonstrated in intact purified virions.

Purified vaccinia virions disintegrated by alkali, by a certain kind of protease (e.g., trypsin), and by autolysis (without an enzyme) release precipitating antigens (144). Purified intact vaccinia virus particles produce no precipitin line when reacted with a homologous antiserum (136). A soluble fraction, obtained from pepsin-treated purified vaccinia viruses and injected into rabbits, elicits the production of neutralizing (Nt), precipitating, complement-fixing (CF), and HAI antibodies (84).

Soluble antigens. Soluble antigens are viral antigens that are released from infected cells during the course of infection, and they are separate from the infectious virions. The soluble antigen fraction can be separated into a high-molecular-weight group (> 200,000) and a low-molecular-weight group (50,000–100,000) (22). The soluble antigen fraction, including the LS antigens (25), is composed of precipitating, CF antigens (30), and "serum-blocking" antigen (Nt-blocking antigen) (5). Rabbits immunized with soluble antigens (virus free) respond by producing Nt antibody (4) and also precipitating, CF, and HAI antibodies (84).

Poxvirus strains in the orthopoxvirus group have been differentiated by comparison of precipitin lines formed by reaction of a specific strain's soluble antigens with homologous antiserum (51, 121). Recently, qualitative differences in the soluble antigens of vaccinia, variola, and monkeypox viruses have been observed by use of absorbed monospecific antisera (44, 53, 77).

Hemagglutinin. Hemagglutinin produced by the poxviruses of the orthopoxvirus group during their infection of cells is separate from the infectious virions and the soluble antigens. Vaccinia hemagglutinin has been shown to be derived from the plasma membrane of the infected cells (15) and, therefore, is probably a product of disrupted plasma membrane modified by viral infection. This view is supported by the fact that soon after cells are infected with vaccinia-variola group poxviruses, hemagglutinin is detectable at the cell surface by the use of a plaque-hemadsorption technique (108), which identifies the cells infected with the poxviruses. Hemagglutinin particles are pleomorphic and measure about 50 nm in diameter (98). Hemagglutinin extracted from heavily infected CAMs and RK 13 cells treated with ether-ethanol has been observed to have a lipid component that possesses HA activity and a protein component that does not possess the HA activity but possesses the antibody-blocking activity (126). Furthermore, the lipid component used to immunize rabbits does not produce HAI antibody, but the protein component does (84). The protein component has been identified as comprising 3 specific glycoproteins (61).

Extracellular and intracellular viral antigens. It has been observed that intracellular rabbitpox virus is neutralized by antiserum produced against live rabbitpox virus and by antiserum produced against inactivated vaccinia virus but that extracellular rabbitpox virus is neutralized only by the antiserum produced against the live rabbitpox virus (4). Thus, an antigenic difference of extracellular and intracellular poxvirus was first observed. The extracellular poxvirus differs from the intracellular poxvirus in that the former possesses an outer envelope that is probably derived from the host cell membrane. This envelope was recently found to possess HA activity (113).

Preparation of Immune Serum

Vaccinia virus antiserum

Vaccinia virus seed can be obtained from any smallpox vaccine (freeze-dried calf lymph). However, if the vaccinia virus is to be used for a purpose other than routine diagnostic work, an established laboratory strain of vaccinia virus should be used. Vaccinia virus strains from easily available vaccines are the New York Board of Health Strain in the Wyeth smallpox vaccine, Dryvax, in the United States and in the Connaught smallpox vaccine in Canada and the Lister (or Elstree) strain in the Lister Institute smallpox vaccine in the United Kingdom and many other European countries. A reconstituted smallpox vaccine usually has a titer of about $10^{8.0}$ pock-forming units/ml on CAMs of 12-day-old chicken embryos. The reconstituted vaccine is diluted 1:10 with a TC maintenance medium, and 1 ml of this diluted vaccine suspension is placed in a 1-liter bottle containing a confluent growth of primary rabbit kidney (PRK) TC with a medium containing 10% inactivated normal rabbit serum for growth and 2% of the same serum for maintenance. A $3+$ to $4+$ cytopathic effect (CPE) can be observed in 2-3 days of incubation at 36 C. The culture medium is then discarded; the cells are scraped and resuspended in 10 ml of McIlvaine buffer, pH 7.4, and frozen and thawed through 3 cycles. This viral material has a titer of about $10^{8.0}$ pock-forming units/ml on CAM. It is then mixed with an equal volume of Freund complete adjuvant.

Each prebled rabbit (older than 6 months) is inoculated in both front footpads, each with 0.3 ml of the mixture. One milliliter is inoculated sc in the right hind quarter. A 1-ml booster of viral immunogen is given intramuscularly (im) in the hind quarter at 20 days. The rabbit is exsanguinated 14 days after the booster. The serum usually has a CF titer of 1:512-1:1024, an HAI titer of 1:320-1:1280, and a precipitation titer of 1:4-1:8.

Variola virus and whitepox virus antiserum

Variola and whitepox viruses can be adapted to grow in PRK cells in 2-3 passages (37) and in rabbit kidney stable cell line, RK-13 (100). The infected cultures contain $10^{5.0}$-$10^{6.0}$ pock-forming units/ml. Variola virus adapted to grow in the PRK cells can then be inoculated into rabbits as described for vaccinia virus.

Monkeypox virus antiserum

Monkeypox virus grown in PRK can be used as an immunogen. Producing monkeypox virus antiserum in rabbits is easier than producing variola or vaccinia antiserum in these same animals because they become ill from the infection. A 0.5-ml volume of a monkeypox virus TC fluid (with a titer of at least 10^6 pock-forming units/ml) inoculated either intradermally (id) or sc can cause a generalized illness in a rabbit (6 months or more of age) in about 3-4 days, and furthermore, the rabbit will show secondary exanthems throughout its body. The rabbit recovers in 10-14 days. A 1-ml booster inoculation of the monkeypox virus TC suspension is given im on day 14 after the initial incculation, and the rabbit is exsanguinated 7 days later.

Orf virus antiserum

Orf virus is grown in ovine kidney cell cultures with use of Eagle medium containing 10% normal ovine serum as a growth medium and Eagle medium containing 2% ovine serum as a maintenance medium. When the CPE is observed to be $3+$ to $4+$ after 3-5 days of incubation at 36 C, the culture is frozen and thawed through 3 cycles. The virus in culture of human embryonic lung fibroblasts (HELF) will measure about $10^{4.5}$ mean tissue culture infective doses (TCID$_{50}$)/ml. A 3-month-old lamb is prepared for immunization by clipping of the wool over areas 10 × 10 cm on the left and right upper front legs. The left leg area is shaved, scarified with a 20-gauge needle point, and swabbed with the orf virus TC. Without shaving or scarification, the right leg area is inoculated sc with 1.5 ml of the viral TC. Lesions develop on the inoculated areas in 12–14 days. Booster inoculations of 5 ml administered im in the hind quarter are given on the days 46 and 60 after the initial inoculation. The lamb is exsanguinated on day 68. The CF and Nt antibodies titers are about 1:128.

Milker's nodule virus antiserum

Milker's nodule virus is grown in bovine embryonic kidney cell cultures, and the virus culture is prepared as described for orf virus (except fetal calf serum is used instead of ovine serum). A viral culture containing about $10^{4.5}$ TCID$_{50}$/ml in HELF is used to immunize a 3-month-old calf. Five milliliters of the virus culture is homogenized with an equal volume of Freund complete adjuvant and inoculated im into the hind right quarter. A similar inoculum is given 2 weeks later, and an additional inoculum is given at weekly intervals for 4 weeks. The animal is exsanguinated 1 week after the sixth inoculation. The CF and Nt antibody titers of the serum are about 1:64.

Tanapox virus antiserum

Tanapox virus immunogen is produced in either African green monkey kidney (AGMK) cell cultures or HELF cultures. The titer obtained is about 10^5 plaque-forming units/ml as determined in AGMK or HELF cultures. The virus culture is mixed after 3 cycles of freezing and thawing with an equal volume of Freund complete adjuvant and is inoculated into rabbits as described for the production of vaccinia virus antiserum. The Nt antibody titer of the serum is about 1:1000–1:2000. The antiserum is not suitable for the CF test when the viral antigen contains monkey or human cells.

Molluscum contagiosum virus antiserum

Production of antiserum for molluscum contagiosum virus in animals has been difficult because the in vitro production of the virus for immunogen has been difficult. Several investigators have reported growing at least some strains of molluscum contagiosum virus in TC (21, 47, 118), but others have reported observing no reliable evidence of viral replication to maturity in cell cultures despite CPE (116). Mitchell has reported experimental production of anti-molluscum contagiosum virus (CF antibody) in humans (89). Using as immunogen a suspension of molluscum contagiosum virus lesions treated with formaldehyde (0.2%), he inoculated sc a patient with a history of a 6-month-old infection by molluscum contagiosum virus. The patient, who previously had had no CF antibody, responded with 1:8 CF antibody titer after 4 inoculations.

Collection, Preparation, and Shipment of Specimens

Precautions for handling smallpox specimens

Since the last case of variola major occurred in Bangladesh in October 1975, the entire continent of Asia has been assumed to be free of smallpox. At present the only known cases of the disease in humans are in Somalia. In the context of the certain eventual global eradication of human smallpox, there are 4 sources of possible reintroduction of variola virus into the human population. These sources could include animal reservoirs, variolators' specimens, residual smallpox scabs in patients' houses, and variola virus stocks in various laboratories throughout the world. Conferees at a meeting sponsored by the World Health Organization (WHO) in 1976 on monkeypox and related poxviruses concluded that no evidence available thus far indicated the existence of an animal reservoir of smallpox. Failure to isolate smallpox virus on CAM and TC from 31 specimens collected in 1976 from variolators in Afghanistan, Ethiopia, and Pakistan (Nakano, J.H., unpublished observations) tends to negate the possibility of reintroduction of variola virus from variolators' specimens. Smallpox scabs in patients' houses also appear to be of no epidemiologic importance as a source of viable virus. It seems, therefore, that variola virus stocks currently stored in laboratories may be the only significant source for reintroduction of variola virus into the human population. It is clear that any such stocks, if retained, should be used only under conditions of strict containment.

To prevent the occurrence of any disaster contributed by these virus stocks, the 30th World Health Assembly (1977) has recommended that variola virus be retained only under the strictest conditions to ensure maximal safety. In August 1977, WHO convened a group of expert consultants to consider safety standards for the maintenance and use of variola virus in laboratories. Their essential recommendations for safety follow:

1. A laboratory where variola virus is used must be constructed to provide the strict physical containment necessary and must be operated in such manner as to prevent inadvertent dissemination of variola virus. The laboratory must be either in a separate building, or in a controlled area within a building, isolated from all other areas of the building. Access to the laboratory must be strictly controlled to exclude entry of unauthorized persons. (In all, 15 restrictions were presented in the definition of an acceptable containment system.)

2. Authorized persons must have *valid* smallpox vaccination within the previous 3 years.

3. Only WHO Collaborating Centers should maintain variola virus, and assurance should be given that a representative group of variola strains will be retained for the future. The recommended WHO Collaborating Centers are

a) Viral Exanthems Branch, Virology Division, Bureau of Laboratories, CDC, USA Department of Health, Education, and Welfare, Atlanta, Georgia, 30333, USA.

b) Laboratory of Smallpox Prophylaxis, Research Institute of Virus Preparations, Moscow, USSR.

c) Virology Department, the Wright-Fleming Institute of Microbiology, St. Mary's Hospital Medical School, London, United Kingdom.

d) Poxvirus Laboratory, Department of Enteroviruses, National Institute of Health, Tokyo, Japan.

e) Rijks Institut voor de Volksgezondheid, Bilthoven, the Netherlands (only for smallpox vaccine).

The Viral Exanthems Branch, CDC, Atlanta, and the Laboratory of Smallpox Prophylaxis, Moscow, will continue as the principal WHO centers for diagnosis of suspected human smallpox cases as well as for research; the other WHO centers will be primarily engaged in research.

4. Variola virus is the only orthopoxvirus recognized as a highly dangerous pathogen, but because whitepox virus is currently indistinguishable from variola virus, it too must be subject to biocontainment measures.

Since monkeypox, vaccinia virus, and the other orthopoxviruses pose no major public health danger, the only precautions required for their handling is smallpox vaccination every 3 years; elaborate containment measures, like those for variola and whitepox viruses, are not considered necessary.

5. For security, storage containers of variola and whitepox viruses must be locked when not in use and for biocontainment, storage and handling of these viruses must be subject to the strict physical containment requirements mentioned above.

Collection of specimens

Any case of suspected smallpox should be investigated immediately by competent health staff, and if the diagnosis of smallpox is still suspected, national health authorities and the WHO should be notified immediately. Any specimens suspected of containing smallpox virus should be forwarded either to CDC, Atlanta, or the Research Institute of Virus Preparations, Moscow, for definitive confirmation.

Laboratory diagnostic results can only be as good as the specimens submitted. The greater the quantity of materials submitted, the more dependable are negative results.

Specimens for virologic diagnosis

Variola, vaccinia, monkeypox, and cowpox specimens.

1. Pre-eruptive stage—Blood collected with sterile anticoagulant can be used as a source of virus, particularly variola virus.

2. Maculopapular rash stage—Cleanse skin with an alcohol sponge, scrape at least 6 lesions with a No. 11 or No. 12 scalpel blade and make thick smears on 4 glass slides. Do not heat treat or fix smears in any way.

3. Vesicular-pustular rash stage—Remove vesicle or pustule dome from 10 lesions with a No. 11 scalpel blade or forceps, and place them in a screw-capped vial. Collect as much vesicular or pustular fluid as possible in 3 or 4 capillary tubes (fill at least to a height of 10 mm). Place the capillary tubes into a screw-capped tube or vial. Scrape the base of the lesions, and make thick smears of the material on glass slides as described above. Make at least 4 slides. The smears should occupy only a small area of the slide but should be as thick as possible.

4. Crusting stage—Remove as many scabs as possible (up to 12) and place in a screw-capped vial. For vaccinia and cowpox only fragments of crusts may be obtainable.

Fulminating (hemorrhagic) smallpox cases. In fulminating smallpox cases where appropriate skin lesions may not be found, autopsy specimens should be collected, including clotted blood, sections of the lungs, liver, spleen, and kidneys. These should be frozen immediately or kept on ice if they can be delivered to the testing laboratory within 24 hr. Do not fix the specimens in formaldehyde solution.

Orf and milker's nodule. Collect vesicular fluid, crusts, and fragments of crusts as described above.

Tanapox. Collect crusts, if present, and biopsies of the lesions and place in a screw-capped vial.

Molluscum contagiosum. Collect expelled material from the lesions on swab tips, or transfer the material directly into a screw-capped vial with an applicator stick or a No. 12 scalpel blade.

Specimens for serologic diagnosis

Collect an acute-phase blood specimen (at least 10 ml) as early as possible during the illness and a convalescent-phase blood specimen (at least 10 ml) 3–4 weeks after the onset of the rash. Serum need not be separated from the clot if the blood can be delivered to a testing laboratory within 24 hr. Otherwise, separate the serum from the clot, and store it at -20 C.

Packing and shipping of specimens

Place serologic or virologic specimens in a primary container (screw-capped vial or jar), and close and seal it securely with waterproof tape. Enclose the primary container in a durable, watertight secondary container, with enough nonparticulate absorbent material (such as a paper towel) in the space at the top, bottom, and sides between the primary and secondary containers so that the entire content of the primary container would be absorbed if it should break or leak. Place each set of double containers in an outer shipping container constructed of corrugated fiberboard, cardboard, or other material of equivalent strength. Enclose a copy of the laboratory record or other identifying information between the secondary container and the outer shipping container. When smallpox specimens are shipped, the outer shipping container should be placed in a cardboard box measuring at least $26 \times 26 \times 39$ cm so that the shipment is less likely to be lost because of small size. Affix a "Shipper's Certificate for Restricted Articles" to the outer shipping container of a smallpox specimen, as required by the Air Transportation Association. This applies to all shipments, domestic or foreign. For information and transportation of smallpox specimens in the United States, also affix to the outer container an "authorizing permit" issued by the Office of Biohazard, CDC, Atlanta, Georgia 30333, and an "etiologic agents" label.

Before shipping smallpox specimens, inform the receiver. Transport smallpox specimens by special air transportation system, registered mail, or an equivalent system which provides for the receiver to be notified immediately upon their arrival.

Smears, vesicular fluid, and crusts can be shipped without refrigeration if prompt delivery is expected. However, autopsy materials and serologic specimens (sera) should be stored and shipped frozen.

Laboratory Diagnosis

Direct examination of clinical material for virus identification

Identification of virions by electron microscopy

Clinical materials such as vesicular fluid, crusts, scrapings, and exudate smears can be easily prepared for examination by EM. Reagents and equipment necessary are a) 400-mesh grids coated with Formvar, b) 2% sodium phosphotungstate (pH 7.0), c) phosphate buffer, pH 7.2 (0.01 M), d) wax-coated glass slides prepared by dipping the slides into melted paraffin wax (Parafilm can be substituted for the waxed slides), e) platinum-tipped forceps, f) glass capillary tubes with rubber microbulbs, and g) plastic Petri dishes (60 mm in diameter) lined with filter paper of appropriate size.

Preparation of specimens and grids. Crusts are ground with phosphate buffer (about 0.3–0.5 ml of buffer for each 5-mm diameter scab) in a thick-walled glass tissue grinder. A suspension prepared in this manner is considered undiluted, and 2 drops of the suspension are placed side by side on a wax-coated glass slide. An equal-sized drop of the buffer is placed close to the second drop of the crust suspension, and the 2 are mixed well with a capillary tube equipped with a rubber microbulb. This mixture is considered to be a 1:2 dilution. Further 2-fold dilutions, through 1:8, are made in the same manner, by mixing 1 drop of suspension and 1 drop of buffer.

For fixing and staining the specimen on an EM grid, a drop of 2% sodium phosphotungstate is placed on another section of the wax-coated slide. Two EM grids coated with Formvar are placed coated-side down in the 1:8 dilution of crust suspension, allowed to float for 30 sec, and then transferred to the drop of 2% sodium phosphotungstate, again coated-side down. The grids are allowed to float an additional 30–60 sec and then placed coated side up on a filter paper lining the petri dish. Two grids are prepared in the same manner from each of the other dilutions (1:4, 1:2, and undiluted). The areas of the paper where the various grids are placed are marked 1:8, 1:4, etc.

Each capillary tube of vesicular fluid is expelled by a capillary bulb (after the sealed ends are removed) onto a wax-coated slide—2 drops on the slide, one of which is diluted 1:2 with buffer in the same manner as with the crust suspensions. Vesicular fluid is usually diluted through 1:4. Grids are prepared as for a crust suspension.

Fluid collected as a smear on a glass slide is softened first with 2 drops of the buffer, and a suspension is made by sucking and expelling with a capillary tube and microbulb. A pooled suspension made from 3 to 4 smears from the same patient is then used without further dilution to prepare grids.

Since grids and their containers are prepared and handled in a smallpox biocontainment area, both must be decontaminated before they are taken out of the area for the grids to be examined by EM. This is accomplished by filling a small plastic container 15 mm in diameter with 10 drops of concentrated formaldehyde solution (37%) and placing it in a 60-mm Petri dish containing the prepared grids. The Petri dish is covered, placed in a larger (150-mm) uncovered Petri dish containing a shallow volume of 5% sodium hypochlorite, and exposed in a pass-through box for 30 min to an ultraviolet light (General Electric Germicidal Lamp (G15T8), 15 W, with a specification of 2.95 W/ft^2 at the exposure distance of 5 cm) at a distance of 2.5 cm. The temperature in the box reaches 45 C. At the end of the 30-min exposure period, the top cover of the small Petri dish is removed and placed top-side down in the sodium hypochlorite solution beside the bottom part of the small Petri dish and is exposed for an additional 15 min. At this time the 60-mm Petri dish is covered with a sterile lid and taken out of the pass-through box.

Examination by EM. The grids are examined for density at a magnification of about 2,000–3,000. An overly dense grid indicates that the material put on the grid was too concentrated, and a very thin grid indicates that the material was too diluted (probably because the amount of specimen available was not sufficient to make a suspension of satisfactory concentration).

Grids found to have a satisfactory density are scanned at a magnification of 10,000–20,000. When a virion is found, its detailed structure is examined at a magnification of 50,000–184,000.

Poxvirus virions with a beaded or filamentous mulberry-like surface are termed "M" form and those with a capsule are termed "C" form (135). Figures 10.1–10.8 show the M and C forms of virions of vaccinia, variola, monkeypox, molluscum contagiosum, Tanapox, milker's nodule, and orf. Figure 10.4 shows only the M form for whitepox virus. More M forms usually are found in the preparations from vesicular fluid, and more C forms in those from crusts. Poxvirus virions permitting no penetration of stain, e.g., 2% potassium phosphotungstate or 1% uranyl acetate, appear as the M form, and virions permitting stain penetration appear as the C form. Specimens with a greater degree of dryness before staining contain a greater percentage of C-form virions, and also stained preparations which have been held longer before examination contain a greater percentage of the C forms (135).

Interpretation and differential diagnosis. EM is probably the most dependable and rapid laboratory diagnostic method available for smallpox, provided that an adequate amount of appropriate specimen is collected as described on pages 275–276. When a strongly suspected case of smallpox (especially with supportive epidemiologic evidence) occurs in a country without endemic smallpox, every effort should be made to have the specimens tested at a competent virologic laboratory where an EM, an experienced person to carry on laboratory diagnosis of smallpox, and an adequate biocontainment system (see pages 274–275) are available.

Clinically, chickenpox is the disease most often confused with smallpox. Specimens from patients suffering from either disease can be quickly identified by EM. The specimen from a chickenpox patient should show herpes-like virus particles, and the specimen from a smallpox patient should show poxvirus particles as shown in Figures 10.2a and 10.2b.

In examining grids by EM, one must differentiate nonvirus particles that resemble poxvirus or herpesvirus from the real virus particles. A number of nonvirus particles resemble the M and the C forms of poxvirus and the core of herpesvirus. Vesicular fluid from chickenpox patients predominantly shows the enveloped herpesvirus, and crusts predominantly show the core. If during an examination by EM a particle is found that is not typical, the specimen should be examined more closely and a typical virus particle that can positively be identified will usually be found. Reference to a printed picture of an atypical particle is often useful for making the decision. Photographic illustrations of some nonvirus particles that can be mistaken for poxvirus particles are shown in a report by Nakano (97).

What is the reliability of EM for the detection of poxviruses in specimens collected from patients with suspected smallpox? Of the specimens from over 5,000 patients examined at CDC since 1966, 758 were identified as variola and 25 as human monkeypox (omitting specimens from patients diagnosed as having monkeypox by serologic or epidemiologic evidence) by a combination test system of EM, culture by chicken CAM, agar gel precipitation (AGP), and TC. Of the 783 positive specimens identified by all methods combined, 765 or 97.7% could have been detected by EM alone. Undoubtedly, more of the negative specimens would have been found positive for poxvirus by EM if an adequate quantity of all specimens had been collected.

Examination of specimens by EM can differentiate variola virus from chickenpox, orf, and milker's nodule viruses but cannot differentiate it from vaccinia, monkeypox, whitepox, cowpox, Tanapox, and molluscum contagiosum virus.

Variola cannot be differentiated clinically from human monkeypox (although human monkeypox is generally milder and rarely causes infection in unprotected close contacts). These infections can be differentiated only by biological genetic marker tests and immunologic tests. Variola can generally be differentiated from vaccinia, cowpox, Tanapox, molluscum contagiosum, and milker's nodule on the basis of clinical and epidemiologic findings.

The percentage of positive poxvirus identifications by EM is much less for vaccinia virus infection than for variola and human monkeypox. Of 61 positive specimens for vaccinia virus by CAM, only 41 (67%) were positive by EM at CDC.

For specimens from clinically diagnosed human orf, EM results were positive in 33 of 41 (82.5%), and TC results were positive in 12 of 41 (29.2%); for ovine orf EM results were positive in 12 of 14 (86.0%), and TC results were positive in 9 of 14 (64.2%) (94). For specimens from persons clinically diagnosed as having milker's nodule (pseudocowpox), EM results were positive in 14 of 14 (100%), and TC results were positive in 8 of 15 (53.3%) (1 case of the 15 was not examined by EM). For crust specimens from bovine teats of clinically diagnosed pseudocowpox, EM results were positive in 50 of 82 (73.0%), and TC results were positive in 32 of 82 (39.0%) (94). Examination by EM of specimens from orf and milker's nodule is more effective in laboratory diagnosis than is virus isolation in TC.

Because the lesions of Tanapox in humans are generally unique, a positive diagnosis may be made by detection of poxvirus particles by EM, provided that there is supportive epidemiologic evidence (monkey association). However, when the case history and epidemiologic evidence are scanty, as in occasional cases in equatorial Africa, isolation of the virus and appropriate serologic tests are required.

Diagnosis of molluscum contagiosum can be verified by EM demonstration of poxvirus particles because of the disease's unique clinical manifestation.

Identification of virus particles in stained smears by light microscopy

If EM is available, examination by light microscope is not needed. Two staining techniques, the Gutstein method and the Moroson silver method modified by Gispen, are described by Downie and Kempe (33) and can be used for identifying stained elementary bodies of the poxviruses in the orthopoxvirus group and orf or contagious pustular dermatitis virus (86).

Identification of viral antigens by immunoserology

Agar gel precipitation test
1. Vaccinia virus antiserum—This serum is prepared in rabbits as described on pages 271–272. Human serum collected during the convalescent phase of smallpox should not be substituted for hyperimmune antivaccinia rabbit serum as a testing reagent because the human serum may contain antibodies other than those against the orthopoxviruses; in this case, precipitin lines other than those against the orthopoxviruses may be observed and may confuse the diagnosis.

Vaccinia virus antiserum reacts against every virus in the orthopoxvirus group.

2. Positive control antigen—Obtain 20 CAM confluently infected with Wyeth smallpox vaccine strain of vaccinia virus, and homogenize them for 3 min at full speed in a 250-ml Sorvall Omnimixer cup (with the cup immersed in an ice-water bath). Add 20 ml of sterile phosphate-buffered saline (PBS), and homogenize the mixture for an additional 2 min. Add 1 part of Genetron 113 to 3 parts of the homogenate, and homogenize for another 3 min. Centrifuge the mixture at 800 × g for 10 min, and draw off and save the supernatant fluid. To 9 parts of this supernatant fluid, add 1 part of 0.01% trypsin (final concentration of the trypsin, 0.001%). Place the mixture in an incubator at 36 C for 1 hr. Concentrate the mixture to a final volume of 20 ml by dialyzing it against 20 M polyethylene glycol. Distribute the concentrated mixture in 1-ml portions and store at −20 C.

Prepare normal CAM control antigen in the same manner by starting with 20 uninfected CAM.

3. Preparation of an AGP test system—Precoat glass slides with frosted ends with 0.2% purified agar melted in distilled water. The frosted area is used for writing the identification. Draw a line between the frosted and the clear section of the slide with a marking pen containing a fast-drying oil-base paint. The slightly raised line prevents the melted agar from running into the frosted area. Melt previously prepared 1% purified agar (prepared in distilled water containing 1:10,000 of thimerosal), and carefully deliver and spread 1.5 ml of the melted agar onto the entire clear area of the slide. A layer of agar about 2 mm thick is formed. Place a plastic template over the hardened agar, and punch out wells in the agar. (The template has a pattern with a centrally located round hole surrounded by 6 round holes. The holes are 4 mm in diameter with 5 mm between the centers.) Remove the punched well cores in the agar by suction with a Pasteur pipette attached to a vacuum line on a portable electric vacuum pump.

4. *Test procedure*—For the AGP test use the suspension of specimens prepared for EM examination without further dilution. Carefully add the specimen suspension to the wells located at the 12 o'clock and 6 o'clock positions, without letting them overflow. Fill the well at the 2 o'clock position with the positive control vaccinia virus antigen and the well at the 4 o'clock position with normal rabbit serum. Fill the central well with the anti-vaccinia rabbit serum. Place the slide in a humid chamber, and incubate it at 35 C.

5. *Interpretation*—Several precipitin lines (positive reaction) will occur within 2-4 hr between the wells containing the specimen and the center well containing the vaccinia antiserum if the specimen is from lesions of smallpox, vaccinia, human monkeypox, cowpox, or whitepox, but not of orf, milker's nodule, Tanapox, or molluscum contagiosum.

At least one of the precipitin lines formed between the wells containing the specimen and the vaccinia antiserum must fuse or join the precipitin lines formed between the wells for the positive control vaccinia antigen and the vaccinia antiserum. (Note that pustular specimens sometimes produce a line against a normal rabbit serum.)

A specimen found negative on first testing may be positive when re-tested with antivaccinia rabbit serum diluted 1:2, 1:4, and 1:8 because of a more optimal antigen-antibody proportion.

In evaluating at the CDC the reliability of the AGP test for detecting variola and monkeypox virus antigens, we found that 783 of more than 5,000 specimens from patients with suspected smallpox were positive for variola or monkeypox by a combination test system (EM, AGP, CAM, and TC), but only 589 or 75.2% were positive by the AGP test alone. Again, the major reason for false-negative results was inadequate amount of specimen for testing. Another reason could have been degeneration of soluble precipitating antigen caused by prolonged exposure of some specimens to high ambient temperatures during shipment. Heating crust extracts at 60 C for 15 min has resulted in greatly weakened AGP reactions (38).

In attempts to detect orf antigen by AGP, 275 (63%) of 360 experimentally produced orf scabs in lambs were positive (120); and in a natural outbreak in lambs with clinical orf, 31% were positive (120).

Tanapox virus antigen can be identified by the AGP test (31, 32), but the test's reliability for diagnosis of the disease is still unmeasured.

Although the antibody assay by the AGP test has been tried for molluscum contagiosum, more work is needed to find out how well this test can identify the viral antigen for diagnosis.

6. *Specific identification of variola, vaccinia, and monkeypox viruses*— The AGP as described above cannot differentiate the poxviruses in the orthopoxvirus group. However, a more specific AGP test using monospecific

antisera prepared by selective absorption of heterologous antibodies has been developed which makes it possible to identify variola, vaccinia, and monkeypox viruses (44, 53).

Immunofluorescence (FA) test. Both the direct and indirect methods of FA can be used for identifying specific poxvirus antigens. A detailed description of the 2 methods is found elsewhere in this book (Chap 4) or refer to Emmons and Riggs (40).

Some investigators have recommended the FA technique for diagnosis of smallpox (93, 109), but under actual field-testing conditions results with this technique ranged from false positive to false negative (39, 69, 78). An investigation at the CDC (106) to evaluate the accuracy of smallpox diagnosis by FA revealed no *false-negative* FA staining in smear specimens of *continuously frozen* vesicular or pustular fluids from 50 smallpox patients and no *false-positive* FA staining for smallpox in smears from 10 varicella patients, but the test was not reliable unless the specimens were kept frozen after collection. Nonspecific staining occurred in specimens stored more than 7 days without freezing.

In a recent investigation in India to evaluate the FA technique for diagnosis of smallpox, Kitamura et al (70) found no *false-negative* FA reactions for smallpox in 50 clinically verified smallpox patients, and no *false-positive* FA staining for smallpox in 4 clinically verified varicella patients. However, of 20 patients with questionable diagnosis of smallpox, varicella, measles, or an unidentified skin disease from whose specimens variola virus was not isolated, 3 patients had specimens which gave FA-positive staining for smallpox. These 3 patients were proven not to have smallpox by clinical and epidemiologic evidence. Therefore, the authors contended that the specimens from 15% of these patients gave false FA-positive reactions for smallpox.

In Bangladesh, where smallpox was endemic in 1975, FA tests on specimens from patients with smallpox or with suspected smallpox were performed by a field laboratory (Stanley O. Foster, MD, CDC, personal communication). Some of the specimens tested by FA were sent to CDC for examination by EM. All of the specimens from 11 clinically certain smallpox patients had been FA positive for smallpox in Bangladesh, and these specimens were all positive for poxvirus by EM at CDC. However, specimens from 7 patients verified by second visits to have either a non-smallpox skin disease, scabies, or boils were also FA positive for smallpox in Bangladesh, but EM negative for either poxvirus or varicella virus at CDC (Nakano, unpublished observations).

The FA test results from these 2 studies suggest that the test does not give false-negative results for specimens of smallpox patients but may give false-positive results for specimens of patients with some non-smallpox skin diseases.

The FA test can be used for detecting FA-positive specimens from suspected smallpox patients, but only for screening purposes until the problem of the false-positive results is solved. It is urged that any specimens from a highly suspected case of smallpox be sent to WHO Collaborating Center for Smallpox and Other Poxvirus Infections, located either at CDC, Atlanta,

GA 30333, or at the Laboratory of Smallpox Prophylaxis, Research Institute of Virus Preparations, Moscow, USSR for confirmation.

Although the FA test has been used to detect viral antigens of viruses other than variola in the orthopoxvirus group, its reliability for diagnosis by testing field specimens, e.g., crust is not known because very few such specimens have been tested.

Orf and molluscum contagiosum viruses in TC (21) have been identified by FA without any problem, but a dependable identification of these viruses in field specimens has still not been determined, nor has its reliability for the diagnosis of milker's nodule and Tanapox in field specimens been demonstrated.

CF test. The CF test is more sensitive than the AGP test for identifying poxvirus antigens but is not preferred over EM for smallpox diagnosis.

The recommended CF test procedure is the microtiter technique described elsewhere in this book (Chap 1). A specimen suspension (unknown antigen) in saline, diluted 2-fold to 1:128, is block titrated against a specific antiserum that has been previously tested and shown to have a high CF titer against a known vaccinia virus antigen. The serum is diluted 2-fold to its end titer. If the reagent serum, blocked against an unknown antigen diluted greater than 1:2 or 1:4, shows a CF titer as high or almost as high as that obtained when the serum is tested against a known positive vaccinia virus antigen, the reaction is considered to be specific, provided that the unknown antigen shows no anticomplementary reaction.

Antiserum containing antibody against a human tissue, human cell line, or human serum should not be used when human specimens are tested.

Smears made from fluid of papules, vesicles, and pustules on 3 slides are suspended in 1 ml of saline solution. Fluid collected in capillary tubes is diluted 1:10 with saline solution. The suspensions are allowed to stand at room temperature for 1 hr and centrifuged at $450 \times g$ for 15 min. The clear supernatant fluid is used for testing.

Before crusts are tested, lipoidal material should be extracted with ether by the following method. One crust dried by calcium chloride or phosphorus pentoxide in a dessicator for 4 hr is ground and allowed to stand in 5 ml of ether for 30 min. The ether is pipetted off, and the residual ether is evaporated. A 1% suspension is made by adding saline solution and is allowed to stand for 2 hr. The suspension is centrifuged at $450 \times g$ for 15 min, and the clear supernatant fluid is used for testing.

The CF test is also used to identify the viral antigens for orf virus (41, 120) and for Tanapox virus (103). Although the CF test has been used only for antibody assays in milker's nodule and molluscum contagiosum, it can probably be used also for viral antigen identification of these viruses.

Isolation and identification of poxviruses by culturing

CAM of embryonated chicken eggs. All poxviruses in the orthopoxvirus group, including variola, vaccinia, monkeypox, whitepox, and cowpox viruses, can be isolated on CAM; many of these can also be identified by their characteristic growth on the CAM. Orf, milker's nodule, Tanapox, and molluscum contagiosum viruses differ from orthopoxviruses in that they cannot grow on CAM. Varicella virus (in the herpesvirus group), the etiologic agent of chickenpox, which is sometimes clinically confused with smallpox, also does not grow on CAM, but the herpes simplex virus does.

1. Preparation of eggs—General instructions for handling eggs are found elsewhere in the book (Chapter 1). For photographic demonstration of egg preparation for CAM inoculation, consult the WHO *Guide to the Diagnosis of Smallpox for Smallpox Eradication Programmes* (141).

The eggs should be obtained from an egg producer who has a healthy flock. Eggs exposed to sunlight or heat have reduced fertility. Those not incubated immediately after receipt should be stored at cool room temperature to deter embryo development.

Fertile chicken eggs must be incubated at 38–39 C for 11–13 days to be useful for isolating and identifying the poxviruses of variola, vaccinia, monkeypox, whitepox, and cowpox. Lower incubation temperatures can have the same effect as shorter incubation time and render the CAM less sensitive or totally insusceptible to poxvirus growth when the eggs are used at the recommended time of 12 days.

2. "Dropping" the CAM—The embryonated eggs are placed blunt end up in a rack, and a small hole is made by a hand punch in the shell membrane of each egg in the area over the air space. While each egg is being candled to determine the embryo's viability, a second small hole is made with a hand punch through the shell, but not through the shell membrane, at a spot over the CAM in an area without large blood vessels. The shell dust is blown away from the CAM hole, and a drop of sterile PBS, pH 7.2, is placed over the CAM hole. A sterile tip of a bent, disposable blood lancet is inserted through the drop of PBS, and the shell membrane is torn. As this happens the PBS droplet is drawn inside, and the CAM falls. The eggs are candled to confirm the formation of a new air space above the dropped CAM. If the CAM has not dropped, a slight suction is applied with a rubber bulb placed over the hole at the blunt end of the egg. If the CAM still does not drop, discard the egg. Inoculate the eggs within 6 hr.

3. Preparation and inoculation of specimen—Blood collected with sterile anticoagulant is centrifuged at $450 \times g$. The plasma and the buffy coat (layer of leukocytes) are separately drawn off, and each is diluted 1:2 with dilute McIlvaine buffer (0.0038 M of phosphate, pH 7.6) containing antibiotics.

Preparation of dilute McIlvaine buffer follows:

1. Solution A = citric acid 0.1 M $CH_3C_6O_7 \cdot H_2O$.
2. Solution B = Na_2HPO_4, 0.2 M (28.392 g/liter of water).
3. Combine 63.5 ml of solution A and 936.5 ml of solution B for a stock solution with a pH of 7.6; sterilize by membrane filtration.
4. To prepare dilute McIlvaine buffer with 0.0038 M phosphate, dilute 1 ml of the above stock with 49 ml of sterile distilled water. Add enough antibiotics to give a final concentration of 500 units of penicillin, 500 µg of streptomycin, and 250 units of neomycin per ml.

The plasma and the leukocyte suspensions are inoculated separately, each into a set of 4 eggs. Each egg is inoculated with 0.1 ml of the specimen directly onto the CAM by a disposable tuberculin syringe equipped with a 25-gauge, 1.6-cm needle.

The vesicular fluid, smear, and scab suspensions prepared for the EM grids are used to inoculate eggs. Each suspension is diluted 1:10, 1:1000, and 1:10,000 with McIlvaine buffer (containing antibiotics) in an attempt to get isolated pocks for better pock morphology characterization and for quantitation of the viruses. Four eggs are inoculated with each dilution as described above and rocked for better distribution of the inoculum over the CAM. The holes in the shell are sealed with plastic cement.

The inoculated eggs are incubated at 35 C instead of 36–37 C to avoid the growth inhibitory effect of the supraoptimal temperatures. The eggs are usually incubated for 72 hr. (Note that 3- or 4-dozen eggs placed in a conventional-style incubator can raise its temperature by 0.6–1 C, and that 20- or 30-dozen eggs can raise its temperature by about 1.5 C.)

The susceptibility of each lot of embryonated eggs should be monitored by inoculating some with house-standard vaccinia and variola virus. (The control viruses should be inoculated after the test specimens have been inoculated to avoid cross-contamination). The monitoring is necessary because we have found that at times, especially during the summer months, the susceptibility of CAM to variola, vaccinia, monkeypox, and herpes simplex viruses can decrease. The decreased susceptibility is easily detected by our house-standard vaccinia virus. The ranges of susceptibility are no growth of vaccinia virus pocks, growth of atypically small vaccinia virus pocks, growth of vaccinia virus pocks, and no reduction in size but with titer lower than usual by 0.5–1.0 logs.

4. Harvesting of infected CAM—Inoculated eggs should be harvested in a containment cabinet, and the cabinet should be decontaminated after each lot is harvested. A separate set of sterile forceps and scissors is used for each specimen. When an early result is desired, 1 or 2 eggs are opened at 48 hr instead of 72 hr, and the CAM are examined.

For harvesting hold the egg with the inoculated side up, insert sharp-pointed scissors into the hole in the blunt end, and cut the shell along the horizontal axis completely around the egg. The lower half, containing the yolk and embryo, is allowed to drop into a discard pan. The inoculated CAM adhering to the top half of the egg shell is removed with forceps and placed in a large Petri dish containing sterile saline. The CAM from each dilution are deposited in 1 Petri dish. The CAM in the dishes are taken out of the containment cabinet and examined for pocks with a magnifying glass under a strong light. The Petri dishes containing the CAM are placed on a wet, black, counter top to allow the pocks to be clearly discerned.

5. Interpretation—The viruses of variola, vaccinia, monkeypox, whitepox, and cowpox and the herpes simplex viruses types 1 and 2 are differentiated by the morphologic characteristics of the pocks that they produce on the chicken CAM. Viruses of varicella-zoster, orf, milker's nodule, Tanapox, and molluscum contagiosum do not grow on CAM.

The vaccinia virus pocks at 72 hr of incubation (Fig 10.9) are 3–4 mm in diameter and flattened, with central necrosis and ulceration and sometimes with slight hemorrhagic appearance. Figure 10.10 shows 1 vaccinia virus pock in CAM, examined at approximately 10X. The erythrocytes are not apparent in this picture; when they are present, they are in the surface layer of the CAM and not in the pock proper.

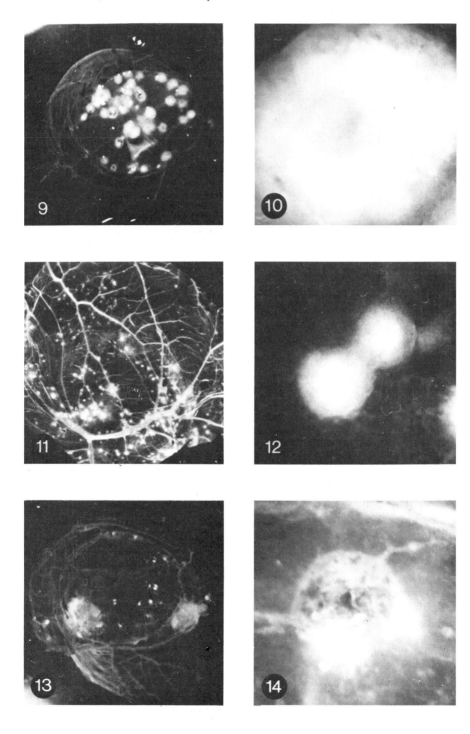

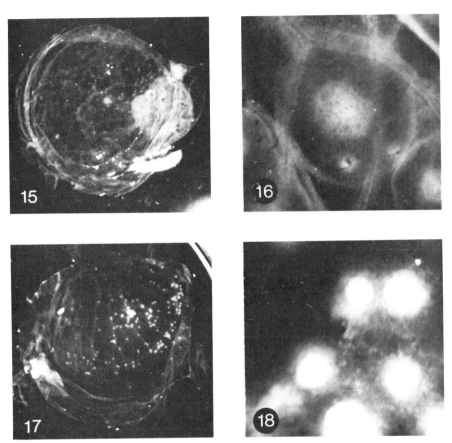

Figure 10.9—Vaccinia virus pocks on CAM.

Figure 10.10—One vaccinia virus pock on CAM, examined at approximately 10X.

Figure 10.11—Variola virus pocks on CAM.

Figure 10.12—Two variola virus pocks on CAM, examined at approximately 10X. Note the sunny-side-up egg appearance.

Figure 10.13—Numerous cowpox virus pocks on CAM. Note the hemorrhagic appearance.

Figure 10.14—One cowpox virus pock on CAM, examined at approximately 10X. Note the clusters of erythrocytes.

Figure 10.15—Monkeypox virus pocks on CAM. Note some pocks with central "punched-out" crater.

Figure 10.16—One monkeypox virus pock on CAM, wedged among the blood vessels. This is one of the several pock morphologies shown by the monkeypox virus. Note the cluster of erythrocytes represented by dark spots. Magnification approximately 10X.

Figure 10.17—Whitepox virus, strain Chimp-9 pocks on CAM.

Figure 10.18—Whitepox virus, strain Chimp-9 pocks on CAM, Magnification, approximately 10X. Note the morphologic similarity of these pocks and the pocks shown in Figure 10.12.

At 72 hr of incubation the variola virus pocks (Fig 10.11) are about 1 mm in diameter, grayish-white to white, opaque, convex or dome-shaped, raised above the CAM surface, round, regular, smooth on the surface, and not hemorrhagic; when examined at approximately 10X (Fig 10.12), they may have a halo around the opaque central area and appear like a fried "sunny-side-up" egg.

The cowpox virus pocks at 72 hr of incubation (Fig 10.13) are about 2-4 mm in diameter, flattened, and rather round and have a bright red central area; when examined at approximately 10X (Fig 10.14), the erythrocytes are accumulated in the pock proper instead of in the top layer cells of the CAM.

The monkeypox virus pocks on CAM at 72 hr of incubation (Fig 10.15) are about 1 mm in diameter, flat, and ridged along the periphery. Some have a crater in the center appearing as a punched-out hole, and some have a central hemorrhagic area caused by the erythrocytes clustered in the surface layer of the CAM, not in the pock proper, with pocks growing below the CAM surface. The characteristic hemorrhagic appearance of the monkeypox virus pocks on the CAM is sometimes not seen when the inoculated eggs are incubated at a temperature higher than 35.5 C. Figure 10.16 shows only the hemorrhagic monkeypox virus pocks. When the pocks in Figure 10.15 are examined carefully, some with the punched-out appearance can be seen.

At 72 hr of incubation the whitepox virus pocks (Figs 10.17 and 10.18) are very similar to those of variola virus. No differentiation can be made.

At 72 hr the herpes simplex virus type 1 pocks are pinpoint size, not raised, not opaque, and not regularly shaped; and when many are present, they are in lattice-work arrangement. The type 2 virus pocks are about 1 mm in diameter, white, flat, and irregular in shape and size. The pocks of the 2 herpes virus types are differentiated fairly easily from the variola virus pocks. If there is any doubt about the identity of the virus forming the pocks, the pocks can be ground and examined by EM or the AGP or CF test. A larger number of pictures showing various pock morphologies on CAM can be found elsewhere (96).

Several factors probably contribute to the reduced susceptibility of the CAM for the poxviruses. Some of these are use of eggs from a different flock, use of unusual antibiotics in the flock, presence of viral infection in the flock causing infection of the embryo and consequent interference, use of lower temperature for the preinoculation incubation of the eggs, lack of sufficient humidity during the preinoculation incubation period, use of a buffer with an excessively high salt concentration for diluting specimens, and incubation of the inoculated eggs at supraoptimal temperatures.

6. *Reliability*—The CAM culturing method is effective for isolating variola, human monkeypox, and vaccinia viruses. Of over 5,000 specimens collected from patients with suspected smallpox and human monkeypox and tested with a combined testing system at CDC, 783 were positive for variola or human monkeypox. Of the 783 positive specimens, 704 (89.9%) were positive by CAM alone. The percentage of positive isolations could have been greater if many of the specimens had not been in transit for a long

time under inadequate refrigeration. Specimens were sometimes in transit for 2-4 weeks and occasionally for 2 months at high ambient temperatures.

Isolation of poxviruses by TC. Detailed description of TC methods is given elsewhere in this book (Chap 3).

The use of TC for isolation is a necessary alternative for the CAM isolation method because of unpredictable insensitivity of the CAM. In addition, a virus particle already identified as a poxvirus by EM requires further identification by isolation and characterization.

The same specimen suspensions prepared for the examination by EM are used for inoculating TC. Each suspension is diluted 1:2 with McIlvaine buffer containing 4,000 units of penicillin, 2,000 μg of streptomycin, and 2,500 units of neomycin sulfate, usually inoculated into 3 TC tubes (0.1 ml/ tube) and incubated at 35.5 C. The inoculated TC are examined daily for signs of CPE. Those which fail to show CPE are observed for 10-12 days. Results of a test are not declared negative unless second passage cultures also incubated 10-12 days fail to show CPE.

1. Isolation of viruses of variola, vaccinia, monkeypox, whitepox, and cowpox—All of the human viruses in the orthopoxvirus group, including the 5 viruses above, can grow on most human and nonhuman primate cell cultures. Many of these viruses can also grow on TC derived from other animals such as rabbit, mouse, and hamster. For routine isolations, however, TC of HELF, infant foreskin fibroblast, primary rhesus monkey kidney cells (PMKC), and Vero cells (a stable line of AGMK cells) are recommended. Vaccinia, monkeypox, and cowpox viruses in TCs cause the cells to fuse and fall apart, forming large plaques (2-6 mm) and a mesh-work of cytoplasmic bridging in 1-3 days. Variola and whitepox viruses cause cell fusions and multinucleated foci; usually hyperplastic clumping of cells occurs in 1-3 days, but the plaques formed are small (1-3 mm) compared with those of vaccinia, monkeypox, and cowpox viruses.

Although human monkeypox virus infection is clinically similar to smallpox, one can differentiate the virus itself from smallpox virus by culturing it in a special cell line of embryonic pig kidney (81). Monkeypox virus does not cause CPE in this cell culture, but variola virus does.

One can more definitively identify variola, whitepox, vaccinia, monkeypox, and cowpox viruses isolated in cell cultures by subculturing them on CAM and observing their specific pock morphology. However, variola virus cannot be differentiated from whitepox virus by this method or any other method. (See pages 285-288 for further discussion on the identification of variola and whitepox viruses.) Because of the close antigenic relationship of the 5 viruses, no *simple* immunologic method can specifically identify them. However, a special immunoprecipitation test with monospecific absorbed serum can differentiate variola, vaccinia, and monkeypox viruses from each other (page 281).

2. Isolation of orf and milker's nodule viruses—Orf virus grows well in ovine cells such as embryonic ovine kidney cells and grows more slowly in primary human amnion cells and in secondary monkey kidney cells (95). Orf viruses from human infections can be isolated in bovine cells, but orf viruses from ovine infections do not grow initially in bovine cells (94). At CDC some strains of orf (from humans) have been isolated in PMK, and isolates growing in ovine cells have also been found to grow in HELF.

Milker's nodule virus grows well in bovine cells (48, 91), and after 1 passage, the virus grows well in WI-26 (48) and BSC-1 (91). Most strains can also be isolated in ovine cells (94). At CDC an isolate has been found to grow in HELF.

3. Isolation of Tanapox virus—The first passage of Tanapox virus may take more than 10 days to show CPE in human thyroid cells, but once the growth is established, the virus can be subcultured on human amnion cells, HEp-2, and WI-38. It also grows in primary cell cultures of vervet monkey kidney, patas monkey kidney, and Vero (36). At CDC it has been grown in HELF and primary AGMK cells.

4. Isolation of molluscum contagiosum virus—Although CPE has been reported to occur in primary human amnion cells (21), human foreskin fibroblasts (101), monkey kidney cells, and FL cells (a stable line of human amnion cells) (118), no permanent virus growth in TC had been established until recently when some strains of molluscum contagiosum virus were reported to have been isolated and subcultured in FL cells (47).

Isolation of poxviruses in animals. No animals have been routinely used to isolate any of the poxviruses mentioned in this chapter. However, monkeys can be inoculated with specimens to isolate variola, whitepox, and monkeypox viruses. Except for Asiatic monkeys, most animals are not susceptible to Tanapox virus. No animals have been known to be experimentally infected with molluscum contagiosum virus, but 8 captive chimpanzees (28) have been found to be naturally infected.

Characterization of orthopoxviruses by biologic genetic markers

Dermal reaction in New Zealand white rabbits

This test is useful in differentiating monkeypox virus from variola virus and cowpox virus from most vaccinia strains.

A 0.1-ml volume of monkeypox virus with a titer of 10^2 pock-forming units/0.1 ml inoculated id into rabbits produces a local hemorrhagic lesion about 15 mm in diameter. A generalized illness is also produced with secondary "satellite" exanthems. An inoculum of variola virus with a titer of 10^5 pock-forming units/0.1 ml produces a reaction that is hardly visible. The Wyeth strain of vaccinia virus, unlike other vaccinia virus strains, also produces only a weak reaction.

Cowpox virus inoculated similarly into rabbits produces a hemorrhagic skin reaction, as does monkeypox virus. Most vaccinia virus strains (except Wyeth strain) produce papules and some necrosis but do not produce a hemorrhagic reaction.

Suckling mouse virulence test by footpad inoculation

The suckling mouse virulence test also differentiates monkeypox virus and variola virus. An inoculum of 0.01 ml of monkeypox virus with a titer of 10^2 pock-forming units/0.1 ml injected into 1 hind footpad of 1-day-old mice produces generalized infection and virtually 100% mortality by the seventh day. A variola virus inoculum with a titer of 10^5 pock-forming units/0.1 ml produces only local infection of the limbs and occasional runting.

Reproductive capacity of poxviruses at supraoptimal temperatures

Variola major virus and certain variola minor viruses can be differentiated by their growth on chicken CAM at 38.3 C (105). Variola major virus grows at 38.3 C; however, variola minor virus from South America does not, and most variola minor virus strains from Botswana and Ethiopia do (Professor K.R. Dumbell, personal communication). Monkeypox virus grows at 41 C, but cowpox virus does not.

Characterization of poxviruses by comparison of their polypeptide components

By using a sodium dodecyl sulfate-polyacrylamide gel electrophoresis system, investigators have obtained a characteristic viral protein pattern for each poxvirus strain. The patterns for variola, vaccinia, and monkeypox viruses can be identified and differentiated (7, 45), but those for variola virus and whitepox virus cannot.

Serologic diagnosis

Serologic methods are certainly not suited for quick and accurate diagnosis of smallpox; however, when no specimen for virologic testing is available, serologic methods are the only alternative. For Nt, HAI, and CF tests, a 4-fold rise in titer between serum specimens collected in the acute and convalescent phases of illness is considered adequate evidence of clinically and epidemiologically supported smallpox infection. However, only a single serum specimen taken late in the illness or during convalescence may be all that is available; interpretation of the results of various serologic tests on such a specimen will be given later in each test section.

Although serologic tests cannot be used for quick and accurate diagnosis, they are useful for general serologic surveys, for special serologic surveys to establish the fact of and the date of past epidemic experience, and in studies of vaccination responses. They can also be used to establish the existence of subclinical infection in individuals. Note, however, that the antigens of the viruses in the orthopoxvirus group (e.g., variola, whitepox, vaccinia, monkeypox, and cowpox viruses, are so closely related that the serologic tests cannot definitively identify each viral infection.

Neutralization test

Availability of the Nt test to assay antibody is decided by whether the etiologic poxvirus can grow in TC or on CAM. A method for neutralizing virus of the orthopoxvirus group with use of CAM is described by Boulter (16) and will not be repeated here. However, an Nt method in which a TC (LLC-Mk2) is used to assay Nt antibody on the basis of 50% plaque reduction of vaccinia virus will be described.

LLC-Mk2, a stable rhesus monkey kidney cell line, is grown in the 24 wells of Linbro model FB 16-24 TC plates as shown in Figure 10.19. A virus control (pretitered) is incubated (same as the test mixture) and inoculated onto the monolayer to form 30–60 plaques per well; this establishes the 100% plaque breakthrough base. Mixtures of the pretitered virus stock and each of the dilutions of a serially diluted test serum incubated and inoculated onto the monolayers in the wells show the plaque-reducing effect of the serum as demonstrated in Figure 10.19.

Tissue culture system. One milliliter of LLC-Mk2 cell suspension containing 50,000 cells/ml in Eagle minimal essential medium (MEM) with 10% fetal calf serum is dispensed into each of the 24 wells in a Linbro plate. Plates with dispensed cell suspensions are covered, stacked, and incubated at 35.5 C in a CO_2 incubator. A confluent cell monolayer develops in each of the wells in about 3 days. Then the growth medium is replaced with a fresh maintenance medium (MEM without serum). The cell monolayers are inoculated on the fifth day after the medium has again been replaced by a fresh maintenance medium.

Stock vaccinia virus for Nt. This stock vaccinia virus is composed of mostly intracellular vaccinia virus with "Nt antibody-blocking" soluble antigen (5) removed.

Inoculate HELF cells (ten 32-oz bottles) with vaccinia virus. For seed virus, use Wyeth smallpox vaccine previously grown in a cell culture since Wyeth vaccine directly inoculated is toxic to TC. Harvest the cells when the CPE is 3+ to 4+. Scrape the cells off the bottle surface, pool, and centrifuge at $800 \times g$ for 20 min. Remove the supernatant fluid, and reconstitute the cells with 20 ml of tris (hydroxymethyl)-aminomethane (Tris) buffer (0.04 M, pH 7.5). Freeze and thaw the cells in 3 cycles. Centrifuge the mixture at $96,000 \times g$ through 12 ml of 40% sucrose cushion for 1 hr at 4 C. Reconstitute the partially purified (about 80%) virus sediment with 20 ml of Tris buffer. Add 30 ml of glycerol to make a final glycerol concentration of 60%, and store the virus suspension at −20C.

Serum dilution. Test sera, a positive control serum, and a negative control serum are serially 2-fold diluted, starting with 1:4 and ending with 1:1,024. The starting dilution of 1:4 is made by addition of 0.2 ml of undiluted serum to 0.6 ml of diluent (Tris buffer 0.02 M, pH 7.5). Sera diluted 1:4 are inactivated at 56 C for 30 min and then are further diluted. The diluted sera are stored at 4 C until used.

Virus dilution. The stock virus (described in the section above) diluted appropriately with Tris-skim-milk-antibiotic solution to yield about 30 plaque-forming units/0.1 ml, This working dilution is determined by prior titration under the test conditions.

The Tris-skim-milk-antibiotic solution is Tris (0.02 M, pH 7.5), 20% skim milk (100% skim milk = 10 g of Difco skim milk/100 ml of distilled water), 2.5X concentration of both penicillin and streptomycin usually used for TC.

Titration of the working virus dilution. Titrate the stock virus to establish the virus concentration of the working dilution. Also make a dilution with a 10 times greater concentration of virus than the working dilution, and a dilution with a 10 times lesser concentration of virus than the working dilution. A volume of 0.6 ml of each of the virus dilutions is mixed with 0.6 ml of Tris buffer (0.02 M, pH 7.5). Incubation and inoculation procedures are exactly like those of the test mixtures.

Serum-virus mixture, inoculation, and incubation. Add 0.6 ml of the working virus dilution to a tube containing 0.6 ml of each dilution of a serum. Mix by vigorously shaking each rack holding the tightly stoppered tubes containing the virus-serum mixture, and incubate for 24 hr at 35.5 C.

Remove medium from the plates containing the cell monolayers, and add 1 ml of fresh MEM without serum to each well. Inoculate 0.2 ml of the serum-virus mixture, virus control, or working virus dilutions to each well of a 3-well set. Incubate the inoculated plates at 35.5 C for 40–44 hr in a CO_2 incubator. Avoid longer incubation because unwanted secondary plaques will occur.

Staining cell monolayers and counting plaques. Add 0.2 ml of 0.3% crystal violet-formalin solution (1.3 g crystal violet dissolved in 50 ml of 95% ethanol, with 300 ml of 37% formaldehyde added and the volume brought to 1 liter with distilled water) directly into each well, without discarding the medium. The cells will not stain if the crystal violet-formalin solution is used alone because of the low pH. Allow the cells to stain for 15–30 min, pour off the medium-stain mixture, and allow the residual fluid to drain from the plates by placing them upside down on a paper towel. Plaques are counted with a dissecting microscope at 10X magnification.

The stained plate (Fig 10.19) demonstrates that the positive serum allows no plaque breakthrough at the serum dilution of 1:10; a few plaques break through at 1:40, a few at 1:60, and more at 1:640, whereas the negative serum shows no reduction in plaque breakthrough at 1:10, 1:40, or 1:160.

Determination of Nt titers from 50% plaque reductions. Calculate the percentage of plaque breakthrough for each serum dilution, and plot this on a probit graph paper, showing the percentages of plaque breakthrough on the ordinate axis and the serum dilutions in negative log_{10} on the abscissa. A best-fitting straight line is drawn through the points, and a vertical line is dropped from the intersection of the plot line; the 50% probit graph line determines the serum dilution end point that gives the 50% plaque reduction.

Interpretation. Nt antibody for smallpox and other diseases caused by the poxviruses in the orthopoxvirus group are usually detected in the latter part of the first week and during the second week after onset. The antibody may persist for a number of years.

Many factors can cause discrepancies in Nt antibody titers. Some of these include use of different cell systems, use of test serum without inactivation, variation in the incubation time for the serum-virus mixture, and presence of excessive Nt antibody-blocking soluble antigen. Even when the test is performed in 1 laboratory but at different times, a titer for a serum can vary from 1:500 to 1:2000. Therefore, a positive control serum that usually has a titer of about 1:1000 should be included in each testing. If the titer of this serum is <1:500 or >1:2000, the test should be repeated for better dependability.

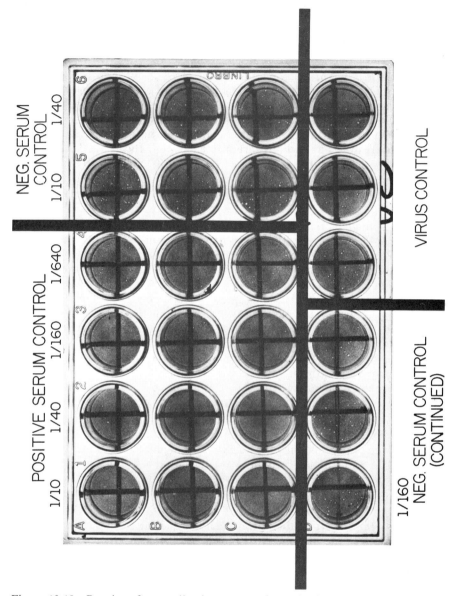

Figure 10.19—Results of neutralization test performed with Linbro model FB16-24TE plate, LLC-MK$_2$ tissue culture, and plaque reduction. Note the gradual increase in plaque breakthrough for the positive serum, showing none at 1:10, very few at 1:40, very few at 1:60 and about 26 plaques per 3 wells at 1:640. The negative serum shows no plaque reduction from 1:10 through 1:160.

Even with a very potent homologous serum, poxviruses generally show a residual plaque breakthrough of about 10%.

The virus stock used in this test is not appropriate for determining the anti-extracellular virus Nt antibody as described by Appleyard et al (3).

Since vaccinia virus is antigenically closely related to other poxviruses of the orthopoxvirus group, it can be used to detect antibody to variola, monkeypox, whitepox, and cowpox. (Note that a routine assay of antibody is orthopoxvirus group specific, not specific for each species, e.g., variola.)

When paired sera, taken from a smallpox patient during the acute and the convalescent stages of disease, show a 4-fold rise in titer, a positive serologic diagnosis can be made without problem. However, when only 1 serum specimen was taken from a patient sometime after the onset of a rash, and it shows only a moderate Nt antibody titer (<1:1000), the diagnosis by serology becomes difficult, especially if the patient had been vaccinated several months before. However, Nt titer of >1:1000 in such a serum specimen is probably significant, provided that the Nt test used was the one described above.

Takabayashi and McIntosh (127) and Nishimura et al (104) reported that addition of fresh, uninactivated normal guinea pig serum (of which the active component is complement) to the virus-antibody mixture in a vaccinia Nt test enhanced or potentiated the Nt titers of human serum. Takabayashi and McIntosh (127) also reported that the enhancement was more marked in human serum obtained in the first week after the primary vaccination (20- to 150-fold) than in serum from immune adults or from cord blood (4- to 25-fold). They further found that the potentiating effect of fresh normal guinea pig serum was evident to a dilution of about 1:176, but they used the serum at dilutions of 1:11–1:22. In our unpublished work we found that although addition of fresh normal guinea pig serum increased the specific Nt titers 10- to 20-fold in serum from revaccinated humans, it also nonspecifically reduced the vaccinia virus plaque production in monkey kidney cell monolayers by 50–75%. The maximal potentiating effect of fresh guinea pig serum was evident to a dilution of 1:320, but the serum was used arbitrarily at dilutions of 1:40–1:100. Lots of fresh guinea pig sera stored at −70 C maintained their potentiating effect for 6 months.

Tests with guinea pig serum as a potentiator can give titers 20- to 150-fold, 4- to 25-fold or 10- to 20-fold greater than titers in the same tests without the potentiator. The fold increase depends on whether an "early serum" or a "late serum" has been taken and on the degree of effectiveness of the potentiating factor in the guinea pig serum. Because our experience in interpretation of test results is based on the titers previously obtained without a potentiator, we are not able to interpret with confidence the potentiated titers, which can range from 4- to 150-fold greater. For example, when the diagnosis by serology depends upon only 1 serum specimen taken from a smallpox patient sometime after the onset of a rash, a titer of 1:1000 obtained by a test using a potentiator does not have the same diagnostic significance as that obtained by a test without a potentiator. Therefore, until experience provides familiarity with the high titers obtained with the potentiators and a basis for evaluating their significance is developed, the method should be used in a restricted manner, limited to detecting low Nt titers or early Nt antibody (produced by primary vaccinees) composed mostly of IgM (usually considered to be less avid in binding with viruses).

The use of anti-gamma globulin in the assay of Nt antibody to vaccinia virus has been reported by Majer and Link (76) and Weeke-Luttmann (133). This method is useful in neutralizing the persistently unneutralizable residual (about 10%) poxvirus particles. When specific IgM and IgG antisera are used, this method is also useful in identifying the presence of the IgM and the IgG portions of the Nt vaccinia virus.

For orf the Nt test must be done in an HELF or ovine TC with an orf virus stock. For milker's nodule the Nt must be done in a HELF or bovine TC with a milker's nodule virus stock.

The Nt test for Tanapox is performed in a primary AGMK cell or HELF tissue culture with a Tanapox virus stock. Results are positive if a blood specimen of a patient with appropriate clinical and epidemiologic history has detectable antibody.

At present, no Nt test is available for molluscum contagiosum.

Reproducibility of Nt test results. In a study to compare the antibody responses by 4 smallpox vaccines administered in various doses by different routes, 20 duplicate sera were tested in 4 different laboratories (14) with a standardized Nt test. The results follow: 67% of the duplicate sera tested had titers that varied less than 3-fold, 26% varied more than 3-fold but less than 10-fold, and 7% varied more than 10-fold. Thus, a titer by an Nt test for poxviruses should not be considered an absolute quantitation, but only an approximation.

Hemagglutination inhibition test

A standard microtiter procedure for the HAI test is described elsewhere in this book (Chap 26), but methods for preparing HAI reagents for the orthopoxvirus group are described below.

Chicken erythrocytes. Since only about 50% of the chicken population has erythrocytes that can be agglutinated by vaccinia hemagglutinin, samples of erythrocytes from several chickens must be pretested. Obtain 5–10 ml of blood from several 7- to 14-month-old Newton white roosters. After washing the erythrocytes from each rooster 3 times with PBS, (pH 7.2) by centrifugation, prepare a 0.5% erythrocyte suspension from each chicken. Set up the standard HA titration for each chicken erythrocyte suspension, using a known positive HA vaccinia virus antigen. Only chickens whose erythrocytes agglutinate with the HA antigen at a ≥ 1:64 dilution or greater are reserved for future use, and others are discarded.

For preparing an erythrocyte suspension for the HAI test, collect 50 ml of blood from an approved rooster, and mix the blood in a bottle at a ratio of 1 part of blood to 4 parts of Alsever solution. The blood can then be stored in a refrigerator for 2 weeks unless the blood cells become excessively fragile and hemolyzed. Blood can be collected from the same rooster as often as every 2 weeks.

The erythrocytes are washed 3 times with PBS (pH 7.2) by centrifugation at $900 \times g$ for 10 min in graduated conical centrifuge tubes (15 ml); the buffy coat formed is removed after each wash. After the third wash, read the packed cell volume and resuspend the erythrocytes in PBS to make a 50% suspension. Prepare a fresh 50% erythrocyte suspension daily; from this 50% erythrocyte suspension, the working dilution of 0.5% erythrocyte suspension is standardized.

Treatment of serum to remove nonspecific hemagglutinin. Make a 1:5 initial dilution of a test serum by adding 0.1 ml of the serum to 0.4 ml of PBS; add 0.05 ml of the 50% chicken erythrocytes and agitate gently. Incubate for 1 hr at 4 C with occasional agitation. Centrifuge at 4 C at $900 \times g$ for 20 min. Recover the supernatant fluid with a Pasteur pipette, and determine the fluid's HAI antibody titer.

Vaccinia HA antigen. Inoculate each of eight 1-liter bottles containing confluent BHK-21 cell monolayers with 2 ml of the vaccinia-infected cell culture with a titer of 10^6 $TCID_{50}/0.1$ ml. Allow the virus to absorb at 35 C for 1 hr, and add 50 ml of Eagle MEM with 0.4% bovine albumen. Harvest the cells by scraping them from the bottle surface when they show $3+$ to $4+$ CPE. Centrifuge at $450 \times g$ for 15 min, and discard the supernatant fluid. Suspend and pool the sedimented cells in 30 ml of reticulocyte swelling buffer (RSB, 0.01 M Tris-HCL, 0.01 M NaCl, 0.0015 M $MgCl_2$, pH 7.8; the solution is made by mixing 20 ml of 0.5 M Tris-HCL, pH 7.8, 2 ml of 5 M NaCl, and 1.5 ml of 1.0 M $MgCl_2$ and adding distilled water to a final volume of 1 liter).

Centrifuge at $450 \times g$ for 15 min, and discard the supernatant fluid. Resuspend the cell sediment again in 30 ml of RSB, centrifuge at $450 \times g$ and discard the supernatant fluid. After the cells have been washed twice in the above manner, resuspend the cells in 8 ml of RSB, and leave the suspension overnight at 4 C to swell the cells. Rupture the cells in the suspension by 20–30 strokes with a Dounce homogenizer. Centrifuge at $70 \times g$ for 15 min to pellet the nuclei and cell debris. Save the supernatant fluid. Repeat the treatment of the sediment by Dounce homogenizer if many intact cells still remain by resuspending the sediment in 8 ml of RSB and subjecting it to another 20–30 strokes. Again centrifuge the suspension at $70 \times g$ for 15 min to pellet the nuclei and cell debris. Combine the 8 ml of supernatant fluid and the previously saved 8 ml of supernatant fluid, and discard the sediment. Centrifuge the 16 ml of supernatant fluid at $96,000 \times g$ for 45 min. Resuspend the sediment in 20 ml of RSB, and add enough thimerosal to give a final concentration of 1:10,000. Perform HA and HAI tests for final evaluation. (The antigen is lyophilized and stored at 4 C).

Interpretation. The HAI test is useful for assay of antibodies produced against variola, whitepox, vaccinia, monkeypox, and cowpox viruses, but because of a high degree of cross-reaction among the viruses of the orthopoxvirus group (including these 5 poxviruses) in this test, it alone is not adequate for specific disease diagnosis. However, it is useful for specific diagnosis when supplemented by adequate clinical and epidemiologic information.

The HAI test cannot be used to assay antibodies to orf, milker's nodule, Tanapox, and molluscum contagiosum viruses because these viruses do not hemagglutinate.

If 2 HA units are used in the HAI test, an HAI titer of 1:5 is essentially negative. A titer of 1:10 is considered positive.

HAI antibody is probably the earliest antibody produced after an infection by a virus of the orthopoxvirus group, and it persists for several months at a high titer. It may persist for several years at a low titer.

In smallpox patients HAI antibody is detectable within 4–7 days after infection and reaches a maximal titer in the second week. The HAI antibody titer is generally greater than 1:80 and in some individuals may be greater than 1:1000. However, if a titer >1:1000 is found in a serum specimen from Africa that has been in transit for several weeks without adequate refrigeration, one must suspect the high titer to be partially nonspecific and must treat the serum (see below) and retest. Often a titer of 1:1280 before treatment can be reduced to 1:160 after treatment, with positive control serum showing no reduction in titer after similar treatment. Extremely high nonspecific HAI titers in human serum collected during autopsies have been reported (43).

Serologic diagnosis of smallpox or human monkeypox can become complicated if the patient had been vaccinated, because in some vaccinated individuals the titer can be as high as 1:320.

Periodate treatment of serum to remove nonspecific HA inhibitors. This is a modification of serum treatment by periodate reported by the WHO (140).

Prepare fresh M/90 solution of KIO_4 (do not substitute $NaIO_4$) by dissolving 0.256 g of KIO_4 in 100 ml of PBS that is constantly stirred by a magnetic stirrer. (Do not use heat). Use this solution within a few hours after preparation. Prepare 3% glycerol in PBS (may be stored in a refrigerator for a few weeks).

To 0.1 ml of serum in a test tube, add 0.3 ml of the M/90 KIO_4 solution, and leave at room temperature for at least 15 min for the oxidation reaction. Add 0.1 ml of the 3% glycerol-PBS solution, and leave at room temperature for at least 15 min to stop the oxidation reaction. Add 0.05 ml of the 50% chicken erythrocytes, and leave at 4 C for 1 hr (for the removal of nonspecific hemagglutinin). Centrifuge at $450 \times g$ for 10 min, and transfer the supernatant fluid to another tube. The serum dilution is considered to be 1:5. Inactivate the 1:5-diluted serum at 56 C for 30 min, proceed with further dilution of the serum, and test for HAI antibody. This treatment removes the nonspecific HA inhibitors and also the nonspecific hemagglutinin in the serum.

A kaolin absorption method used by some workers to remove nonspecific inhibitors has been found at CDC to be unsuitable, at least for the HAI test, because it removes the specific antibody. The kaolin method reduces our positive control serum titer as much as 4-fold, but the periodate method seems to have no such effect.

Reproducibility of HAI test results. Twenty duplicate sera were tested by 5 different laboratories using a standardized HAI test (14); 73% of the duplicate sera were found by all 5 laboratories to have the same titer, 22% had titers different by only 2-fold, and 5% had titers different by 4-fold or more. That 95% of the results obtained by the 5 laboratories showed the HAI titers to differ by only 2-fold or less indicates that the test gives reproducible results.

Complement fixation test

A microtiter CF method is described elsewhere in this book (Chapter 1). The CF antigen used is the same as that prepared for the HA antigen (pages 25-29).

Interpretation. CF antibody usually does not appear in smallpox patients until the second week after the infection, and the titers usually reach a higher level in patients with previous vaccination than in those without previous vaccination. However, more than 50% of serum specimens from unvaccinated smallpox patients examined after the eighth day of onset were found to be negative for CF antibody (35). Thus, when used alone, the CF test has only limited diagnostic value because only the positive results are useful.

After vaccination or revaccination, the CF antibody titer is usually less than 1:64; however, in smallpox patients the titer can be as high as 1:640 or 1:1280 (33).

Positive CF test results for orf and milker's nodule in serum from humans constitute adequate evidence for diagnosing these diseases because humans are usually not expected to have any antibody against these viruses. However, negative CF test results do not necessarily rule out the infections.

The CF test can be used to diagnose Tanapox in humans (42), but with the same reservation as above for negative results.

CF antibody against molluscum contagiosum virus can be detected in patients with molluscum contagiosum (79), but its usefulness in diagnosis is still debatable.

Serum sent from Africa, India, and Bangladesh and received at CDC after being in transit for several weeks or months without adequate refrigeration have often shown anticomplementary (AC) reaction and, therefore, have required special treatment (see below).

Treatment of serum to remove anticomplementary (AC) reaction. The following carbon dioxide treatment was reported in the WHO Technical Report (140):

To 0.1 ml of serum add 0.8 ml of sterile distilled water. Drop in a piece of dry ice about 6 mm in diameter, and allow it to bubble until it has completely disappeared. Centrifuge the mixture at $800 \times g$ for 10 min at 4 C. Decant the supernatant fluid into another tube and discard the sediment. Add 0.1 ml of NaCl, 8.5% (10X physiologic saline) to the supernatant fluid. The starting dilution of the serum is 1:10. Inactivate the 1:10 diluted serum at 56 C for 30 min.

The carbon dioxide treatment removes the AC activity completely or to the extent that the AC activity does not interfere with the interpretation of the CF titers. The treatment does not reduce the CF titer of a positive control serum.

CF testing of serum immune globulin such as vaccinia immune globulin and zoster immune globulin always presents a problem because of the presence of a very high AC activity. The AC titer is usually almost as high as or higher than the specific antibody titers. The carbon dioxide treatment usually does not reduce or eliminate the AC reaction in these specimens. A modification described by Miller (88) of the kaolin adsorption method described for arbovirus study (56) is recommended. Although some loss of specific CF titer occurs by this method (usually about 2-fold), the method does reduce or eliminate the AC activity (titers as high as 1:1280 or higher). Although this method is satisfactory for immune globulin with high protein content (16.5%), it is not recommended for most serum specimens. The procedure follows:

To 0.1 ml of 16.5% globulin solution, add 0.9 ml of gelatin-veronal buffer, pH 7.3–7.4 (Mayer) (110), add 1 ml of a 25% wt/vol slurry of Fisher kaolin (acid-washed), and mix the 2 solutions vigorously for 30 sec. Then let the mixture sit for exactly 5 min. Mix vigorously again for 30 sec, and let it sit again for 5 min. Continue the mixing and standing for a total of 20 min and 5 cycles. Immediately centrifuge the mixture at $450 \times g$ for 10 min, and remove the supernatant fluid for CF antibody assay. Discard the pellet. The final dilution of the specimen in this step is 1:20. Proceed with further dilution, and perform a standard microtiter CF antibody assay (110).

Agar gel precipitation test

Preparation of antigen. Vaccinia virus antigen for detecting precipitating antibody in smallpox, vaccinia, monkeypox, and cowpox is prepared as described on page 280.

Specific antigens for orf, milker's nodule, and Tanapox precipitating antibody assays are made from TC of the specific viruses.

Antigen for molluscum contagiosum is made from lesions collected from patients.

Procedure. The test is carried out as described on page 280.

Interpretation. The method for observing the precipitin lines in the assay for antibody is the same as that used in the test for antigens. Serum from unvaccinated smallpox patients are less likely to be positive. As with CF antibody precipitating antibody is not detected in every clinically positive case of variola, vaccinia, monkeypox, orf, milker's nodule (112), Tanapox, and molluscum contagiosum; therefore, the negative results do not necessarily rule out the infections.

Radioimmunoassay (RIA)

Antibody assays by RIA for variola, vaccinia, and monkeypox have been found to be dependable (145). The RIA detects antibodies produced against variola and vaccinia viruses (145) and also monkeypox virus (60) almost as early as the HAI test does. The method also measures antibodies that are as long-standing as those measured by the Nt test.

This method cannot be performed routinely in many laboratories because it requires elaborate equipment. However, where facilities permit, it can probably replace the Nt test and can be a valuable tool for large-scale serologic surveys.

Immunofluorescence test

An indirect method of FA is used to assay antibody against an antigen made of vaccinia virus infected BHK-21 cells (54). This method, like the

RIA, can measure antibodies to variola, vaccinia, and monkeypox and also detects antibodies that have persisted for at least 10 years.

Although FA assay of antibody for molluscum contagiosum has been successful (21, 118), experience has been insufficient to evaluate its dependability.

The FA test has not been used to assay orf and milker's nodule antibody, but since it identifies the viral antigen of orf, antibody assay appears feasible.

Identification of specific variola, vaccinia, and monkeypox antibodies

Routine serologic tests are inadequate to make a specific laboratory diagnosis of variola, monkeypox, or vaccinia when only sera collected after the appearance of rash are available. However, recently an FA test (54) and an RIA test (60) have been developed to determine specifically whether a person has had one of these infections at some time in the past. The individual's serum is selectively absorbed with vaccinia, variola, or monkeypox antigen. The portion of the antibody that is not absorbed reacts specifically with vaccinia, variola, or monkeypox virus and is detected by FA or RIA. For example, when a convalescent-phase serum specimen from a person infected with monkeypox virus is absorbed with vaccinia antigen, RIA reveals very little reaction with vaccinia or variola virus antigen but shows significant reaction with monkeypox virus antigen. When a serum from a smallpox patient is similarly absorbed, RIA reaction is greatest against variola antigen. When a serum from a vaccinee is so treated, RIA reaction is not significant against any of the 3 virus antigens.

Brief laboratory diagnostic scheme

I. A suspected case of smallpox or of human monkeypox virus infection with supportive epidemiologic and clinical histories.

A. EM: herpes-like virus = chickenpox, or herpes simplex infection.

B. EM: poxvirus = presumptive smallpox or monkeypox virus infection, depending on the epidemiologic history.

    1. CAM: definite identification of variola virus.

    2. CAM: definite identification of monkeypox virus.

    3. Rabbit dermal test: support identification of monkeypox virus.

    4. Suckling mouse footpad test: support identification of monkeypox virus.

C. EM: negative for virus; if an adequate amount of specimen (especially crusts) was collected, the infection is probably not smallpox or monkeypox.

    1. AGP: for further support.

    2. CAM: for further support.

    3. TC: for further support.

    4. Serum: for further support (against vaccinia virus antigen).

(If all the supportive tests are negative, the infection is not smallpox or monkeypox, provided that the virologic tests are performed with an adequate amount of comparatively fresh specimen. The serologic test results may or may not influence the final diagnosis.)

II. A suspected case of vaccinia infection with supportive epidemiologic and clinical histories.

A. EM: poxvirus = presumptive vaccinia virus infection. CAM: definite identification = vaccinia virus.

B. EM: herpes-like virus = herpes simplex virus. CAM: definite identification = herpes simplex virus..

C. EM: negative for virus = can still be vaccinia or herpes simplex infection.

1. CAM: definite identification = vaccinia virus.

2. CAM: definite identification = herpes simplex virus.

3. CAM: negative = diagnosis unknown, can still be vaccinia infection.

4. TC: for further support = negative result does not rule out the infection.

5. Serum: for further support = if serologic reactions (HAI, CF, Nt) are negative for vaccinia virus antigen, the infection is not vaccinia; if serologic reactions are moderate without previous smallpox vaccination, the infection is probably vaccinia, but with previous vaccination the infection is not confirmed; if serologic reactions are high, with or without previous vaccination, the infection is probably vaccinia.

III. A suspected case of cowpox infection with or without association with cattle, with supportive clinical history.

A. EM: poxvirus similar to vaccinia = cowpox or vaccinia.

1. CAM: definite identification = cowpox virus.

2. CAM: definite identification = vaccinia virus.

B. EM: negative for virus = does not rule out the infection.

1. CAM: for further support = lack of isolation does not rule out the infection.

2. TC: for further support = lack of isolation does not rule out the infection.

3. Serum: for further support = negative serologic reactions (HAI, CF, Nt) rule out infection by cowpox or vaccinia virus; moderate serologic reactions, with previous smallpox vaccination, do not confirm the infection, but without previous vaccination, they can confirm the infection; high serologic reactions confirm infection by cowpox or vaccinia virus.

IV. A suspected case of orf infection associated with sheep or goat, supportive clinical history.

A. EM: poxvirus characteristic of orf virus = orf infection. TC: for further support.

B. EM: negative for virus = does not rule out the infection.

1. TC: for further support = negative isolation does not rule out the infection.

2. Serum: for further support = positive CF, Nt, or AGP test indicates the infection; negative CF or AGP test does not rule out the infection: experience inadequate to interpret negative Nt test.

V. A suspected case of milker's nodule associated with cattle and supportive clinical history.

A. EM: poxvirus characteristic of milker's nodule virus = milker's nodule. TC: for further support.

B. EM: negative for virus = does not rule out the infection.

1. TC: for further support = negative isolation does not rule out the infection.

2. Serum: for further support = positive CF, Nt, or AGP test confirms the infection; negative CF or AGP test does not rule out the infection; experience insufficient to interpret negative Nt test.

VI. A suspected case of Tanapox infection with supportive epidemiologic and clinical histories.

A. EM: poxvirus = Tanapox infection. TC: for further support.

B. EM: negative for virus = positive diagnosis of Tanapox infection highly improbable.

1. TC: for further support.

2. Serum: for further support = positive Nt, CF, or AGP test confirms the infection; negative CF or AGP test probably does not rule out the infection; negative Nt test probably rules out the infection.

VIII. A suspected case of molluscum contagiosum with supportive epidemiologic and clinical histories.

A. EM: poxvirus = molluscum contagiosum.

B. EM: negative for virus = positive diagnosis of molluscum contagiosum highly improbable.

References

1. ANDREWS CH and HORSTMANN DM: The susceptibility of viruses to ethyl ether. J Gen Microbiol 3:290–297, 1949

2. ANTHONY RL, TAYLOR DL, DANIEL RW, COLE JL, and McCRUMB FR JR: Studies of variola virus immunity in smallpox. I. Variola virus hemagglutinins. J Infect Dis 121:295–302, 1970

3. APPLEYARD G, HAPEL AJ, and BOULTER EA: An antigenic difference between intracellular and extracellular rabbitpox virus. J Gen Virol 13:9–17, 1971

4. APPLEYARD G and WESTWOOD JCN: Protective antigen from the pox-viruses. II. Immunization of animals. Br J Exp Pathol 45:162–173, 1964

5. APPLEYARD H, ZWARTOUW HT, and WESTWOOD JCN: A protection antigen from the pox-viruses. I. Reaction with neutralizing antibody. Br J Exp Pathol 45:150–161, 1964

6. ARITA I and HENDERSON DA: Monkeypox and whitepox viruses in West and Central Africa. Bull WHO 53:347–353, 1976

7. ARITA M and TAGAYA I: Structural polypeptides of several strains of orthopoxvirus. Microbiol Immunol 21:343–346, 1977

8. BARDELL D: Smallpox during the American war of independence. Am Soc Microbiol News 42:526–530, 1976

9. BAXBY D: Identification and interrelationship of the variola vaccinia subgroup of poxviruses. Progr Med Virol 19:215–246, 1975

10. BAXBY D: Is cowpox misnamed? A review of ten human cases. Br Med J 1:1379–1380, 1977

11. BECKER FT: Milker's nodules. J Am Med Assoc 115:2140–2144, 1940

12. BEDSON HS and DUCKWORTH MJ: Rabbitpox: an experimental study of the pathways of infection in rabbits. J Pathol Bacteriol 85:1–20, 1963

13. BEDSON HS, DUMBELL KR, and THOMAS WRG: Variola in Tanganyika. Lancet 2:1085–1088, 1963
14. BENESON AB, CHERRY JD, McINTOSH K, CONNOR JD, ALLING DW, NAKANO J, ROLFE UT, SCHANBERGER JE, TODD WA, DeCASTRO F, HORVATH FL, BAIRAN A, PHILLIPS IA, GALASSO GJ, and MATTHEIS MJ: Clinical and serologic study of four smallpox vaccines comparing variations of dose and route of administration. Basic study and laboratory standardization. J Infect Dis 135:135–144, 1977
15. BLACKMAN KE and BUBEL HC: Origin of the vaccinia virus hemagglutinin. J Virol 9:290–296, 1972
16. BOULTER EA: The titration of vaccinial neutralizing antibody on chorioallantoic membranes. J Hyg 55:502–512, 1957
17. BRAS G: The morbid anatomy of smallpox. Docum Med Geograph Trop 4:303–351, 1952
18. BREMAN JG, NAKANO JH, COFFI E, GODFREY H, and GANTUN JC: Human poxvirus disease after smallpox eradication. Am J Trop Med Hyg 26:273–281, 1977
19. BROWN ST and WEINBERGER J: Molluscum contagiosum: sexually transmitted disease in 17 cases. J Am Vener Dis Assoc 1:35–36, 1974
20. CASSEY HW, WOODRUFF JM, and BUTCHER WI: Electron microscopy of a benign epidermal pox disease of rhesus monkeys. Am J Pathol 51:431–446, 1967
21. CHANG TW and WEINSTEIN L: Cytopathic agents isolated from lesions of molluscum contagiosum. J Invest Derm 37:433–439, 1961
22. COHEN GH and WILCOX WC: Soluble antigens of vaccinia infected mammalian cells. I. Separation of virus-induced antigens into two classes on the basis of physical characteristics. J Bacteriol 92:678–686, 1966
23. COLLIER LH, McCLEAN D, and VALLET L: The antigenicity of ultraviolet irradiated vaccinia virus. J Hyg 53:513–534, 1955
24. COSTRUCCI G, McKERCHER DG, CHILLI V, ARANCIA G, and NAGIONALI C: Characteristics of a paravaccinia virus from cattle. Arch Gesamte Virusforsch 29:315–330, 1970
25. CRAGIE J and WISHART FO: Studies on the soluble precipitable substances of vaccinia. J Exp Med 64:819–830, 1936
26. CRANDELL RA, CASEY HW, and BRUMLOW WB: Studies of a newly recognized poxvirus of monkeys. J Infect Dis 119:80–88, 1969
27. DIXON CW: Smallpox. J and A Churchill, Ltd, London, 1962, 512 pp
28. DOUGLAS JD, TANNER KN, PRINE JR, VAN RIPER DC, and DERWELIS SK: Molluscum contagiosum in chimpanzees. J Am Vet Med Assoc 151:901–904, 1967
29. DOURMASHKIN R and BERNHARD W: A study with the electron microscope of the skin tumour of molluscum contagiosum. J Ultrastruct Res 3:11–38, 1959
30. DOWNIE AW and DUMBELL KR: Poxviruses. Ann Rev Microbiol 10:237–252, 1956
31. DOWNIE AW and ESPÀNA C: Comparison of tanapox virus and yaba-like viruses causing epidemic disease in monkeys. J Hyg 70:23–32, 1972
32. DOWNIE AW and ESPÀNA C: A comparative study of tanapox and yaba viruses. J Gen Virol 19:37–49, 1973
33. DOWNIE AW and KEMPE CH: Poxviruses In Diagnostic Procedures for Viral and Rickettsial Infections, 4th edition, Lennette EH and Schmidt NJ (eds), Am Public Health Assoc, Inc, New York 1969, pp. 281–320
34. DOWNIE AW, McCARTHY K, McDONALD A, MacCALLUM FO, and MACRAE AD: Virus and virus antigen in blood of smallpox patients. Their significance in early diagnosis and prognosis. Lancet 2:164–166, 1953
35. DOWNIE AW, ST VINCENT L, GOLDSTEIN L, RUO AR, and KEMPE CH: Antibody response in non-haemorrhagic smallpox patients. J Hyg 67:609–618, 1969
36. DOWNIE AW, TAYLOR-ROBINSON CH, CAUNT AE, NELSON GS, MANSON-BAHR PEC, and MATTHEWS TCH: Tanapox: a new disease caused by a pox virus. Br Med J 1:363–368, 1971
37. DUMBELL KR and BEDSON HS: Adaptation of variola to grow in the rabbit. J Pathol Bacteriol 91:459–465, 1966
38. DUMBELL KR and NIZAMUDDIN MD: An agar precipitation test for the laboratory diagnosis of smallpox. Lancet 1:916–917, 1959
39. EL-GANGOURY ALA: Evaluation of the fluoreseent antibody technique for the diagnosis of smallpox. J Clin Pathol 20:879–882, 1967
40. EMMONS RW and RIGGS JL: Application of immunofluorescence to diagnosis of viral in-

fections, *In* Methods in Virology, Maramoseh K, Thompson B, and Korrowski H (eds), Vol. 6, Academic Press, New York, 1977, pp 1-28

41. ERICKSON GA, CABREY EA, and GUSTAFSON GA: Generalized contagious ecthyma in a sheep rancher: diagnostic consideration. J Am Vet Med Assoc 166:262-263, 1975

42. ESPANA C: A pox disease of monkeys transmissible to man *In* Medical Primatology Proceedings 2nd Conf Exp Med Surg Primatol, S. Karger, Basel, 1971, pp 694-708

43. ESPMARK JA and MAGNUSSON B: A non-specific inhibitor to vaccinia haemagglutination in post mortem human sera. Act Pathol Microbiol Scandinav 62:595-599, 1964

44. ESPOSITO JJ, OBIJESKI JF, and NAKANO JH: Serological relatedness of monkeypox, variola and vaccinia viruses. J Med Virol 1:35-47, 1977

45. ESPOSITO JJ, OBIJESKI JF, and NAKANO JH: The virion and soluble antigen proteins of variola, monkeypox and vaccinia viruses. J Med Virol 1:95-110, 1977

46. ESPOSITO JJ, OBIJESKI JF, and NAKANO JH: Orthopoxvirus DNA: strain differentiation by electrophoresis of restriction endonuclease fragmented virion DNA. Virology 89:53-66, 1968

47. FRANCIS RD and BRADFORD HB JR: Some biological and physical properties of molluscum contagiosum virus propagated in cell culture. J Virol 19:382-388, 1976

48. FRIEDMAN-KIEN AE, ROWE WP, and BANFIELD WG: Milker's nodules: isolation of a poxvirus from human case. Science 140:1335-1336, 1963

49. FOSTER SO, BRINK EW, HUTCHINS DL, PIFER JM, LOURIE B, MOSER CR, CUMMINGS EC, KUTEYI OEK, EKE REA, TITUS JB, SMITH EA, HICKS JW, and FOEGE WH: Human monkeypox. Bull WHO 46:569-576, 1972

50. FULGINITI VA: Poxvirus diseases *In* Practice of Pediatrics, Kelley VC (ed), Vol II, Part 2. Harper and Row, Hagerstown, Maryland, 1976, pp 1-21

51. GISPEN R: Analysis of pox virus antigens by means of double diffusion. A method for direct serological differentiation of cowpox. J Immunol 74:134-141, 1955

52. GISPEN R and BRAND-SAATHOF B: "White" poxvirus strains from monkeys. Bull WHO 46:585-592, 1972

53. GISPEN R and BRAND-SAATHOF B: Three specific antigens produced in vaccinia, variola, and monkeypox infections. J Infect Dis 129:289-295, 1974

54. GISPEN R, HUISMAN J, BRAND-SAATHOF B, and HEKKER AC: Immunofluorescence test for persistent poxvirus antibodies. Arch Gesamte Virusforsch 44:391-395, 1974

55. HALL AS and McNULTY WP: A contagious pox disease in monkeys. J Am Vet Med Assoc 151:833-838, 1967

56. HAMMON WM and SATHER GE: Arboviruses *In* Diagnostic Procedures for Viral and Rickettsial Infections. Lennette EH and Schmidt NJ (eds), 4th edition, Am Public Health Assoc, Inc, NY, 1969, pp 227-280

57. HEDSTRÖM KG: Effect of live and inactivated vaccinia virus preparations on production of antibodies in animals. International Symposium on Smallpox Vaccine, Bilthoven, 1972; Symp Series Immunobiol Standard, Reamey RH and Cohen H (eds), S Karger, Basel, 1973, pp 61-67

58. HODGSON-JONES IS: Orf in London. Br J Med J 1:795-796, 1951

59. HOLOWCZAK JA and JOKLIK WK: Studies on the structure proteins of vaccinia virus 1. Structural proteins of virion and cores. Virology 33:717-725, 1967

60. HUTCHINSON HD, ZIEGLER DW, WELLS DE, and NAKANO JH: Differentiation of variola, monkeypox and vaccinia antisera by radioimmunoassay. Bull WHO Vol 55, 1977

61. ICHIHASHI Y: Vaccinia-specific hemagglutination. Virology 76:527-538, 1977

62. INTERNATIONAL COMMITTEE ON TAXONOMY OF VIRUSES: Classification and Nomenclature of Viruses, Fenner (ed), S Karger, Basel, 1976

63. IRONS JV, SULLIVAN TD, COOK EBM, COX GW, and HALE RA: Outbreak of smallpox in the lower Rio Grande valley of Texas in 1949. Am J Public Health 43:25-29, 1953

64. JENNER E: An inquiry into the causes and effects of the variolae vaccinae, a disease discovered in some of the western counties of England, particularly Gloucestershire and known by the name of the cowpox. Printed for the author by Sampson Low, No. 7, Berwick Street, Soho, 1798. Republished by Cassell and Comp, Limited, London, 1896

65. JENNER E: Further observations on the variolae vaccinae. Sampson Low, London, 1799

66. JOKLIK WK: The poxviruses. Bacteriol Rev 30:33-66, 1966

67. KAHN C: History of smallpox and its prevention. Am J Dis Child 106:597-609, 1963

68. KAPLAN C and MURRAY HGS: The preparation of a stable potent dried smallpox vaccine *In* Extrait des Compte-rendu du Symposium sur la Vaccination Antivariolique, Lyon 6/9 Decembre 1962, pp 1-5

69. KIRSCH D and KISSLING R: The use of immunofluorescence in the rapid presumptive diagnosis of variola. Bull WHO 29:126-128, 1963

70. KITAMURO T, AOYAMA Y, KURATA T, ARITA, M, and IMAGAWA Y: Virological studies of smallpox in endemic area. I. Evaluation of immunofluorescence staining as a rapid diagnostic procedure in the field. Jpn J Med Sci Biol 30:215-227, 1977

71. LADNYJ ID, ZIEGLER P, and KIMA E: A human infection caused by monkeypox virus in Basankusu Territory, Democratic Republic of the Congo. Bull WHO 46:593-597, 1972

72. LANE JM, MILLAR JD, and NEFF JM: Smallpox and smallpox vaccination policy. Annu Rev Med 22:251-272, 1971

73. LANE JM, RUBEN FL, NEFF JM, and MILLAR JD: Complication of smallpox vaccination, 1968. National surveillance in the United States. N Engl J Med 281:1201-1208, 1969

74. LEAVELL UW JR, MCNAMARA MJ, MUELLING R, TALBERT WM, RUCKER RC: Orf, report of 19 human cases with clinical and pathological observations. J Am Med Assoc 204:657-664, 1968

75. LENNETTE EH: Perspectives in virology: vaccinations *In* Perspectives in Virology, IX, Antiviral Mechanism, Pollard M (ed), Academic Press, New York, 1975, pp 1-8

76. MAJER M and LINK F: Studies of the non-neutralizable fraction of vaccinia virus. Clin Exp Immunol 7:283-291, 1970

77. MALTSEVA NN and MARENNIKOVA SS: A method for serological differentiation of closely related poxviruses. Acta Virol 20:250-252, 1976

78. MALTSEVA NN and NISHANOV RA: Application of the fluorescent antibody method for rapid diagnosis of diseases caused by poxviruses. J Hyg Epid Microbiol Immunol 20:214-220, 1976

79. MANUEL FR: How common is molluscum contagiosum? Can Med Assoc J 114:999, 1976

80. MARENNIKOVA SS and SHELUHINA EM: White rats as a source of pox infection in carnivora of the family felidae. Acta Virol 20:442, 1976

81. MARENNIKOVA SS, SELUHINA EM, MAL'CEVA NN, CAMESKJAN KL, and MACEVIC GR: Isolation and properties of the causal agent of a new variola-like disease (monkeypox) in man. Bull WHO 46:599-611, 1972

82. MARENNIKOVA SS, SELUHINA EM, MAL'CEVA NN, and LADNYJ ID: Poxviruses Isolated from clinically ill and asymptomatically infected monkeys and a chimpanzee. Bull WHO 46:613-620, 1972

83. MARENNIKOVA SS, SHELUKHINA EM, and SHENKMAN LS: "White-wild" (variola-like) poxvirus strains from rodents in Equatorial Africa. Acta Virol 20:80-82, 1976

84. MARQUARDT J: Presence of hemagglutinin in the vaccinia virion. Arch Gesamte Virusforsch 35:133-142, 1971

85. MCCLEAN D: The antigenicity of vaccinia virus inactivated with alcohol. J Pathol Bacteriol 57:261-265, 1945

86. MCDONALD A: Complement-fixation tests in the diagnosis of contagious pustular dermatitis infection in man. J Pathol Bacteriol 63:758-761, 1951

87. MCNULTY WP JR, LOBITZ WC JR, HU F, MARUFFO CA, and HALL AS: A pox disease in monkeys transmitted to man. Arch Dermatol 97:286-293, 1968

88. MILLER WJ: Personal communication, Merck Institute for Therapeutic Research, West Point, PA

89. MITCHELL JC: Observations on the virus of molluscum contagiosum. Br J Exp Pathol 34:44-49, 1953

90. MOORE RM JR: Human orf in the United States, 1972. J Infect Dis 127:731-732, 1973

91. MOSOVICI C, COHEN EP, SANDERS J, and DELONG SS: Isolation of a viral agent from pseudocowpox disease. Science 141:915-916, 1963

92. MOSS B: Reproduction of poxviruses *In* Comprehensive Virology, Fraenkel-Conrad H and Wagner RR (eds), Vol 3, Plenum Press, New York, 1974, pp 405-474

93. MURRAY HGS: The diagnosis of smallpox by immunofluorescence. Lancet 1:847-848, 1963

94. NAGINGTON J: The growth of paravaccinia viruses in tissue culture. Vet Rec 82:477-482, 1968

95. NAGINGTON J and WHITTLE CH: Human orf. Isolation of the virus by tissue culture. Br Med J 2:1324–1327, 1961

96. NAKANO JH: Comparative diagnosis of poxvirus diseases *In* Comparative Diagnosis of Viral Diseases, Vol I, Part A, Human and Related Viruses, Kurstak E and Kurstak C (eds), Academic Press, New York, 1977

97. NAKANO JH and BINGHAM PG: Smallpox, vaccinia, and human infection with monkeypox viruses, *In* Manual of Clinical Microbiology, 2nd edition, Lennette EH, Spalding EH, and Truant JP (eds), Am Soc Microbiol, Washington, DC, 1974, pp 782–794

98. NEFF BJ, ACKERMAN WW, and PRESTON RE: Studies of vaccinia hemagglutinin obtained from various vaccinia infected tissues. Density gradient centrifugation and electron microscopy. Proc Soc Exp Biol Med 118:664–671, 1965

99. NEFF JM, LANE JM, PERT JH, MOORE R, MILLAR JD, and HENDERSON DA: Complication of smallpox vaccination. I. National survey in the United States, 1963. N Engl J Med 276:125–132, 1967

100. NETTER R and PIAT A: Essais de culture de quatre souches de virus varioliques sur cellules RK13 et BHK21. Ann Inst Pasteur Paris 116:820–826, 1969

101. NEVA FA: Studies on molluscum contagiosum. Observations on the cytopathic effect of molluscum suspensions in vitro. Arch Intern Med 110:720–725, 1962

102. NICHOLAS AH: A poxvirus of primates. I. Growth of the virus in vitro and comparison with other poxviruses. J Natl Cancer Inst 45:897–905, 1970

103. NICHOLS AH: A poxvirus of primates. II. Immunology. J Natl Cancer Inst 45:907–914, 1970

104. NISHIMURA C, NOMURA M, KITAOKA M, TAKEUCHI Y, and KIMURA M: Complement requirement of the neutralizing antibody appearing after immunization with smallpox vaccine. Jpn J Microbiol 12:256–259, 1968

105. NIZAMUDDIN M and DUMBELL KR: A simple laboratory test to distinguish the virus of smallpox from that of alastrim. Lancet 1:68–69, 1961

106. NOBLE J JR and LOGGINS MS: Accuracy of smallpox diagnosis by immunofluorescence with a purified conjugate. Appl Microbiol 19:855–861, 1970

107. OBIJESKI JF, PALMER EL, GAFFORD LG, and RANDALL CC: Polyacrylamide gel electrophoresis of fowlpox and vaccinia virus proteins. Virology 51:512–516, 1973

108. ODA M: Plaque-hemadsorption technique for the detection of non-hemagglutinating vaccinia virus. Virology 23:432–434, 1964

109. OLDING-STENKVIST E, GRANDIEN M, and ESPMARK A: Early diagnosis of virus-caused vesicular rashes by immunofluorescence on skin biopsies. II. Poxvirus (vaccinia). Scand J Infect Dis 8:129–137, 1976

110. PALMER DF, CASEY HL, OLSEN JR, ELLER VH, and FULLER JM: A Guide to the Performance of the Standardized Diagnostic Complement Fixation Method and Adaptation to Micro Test. US Dept HEW, Center for Disease Control, Atlanta, Ga. 30333, 1st edition, 1969

111. PALMQUIST EE: The 1946 smallpox experience in Seattle. Can J Public Health 38:213–218, 1947

112. PAPADOPOULOS OA, DAWSON PS, HUCK RA, and STUART P: Agar gel diffusion studies of paravaccinia viruses. J Comp Pathol 78:219–225, 1968

113. PAYNE LG and NORRBY E: Presence of haemagglutinin in the envelope of extracellular vaccinia virus particles. J Gen Virol 32:63–72, 1976

114. PIRIE GD, BISHOP PM, BURKE DC, and POSTLETHWAITE R: Some properties of purified molluscum contagiosum virus. J Gen Virol 13:311–320, 1971

115. PLOWRIGHT W and FERRIS RD: Ether sensitivity of some mammalian poxviruses. Virology 7:357–358, 1959

116. POSTLETHWAITE R: Molluscum contagiosum. A review. Arch Environ Health 21:432–452, 1970

117. PRECAUSTA P and STELLMAN C: Isolation and comparative study in vitro of five strains of contagious ecthyma of sheep. Zentralbl Veterinaermed Reihe B 20:340–355, 1973

118. RASKIN J: Molluscum contagiosum. Tissue culture and serologic study. Arch Derm. 87:552–559, 1963

119. ROBERTS JA: Histopathogenesis of mousepox. I. Respiratory infection. Br J Exp Pathol 43:451–461, 1962

120. ROMERO-MERCADO CH, McPHERSON EA, LAING AH, LAWSON JB, and SCOTT GR: Virus particles and antigens in natural orf. Arch Gesamte Virusforsch 40:159-160, 1973
121. RONDLE CJM and DUMBELL KR: Antigens of cowpox virus. J Hyg 60:41-49, 1962
122. ROUHANDEH H, ENGLER R, TABER M, FOUAD A, and SELLS LL: Properties of monkey pox virus. Arch Gesamte Virusforsch 20:363-373, 1967
123. SCHOCH A: Sheep pox infection in man. Arch Derm Syph 39:1040-1041, 1939
124. SHELUKHINA EM, MALTSEVA NN, SHENKMAN LS, and MARENNIKOVA SS: Properties of two isolates (MK-7-73 and MK-10-73) from wild monkeys. Br Vet J 131:746-748, 1975
125. SHIEK W: Wirtszellbedingte dichteunterschiede des intra- und extraviralen vakzinevirus— hämagglutinins. Arch Gesamte Virusforsch 46:325-333, 1974
126. SMITH EC, PROTT BC, and BAXBY D: In vitro dissociation and reconstitution of poxvirus hemagglutinin. J Gen Virol 18:111-118, 1973
127. TAKABAYASHI K and McINTOSH K: Effect of heat-labile factors on the neutralizations of vaccinia virus by human sera. Infect Immun 8:582-589, 1973
128. TRUEBLOOD MS and CHOW TL: Characterization of agents of ulcerative dermatosis and contagious Ecthyma. Am J Vet Res 24:47-51, 1963
129. TUDOR V and STRATI I: Smallpox: Cholera (English edition) Abacus Press, Tunbridge Wells, Kent, 1977
130. TURNER GS and KAPLAN C: Observation on photodynamic inactivation of vaccinia virus and its effect on immunogenicity. J Hyg 63:395-410, 1965
131. VON MAGNUS P, ANDERSEN EK, PETERSEN KB, and BIRCH-ANDERSEN A: A pox-like disease in cynomolgus monkeys. Acta Pathol Microbiol Scand 46:156-176, 1959
132. WARREN J: Other infections In Viral and Rickettsial Infections of Man, Horsfall FL Jr and Tamm I (eds), 4th edition, JB Lippincott Co., Philadelphia, PA, 1965
133. WEEKE-LUITMANN M: Steigeruns der neutralisation von vaccinia-virus durch anti-globulin. Arch Gesamte Virusforsch 31:28-32, 1970
134. WEINSTEIN I: An outbreak of smallpox in New York City. Am J Public Health 37:1376-1384, 1947
135. WESTWOOD JC, HARRIS WJ, ZWARTOUW HT, TITMUSS DHJ, and APPLEYARD G: Studies on the structure of vaccinia virus. J Gen Virol 34:67-78, 1964
136. WESTWOOD JCN, ZWARTOUW HT, APPLEYARD G, and TITMUSS DHJ: Comparison of the soluble antigens and virus particle antigens of vaccinia. J Gen Microbiol 38:47-53, 1965
137. WILCOX WC and COHEN GH: The poxvirus antigens In Current Topics in Microbiology and Immunology 47:1-19, 1969
138. WINSLOW OE: A destroying angel: the conquest of smallpox in colonial Boston. Houghton Mifflin Co, Boston, 1974
139. WOODROOFE GM and FENNER F: Serological relationship within the poxvirus group: an antigen common to all members of the group. Virology 16:334-341, 1962
140. WORLD HEALTH ORGANIZATION: Expert Committee on Respiratory Virus Disease, First Report. WHO Tech Rep Ser No. 170:40-41, 1959
141. WORLD HEALTH ORGANIZATION: Guide to the Laboratory Diagnosis of Smallpox for Smallpox Eradication Programmes. WHO Geneva, 1969, 46 pp
142. WORLD HEALTH ORGANIZATION: Expert Committee on Smallpox Eradication. WHO Tech Rep Ser No 493:24-27, 1972
143. WORLD HEALTH ORGANIZATION: Weekly Epidemiological Record. WHO, Geneva 53:9-20, 1978
144. ZWARTOUW HI, WESTWOOD JCN, and HARRIS WJ: Antigens from vaccinia virus particles. J Gen Microbiol 38:39-45, 1965
145. ZIEGLER DW, HUTCHINSON HD, KAPLAN JP, and NAKANO JH: Detection by radioimmunoassay of antibody in human smallpox patients and vaccinees. J Clin Microbiol 1:311-317, 1975

CHAPTER 11

HERPES SIMPLEX VIRUS TYPES 1 AND 2 AND HERPESVIRUS SIMIAE

William E. Rawls

Introduction

The herpesvirus group consists of a large number of viruses which are wide spread in nature. Humans serve as the reservoir for 5 members of the group: herpes simplex viruses (HSV) type 1 and type 2; cytomegalovirus; varicella-zoster (V-Z) virus; and Epstein-Barr (EB) virus. Occasionally, infection of humans by herpesviruses of other vertebrates can occur and these infections may produce clinical illness. Herpesvirus simiae (herpes B virus) is especially significant in this regard since the disease in man is commonly fatal. In this chapter, the 2 types of HSV and herpesvirus simiae are dealt with separately.

Herpes Simplex Virus Types 1 and 2

History

Certain clinical entities associated with HSV infections have been delineated in the medical literature for several centuries (114). Gruter (85) and Lowenstein (136) are credited with the initial successful isolation of HSV. In these experiments, material collected from patients with human herpetic keratitis and of herpes labialis was found to produce specific lesions on the corneas of rabbits.

The observations that most adults had neutralizing antibodies to the virus and that only those adults with antibodies developed recurrent herpes (4) led some investigators to doubt the infectious agent as a causative factor in herpes labialis. The etiologic role of HSV in acute gingivostomatitis of children was clearly demonstrated in the late 1930s (45), and the concept of virus latency with recurrence was introduced as an explanation for recurrent herpes labialis (28). It is now recognized that HSV does not differ basically from other infectious agents with respect to the primary infection of susceptible hosts. However, unlike many agents the viruses often remain latent after the manifestations of the initial infections subside, and recurrent lesions may be produced with reactivation of the latent virus. The virus remains latent in the ganglion of sensory nerves (12–14, 177).

An appreciation for the diversity of clinical presentations of primary HSV infections became apparent with the demonstration of the role of the virus in eczema herpeticum (205, 223) and in vulvovaginitis (239). Work by Gallardo defined the role of the virus in keratoconjunctivitis (71). Isolation of HSV from diseased brain tissue demonstrated its importance in encephalitis (247), and it has recently been shown that type 2 virus causes aseptic meningitis, especially in adults (264).

Isolates of HSV were thought, until recently, not to display significant antigenic differences. In 1961, Schneweis and Brandis (216) reported substantial differences between strains which could be detected by a neutralization test. It was subsequently found that the anatomic site of isolation correlated with the antigenicity of the virus; isolates from genital sites fell into one group while isolates from nongenital sites tended to fall into another group (48). Genital isolates were also found to differ significantly from nongenital isolates in a number of biological and biochemical properties (153). The viruses associated with nongenital sites are usually type 1 viruses while the venereally spread viruses associated with genital lesions are usually type 2 viruses. An expanded interest in HSV type 1 and type 2 has arisen from observations suggesting an etiologic association between type 2 virus and squamous cell carcinoma of the cervix (168, 188).

Clinical aspects

While infections with either type 1 or type 2 HSV may be inapparent (27, 222), infections by these viruses are sometimes quite severe and occasionally they may be fatal. Among the factors which influence the severity of the infection is the immune status of the individual. Prior infection with one type of virus tends to limit the extent of tissue damage associated with a second infection by the same or other virus type (1, 118). Furthermore, in patients with defects in cell-mediated immunity, the infections are frequently quite severe or prolonged (56, 112, 133, 149, 211, 263).

Latency commonly follows infection with either type 1 or type 2 HSV. Population surveys indicate that 37–46% of young adults experience recurrent herpes labialis (51, 84). The occurrence of recurrent herpes does not appear uniformly in the population (51). For herpes genitalis, as many as two-thirds of the patients may suffer from recurrence (31). A variety of lesions may result from reactivation of the viruses, and lesions associated with recurrences in an individual are often similar to those experienced with past recurrent episodes. Type 1 HSV has been repeatedly recovered from trigeminal ganglia while type 2 HSV has been recovered from sacral ganglia (12, 13, 15, 177). Thus, the virus appears to reside in the nerve root ganglion during latency. Nonspecific factors such as cold, fever, menses, emotional stress, sunlight, and trauma appear to precipitate recurrent episodes (114). While a number of hypotheses have been put forth to explain the processes involved in recurrence (97, 126, 260), the mechanisms of latency and activation of the viruses-remain poorly understood.

Mode of transmission

Both type 1 and type 2 HSV are spread by the exchange of contaminated secretions from an infected individual to a susceptible host. The usual source of virus is an individual who has recurrent lesions or who may be secreting virus but does not have a clinically apparent lesion. For HSV type 1, spread is by oral-respiratory secretions while HSV type 2 is usually transmitted venereally (113, 175, 191). Neither virus displays significant seasonal variation in incidence of infections.

Primary infections by HSV type 1 tend to occur early in life in small foci such as family or in an institution. Most individuals are infected during the first 6 years of life in environments associated with lower socioeconomic conditions (222). The same pattern is not observed in upper socioeconomic settings, where a considerable proportion of the population may escape infection in the first decade of life (16, 240, 265); primary infections with HSV type 1 are observed not uncommonly in young adults with this social background (79).

The age-specific incidence of HSV type 2 is similar to that observed for venereal diseases (156); highest rates are observed late in the second decade and in the third decade of life (113, 191, 295). The occurrence of the disease correlates with sexual activity, and the virus has been isolated most readily from prostitutes and from patients attending venereal disease clinics. The primary infections with HSV type 2 tend to be more severe among patients who have not previously been infected with HSV type 1; thus, clinical illness from type 2 infections is relatively more frequent among those from upper socioeconomic classes.

The incubation period ranges from 2 to 11 days for both viruses, and peak incubation time is 6–7 days. Virus is shed in secretions for 3–4 weeks following a primary infections, while virus shedding associated with recurrent lesions is usually limited to 3–5 days (1). Vesicular fluid is very rich in infectious virus.

Clinical manifestations

Mouth and lips. A variety of clinical illnesses may be caused by HSV types 1 and 2. The most common portal of entry for HSV type 1 is the oral cavity, and acute gingivostomatits is a readily recognized manifestation of the infection (45). In this disease, the initial lesions appear as vesicles on the mucous membranes; however, the vesicles quickly evolve into grayish-yellow patches of shallow ulcers. Inflammation and ulceration of the gums and other mucous membranes of the mouth may become extensive. Cervical lymphadenopathy, fever, malaise, and diarrhea may accompany the illness. The disease is self-limited and the lesions resolve in about 2–3 weeks. The gingival component of the illness is not always predominant, in which case the infection may manifest as rhinitis, tonsillitis, pharyngitis, or scattered oral ulcers (30, 55, 79, 228). Extension of the disease process onto the esophogeal and laryngeal mucosa appears to occur uncommonly in the immunologically competent individuals, and not uncommonly in individuals with comprised immune responsiveness (149, 163, 164).

Recurrent herpes labialis, the most common manifestation of HSV type 1, usually involves the mucocutaneous junction of the lip. A burning or sense of irritation often heralds the onset of a lesion, and red papules appear within a few hours. The papules become a cluster of thin-walled vesicles which subsequently rupture leaving a dark crust. The lesions heal in about 4–7 days, and healing is without residual scarring. Recurrences are often located in the same area of the lip as previous lesions.

Eye. Primary infections of the eye beyond the newborn period are almost always caused by HSV type 1 (160). This initial infection is characterized by a unilateral follicular conjunctivitis, preauricular lymphadenopathy, and involvement of the corneal epithelium which may produce corneal opacities. Once specific immunity develops, follicular lesions of the conjunctiva rarely develop. Recurrent infections of the eye are not rare, and keratitis is the major manifestation. Infections of the superficial layers of the cornea give rise to dendritic ulcerations. Extension of the lesions to deeper layers of the eye produces a disciform keratitis and destruction of stromal fibers, which leads to scar formation and visual impairment. Virus can be readily isolated from cases of primary follicular conjunctivitis and from recurrent cases with dendritic ulcerations; however, virus is not readily detected in corneal scrappings of cases with stromal keratitis (38, 88, 288, 298).

Central nervous system. Involvement of the central nervous system is an uncommon complication of HSV infections. When it occurs, HSV type 1 infections are manifest as encephalitis while type 2 infections are manifest as aseptic meningitis. Herpetic encephalitis is one of the most common forms of severe encephalitis in adults (111, 146). The virus causes an acute necrosis of tissues in the frontal or temporal lobes which may result in localized neurologic abnormalities. These localized abnormalities superimposed upon general features of encephalitis such as fever, headache, nuchal rigidity, coma, and seizures permit the diagnosis of herpetic encephalitis to be considered on the basis of clinical findings. The course of the disease is rapid, and the majority of patients die within 2–3 weeks; partial paralysis and mental retardation are not uncommon among survivors (168).

Recently, it has become apparent that meningitis may be a complication of infections with HSV type 2 (40, 90, 96, 107, 238, 252, 264, 295). The disease is most prevalent in young adults and has been observed more among females than among males. The major symptoms are photophobia, headache, and meningismus. The course of the disease is benign and self-limited. Recurrent symptoms of meningeal irritation have been reported. In a number of the cases, an active infection of the genitalia with HSV type 2 is clinically apparent. Recurrence of genital lesions may be accompanied by neuralgia in these patients as well as in patients whose initial infection is not complicated by overt meningitis (98).

Skin. HSV does not appear to be able to penetrate healthy intact skin; however, diseased or traumatized skin can serve as a portal of entry. Eczema herpticum (Kaposi varicelliform eruption) is characterized by the development of a vesicular eruption in the eczematous areas of the skin of patients with atopic eczema (205, 223, 287). Other dermatoses such as Darier disease may also underlie the unusually widespread involvement of the skin by the virus (46, 106). Thermal injury predisposes patients to widespread HSV infections, and in some of these cases there may be systemic spread of the virus and a fatal outcome (163).

Lacerations or abrasions of healthy skin may provide portals for entry for HSV. A local lesion develops which vesiculates; lymphangitis and lymphoadenopathy may develop proximal to the lesion. An example of this form of infection is herpes paronychia (herpetic whitlow) which is especially common among persons in the medical, nursing, and dental professions (200, 257). Herpes gladiatorum is another form of the infection resulting from HSV contamination of abrasions acquired while wrestling (224, 286).

Genitalia. Genital infections in individuals without prior exposure to either type of HSV may be characterized by extensive vesicles and/or ulcerations of the mucous membranes and skin of the genitalia (118). Fever, inguinal lymphadenopathy, and dysuria, especially in women, may accompany the local lesions (196). Most infections are less severe, and in women the lesions may be confined to the cervix where they are asymptomatic (27, 153). In males the disease is characterized by vesicular eruptions on the glands, prepuce, or shaft of the penis (31). Recurrent lesions are fewer in number and of shorter duration than lesions associated with primary infections (1, 190). Both type 1 and type 2 HSV may produce genital lesions which are clinically indistinguishable. The proportion of cases of herpes genitalis caused by type 1 HSV varies from about 7% to almost 50% (31, 118, 160, 242, 295).

Generalized infections. Severe generalized infections with either type of HSV are normally confined to the newborn period or to patients with immunologic deficiencies. Type 2 HSV acquired during passage through the birth canal accounts for most cases of newborn disease, but a similar disease accompanies type 1 HSV infections acquired from other sources (157, 289). Some infections acquired in the newborn period are confined to one or a few organ systems such as skin, eyes, or central nervous system. However, dissemination of the virus to multiple organs including the liver and adrenals is not uncommon, and these infections are frequently fatal. It has been postulated that the newborn infant is immunologically immature and cannot limit the spread of the virus.

Systemic dissemination of the virus also occurs in some patients infected with the viruses beyond the newborn period (162). Almost all of these patients have conditions associated with abnormal immunologic functions. These conditions include certain inherited immunodeficiency diseases (211), malnutrition (17, 263) immunosuppressive therapy (162), hematologic malignancies (149), and burns (163). Rarely, systemic spread occurs in adult patients with no apparent underlying cause (114). These patients may have skin eruptions which are varicella-zoster like, hepatitis, tracheobronchitis or esophagitis.

Pathology

The basis for the pathologic changes observed with herpesvirus infection is the virus-induced alterations of the infected cells and the accompanying inflammatory response. In the skin, the characteristic vesicle is the result of acantholysis of parabasal and intermediate cells of the epithelium. The floor of the vesicles consists of naked papillae of the corium, and an intact superficial layer of cornified epithelial cells covers the vesicle. At the edges of the lesion the cells infected by the virus can be identified by certain characteristic changes. These changes include multinucleated giant cell formation, ballooning of the cell, degeneration of the cell nucleus, and the presence of characteristic intranuclear inclusion bodies. The vesicle contains a fibrinous fluid in which leukocytes, multinucleated giant cells, and swollen epidermal cells are found. The corium beneath the lesion contains an infiltrate of inflammatory cells, but the cells of the corium are not destroyed and the lesions heal without scarring. The lesions of mucous membranes are similar to those which develop in the skin, except the vesicle roof is much thinner and there is an early loss of vesicle fluid.

Necrosis is characteristically found in deeper tissues infected by HSV. In fatal disseminated infections, coagulation necrosis of the liver, adrenals, lungs, and spleen is not uncommonly observed. Cells containing intranuclear inclusions are observed at the periphery of the necrotic areas in most cases. The brains of fatal cases are usually congested with foci of soft, friable discolorations. The most pronounced changes are observed in the cerebral cortex, especially in the frontal and temporal lobes. Areas of necrosis are observed in both the gray matter and the white matter. The nuclei of oligodendrocytes and neurons may contain typical inclusion bodies, but these are often absent. Widespread infiltration of the leptomeninges by mononuclear inflammatory cells is a common feature as is scattered perivascular hemorrhages.

The immune response of the host appears to be important in the pathogenesis of the lesions induced by HSV. Primary lesions in the immunologically naive patient are more extensive, and the base of the lesion is less raised and erythematous than in the recurrent lesions. While antibodies may contribute to pathogenesis of the lesions through antigen-antibody complex formation (145), humoral immunity appears to play a minor role in limiting virus infection at local sites (47). Clinical and experimental observations on the severity and course of lesions among patients and laboratory animals with abnormal cell-mediated immune functions indicate the importance of this system in recovery. *In vitro* studies have demonstrated the ability of peripheral blood leukocytes to limit the spread of HSV from cell to cell (131), and this function appears to be mediated through interferon (8, 86, 132). In addition, HSV-infected cells can be lysed *in vitro* by lymphocytes (35, 206, 255) and by antibodies and blood leukocytes (185, 230, 261). Whether these mechanisms are operative *in vivo* has yet to be determined.

Description and Nature of the Agents

General architecture

There is general similarity of the structure of members of the herpesvirus group. HSV type 1 has been the most extensively studied member of the group, and the description which follows is derived mostly from data obtained in studies of this virus. The virion is composed of an icosahedral nucleocapsid with a core containing DNA, and the nucleocapsid is surrounded by an envelope. The diameter of the complete virus particles ranges from 110 to 220 nm (115). The nucleocapsid is an icosahedron formed by 162 capsomeres with the shape of long hollow prisms, and its average diameter is 95–105 nm.

The core of the virus contains the nucleoprotein (52) and has a diameter of 75 nm. It appears as an electron-dense toroid surrounding a less-dense central structure (69). With special techniques, coiled filamentous structures have been found on the surface of the core which could correspond to the viral nucleoprotein (198). Two other shells have been noted in the space between the core and the icosahedral capsid (197, 198); more recently this space with ill-defined structures has been referred to as the "peri-core" (199).

In the mature particle, the nucleocapsid is enveloped by a membrane, and by electron microscopy the membrane appears as a 3-layered structure similar to the membranes of cells. The virus obtains this membrane as the nucleocapsid buds out of the nucleus through the inner lamella of the nuclear membrane into the perinuclear cysternae (41, 42, 197, 219, 220). Type 2 HSV appears to also obtain its envelope by budding through other membranes inside the cell (41, 220). Structures thought to represent virus-specific surface proteins are observed on the outer surfaces of membranes through which the viruses bud (42, 250). Between the membrane and the nucleocapsid is a space filled with an amorphous material (198). The intact virus particle has a buoyant density of 1.271 g/cm^3 in cesium chloride (194).

Chemical composition

Obtaining highly purified preparations of HSV is difficult, and thus estimations of the chemical composition of the virus are open to question. One estimate reported that HSV contains 70% protein, 22% phospholipids, 1.5% carbohydrate, and 6.5% DNA (210).

Deoxyribonucleic acid

Knowledge regarding the DNA of HSV types 1 and 2 has expanded rapidly in recent years. The genome is a linear, double-stranded, single DNA molecule with a molecular weight of slightly less than 1×10^8 (18, 66). A buoyant density of about 1.726 g/cm^3 has been reported for type 1 and 1.728 g/cm^3 for type 2 (80, 120). These buoyant density values have been used to estimate the base composition of the DNA; a G-C content of 67% has been estimated for HSV type 1 and 69% for type 2 (80, 12). These values correlate with those obtained using the melting profile of viral DNA (66, 82). This relatively high G-C content allows the separation of viral DNA from cellular DNA using isopycnic density gradient centrifugation.

A striking feature of the viral DNA is that following denaturation the DNA appears as a heterogenous population of single-stranded fragments shorter than the size of the intact viral DNA (82, 290). This has been interpreted as indicating the presence in the DNA of single-strand nicks, gaps, or some kind of alkaline-labile bonds. Recently, it has been shown that these nicks or gaps are randomly located in the DNA and they can be enzymatically repaired *in vitro* (104).

The molecular organization of the HSV type 1 DNA has been approached using different restriction endonucleases (36, 92, 93, 235, 292, 293). Different laboratories have reported full cleavage maps for HSV type 1 (92, 93, 234, 291). Electron microscopic studies of HSV type 1 DNA digested with lambda 5' exonuclease and allowed to self-anneal (227) have shown the presence of terminally redundant sequences. These sequences constituted about 0.5% of the genome. Similar studies using single-stranded DNA before and after reassociation suggest that larger pieces of the terminal sequences are repeated internally in the genome but in an inverted form (89). These terminal and internal inverted sequences are encompassed by 2 segments of unique nonrepetitive sequences: a short one (S) and a long one (L). The existence of these repetitive internally inverted sequences and of the L and S segments seem to be characteristic of several members of the herpesvirus group. The S segment represents about 20% of the genome, and the L segment accounts for the other 80%. It has been suggested that internal intramolecular recombination between the inverted redundant sequences as well as intermolecular recombination between these sequences could generate inversions of the S and L segments leading to 4 possible arrangements of the genes in the HSV genome (227). Little is presently known about the gene order on the viral DNA. Using temperature-sensitive mutants, some mutations have been ordered in a linkage map for both type 1 and type 2 HSV (212). It also appears possible to map structural genes using the parallel characterization of the DNA and polypeptides of intertypic recombinants. Thus, knowledge regarding the coding functions of the DNA should expand rapidly. Purified preparations of HSV DNA are infectious (83, 125, 227).

Proteins

A total of 33 polypeptides have been identified in purified preparations of HSV type 1. Rapid posttranslation cleavage of precursor polypeptides in their production has not been detected, but the precursor-product relation between some of the virion proteins cannot be completely ruled out at present (198). As many as 8 of the structural polypeptides are glycosylated (248, 249). The glycoproteins are associated with the virus envelope. Eight of the virion polypeptides are in the capsids of mature virions (77). Incomplete capsids and unenveloped capsids extracted from the nuclei of infected cells seem to contain additional polypeptides. Six of the virion proteins are phosphorylated (78). The existence of one virus polypeptide with a high content of arginine was reported (167), but this has not been confirmed and the presence of a core-associated basic protein in the virus seem unlikely (198). Instead, polyamines which have been shown to be present in the virion could be the basic components associated with the DNA (76). All the virion polypeptides are virus specific in the sense that no normal cellular polypeptides are found in the virus.

Lipids

The lipids of the virion are exclusively associated with the outer enveloping membrane and most likely are provided by the host cell. A similarity in the phospholipid composition of the outer envelope of the virus and the nuclear membrane of host cells has been reported (22).

Resistance

Storage

HSV types 1 and 2 are relatively thermolabile, and the viruses are customarily stored in the frozen state (-70 C or less). Preservation is aided by the addition of proteins, and animal serum at 10% concentrations, egg yolk at 0.1% concentrations, gelatin at 0.5% concentrations, nutrient broth and skim milk have all been advocated as additives. The loss of infectivity is not simply due to the absence of protein since purified virus suspended in distilled water and 0.25 M sucrose is relatively stable when compared to virus resuspended in allantoic fluid (see Ref 268). It has also been found that viruses suspended in 1 M Na_2SO_4 or Na_2HPO_4 are stabilized. Infectious virus produced in tissue cultures is usually maintained by freezing the virus suspended in culture medium containing 2% serum at -70 C.

Virus infectivity in animal tissues or chorioallantoic membranes has been maintained by storing the material in 50% glycerol. In glycerol, infectious virus has been recovered from tissues after storage for 6 months at 4-8 C and 18 months at -20 C. Lyophilization is another effective method of preparing virus for storage at 4-8 C.

Physical agents

Heat degrades the viruses, and the rate of loss of infectivity depends upon the environmental conditions and the temperature. In tissue culture medium the half-life of HSV is about 1.5 hr at 37 C and about 3-4 hrs at 30 C. The viruses are more stable when suspended in distilled water than in molar solutions of divalent cations ($Mg++$ or $Ca++$) or in Earle salt solution (276). Exposure of HSV to 1 M NaCl does not alter survival in 140 min at 4 C, and there is no evidence that osmolarity of the suspending fluids influences the degradation of the virus. In fact, 2 M $Na+$ has been reported to increase the stability of HSV at 37 C (276).

Type 1 HSV was found to be relatively stable at pH 5.5-9.5 in experiments carried out at 26 C with virus suspended in tissue culture fluids; below pH 4 or above pH 10.5 infectivity was rapidly lost. In the presence of radiant energy, HSV is rapidly inactivated: 50% loss in 5-7 sec of ultraviolet light and 90% loss upon exposure to 1200 r of x-ray for 2 min (183). Gamma radiation destroys infectivity (180). HSV can be rendered sensitized to light by photosensitizing dyes. Toluidine blue, proflavin, or neutral red at 10^{-4}M in suspensions of dye-free virus preparations renders HSV sensitive to light at pH 9 and 37 C; exposure to light for 30 sec completely inactivated over 10^6 infectious units/ml (277). Photosensitization has been advocated as a method of therapy.

Chemicals

Virus suspensions are readily destroyed by organic solvents such as ether, chloroform and alcohol. However, lyophilized virus is relatively resistant to absolute alcohol and ether. Phenol at 5% concentration abolishes all infectivity after 18 hr at 4 C, and the virus is readily inactivated by 1:1000 potassium permanganate, 10^{-2}M formaldehyde, 10^{-3}M iodine, and 10^{-4}M or greater concentrations of lead, silver, gold, cadmium, and mercury (225). Quaternary ammonium cationic detergents such as cetyl pyridinium chloride (Ceepryn) and benzalkonium chloride (Zephiran) are virocidal at concentrations of 1:10,000 (268). A number of quinone derivatives inactivate herpesviruses (225) as does beta-propiolactone. The viruses are also destroyed by 0.1% merthiolate. Exposure of virus preparations to fluorocarbon (Freon 112 n-heptane) in an Omnimix for 5 min at 4 C did not reduce virus titer immediately, but repeated treatment or storage of treated preparations resulted in substantial loss of infectivity (268). Incubation of HSV type 1 and type 2 at 37 C with sodium p-chloromercuribenzoate or chlorhexidine gluconate inactivated the viruses; however, the viruses were not equally susceptible, and type 1 and type 2 could be differentiated using chlorhexidine gluconate (229).

HSV types 1 and 2 are inactivated by a number of proteolytic enzymes. In 1 hr at 37 C and pH 7.0-7.2, 10^5 infectious units/ml of virus were lost in the presence of 1 μg/ml of chymotrypsin, 5 μg/ml papain, 5 μg/ml protease, and 100 μg/ml aminopeptidase. Alkaline phosphatase (10 μg/ml) also destroyed infectivity while lysozymes, hyaluronidase, purified sialidase, and adenosine triphosphatase had no effect (268).

Bile and egg white have been used to inactivate the virus at 36 C (297), and an inhibitor thought to be identical with the properdin system has been reported in rat serum (59). Attachment of the virus onto cells can be prevented with synthetic polyanions and heparin (151, 152, 272). Tannic acid or flavonols at concentrations of 300 μg/ml have also been found to reduce virus infectivity when incubated at 26 C for 2 hr (19).

Antigenic composition

Numbers of immunotypes

There are two types of HSV that can be distinguished antigenically and biologically (154, 160). The two virus types share cross-reacting antigens, and the reactivity of the viruses with heterologous antiserum is greater than that observed for serotypes within most virus groups (196). However, the buoyant densities of the DNA of type 1 and type 2 HSV are 1.726 and 1.728 g/cm^3, respectively, (80, 120) and only about half of the DNA molecules of the two viruses are homologous (121, 218). The viruses differ in their ability to form plaques in chick embryo cells (58, 137), in the size of pocks produced on the chorioallantoic membranes of hens eggs (155, 178), and in their ability to replicate at different temperatures (134). Deoxynucleosides block the cytopathogenic effect (CPE) induced by type 2 HSV but not that induced by type 1 (119), and different feulgen-deoxyribonucleic acid hydrolysis patterns have been noted in cells infected with type 1 and type 2 viruses (271). Antigenic differences have been demonstrated by neutralization test (174, 216), immunofluorescence, (74, 158) immunodiffusion, and immunoelectrophoresis (110, 217). Thus, the detectable antigenic differences combined with the structural and biologic differences clearly indicate that two types of virus exist.

Within each type, considerable variability may be observed in the biologic property examined (178). Strain differences in CPE are not rare, and strains which produce syncytium or giant cells instead of rounding of individual cells are occasionally isolated. Such strains tend to emerge upon tissue culture passage but are sometimes observed among viruses isolated directly from lesions. In addition, it has been shown that some alteration of antigenicity may be associated with tissue culture propagation (87).

Description of various antigens

The herpesviruses are relatively complex, and a number of antigens and enzymes are coded for by the viral genomes (122, 160). Of the many virus-specific polypeptides identified by polyacrylamide gel electrophoresis of cells infected by HSV type 1 or 2, only a few have been examined with respect to antigenicity. By gel diffusion, 7–12 precipitin lines have been reported (269, 281). More recently, attempts have been made to identify the role of the proteins in the immune response to the virus (37, 182, 233, 249, 274). A protein with a molecular weight of about 131,000 and readily solubilized from cells infected with either virus, induces antibodies that react with both type 1 and type 2 antigen preparations. These antibodies weakly neutralize both virus types (182), and the antigen may be similar to major cross-reacting antigen detected by human serum (237). Two high molecular weight glycoproteins which induce antibodies capable of neutralizing both virus types can be extracted from infected cells with nonionic detergent (274). The major glycoprotein of HSV type 1 has a molecular weight of 131,000 and induces a type-specific antibody capable of virus neutralization. Two type-specific antigens can be extracted from cells infected with type 2 HSV. In addition to these two type-specific antigens extracted with nonionic detergent, an antigen specific for HSV type 2 can also be obtained which is water soluble; antibodies to the water soluble antigen do not neutralize the virus, while antibodies to the other two antigens are capable of neutralizing type 2 virus (274). While antibodies to the various antigens appear after infection, purified preparations of the antigens have not yet been utilized for diagnostic purposes.

In examining the association between HSV type 2 and cervical carcinoma, serum from women with cervical cancer was found to react with antigens induced by type 2 HSV, and the antibody activity to these antigens did not correlate with virus neutralizing activity of the serum. One antigen detectable 4 hr after infection of cells has been called AG-4. The antigen is a protein with a molecular weight of about 161,000 and appears to be incorporated as a minor component in mature virions (7). Antibodies to AG-4 have been detected by a quantitative complement-fixation test and detectable levels of antibody activity have been reported primarily in patients bearing active cervical neoplasms. A second antigen has been prepared from membranes of cells infected by HSV type 2. Membranes were obtained from cells 24 hr after infection, and the antigen was liberated from the membranes by sonication. Purification of the sonicate by polyacrylamide gel electrophoresis yielded an antigen (HSV-TAA) with a molecular weight of about 40–60,000 that could be eluted from the gels (101). Antibodies to this antigen have been found in serum of patients with active or treated squamous cell carcinomas of the cervix or of the head and neck (101). The major polypeptide synthesized within 4–6 hr after infection by type 2 has also served as an antigen to detect antiviral antibodies (5). This polypeptide, with a molecular weight of 143,000 was radiolabeled and used in an immunoprecipitation test to quantitate antibodies in human serum; quantitatively greater amounts of antibodies were found in serum of women with cervical cancer than in serum of control women (144).

The antigenicity of subunits of the viruses has been examined with respect to serologic diagnosis. Preparations of envelope, capsids, and soluble antigens of HSV type 1 and type 2 were prepared by density gradient centrifugation (139). The subunit preparations do not appear to provide any distinct advantage as diagnostic reagents over crude antigens (10).

Pathogenicity in animals

Both type 1 and type 2 HSV infect a wide variety of laboratory animals. Earlier studies dealing with the pathogenicity of the viruses in animals have been reviewed by Nahmias and Dowdle (154). While animals are now seldom used for diagnostic purposes, they are used to study the mechanisms of recurrence (259, 260), various aspects of immunologic reactivity (35, 184, 201), oncogenicity (169, 284), and effectiveness of putative therapeutic agents.

Newborn mice develop fatal infections regardless of the route of injection; however, in adult animals fatal encephalitis is consistently observed only following intracerebral infection. Peripheral inoculation of a number of animal species may result in an ascending myelitis and ultimately fatal encephalitis. Among the animals which develop fatal infections are mice, hamsters, cotton rats, and owl monkeys. Localized lesions develop at the site of inoculation in rabbits, guinea pigs, and cebus monkeys. Cornea inoculation of rabbits produces a keratoconjunctivitis similar to that seen in humans. A similar lesion can be produced in guinea pigs.

Growth in tissue culture

Replicative cycle

A feature of HSV types 1 and 2 is their ability to infect a wide variety of animals and animal cells grown in culture. Replication of the viruses has been examined in a number of cell systems, and the duration of successive steps in the replication cycle depends upon the type of cell, the virus strain, and the multiplicity of the infection. The general features of the replicative cycle can be illustrated by type 1 infection of HEp-2 cells in which virus DNA synthesis begins about 3 hr after infection and new progeny virus is detectable 3 hr later. The duration of a complete cycle is about 12–18 hr, and between 10^3 and 10^5 virus particles are produced per cell; only about 1 in 100 to 1 in 1000 particles are infectious.

Viropexis and fusion to the host cell membrane are two proposed mechanisms for entry of attached virus into the cell. Viropexis entails the movements of the virus into the cell by pinocytosis in which case the virus appears in the cytoplasm in a vacuole. The second proposed mechanism of entry involves the fusion of the virus envelope with the host cell membrane, and the nucleocapsid is released directly into the cytoplasm (42, 135, 136). Active macromolecular synthesis does not seem to be required for the movement of the viral DNA to the cell nucleus where replication begins with RNA transcription from the parental DNA (195, 275). The transcription appears to be facilitated by cellular RNA polymerase II (2, 23).

The DNA is not transcribed synchronously throughout the replicative cycle. About 45% of the genome is transcribed 2 hr after infection, but almost 50% is transcribed 8 hr after infection (67). Not all of the transcribed sequences are produced in the same abundance; both the 2-hr and 8-hr transcripts represent 2 classes differing in their abundance (65). In the nucleus the virus transcripts range in size from 10S to more than 60S, while the RNA associated with polysomes range in size from 10S to 35S (275). By competition hybridization it was shown that about 80% of the nucleotide sequences present in the heterogenous, high-molecular-weight nuclear RNA are also represented in the smaller nuclear RNA and in the polyribosomal RNA. At least a portion of the transcribed RNA is polyadenylated at the 3′ end and capped at the 5′ end (14, 231, 232).

The synthesis of viral proteins takes place exclusively in the cytoplasm of the infected cells, and some of these proteins find their way into the nucleus where virus assembly occurs. The viral DNA has enough coding capacity for as many as 5.5×10^4 amino acids, and it should be able to code for about 50 polypeptides with an average length of 10^3 amino acids. Using electrophoretic techniques of high resolution, as many as 49 putative HSV type 1 specific polypeptides were identified in infected cells (102). In HSV type-2 infected cells, 57 virus-specific polypeptides have been identified (181). Of the type 1 polypeptides, 23 could be correlated in their electrophoretic mobility with virion structural proteins, 15 were classified as nonstructural, and for the rest the classification was uncertain (102). Rapid posttranslational cleavage does not seem to occur in cells infected with HSV type 1, and the most extensive changes that some of the virus-specific proteins undergo seem to be the phosphorylation and glycosylation (248).

The synthesis of the viral proteins is regulated (103). Immediately after the removal of drugs that inhibit protein synthesis, infected cells translate certain virus-specific polypeptides called "alpha" proteins. They include a few nonstructural proteins and one minor structural polypeptide (VP-4). The messenger (m) RNAs coding for these proteins are accumulated during incubation of the cells in the presence of the inhibitors of protein synthesis. A second group of polypeptides called "beta" protein then appear, and the rate of synthesis of these proteins increases as the rate of the production of the alpha proteins decreases. This group includes most of the nonstructural proteins and a few minor structural polypeptides. Later in the replicative cycle, the rate of synthesis of these polypeptides also decreases. The decline in the rate of the synthesis of the beta polypeptides is associated with the increase in the production of a third group of virus-specific proteins or "gamma" proteins which include the major structural proteins. Inhibitors of DNA synthesis will greatly reduce the synthesis of the gamma proteins while not affecting alpha protein synthesis or preventing the decline in the synthesis of beta proteins. These findings fit the "cascade regulation" model of genome expression. According to this model, mRNA for alpha proteins are transcribed soon after infection and these proteins subsequently promote the transcription of mRNA for beta proteins. Beta proteins promote the replication of viral DNA and inhibit transcription of further alpha mRNA. The gamma proteins are synthesized after DNA synthesis, and these proteins also inhibit the further production of beta proteins.

The core and the capsid of the virus are assembled in the nucleus. The virus buds from the nuclear membrane. Mature virions can be visualized in vacuoles within the cytoplasm or within the endoplasmic reticulum. During replication of the virus, synthesis of host cell macromolecules is dramatically altered. Cellular DNA synthesis decreases 2 hr after infection and is shut off completely by 7 hr after infection. Host cell RNA synthesis stops, and there is a dramatic decrease in host cell protein synthesis about 2–3 hr after infection. With a high multiplicity of infection, extensive cytologic changes ensue which can be seen microscopically within 6 hr after infection.

Uses of tissue culture

HSV types 1 and 2 grow in a wide variety of tissue culture cells. However, not all types of cells are equally efficient in supporting virus replication, and abortive infections of the viruses have been noted in certain cell systems. The abortive infection may be strain associated as has been demonstrated for the MP strain of HSV type 1 which does not replicate in canine kidney cells. Virus penetration occurs and viral DNA and proteins are made, but the progeny virus particles are not enveloped (251). An abortive cycle with similar characteristics has been observed in adult mouse macrophages infected with HSV type 1 (258). The abortive infection in certain cells may be type specific; newly isolated strains of HSV type 1 produce very low yields of progeny virus in primary chick embryo cells, while HSV type 2 isolates grow in these cells (137). The temperature of incubation is a critical factor in virus replication, and abortive replication occurs at elevated temperatures. Partial inactivation of the viruses by ultraviolet (UV) irradiation results in abortive cycles in some of the infected cells, and under these conditions a fraction of the cells may be biochemically (150) or oncogenically transformed (49).

Both primary cell cultures and established cell lines have been used extensively for the diagnosis of herpetic infections. Primary rabbit kidney cells (38, 265, 268), human embryonic kidney cells (90, 143, 262), human amnion cells (31, 38, 206), human diploid fibroblasts (1, 20, 27, 29, 33, 94, 99, 143, 162, 253, 262, 288), and African green monkey kidney cells (29, 90) have all been found suitable for virus isolation and for preparation of diagnostic reagents. Established cell lines of rabbit kidney (RK-13) (236), baby hamster kidney (BHK-21) (241, 288), monkey kidney (Vero) (185, 262), and mouse fibroblasts (L-cells), as well as HeLa cells (94, 99, 143) and HEp-2 cells, (6, 29, 90) have all been used for diagnostic purposes. Extensive surveys comparing the relative sensitivity of all of the various cell types for virus isolation have not been carried out, but where examined, human embryonic kidney cells and human diploid fibroblasts were found to be slightly superior. Of the established cell lines, Vero cells have been found to be suitable in the experience of the author. Cells grown in culture are the substrate of choice for isolating viruses from clinical specimens, for preparing and assaying virus stocks, and for preparing antigens used in serologic tests. Although the description of procedures in this chapter primarily include Vero cells, one of the cell types mentioned above may also be used.

Two forms of CPE are observed. The most common begins with cytoplasmic granulation after which the cells become enlarged or ballooned. These macrocytes then become rounded, take on a refractile appearance, and undergo lytic degeneration. The second type of CPE is the formation of multinucleated giant cells. This results from virus-induced fusion of cell membranes with the migration of nuclei in the fused cells into aggregates. The formation of these structures, also called polykaryocytes, is dependent upon the genetic constitution of the virus strain, the cell type, and the tissue culture conditions (179).

Virus stocks can be prepared by infecting monolayers of Vero cells grown in a suitable size flask. At a multiplicity of infection of about 1–3 infectious units per cell, progeny virus appear from 6 to 8 hr after infection, and maximum virus titers are obtained about 20 hr after infection. At this time most of the virus is cell associated and can be released by disrupting the cells. This can be accomplished by rapid freeze-thawing or by sonication. The yields of infectious virus are generally less from cells infected with type 2 virus than from those infected with type 1. Repeated passage of either virus type at high multiplicities of infection may result in the production of defective viruses which will result in stocks of low titer.

Preparation of Immune Serum

The antibody responses to HSV types 1 and 2 are similar to those seen with other viruses in that the initial response following a primary infection contains appreciable quantities of IgM antibodies. The IgM antibodies do not normally persist for long periods, although 19S antibodies to the viruses have been detected in late-phase serum obtained from immunized animals (see review 87). Appreciable quantities of IgM antibodies do not normally persist in human serum, and the demonstration of IgM antibodies to the viruses in serum or cerebrospinal fluid constitutes presumptive evidence of a recent primary infection. The antibody response in animals may vary considerably both in quantity and quality within and between species. In addition, antibodies from different animal species may be directed toward different antigenic determinants of the virus. Thus, the particular use of the antiserum should be taken into consideration when selecting the animal species to be immunized, the method of immunization, and the time after immunization when blood is collected (87).

Rabbits are the animals of choice for preparation of antiserum needed in a diagnostic laboratory. The specificity of the antiserum can be improved by preparing the antigens in rabbit kidney cells. Kidneys are removed from 3-week-old rabbits and trypsinized, and the monodispersed cells are seeded in large culture flasks in Eagle medium containing 10% fetal bovine serum. When the monolayers are confluent, they are rinsed twice with phosphate-buffered saline (PBS) and refed with Eagle medium containing 5% normal rabbit serum which has been heat inactivated at 56 C for 30 min. The cultures are incubated for 48 hr at 37 C, and then the monolayers are infected by removing the medium and adding 0.1–1 plaque-forming units (pfu) of virus per cell in a small volume. Virus is allowed to adsorb 1–2 hr at 37 C after which excess virus is removed by 2 washes with PBS, and the cultures are refed with Eagle medium containing 2% normal rabbit serum. The cultures are incubated until 3+ to 4+ CPE develops (24–48 hr), and the cells are scraped into the medium using a rubber policeman. The suspended cells are then sedimented by centrifugation at $200 \times g$ for 10 min, and sufficient supernatant fluid is removed to make a 10–20% cell suspension from the pelleted cells. The cells are then ruptured by 3 cycles of freezing and thawing or by sonic oscillation, and the preparation may be used immediately or stored at − 20 C. The rabbits should be initially injected with 1 ml of antigen which has been exposed to UV light to avoid loss of animals from herpetic encephalitis. The antigen is pipetted into a 60-mm plastic Petri dish, and the open dish is exposed to UV light at a distance of about 12 inches for 5 min. This treatment inactivates most infectious virus without destroying antigenicity. The antigen is then aspirated into a syringe and injected intraperitoneally into the rabbit. Ten days later the rabbit is injected intramuscularly with 1 ml of antigen mixed with an equal amount of complete Freund adjuvant. At 2-week intervals the rabbit should be given 2 additional injections of antigen with adjuvant. Serum is collected 2 weeks after the last injection. Micro-neutralization titers of 1:500–1:1000 are commonly attained with this method (226). Lower-titer antiserum can be obtained from infected rabbits by way of corneal or skin scarification using virus stocks available in the laboratory. The animals are bled 4–6 weeks after initiation of the infection. The antibody response of the rabbits is variable, and some of the animals may be lost from encephalitis; thus, it may be necessary to infect a number of animals in order to obtain a suitable antiserum (268).

Antiserum may also be prepared in guinea pigs. Antigen containing infectious virus is mixed with complete Freund adjuvant and injected in 0.1-ml amounts into the footpads of the animals. Preparation of antigen in guinea pig cells reduces antibody formation to tissue culture components. The animals are bled 4–6 weeks after injection, and neutralization titers in the range of 1:100–1:300 can usually be obtained (268). Antiserum prepared in guinea pigs has been reported to be superior to rabbit antiserum in differentiating HSV type 1 from type 2.

Collection and Preparation of Specimens for Laboratory Diagnosis

Precautions

HSV type 1 and type 2 do not constitute an unusual hazard to laboratory workers, and the precautionary measures generally used in handling viruses will suffice. Accidental contamination of an open wound or inadvertent inoculation may cause a local herpetic lesion, and persons with skin diseases such as atopic eczema should avoid working with the virus.

Sources of material and collection of specimens for virus isolation

As with other viruses, the probability of isolating HSV decreases with time after the lesions develop. Greatest isolation rates are obtained from vesicle fluid, and the rates decrease as the ulcerative phase of the lesion becomes crusted and resolves. Thus, the specimens should be collected as soon as possible in the course of the illness.

Isolation rates are also influenced by the duration between collection of specimens and inoculation of the specimens into a tissue culture substrate. This interval should be as short as conveniently possible. The loss of virus infectivity is reduced if the specimen can be transported and maintained at 4 C in a suitable medium. Storage of the specimen for more than a few hours at 4 C may result in the complete loss of infectivity in specimens containing small amounts of virus. Specimens which cannot be processed within a few hours should be stored at -70 C.

Special transport media. These have been reported to stabilize the virus and reduce loss in clinical specimens (26, 159). One of these media is prepared by dissolving 4 g of NaCl, 0.2 g of KC1, and 1.7 g of K_2PO_4 in 500 ml of distilled water and adding 10 g of charcoal (Colab; Chicago, Ill.). In another 500 ml of distilled water, 4 g of agarose (Fisher Co.) is dissolved by heating. The 2 solutions are combined and autoclaved. When the mixture has cooled to 40 C, it is dispensed into sterile tubes (159). The other medium contains bentonite instead of charcoal and agarose (24). Antibiotics (pencillin 1000 u/ml, streptomycin 1000 μm/ml, and mycostatin 1000 units) added to the cooled medium may help suppress bacterial and mycotic contamination in the specimen. Special transport medium is not critical for virus isolation, and nutrient broth, balanced salt solution with 10% serum, or tissue culture medium with 10% serum are usually satisfactory. If none of the above preparations is available, distilled water can be used.

Vesicle fluid. This can be aspirated from a mature vesicle with a 26 or 27 gauge needle attached to a tuberculin syringe. The lesion is carefully cleansed with 70% ethanol, and the needle is inserted into the edge of the vesicle with the bevel up. The plunger of the syringe is carefully withdrawn as the needle is inserted. The material aspirated is immediately injected into diluent, and the syringe and needle are rinsed by aspirating and expelling about 0.2 ml of diluent. Virus in the fluid can also be obtained by lifting the top from the vesicle and catching the fluid in a cotton swab.

Swabs of herpetic ulcers. Sterile swabs are firmly rubbed against the ulcer and then immediately immersed in diluent or transport medium. The swab is swirled vigorously, and then excess fluid is removed by pressing the swab against the side of the tube. A volume of 1–2 ml of fluid is normally placed in the tubes.

Saliva. Saliva is collected in sterile glass containers and processed immediately or transferred to a tube and stored at −70 C.

Cerebrospinal fluid. No special processing is required for cerebrospinal fluid, which is usually collected aseptically. The fluid may be inoculated directly onto monolayers of tissue culture cells, or the cells in the cerebrospinal fluid can be sedimented by centrifugation at $200 \times g$ for 10 min and resuspended in diluent. Both the fluid and resuspended cells can be used as inoculum.

Tissues. Specimens of organs obtained at autopsy or at surgery should be collected as aseptically as possible. It is recommended that these samples be processed as soon as possible in which instance they should be immersed in sterile diluent and sent immediately to the laboratory. Viruses in neural tissue may only be isolated in some cases by cultivating viable cells in tissue culture either alone or with another type of cell susceptible to the virus (12, 15). If the specimens must be stored, it has been recommended that they be kept in a sterile solution of neutral 50% glycerol in saline at −20 C or placed in a sterile container and frozen at −70 C.

Sampling for serologic diagnosis

Paired samples are required for serologic diagnosis, and the initial blood sample should be collected as early in the course of the illness as possible. The second sample should be collected 2–3 weeks later. The samples are collected aseptically, a clot is allowed to form at 37 C or room temperature, and then the specimen can be held overnight at 4 C. The serum separated from the clot should be stored at −20 C.

Sampling for microscopy

Light microscopy. Cells with changes characteristic of HSV infection are present in greatest numbers at the base of vesicle or ulcer; they decrease in numbers as the lesion heals. Specimens for light microscopy are collected by lifting the top of the vesicle, if present, and scraping cells from the base of the ulcer with a scapel or a curette. Cells can be carefully scraped from diseased cornea in a similar manner. The cells are smeared on a microscope slide and fixed in methanol.

Immunofluorescence examination. Specimens are obtained as described for light microscopy, but the smeared cells are dried and fixed for 10 min with cold acetone. Virus antigens can also be detected in biopsy specimens by immunofluorescence (FA) (166). The biopsy is quick frozen, 6-μ sections are cut and placed on microscope slides after which they are air dried and fixed in acetone. Cells in samples of cerebrospinal fluid may be examined by FA. The cells are sedimented by centrifugation at $200 \times g$ for

10 min, after which they are resuspended in a small amount of PBS and placed on a microscope slide. The cells are then air dried and fixed in acetone.

Electron microscopy. For electron microscopic (EM) examination, vesicle fluid is aspirated with a small-gauge needle attached to a tuberculin syringe and expressed into a small amount (0.1 ml) of distilled water. Scrapings from the base of herpetic ulcers or lesion crust placed in a small volume of water may also be shown to contain virus by EM.

Laboratory Diagnosis

Identification of HSV type 1 or type 2 in material obtained from diseased tissues represents the preferred method of establishing a diagnosis. The presence of the virus in the lesion can be inferred by examination of stained cells by light microscopy or by visualizing herpesvirus particles by EM. A firmer diagnosis can be made by demonstrating HSV-specific antigens in cells obtained from the lesions or by isolating the viruses from the lesions.

The diagnosis of the first infection of an individual with either type 1 or 2 virus can be readily established by demonstrating a ≥4-fold rise in antibodies to the viruses in paired sera. The presence of antiviral antibodies of the IgM class in convalescent-phase serum or in cerebrospinal fluid also provides presumptive evidence of a herpetic infection (75, 124, 214). However, among patients who have previously been infected with either type 1 or type 2 virus, a characteristic antibody reponse may not always follow a recurrent infection (47) or an infection with the second type of virus (140, 243). Thus serologic diagnosis of other than the initial primary infection may be difficult (111).

Direct examination

Light microscopy

To detect virus-infected cells by light microscopy, cells are carefully scraped from the base of the lesion. The cells are smeared onto a clear microscope slide, air dried, fixed with methanol, and stained with Wright or Giemsa preparations. Cells actively infected with virus may be identified by a ''ballooning'' cytoplasm and by the fusion of the cells into multinucleated giant forms. Biopsy specimens of skin lesions or of other diseased tissues often show similar changes when stained with hematoxylin and eosin. In addition, Cowdry type A inclusion bodies are sometimes observed in the infected cells (39), but these inclusions are not invariably present (298). The intranuclear type A inclusions are more easily found in deep tissues than in superficial ones, and their presence or absence may be dependent upon the methods of fixing and staining the specimens (135). Identification of virus-infected cells in cervical smears stained according to the Papanicolaou method may detect type 2 infections of women (153, 161, 266). The cellular changes described above are not unique to HSV type 1 or type 2 but may also be induced by other members of the herpesvirus group such as varicella-zoster virus (V-Z). In addition, detecting virus-induced changes by light microscopy has been found to be less sensitive than methods in which viral antigens are detected or in which virus is isolated from lesions.

Electron microscopy

Herpesviruses as the cause of vesicular lesions can be rapidly differentiated from other viruses by electron microscopic examination of vesicle fluid. Vesicle fluid carefully aspirated from the vesicles may be examined directly or placed in 1 or 2 drops of distilled water. A small amount of the sample is placed on a grid and blotted with filter paper. A drop of neutral phosphotungstic acid (3% in distilled water) is added to the grid, which is again blotted. The specimen should then be examined in the electron microscope where typical herpesvirus particles will be seen if the lesions are caused by HSV types 1 or 2 or V-Z. The greatest concentrations of virus particles are in vesicle fluid where up to 3×10^9 particles/ml of fluid may be found (245). Virus particles can also be found by EM examination of thin sections of fixed tissues (91). This technique, however, is time consuming and offers no advantage over other methods of diagnosis in most cases.

Immunofluorescent examination

Demonstrating viral antigens in cells obtained from the lesion is presently the method of choice for direct examination. Where studied, FA has been found to be as sensitive as virus isolation (25, 43, 73, 99, 117, 166, 204, 256, 262, 270, 273, 298). The success of the method requires the collection of specimens which contain sufficient numbers of cells for adequate examination. Cells are carefully scraped from the base of the skin lesions or from the cornea in the case of eye infections. The cells are smeared onto a clean microscope slide, allowed to air dry, and then are fixed for 10 min with cold acetone. After excess acetone has evaporated, the slides are washed with PBS, pH 7.2, and smeared cells are covered with appropriately diluted anti-virus immunoglobulin labeled with fluorescein isothiocyanate (32). The slides are incubated for 30 min at 37 C in a humid atmosphere, and then excess antibody is removed by 3 washes with PBS. A coverslip is mounted over the cells, and the slide is examined using a fluorescence microscope. Multiple yellow or yellow-green fluorescing cells are usually found in postive smears. The test should include slides of cells known to contain viral antigens as well as cells not containing viral antigen for positive- and negative-control purposes. It is possible to store the fixed cells at -20 C without appreciable loss of antigenic activity, thus making it possible to perform the test on batches of accumulated specimens. Unless adsorbed with heterologous virus antigen, most antiserum prepared against either type 1 or type 2 virus will react to antigens of either virus type. The use of unadsorbed antiserum conjugate will not usually differentiate which type of virus has caused the lesion.

Biopsing lesions enhances the probability of obtaining an adequate specimen (166). Four to 6 μ cuts from frozen specimens can be placed on slides, air dried, fixed with acetone, and then stained with conjugated antiserum as described above. Tissues fixed in formalin and sectioned in paraffin maintain some viral antigenicity. These sections can be deparaffinized with xylene and rehydrated with saline prior to staining.

A major diagnostic problem is confronted with patients with suspected herpes meningitis or encephalitis. While virus can be isolated from the spinal fluid in some cases of meningitis, it is not usually possible to isolate the virus from this source in cases of encephalitis. Application of the FA technique to cells sedimented from cerebrospinal fluid specimens or to brain biopsy may prove fruitful (43, 262, 270). It should be noted that other techniques for detecting viral antigens have been successfully applied to brain biopsy specimens. These include the use of immunoperoxidase (21) and a radioimmunoassay (RIA) (60).

Virus isolation and identification of isolates
Isolation in tissue culture

While HSV type 1 and type 2 can be isolated in an number of different laboratory animals as well as embryonated hen's eggs (154, 268), cells grown in tissue culture are considered the method of choice by most diagnostic virologists. As indicated in the section on virus replication, the viruses grow readily in a number of primary and established cell culture systems, and the system selected depends, in part, upon the personal choice and availability of the types of cells. Primary cultures of rabbit kidneys are easily prepared and sensitive but are of little value in isolating viruses other than HSV from human specimens. Cells of human or primate origin have been found useful either as primary cultures or in the form of established cell lines. On the basis of broad usefulness with respect to other viruses, ease of handling and sensitivity to the herpesviruses, human embryonic kidney (HEK) cells and human embryonic lung (HEL) fibroblasts are among the more convenient cells for use in the diagnostic laboratory (94, 143). Of the established cell lines, Vero cells are recommended for isolating type 1 and type 2 virus.

The cells are seeded into appropriate tissue culture tubes, and when the cells form confluent monolayers the medium is drained from 4 tubes. About 0.1 ml of the clinical specimen is inoculated into each of 2 tubes, and the other 2 tubes serve as uninoculated controls. The cultures are incubated for 1 hr at 37 C to allow the virus to adsorb. After adsorption, 1 ml of Eagle medium containing 2% fetal bovine serum and antibiotics is added, and the cultures are again incubated at 37 C. The cultures are then observed daily for CPE. In HEL, HEK, and Vero cells, typical CPE may be detected within 24 hr when vesicular fluid is used as the inoculum. Most isolates produce CPE within 3–4 days, and it is rarely productive to observe the cultures beyond 7 days (89, 94, 95). Passage of lysates of inoculated cultures to new cell monolayers is not usually productive; however, exceptions have been reported. If no CPE has developed by 7 days, the cultures are frozen and thawed 3 times using an alcohol-dry ice bath, and 0.1 ml of the lysates is used as inoculum for new monolayers of cells. The procedure used for the inoculation of cultures with the clinical specimen is repeated.

The time required to produce CPE and the extent of CPE depends upon the amount of virus in the inoculum. Vesicle fluid rich in virus may produce extensive CPE within 24 hr, while throat or vaginal swabs obtained from asymptomatic patients may contain very little virus. With few infectious particles in the inoculum, a rounding of scattered cells is initially observed, and over the next few days there is a rapid increase in the number of cells showing CPE. The infected cells typically round up and take on a refractile appearance. Occasionally, infected cells fuse to produce multinucleated giant cells (polykaryocytes). The CPE may be confined to foci which have an area in the center with no cells and a rim of rounded cells around the clear area. There is an enlargement of the foci with time, and the entire monolayer is eventually destroyed. In other instances, scattered cells with CPE are observed, and the monolayer tends to be destroyed more rapidly and more evenly. The CPE produced by type 1 and type 2 virus is somewhat characteristic in each cell type used, and with experience the nature of the isolate can be suspected by observing the development of the CPE (48, 123, 176, 241). It should be noted that inoculation of high concentrations of V-Z may produce CPE changes quite similar to the advanced CPE produced by HSV type 1 or type 2.

Assays of virus preparation

Preparations of HSV types 1 and 2 may be assayed by determining the dilution that is lethal to adult or suckling mice inoculated intracerebrally or intraperitoneally, respectively (268). The viruses may also be titered by inoculating 0.05 ml of dilutions of the virus preparations onto the chorioallantoic membrane of 12-day-old eggs and then counting the pocks which develop after 48 hr of incubation at 37 C (268). However, these methods are more cumbersome and tend to be less reliable than assays performed in cells grown in tissue culture.

Tissue culture infectious dose 50 (TCID$_{50}$). The TCID$_{50}$ may be determined using cells grown in culture tubes or in microtiter plates. To assay virus in culture tubes, the tubes are seeded with 1×10^5 Vero cells suspended in 1 ml of Eagle medium supplemented with 10% fetal bovine serum. The tubes are incubated in slanted racks at 37 C, and suitable monolayers develop in 2–4 days. Tenfold dilutions, 10^{-1} to 10^{-7}, of the virus preparation are made in Eagle medium containing 2% fetal bovine serum. The medium is drained from the tubes, and each of 4 tubes are inoculated with 0.1 ml of each dilution of the virus; only 10^{-4} to 10^{-7} need be inoculated for most preparations. After adsorption for 1 hr at room temperature, 1 ml of Eagle medium with 2% fetal bovine serum is added to each tube. The tubes are incubated at 37 C and examined for CPE after 5 days of incubation. The TCID$_{50}$ endpoint is calculated from the distribution of cultures showing typical virus CPE.

Assays are carried out in microtiter plates by adding 0.05 ml of each virus dilution to 6 wells of the plate. Vero cells are suspended in Eagle medium containing 10% fetal bovine serum at a concentration of 3×10^5 cells/ml. Each well of the plate receives 0.05 ml of the cell suspension. For control purposes, a row of wells is included which receives 0.05 ml of cells and 0.05

ml of medium instead of virus. The plates are covered and incubated at 37 C in a 5% CO_2 in air atmosphere for 5 days, after which the monolayers in the wells are examined for CPE with the aid of an inverted microscope. An alternative to examining the monolayers microscopically is to stain the monolayers and score them macroscopically. To do this, the plate covers are discarded, and the plates are immersed for 1 min in a solution of 5% formalin in PBS, pH 7.2. The cells are then stained by immersing the plates in a crystal violet solution (1.3 g crystal violet dissolved in 50 ml of 95% ethanol and diluted to 1 liter with 5% formalin in PBS). Wells containing intact monolayers stain blue, while wells in which the virus destroyed the cells do not stain and appear clear. The $TCID_{50}$ of the virus preparation is calculated from the wells scored as CPE positive or absence of staining with crystal violet.

Plaque assays. Quantitation of virus by plaque formation in monolayers of several cell types has been described (109, 187, 209, 214, 282). Agar, agarose, methylcellulose (Methocel), and antiviral antibodies present in human gamma globulin have all been used in the assays to prevent the spread of progeny virus. The agar preparations used for plaque assays of other viruses has an inhibitory effect on plaque formation by HSV type 1 and 2. This inhibition can be overcome by adding protamine to the overlay medium. Agarose is not inhibitory at a concentration of 0.5%.

Confluent monolayers of Vero cells grown in 60- × 15-mm plastic Petri dishes incubated in a 5% CO_2 in air atmosphere provide a suitable substrate. The assay is performed by making 10-fold dilutions of the virus stock in Eagle medium supplemented with 2% fetal bovine serum. The growth medium is aspirated from the cell monolayers, and 0.2 ml of the appropriate virus dilutions is added to the plates; duplicate plates are inoculated for each dilution tested. (The dilutions to be tested can be estimated from the anticipated titer of the stock; i.e., a stock thought to contain about 1×10^6 pfu/ml will yield about 2 plaques at 10^{-5} dilution, 20 plaques at 10^{-4} dilution and 200 plaques at 10^{-3} dilution. This stock would be assayed at 10^{-3}, 10^{-4} and 10^{-5}). After adding the inoculum, the plates are incubated at 37 C for 1 hr in 5% CO_2 in air atmosphere, and then the monolayers are overlaid with 4 ml of an agar overlay. The overlay consists of Eagle MEM containing 1% agar, 5% fetal bovine serum, 40 mg/100 ml protamine sulfate, and antibiotics. The temperature of the agar is adjusted to 43–44 C before being added to the plates which are then placed at room temperature until the agar solidifies. The plates are incubated at 37 C for 3 days, after which the agar overlays are carefully removed and the cells are fixed and stained with ethanol-formalin-acetic acid solution containing 1% crystal violet (20 parts 70% ethanol, 2 parts formalin, and 1 part acetic acid). Excess fixative is removed after about 2 min. The monolayers are then rinsed with tap water, and the plaques are counted. Multiplication of the average numbers of plaques on the duplicate plates by 5 times the reciprocal of the dilution inoculated onto these plates gives the pfu/ml of the original virus preparation.

Alternate methods to the above technique include addition of a second agar overlay containing 1:10,000 dilution of neutral red. The plates with the second overlay are incubated overnight at 37 C, after which they are examined for white areas of virus-infected cells which do not take up the neutral red. Instead of agar, medium supplemented to a final concentration of 1:100 with human gamma globulin may be added to the plates after the adsorption period. The antibodies present in the globulin preparation prevent secondary plaque formation but do not prevent cell-to-cell spread of the virus. The medium is aspirated from the plates after 3 days of incubation, and the monolayers are fixed and stained with 1% crystal violet. Methocel hardens upon warming, and it may also be used as a semisolid overlay instead of agar by adding Methocel to culture medium at a final concentration of 1.5%. The medium is chilled and applied with a chilled pipette. Visualization of the plaques is possible using neutral red or by chilling the plates, removing the Methocel, and staining the monolayers with crystal violet.

Identification of isolates

The clinical lesions produced by HSV type 1 and type 2 are essentially indistinguishable with respect to pathogenesis and histologic features. As a generality, lesions below the waist are usually caused by HSV type 2, while those above the waist are caused by HSV type 1. However, type 1 HSV is sometimes isolated from genital lesions, and type 2 HSV is occasionally isolated from lesions above the waist. The isolates from clinical specimens may be identified simply as HSV, or they may be identified according to type depending upon the particular needs of the clinician. Typing may be accomplished by taking advantage of certain biologic differences of the 2 virus types or by immunologic methods.

Typing by replications in chick embryo (CE) cells. It has been observed that type 2 isolates replicate in CE cells, while the replication of type 1 isolates is abortive (58, 137). This observation has been used to identify isolates using plaque formation (58, 283) or by looking for CPE in CE cells grown in microtiter plates (165, 296). To perform the test in microtiter plates, chick embryo cells are obtained from 9- to 10-day-old chick embryos by trypsinization. Monodispersed Vero cells are also prepared. The stock of the isolate to be typed is diluted in 10-fold steps in MEM to 10^{-5}. Diluted virus (0.05 ml) is delivered to 2 wells per dilution in each of 2 microtiter plates. The wells of 1 plate are then seeded with 0.1 ml of $1.5 + 10^6$ CE cells/ml, and the wells of the other plate are seeded with 0.1 ml of $5 + 10^5$ Vero cells/ml. Control wells containing cells and no virus are included in each plate. The plates are covered with sterile plastic lids and incubated at 37 C in a 5% CO_2 in air atmosphere for 3 days. The plates are then immersed for 1 min in a 5% formalin solution in PBS, pH 7.2, followed by immersion of the plates in a solution of crystal violet (1.3 g of crystal violet dissolved in 50 ml of 95% ethanol and diluted to 1 liter with 5% formalin in PBS). The plates are then washed with tap water, and the wells containing intact monolayers are determined by direct examination. Type 2 isolates are characterized by destruction of monolayers of CE and Vero cells at comparable dilutions of the stock. The destruction of Vero cells at 2 $\log_{10}$ dilutions greater than the destruction of CE cells indicates that the isolate is type 1.

Identification of isolates by immunologic means. A high-titer antiserum to either type 1 or type 2 virus contains sufficient cross-reacting antibody to allow the identification of an isolate of HSV using a variety of immunologic techniques. A neutralization (Nt) test using a known amount of virus and antibody in excess provides a convenient method. A stock of the isolate is assayed as described above and 50–100 $TCID_{50}$ (or about 100 pfu) in 0.5 ml is mixed with 0.5 ml of a 1:16 dilution of the herpesvirus antiserum which has a titer of 1:100 or greater. An equal amount of virus is mixed with a 1:16 dilution of normal rabbit serum. The mixtures are allowed to stand at room temperature for 1 hr, after which they are assayed for surviving virus by plaque assay or by inoculating cell monolayers in culture tubes and observing the cells daily for CPE. A clear difference in the appearance of CPE or number of plaques in cultures inoculated with virus and antiserum when compared to cultures inoculated with virus and normal serum identifies the isolate as one of the HSV. For practical purposes it is often possible to use the virus isolate at a 1:10 dilution of stock instead of performing an initial virus titration; however, spurious negative test can result from the use of unusually high-titer virus stocks.

   Typing by immunologic test. Isolates can be typed by using antiserum at dilutions which react with the homologous virus type but not with the heterologous type or by determining the relative antibody titers of known type 1 and type 2 antisera against the isolate. Alternatively, the antiserum can be made specific by adsorption with antigen of the heterologous virus type.

   A number of immunologic methods have been used to differentiate between type 1 and type 2 viruses. The analysis of kinetics of Nt (216) and endpoint Nt tests (174, 253) have been used, as have FA (64, 89, 128, 158, 273) and solid-phase RIA (60, 175). The inhibition of passive hemagglutination has been shown to be a rapid and effective method for typing isolates (11, 217). In addition, the immunoperoxidase method (20, 110) has been applied to the problem of differentiating between two virus types. Each method has certain advantages, and the method selected depends upon personal preference. Of the described methods, FA has been most widely used and, along with solid-phase RIA, is detailed here. The technical aspects of other methods are described in the literature cited or can be derived from the methods of measuring antibodies as described below.

   Typing by immunofluorescence. The antigens used for FA consist of virus-infected cells which can be grown on coverslips or prepared in standard tissue culture vessels and placed on microscope slides. To prepare antigen by the latter method, monolayers of Vero cells in culture tubes or tissue culture flasks are inoculated with virus. The cultures are incubated at 37 C, and the cells are removed from the surface of the culture vessel by trypsinization when 3+ to 4+ CPE develops. The cells are sedimented from the trypsinizing solution by centrifugation at $200 \times g$ for 10 min, and the cell pellet is resuspended to a concentration of about 1×10^6 cells/ml in PBS supplemented with 2% fetal calf serum. Approximately 0.05 ml of the cell suspensions are spotted on marked areas of microscope slides. The spots are air dried and then fixed for 10 min in cold acetone. After rinsing with PBS, pH 7.2, the slides are ready for immediate use or they may be stored at −20 C and used at a later date.

   Antiserum for typing of isolates can be obtained commercially or prepared as described below. The antiserum may be used as the source of intermediate antibody in the indirect FA assay, or the IgG from the antiserum can be conjugated with fluorescein isothiocyanate (32) and serve as the reagent for direct FA. Antiserum of superior quality is needed for direct FA, and more reagent is required than in the indirect method. Since considerable variability in the degree of cross-reactivity has been observed among antisera, it may be necessary to screen several sera to find the one that most readily distinguishes between the two types of virus.

To determine the reactivity of an unadsorbed serum, 2-fold dilutions from 1:20 to 1:640 are prepared in PBS. One drop of each dilution is placed on a spot on a slide containing type 1 antigen, and 1 drop of each dilution is likewise placed on a spot containing type 2 antigen. The serum dilutions should also be placed on spots of control antigen consisting of uninfected Vero cells treated the same as infected cells. After 30 min of incubation at 37 C in a humid atmosphere, the slides are washed 3 times in PBS, and a drop of fluorescein-conjugated IgG is added to the immunoglobulin of the serum used in the intermediate reaction. The appropriate dilution of the conjugate is determined by preliminary block titrations. The slides are washed 3 times with PBS after a second incubation period of 30 min at 37 C. Coverslips are then mounted over the spots using a glycine buffer and examined in a fluorescence microscope. In the direct reaction, the conjugated anti-HSV IgG is diluted 2-fold, from 1:5 to 1:160 and reacted as described above. The slides are washed and prepared for examination after a single 30-min period. A dilution of serum can usually be found at which intense fluorescence is observed in cells infected with one type of virus, while little or no staining is observed in cells infected with the other virus type. This dilution of reagent can then be used to stain cells infected with unknown isolates. Antiserum prepared against type 1 viruses usually provide a greater differential in reactivity to the two viruses than does antiserum prepared against type 2 virus. Instead of determining serum dilutions that differentiate between virus types, absorbed antiserum can be used, in which case only titrations against known antigens are required to determine the optimum working dilution, after it has been established that cross-reacting heterotypic antibodies have been effectively removed. The technique for absorbing the antiserum is described below.

Unknown isolates are typed by spotting infected cells on microscope slides and fixing the cells as described above. Uninfected cells and slides containing known HSV type 1 and known HSV type 2 antigens are included in the test for control purposes. The antigens are then stained with the appropriate dilution of an antiserum that will distinguish between the types of virus or with cross-adsorbed reagents.

Preparation of type-specific antiserum by adsorption. Monolayers of Vero cells in large culture flasks or roller bottles are infected with approximately 1 $TCID_{50}$ of virus per cell and incubated at 37 C. When 4+ CPE develops (24–48 hr) the cells are scraped into the culture medium with a rubber policeman. The cells are then pelleted by centrifugation at 200 × g for 10 min, and sufficient PBS, pH 7.2, is added to make a 10% cell suspension. The cells are disrupted by 3 cycles of freezing and thawing; this antigen may be used immediately for adsorption or may be stored frozen. Antiserum to HSV type 1 is made monospecific by absorption with type 2 antigen, and type 2 antiserum is made monospecific by absorption with type 1 antigen. To 0.5 ml of the heterologous virus antigen is added 0.5 ml of undiluted antiserum plus 4 ml of PBS to give a 1:10 dilution of the serum. The antigen-antibody mixture is incubated for 1 hr at 37 C and then overnight at 4 C. Complexes of antigen and antibody are removed by centrifugation at 80,000 × g for 1 hr, and the supernatant fluid should contain the type-specific antibody. The type-specific preparation should be tested against viral antigens of the virus type used for adsorption to assure the adequacy of adsorption. A second adsorption with 0.5 ml of antigen may be needed, but care should be taken to keep further dilution of the antiserum to a minimum.

Typing by solid-phase radioimmunoassay. Solid-phase RIA has been found to be applicable for typing virus isolates (60, 175) and for detecting HSV antigens in specimens obtained from lesions (60). Because of the greater sensitivity of this method, it has a distinct advantage in terms of requiring very small amounts of typing serum. This makes it economically possible to utilize serum made monospecific by absorption. The antigen for the assay can be prepared in 1-dram vials (60), or the antigen can be adsorbed onto imitation pearls (246). Sterile 1-dram vials are seeded with about 5×10^4 HEL fibroblasts or Vero cells suspended in 1 ml of MEM containing 10% fetal bovine serum. After 1–2 days of incubation at 37 C, about 1×10^5 infectious units of virus in 0.1 ml are added to the vials which are incubated for an additional 24 hr. The medium is then aspirated, and the monolayers are rinsed with 1 ml of distilled water and immediately fixed for 20 min with acetone. This antigen source can be used immediately or stored frozen at − 70 C (60).

Antigen for adsorption onto imitation pearls is prepared by infecting monolayers of cells grown in culture tubes or in tissue culture flasks. When 3+ to 4+ CPE is evident, the cells are scraped into the growth medium and washed once in PBS. The cells are then resuspended in PBS to a concentration of about 10^6 cells per ml and ruptured by freezing-thawing and/or sonication. The pearls (Grieger of Pasadena, Calif., W773-6), are rinsed twice with distilled water and then placed in the antigen preparation for 1 min at 4 C. Six to 9 pearls are sensitized in the antigen preparation of the unknown (about 100 pearls can be sensitized before exhausting the antigen preparations) (172). The pearls are removed from the antigen preparation with forceps and dipped 6 times in a beaker containing 150 ml of PBS and then dipped 6 times in a second beaker of PBS. The sensitized pearls are ready for immediate use in the RIA.

The antiserum used in this assay is similar to those described for immunofluorescence, and adsorption can be carried out as described above. The antiserum is titrated against known type 1 and type 2 virus antigens to determine the appropriate dilutions to use in the assay for typing unknowns. The test is carried out on antigens in vials by adding 0.2 ml of the typing serum, appropriately diluted in PBS, pH 7.2, to duplicate vials containing the unknown antigens (60). For control purposes, vials containing known HSV type 1 and type 2 antigens, as well as vials containing uninfected cell antigen should be treated similarly. The antibodies are allowed to react with the antigens for 2 hr at 37 C or overnight at 4 C, after which excess antiserum is aspirated, and the vials are washed 3 times with 3 ml of PBS. An immune globulin preparation containing antibodies to the IgG in the typing serum is labeled with ^{125}I by the chloramine T method (141). The ^{125}I-labeled immune globulin in PBS containing 1% bovine serum albumin is added to the vials (the amount added depends upon the labeling conditions and the potency of the anti-IgG serum. For example, labeling with ^{125}I in carrier free form at 500 μCi/mg of protein should yield a reagent that can be added as 4×10^4 counts per minute (cpm) in 0.1 ml). The reaction with the ^{125}I-labeled IgG is allowed to continue for 1–2 hr at room temperature, after which excess reagent is aspirated and the vials are washed 3 times with 3 ml of PBS. The residual cpm of ^{125}I bound to the antigen are assayed in a gamma counter. The mean cpm of duplicate samples of the unknown treated with one of the typing sera should be in clear excess of the cpm in vials containing control cells and should be similar to the cpm of one of the known antigens.

Pearls to which antigens are adsorbed are immersed in 0.5 ml of appropriately diluted typing serum; the serum is diluted in PBS with 1% bovine serum albumin (172). After 1 hr at room temperature or overnight at 4 C, the pearls are removed with forceps and dipped 6 times in 150 ml of PBS and 6 additional times in a second beaker of PBS. Each pearl is then incubated in 1 ml of appropriately diluted ^{125}I-labeled anti-IgG. After 1 hr at room temperature, the pearls are again washed in PBS, placed in an appropriate container, and assayed for radioactivity in a gamma counter. An excess of ^{125}I bound to the pearls containing the unknown antigen and reacted with one of the typing serum should match one of the known antigens reacted with that serum.

Serologic diagnosis

General considerations

Assays for antibodies to HSV type 1 and type 2 may be of value in providing laboratory confirmation of an initial infection by either virus type. The demonstration of a >4-fold rise in antibodies to the virus in paired acute- and convalescent-phase sera indicates an infection by one of the viruses. The antibodies reach peak titers about 4–6 weeks after the initial infection and, while the titers of antibody may decline to undetectable levels, they usually persist at relatively stable levels. An IgM response accompanies the initial virus infection, and IgM antibodies to type 1 and type 2 virus persist for about 8 weeks (124). In an individual with pre-existing antibodies, recurrence or reinfection with the same or different virus type does not produce dramatic changes in antibody titers. Serologic confirmation of recurrence (47) and/or infection with a second type of virus is, therefore, not always easy (190).

Of special consideration is the problem of diagnosing HSV infections of the central nervous system (111). In this regard, analysis of cerebrospinal fluid (CSF) for antibody activity may be beneficial. Antibodies in the CSF may result from serum antibodies crossing the blood-brain barrier at a site of inflammation, or they may be produced locally within the central nervous system (183). Analysis of paired CSF samples obtained during the course of the illness for a rise in antibodies to the virus or detection of high levels of antibodies to the virus in the CSF in relation to serum antibody levels may be of diagnostic value (29, 44, 62, 129, 130, 138, 173). Low levels of antibodies to the virus are present in the CSF of many patients (208), so the detection of antibodies in a single CSF sample is of little diagnostic value.

Serologic assays have also been used in epidemiologic studies to detect past infections with the viruses and to investigate an association between HSV type 2 and squamous cell carcinoma of the cervix. The information available suggests that women with excess antibody activity to HSV type 2 are at greater risk of developing carcinoma of the cervix than are women with lower titers of antibodies to the virus (192). In theory, quantitation of antibodies to HSV type 2 should be useful in identifying women at an increased risk of developing cervical cancer. However, the antibody assay systems used to date have not been sufficiently discriminatory or have been too technically demanding for general use in a diagnostic laboratory.

Techniques available

A wide variety of tests have been used to detect antibodies to HSV type 1 and type 2 antigens. Tests to measure neutralizing antibodies to the viruses include various combinations of constant virus-varying serum concentrations, constant serum-varying virus concentrations, and kinetic analysis of neutralization with assays for surviving virus being carried out in animals, eggs, or cells grown in tissue culture (268). The antibodies involved in neutralization also react with the surface of virus-infected cells, and these antibodies have been assayed by indirect FA using viable cells (244), lysis of infected cells by antibody and complement (140, 243), as well as lysis of the cells by antibody-dependent cellular cytotoxicity (230, 261). In addition to Nt antibodies, antibodies are produced to a number of virus-induced antigens. Antibodies to antigens within fixed cells have been quantitated by indirect FA (33, 89, 124, 127, 130) and by solid-phase radioimmunoassay (62, 171, 172). Soluble antigens prepared from virus-infected cells have been used to measure antibodies by complement fixation (CF) (6, 70, 100), immunodiffusion (217, 269), immunoprecipitation (5, 173), indirect hemagglutination (10, 129, 217), and immune adherence hemagglutination.

The two types of virus share cross-reacting antigens, and an appreciable amount of antibody produced in response to an initial infection is to the shared antigens. Serologic confirmation of an infection with either virus type requires only that a significant rise in antibody titer be demonstrated, which can be done by the CF test (70). Differentiation of an infection as type 1 or type 2 is more difficult and requires the determination of relative antibody activity to the 2 viruses or the detection of virus-specific antibody. The standard CF test does not have the sensitivity needed to differentiate between the antibody responses to type 1 and type 2 viruses, and more sensitive techniques are required.

A degree of antigenic cross-reactivity exists between the two types of HSV and V-Z (116, 202). Patients infected with V-Z who have had past herpetic infections may have a rise in antibody titers to antigens of HSV type 1 and type 2. A similar type of rise in titer to V-Z may occur in patients infected with HSV type 1 or type 2. The heterotypic responses have been observed using FA, Nt, and CF tests (213, 215). Thus, in atypical clinical cases of vesicular eruptions, paired sera should be tested against antigens of both viruses. The antibody titer rise to the infecting virus frequently exceeds the heterologous antibody rise.

Complement-fixation (CF) test. The CF test has become an established technique for detecting a significant rise in antibodies during herpetic infections. The antigen preparations used in diagnostic laboratories contain multiple antigens, but it is seldom necessary to carry the antigen through purification steps. If partial purification of the antigen is desired, it can be performed by column chromatography using calcium phosphate or DEAE-cellulose. The preferential adsorption of the viruses on aluminum and calcium salts may also serve as a method of obtaining a degree of purification of the viruses from the antigens (278). In addition, virus envelope, capsid, and soluble components produced in infected cells have been separated by differential sedimentation and used as antigens in the CF test (139). The evidence available suggests that the partially purified antigens offer no distinct advantage over the standard antigen preparations (10).

Special CF antigens have been used in seroepidemiologic investigations examining the association between HSV type 2 and cervical carcinoma. One such antigen is a soluble antigen called AG-4, and antibodies to this antigen have been reported in the serum of women with active neoplastic lesions of the cervix (6). Another antigen has been prepared by solubilizing proteins from membranes of virus-infected cells using sonication. These proteins were then concentrated and separated from other proteins by gel electrophoresis. The proteins eluted from the center of the gels served as antigens to detect antibodies which were found primarily among patients with squamous cell carcinoma of many sites including the cervix (100).

Special handling of standard CF antigen by adsorption of cross-reacting antigens with rabbit antiserum to heterologous virus has been described for the detection of type-specific antibody. After exhaustive adsorption, the adsorbed antigen was used in a CF test to detect type specific antibodies (236). Since these antigens have not yet received widespread acceptance in diagnostic laboratories, they are not detailed here.

Preparation of antigen. Tissue culture systems have largely replaced eggs and suckling mice brains as a source of CF antigen for routine use (268). To prepare the antigen, monolayers of Vero cells are grown in 150-cm^2 tissue culture flasks. The growth medium is drained from the confluent monolayers, and 1 ml of virus stocks containing about 10^7 infectious units/ml is added to the monolayer. After adsorption for 1 hr at room temperature, 50 ml of maintenance medium is added to each flask, which is then incubated at 37 C. Extensive CPE will develop within 24–48 hr, at which time the cells are scraped into the medium. The cells are then pelleted by centrifuged at $200 \times g$ for 10 min, washed once with PBS, and resuspended in Veronal buffer at a concentration of about 10^8 cells/ml. The cells are then disrupted by 3 cycles of freezing and thawing or by sonication. The preparation is clarified by centrifugation at 1000 rpm for 5 min, and supernatant fluid may be used immediately as antigen or stored frozen. Cells not infected with virus are handled similarly and serve as control antigen.

The test is carried out most economically in microtiter U-plates. A box titration of the antigen is initially carried out against a known antiserum. Dilutions are made in Veronal-buffered saline (VBS) containing 0.1% gelatin. An 0.025-volume of diluent is placed in each well with a calibrated microtiter dropper (Cooke Laboratories). To the first well of each row is added 0.025 ml of antigen, thus producing a 1:2 dilution. Serial 2-fold dilutions are then made using 0.025 microdiluters. The antiserum is heated for 30 min at 56 C and diluted separately from 1:10 to 1:640 in the diluent; then 0.025 ml of each dilution is added to each well of a row. The antigen-antibody mixtures are incubated for 15 min at room temperature, and then 0.05 ml of guinea pig serum diluted to contain 5 hemolytic units per 0.05 ml is added to each well. (It is necessary to measure the complement activity in the stock guinea pig serum prior to setting up the test). The U-plates are then covered and incubated for 15–18 hr at 4 C. The sheep erythrocytes (RBC) to be used as indictors of unfixed complement are washed in VBS until the supernatant fluid is clear, and their concentration is adjusted to 2.5% (v/v packed cells). An equal volume of hemolysin is added to sensitize the cells. (The hemolysin must have been previously titrated to determine the optimal concentration). After 20 min at room temperature 0.025 ml of sensitized RBC is added to each well of the plates. The unfixed complement will lyse the sensitized cells upon incubation of the plates for 1 hr at 37 C. Antigen plus diluent, antiserum plus diluted control, antigen plus antiserum, and a complement titration are included in the test to assure specificity of the reactions and the adequacy of the complement concentration. The degree of hemolysis is recorded on a 0-4 scale with 4 meaning no hemolysis and 0 meaning total hemolysis. The dilution of antigen and antiserum producing 2 or greater degrees of hemolysis is taken as 1 unit. To test an unknown serum, the serum is heat inactivated at 56 C for 30 min and diluted in serial 2-fold steps in the U-plates in 0.025-ml volumes. The antigen is diluted to contain 4 units, and 0.025 ml is added to each well. The test is then completed as described above. The antibody titer is that dilution which produces a 3 + or greater degree of CF.

Neutralization test. Nt antibodies to HSV type 1 and type 2 can be readily detected by mixing virus and serum together in various combinations and then assaying for surviving virus. Both the rate of antibody binding and antibody concentration are measured in kinetic assays. These tests are performed by mixing a known amount of virus with a single dilution of serum and then removing a sample of the reaction mixture at intervals. The virus-antibody reaction in the sample is immediately stopped by dilution, after which surviving virus is assayed (188). Antibody activity is expressed as a K-value which is derived by a formula assuming the neutralization to be a first-order reaction. Quantitation of antibody activity to HSV type 1 or type 2 in the same serum sample has been done by independently testing the two viruses or by using a mixture of the two viruses and then assaying for surviving virus in a system where the two viruses produced morphologically distinct plaques (203). Kinetics of Nt assays are demanding and have limited usefulness in diagnostic laboratories.

Methods involving a constant dose of virus with varying dilutions of serum are most commonly used for antibody quantitation. Serial 2-fold dilutions, 1:8–1:256, of the serum are made, and HSV type 1 or type 2 is added to each serum dilution so that there is approximately 50–100 infectious units of virus per 0.1 ml of reaction mixture. The serum-virus mixtures are held for 1 hr at room temperature or 4 C and then assayed for surviving virus. This is commonly done by the plaque-counting method or by inoculating cells in cultures and observing for CPE (189). Surviving virus may also be assayed by pock formation on the chorioallantoic membrane of eggs or by injecting suckling mice intracerebrally (268). Among these various possible combinations, the microneutralization test has sufficient merits in terms of economy of reagents and ease of performance to be considered the method of choice (174, 189, 253).

The microneutralization test is carried out using microtiter plates which are suitable for tissue culture. The test serum is diluted 1:10–1:640 in Eagle medium containing 2% fetal bovine serum. The virus stocks are diluted in the same medium to a concentration of 5×10^4 infectious units/ml. To 0.45 ml of each serum dilutions is added 0.05 ml of the diluted virus, after which the virus-serum mixtures are mixed well and held for 1 hr at 4 C. The cell substrate, i.e. secondary rabbit kidney cells or Vero cells, are trypsinized from large culture flask and the monodispersed cells are resuspended in Eagle medium containing 10% fetal bovine serum; the cell concentrations are adjusted to about 3×10^5/ml. To each well of the microtiter plate is added 0.05 ml of the cell suspension, and 0.05 ml of each virus-serum mixture is added to 6 wells of the plate. If antibodies to both viruses are assayed, the serum dilutions are divided into 2 sets of 0.45 ml, and to one series is added HSV type 1 while HSV type 2 is added to the other series; under these circumstances the second 6 wells of the row of microtiter plates receive 0.05 ml of the second virus-serum mixture. The plates are covered and incubated at 37 C for 3 days in a humid atmosphere of 5% CO_2 in air. At the end of the incubation period, the monolayers of each well are examined with an inverted microscope, and the degree of CPE is recorded. In each microtiter plate, wells should be included which contain cells plus 0.05 ml of diluent, wells which contain cells plus 0.05 ml of the test serum diluted 1:10, and cells plus 0.05 ml of virus mixed with diluent instead of serum. Destruction of fewer than 50% of the cells by a virus-serum mixture when compared with 100% destruction in the virus control wells is taken as evidence of neutralizing activity, and the serum dilution that shows antibody activity in 50% of the wells, as estimated by the method of Reed and Muench, is recorded as the antibody titer (189). A modification of the microneutralization technique has been described in which the microtiter plates are incubated for 5 days, after which the covers of the plates are discarded and the cells are stained. This is accomplished by immersing the plates for 1 min in a solution of 5% formalin in PBS, pH 7.2, and then immersing the plates in a solution of crystal violet. The plates are then washed with tap water, and the wells containing intact monolayers can be read directly without the use of a microscope (253).

Hemadsorption test. The adsorption of RBC to the surface of cells infected with HSV provides the basis for 2 assays of antiviral antibodies. Cells infected with the viruses develop receptors for the Fc portion of immunoglobulins, and sheep RBC coated with rabbit anti-sheep RBC antibodies adsorb onto the surface of infected cells (279, 280). The Fc receptors appear about 5-6 hours after infection and persist throughout the replicative cycle (285). Pretreatment of infected cells with antiserum to the viruses 2 hr prior to the addition of the antibody-coated RBC will inhibit the hemadsorption. Titers of antiserum which inhibit hemadsorption can be determined by analysis of serial dilutions of the test serum, and the hemadsorption-inhibition titers are similar to those obtained by standard Nt test.

Mixed hemadsorption can also be used to quantitate antibodies on the surface of virus-infected cells (53, 54). In this reaction, antiviral immunoglobulins are reacted with the infected cells, and immunoglobulins of the same species are used to coat RBC. Antibodies against the species of immunoglobulins are then used to bind the coated RBC to the immunoglobulins on the infected cells. The test is performed by seeding cells in 200-ml widemouth milk-dilution bottles. GMK-AH1 cells grown in MEM with 10% calf serum have been shown to be satisfactory (34, 51); however, most cells supporting virus replication should work equally well. When the cell monolayers are confluent, they are inoculated with 10^6 infectious units of virus, and medium No. 199 with 2% calf serum is added after virus adsorption is complete. The medium is removed after 20 hr of incubation at 37 C, and the monolayers are overlaid with 12 ml of 1% Difco agar in Eagle medium with 2% calf serum. Filter paper disks, 5 mm in diameter, are soaked in a 1:10 dilution of the serum to be tested and placed on the agar. The bottles are held at room temperature for 48 hr at which time the agar layer is removed and the indicator RBC are added. The indicator cells are allowed to react for 1 hr, after which unattached RBC are removed and the diameter of the hemadsorption zones are measured. The indicator cells are prepared by mixing 2% sheep RBC with an appropriate dilution of heat-inactivated anti-sheep RBC prepared in a cynomolgus monkey or some other primate. After 1 hr, the RBC are washed in PBS and resuspended in heat-inactivated antihuman IgG which has been appropriately diluted in PBS. An additional incubation for 1 hr followed by removal of unbound antibody by washing provides the indicator RBC (57). A zone diameter of 10 mm or more is considered positive, and the diameter of the zone is linearly related to the logarithm of the antibody concentration (54). All serum samples should be simultaneously tested on uninoculated cell control monolayers. The sensitivity of the mixed hemadsorption test appears to be similar to that of the standard Nt test. The size of the zones of hemadsorption tend to be larger on monolayers of cells infected with the same virus type that caused patients infection than on monolayers infected with the heterologous virus type (34).

Indirect hemagglutination test. Unlike a number of viruses, the herpesviruses do not directly agglutinate RBC. However, the RBC can be sensitized with viral antigens and can then be agglutinated in the presence of antibodies to the viral antigens (221). Indirect hemagglutination of sensitized

RBC has been used to quantitate both cross-reacting (68) and type-specific antibodies (9, 24, 217) to HSV type 1 and type 2.

Antigens for the test are prepared in monolayers of diploid human fetal fibroblasts. Monolayers of cells in large culture flask (150 cm^2) are infected with about 10^6–10^7 infectious units of either HSV type 1 or type 2. After adsorption for 1 hr at room temperature, 40 ml of Eagle medium with 2% fetal bovine serum is added to the cultures, which are incubated at 37 C until 3+ to 4+ CPE develops. The cells are then freed from the surface using a rubber policeman or glass beads and pelleted from the medium by centrifugation at 200 × g for 10 min. The packed cells are resuspended in PBS to give a 10% suspension. The cells are then ruptured by 3 cycles of freezing and thawing or sonication, after which the preparation is clarified by centrifugation at 200 × g for 10 min. The supernatant fluid serves as the antigen source and can be stored at −70 C.

The antigen is bound to RBC treated with tannic acid. Sheep RBC collected in sterile 3.8% sodium acetate or Alsever solution are aged for 1–6 weeks at 4 C. The cells are washed 3 times with phosphate buffer, pH 7.2 (made by mixing 175 ml of 0.15 M NaCl with 9.5 ml of 0.15 M Na$_2$HPO$_4$ and 3.0 ml of 0.15 M NaH$_2$PO$_4$). Attempts are made to aspirate the buffy coat layer during the washing process, and after the third centrifugation, the cells are resuspended to a concentration of 2.5% in PBS, pH 7.2. Tannic acid (reagent grade) is diluted in PBS within 1 hr of use, and the optimal dilution, which should be determined for each fresh batch of cells, is usually between 1:20,000 and 1:160,000. Equal volumes of the tannic acid solution and the 2.5% suspension of RBC are mixed and held at 37 C for 10 min. The cells are then pelleted at 1000 rpm for 10 min and washed once with PBS, pH 7.2. The cells are then resuspended to a 2.5% concentration in a phosphate buffer, pH 6.7 (made by mixing 100 ml of 0.15 M NaCl with 100 ml of a buffer composed of 32.3 ml of 0.15 M Na$_2$HPO$_4$ and 67.7 ml of 0.15 M KH$_2$PO$_4$). The cells should be used when freshly prepared; however, they can be fixed with gluteraldehyde and stored at −60 C (170). The tanned RBC are sensitized by mixing equal volumes of 2.5% tanned cells and virus antigen appropriately diluted in the pH 6.7 PBS. After 30 min incubation at room temperature the cells are centrifuged at 200 × g for 10 min and washed twice with a diluent containing 1% normal rabbit serum, which is free of sheep RBC agglutinins (1 part serum and 99 parts PBS, pH 7.2). The cells are finally diluted to 1% in this diluent. The optimal dilution of antigen to be used for sensitization of the tanned cells is determined in a box titration in which cells sensitized with varying dilutions of the antigen are tested against a known positive antiserum. The optimal antigen dilution is the one which gives the highest antibody titer.

To perform the indirect hemagglutination test, the serum to be tested is diluted 1:8 in the 1% normal rabbit serum diluent (NRSD). In microtiter U-plates, the serum is further 2-fold diluted to 1:4096 in 0.05-ml volumes of NRSD. Each serum is diluted in duplicate, and to each well of 1 dilution series is added 0.025 ml of cells sensitized with HSV type 1 antigen while 0.025 ml of cells sensitized with HSV type 2 antigen is added to the second dilution series. The plates are then sealed with clear tape, mixed well, and allowed to set at room temperature for 2–3 hr. The antibody titer is determined by examining the plates and finding that serum dilution where agglutinated cells produce a thin layer which covers 80% or more of the bottom of the well. Separate endpoints are recorded for cells sensitized with type 1 and with type 2 antigen.

The inhibition of the agglutination by the antigens used to sensitize the cells has been advocated as a means of detecting type-specific antibody (11, 24, 217). This test is performed on serum after the antibody titer has been determined as described above. The serum is diluted to contain 16 units of antibody, i.e., the antibody titer divided by 16. Then 0.05 ml of this serum dilution is placed in the first well of 3 rows of the microtiter plate which will receive HSV type 1 sensitized cells. The first well of 3 rows of a plate which will receive HSV type 2 sensitized cells are also filled with 0.05 ml of diluted test serum. Known positive type 1 and positive type 2 sera appropriately diluted to contain 16 units are included in the test. To one of the wells in each series of 3 is added 0.05 ml of type 1 virus inhibiting antigen; the second well receives 0.05 ml of type 2 virus antigen, and the third well receives 0.05 ml of control cell antigen. The inhibiting antigens can be the same preparations used to sensitize the tanned RBC, and the dilution to be used is predetermined by examining the ability of different dilutions of the antigens to inhibit agglutination by known serum. After mixing the solutions, the plates are incubated for 30 min at room temperature. The remaining wells of each row are then filled with 0.05 ml of NRSD, and contents of the first wells are serially 2-fold diluted with 0.05-ml microdiluters. Cells sensitized with type 1 and with type 2 antigens are then added to the appropriate rows, and the plates are sealed with clear tape. After mixing and incubation at room temperature for 2–3 hr, the plates are examined for agglutination.

Serum containing HSV type 1 specific antibodies show agglutination of type 1 sensitized RBC after treatment with type 2 inhibiting antigen but not after treatment with type 1 inhibiting antigen; both inhibiting antigens abolish the ability of the serum to agglutinate type 2 sensitized RBC. The reverse occurs for serum containing type 2 specific antibodies, i.e., no agglutination of type 1 sensitized RBC after treatment with either inhibiting antigen and agglutination of type 2 sensitized RBC after treatment with type 1 inhibiting antigen. If the inhibiting antigens remove all agglutinating activity to cells sensitized with either antigen, the serum is considered untypable. Some serum contains type-specific antibodies to both virus types in which case treatment with heterologous antigens does not abolish the ability of the serum to agglutinate the sensitized cells; sensitized RBC are agglutinated by serum treated with type 2 inhibiting antigen, and the same serum treated with type 1 inhibiting antigen agglutinates type 2 sensitized RBC. In all cases, treatment with control antigen should not influence the ability of the serum to agglutinate the sensitized cells, and the treatment by the inhibiting antigen is not adequate if the antigen does not inhibit agglutination of RBC sensitized with the same antigen type used for inhibition.

Immune adherence hemagglutination. This test is based upon the agglutination of human type O RBC by antigen, antibody, and complement through a C3 receptor on the RBC. The assay has the simplicity and economy of the CF test but is more sensitive (105). The test is performed by heat inactivating the serum samples and preparing, in duplicate, serial 2-fold dilutions beginning at 1:8 in VBS supplemented with 0.1% bovine serum albumin (BSA). The dilutions are made in microtiter U-plates (Cooke Co.) in volumes of 0.025 ml/well. Each well of one series of dilutions receives 0.025 ml of optimally diluted viral antigen, while the wells in the other series receives 0.025 ml of control antigen diluted similarly. The antigens are diluted in BSA-VBS, and the optimal dilution is predetermined by checkerboard titration of the antigen against a reference antiserum. Plates containing the serum-antigen mixtures are carefully agitated to assure thorough mixing and then incubated overnight at 4 C in a humid chamber. Guinea pig serum is then added as a complement source; the serum is diluted in BSA-VBS to an appropriate dilution predetermined by checkerboard titration of complement against optimal serum-antigen mixtures, and 0.025 ml is added to each well. After mixing, the plates are incubated at 37 C for 40 min, and 0.025 ml of a dithiothreitol (DTT) solution is then added. (This solution is prepared in BSA-VBS containing 40 mM EDTA by adding DTT to a concentration of 3 mg/ml). Finally, 0.025 ml of 1% suspension of human type O Rh$^+$ RBC is added to each well, and after mixing, the plates are left at room temperature for 1–2 hr to allow agglutination pattern to develop. The wells in which 50% or more of the bottom is covered by agglutinated cells is considered positive, and the highest dilution positive for agglutination is taken as the antibody titer.

An important aspect of the test is the source of the RBC since there is considerable variation in the ability of type O Rh$^+$ RBC from different donors to adhere to the antigen-antibody-complement complexes. It is advisable to screen a number of donors to find the most suitable ones and to perform a block titration with known positive reagents with each new batch of RBC. The RBC are collected in Alsever solution and can be stored at 4 C for 1 week. Prior to use, the RBC are washed twice with 40 mM EDTA in BSA-VBS, and the final cell pellet is resuspended to 1% in the same solution. Each test should include, in addition to control antigen, known-positive and -negative sera.

Indirect immunofluorescence. The antibody titers derived by this method are slightly higher than those obtained by Nt test. The technique has been used to assay antibodies to antigens on the surface of viable cells as well as intracellular antigens. Measuring antibodies to intracellular antigens is more practical from the diagnostic point of view since a large supply of antigen can be prepared at one time and stored frozen, while a fresh source of antigen is required each time the assay for antibodies to antigens at the cell surface in carried out.

Suitable cells, such as Vero cells, grown in large tissue culture flasks and infected with HSV type 1 or type 2 serve as antigen. When the 2+ to 3+ CPE has developed, the cells are removed from the surface of the culture vessel mechanically or with trypsinization, and the cells are pelleted by centrifugation at 200 × *g* for 10 min. The cells are resuspended in PBS to about 10^6 cells/ml, and 0.05-ml amounts are placed within etched circles on microscope slides. The slides are air dried, fixed in cold acetone for 10 min, and rinsed in PBS, pH 7.2. The serum is diluted in serial 2-fold steps from 1:10 to 1:640 in PBS, and a drop of each dilution is added to an area of fixed cells. The slides are incubated at 37 C for 30 min in a moist atmosphere, rinsed well with PBS, and then stained with appropriately diluted fluorescein-conjugated antihuman globulin which can be obtained commercially. The stained cells are mounted in buffered-glycerol saline and examined for fluorescence. The titer is taken as the highest serum dilution that produces distinct fluorescence in infected cells when compared with uninfected cells. The titers of antibody to HSV type 1 and type 2 can be determined for a serum sample by simultaneously testing each serum dilution against type 1 infected cells and against type 2 infected cells. As with Nt assays, the relative titers to the two viruses may be indicative of the type of infection experienced in the past (89).

Solid-phase radioimmunoassay. A major advantage of the solid-phase RIA is its high degree of sensitivity (61, 172). Viral antigens are fixed to a solid substrate, and the human immunoglobulins binding to the antigens are quantitated with ^{125}I antihuman IgG. To perform the test, antigens are prepared on solid substrates as described above under the description of typing isolates. Quantitation of antibody requires the testing of 6 serial 0.5 $\log_{10}$ dilutions of the serum beginning at 1:100. The dilutions are made in PBS containing 1% BSA. The test is carried out on antigen fixed in vials (61) by adding 0.2 ml of each serum dilution to vials containing viral antigen or control antigen derived from uninfected cells. After overnight incubation at 4 C, unreacted antibody is aspirated, and the monolayers are washed twice with 3 ml of PBS. About 0.1 ml of ^{125}I-labeled antihuman globulin containing 40,000–50,000 cpm is added to each vial. The vials are then incubated for 1–2 hr at room temperature, washed 3 times with 3 ml of PBS, and counted in a gamma counter. The reciprocal of the highest dilution of serum which yields a significantly greater degree of radioactivity in the vials containing viral antigen than in vials containing control antigen is taken as the antibody titer. Antibodies may also be quantitated by testing the serum dilutions against antigen fixed on imitation pearls (172) instead of using antigen in vials.

Type-specific antibodies can be detected by this technique after adsorbing serum (61, 63). Antigens for adsorption are prepared by growing cells in large tissue culture vessels. When confluent the monolayers are infected with about 0.1 infectious units/per cell, and the cultures are incubated 2–3 days, at which time 3+ to 4+ CPE has developed. The cells are dislodged from the vessel surface and then pelleted from the medium by centrifugation at 200 × g for 10 min. The cell pellets are washed once with PBS, and the resulting cell pellets are stored frozen at −70 C. Cells infected with type 1, with type 2, and uninfected cells are so prepared. To detect type-specific antibody, the serum sample is diluted 1:1000 and divided into 3 samples of 1.2 ml each. To one sample is added 10 μl of type 1 cell pack antigen, to a second sample is added 10 μl of type 2 cell pack antigen, and to the third is added 10 μl of control antigen. The antigen-serum mixtures are incubated for 30 min at 37 C and then overnight at 4 C with constant agitation. The samples are then centrifuged at 80,000 × g for 1 hr, and the supernatant fluids are tested in the RIA as described above against type 1, type 2, and uninfected cell antigens. The adequacy of adsorption is attested to when adsorption by the viral antigens removes all activity when tested against the same virus type. Failure of adsorption to remove binding to the heterologous antigen indicates specific antibody to the virus type against which the adsorbed sample was tested; i.e., if serum adsorbed with type 1 reacts with type 2 antigen, type 2 antibodies are present, etc. The quality of the ^{125}I-labeled anti-human globulin is of importance. Serum of good quality can be obtained commercially (Antibodies Inc., Davis, Calif.).

Assays of cell-mediated immunity

Underlying deficiencies of cell-mediated immunity may give rise to prolonged and/or severe infections with HSV (50, 186). Assessment of cell-mediated immunity to the viruses may thus be of value in evaluating certain patients with herpetic lesions (50). The cutaneous delayed hypersensitivity response to antigen injected intradermally has been used as an *in vivo* test of cell-mediated immunity (3, 108, 207). Several *in vitro* assays which correlated with delayed hypersensitivity have also been used to assess cell-mediated immunity. These include antigen-stimulated blastogenesis of lymphocytes (50, 86, 201, 254, 255, 294), lymphocyte-mediated cytotoxicity (206, 294, 255, 267), the production of macrophage-migration inhibitory factor (72, 294), and antigen stimulation of interferon production (86, 186).

Cutaneous delayed hypersensitivity

Antigens for this test have been prepared from chorioallantoic membranes, amniotic fluid, or allantoic fluid of infected eggs (268). A more convenient method is to prepare the antigens in cultures of primary rabbit kidney cells (3). Monolayers of the cells are infected with the virus and incubated in the presence of serum-free culture medium. After extensive CPE develops, the supernatant fluid is removed and heated at 56 C for 1 hr to destroy virus infectivity. The fluid is then centrifuged for 1 hr at 105,000 × g, and the pellet is resuspended in PBS to one-tenth the original volume (268). Control antigen is prepared similarly from monolayers of uninfected cells which are incubated for 7 days at 37 C in serum-free medium. The antigen is tested to confirm the complete inactivation of the virus, and the antigens are stored frozen. The test is performed by injecting 0.1 ml of the test and control antigens intradermally on the volar surfaces of the forearms. The sites of injection are examined 24–36 hr later, and induction of erythema ≥5 mm at the site of the injection of the test antigen, but not at the site of control antigen injection, indicates past infection and suggests intact cell-mediated immunity to the virus.

In vitro assays

The different *in vitro* assays do not appear to yield identical data. For example, groups of patients with recurrent herpetic infections have been described in which comparatively normal blastogenic responses were found despite decreased lymphocytotoxicity responses (255, 294) and depressed migration inhibitory factor production (294). However, the use of a single assay system is usually adequate for assessing the specific cell-mediated immune reactivity to the viruses. Induction of lymphocyte blastogenesis by viral antigen is technically simple and can be used for this purpose. A second method which may be selected for use in a diagnostic laboratory is the production of interferon by immune mononuclear cells upon exposure to the viral antigens (86, 186).

Antigen for the assays is prepared in monolayers of cells grown in flasks. The growth medium is removed and the cells are infected with about 1 infectious unit per cell, and after adsorption the monolayers are covered with about 40 ml of Eagle medium containing 10% fetal bovine serum. The cultures are incubated at 37 C for 1-2 days, at which time 50-75% of the cells show CPE. The cultures are quickly frozen at −70 C, thawed, and the cellular debris is removed by centrifugation at 1000 rpm for 15 min. The supernatant fluid is then centrifuged at 80,000 × g for 1 hr, and the pellet is resuspended in 10 ml of sterile PBS. After destroying virus infectivity by heating for 1 hr at 56 C, the antigen is dispensed in 1-ml amounts and stored at −70 C. Control antigen is prepared by processing uninfected cell monolayers in a similar manner.

Basically, the test consists of mixing antigen with peripheral blood lymphocytes and then measuring DNA synthesis by assessing the uptake of ^{3}H thymidine into DNA. The assay may be run on blood mononuclear cells partially purified on Ficoll-Hypaque gradients (86) or on whole blood (50). To perform the whole blood assay in microtiter plates, blood is collected in heparin from the patient and diluted 1:10 in medium RPMI 1640 supplemented with antibiotics (penicillin 1000 units/ml and streptomycin 100 μg/ml). One-tenth milliliter of the diluted blood is added to the wells of the microtiter plates. Virus and control antigens are diluted in medium, and 0.1 ml of each dilution is added to triplicate wells. Optimal concentrations of antigen should be determined in a preliminary assay using cells from a person known to have been infected in the past with the virus. Three concentrations of virus are normally used in each assay, i.e., 1:4, 1:16, and 1:64 of stock antigens. To assess the viability of the cells, appropriately diluted phytohemagglutinin (PHA-P, Difco) in 0.1 ml-amounts should be added to 3 wells in a separate plate. The plates are incubated at 37 C in a 5% CO_2 air atmosphere. The plates containing the PHA are incubated 3 days, while the plates containing the viral and control antigens are incubated 6 days.

Blastogenesis is assessed by adding 0.1-0.2 μCi of ^{3}H-thymidine to each well and incubating the plates an additional 5-6 hr. The cells are frozen and thawed, and the contents of the wells are aspirated and placed onto Whatman glass fiber filter papers (GFA-3). The harvesting can be greatly facilitated by using a multiple automatic sample harvester (MASH, Microbiological Associates). After carefully washing unincorporated radioactivity from the filter papers with saline, the filters are dried at 150 C for 2 hr and placed in scintillation vials containing 0.5 ml NCS tissue solubilizer (Nuclear, Chicago) and 10 ml of scintillation fluid. The radioactivity in the vials is quantitated in a scintillation counter and the average cpm of triplicate samples are calculated. The index of virus stimulation is calculated by dividing the cpm for the virus antigen dilution giving maximum incorporation by the cpm for that dilution of control antigen. Stimulation indexes of 1 are normally obtained in patients not previously infected, while values of 1.5 or higher are observed in patients with past infections. The absence of stimulation by viral antigens is meaningful only if a clear stimulation is observed in cultures containing an optimal concentration of PHA.

References

1. ADAMS HG, BENSEN EA, ALEXANDER ER, VONTVER LA, REMINGTON MA, and HOLMES KK: Genital herpetic infection in men and women: clinical course and effect of topical application of adenine arabinoside. J Infect Dis 133:151-159, 1976
2. ALWINE J, STEINHART WL, and HILL CW: Transcription of herpes simplex type 1 DNA in nuclei isolated from infected HEp-2 and KB cells. Virology 60:302-307, 1974
3. Anderson WA and KILBOURNE ED: A herpes simplex skin test. Diagnostic antigen of low protein content from cell culture fluid. J Invest Dermatol 37:25-28, 1961
4. ANDREWES CH and CARMICHAEL EA: A note on the presence of antibodies to herpesvirus in post-encephalitic and other human sera. Lancet 1:857-858, 1930
5. ANZAI T, DREESMAN GR, COURTNEY RJ, ADAM E, RAWLS WE, and BENYISH-MELNICK M: Antibody to herpes simplex virus type 2 induced nonstructural proteins in women with cervical cancer and in control groups. J Natl Cancer Inst 45:1051-1059, 1975
6. AURELIAN L: VIRIONS AND ANTIGENS OF HERPESVIRUS TYPE 2 IN CERVICAL CARCINOMA. CANCER RES 33:1539-1547, 1973
7. AURELIAN L and STRNAD BC: Herpesvirus type 2—related antigens and their relevance to humoral and cell-mediated immunity in patients with cervical cancer. Cancer Res 36:810-820, 1976
8. BABIUK LA and ROUSE BT: Immune interferon production by lymphoid cells: role in the inhibition of herpesviruses. Infect Immun 13:1567-1578, 1976
9. BACK AF and SCHMIDT NJ: Indirect haemagglutinating antibody response to herpesvirus hominis types 1 and 2 in immunized laboratory animals and in natural infections of man. Appl Microbiol 28:392-399, 1974
10. BACK AF and SCHMIDT NJ: Reactivity of envelope, capsid and soluble antigens of herpesvirus hominis type 1 and 2 in the indirect hemagglutination test. Infect Immun 10:102-106, 1974
11. BACK AF and SCHMIDT NJ: Typing herpesvirus hominis antibodies and isolates by inhibition of the indirect hemagglutination reaction. Appl Microbiol 28:400-405, 1974
12. BARINGER JR and SWOVELAND P: Recovery of herpes simplex virus from human trigeminal ganglions. N Engl J Med 288:648-650, 1973
13. BARINGER JR: Recovery of herpes simplex virus from human sacral ganglions. N Engl J Med 291:828-830, 1974
14. BARTOSKI M and ROIZMAN B: RNA synthesis in cells infected with herpes simplex viruses. XIII. Differences in the methylation patterns of viral RNA during the reproductive cycle. J Virol 20:583-588, 1976
15. BASTIAN FO, RABSON AS, LEE CL, and TRALKA TJ: Herpesvirus hominis: isolation from human trigeminal ganglion. Science 178:306-307, 1972
16. BECKER WB: The epidemiology of herpesvirus infection in three racial communities in Capetown. S Afr Med J 40:109-111, 1966
17. BECKER WB, KIPPS A, and MCKENZIE D: Disseminated herpes simplex virus infections. Its pathogenesis based on virological and pathological studies in 33 cases. Am J Dis Child 115:1-8, 1968
18. BECKER Y, DYM H, and SAROV I: Herpes simplex virus DNA. Virology 36:184-192, 1968
19. BELADI I, PUSZTAI R, and BAKAI M: Inhibitory activity in tannic acid and flavonols on the infectivity of herpesvirus hominis and herpesvirus suis. Naturwissenschaften 52:402, 1965
20. BENJAMIN DR: Rapid typing of herpes simplex virus strains using the indirect immunoperoxidase method. Appl Microbiol 28:568-571, 1974
21. BENJAMIN DR, RAY CG: Use of immunoperoxidase on brain tissues for the rapid diagnosis of herpes encephailitis. Am J Clin Pathol 64:472-476, 1975

22. BEN-PORAT T and KAPLAN AS: Phospholipid metabolism of herpesvirus infected and uninfected rabbit kidney cells. Virology 45:252–264, 1971
23. BEN-ZEEV A, ASHER Y, and BECKER Y: Synthesis of herpes simplex virus-specified RNA by an RNA polymerase II in isolated nuclei *in vitro*. Virology 71:302–311, 1976
24. BERNSTEIN MT and STEWART JA: Method for typing antisera to herpesvirus hominis by indirect hemagglutination inhibition. Appl Microbiol 21:680–684, 1971
25. BIEGELEISON JZ. JR, SCOTT LV, and LEWIS V JR: Rapid diagnosis of herpes simplex virus infection with fluorescent antibody. Science 129:640–641, 1959
26. BISHAI FR and LABZOFFSKY NA: Stability of different viruses in a newly developed transport medium. Can J Microbiol 20:75–80, 1974
27. BOLOGNESE RJ, CORSON SL, FUCCILLO DA, TRAUB R, MODER F, and SEVER JL: Herpesvirus hominis type II infections in asymptomatic pregnant women. Obstet Gynecol 48:507–510, 1976
28. BURNET FM and WILLIAMS SW: Herpes simplex: a new point of view. Med J Aust 1:637–642, 1939
29. CARROLL JF and BOOSS J: Cerebrospinal fluid IgG level in herpes simplex encephalitis. J Am Med Assoc 236:2092–2093, 1976
30. CESARIO TC, POLARD JD, WULFF H, CHIN TDY, and WENNER HA: Six years experience with herpes simplex virus in a children's home. Am J Epidemiol 90:416–422, 1969
31. CHANG TW, FIUMARA NJ, and WEINSTEIN L: Genital herpes. Some clinical and laboratory observations. J Am Med Assoc 229:544–545, 1974
32. CHERRY WB: Immunofluorescence techniques *In* Manual of Clinical Microbiology, Lennette EH, Spaulding EH, and Truant JP (eds) Washington, D.C., Am Soc Microbiol, 1974, pp 29–44
33. CHO CT, FENG, KK, BRAHMACUPTA N, and LUI C: Immunofluorescent staining for the measurement of antibodies to herpesvirus hominis. J Infect Dis 132:311–315, 1975
34. CHRISTENSON B and ESPMARK A: Long-term follow-up studies on herpes simplex antibodies in the course of cervical cancer. II. Antibodies to surface antigen of herpes simplex virus infected cells. Int J Cancer 17:318–325, 1976
35. CLANCY R, RAWLS WE, and JAGANNATH S: Appearance of cytotoxic cells within the bronchus following local infection with herpes simplex virus. J Immunol 119:1102–1105, 1977
36. CLEMENTS JB, CONTINI R, and WILKIE J: Analysis of herpesvirus DNA substructure by means of restriction endonucleases. J Gen Virol 30:243–256, 1976
37. COHEN GH, DELEON MP, and NICHOLS C: Isolation of a herpes simplex virus specific antigenic fraction which stimulates the production of neutralizing antibody. J Vriol 10:1021–1030, 1972
38. COLEMAN VR, THYGESON P, DAWSON P, and JAWETZ EL: Isolation of virus from herpetic keratitis. Influence of idoxuridine on isolation rate. Arch Opthal 81:22–24, 1969
39. COWDRY EV: Problem of intranuclear inclusion in virus diseases. Arch Pathol 18:527–542, 1934
40. CRAIG CP and NAHMIAS AJ: Different patterns of neurologic involvement with herpes simplex virus types 1 and 2: isolation of herpes simplex virus type 2 from the buffy coat of two adults with meningitis. J Infect Dis 127:365–372, 1973
41. DARLINGTON RW and MOSS LH: Herpesvirus envelopment. J Virol 2:48–55, 1968
42. DARLINGTON RW and MOSS LH: The envelope of herpesvirus. Prog Med Virol 11:16–45, 1969
43. DAYAN AD and STOKES MI: Rapid diagnosis of encephalitis by immunofluorescent examination of cerebrospinal fluid cells. Lancet 1:177–179, 1973
44. DIEBEL R and SCHRYNER GD: Viral antibody in the cerebrospinal fluid of patients with acute central nervous system infections. J Clin Microbiol 3:397–401, 1976
45. DODD K, JOHNSTON LM, and BUDDINGH GJ: Herpetic stomatitis. J Pediatr 12:95–102, 1938
46. DOEGLAS HM and MOOLHUYSEN TM: Kaposi's varicelliform eruption. Two cases caused by herpesvirus hominis infection complicating Darier's disease. Arch Dermatol 100:592–595, 1969
47. DOUGLAS RG JR and COUCH RB: A prospective study of chronic herpes simplex virus infection and recurrent herpes labialis in humans. J Immunol 104:289–295, 1970

48. DOWDLE WR, NAHMIAS AJ, HARWELL RW and PAULS FP: Association of antigenic type of herpesvirus hominis with site of viral recovery. J Immunol 99:974–980, 1967

49. DUFF R and RAPP F: Properties of hamster embryo fibroblasts transformed *in vitro* after exposure to ultraviolet irradiated herpes simplex virus type 2. J Virol 8:469, 1971

50. EL ARABY II, CHERNESKY MA, RAWLS WE, and DENT PB: Depressed herpes simplex virus induced lymphocyte blastogenesis in individuals with severe recurrent herpes infections. Clin Immunol Immunopathol 9:253–263, 1978

51. EMBEL JA, STEPHENS RG, and MANUEL RR: Prevalence of recurrent herpes labialis and aphthous ulcers among young adults on six continents. Can Med Assoc J 113:627–630, 1975

52. EPSTEIN MA: Observations on the fine structure of mature herpes simplex virus and on the composition of its nucleoid. J Exp Med 115:1–12, 1962

53. ESPMARK JA: Rapid serological typing of herpes simplex virus and titration of herpes simplex antibody by the use of mixed hemadsorption—a mixed antiglobulin reaction applied to virus infected tissue cultures. Arch Gesamte Virusforsch 17:89–97, 1965

54. ESPMARK JA and FAGRAEUS A: Identification of the species of origin of cells by mixed hemadsorption: a mixed antiglobulin reaction applied to monolayer cell cultures. J Immunol 94:530–537, 1965

55. EVANS AS and DICK EC: Acute pharyngitis and tonsillitis in University of Wisconsin students. J Am Med Assoc 190:699–708, 1964

56. EVANS DI and HOLZEL A: Immune deficiency state in a girl with eczema and low serum IgM. Possible female variant of Wiskott-Aldrich syndrome. Arch Dis Childhood 45:527–533, 1970

57. FAGRAEUS A, ESPMARK JA and JONSSON J: Mixed haemadsorption: a mixed antiglobulin reaction applied to antigens on a glass surface. Immunology 9:161–175, 1965

58. FIGUEROA ME and RAWLS WE: Biological markers for differentiation of herpesvirus strains of oral and genital origin. J Gen Virol 4:259–267, 1969

59. FINKELSTEIN RA, ALLEN R, and SULKIN SE: Inhibition of herpes simplex virus by normal serum: Its relationship to the properdin system. J Infect Dis 104:184–192, 1959

60. FORGHANI B, SCHMIDT NJ, and LENNETTE EH: Solid phase radioimmunoassay for identification of herpesvirus hominis types 1 and 2 from clinical materials. Appl Microbiol 28:661–667, 1974

61. FORGHANI B, SCHMIDT NJ, and LENNETTE EH: Solid phase radioimmunoassay for typing herpes simplex viral antibodies in human sera. J Clin Microbiol 2:410–418, 1975

62. FORGHANI B, SCHMIDT NJ, and LENNETTE EH: Sensitivity of a radioimmunoassay method for detection of certain viral antibodies in sera and cerebrospinal fluids. J Clin Microbiol 4:470–478, 1976

63. FORGHANI B, KLASSEN T, and BARINGER JR: Radioimmunoassay of herpes simplex virus antibody: Correlation with ganglionic infection. J Gen Virol 36:371–375, 1977

64. FRASER CE, MELENDEZ LV, and SIMEONE T: Specificity differentiation of herpes simplex virus types 1 and 2 by indirect immunofluorescence. J Infect Dis 130:63–66, 1974

65. FRENKEL N and ROIZMAN B: Ribonucleic acid synthesis in cells infected with herpes simplex viruses: Control of transcription and of RNA abundance. Proc Nat Acad Sci USA 68:2654–2658, 1972

66. FRENKEL N and ROIZMAN B: Separation of the herpesvirus DNA on sedimentation in alkaline gradients. J Virol 10:565–572, 1972

67. FRENKEL N, SILVERSTEIN S, CASSAI ER, and ROIZMAN B: RNA synthesis in cells infected with herpes simplex virus. VII. Control of transcription and of transcript abundancies of unique and common sequences of herpes simplex 1 and 2. J Virol 11:886–892, 1973

68. FUCCILLO DA, MODER FL, CATALANO LW JR, VINCENT MM, and SEVER JL: Herpesvirus hominis types I and II: A specific microindirect hemagglutination test. Proc Soc Exp Biol Med 133:735–739, 1970

69. FURLONG D, SWIFT H, and ROIZMAN B: Arrangement of herpesvirus deosyribonucleic acid in the core. J Virol 10:1071–1074, 1972

70. GAJDUSEK DC, ROBBINS ML, and ROBBINS FC: Diagnosis of herpes simplex infections by the complement-fixation test. J Am Med Assoc 149:235–240, 1952

71. GALLADO E: Primary herpes simplex keratitis: clinical and experimental study. Arch Ophthalmol 30:217–220, 1943

72. GANGE RW, DE BATS A, PARK JR, BRADSTREET CM, and RHODES EL: Cellular immunity and circulating antibody to herpes simplex virus in subjects with recurrent herpes

simplex lesions and controls as measured by the mixed leukocyte migration inhibition test and complement fixation. Br J Dermatol 93:539–544, 1975

73. GARDNER PS, McQUILLIN J, BLACK MM, and RICHARDSON J: Rapid diagnosis of herpesvirus hominis infections in superficial lesions by immunofluorescent antibody technique. Br Med J 4:89–92, 1968

74. GEDER L, SKINNER GRB: Differentiation between type 1 and type 2 strains of herpes simplex virus by an indirect immunofluorescent technique. J Gen Virol 12:179–182, 1971

75. GERNA G, and CHAMBERS RW: Rapid detection of human cytomegalovirus and herpesvirus hominis IgM antibody by the immunoperoxidase technique. Intervirology 8:257–271, 1977

76. GIBSON W and ROIZMAN B: Compartmentalization of spermine and spermidine in herpes simplex virion. Proc Natl Acad Sci USA 68:2818–2821, 1971

77. GIBSON W and ROIZMAN B: Proteins specified by herpes simplex virus. VIII. Characterization and composition of multiple capsid forms of subtypes 1 and 2. J Virol 10:1044–1052, 1972

78. GIBSON W and ROIZMAN B: Proteins specified by herpes simplex virus. X. Staining and radiolabeling properties of B-capsid and virion proteins in polyacrylamide gels. J Virol 13:155–165, 1974

79. GLEZEN WP, FERNOLD GW, and LOHR JB: Acute respiratory disease of University students with special reference to the etiologic role of herpesvirus hominis. Am J Epidemiol 101:111–121, 1975

80. GOODHEART CR, PLUMMER G, and WANER JL: Density differences of DNA of human herpes simplex viruses, types I and II. Virology 35:473–475, 1968

81. GRAFSTROM RH, ALWINE JC, STEINHART WL, HILL CW, and HYMAN RW: The terminal repetition of herpes simplex virus DNA. Virology 67:144–157, 1975

82. GRAHAM BJ, LUDWIG H, BRONSON DL, BENYESH-MELNICK M, and BISWAL N: Physicochemical properties of the DNA of herpesviruses. Biochem Biophys Acta 259:13–23, 1972

83. GRAHAM FL, VELDHUISEN G, and WILKIE NM: Infectious herpesvirus DNA. Nature (London) New Biol 245:265–266, 1973

84. GROUT P and BARBER VE: Cold sores an epidemiological survey. J R Coll Gen Pract 26:428–434, 1976

85. GRUTER W: Experimentelle und klinische untersuchungen uber den sogenannten Herpes corneae. Ber Versamml Dtsch Ophth Ges 42:162–167, 1920

86. HAAHR S, RASMUSSEN L, and MERIGAN TC: Lymphocyte transformation and interferon production in human mononuclear cell microcultures for assay of cellular immunity to herpes simplex virus. Infect Immun 14:47–54, 1976

87. HAMPAR B and MARTOS LM: Immunological relationships In The Herpesviruses, Kaplan AS (ed) New York, Academic Press, 1973, pp 221–259

88. HANNA L, JAWETZ E, and COLEMAN VR: Studies of herpes simplex. VIII. The significance of isolating simplex virus from the eye. Am J Ophthalmol 43:126–131, 1957

89. HANNA L, KESHISHYAN H, JAWETZ F, and COLEMAN VR: Diagnosis of herpesvirus hominis infections in a general hospital laboratory. J Clin Microbiol 1:318–323, 1975

90. HARFORD CG, WELLINGHOFF W, and WEINSTEIN RA: Isolation of herpes simplex virus from the cerebrospinal fluid in viral meningitis. Neurology 25:198–200, 1975

91. HARLAND WA, ADAMS TH, and McSEVENEY D: Herpes simplex particles in acute necrotising encephalitis. Lancet 2:581–582, 1967

92. HAYWARD GS, FRENKEL N, and ROIZMAN B: Anatomy of herpes simplex virus DNA. Strain differences and heterogeneity in the locations of restriction endonuclease cleavage sites. Proc Natl Acad Sci USA 72:1768–1772, 1975

93. HAYWARD GS, JACOB RJ, WADSWORTH SC, and ROIZMAN B: Anatomy of herpes simplex virus DNA: Evidence for four populations of molecules that differ in their relative orientations of their long and short components. Proc Nat Acad Sci USA 72:4243–4247, 1975

94. HERRMANN EC JR: Experiences in laboratory, diagnosis of herpes simplex, varicella-zoster, and vaccinia virus infections in routine medical practice. Mayo Clin Proc 42:744–753, 1967

95. HERRMANN EC JR: Rates of isolation of viruses from a wide spectrum of clinical specimens. Am J Clin Pathol 57:188–194, 1972

96. HEVRON JE JR: Herpes simplex virus type 2 meningitis. Obst Gynecol 49:622-624, 1977
97. HILL TJ and BLYTH WA: An alternative theory of herpes simplex recurrence and a possible role for prostaglandins. Lancet I:397-399, 1976
98. HINTHORN DR, BAKER, LH, ROMIG DA, and LIU C: Recurrent conjugal neuralgia caused by herpesvirus hominis type 2. J Am Med Assoc 236:587-588, 1976
99. HITCHOCK G, RANDELL PL, and WISHART MM: Herpes simplex lesions of the skin diagnosed by the immunofluorescence technique. Med J Aust 2:280-284, 1974
100. HOLLINSHEAD AC, LEE O, CHRETIEN PB, TARPLEY JL, RAWLS WE, and ADAM E: Antibodies to herpesvirus nonvirion antigens in squamous carcinoma. Science 182:713-715, 1973
101. HOLLINHEAD AC, CHRETIEN PB, LEE OB, TARPLEY JL, KERNEY SE, SILVERMAN NA, and ALEXANDER JC: In vivo and in vitro measurements of the relationship of human squamous carcinomas to herpes simplex tumor-associated antigens. Cancer Res 36:821-828, 1976
102. HONESS RW, and ROIZMAN B: Proteins specified by herpes simplex virus. XI. Identification and relative molar rates of synthesis of structural and nonstructural herpes polypeptides in the infected cells. J Virol 12:1347-1365, 1973
103. HONESS RW and ROIZMAN B: Regulation of herpesvirus macromolecular synthesis. I. Cascade regulation of the synthesis of three groups of viral proteins. J Virol 14:8-19, 1974
104. HYMAN RW, OAKES E, and KUDLER L: In vitro repair of the pre-existing nicks and gaps in herpes simplex virus DNA. Virology 76:286-294, 1977
105. ITO M, and TAGAYA I: Immune adherence hemagglutination test as a new sensitive method for titration of animal virus antigens and antibodies. Jpn J Med Sci 19:109-126, 1966
106. IZUMI A and GOLDSCHMIDT H: Herpes simplex infection complicating Darier's disease. Caused by type 1 herpesvirus hominis. Arch Dermatol 102:650-653, 1970
107. JARRATT M and HUBLER WR JR: Herpes genitalis and aseptic meningitis. Arch Dermatol 110:771-772, 1974
108. JAWETZ E, COLEMAN VR, and ALLENDE MF: Studies on herpes simplex virus. II. A soluble antigen of herpes virus possessing skin-reactive properties. J Immunol 67:197-205, 1951
109. JAWETZ E, SCHULTZ R, COLEMAN V, and OKUMOTO M: Studies of herpes simplex XI. The antiviral dynamics of 5-Iodo-2-deoxyuridine in vivo. J Immunol 95:635-642, 1965
110. JEANSSON S: Differentiation between herpes simplex virus types 1 and type 2 strains by immunoelectroosmophoresis. Appl Microbiol 24:96-100, 1972
111. JOHNSON RT, OLSON LC, and BUESCHER EL: Herpes simplex virus infections of the nervous system. Problems in laboratory diagnosis. Arch Neurol 13:260-264, 1968
112. JORDON SW, MCLAREN LC, and CROSBY: Herpetic tracheobronchitis. Cytologic and virologic detection. Arch Intern Med 135:784-788, 1975
113. JOSEY WE, NAHMIAS AJ, NAIB ZM: The epidemiology of type 2 (genital) herpes simplex virus infections. Obstet Gynecol Survey 27:295-302, 1972
114. JUEL-JENSEN BE and MACCALLUM FO: Herpes simplex, varicella and zoster. Clinical manifestations and treatment. JB Lippincott Co, Philadelphia, 1972, pp 1-194
115. KAPLAN AS: Herpes simplex and pseudorabies viruses In Virology Monographs, Springer Verlag, New York, 1969
116. KAPSENBERG JG: Possible antigen relationship between varicella zoster virus and herpes simplex virus. Arch Gesamte Virusforsch 15:67-73, 1964
117. KAUFMAN HE: The diagnosis of corneal herpes simplex infection by fluorescent antibody staining. Arch Ophthamol 64:382-384, 1960
118. KAUFMAN RH, GARDNER HL, RAWLS WE, DIXON RE, and YOUNG RL: Clinical features of herpes genitalis. Cancer Res 33:1446-1451, 1973
119. KELMAN AD, CAPOZZA FE, and KIBRICK S: Differential action of deoxynucleosides on mammalian cell cultures infected with herpes simplex virus types 1 and 2. J Infect Dis 131:452-455, 1975
120. KIEFF ED, BACHENHEIMER SL, and ROIZMAN B: Size, composition, and structure of deoxyribonucleic acid of herpes simplex virus subtypes 1 and 2. J Virol 8:125-132, 1971

121. KIEFF E, HOYER B, BACHENHEIMER SL, and ROIZMAN B: Genetic relatedness of type 1 and type 2 herpes simplex viruses. J Virol 2:738-745, 1972

122. KIT S and DUBBS DR: Enzyme induction by viruses. Monogr Virol, Vol. 2 (Karger Basel) 1969

123. KLEGER B and PRIER JE: Herpes simplex infection of the female genital tract. II. Association of cytopathic effect in cell culture with site of infection. J Infect Dis 120:376-378, 1969

124. KURTZ JB: Specific IgG and IgM antibody responses in herpes simplex virus infections. J Med Microbiol 7:333-341, 1974

125. LANDO D and RYHNER M-L: Pouvoir infectieux due DN d'herpesvirus hominis en culture cellulaire. CR Acad Sci Ser D 269:527-530, 1969

126. LEHNER T, WILTON JM, and SHILLITOE EJ: Immunological basis for latency, recurrences of putative oncogenicity of herpes simplex virus. Lancet 2:60-62, 1975

127. LEINIKKI P: Immunofluorescent assay of herpesvirus type 1 and type 2 antibodies in rabbit and human sera. Arch Gesamte Virusforch 35:349-355, 1971

128. LEINIKKI P: Typing of herpesvirus hominis strains by indirect immunofluorescence and biological markers. Acta Pathol Microbiol Scand Sect B 81:65-69, 1973

129. LERNER AM, LAUTER CB, NOLAN DC, and SHIPPERY MJ: Passive hemagglutinating antibodies in cerebrospinal fluids in herpesvirus hominis encephalitis. Proc Soc Exp Biol Med 140:1460-1466, 1972

130. LEVENTON-KRISS S, RANNON L, and JOFFE R: Fluorescence and neutralizing antibodies to herpes simplex virus in the cerebrospinal fluid of patients with central nervous system disease. Isr J Med Sci 12:553-559, 1976

131. LODMELL DL, NIWA A, HAYASHI K, and NOTKINS AL: Prevention of cell to cell spread of herpes simplex virus by leukocytes. J Exp Med 137:706-720, 1973

132. LODMELL DL and NOTKINS AL: Cellular immunity to herpes simplex virus mediated by interferon. J Exp Med 140:764-778, 1974

133. LOGAN WS, TINDALL JP, and ELSON ML: Chronic cutaneous herpes simplex. Arch Dermatol 103:606-614, 1971

134. LONGSON M: A temperature marker test for the differentation of strains of herpesvirus hominis. Ann Inst Pasteur 120:699-708, 1971

135. LOVE R and WILDY P: Cytochemical studies of the nucleoproteins of HeLa cells infected with herpesvirus. J Cell Biol 17:237-254, 1963

136. LOWENSTEIN A: Aetiologische Unterschungen uber den fieberhaften herpes. Muench Med Wochenschr 66:769-770, 1919

137. LOWRY SP, MELNICK JL, and RAWLS WE: Investigation of plaque formation in chick embryo cells as a biological marker for distinguishing herpes virus type 2 from type 1. J Gen Virol 10:1-9, 1971

138. MACCALLUM FO, CHINN IJ, and GOSTLING JVT: Antibodies to herpes-simplex virus in the cerebrospinal fluid of patients with encephalitis. J Med Microbiol 7:325-331, 1974

139. MARTIN ML, PALMER EL, and KISSLING RE: Complement-fixing antigens of herpes simplex virus types 1 and 2: reactivity of capsid envelope and soluble antigens. Infect Immun 5:248-254, 1972

140. McCLUNG H, SETH P, and RAWLS WE: Relative concentrations in human sera of antibodies to cross-reacting and specific antigens of herpes simplex virus types 1 and 2. Am J Epidemiol 104:192-201, 1976

141. McCONALEY PJ and DIXON FJ: A method of trace iodination of protein for immunologic studies. Int Arch Allergy 29:185-189, 1966

142. McINDOE WA and CHURCHOUSE MJ: Herpes simplex of the lower genital tract in the female. Aust NZ J Obstet Gynecol 12:14-23, 1972

143. McSWIGGAN DA, DAROUGAR S, RAHMAN AF, and GIBSON JA: Comparison of the sensitivity of human embryo kidney cells, HeLa cells, and WI-38 cells for the primary isolation of viruses from the eye. J Clin Pathol 28:410-413, 1975

144. MELNICK JL, COURTNEY RJ, POWELL KL, SCHAFFER PA, BENYISH-MELNICK M, DREESMAN GR, ANZAI T, and ADAM E: Studies on herpes simplex virus and cancer. Cancer Res 36:845-856, 1976

145. MEYERS RL and PETTIT TH: The pathogenesis of corneal inflammation due to herpes simplex virus. I. Corneal hypersensitivity in the rabbit. J Immunol 111:1031-1042, 1973

146. MILLER JD and ROSS CAC: Encephalitis: a four year survey. Lancet I:1121–1126, 1968
147. MIYAMOTO K and MORGAN C: Structure and development of viruses as observed in the electron microscope XI. Entry and uncoating of herpes simplex virus. J Virol 8:910–918, 1971
148. MORGAN C, ROSE HM, and MEDNIS B: Electron microscopy of herpes simplex virus I. Entry. J Virol 2:507–516, 1968
149. MULLER SA, HERRMANN EC JR, and WINKELMANN RK: Herpes simplex infections in hematologic malignancies. Am J Med 52:102–114, 1972
150. MUNYON W, KRAISELBURD E, DAVIS D, and MANN J: Transfer of thymidine kinase to thymidine kinaseless L cells by infection with ultraviolet-irradiated herpes simplex virus. J Virol 7:813–820, 1971
151. NAHMIAS AJ and KIBRICK S: Inhibitory effect of heparin on herpes simplex virus. J Bacteriol 87:1060–1066, 1964
152. NAHMIAS AJ, KIBRICK S, and BERNFELD P: Effect of synthetic and biological polyanions on herpes simplex virus. Proc Soc Exp Biol Med 115:993–996, 1964
153. NAHMIAS AJ, NAIB ZM, JOSEY WE, and CLEPPER AC: Genital herpes simplex infection: Virologic and cytologic studies. Obstet Gynecol 29:395–400, 1967
154. NAHMIAS AJ and DOWDLE WR: Antigenic and biologic differences in herpesvirus hominis. Prog Med Virol 10:110–159, 1968
155. NAHMIAS AJ, DOWDLE WR, NAIB ZM, HIGHSMITH A, HARWELL RW, and JOSEY WE: Relation of pock size on chorioallantoic membrane to antigenic type of herpesvirus hominis. Proc Soc Exp Biol Med 127:1022–1028, 1968
156. NAHMIAS AJ, DOWDLE WR, NAIB ZM, JOSEY WE, McLOVE D, and DOMESCIK G: Genital infection with type 2 herpesvirus hominis. A commonly occurring venereal disease. Br J Vener Dis 45:294–298, 1969
157. NAHMIAS AJ, ALFORD CA, and KORONES SB: Infection of the newborn with herpesvirus hominis. Advan Pediat 17:185–226, 1970
158. NAHMIAS A, DELBUONO I, PIPKIN J, HULTON K, and WICKLIFFE C: Rapid identification and typing of herpes simplex virus types 1 and 2 by a direct immunofluorescence technique. Appl Microbiol 22:455–458, 1971
159. NAHMIAS A, WICKLIFFE C, PIPKIN J, LEIBOVITZ A, and HUTTEN R: Transport media for herpes simplex virus types 1 and 2. Appl Microbiol 22:451–454, 1971
160. NAHMIAS AJ and ROIZMAN B: Infection with herpes simplex viruses 1 and 2. N Eng J Med 289:667–674, 719–725, 781–789, 1973
161. NAIB ZM, NAHMIAS AJ, and JOSEY WE: Cytology and histopathology of cervical herpes simplex infection. Cancer 19:1026–1031, 1966
162. NARAQI S, JACKSON GG, and JONASSON OM: Viremia with herpes simplex type 1 in adults. Four nonfatal cases, one with features of chicken pox. Ann Intern Med 85:165–169, 1976
163. NASH G and FOLEY FD: Herpetic infection of the middle and lower respiratory tract. Am J Clin Path 54:857–863, 1970
164. NASH G and ROSS JJ: Herpetic esophagitis. A common cause of esophageal ulceration. Hum Pathol 5:339–345, 1974
165. NORDLUND JJ, ANDERSON C, HSUNG GD, and TENSER RB: The use of temperature sensitivity and selective cell culture systems for differentiation of herpes simplex virus types 1 and 2 in a clinical laboratory. Proc Soc Exp Biol Med 155:118–123, 1977
166. OLDING-STENKVIST E and GRANDIEN M: Early diagnosis of virus-caused vesicular rashes by immunofluorescence on skin biopsies I. Varicella, zoster and herpes simplex. Scand J Infect Dis 8:27–35, 1976
167. OLSHERSKY V and BECKER Y: Herpes simplex virus structural proteins. Virology 40:948–960, 1970
168. OLSON LC, BUESCHER EL, ARTENSTEIN MS, and PARKMAN PD: Herpesvirus infections of the human central nervous system. N Engl J Med 277:1271–1277, 1967
169. PALMER AE, LONDON WT, NAHMIAS AJ, NAIB ZM, TUNCA J, FUCCILLO DA, ELLENBERG JH, and SEVER JL: A preliminary report on investigation of oncogenic potential of herpes simplex virus type 2 in Cebus monkeys. Cancer Res 36:807–809, 1976
170. PALMER DF, CAVALLERO JJ, HERRMANN K, STEWART JA, and WALLIS KW: A procedural guide to the serodiagnosis of toxoplasmosis rubella, cytomegalic inclusion disease, herpes simplex In Immunology Series, Wallis KW (ed), No. 5 Center for Disease Control, Atlanta, Ga., pp 23–26

171. PARKINSON AJ and KALMAKOFF J: Detection of virus specific immunoglobulins using a doubly labeled fluorescein-^{125}I antibody. J Clin Microbiol 3:637-639, 1976
172. PATTERSON WR and SMITH KO: Improvements of a radioimmunoassay for measurement of viral antibody in human sera. J Clin Microbiol 2:130-133, 1975
173. PAULI G and LUDWIG H: Immunoprecipitation of herpes simplex virus type 1 antigens with different antisera and human cerebrospinal fluids. Arch Virol 53:139-155, 1977
174. PAULS FP and DOWDLE WR: A serologic study of herpesvirus hominis strains by microneutralization tests. J Immunol 98:941-947, 1967
175. PIRAINO FF, SEDMAK G, ALTSHULER C, and PIERCE R: Rapid antigenic typing of herpesvirus hominis isolates on the surface of infected cells by kinetic binding of ^{125}I labeled HV I antibodies. Am J Clin Pathol 62:581-590, 1974
176. PLUMMER G, WANER JL, and BOWLING CP: Comparative studies of type 1 and type 2 herpes simplex viruses. Br J Exp Path 49:202-208, 1968
177. PLUMMER G: Isolation of herpesviruses from trigerminal ganglia of man, monkeys and cats. J Infect Dis 128:345-347, 1973
178. PLUMMER G, GOODHEART CR, MUYAGI M, SKINNER GRB, THOULESS ME, and WILDY P: Herpes simplex viruses: discrimination of types and correlation between different characteristics. Virology 60:206-216, 1974
179. POSTE G: Virus-induced polykaryocytosis and the mechanism of cell fusion. Advanc Virus Res 16:303-356, 1970
180. POLLEY JR: Preparation of non infective soluble antigens with gamma radiation. Can J Microbiol 7:135-139, 1961
181. POWELL KL and COURTNEY R: Polypeptide synthesized in herpes simplex virus type 2 infected HEp-2 cells. Virology 66:217-228, 1975
182. POWELL KL and WATSON DH: Some structural antigens of herpes simplex virus type 1. J Gen Virol 29:167-178, 1975
183. POWELL WF: Radiosensitivity as an index of herpes simplex virus development. Virology 9:1-19, 1959
184. RAGER-ZISMAN B and BLOOM BR: Immunological destruction of herpes simplex virus I infected cells. Nature 251:542-543, 1974
185. RAMSHAW IA: Lysis of herpesvirus infected cells by immune spleen cells. Infect Immun 11:767-769, 1975
186. RAND KH, RASSMUSSEN LE, POLLARD RB, ARVIN A, and MERIGAN TC: Cellular immunity and herpesvirus infections in cardiac-transplant patients. N Engl J Med 296:1372-1377, 1977
187. RAPP F: Variants of herpes simplex virus: Isolation, characterization and factors influencing plaque formation. J Bacteriol 86:985-991, 1963
188. RAWLS WE, TOMPKINS WAF, FIGUEROA ME, and MELNICK JL: Herpesvirus type 2: association with carcinoma of the cervix. Science 161:1255-1256, 1968
189. RAWLS WE, IWAMOTO K, ADAM E, and MELNICK JL: Measurement of antibodies to herpesvirus types 1 and 2 in human sera. J Immunol 104:599-606, 1970
190. RAWLS WE, GARDNER HL, FLANDERS RW, LOWRY SP, KAUFMAN RH, and MELNICK JL: Genital herpes in two social groups. Am J Obstet Gynecol 110:682-689, 1971
191. RAWLS WE and GARDNER HL: Herpes genitalis: venereal aspects. Clinic Obstet Gynecol 15:912-918, 1972
192. RAWLS WE, GARFIELD CH, SETH P, and ADAM E: Serological and epidemiological considerations of the role of herpes simplex virus type 2 in cervical cancer. Cancer Res 36:829-835, 1976
193. ROBERTS-THOMSON PJ, ESIRI MM, YOUNG AC, and MACLENNAN IC: Cerebrospinal fluid immunoglobulin quotents, kappa/lambda ratios, and viral antibody titers in neurological disease. J Clin Pathol 29:1105-1115, 1976
194. ROIZMAN B and ROANE PR JR: A physical difference between two strains of herpes simplex virus apparent on sedimentation in cesium chloride. Virology 15:75-79, 1961
195. ROIZMAN B, BACHENHEIMER AL, WAGNER EK, and SAVAGE T: Synthesis and transport of RNA in herpesvirus infected mammalian cells. Cold Spring Harbor Symp Quant Biol 35:753-771, 1970
196. ROIZMAN B, KELLER JM, SPEAR PG, TERNI M, NAHMIAS AJ, and DOWDLE WR: Variability, structural glycoproteins, and classification of herpes simplex viruses. Nature 227:1253-1254, 1970

197. ROIZMAN B and SPEAR P: Herpesviruses *In* Ultrastructure of Animal Viruses and Bacteriophages: An Atlas. Dalton AJ and Magenan F (eds) Academic Press, New York, 1973, pp 83-107

198. ROIZMAN B and FURLONG D: The replication of herpesviruses *In* Comprehensive Virology Frenkel-Conrat H and Wagner RR (eds) Plenum Press, New York, 1974, pp 229-403

199. ROIZMAN B, SPEAR PG, and KIEFF E: Herpes simplex viruses I and II. A biochemical definition *In* Perspectives in Virology, Pollard M (ed) 8:129, 1974

200. ROSATO FE, ROSATO EF, and PLOTKIN SA: Herpetic paronychia—an occupational hazard of medical personnel. N Engl J Med 283:804-805, 1970

201. ROSENBERG GL, FARBER PA, and NOTKINS AL: *In vitro* stimulation of sensitized lymphocytes by herpes simplex virus and vaccinia virus. Proc Natl Acad Sci USA 69:756-760, 1972

202. ROSS CAC, SUBAK-SHARPE JH, and FERRY P: Antigenic relationship of varicella-zoster and herpes simplex. Lancet 2:708-711, 1965

203. ROYSTON I and AURELIAN L: The association of genital herpesvirus with cervical atypia and carcinoma *in situ*. Am J Epidemiol 91:531-538, 1970

204. RUBIN SJ, WENDE RD, and RAWLS WE: Direct immunofluorescence test for the diagnosis of genital herpesvirus infections. Appl Microbiol 26:373-375, 1973

205. RUCHMAN I, WELSH AL, and DODD K: Kaposi's varicelleform eruption. Isolation of the virus of herpes simplex from the cutaneous lesions of three adults and one infant. Arch Derm Syph 56:846-863, 1947

206. RUSSELL AS, PERCY JS, and KOVITHAVONGS T: Cell-mediated immunity to herpes simplex in humans: lymphocyte cytotoxicity measured by ^{51}Cr release from infected cells. Infect Immun 11:355-359, 1975

207. RUSSELL AS: Cell mediated immunity to herpes simplex in man. Am J Clin Pathol 60:826-830, 1973

208. RUSSELL AS, and SAERTRE A: Antibodies to herpes simplex virus in "normal" cerebrospinal fluid. Lancet 1:64-65, 1976

209. RUSSELL WC: A sensitive and precise plaque assay for herpesvirus. Nature 195:1028-1029, 1962

210. RUSSELL WC, WATSON DH, and WILDY P: Preliminary chemical studies on herpesvirus. Biochem J 87:26-27, 1963

211. ST GEME JW JR, PRINCE JT, BURKE BA, GOOD RA, and KRIVET W: Impaired cellular resistant to herpes-simplex virus in Wiskott-Alrdich syndrome. N Engl J Med 273:229-234, 1965

212. SCHAFFER PA: Genetics of herpesviruses: A review. Second International Symposium on Oncogenesis and Herpesviruses Nuremberg, Fed. Rep. of Germany, 1974, Int. Agency for Res. on Cancer, Lyon, France, 1975, pp 195-217

213. SCHMIDT NJ, LENNETTE EH, and MAGOFFIN RL: Immunological relationship between herpes simplex and varicella-zoster virus demonstrated by complement fixation, neutralization and fluorescent antibody tests. J Gen Virol 4:321-328, 1969

214. SCHMIDT NJ, FOGHANI B, and LENNETTE EH: Type specificity of complement-requiring and immunoglobulin M neutralizing antibody in initial herpes simplex virus infections of humans. Infect Immun 12:728-732, 1975

215. SCHMIDT NJ, DENNIS J, and LENNETTE EH: Complement-fixing reactivity of varicella-zoster virus subunits antigens with sera from homotypic infections and heterotypic herpes simplex virus infections. Infect Immun 15:850-854, 1977

216. SCHNEWEIS KE and BRANDIS H: Typen differenzen beim herpes simplex virus. Zentralbl. Bakteriol Parasitenkol Infektionskr 183:556-558, 1961

217. SCHNEWEIS KE and NAHMIAS AJ: Antigens of herpes simplex virus type 1 and 2—immunodiffusion and inhibition passive hemagglutination studies. Z Immunitaetsforsch 141:471-487, 197

218. SCHULTE-HOLTHAUSEN H and SCHNEWEIS KE: Differentiation of herpes simplex virus serotypes 1 and 2 by DNA-DNA hybridization. Med Microbiol Immunol 161:279-285, 1975

219. SCHWARTZ J and ROIZMAN B: Concerning the egress of herpes simplex virus from infected cells: Electron and light microscope observations. Virology 38:42-49, 1969

220. SCHWARTZ J and ROIZMAN B: Similarities and differences in the development of laboratory strains and freshly isolated strains of herpes simplex virus in HEp-2 cells: electron microscopy. J Virol 4:879–889, 1969

221. SCOTT LV, FELTON FG, and BARNEY JA: Hemagglutination with herpes simplex virus. J Immunol 78:211–213, 1957

222. SCOTT TFM: Epidemiology of herpetic infections. Am J Ophthal 43:134–147, 1957

223. SEIBERBERG S: Zur aetiology der pustulosis vacciniformis acuta. Schweiz Z Allg Path Bakt 4:398–401, 1941

224. SELLING B and KIBRICK S: An outbreak of herpes simplex among wrestlers (herpes gladiatorum). N Engl J Med 270:979–982, 1964

225. SERY TW and FURGIUELE FP: The inactivation of herpes simplex virus by chemical agents. Am J Ophthalmol 51:42–57, 1961

226. SETH P, RAWLS WE, DUFF R, RAPP F, ADAM E, and MELNICK JL: Antigenic differences between isolates of herpesvirus type 2. Intervirology 3:1–14, 1974

227. SHELDRICK P and BERTHELOT N: Inverted repetitious in the chromosome of herpes simplex virus. Cold Spring Harbor Symp Quant Biol 39:667–678, 1974

228. SHERIDAN PJ and HERRMANN EC JR: Intraoral lesions of adults associated with herpes simplex virus. Oral Surg Oral Med Oral Pathol 32:390–397, 1971

229. SHINKAI K and YOSHIDA Y: Different sensitivities of type 1 and type 2 herpes simplex virus to sodium p-chloromercuribenzoate and chlorhexidine gluconate. Proc Soc Exp Biol Med 147:201–204, 1974

230. SHORE SL, NAHMIAS AJ, STARR SE, WOOD PA, and McFARLIN DE: Detection of cell-dependent cytotoxic antibody to cells infected with herpes simplex virus. Nature 251:350–352, 1974

231. SILVERSTEIN S, BACHENHEIMER SL, FRENKEL N, ROIZMAN B: The relationship between post transcriptional adenylaton of herpesviruses RNA and mRNA abundance. Proc Natl Acad Sci USA 70:2101–2104, 1973

232. SILVERSTEIN S, MILLETTE R, JONES PR, and ROIZMAN B: RNA synthesis in cells infected with HSV. XII. Sequence complexity and properties of RNA differing in extent of adenylation. J Virol 18:977–991, 1976

233. SIM C and WATSON DH: The role of type specific and cross reacting structural antigens in the neutralization of herpes simplex virus types 1 and 2. J Gen Virol 19:217–233, 1973

234. SKARE J and SUMMERS WC: Structure and function of herpesvirus genomes. II. EcoRI, XbaI, and Hind III endonuclease cleavage site on herpes simplex virus type 1 DNA. Virolology 76:581–595, 1977

235. SKARE J, SUMMERS WP, and SUMMERS WC: Structure and function of herpesvirus genomes. I. Comparison of five HSV-1 and two HSV-2 strains by cleavage of their DNA with EcoRI restriction endonuclease. J Virol 15:726–732, 1975

236. SKINNER GR, HARTLEY CH, and WHITNEY JE: Detection of type-specific antibody to herpes simplex virus type 1 and 2 in human sera by complement-fixation test. Arch Virol 50:323–333, 1976

237. SKINNER GRB, TAYLOR J, and EDWARDS J: Precipitating antibodies to herpes simplex virus in human sera: prevalence of antibody to common antigen (Band II). Intervirology 4:320–324, 1974

238. SKOLDENBERG B, JEANSSON S, and WOLONTIS S: Herpes simplex virus type 2 and acute aseptic meningitis. Clinical features of cases with isolation of herpes simplex virus from cerebrospinal fluids. Scand J Infect Dis 7:227–232, 1975

239. SLAVIN HB and GAVETT E: Primary herpetic vulvovaginitis. Proc Soc Exp Biol Med 63:343–345, 1946

240. SMITH IW, PENTHERER JF, and MacCALLUM FO: The incidence of herpesvirus hominis antibody in the population. J Hyg 65:395–408, 1967

241. SMITH IW, PEUTHERER JF, and ROBERTSON DHH: Characterization of genital strains of herpesvirus hominis. Br J Vener Dis 49:385–390, 1973

242. SMITH IW, PEUTHERER JF, and ROBERTSON DH: Virological studies in genital herpes. Lancet 2:1089–1090, 1976

243. SMITH JW, ADAM E, MELNICK JL, and RAWLS WE: Use of the ^{51}Cr release test to demonstrate patterns of antibody responses in humans to herpesvirus types 1 and 2. J Immunology 109:554–564, 1972

244. SMITH JW, LOWRY SP, MELNICK JL, and RAWLS WE: Antibodies to surface antigens of herpesvirus type 1 and 2 infected cells among women with cervical cancer and control women. Infect Immun 5:305-310, 1972

245. SMITH KO and MELNICK JL: Recognition and quantitation of herpesvirus particles in human vesicular lesions. Science 137:543-544, 1962

246. SMITH KO, GEHLE WD, and McCRACKEN AW: Radioimmunoassay techniques for detecting naturally occurring viral antibody in human sera. J Immunol Methods 5:337-344, 1974

247. SMITH MG, LENNETTE EH, and REAMES HR: Isolation of the virus of herpes simplex and the demonstration of intranuclear inclusions in a case of acute encephalitis. Am J Pathol 17:55-68, 1941

248. SPEAR PG and ROIZMAN B: Proteins specified by herpes simplex virus. IV. The site of glycosylation and accumulation of viral membrane proteins. Proc Natl Acad Sci USA 66:730-737, 1970

249. SPEAR PG and ROIZMAN B: Proteins specified by herpes simplex virus. V. Purified and structural proteins of the herpesvirion. J Virol 9:143-159, 1972

250. SPRING SB, ROIZMAN B, and SCHWARTZ J: Herpes simplex virus products in productive and abortive infection. II. Electron microscopic and immunologic evidence for failure of virus envelopment as a cause of abortive infection. J Virol 2:384-392, 1968

251. SPRING SB, ROIZMAN B, and SCHWARTZ J: Herpes simplex virus products in productive and abortive infection II. Electron microscopic and immunological evidence for failure of virus envelopment as a cause of abortive infection. J Virol 2:384-392, 1968

252. STALDER H, OXMAN M, DAWSON DM, and LEVIN MJ: Herpes simplex meningitis: isolation of herpes simplex virus type 2 from cerebrospinal fluid. N Engl J Med 289:1296-1298, 1973

253. STADLER H, OXMAN MN, and HERRMANN KL: Herpes simplex virus neutralization: a simplification of the test. J Infect Dis 131:430-432, 1975

254. STARR SE, KARATELA SA, SHORE SL, DUFFEY A, and NAHMIAS AJ: Stimulation of human lymphocytes by herpes simplex virus antigens. Infect Immun 11:109-112, 1975

255. STEELE RW, VINCENT MM, HENSEN SA, FUCCILLO DA, CHAPA IA, and CANALES L: Cellular immune responses to herpes simplex virus type 1 in recurrent herpes labialis: *In vitro* blastogenesis and cytotoxicity to infected cell line. J Infect Dis 131:528-534, 1975

256. STENKVIST EO and BREGE KG: Application of immunofluorescent technique in the cytologic diagnosis of human herpes simplex keratitis. Acta Cytol 19:411-414, 1975

257. STERN H, ELEK SD, MILLER DM, and ANDERSON HF: Herpetic Whitlow, a form of cross-infection in hospitals. Lancet 2:871-874, 1959

258. STEVENS JG and COOK ML: Restriction of herpes simplex virus by macrophages. An analysis of the cell-virus interaction. J Exp Med 133:19-38, 1971

259. STEVENS JG, NEWBURN AB, and COOK ML: Latent herpes simplex virus from trigeminal ganglia of rabbits with recurrent eye infection. Nature (London) New Biol 235:216-217, 1972

260. STEVENS JG and COOK ML: Maintenance of latent herpetic infection: an apparent role for antiviral IgG. J Immunol 113:1685-1693, 1974

261. SUBRAMANIAN T and RAWLS WE: Comparison of antibody-dependent cellular cytotoxicity and complement-dependent antibody lysis of herpes simplex virus-infected cells as methods of detecting antiviral antibody in human sera. J Clin Microbiol 5:551-558, 1977

262. TABER LH, BRASIER F, COUCH RB, GREENBERG SB, JONES D, and KNIGHT V: Diagnosis of herpes simplex virus infection by immunofluorescence. J Clin Microbiol 3:309-312, 1976

263. TEMPLETON AC: Generalized herpes simplex in malnourished children. J Clin Pathol 23:24-30, 1970

264. TERNI M, CARCCIALANZA D, CASSAI E, and KIEFF E: Aseptic meningitis in association with herpes progenitalis. N Engl J Med 285:503-504, 1971

265. TERZIN AL, MASIC MG: Age-specific incidence of neutralization antibodies of herpes simplex virus. J Hyg 77:155-160, 1976

266. THIN RN, ATIA W, PARKER JD, NICOL CS, and CANTI G: Value of papanicolaou—stained smears in the diagnosis of trichomoniasis, candidiasis, and cervical herpes simplex virus infection in women. Br J Vener Dis 51:116-118, 1975

267. THONG YH, VINCENT MM, HENSEN SA, FUCCILLO DA, ROLA-PLESZCZYNSKI M, and BELLANTI JA: Depressed specific cell-mediated immunity to herpes simplex virus type 1 in patients with recurrent herpes labialis. Infect Immun 12:76-80, 1975

268. TOKUMARU T: Herpesviruses, herpesvirus hominis, herpesvirus simiae, herpesvirus suis, *In* Diagnostic Procedures for Viral and Rickettsial Infections Lennette EH and Schmidt NJ (eds) Am Public Health Assoc Inc, New York, 1969, pp 641-700

269. TOKUMARU T: Studies of herpes simplex virus by the gel diffusion technique. II. The characterization of viral and soluble precipitating antigens. J Immunol 95:189-195, 1965

270. TOMLINSON AH, CHINN IJ, and MacCALLUM FO: Immunofluorescence staining for the diagnosis of herpes encephalitis. J Clin Pathol 27:495-499, 1974

271. TRUSAL LR, ANTHONY A, and DOCHERTY JJ: Differential feulgen-deoxyribonucleic acid hydrolysis patterns of herpes simplex virus type 1 and 2 infected cells. J Histochem Cytochem 23:283-288, 1975

272. VAHERI A and PENTTINEN K: Effect of polyphlorogucinol phosphate, an acid polymer, on herpes simplex virus. Ann Med Exp Biol Fenn 40:334-341, 1962

273. VESTERGAARD BF and THYBO H: Rapid diagnosis and typing of herpesvirus hominis by the fluorescent antibody method. Scand J Infect Dis 6:113-116, 1974

274. VESTERGAARD BF, BJERRUM OJ, NORRILD B, and GRAUBALLE PC: Crossed immuno-electrophoretic studies of the solubility and immunogenicity of herpes simplex virus antigens. J Virol 24:82-90, 1977

275. WAGNER EK and ROIZMAN B: RNA synthesis in cells infected with herpes simplex viruses II. Evidence that a class of viral mRNA is derived from a high molecular weight precursor synthesized in the nucleus. Pro Natl Acad Sci USA 64:626-633, 1969

276. WALLIS C, YANG C, and MELNICK JL: Effect of cations on thermal inactivation of vaccinia, herpes simplex and adenoviruses. J Immunol 89:41-46, 1962

277. WALLIS C and MELNICK JL: Photodynamic inactivation of animal viruses: a review. Photochem Photobiol 4:159-170, 1965

278. WALLIS C and MELNICK JL: Concentration of viruses on aluminum and calcium salts. Am J Epidemiol 85:459-468, 1967

279. WATKINS JF: Adsorption of sensitized sheep erythrocytes to HeLa cells infected with herpes simplex virus. Nature 202, 1364-1365, 1964

280. WATKINS JF: The relationship of the herpes simplex haemadsorption phenomenon to the virus growth cycle. Virology 26:746-753, 1965

281. WATSON DH, SHEDDEN WIH, ELLIOT A, TETSUKA T, WILDY P, BOURGAUX-RAMOISY P, and GOLD E: Virus specific antigens in mammalian cells infected with herpes simplex virus. Immunology 11:399-408, 1966

282. WENTWORTH BB and FRENCH L: Plaque assay to herpesvirus hominis on human embryonic fibroblasts. Proc Soc Exp Biol Med 131:588-592, 1969

283. WENTWORTH BB and ZABLOTNEY SL: Efficiency of plating on chick embryo cells and kinetic neutralization of herpesvirus hominis strains. Infect Immun 5:377-382, 1972

284. WENTZ WB, REAGAN JW, and HEGGIE AD: Cervical carcinogenesis with herpes simplex virus, type 2. Obstet Gynecol 46:117-121, 1975

285. WESTMORELAND D and WATKINS JF: The IgG receptor induced by herpes simplex virus; studies using radiolabel IgG. J Gen Virol 24:167-178, 1974

286. WHEELER CE JR and CABANISS WH JR: Epidemic cutaneous herpes simplex in wrestlers (herpes gladiatorum) J Am Med Assoc 194:933-997, 1965

287. WHEELER CE JR and ABELE DC: Eczema herpeticum, primary and recurrent. Arch Dermatol 93:162-173, 1966

288. WHITE DO, SHEW MA, HOWSMAN KG, and ROBERTSON IF: Herpes simplex virus infection of the cornea. Med J Aust 2:59-63, 1968

289. WHITLEY RJ, CHIEN LT, and ALFORD CA JR: Neonatal herpes simplex virus infection. Int Ophthalmol Clin 15:141-149, 1975

290. WILKIE N: The synthesis and substructure of herpesvirus DNA; the distribution of alkali-labile single stranded interruption in HSV-1 DNA. J Gen Virol 21:453-467, 1973

291. WILKIE NM: Physical maps for HSV-1 DNA for restriction endonucleases Hind III, Hpa-I and X bad. J Virol 20:222-233, 1976

292. WILKIE NM, CLEMENTS JB, MacNAB JCM, and SUBAK-SHARPE JH: The structure and biological properties of herpes simplex DNA. Cold Spring Harbor Symp Quant Biol 39:657-666, 1974

293. WILKIE NM and CORTINI R: Sequence arrangement in HSV-1 DNA: identification of terminal fragments in restriction endonucelase digests and evidence of inversions in redundant and unique sequences. J Virol 20:211-221, 1976

294. WILTON JMA, IVANYI L, and LEHNER T: Cell-mediated immunity in herpesvirus hominis infections. Br Med J 1:723-726, 1972

295. WOLONTIS S and JEANSSON S: Correlation of herpes simplex virus types 1 and 2 with clinical features of infection. J Infect Dis 135:28-33, 1977

296. YANG JPS, CHIANG WT, GALE JL, and CHEN NST: A chick embryo cell microtest for typing of herpes virus hominis. Proc Soc Exp Biol Med 148:324-328, 1975

297. YOSHINO K: Infection of one day old fertile hen's eggs with herpes simplex virus. J Immunol 76:301-307, 1956

298. ZARTESNA NS, MURAVIEVA TV, VINOGRADOVA VL, SHUBLADZE AK, MAENSKAYA TM, KASPAROV AA, and RZHECHCTSKAYA OV: Comparative evaluation of methods for laboratory diagnosis of herpetic eye disease. Am J Ophthalmol 75:997-1003, 1973

HERPESVIRUS SIMIAE

Herpesviruses are common among nonhuman primates, and over 21 different herpesviruses have been isolated from different species of monkeys and apes (1, 40). Of the known nonhuman primate herpesviruses, herpesvirus simiae is of special interest since it may infect man and produce a fatal illness. Sabin and Wright, in 1934, isolated the virus from the brain of a patient who died 18 days after being bitten by a monkey, *Macaca mulatta* (53). The virus is a natural parasite of Asian monkeys of the genus *Macaca* (1, 23, 40). Human cases of infection by the virus have been periodically observed since the initial case was reported, and the majority of the cases have been fatal (18). Individuals handling monkeys or working with tissue and cells derived from monkeys are at risk of becoming infected.

Clinical aspects in humans

The virus is usually acquired from a monkey bite or contact with saliva or tissues of monkeys, and symptoms of illness begin 1-3 weeks later. At the site of entry such as the bite wound, an erythematous vesicular lesion may develop. Signs and symptoms related to organ systems other than the nervous system may predominate early in the illness. Acute abdominal pain and diarrhea, vesicular pharyngitis with severe sore throat, urinary retention, and signs and symptoms of pneumonia have all been reported as forms of presentation of illnesses caused by herpesvirus simiae (38). As the illness progresses, signs of ascending myelitis with paralysis of the lower extremities become evident. As the paralysis ascends, cranial nerves may be affected and diplopia is a common symptom. The patient may develop respiratory failure when the brain stem becomes involved, and asphyxia from respiratory paralysis is a common cause of death. The predominance of nervous system symptoms correlates with the extent of damage of the spinal cord and brain stem and the distribution of virus found in specimens collected at post mortem examination. Vesicular skin eruptions may occasionally be found in examination of the patient (25). The illness has been fatal in 85% of the cases reported in the literature, and those who survive the illness have been left with residual neurologic defects (9, 25).

Clinical aspects in rhesus monkeys

The host-virus relationship between herpesvirus simiae and rhesus monkeys appears to be similar to that between herpes simplex virus (HSV) type 1 and humans. The manifestations of infection are usually limited to mucosal and cutaneous lesions without severe systemic or brain and spinal cord involvement. Thus, the disease is recognized by the presence of small vesicles or ulcers on the mucous membranes of the oral cavity or at the mucocutaneous junction of the lips. These lesions evolve in a manner similar to those of herpes simplex lesions, i.e., vesicles to ulcers which crust and heal without scarring in 1–2 weeks. The primary infections are followed by latency of the virus which can be isolated from trigeminal ganglia (8, 64). The lesions may be confined to the oral cavity, but not uncommonly lesions containing cells with typical herpesvirus inclusion bodies are also found elsewhere on the body, and these are thought to be caused by contaminating scratches or bites with virus-containing saliva (34). The virus also infects the eye producing a nonbacterial keratoconjunctivitis, and herpesvirus simiae has been repeatedly isolated from the brains of monkeys (17, 28).

The prevalence of herpesvirus simiae among *M. mulatta* has been found to vary with age and with the conditions in which the monkeys live. Monkeys reared in closed colonies are rarely infected (20), while evidence of infection in monkeys captured from their natural habitat varies with the place of origin of the animals. Evidence of past infection was found to increase from 11.2% at 1 year of age to 33% at 3 years of age and over in a study of 669 monkeys (46). The overall occurrence of infections has been reported to be 4.2% and 16.6% among rhesus monkeys captured in India and China, respectively (46), 35% among *M. irus* captured in the Phillipines and Thailand (21), and 72% among those from Indonesia (67). Antibodies to HSV, that probably represent cross-reacting antibodies induced by herpesvirus simiae, were found among 6% of newly captured bonnet monkeys by Christopher et al and 11.4% of bonnet monkeys held in captivity 1–8 weeks also had antibodies (16). An increase in the occurrence of antibodies has been found among captured monkeys held in closed colonies (27) since 10% of monkeys had antibodies soon after capture but 60–70% of monkeys held in colonies were found to have antibodies (30). Clinical illness was observed in 2.3% of 14,400 monkeys held in a large colony. Infections have been observed among monkeys more often in October and less often in the spring (33).

Pathology in humans (38, 45, 60)

The major changes are found in the central nervous system (CNS), where increased vascular markings can be seen on gross inspection of the spinal cord, cerebellum, pons, and cerebrum. Inflammatory changes are often evident on inspection of the leptomeninges. On microscopic examination, intranuclear inclusions are found in nerve cells of the cord. Foci of degeneration may be found in the white matter of the tracts, and glial reactions are not marked. Marked infiltration of the walls of arteries and veins with perivascular infiltration and extravasation of erythrocytes are seen in some areas. In addition to changes in the CNS, foci of congestion and extravasation of erythrocytes into the alveoli of the lungs may be observed. Evidence of mild interstitial hepatitis may be found upon examining the liver, while the heart may show focal infiltration of mononuclear cells in the myocardium and epicardial fat. Petechial hemorrhages in the epicardium may also be observed.

Pathology in rhesus monkeys

The mucocutaneous lesions of herpesvirus simiae in monkeys are pathologically indistinguishable from those of their counterpart HSV in man (55).

The pathologic features of disease induced by experimental inoculation of herpesvirus simiae into rhesus monkeys have been described (55, 56). Following intracerebral inoculation there is an intense reaction in the meninges, and the reaction extends from the site of inoculation. A fibrous exudate which contains relatively few inflammatory cells characterizes the reaction over tissue showing changes of acute destruction. The meningeal vessels may be involved, and the virus produces necrosis of the adventitia and muscular coat of the vessel walls. A polymorphonuclear infiltration occurs around the diseased vessels and, in areas of lesser involvement, cells with nuclear inclusions may be seen. The brain matter appears to be infected by direct extension of the virus along the sheath of the penetrating vessels, and the extension is to seldom more than the second layer of the cortex. Occasionally, widespread hemorrhagic necrosis, vascular thrombosis, and edema may be observed in the cerebrum. The spaces of Virchow-Robin may be filled with elements of adventitial proliferation, and the nerve cells may degenerate into structureless masses. Intranuclear inclusions in glial cells may be seen.

Intraperitoneal inoculation produces an acute exudative peritonitis. Involvement of blood vessels with thrombus formation appears to be the basic lesion. Multiple organs are involved, and focal necrosis of the liver, spleen, adrenals, kidneys, and ovaries is observed. Severe changes resembling those seen in bacterial pneumonia are observed in the lungs of animals inoculated intraperitoneally or after aerosol exposure. Spontaneous simian giant cell pneumonia (Wartin-Finkeldey type) has been observed with coexistent herpesvirus simiae infection and may represent changes induced by virus infection of the lower respiratory tract (59).

Pathology in rabbits

The virus is more neurotropic in rabbits than in monkeys (55-57). Following intracerebral inoculation there is less vascular necrosis, less meningeal involvement, and a greater degree of destruction of nerve cells in rabbits than in monkeys. In the rabbits, inclusion bodies are found quite extensively in both glial cells and neurons, and the inclusions are particularly numerous in the basal ganglia. When virus is injected at a peripheral site, the lesions are characterized by vascular changes and local necrosis. Unlike monkeys, peripheral inoculation of rabbits leads to CNS involvement, and the virus reaches the CNS by ascending the peripheral nerves. The nerves are found to have slight to moderate infiltration of polymorphonuclear leukocytes in the bundles and some glial proliferation; these forming cells are destroyed by the virus so that there is no persisting hypercellularity. As areas of the nervous system become infected, the neurons go through a stage of intranuclear inclusion formation followed by necrosis. Neuronophagia and cellular infiltration are not associated with the destructive process.

Virus injected intramuscularly produces local necrosis of muscle cells initially, but as the disease progresses there is involvement of nerves and of the walls of blood vessels. Within 2-3 days the virus spreads along the nerve to the spinal cord. Signs of disease become apparent 3-4 days after the virus reaches the spinal cord.

Description and Nature of the Agent

Size and shape

The morphologic characteristics of herpesvirus simiae are essentially the same as those of HSV (51, 52, 58), and the 2 viruses cannot be distinguished by electron microscopic examination. By electron microscopy of sections of virus-infected cells, mature particles were found to have a diameter of about 130-180 nm (51). This size estimate is in agreement with a diameter of 100-150 nm estimated by filtration of virus through Gradocol membranes (19) and the estimate of 125 nm derived from sedimentation characteristics of the virus (54).

In an earlier report, the appearance and development of virus in infected monkey kidney cells were studied by electron microscopic examination of sections. Characteristic virus particles were first noted in the marginated chromatin of the nucleus 10-14 hr after inoculation of the cultures. These particles were from 60-130 nm in diameter, and they were surrounded by a dense membrane. In later stages of infection, there were 100- to 180-nm double-membraned particles in the nucleoplasm, while both types of particles were seen in the cytoplasm of the cell. Some of the cells with nuclear margination had particles attached to or embedded in the cell membrane. Most of the particles associated with the cell membrane were 130-180 nm in diameter (51). Subsequent studies (52, 58) have in general confirmed these findings and have reported that some strains of virus may show particles in crystalline arrays in the nucleus (58). It is also apparent that the mature virus particle acquires the outer membrane from the nuclear membrane during the process of evagination into the cytoplasm (52, 58).

Chemical composition

Very little information is available with respect to the chemical composition of the herpesvirus simiae. It is assumed that its composition is similar to that of other members of the herpesvirus group and the inhibition of growth of herpesvirus simiae in infected rabbit cornea by 5 iodo-2'-deoxyuridine is compatible with the assumed DNA nature of the genome (3).

Resistance

Herpesvirus simiae is more stable than HSV. Virus in brain tissues can be preserved in 15% or 50% glycerol at -20 C. The virus suspended in tissue culture fluid which contains serum is quite stable, and stocks containing over 10^6 $TCID_{50}$ were found not to lose significant infectivity when held at 4 C for 8 weeks. Storage of such a virus preparation at 40 C for 2 weeks resulted in a complete loss of infectivity. It is of interest that stocks frozen at -20 C or at -70 C and thawed once lost 2 logs of infectious virus, but the titer was preserved thereafter for at least 63 days (37). The virus is inactivated at 55–60 C within 30 min, but this period of time was not adequate to completely destroy virus held at 50 C (30).

A number of chemicals and enzymes destroy herpesvirus simiae. Peracetic acid at an 0.02 M solution destroys 7 logs of virus in 5 min at room temperature. A stock solution of 40% is prepared, and a 2% solution of the stock retains viricidal properties for 1 week at room temperature. This solution can be used on glass, plastics, stainless steel, and other surfaces in the laboratory, but the substances cannot be used as a viricidal agent in the tissue culture medium (36). β-propiolactone and lysol have both been found to inactivate the virus.

A 1:16,000 dilution of formaldehyde (0.025 mg/ml) reduced infectivity of virus suspended in tissue culture medium from about 10^7 to undetectable levels in 4 days at 36 C (32). Concentrations of 0.5 mg/ml destroys comparable amounts of virus in 4 hr at 37 C (12). Attempts have been made to use formaldehyde inactivated virus to induce antibodies to the virus. Difficulty was experienced by some investigators in finding a concentration of formaldehyde that would destroy infectivity but not antigenicity (12, 30, 41, 48). However, Hull et al (32) were successful in preparing a noninfectious antigen using 1:400 formalin and exposing the virus for 96 hr at 37 C.

Herpesvirus simiae is inactivated at 37 C by 2×10^{-4} moles/ml solution of aluminum chloride (65). Glyoxal and kethoxal at concentrations of 0.05 mg/ml were found to completely inactivate the virus (12). Virus infectivity is also reduced upon incubation for 1 hr at 37 C at pH 7.0-7.2 with 10 $\mu g/ml$ of trypsin, 5 $\mu g/ml$ of chymotrypsin, 0.5 $\mu g/ml$ of papain, and 50 $\mu g/ml$ of protease. The enzymes and alkaline phosphatase also inactivate the virus when the enzymes are used at concentrations of 10 $\mu g/ml$. As with HSV, the adsorption of herpesvirus simiae onto cells in tissue culture is inhibited by heparin at concentrations of 10 $\mu g/ml$ (5).

The virus is sensitive to ultraviolet light with kinetics of inactivation similar to those of HSV. The sensitivity of the virus to beta irradiation has also been examined using a Van de Graaf electron accelerator (12). Infectivity in a stock containing 10^7 pfu/ml was completely lost when the stock was exposed frozen, -70 C, to 3×10^6 r. Fewer rads were required to inactivate the virus when exposure took place at higher temperatures (4).

Antigenic composition

The antigenic composition of herpesvirus simiae has not been examined in detail. Most of the information available has been derived from studies designed to assess shared antigens with other members of the herpesvirus group. Cross-neutralization has been observed between herpevirus simiae and HSV (11, 32, 61, 66), but not between herpesvirus simiae and pseudorabies virus (47, 66) or between herpesvirus simiae and equine herpes types 1 and 2 and infectious bovine rhinotracheitis virus (47). Antiserum to herpesvirus simiae neutralizes HSV and herpesvirus simiae equally well, while antiserum to HSV neutralizes the heterologous virus at much lower titers than homologous virus. These observations suggest that antigenic determinants are shared on the surface of the viruses.

Cross-reactivity is also observed using complement-fixation tests (26). The antigens in this reaction may be the same as those detected by neutralization; however, additional antigens are probably involved. Using antiserum to HSV, Watson et al (66) identified 3 immunoprecipitin bands in preparations of cells infected with herpesvirus simiae. The bands formed lines of identity by immunodiffusion with antigens derived from HSV-infected cells. Thus, at least 3 antigens of herpesvirus simiae and HSV are shared.

It is not clear whether or not all isolates of herpesvirus simiae are antigenically identical. Evidence for heterogenicity of herpesvirus simiae was presented by Vizoso (63), and Prier and Goulet (31) reported differences between strains of virus with respect to neutralization. They reported that antiserum to the Sabin strain of virus failed to neutralize the 3088 strain, while antiserum to 3088 neutralized both strains of virus. Plummer (47) examined 2 strains (W and S) and found them to be equally cross-neutralized. Clearly, more data are required to resolve this issue.

Pathogenicity in eggs, animals, and tissue culture

Herpesvirus simiae replicates readily in cells grown in tissue culture, and the cell types used for HSV can be used to isolate herpesvirus simiae. The established monkey kidney cell lines LLC-MK$_1$ and LLC-MK$_2$ (31) as well as Vero (64) have been used to propagate the virus. Studies have also been carried out in rat embryo cells (39). Of special interest is the ability of primary rhesus monkey kidney cells to readily support the growth of the virus, since HSV does not grow well in these cells. Growth in these cells can be used for biological differentiation of the 2 viruses.

The cytopathogenic effect (CPE) induced by herpesvirus simiae is very similar to that observed in cells infected by HSV. Cytoplasmic granulation, enlargement, and rounding of the cells are observed initially; these changes are followed by ballooning degeneration and necrosis. In addition, syncytial giant cells are formed by some strains, and this is dependent upon the cell type. A giant-cell response is commonly observed in monkey cells, while a rounding of cells with occasional giant cells is observed in rabbit kidney cells. Two strains were isolated and CPE was examined in monkey kidney cells, KB cells, and in a variety of tissue culture lines (24). One strain produced syncytial giant cells, while the other strain produced the round cell type of CPE. In HeLa cells both strains formed syncytia; however, virus harvested from HeLa cells were found to produce their original type of CPE when passed back to KB cells. These observations are similar to those of HSV and indicate that polykarocytosis depends upon the genetic composition of the virus and a suitable cell type.

The virus can be isolated by intracerebral inoculation of the specimen into suckling mice or hamsters (49, 64). However, mice are less susceptible to infection with this virus than to HSV (53). Adult mice are normally not susceptible, although it has been reported that the virus can be adapted to adult mice (50). The rabbit, monkey, and guinea pig have all been infected by inhalation of virus suspended in an aerosol, and rabbits were found to be the most susceptible in this study (15). Rabbits injected subcutaneously develop a necrotic skin lesion at the site of injection and an ascending paralysis. The skin lesion is different from that induced by HSV, and it has been suggested that the lesions are sufficiently characteristic to distinguish between the 2 viruses (64).

Embryonated hens' eggs are relatively resistant to herpesvirus simiae until the virus has been adapted by several passages. Greatest success has been obtained by inoculating the virus into the amniotic cavity of 11-day-old eggs. The embryos die, but only low titers of virus are removed. Infection of the chorioamniotic membrane produces pocks in 48 hr that are similar in size and morphology to those induced by HSV (2, 10).

Preparation of Immune Serum

Rabbits and guinea pigs

Antiserum can be prepared in these laboratory animals using inactivated virus. Virus stocks prepared in cell cultures are treated with 1:4000 formaldehyde (0.25 mg/ml) for 48 hr at 37 C and stored, without neutralization with bisulfite, at 5 C. Doses of 5 ml of the inactivated virus preparations are given intraperitoneally 3 times a week for 4 weeks, and the animals are bled 1 week after the last infection. Neutralizing titers of about 1:16 have been obtained using this procedure in rabbits (48), while somewhat higher titers were reported when a similar schedule was used in guinea pigs (32). The injection of live virus into animals that had been immunized with inactivated virus has been reported to increase antibody titers (2).

Monkeys

Antiserum with neutralizing titers of better than 1:100 can be obtained by injecting rhesus monkeys with live virus (7, 47). Virus grown in monkey kidney cells is injected intramuscularly either as a single injection or as 3 injections given 4 weeks apart. Serum is collected about 6 weeks after a single injection or 3 weeks after the last of multiple injections.

Horses

Large volumes of high-titer antiserum can be prepared in horses (13). Virus is grown in rabbit kidney cells, and 0.5 ml of live virus is inoculated subcutaneously along with 1 ml of virus intramuscularly. Two weeks after the initial inoculation, a series of booster inoculations are given subcutaneously in the neck in volumes of 5, 50, and 100 ml, respectively, 3 times a week. A total of 2,000 ml was given in the report describing the procedure, and this was equivalent to 2×10^{11} pfu of virus (13). Antiserum with a titer of 1:2048 as determined by neutralization of 500 pfu/ml of virus was obtained by this method. Immune gamma globulin could be prepared from the antiserum since the serum was found to be protective for infected rabbits. The horses did not become ill and did not secrete virus in their saliva (13).

Sheep

Immune serum with neutralizing titers >1:128 and which was usable for immunofluorescence has been prepared in sheep (6). Rabbit kidney cells were grown in tissue culture, infected with virus, and then monodispersed after CPE developed. A 0.05-ml dose of a suspension of the infected cells was given subcutaneously, and 1.0 ml of cells was injected 3 weeks later by the same route. This was followed by injection of 2–10 ml every 2–3 days for several weeks. Further doses of 5–20 ml were given over the next 4–6 months.

Collection and Preparation of Specimens for Laboratory Diagnosis

Precautions

Herpesvirus simiae is potentially hazardous to laboratory workers, and great care should be exercised when handling the virus. Apart from the danger of becoming infected through monkey bites, the virus may enter the body through cuts or minor abrasions of the skin. It has been possible to infect monkeys and rabbits with aerosolized virus, and the potential danger exists of acquiring the virus in the laboratory by a similar means. The material known or thought to contain the virus should be handled in facilities constructed for biohazards. Operations should be carried out in a suitable biohazard hood; the worker should wear gloves, a gown, and eye protectors. Manipulation of virus-containing material should always be carried out by manual pipetting or by using plastic disposable syringes. Material contaminated with the virus should be carefully sealed in plastic bags and autoclaved before discarding. For storage, the virus should be sealed in ampules which should be kept in a separate metal container at $-70°$ C. Laboratory animals infected with the virus should be kept in isolator units and handled with care when specimens are obtained.

While most infections in humans have resulted from direct contact with monkeys (44), the possibility exists that exposure to the virus can occur during the routine handling of monkey kidney tissue cultures. About 0.1% of the kidney tissue cultures derived from 6,152 monkeys were found to contain herpesvirus simiae (46), and Hull et al (29) found 20 strains of herpesvirus simiae among the 960 virus isolates obtained from various monkey tissues.

Wounds from monkey bites should be immediately cleaned by scrubbing with soap and water. A local antiseptic such as iodine should then be applied and, if possible, the person should be passively immunized (35). Passive immunization has been shown to be effective in experimental animals (4, 13); however, its efficacy in humans has not been established. Human gamma globulin preparations have been found to contain reasonable titers of neutralizing antibodies to herpesvirus simiae (62), and this material or monkey immune serum may be used. The wound site should be infiltrated with about 1 ml of the immune globulin, and 5 ml should be inoculated into the muscles of the same limb. A serum sample should be collected prior to injecting the immune globulin, and this sample should be stored for future use in serologic test if the need arises. Testing of the saliva of the monkey for virus and serum for antibodies to the virus can aid in estimating the risk of the person's developing illness.

Sources of material and collection of specimens

The virus has usually been isolated from material obtained post mortem in human cases. Virus in brain tissue can be preserved in 50% glycerol at −20 C if the specimen is to be stored before processing. Antemortem, the virus can be isolated from vesicular lesions which may develop at the site of the bite. Samples from these lesions can be collected by aspirating the fluid from the vesicle with a fine needle and a tuberculin syringe or by collecting material from the lesion with a cotton swab and agitating the swab in 1 ml of a suitable transport medium or culture medium. The handling and shipping of specimens containing herpesvirus simiae are essentially the same as those described above for HSV.

Laboratory Diagnosis

Virus isolation

Tissue culture

The method of choice is to isolate the virus in cells grown in tissue culture. A wide variety of cells have been shown to support replication of the virus, and these include primary and continous rabbit kidney cell lines, HeLa cells, primary human amnion and FL cell line, and primary chick embryo fibroblasts, as well as primary and continous monkey kidney cell lines. The virus rapidly produces CPE in the cells, and the CPE is essentially the same as that produced by HSV. Primary monkey kidney supports the replication of herpesvirus simiae much better than that of HSV, and this fact may aid in distinguishing between the 2 viruses.

Animal host

The virus may also be isolated by injecting specimens intracerebrally into suckling mice or hamsters which will develop a fatal illness. However, rabbits are highly susceptible to the virus regardless of the route of inoculation.

The local lesion of rabbits injected intradermally may appear as a small papule or as an inflamed area of induration 2–3 cm in diameter with a central zone of necrosis. Specimens containing few infectious particles may require an incubation period as long as 10–12 days before the local lesion develops which is in contrast to HSV where a maximal incubation period of 4–5 days is required. With greater concentrations of the virus, the lesion evolves more rapidly, but the central necrosis produced by herpesvirus simiae is not normally found in lesions produced by HSV. After the development of the local lesion, a flaccid paralysis occurs, and the paralysis is sometimes preceded by a sudden extension of the skin lesion. Injection of 0.5 ml of virus-containing specimen into the calf muscle of 1 hind leg leads to a flaccid paralysis of both hind extremities after an incubation period of 6–7 days. Intravenous injection may result in fever after 6–7 days, and the temperature may then drop to subnormal levels. On the eighth day, paralysis of all the extremities develops, and encephalitic signs such as tremors or salivation may accompany the paralysis. Death usually occurs about the tenth day after intravenous inoculation.

The cotton rat has been found to be as susceptible to the virus as the rabbit. Intracerebral or intraperitoneal inoculation of the virus leads to CNS disease with ataxia and prostration after an incubation period of 4–6 days (42).

Identification of the isolate

The virus is identified by neutralization test. A stock of the isolate is assayed in tubes containing monolayers of cells or by plaquing on monolayers of cells grown in flasks or Petri dishes. These assays are performed in essentially the same manner as those described for HSV except that protamine sulfate is not required in the agar overlay medium. The isolate is diluted in culture medium to contain about 500 infectious units of virus in 0.5 ml and mixed with appropriately diluted antiserum to herpesvirus simiae, The mixture is incubated at 37 C for 1 hr, and then assayed for surviving virus. Controls should include tubes receiving preimmune serum and antiserum to HSV. If the virus is herpesvirus simiae, it will be neutralized by antiserum to this virus but not by antiserum to HSV; if the isolate is neutralized well by both antisera it is HSV.

Serologic Diagnosis

It is frequently not possible to isolate virus from patients prior to postmortem examination; thus, serologic diagnosis is the means available to establish an antemortem diagnosis (9). Patients not uncommonly have pre-existing antibodies to HSV; thus, in infected patients a rise in titers to HSV is observed along with the appearance and rise in antibody titers to herpesvirus simiae. Increases in antibody activity are observed 2–3 weeks after the onset of illness and, with time, the ratio of antibody titers to herpesvirus simiae over titers to HSV approach unity. This appears to be true for antibodies measured by virus Nt (9, 25) or by CF (26). It is also possible to make a presumptive diagnosis by quantitating antibody activity to the 2 viruses in serially collected samples of cerebrospinal fluid (9).

Neutralization test

The Nt test is the method of choice for measuring antibodies, and higher titers have been obtained using the plaque-reduction test as compared with neutralization of CPE in monolayers in tube cultures (61, 62). Antibodies have also been quantitated using a microneutralization assay (26). In all instances, the assays are technically performed in the same manner as described for HSV.

A technique has been described whereby the Nt test can be carried out in tubes with minimal exposure of the worker to the dangerous herpesvirus simiae. Monolayers of cells are grown in culture tubes which are incubated in slanted racks. The monolayers form on the side of the tube, and the tubes are marked on the side containing the monolayers. The serum to be tested is appropriately diluted in tissue culture medium, and 0.5 ml of diluted serum is added to tubes from which the spent medium has been removed. Four tubes are used for each serum dilution. Stock virus is then diluted in tissue culture medium to a concentration of about 100–200 infectious units/ 0.5 ml. The tubes containing the diluted serum are placed in a slanted rack with the cell monolayers up, and 0.5 ml of diluted virus is added to each tube. The tubes are then stoppered, and the rack is incubated for 2 hr at 37 C in a slanted position with the serum-virus mixtures on the bottom side of the tube opposite the monolayers. After incubation, the tubes are rotated so that the monolayers are down and covered by the virus-serum mixture. Control tubes containing virus plus 0.5 ml of medium only are included in the test. The tubes are observed for CPE, and the endpoints of neutralization are estimated by comparing the degree of CPE in the tubes containing the different dilutions of test serum with the CPE in control tubes.

Complement-fixation test

Antigen for CF is prepared in monolayers of primary rabbit kidney cells grown in 32-oz culture flasks. The cells are infected with the virus and incubated approximately 48 hr, at which time 2+ to 3+ CPE is evident. The medium is carefully removed, and the monolayers are washed once with 10 ml of saline buffered at pH 9 with 0.05 glycine-NaOH. The cells are then scraped into 10 ml of this buffer and ruptured by freeze-thawing or sonication. The material is then centrifuged at $200 \times g$ to remove all debris, and the supernatant fluid which contains the antigen is dispensed and stored frozen. Control antigen is prepared by treating uninfected cells in a similar manner. The CF test is carried out in the usual fashion. Antibodies detected by CF are not specific for herpesvirus simiae since they cross-react with HSV antigens (26).

Cross-reactions between herpesvirus simiae and HSV

The cross-reactions observed between these two viruses in Nt tests deserves comment since they have practical implications. Antiserum to herpesvirus simiae neutralizes HSV at titers equal to or greater than the Nt titers for the homologous virus (22, 26, 47). This observation has been utilized in examining monkey serum for past infections with herpesvirus simiae by using the less dangerous HSV as antigen in the Nt test. The reverse relationship is less marked in that herpesvirus simiae is neutralized poorly by antibodies to HSV. However, heterotypic reactions to herpesvirus simiae are seen in human serum (14, 26, 62) which must be taken into account when attempting to diagnose cases of herpesvirus simiae in humans by serologic means. The heterotypic response is seen primarily in serum with high titers of antibodies to HSV. In a study by Cabasso et al (14) the heterotypic response to herpesvirus simiae was found to increase with age irrespective of chances of exposure to herpesvirus simiae. The ratio of mean titers to HSV and herpesvirus simiae was 0 to 0, 1:22 to 0, 1:48 to 1:7, 1:88 to 1:24, respectively, for the various age groups of serum studied. Antibodies to HSV in high titers do not seem to be of value in preventing a fatal infection by herpesvirus simiae in humans (43).

References

1. BARAHONA H, MELENDEZ LV, and MELNICK JL: A compendium of herpesviruses isolated from non-human primates. Intervirology 3:175-192, 1974
2. BENDA R: Active immunization against infection caused by B virus (herpesvirus simiae). 2. Dynamics of neutralizing antibodies in rabbits immunized with inactivated vaccine and challenged with live virus. Attempts to obtain highly active antiserum against B virus. J Hyg Epidemiol Microbiol Immunol 9:487-499, 1965
3. BENDA R: Attempt at inhibiting B virus (herpesvirus simiae) growth in rabbits by 5-iodo-2'-deoxyuridine. Acta Virol 9:556, 1965
4. BENDA R: Active immunization against infection caused by B virus (herpesvirus simiae). 3. Immunoprophylaxis of inhalation infection in rabbits. J Hyg Epidemiol Microbiol Immunol 10:105-108, 1966
5. BENDA R: Effect of heparin on B virus multiplication in vitro. Acta Virol 10:376, 1966
6. BENDA R, PROCHAZKA O, CĚRNA L, REHN F, DUBANSKA H, and HRONOVSKY V: Demonstration of B virus (herpesvirus simiae) by the direct fluorescent antibody technique. Acta Virol 10:149-154, 1966
7. BLACK FL and MELNICK JL: Microepidemiology of poliomyelitis and herpes B infections. Spread of the virus within tissue culture. J Immunol 74:236-242, 1955
8. BOULTER EA: The isolation of monkey B virus (Herpesvirus Simiae) from the trigeminal ganglia of a healthy seropositive rhesus monkey. J Biol Stand 3:279-280, 1975
9. BRYAN BL, ESPANA CD, EMMONS RW, VIJAYAN N, and HOEPRICH PD: Recovery from encephalomyelitis caused by herpesvirus simiae. Report of a case. Arch Intern Med 135:868-870, 1975
10. BURNET FM, LUSH D, and JACKSON AV: The propagation of herpes B and pseudorabies viruses on the chorioallantois. Aust J Exp Biol Med Sci 17:35-40, 1939
11. BURNET FM, LUSH D, and JACKSON AV: The relationship of herpes and B viruses; immunological and epidemiological considerations. Aust J Exp Biol Med Sci 17:41-51, 1939
12. BUTHALA DA: Studies on herpesvirus simiae (B virus): inactivation and attempts at vaccine production. J Infect Dis 111:95-100, 1962
13. BUTHALA DA: Hyperimmunized horse anti-B virus globulin: preparation and effectiveness. J Infect Dis 111:101-106, 1962
14. CABASSO VS, CHAPPELL WA, AVAMPATO JE, and BITTLE JL: Correlation of B virus and herpes simplex virus antibodies in human sera. J Lab Clin Med 70:170-178, 1967

15. CHAPPELL WA: Animal infectivity of aerosols of monkey B virus. Ann NY Acad Sci 83:931-934, 1960
16. CHRISTOPHER S, JOHN TJ, and FELDMAN RH: Virus infections of bonnet monkeys. Am J Epidemiol 94:608-611, 1971
17. DANIEL MD, GARCIA FG, MELENDEZ LV, HUNT RD, O'CONNOR J, and SILVIA D: Multiple herpesvirus simiae isolation from a rhesus monkey which died of cerebral infarction. Lab Anim Sci 25:303-308, 1975
18. DAVIDSON WL and HUMMELER K: B virus infection in man. Ann NY Acad Sci 85:970-979, 1960
19. DEROBERTIS E: An electronmicroscope analysis of nerves infected with the B virus. J Exp Med 90:291-296, 1949
20. DIGIACOMO RF, and SHAH KV: Virtual absence of infection with herpesvirus simiae in colony reared rhesus monkeys (Macaca malatta) with a literature review on antibody prevalence in natural and laboratory rhesus populations. Lab Anim Sci 22:61-67, 1972
21. ENDO M, KAMIMURA T, KUSANO N, KAWAI K, et al: Etude du virus B au Japon. II. Le premier isolement du virus B au Japon. Jpn J Exp Med 30:385-392, 1960
22. ENDO M, KAMIMURA T, AOYAMA Y, HAYASHIDA T, et al: Elude du virus Ba au Japon. I. Recherche des anticorps neutralisant le virus B chez les singes d'origine japonaise et les singes strangers importes au Japon. Jpn J Exp Med 30:227-233, 1960
23. ESPANA C: Herpesvirus simiae infection in Macaca radiata. Am J Phys Anthropol 38:447-454, 1973
24. FALKE D: Isolation of two variants with different cytopathic properties from a strain of herpes B virus. Virology 14:492-495, 1961
25. FURER J, BAZELY P, and BRAUDE AI: Herpes B virus encephalomyelitis presenting as ophthalmic zoster. A possible latent infection reactivated. Ann Intern Med 79:225-228, 1973
26. GARY GW JR and PALMER EL: Comparative complement fixation and serum neutralization antibody titers to herpes simplex virus type 1 and herpesvirus simiae in Macaca mulatta and humans. J Clin Microbiol 5:465-470, 1977
27. GRALLA EJ, CIECURA SJ, and DELAHUINT CS: Extended B virus antibody determination in a closed monkey colony. Lab Anim Care 16:510-514, 1966
28. HARTLEY EG: "B" virus-herpesvirus simiae. Lancet 1:87, 1966
29. HULL RN, MINNER JR, and MASCOLI CC: New virus agents recovered from tissue cultures of monkey kidney cells. III. Recovery of additional agents both from cultures of monkey tissues and directly from tissues and excreta. Am J Hyg 68:31-44, 1958
30. HULL RN and NASH JC: Immunization against B virus infection. I. Preparation of an experimental vaccine. Am J Hyg 71:15-28, 1960
31. HULL RN, CHERRY WR, and TRITCH AJ: Growth characteristics of monkey kidney cells strain LLC-MK$_1$ and LLC-MK$_2$ (NCTC-3196) and their utility in virus research. J Exp Med 115:903-917, 1962
32. HULL RN, PECK FB, WARD TG, and NASH LC: Immunization against B virus infection. II. Further laboratory and clinical studies with an experimental vaccine. Am J Hyg 76:239-251, 1962
33. KEEBLE SA, CHRISTOFINIS GJ, and WOOD W: Natural virus B infection in rhesus monkeys. J Pathol Bacteriol 76:189-199, 1958
34. KEEBLE SA: Virus B infection of monkeys, a disease communicable to man. Vet Res 73:618-621, 1961
35. KLENERMAN L, COID CR, and AOKI FY: Treatment of wounds from animals suspected of carrying neurotropic viruses. Br Med J 3:740-741, 1975
36. KLINE LB and HULL RN: The viricidal properties of peracetic acid. Am J Clin Pathol 33:30-33, 1960
37. KRECH U and LEWIS LF: Propagation of B virus in tissue cultures. Proc Soc Exp Biol Med 87:174-178, 1954
38. LOVE FM and JUNGHERR E: Occupational infection with virus B of monkeys. J Am Med Assoc 179:804-806, 1962
39. MATHEWS J and BUTHALA DA: Studies on herpesvirus simiae (B virus) cell surface reaction to infection. Cornell Vet 53:481-492, 1963
40. MCCARTHY K and TOSOLINI FA: A review of primate herpes viruses. Proc R Soc Med 68:145-150, 1975

41. McLeod DRE, Shimada FT, and Walcroft MJ: Experimental immunization against B virus. Ann NY Acad Sci 85:980-989, 1960
42. Melnick JL and Banker DD: Isolation of B viruses (Herpes Group) from the central nervous system of a rhesus monkey. J Exp Med 100:181-194, 1954
43. Nagler FP and Klotz MA: Fatal B virus infection in a person subject to recurrent herpes labialis. Can Med Assoc J 79:743-745, 1958
44. Perkins FT and Hartley EG: Precautions against B virus infection. Br Med J 2:899-901, 1966
45. Pierce FT, Pierce JD, and Hull RN: B virus: its current significance, description and diagnosis of a fatal human infection. Am J Hyg 68:242-250, 1958
46. Pille ER: Virus B infection in monkeys. Probl Virol 6:542-547, 1960
47. Plummer G: Serological comparison of the herpes viruses. Br J Exp Path 45:135-141, 1964
48. Prier JE and Goulet NR: Preliminary findings concerning the formalin inactivation of herpes B virus. Am J Vet Res 22:1112-1116, 1961
49. Reagan RL, Day WC, Harmon MP, and Brueckner AL: Effect of "B" virus (strain No. 1) in the Syrian hamster. Am J Trop Med 1:987-989, 1952
50. Reagan RL, Day WC, Harmon MP, and Brueckner AL: Adaptation of "B" virus to the Swiss albino mouse. J Gen Microbiol 7:327-328, 1952
51. Reissig M and Melnick JL: The cellular changes produced in tissue cultures by herpes B virus correlated with the concurrent multiplication of the virus. J Exp Med 101:341-351, 1955
52. Ruebner BH, Kevereux D, Roruik M, Espana C, and Brown JF: Ultrastructure of herpesvirus simiae (herpes B virus). Exp Mol Pathol 22:317-325, 1975
53. Sabin AB and Wright AM: Acute ascending myelitis following a monkey bite, with the isolation of a virus capable of reproducing the disease. J Exp Med 59:115-136, 1934
54. Sabin AB: Studies on the B virus. II. Properties of the virus and pathogenesis of the experimental disease in rabbits. Br J Exp Pathol 15:268-279, 1934
55. Sabin AB: Studies on the B virus. III. The experimental disease in Macaca rhesus monkeys. Br J Exp Pathol 15:321-334, 1934
56. Sabin AB and Hurst EW: Studies on the B virus. IV. Histopathology of the experimental disease in rhesus monkeys and rabbits. Br J Exp Pathol 16:133-148, 1935
57. Sabin AB: The nature and rate of centripetal progression of certain neurotropic viruses along peripheral nerves. Am J Pathol 13:615-617, 1937
58. Siegert R: Elektronenoptische untersuchungen uber die kernveranderungen herpes-infizierter zellen. Wien Z Nervenheilkd Deren Grenzgeb 18:159-178, 1960
59. Soto PJ and Deauvelle GA: Spontaneous simian giant cell pneumonia with co-existent B virus infection. Am J Vet Res 25:793-805, 1964
60. Thomas E and Henschel E: Uber die herpes-B-virus-myelitis und encephalitis beim menschen. Deutsch Z Nervenheilkd 181:494-516, 1960
61. Ueda Y, Tagaya I, and Shiroki K: Immunological relationship between herpes simplex virus and B virus. Arch Gesamte Virusforch 24:231-244, 1968
62. Van Hoosier G and Melnick JL: Neutralizing antibodies in human sera to herpesvirus simiae (B virus). Tex Rep Biol Med 19:376-380, 1961
63. Vizoso AD: Heterogeneity in herpes simiae (B virus) and some antigenic relationships in the herpes group. Br J Exp Pathol 55:471-477, 1974
64. Vizoso AD: Recovery of herpes simiae (B virus) from both primary and latent infections in rhesus monkeys. Br J Exp Pathol 56:485-488, 1975
65. Wallis C and Melnick JL: Suppression of adventitious agents in monkey kidney cultures. Tex Rep Biol Med 20:465-475, 1962
66. Watson DH, Wildy P, Harvey BAM, and Shedden WIH: Serological relationships among viruses of the herpes group. J Gen Virol 1:139-141, 1967
67. Zeitlyonok NA, Chumakova MY, Ralph NM, and Goen LS: Distribution area and natural hosts of latent viruses in monkeys. Occurrence of simian vacuolating virus (SV40) and herpesvirus simiae in cynomolgus monkeys in Indonesia. Acta Virol 10:537-541, 1966

CHAPTER 12

VARICELLA AND HERPES ZOSTER

Thomas H. Weller

Introduction

A single virus, now termed varicella-zoster virus (V-Z) or *Herpesvirus varicellae*, is the causative agent of varicella (chickenpox) and of herpes zoster (shingles). Varicella reflects a primary infection, while herpes zoster develops in the immunologically experienced individual. Most, if not all, cases of herpes zoster follow the activation of latent preexisting varicella virus, although the mechanisms remain obscure.

Evidence for a common etiology gradually accumulated. As first noted in 1888 by von Bokay (7), varicella may develop in susceptible children after contact with cases of herpes zoster. Kundratitz (45) inoculated zoster material and produced a varicelliform eruption in a few volunteers. The cutaneous lesions in varicella (91) and in zoster (47) were found to be histopathologically identical. Using extracts of cutaneous lesions, various workers documented an immunologic relationship (2, 8, 56). Attempts to find a susceptible experimental animal were unsuccessful, although inoculation of the monkey testis (65) and of human skin fragments implanted on the embryonated hen egg resulted in focal lesions (6, 33). In 1953, isolation and serial propagation of V-Z was accomplished in cultures of human tissues (94). The agent *in vitro* was cell associated, and transfer of infected cells was essential for serial propagation. The immunologic identity of strains of virus recovered from patients with varicella and herpes zoster was established by fluorescent-antibody techniques (96), by complement fixation, and by neutralization procedures (97). Garland (23) was the first to suggest that zoster reflected activation of a latent varicella virus.

Clinical aspects

Varicella

Transmission. Droplet infection has been assumed to be the usual mode, although virus is rarely demonstrable in nasopharyngeal secretions in contrast to the ease of its recovery from the cutaneous lesions. Contact infection undoubtedly plays a role when an individual with herpes zoster is the index case.

Pathogenesis. The initial site of virus replication is not known. Thereafter, a viremia, possibly intermittent, occurs. Virus is widely disseminated in the body, and focal lesions comparable to those in the skin can develop in the viscera.

Incubation period. The incubation period is usually 14–17 days, with extremes of 10–23 days.

Period of infectivity. The period of infectivity extends from 2 or 3 days before appearance of rash to the time the last crop of cutaneous lesions reaches the pustular stage. Thus the patient is usually noninfectious by the fifth day of the eruption, unless the host response is atypical as reflected by the continuing appearance of new crops of vesicles.

Symptoms. A prodromal period of malaise and fever can precede the eruption, or the characteristic exanthem can be the first overt evidence of infection. The rash is characteristically pleomorphic. This reflects the evolution in the course of hours of individual lesions through the macular, papular, and vesicular stages, as well as the concurrent appearance of successive crops of new lesions over a 2- to 4-day period. The lesions usually appear first and in greatest number on the trunk, and then develop on the neck, face, and the proximal parts of the extremities. While varicella is typically benign, on occasion most of the skin surface can be involved, and the febrile response can be pronounced.

Complications. Secondary bacterial infection of the involved skin is common. Pneumonia can occur, particularly in the adult; in one series of young adults with varicella wherein röntgenologic examinations were performed routinely, 16% showed pulmonary abnormalities (93). Infrequently, varicella pneumonia is fatal (70). Central nervous system involvement can precede, accompany, or follow varicella as a rare complication. Cerebellar ataxia is relatively common and has a good prognosis. An encephalopathy can occur which is characterized by hemorrhagic perivascular infiltration and demyelinization. Glomerulonephritis rarely develops (104).

Herpes zoster

Transmission. In contrast to the epidemic and seasonal nature of varicella, zoster has a random temporal distribution. This epidemiologic characteristic is in accord with the concept that zoster reflects activation of preexisting varicella virus harbored in a latent state by the partially immune host.

Incubation period and pathogenesis. The pathogenesis of zoster is obscure, and the site of viral latency is unknown. The cutaneous lesions are typically unilateral and confined to 1 or more dermatomes related to specific dorsal root or extramedullary cranial nerve ganglia. Virus is assumed to spread peripherally from the involved ganglia along the sensory nerves to the skin.

Often no inciting factors can be established as having triggered the pathologic process in zoster. However, trauma, therapy with drugs such as arsenicals, and the presence of certain malignancies have long been recognized as predisposing influences. Zoster is commonly encountered in recipients of organ transplants who are receiving immunosuppressive therapy; in one series, 8% of renal transplant recipients followed for 2 years developed zoster (64). Immunologic investigations on such patients indicate an unstable viral-host relationship (48). Preeruptive zoster serum has low but demonstrable levels of neutralizing antibody (75). In zoster the neutralizing antibody response is limited to a rise in IgG (46), although immunofluorescence studies show an apparent increase in IgM (11, 66). Lymphocytes from normal adults with a history of varicella respond on exposure to varicella antigens *in vitro;* depressed cellular responsiveness to V-Z antigens has been demonstrated in patients with Hodgkin disease, and in individuals with zoster, but cannot always be correlated with the pattern of viral activity (41, 68, 69). Leukocytes from V-Z immune donors exhibit the capacity to inactivate virus; this capacity is reduced in the early phase of zoster (29). There are observations suggesting that some "immune" adults develop subclinical infections on reexposure, manifested by a rise in titer of neutralizing antibody (11, 15). The epidemiology and pathogenesis of varicella and zoster has recently been reviewed elsewhere (95).

Period of infectivity. The patient with zoster does not disseminate virus as readily as does the individual with varicella. However, vesicles yielding virus can persist longer than in varicella, i.e., 4–7 days after appearance of the rash (31).

Symptoms. Erythematous maculopapular plaques develop over an area of the involved dermatome. Single or confluent clumps of vesicles then appear which evolve to healing crusted lesions over a period of 1–3 weeks. Pain is significant in two-thirds of cases (13). On occasion, severe referred pain developing before the eruption can pose a diagnostic problem. In over 50% of patients, the trunk is the site of the cutaneous eruption, with the cervical and lumbar regions less frequently involved. Of the cranial nerves, the trigeminal, and especially its ophthalmic division, is the most commonly affected. Generalization of the eruption with appearance of scattered varicelliform lesions over the body is not rare. Longitudinal serologic studies of individuals with a predisposition to zoster, i.e., renal transplant recipients, document episodes of pain unaccompanied by an eruption but associated with a rise in antibody (48).

Complications. A small percentage of patients with zoster suffer from an intractable postherpetic neuralgia. With ophthalmic involvement, serious corneal damage can result. Encephalitis can occur and motor paralysis is a recognized complication (35).

Pathology

In the developing cutaneous lesion of varicella, and of zoster, ballooning degeneration of cells occurs in the epidermis and, to a lesser extent, in the corium (Fig 12.1). Intranuclear inclusions appear in many types of cells, and multinucleated giant cells form in which each nucleus contains an inclusion. Fluid collects in the cellular interspaces and lifts the superficial

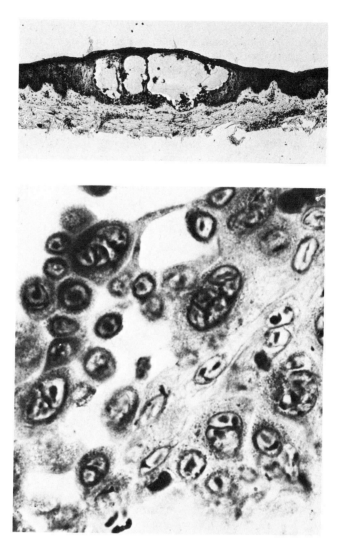

Figure 12.1 Varicella histopathology. Above: vesicle on first day of exanthem. Below: same vesicle showing intranuclear inclusions and multinucleate giant cells (from original preparation of Dr. E. E. Tyzzer, made June 9, 1904). Magnification 830X. (*Source:* T. H. Weller et al in *Harvey Lectures, 1956-1957.* New York: Academic Press, Inc., pp. 230-231.)

cornified layer to form a delicate vesicle. With necrosis of affected cells, the fibrin content of the fluid increases and there is an infiltration of inflammatory cells. In zoster, the cellular infiltrate is predominantly polymorphonuclear in type; the abrupt increase in the number of cells coincides with the appearance of interferon in the vesicle fluid (83). In all patients with varicella, comparable lesions probably develop in the viscera; in fatal cases lesions are found widely distributed in the lungs, liver, and elsewhere (17).

Similar visceral lesions occur in a relatively benign illness in monkeys caused by a distinct, but related, simian varicella virus (99).

Head and Campbell (37) demonstrated that during the eruptive phase of zoster the associated dorsal root ganglion is infiltrated with round cells, and focal hemorrhages with nerve cell destruction occur. Degenerative changes can be traced along sensory nerves to the skin as well as in posterior columns of the cord. There may be a localized leptomeningitis spreading to involve the anterior horns, thus explaining the rare complication of motor paralysis.

Description and Nature of the Agent

Characteristics and classification

Varicella-zoster virus, *Herpesvirus varicellae,* is a member of the *Herpesvirus* group. The propensity for persistence of the herpesviruses in the infected host is dramatically expressed as zoster. All members are ultrastructurally similar and induce intranuclear inclusions. Among the herpesviruses pathogenic for man, *H. hominis* (herpes simplex; HSV) has a limited antigenic relationship with V-Z but lacks the host specificity and the cell association of infectivity *in vitro* that are characteristic of *H. varicellae.* The human cytomegaloviruses (CMV) are more distantly related, if at all. Simian agents that produce varicelliform disease in various monkeys have major antigens in common with *H. varicellae;* however, they differ biologically (20, 99).

Size and shape

Electron microscopic pictures of virus particles derived from cutaneous lesions of varicella (1), or of zoster (50, 102), as well as of the developmental stages of V-Z in infected cells *in vitro* (4), provide information on the structure of the virus particle. The particle is composed of a nucleocapsid about 100 nm in diameter surrounded by concentric membranes with an outer diameter of 160–200 nm. Particles in the nucleus may possess 1 membrane; those in the cytoplasm may have 2 or more. The capsid is icosahedral with 5:3:2 axial symmetry. It consists of 162 short tubular capsomeres arranged around a central core. In contrast to particles from vesicle fluid, extranuclear particles from cells infected *in vitro* often have defective cores or membranes (18).

Chemical composition

H. varicellae is a deoxyribonucleic acid (DNA) virus. The buoyant density of viral DNA derived from infected cell cultures has been reported as 1.717 (26), 1.705 (49), and 1.707 (59). It is to be noted that the composition of V-Z, of necessity, has been investigated using culture-derived materials that contain many defective particles.

Resistance

The difficulties of obtaining cell-free infectious V-Z account for the sparsity of information on resistance to physical agents. We observed that the infectivity of vesicle fluid frozen at -70 C after dilution in sterile neutral fat-free milk was maintained for years (98). Cell-free virus obtained by sonication of infected cells is well preserved at -70 C when frozen in tissue culture medium with fetal calf serum plus sorbitol in a final concentration of 10% (10).

When cultivated *in vitro*, V-Z is intimately cell associated, and maintenance of infectivity is influenced by the condition of the host cell. Gold (30) found that loss of infectivity of infected cells occurred when they were maintained at room temperature for 60 min at a pH under 6.2 or over 7.8. Techniques that preserve cells by freezing maintain the infectivity of cell-associated virus. V-Z infected cells may be stored in liquid nitrogen at -195 C in Eagle medium with 20% calf serum and 15% glycerol (61), or at -70 C in basal Eagle medium with 10% calf serum and 10% dimethyl sulfoxide (76). Preservation of cell-associated virus by lyophilization in a phosphate buffer, sodium glutamate (0.0049 M), and 1% bovine albumin medium provides a source of cell-free virus on reconstitution for neutralization tests (Nt) (38). We now store cell-free V-Z in SPGA solution (39) (0.218 M sucrose, 0.0038 M KHP_2O_4, 0.0072 M K_2HPO_4, 0.0049 M Na glutamate, 1% bovine albumin).

Antigenic composition

Strains of virus from patients with varicella or from zoster are immunologically identical. Antigenic variants of V-Z have not been described. Analysis of concentrated culture-derived virus, after density gradient centrifugation in CsCl or sucrose and gel filtration by double diffusion in agar against a human zoster serum, delineated 5 reactive components (12). One antigen, termed β, was destroyed by ether and by CsCl, and all were labile on exposure to trypsin, urea, and sodium dodecylsulfate. With zoster vesicle fluid as antigen, 3 reaction lines developed in gel-diffusion precipitation tests (88). Comparison of culture-derived V-Z and HSV viral antigens revealed one precipitating antigen in common that gave a reaction of identity and was absorbable by the heterologous reagent (90).

Cells infected *in vitro* with V-Z develop surface or membrane antigens that can be detected by a mixed agglutination test using viral antibody and indicator cells consisting of sheep erythrocytes (RBC) treated successively with monkey anti-sheep red cell serum and goat anti-human globulin serum (40). Antibodies to specific cell membrane antigens can be detected by an indirect immunofluorescence reaction, and these are sensitive indicators of the immune status (103) of adults.

Relatively crude extracts of V-Z infected cultures are customarily used as antigen in complement-fixation (CF) tests. Soluble complement-fixing antigens are demonstrable in vesicle fluid (14) and can be obtained from infected cell cultures. Two soluble and 2 particulate antigens prepared from culture materials by Martin and Palmer exhibited complement-fixing activity (52). Further study of subunit complement-fixing antigens (73) indicates that the capsid component is the most reactive fraction and that in primary V-Z infections the antibody response is primarily to this element.

No hemagglutinin activity has been reported.

Pathogenicity for animals

Common laboratory animals are not susceptible to infection with V-Z. The susceptibility of higher primates has not been explored systematically, although Rivers (65) produced microscopic lesions in the inoculated testes of vervet monkeys. Closely related, but biologically distinct, simian varicella viruses have been isolated from several species of monkeys.

Growth in tissue cultures

Host range. V-Z grows readily in monolayer cultures of human cells of various types, including fibroblastic and epithelial cells (98). Primary or secondary cultures, heteroploid or diploid cell lines can be employed. Growth also occurs in cultures of cells of simian origin, although cells of human origin are preferable. Cell cultures of nonprimate origin are much less susceptible to infection. However, the report that V-Z can be propagated in cells from guinea pig embryos (82) has been confirmed (21, 36, 79). Attempts to propagate V-Z in cultures of rabbit cells were reported as successful with one of several strains of virus examined (85); negative results have been obtained by other investigators (21, 36).

The focal cytopathic process. The cytopathic effect (CPE) in monolayer cultures is characteristically focal. Extension of individual lesions occurs by infection of contiguous cells and is determined by the architecture of the cell sheet. The process is slowed or stopped if uninfected cells are not in intimate contact with infected cells, or if conditions are suboptimal for cell growth and motility. This fact has practical implications. It is common practice to replace "growth" medium with a simple "maintenance" medium at the time tissue cultures are inoculated. Some maintenance systems provide a cellular substrate that is suboptimal for the growth of V-Z.

Infectious material passes from cell to cell. Slotnick and Rosanoff (81), using fluorescent-antibody techniques, visualized antigenic material in cytoplasmic strands that connected cells. Further evidence indicating transfer of infectious material via intercellular connections was obtained by Gold (30). He observed that incorporation of specific antibody in the culture system did not affect virus transfer and established that transfer was accomplished within 30 min. Assessing spread of infection by immunofluorescence methods, Rapp and Vanderslice (62) concluded that 8–16 hr were required for virus to infect neighboring cells.

In cultures of fibroblastic cells, the initial lesion appears as a small group of swollen, glassily refractile cells which contrast sharply with the unaltered outgrowth. Typically, the focus progresses linearly along the long axis of the cells (Fig 12.2). In monolayer cultures of amnion or kidney cells, the foci appear as small plaques of irregularly rounded enlarged cells that are

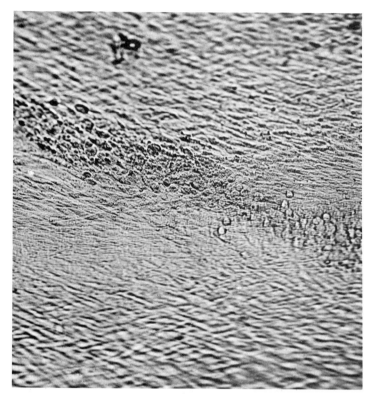

Figure 12.2 Cytopathology of V-Z: changes induced by varicella strain. Focal changes produced in roller cultures of foreskin tissue, fourth passage, seventh day. (*Source:* Weller TH et al: J Exp Med 108:843–868, 1958)

swollen, refractile, and distinct from the unaltered transparent cell sheet. Multinucleated giant cells may develop, and radiating cytoplasmic processes may extend from involved cells. When involved cells are stained and examined all contain intranuclear inclusion bodies (Figs 12.3, 12.4, 12.5). The individual foci gradually increase in size and coalesce until, if conditions are optimal, the whole cell sheet is involved.

Maintenance in serial passage. Isolates are passed by inoculating established cell cultures with viable infected cells. Customarily, for subculture, when a cell sheet shows 50–75% CPE, the fluid medium is removed and infected cells are dislodged with trypsin (86), which yields higher numbers of infected cells than does versene (30). This is accomplished by wetting the cell sheet with 0.25% trypsin in phosphate-buffered saline (PBS), pH 7.5, for 5–20 min; any excess trypsin is then removed, and the dislodged cells are suspended in tissue culture growth medium for inoculation into new cultures.

Preparation of cell-free infectious virus from culture materials. Significant amounts of cell-free infectious virus were first obtained from V-Z infected cultures of human thyroid cells by Caunt (16). Sonication of the in-

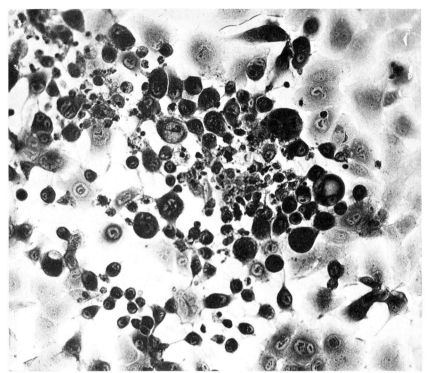

Figure 12.3 Cytopathology of V-Z: changes induced by varicella strain. Small focal lesion in human amnion cell culture, thirty-fourth passage, thirteenth day. Hematoxylin and eosin staining. (*Source:* Weller TH et al: J Exp Med 108:843–868, 1958)

fected thyroid cells for 2 min or less yielded cell-free suspensions containing 10^4–10^5 infectious particles per ml. Brunell (10) obtained cell-free virus from sonicated infected human embryonic lung cultures. The yield was of the order of 0.125–0.72 plaque forming units (pfu) per V-Z infected cell, and it was noted that exposure to trypsin reduced infectivity titers. Using a high multiplicity of infectious particles, i.e., 2×10^6 pfu, or of infected cells, as inocula, Schmidt and Lennette (76) improved the yield of cell-free virus derived from human fetal diploid lung cultures. Infected cells were harvested in culture medium containing 10% sorbitol by shaking with glass beads, and infectious particles were released by sonication for 30 sec. The highest titer of cell-free virus was obtained when cultures were processed 24–36 hr after infection, some 24 hr before the development of advanced cytopathic changes.

Quantitation of virus in vitro. Infected cells (61, 76) and cell-free virus may be titrated by plaque procedures (15, 39, 76) using monolayer cultures of susceptible cells maintained in a CO_2 incubator. With an immunoperoxidase technique, employing a selected zoster convalescent-phase serum (nonreactive with HSV and CMV) and goat anti-human IgG coupled

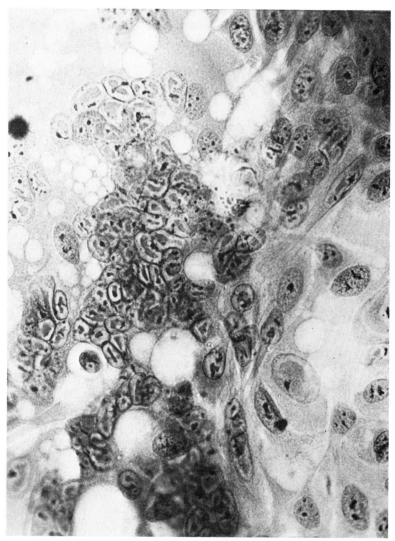

Figure 12.4 Cytopathology of V-Z: changes induced by zoster strain. Edge of syncytial mass, apparently of epithelial origin, packed with nuclei containing
developing inclusions. Culture of foreskin tissue sixth day after inoculation with twenty-fifth-passage virus. Hematoxylin and eosin staining.
700X. (*Source:* Weller TH et al: J Exp Med 108:843–868, 1958)

to horse radish peroxidase as reagents, microplaques 1–2 mm in diameter
can be identified in 72 hr (25). It has been reported that incubation at 31 C
yields more and better-defined plaques (39) than the higher temperatures
customarily used.

Metabolic interactions and inhibitors; variants. The contamination of
cell lines with *Mycoplasma* sp assumes practical significance if the arginine-
requiring *M. arginini* is the contaminant, as V-Z cytopathology is sup-

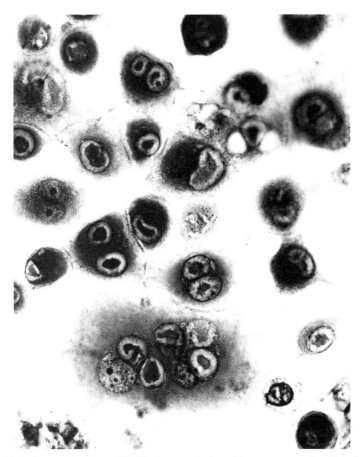

Figure 12.5 Cytopathology of V-Z: changes induced by zoster strain. Detail of cytopathic changes in human amnion cell culture 6 days after inoculation
with second-passage virus. Hematoxylin and eosin staining. 520X.
(*Source:* Weller TH et al: J Exp Med 108:843–868, 1958)

pressed; supportive evidence derives from the fact that cell cultures maintained on arginine-deficient media do not develop V-Z plaques (80).

In heavily infected cultures of human embryonic fibroblasts, significant
amounts of interferon are present 12–24 hr after inoculation. Exposure of a
susceptible cell sheet to human interferon for 24 hr before inoculation reduces the plaque count (3).

Antiviral activity of compounds that interfere with DNA synthesis is
assayed by inhibition of the cytopathic activity of V-Z *in vitro*. Idoxuridine
(5-iodo-2′-deoxyuridine) (60, 63), the first such compound to be examined,
and cytabarine (1-β-D-arabinofuranosylcytosine) have undesirable attributes when used clinically. Adenine arabinoside (Ara-A; 9-β-D-arabinofura-
nosyladenine) is less toxic and appears useful in the treatment of zoster (101). More recently phosphonoacetic acid (53) and rifampin (59) have
been shown to inhibit replication of V-Z *in vitro*.

Attempts by us and by other workers to adapt V-Z by long-term serial propagation *in vitro* and to thus increase yields of cell-free virus have been unsuccessful. Nii and Maeda (57) cloned V-Z isolates grown in Vero cells, and segregated 2 variants on the basis of CPE; one line induced syncytial giant cells.

Preparation of Immune Serum

Use of convalescent-phase human serum

Serum from individuals convalescing from zoster is customarily used for reference and as a reagent for the identification of V-Z. Such serum should be carefully selected in terms of the presence of V-Z antibody in high titer, and the absence, or occurrence in low titer, of antibodies reactive with HSV, CMV, and vaccinia virus.

Preparation of antiserum

In rhesus monkeys. Antiserum can be prepared in monkeys using virus propagated in homologous cells, thus by-passing problems associated with the presence of antibodies to foreign host proteins (78). Monkey kidney cell cultures were grown with 5% normal monkey serum, 0.5% lactalbumin hydrolysate, and Hanks balanced salt solution. The monkey cell cultures were inoculated with infected human fetal diploid kidney cells which were carefully washed to remove residual traces of bovine serum, and the inoculated cultures then maintained on Eagle minimal essential medium (MEM) with Earle salt solution. Monkeys were immunized by 3 biweekly 4-ml intramuscular doses comprising equal parts of infected monkey culture material and an adjuvant consisting of 1 part Arlacel A and 9 parts Standard mineral oil CT 70, and the animals were bled 7–10 days after the last injection.

In rabbits or guinea pigs. Kissling et al (44) prepared antiserum in rabbits or guinea pigs using an antigen derived from heavily infected diploid human fibroblast cultures, disrupted by sonication, and then partially purified by discontinuous sucrose density gradient centrifugation. Antigen, active in the CF reaction, was collected from bands at the 35–60% sucrose interface. To immunize guinea pigs, a series of seven 0.2-ml injections was given intraperitoneally over an 18-day period, and animals were bled 7–10 days after the last injection. Rabbits were inoculated intramuscularly with 2 ml of a mixture of equal parts of antigen and Freund complete adjuvant followed by a 1-ml dose of antigen alone on day 27; they were bled 50 days later.

Collection and Preparation of Specimens for Laboratory Diagnosis

Precautions

Historically, the differential diagnosis of varicella and smallpox has been a source of confusion; resolution of the problem by identification of the etiologic agent was, and is, a diagnostic emergency. Now it appears that smallpox has been eradicated. However, until global eradication is confirmed, the possibility of introduction of smallpox into the United States remains; therefore, unless there are clearcut indications to the contrary, *specimens collected from an individual with a vesiculo-pustular exanthem should be handled as if from a case of smallpox, until proved otherwise.* No laboratory-acquired V-Z infections have been reported.

Procedures for virus isolation

From the cutaneous lesion. The fresh vesicular lesion provides the material of choice for virus isolation; attempts to recover virus from crusted lesions are a waste of time. If the typical pleomorphic eruption of varicella is present, and if material is collected during the first 3 days of exanthematous illness from a lesion containing nonpurulent fluid, isolation of virus is readily accomplished (31, 86, 98). Isolation of virus is rare thereafter unless the host response is atypical. In contrast, in patients with zoster, isolation of virus from persistent vesicles can be accomplished through the seventh day, or possibly later, after appearance of the segmental lesion.

Because some vesicle fluids clot upon collection, immediate dilution is desirable. After gently sponging the fresh lesion with sterile saline, we aspirate the contents with a No. 27 needle and a 0.25-ml syringe containing about 0.05 ml of neutral skim milk. Individual aspirates are pooled by immediately rinsing in a tube containing 1–2.5 ml skim milk. If inoculation of cultures is not feasible immediately, the specimen should be frozen in sealed ampules, preferably at −70 C.

From other sites. With a single exception, repeated attempts to recover V-Z from throat washings have been unsuccessful (31, 55, 100). In uncomplicated cases, viremia is rarely demonstrable (31); in the immunocompromised leukemic child with varicella pneumonia, virus can be isolated from heparinized venous blood (19). Attempts to recover virus from the urine of patients with varicella or zoster have been unsuccessful (54). Virus has been isolated from the cerebrospinal fluid of patients with zoster that have evidence of central nervous system involvement as reflected by a pleocytosis (31).

For isolation of virus from tissues obtained postmortem, 10% suspensions (wt/vol) can be prepared in tissue culture medium by grinding with alundum; the supernatant material obtained after slow centrifugation is employed as the inoculum (17).

Direct immunodiagnosis

While V-Z can be recovered only from vesicle fluid collected prior to pustulation, specific antigen can be demonstrated by agar gel immunodiffusion (92) in vesicle fluid or in crusts from cutaneous lesions extracted in 0.5 ml of Sorenson buffer (pH 8.2). Positive reactions have been obtained as late as 14 days after the onset of varicella and 23 days after the onset of zoster.

Collection of blood for serologic diagnosis

Acute-phase serum should be collected as soon as possible. CF antibody is usually not detectable in specimens collected within 4 days of onset of varicella, but may be present in significant titers in acute-phase serum obtained from patients with herpes zoster. Convalescent-phase specimens should be collected from 2–6 weeks after onset. Titers of CF antibody decline thereafter and may reach nonreactive levels in 6–12 months (32, 87).

Microscopy

Light microscopy. Examination of smears or of biopsies of the fresh cutaneous lesion provides a simple and rapid approach to the important differentiation of lesions produced by the varicella-herpes group of viruses from those produced by agents of the variola-vaccinia group. The presence of multinucleated giant cells and intranuclear inclusions eliminates variola-vaccinia viruses from consideration.

Preparation of material from the cutaneous lesion: The value of the smear technique introduced by Tyzzer has been emphasized by Blank et al (5) who recommend: After gentle sponging of the cutaneous vesicle with alcohol, the delicate roof of the vesicle is carefully incised peripherally and reflected. Excess fluid is removed by gentle blotting. The base of the lesion is gently scraped with a Bard-Parker No. 15 blade, avoiding gross bleeding. Cellular material collected on the edge of the blade is gently spread on a microscope slide and air-dried before transmittal to the laboratory.

Biopsy material: A superficial biopsy across a fresh lesion, including the floor of the vesicle, is adequate. This should be fixed immediately in Bouin or Zenker fluids before being sent to the laboratory. (If there is any question of smallpox the use of frozen-section techniques on unfixed tissues carries the risk of disseminating material that is highly infectious.)

Electron microscopy. For rapid diagnosis vesicular scrapings can be diluted with distilled H_2O, mixed with 3% aqueous phosphotungstic acid, appropriately dried on a specimen grid, and examined for the presence of herpes-type particles (102). However, the examination of stained smears by light microscopy yields comparable information, and either approach suffices only to differentiate agents of the herpes group from those of the variola group.

Immunofluorescence examination. Smears of cellular material collected from the base of vesicular lesions prepared on slides, air-dried, fixed in acetone for 10 min, and again dried can be examined by either direct or indirect fluorescent-antibody (FA) techniques. Multiple smears should be prepared to provide adequate cellular material and to permit essential controls with HSV and vaccinia antisera. Differentiation of the cutaneous lesion of V-Z and of HSV can be accomplished by direct or indirect immunofluorescence of 4-μ cryostat-cut, frozen sections of punch biopsies using appropriately absorbed and labeled human serum (58); biopsies can be kept as long as 24 hr at 4 C before frozen sections are cut, or can be stored frozen at -70 C or in liquid nitrogen.

Laboratory Diagnosis

Direct examination of clinical material

Smears from vesicular lesions, biopsies, or postmortem specimens. The demonstration of multinucleate giant cells with intranuclear inclusions documents that the lesion is of herpesvirus origin (HSV or V-Z), and eliminates variola and vaccinia from consideration. Smears can be fixed with methyl alcohol and stained with dilute buffered Giemsa stain, pH $7.0-7.2$, or less desirably with Wright stain. Examine with the oil immersion lens for multinucleated giant cells. By this technique the intranuclear inclusion is poorly differentiated and may appear as an amorphous purplish mass completely filling the nucleus and replacing the normal nucleolar structure and chromatin network. Routine hematoxylin and eosin staining of tissue sections reveals the typical histopathologic changes induced by members of the herpes group (Fig 12.1), although better differentiation of the intranuclear inclusion will be obtained with Giemsa stain as modified for tissue sections.

Application of immunologic techniques. Application of immunodiffusion or of FA procedures to clinical materials provides a quick answer to the problem of differentiating between V-Z and HSV, if appropriate controls are used.

In one study (92), 92% of 79 vesicle fluid samples and 59% of 49 extracts of crusts obtained from V-Z lesions yielded reactions, usually within 12–24 hr, when examined in a micro agar-gel diffusion system. Tests were performed in 2-mm wells on slides layered with 2.5 ml of melted 0.5% Ionagar No. 2 in Sorenson phosphate buffer (pH 8.2) with 0.1% free protamine. A zoster immune serum, devoid of antibodies to herpes simplex and reconstituted to a tenth of the original volume after concentration by lyophilization, was the reagent. A positive control consisting of culture-produced V-Z antigen was included in each test; the wells were arranged so that a line of identity would form if the unknown sample was reactive. No reaction was obtained with vesicular materials from 20 patients with HSV. If desired, vaccinia antiserum and vaccinia antigen can be included in the reaction pattern.

Material from lesions or cryostat-cut sections of tissues also yield an etiologic diagnosis if FA procedures are applied. The direct method using fluorescein-conjugated antibody from monkeys immunized with V-Z devoid of heterologous host antigens is desirable (78). Cross-reactions with HSV in the indirect method can be eliminated by preabsorption of human V-Z convalescent-phase serum with HSV-infected monkey kidney cells (58). The fact that reactive V-Z antigens in cutaneous lesion biopsies visualized by FA occur primarily in the deeper layers of the epidermis, hair follicles, and sebaceous glands explains why punch biopsies yield more reliable results than do smears of scrapings (58).

Virus Isolation

Isolation in cultured cells

Cultures of human cells provide the optimum substrate for the isolation and propagation of V-Z. Common laboratory animals and the embryonated hen's egg are not overtly susceptible.

A spectrum of cultured cells of human origin, fibroblastic or epithelial in type, and either primary or of an established cell line can be used for the isolation and growth of V-Z. The culture system must satisfy 2 conditions. First, a uniform transparent confluent monolayer of cells is required so that the developing focal lesions of V-Z are readily apparent on microscopic examination. Second, the morphologic integrity, and preferably active growth, of the cell sheet needs be preserved for 14, or better 21, days, the maximal "incubation" period for appearance of foci.

For isolation we prefer primary or low-passage cultures of human fibroblasts derived from embryonic skin-muscle, lung tissue, or preputial tissues. Medium No. 199 provides optimal conditions with 10% irradiated fetal bovine serum, 100 μ/ml of penicillin and 100 μg/ml of streptomycin provides optimal conditions; cultures are rolled at 35 C, and the medium is changed weekly or more often if indicated. Cultures in good condition exhibit numerous mitotic figures 24–28 hr after a change of medium.

Schmidt et al (74) prefer cultures of human fetal diploid cells for the isolation of V-Z. Initiated with Eagle MEM and 10% fetal bovine serum, after inoculation the cultures are maintained on Leibovitz No. 15 medium with 2% fetal bovine serum; the use of Leibovitz medium obviates the need for a change of fluids for 14 days.

Gold (30) examined several cell types and concluded that human amnion cells, maintained on Eagle MEM with 10% calf serum, were preferred because of their consistent susceptibility to infection and because they could be maintained in culture for periods of 3–6 weeks without undergoing spontaneous degeneration.

After inoculation of actively growing monolayer cultures with 0.1–0.2 ml diluted vesicle fluid, focal lesions usually can be detected by microscopic examination between the fourth and seventh day, although initial changes can appear as early as day 3 or as late as day 22. The focal lesions enlarge slowly and gradually increase in number. Cytopathic involvement of as much as 50% of the cell sheet can require days or several weeks to develop, depending on the infectivity of the original inoculum and the cultural conditions. When 20% or more of the cell sheet shows cytopathic changes, subculture is readily achieved by passing a suspension of infected cells obtained by trypsinization.

Identification of isolates

Presumptive identification based on cytopathology. A presumptive identification of V-Z is justified on the basis of the typical persistent focal cytopathic process along with demonstration of multinucleate giant cells and intranuclear inclusions, characteristics that eliminate variola-vaccinia viruses from consideration. To be differentiated are:

1. Herpes simplex virus—The CPE of HSV may be focal for a brief period and similar to that of V-Z, but rapidly spreads to involve all available cells. Further, HSV grows freely in cultures of cells from various laboratory animals, i.e., rabbit or hamster kidney cells, etc., and produces fatal illness in suckling mice.

2. Human cytomegalovirus—In some culture systems the persistent focal lesions of CMV can resemble those of V-Z. CMV produces typical CPE primarily in fibroblastic cells, replicating much less readily than does V-Z in cells of epithelial origin. CMV is not as cell associated as V-Z *in vitro;* virus eventually appears in the fluid phase and generalization of the cytopathic process occurs. However, this characteristic may not be exhibited by some new isolates of CMV for several weeks. Greenish-brown or brown pigment granules may develop in association with the cytopathic foci of CMV, and multinucleate giant cells are not as prominent a feature as with V-Z. Neither CMV nor V-Z produce illness in suckling mice or other rodents.

Specific identification of isolates. Specific identification is accomplished by using infected cells from the culture, or extracts thereof, as antigen in reactions with antibody of known specificity. Because of availability, convalescent-phase serum from patients with zoster is usually employed as the source of antibody; these should be selected in terms of nonreactivity with CMV and HSV antigens, either preexistent or else achieved by absorption with CMV or HSV antigens prior to use. If available, a desirable alternative is the use of V-Z antiserum prepared in monkeys or rabbits (see above). Antiserum prepared in animals with human-cell–derived materials should be preabsorbed with homologous cell extracts before use. In all tests, appropriate controls would include comparable uninfected cells or extracts thereof, cells infected with a known strain of V-Z or extracts thereof, and the use in parallel of an acute-phase or preimmunization serum comparable to the test reagent. Immunofluorescent staining by the direct or indirect method is the most convenient procedure for specific identification; alternatively, the isolate may be used as a source of CF antigen.

1. Identification by immunofluorescent staining—Procedures for identification by direct immunofluorescence were introduced by Schmidt and coworkers (78). (For details of preparation of fluorescein-immunoglobulin conjugates for use in the direct method, see reference 72.) When cytopathic changes involve 30–50% of the culture, cells are harvested by trypsinization from one or more cultures, sedimented by slow-speed centrifugation, resuspended and washed in culture medium, and reconcentrated by gentle centrifugation. A suspension of cells from uninoculated control cultures is prepared in the same manner. Microdrops of suspensions of infected and of control cells are transferred to slides, allowed to dry, fixed with acetone for 10 min, and redried. Preparation of each set in triplicate permits concurrent examination with conjugates specific for V-Z, HSV, and vaccinia viruses. Schmidt (72) recommends that working dilutions of each conjugate be prepared in a 20% suspension of mouse or beef brain tissue in PBS (pH 7.2) to reduce nonspecific staining. To stain, each of the 3 conjugates is layered over a slide bearing an infected smear and a slide with a control smear, and the preparations are incubated in a humidified chamber for 20 min at 35 C.

The slides are then washed for 10 min each in 2 changes of 0.01 M PBS in a Coplin jar, followed by a similar wash in distilled water. After drying, coverslips are applied using buffered glycerol-saline (pH 7.5) to mount, and the slides examined with a fluorescence microscope. If the isolate is V-Z, infected cells show both nuclear and cytoplasmic fluorescence with the V-Z conjugate, uninfected cells are negative, and both infected and uninfected cells are nonreactive with the HSV and vaccinia conjugate. If a CMV conjugate is available, a fourth series done in parallel is desirable.

Indirect immunofluorescent staining can be employed to identify isolates by using acute- and convalescent-phase sera from patients with varicella as reagents (96); in this instance the human serum should contain no or low levels of antibody against HSV, CMV, and vaccinia. (Alternatively, serum from immunized animals can be used, with appropriate conjugates.) Smears of infected and noninfected cells are prepared as described above on duplicate slides. Acute- and convalescent-phase sera are inactivated at 56 C for 30 min and doubling dilutions are made; Schmidt (72) uses a 20% suspension of mouse or beef brain as diluent. Smears are layered with drops of the diluted serum and allowed to react as in the direct test. After thorough washing, the smears are overlayed with a working dilution of anti-human gamma globulin conjugate, also diluted in brain suspension (72), and reincubated for a second 20-min period. They are then washed and mounted as in the direct system and examined. Positive reactions should occur to the established titer with the convalescent-phase serum and infected cells, be negative or reactive only in low titer with acute-phase serum, and both acute- and convalescent-phase sera should be nonreactive with uninfected cells.

2. *Identification by complement fixation*—CF antigen (see below) can be prepared from an isolate, and its identity determined by comparative box titrations that incorporate known antigens and reactive varicella serum devoid of antibody for HSV, CMV, and vaccinia virus. The process requires passage of the isolate to bottle cultures of susceptible cells to obtain sufficient antigen and is time consuming.

Serologic diagnosis

Over the past decade new methods have become available for the serologic diagnosis of V-Z and for the assessment of the immune status of the exposed individual. A limited supply of zoster immune globulin (ZIG) has become available that, if administered in the immediate postexposure period, can prevent or modify varicella in the high-risk patient, i.e., the leukemic or the immunosuppressed. To determine if an exposed patient is susceptible, the widely used varicella CF test has limited applicability. The laboratory needs be informed as to what information is being sought.

Complement-fixation test (CF)

Preparation of antigen. V-Z can be grown in bottle cultures of human fibroblastic cells or of human embryonic kidney cells; the medium should support active growth. The inocula should be of a high order of infectivity that will induce cytopathic involvement of the whole cell sheet in 6–10 days, at which time the medium is removed and the cells are harvested by scraping. After washing and concentration by centrifugation, the infected cells are either suspended in a small volume of Veronal-buffered saline (pH 7.2) (32, 44) or in Hanks balanced salt solution (72) and disrupted by repeated freeze-thawing or sonication; the product constitutes the antigen. Antigen is available commercially. The CF test is customarily carried out in a microtiter system as described in Chapter 1.

Interpretation and limitations. The CF reaction is particularly useful for the serologic confirmation of a primary attack of varicella. Comparison of the titer of serum obtained during the first 5 days of illness with that of a convalescent-phase specimen obtained 2–3 weeks later should show an increase of several-fold. An exception may be the failure of the CF reaction to detect rises in titer in varicella-infected infants (9). CF is less useful in the confirmation of the diagnosis of suspected cases of zoster where a relatively high titer may be observed in the acute-phase specimen with little subsequent rise.

Problems of interpretation can arise due to the antigenic relationship of V-Z and HSV and to responses to the heterologous agent. Individuals who have previously had varicella are particularly prone to exhibit a 4-fold or greater rise in titer of V-Z CF antibody when subsequently infected with HSV and conversely (43, 67, 71, 77, 84). A study of several V-Z viral subunit CF antigens failed to identify a component that exhibited enhanced specificity (73), and would eliminate V-Z-HSV cross-reactions. However, if paired sera are examined by CF concurrently with V-Z and HSV antigens, the response to the homologous agent can sometimes greatly exceed the heterologous response.

The CF reaction is of little use in the evaluation of susceptibility to varicella in the exposed adult. After varicella, the titer of CF antibody declines and may fall below detectable levels in 12 months.

Virus neutralization tests. Difficulties in obtaining supplies of cell-free V-Z preclude the use of Nt tests in routine diagnostic work. If this problem is resolved, recent advances in technique, including the introduction of plaque-reduction methods (15, 77), the demonstration of enhancement of neutralization by incorporation of complement (75), and the rapid visualization of microplaques by immunoperoxidase staining (24, 25), suggest that the neutralization reaction is generally useful.

Immunofluorescence tests

Indirect staining with fixed infected cells. Rises in V-Z antibody titer can be demonstrated by examination of serially diluted acute- and convalescent-phase sera with the indirect FA technique utilizing infected cells from cultures as antigen (77, 78). The method is time consuming, may detect heterologous HSV responses, and is less practical than is CF for routine diagnostic purposes.

The indirect method is useful in the assessment of the immune status of the exposed high-risk subject. In a study of a group of exposed individuals (34), 12 of 51 had no V-Z antibody on indirect FA examination; 9 of the 12 developed varicella, while all 39 reactive individuals were resistant.

Indirect staining of membrane antigen in living cells (FAMA). Detection of V-Z–induced membrane antigen in living infected cells by indirect FA is recommended as a quick and sensitive indicator of immune status, i.e., susceptibility on exposure (103).

To perform the test, embryonic lung fibroblasts are harvested 48 hr after infection in PBS by scraping; the cell concentration is adjusted to 10^5 cells/ml, and 0.025-ml volumes of cells and serum are reacted for 30 min at 25 C in wells of microtiter U-plates; after 3 washings with intervening centrifugation *in situ,* 0.025 ml goat anti-human gamma globulin fluorescein conjugate is added and reacted for 25 min; after 3 additional washings and centrifugations, the cells are suspended in glycerol saline, 9:1, and 10 lambda of cell suspension are transferred to a slide, and a coverslip is added and sealed with nail polish. On examination by fluorescence microscopy, if V-Z antibody is present, cells are outlined with a bright ring; nuclear staining, if present, should be ignored. Retrospective study of serum collected during 2 institutional outbreaks confirmed the finding that individuals with a FAMA titer of $\geq$ 1:2 do not develop varicella on intimate exposure (28).

Other tests

Indirect hemagglutination (IHA). Tanned RBC coated with culture-derived V-Z antigen have been used in IHA tests (22, 51, 89). The method probably will have limited applicability in confirmation of the diagnosis of varicella, as the IHA antibody response may not be detectable for several weeks after onset. However, reactive antibody, once present, is reported as being persistent; the method may be useful in the assessment of the immunologic status of adults.

Immune adherence hemagglutination (IAHA). The IAHA test, recently adapted to the detection of V-Z antibody (27, 42), is an indirect measure of V-Z antigen-antibody union occurring in the presence of complement and fresh human "O" RBC; the union activates the third component of complement (C'3), and the cells agglutinate because of their C'3 receptors. The new procedure utilizes a sonicated culture-derived V-Z antigen that is stable in the frozen state. It is useful for assessment of immune status, and also for the evaluation of antibody content of lots of ZIG.

References

1. ALMEIDA JD, HOWATSON AF, and WILLIAMS MG: Morphology of varicella (chickenpox) virus. Virology 16:353–355, 1962
2. AMIES CR: The elementary bodies of zoster and their serological relationship to those of varicella. Br J Exp Pathol 15:314–319, 1934
3. ARMSTRONG RW and MERIGAN TC: Varicella zoster virus: interferon production and comparative interferon sensitivity in human cell cultures. J Gen Virol 12:53–54, 1971
4. BECKER P, MELNICK JL, and MAYOR HD: A morphologic comparison between the developmental stages of herpes zoster and human cytomegalovirus. Exp Mol Pathol 4:11–23, 1965
5. BLANK H, BURGOON CF, BALDRIDGE GD, MCCARTHY PL, and URBACH F: Cytologic smears in diagnosis of herpes simplex, herpes zoster, and varicella. J Am Med Assoc 146:1410–1412, 1951

6. BLANK H, CORIELL LL, and SCOTT TF MCN: Human skin grafted upon the chorioallantois of the chick embryo for virus cultivation. Proc Soc Exp Biol Med 69:341–345, 1948

7. BOKAY J VON: Über den ätiologischen Zusammenhang der Varizellen mit gewissen Fällen von Herpes zoster. Wein Klin Wochenschr 22:1323–1326, 1909

8. BRAIN RT: The relationship between the viruses of zoster and varicella as documented by the complement-fixation reaction. Br J Exp Pathol 14:67–73, 1933

9. BRUNELL PA: Placental transfer of varicella-zoster antibody. Pediatrics 38:1034–1038, 1966

10. BRUNELL PA: Separation of infectious varicella-zoster virus from human embryonic lung fibroblasts. Virology 31:732–734, 1967

11. BRUNELL PA, GERSHON AA, UDUMAN SA, and STEINBERG S: Varicella-zoster immunoglobulins during varicella, latency, and zoster. J Infect Dis 132:49–54, 1975

12. BRUNELL PA, GRANAT M, and GERSHON AA: The antigens of varicella-zoster virus. J Immunol 108:731–737, 1972

13. BURGOON CF JR, BURGOON JS, and BALDRIDGE GD: The natural history of herpes zoster. J Am Med Assoc 164:265–269, 1957

14. CAUNT AE, RONDLE CJM, and DOWNIE AW: The soluble antigens of varicella-zoster virus produced in tissue culture. J Hyg 59:249–258, 1961

15. CAUNT AE and SHAW DG: Neutralization tests with varicella-zoster virus. J Hyg 67:343–352, 1969

16. CAUNT AE and TAYLOR-ROBINSON D: Cell-free varicella-zoster virus in tissue culture. J Hyg 62:413–424, 1964

17. CHEATHAM WJ, WELLER TH, DOLAN TF, and DOWER JC: Varicella: report of two fatal cases with necropsy, virus isolation, and serologic studies. Am J Pathol 32:1015–1035, 1956

18. COOK ML and STEVENS JG: Replication of varicella-zoster virus in cell culture; an ultrastructural study. J Ultrastruc Res 32:334–350, 1970

19. FELDMAN S and EPP E: Isolation of varicella-zoster virus from blood. J Pediatr 88:265–267, 1976

20. FELSENFELD AD and SCHMIDT NJ: Antigenic relationships among several simian varicella-like viruses and varicella-zoster virus. Infect Immun 15:807–812, 1977

21. FIORETTI A, IWASAKI Y, FURUKAWA T, and PLOTKIN SA: The growth of varicella-zoster virus in guinea pig embryo cells. Proc Soc Exp Biol Med 144:340–344, 1973

22. FURUKAWA T and PLOTKIN SA: Indirect hemagglutination test for varicella-zoster infection. Infect Immun 5:835–839, 1972

23. GARLAND J: Varicella following exposure to herpes zoster. N Engl J Med 228:336–337, 1943

24. GERNA G, ACHILLI G, and CHAMBERS RW: Determination of neutralizing antibody and IgG antibody to varicella-zoster virus and of IgG antibody to membrane antigens by the immunoperoxidase technique. J Infect Dis 135:975–979, 1977

25. GERNA G and CHAMBERS RW: Varicella-zoster plaque assay and plaque reduction neutralization test by the immunoperoxidase technique. J Clin Microbiol 4:437–442, 1976

26. GERSHON A, CASIO L, and BRUNELL P: Varicella-zoster virus: biophysical properties and morphologic observations of a cell-associated herpes-virus. Bacteriol Proc, p 171, 1971

27. GERSHON AA, KALTER ZG, and STEINBERG S: Detection of antibody to varicella-zoster by immune adherence hemagglutination. Proc Soc Exp Biol Med 151:762–765, 1976

28. GERSHON AA and KRUGMAN S: Seroepidemiologic survey of varicella: value of specific fluorescent antibody test. Pediatrics 56:1005–1008, 1975

29. GERSHON AA, STEINBERG S, and SMITH M: Cell-mediated immunity to varicella-zoster virus demonstrated by viral inactivation with human leucocytes. Infect Immun 13:1549–1553, 1976

30. GOLD E: Characteristics of herpes zoster and varicella viruses propagated in vitro. J Immunol 95:683–691, 1965

31. GOLD E: Serologic and virus isolation studies of patients with varicella or herpes-zoster infection. N Engl J Med 274:181–185, 1966

32. GOLD E and GODEK G: Complement fixation studies with a varicella-zoster antigen. J Immunol 95:692–695, 1965

33. GOODPASTURE EW and ANDERSON K: Infection of human skin grafted on the chorioallantois of chick embryos, with the virus of herpes zoster. Am J Pathol 20:447-455, 1944

34. GRANDIEN M, APPELGREN P, ESPMARK A, and HANNGREN K: Determination of varicella immunity by the indirect immunofluorescence test in urgent clinical situations. Scand J Infect Dis 8:65-69, 1976

35. GRANT BD and ROWE CR: Motor paralysis of the extremities in herpes zoster. J Bone Joint Surg 43A:885-896, 1961

36. HARBOUR DA and CAUNT AE: Infection of guinea-pig embryo cells with varicella-zoster virus: Arch Virol 49:39-47, 1975

37. HEAD H and CAMPBELL AW: The pathology of herpes zoster and its bearing on sensory localisation. Brain 23:353-523, 1900

38. HONDO R, SHIBUTA H, and MATUMOTO M: Lyophilization of varicella virus: Arch Gesamte Virusforsch 40:397-399, 1973

39. HONDO R, SHIBUTA H, and MATUMOTO M: An improved plaque assay for varicella virus. Arch Virol 51:355-359, 1973

40. ITO M and BARRON AL: Surface antigens produced by herpesviruses: varicella-zoster virus. Infect Immun 8:48-52, 1973

41. JORDAN GW and MERIGAN TC: Cell-mediated immunity to varicella-zoster virus; in vitro lymphocyte responses. J Infect Dis 130:495-501, 1974

42. KALTER ZG, STEINBERG S, and GERSHON AA: Immune adherence hemagglutination: further observations on demonstration of antibody to varicella-zoster virus. J Infect Dis 135:1010-1013, 1977

43. KAPSENBERG JG: Possible antigenic relationship between varicella-zoster virus and herpes simplex virus. Arch Gesamte Virusforsch. 15:67-73, 1964

44. KISSLING RE, CASEY HL, and PALMER EL: Production of specific varicella antiserum. Appl Microbiol 16:160-162, 1968

45. KUNDRATITZ K: Experimentelle Übertragungen von Herpes zoster auf den Menschen und die Beziehungen von Herpes zoster zu Varicellen. Monatsschr Kinderheilk 29:516-522, 1925

46. LEONARD LL, SCHMIDT NJ, and LENNETTE EH: Demonstration of viral antibody activity in two immunoglobulin G subclasses in patients with varicella-zoster infection. J Immunol 104:23-27, 1970

47. LIPSCHÜTZ B: Untersuchungen über die Ätiologie der Krankheiten der Herpesgruppe (Herpes zoster, Herpes genitalis, Herpes febrilis). Arch Dermatol Syph 136:428-482, 1921

48. LUBY JP, RAMIREZ-RONDA C, RINNER S, HULL, A, and VERGNE-MARINI P: A longitudinal study of varicella-zoster virus infections in renal transplant recipients. J Infect Dis 135:659-663, 1977

49. LUDWIG H, HAINES HG, BISWAL N, and BENYESH-MELNICK M: The characterization of varicella-zoster virus DNA. J Gen Virol 14:111-114, 1972

50. LUTZNER MA: Fine structure of the zoster virus in human skin. J Ultrastruc Res 7:409-417, 1962

51. MANKIKAR SD, PETRIC M, and MIDDLETON PJ: Indirect microhemagglutination test for varicella-zoster antibody determination. Can J Microbiol 22:1245-1251, 1976

52. MARTIN ML and PALMER EL: Complement-fixing antigens produced by varicella-virus in tissue culture. Appl Microbiol 26:410-413, 1973

53. MAY DC, MILLER RL, and RAPP F: The effect of phosphonoacetic acid on the in vitro replication of varicella-zoster virus. Intervirology 8:83-91, 1977

54. MEURISSE EV: Laboratory studies on the varicella-zoster virus. J Med Microbiol 2:317-325, 1969

55. NELSON AM and ST. GEME JW JR: On the respiratory spread of varicella-zoster virus. Pediatrics 37:1007-1009, 1966

56. NETTER A and URBAIN A: Le virus varicello-zonateux. Ann Inst Pasteur 46:17-28, 1931

57. NII S and MAEDA Y: Studies of herpes zoster virus in vitro. I. Isolation of two variants. Biken J 12:219-230, 1969

58. OLDING-STENKVIST E and GRANDIEN M: Early diagnosis of virus-caused vesicular rashes by immunofluorescence on skin biopsies. I. Varicella, zoster, and herpes simplex. Scand J Infect Dis 8:27-35, 1976

59. PLOTKIN SA, FURUKAWA T, and TANAKA S: Growth characteristics of varicella-zoster virus. Fed Proc 33:739, 1974
60. RAPP F: Inhibition by metabolic analogues of plaque formation by herpes zoster and herpes simplex viruses. J Immunol 93:643–648, 1964
61. RAPP F and BENYESH-MELNICK M: Plaque assay for measurement of cells infected with zoster virus. Science 141:433–434, 1963
62. RAPP F and VANDERSLICE D: Spread of zoster virus in human embryonic lung cells and the inhibitory effect of iododeoxyuridine. Virology 22:321–330, 1964
63. RAWLS W, COHEN RA, and HERRMANN EC: Inhibition of varicella virus by 5-iodo-2-deoxyuridine. Proc Soc Exp Biol Med 115:123–127, 1964
64. RIFKIND D: The activation of varicella-zoster virus infections by immunosuppressive therapy. J Lab Clin Med 68:463–474, 1966
65. RIVERS TM: Nuclear inclusions in the testicles of monkeys injected with tissue of human varicella lesions. J Exp Med 43:275–288, 1926
66. ROSS CAC and MCDAID R: Specific IgM antibody in serum of patients with herpes zoster infections. Br Med J 4:522–523, 1972
67. ROSS CAC, SUBAK-SHARPE JH, and FERRY P: Antigenic relationship of varicella-zoster herpes simplex. Lancet 2:708–711, 1965
68. RUCKDESCHEL JC, SCHIMPFF SC, SMYTH AC, and MARDINEY MR: Herpes zoster and impaired cell-associated immunity to the varicella-zoster virus in patients with Hodgkin's disease. Am J Med 62:77–85, 1977
69. RUSSELL AS, MAINI RA, BAILEY M, and DUMONDE DC: Cell-mediated immunity to varicella-zoster antigen in acute herpes zoster (Shingles). Clin Exp Immunol 14:181–185, 1973
70. SARGENT EN, CARSON MJ, and REILLY ED: Roentgenographic manifestations of varicella pneumonia with postmortem correlation. Am J Roentgenol 93:305–317, 1966
71. SCHAAP GJP and HUISMAN J: Simultaneous rise in complement-fixing antibodies against *Herpesvirus hominis* and varicella-zoster virus. Arch Gesamte Virusforsch 25:52–57, 1968
72. SCHMIDT NJ: Varicella-zoster virus *In* Manual of Clinical Microbiology, 2nd edition Lennette EH, Spaulding EH, and Truant JP, (eds) Am Soc Microbiol, Washington, DC 1974
73. SCHMIDT NJ, DENNIS J, and LENNETTE EH: Complement-fixing reactivity of varicella-zoster virus subunit antigens with sera from homotypic infections and heterotypic herpes simplex virus infections. Infect Immun 15:850–854, 1977
74. SCHMIDT NJ, HO HH, and LENNETTE EH: Comparative sensitivity of human fetal diploid kidney cell strains and monkey kidney cell cultures for isolation of certain human viruses. Am J Clin Pathol 43:297–301, 1965
75. SCHMIDT NJ and LENNETTE EH: Neutralizing antibody responses to varicella-zoster virus. Infect Immun 12:606–613, 1975
76. SCHMIDT NJ and LENNETTE EH: Improved yields of cell-free varicella-zoster virus. Infect Immun 14:709–715, 1976
77. SCHMIDT NJ, LENNETTE EH, and MAGOFFIN RL: Immunological relationship between herpes simplex and varicella-zoster viruses demonstrated by complement fixation, neutralization and fluorescent antibody. J Gen Virol 4:321–328, 1969
78. SCHMIDT NJ, LENNETTE EH, WOODIE JD, and HO HH: Immunofluorescent staining in the laboratory diagnosis of varicella-zoster virus infections. J Lab Clin Med 66:403–412, 1964
79. ŠEFČOVIČOVÁ L: Varicella-zoster virus cultivation in cell-cultures of non-primate origin. Acta Virologica 15:171–173, 1971
80. SLACK PM and TAYLOR-ROBINSON D: The influence of mycoplasmas on the cytopathic effect of varicella virus. Arch Gesamte Virusforsch 42:88–95, 1973
81. SLOTNICK VB and ROSANOFF E: Localization of varicella virus in tissue culture. Virology 19:589–592, 1963
82. SÖLTZ-SZÖTS J: Virologische und serologische Untersuchengen beim Herpes zoster. Arch Klin Exp Dermatol 220:105–128, 1964
83. STEVENS DA, FERRINGTON RA, JORDON GW, and MERIGAN TC: Cellular events in zoster vesicles: relation to clinical course and immune parameters. J Infect Dis 131:509–515, 1975

84. SVEDMYR A: Varicella virus in hela cells. Arch Gesamte Virusforsch 17:495–503, 1965
85. TAKAHASHI M and OSAME J: Serial propagation of varicella virus in primary rabbit kidney. Biken J 16:81–84, 1973
86. TAYLOR-ROBINSON D: Chickenpox and herpes zoster. III. Tissue culture studies. Br J Exp Pathol 40:521–532, 1959
87. TAYLOR-ROBINSON D and DOWNIE AW: Chickenpox and herpes zoster. I. Complement fixation studies. Br J Exp Pathol 40:398–409, 1959
88. TAYLOR-ROBINSON D and RONDLE CJM: Chickenpox and herpes zoster. II. Ouchterlony precipitation studies. Br J Exp Pathol 40:517–520, 1959
89. TRLIFAJOVÁ J, RYBA M, and JELINEK J: Indirect hemagglutination reaction (IH)—The method of choice for the detection of anamnestic antibodies to varicella-zoster (VZ) virus. J Hyg Epidemiol Microbiol Immunol 20:101–106, 1976
90. TRLIFAJOVÁ J, SOUREK J, and RYBA M: Antigenic relationship between varicella-herpes zoster and herpes simplex viruses studied by the gel precipitation reaction. Acta Virol 15:293–300, 1971
91. TYZZER EE. The histology of the skin lesions in varicella. Philipp J Sci 1:349–372, 1906
92. UDUMAN SA, GERSHON AA, and BRUNELL PA: Rapid diagnosis of varicella-zoster infections by agar-gel diffusion. J Infect Dis 126:193–195, 1972
93. WEBER DM and PELLECCHIA JA: Varicella pneumonia. Study of prevalence in adult men. J Am Med Assoc 192:572–573, 1965
94. WELLER TH: Serial propagation in vitro of agents producing inclusion bodies derived from varicella and herpes zoster. Proc Soc Exp Biol Med 83:340–346, 1953
95. WELLER TH: Varicella-herpes zoster virus In Viral Infections of Humans, Evans AS (ed) Plenum Medical Book Company, NY, 1976, pp 457–480
96. WELLER TH and COONS AH: Fluorescent antibody studies with agents of varicella and herpes zoster propagated in vitro. Proc Soc Exp Biol Med 86:789–794, 1954
97. WELLER TH and WITTON HM: The etiologic agents of varicella and herpes zoster. Serologic studies with the viruses as propagated in vitro. J Exp Med 108:869–890, 1958
98. WELLER TH, WITTON HM, and BELL EJ: The etiologic agents of varicella and herpes zoster. Isolation, propagation, and cultural characteristics in vitro. J Exp Med 108:843–868, 1958
99. WENNER HA, ABEL D, BARRICK S, and SESHUMURTY P: Clinical and pathogenetic studies of Medical Lake macaque virus infection in cynomologous monkeys (Simian varicella). J Infect Dis 135:611–622, 1977
100. WENNER HA, BARRICK S, ABEL D, and SESHUMURTY P: The pathogenesis of simian varicella virus in cynomologous monkeys. Proc Soc Exp Biol Med 150:318–323, 1975
101. WHITLEY RJ, CHIEN LT, DOLIN R, GALASSO GJ, ALFORD CA JR, (editors) and the collaborative study group: Adenine arabinoside therapy of herpes zoster in the immunosuppressed. NIAID collaborative study. N Engl J Med 294:1193–1199, 1976
102. WILLIAMS MG, ALMEIDA JD, and HOWATSON AF: Electron microscopic studies on viral skin lesions. A simple and rapid method of identifying virus particles. Arch Dermatol 86:290–297, 1962
103. WILLIAMS V, GERSHON A, and BRUNELL PA: Serologic response to varicella-zoster membrane antigens measured by indirect immunofluorescence. J Infect Dis 130:669–672, 1974
104. YUCEOGLU AM, BERKOVICH S, and MINKOWITZ S: Acute glomerulonephritis as a complication of varicella. J Am Med Assoc 202:879–881, 1967

CHAPTER 13

LABORATORY DIAGNOSIS OF CYTOMEGALOVIRUS INFECTIONS

David W. Reynolds, Sergio Stagno,
and Charles A. Alford

Introduction

Cytomegaloviruses (CMV) comprise a group of agents within the herpesvirus family known for their widespread distribution in humans and in numerous other mammals. *In vivo* and *in vitro* infections with these viruses are highly species-specific and result in a characteristic cytopathology of greatly enlarged (cytomegalic) cells containing intranuclear and cytoplasmic inclusions. The old terminology of "salivary gland virus" stems from the frequency with which pathognomonic cytomegalic cells were detected by pathologists in salivary glands of infected children and also of lower animals. Human cytomegalovirus (HCMV) infection has also been termed "cytomegalic inclusion disease" indicating the first etiologic association with a disseminated disease of the newborn.

For many years the diagnosis of CMV infection of humans was entirely dependent on histologic study of postmortem tissues. Diagnosis during life was not achieved until the introduction of exfoliative cytology as a laboratory tool for the detection of pathognomonic cells in the urine of infants with cytomegalic inclusion disease (24, 72). The isolation and propagation *in vitro* of HCMV (94, 107, 137) provided not only a further means of detecting infection during life, but also served as a basis for the development of diagnostic serologic procedures.

Extensive application of these diagnostic tools to human populations has established that CMV infection, largely inapparent, is quite common (64, 135). Moreover, persistent excretion occurs in the face of specific antibody, especially in infancy (61, 73, 75, 112). These findings together with the recent documentation of recurrent episodes of virus excretion in adults (11, 45, 91) indicate the need for caution in interpreting the clinical significance of positive laboratory findings. Still unresolved is the question of whether recurrences represent reactivation of latent or low-grade persistent infection, reinfections or combinations thereof. Central to the resolution of this latter concern is a clear definition of the antigenic and genetic variability of HCMV. Techniques are now available for investigation of this

399

problem (48). Answers from such molecular epidemiologic studies should shed light not only on the relative roles of reactivation and reinfection in transmission but also on the role of strain differences as virulence factors.

Clinical and epidemiologic aspects of infection

Clinical syndromes. The clinical manifestations of HCMV infection vary with the age at acquisition as well as the immune competence of the individual. The great majority of persons acquiring primary infection suffer no acute illness irrespective of age. *Congenital infection* is no exception. Ninety-five percent or more of offspring infected *in utero* have no apparent disease at birth (75, 93, 115). With severe intrauterine infection, death can supervene *in utero* or in the neonatal period; however, even in diseased infants, death is uncommon. Instead they have one or usually more of the following signs or symptoms: jaundice with hepatosplenomegaly, thrombocytopenic purpura, and intrauterine growth retardation. Less commonly, overt organ system involvement includes pneumonitis, microcephaly with or without periventricular calcifications, chorioretinitis, optic atrophy, inguinal hernias (males), and brachial arch abnormalities. Various degrees of psychomotor retardation become manifest in early life in the majority of children with overt disease at birth and sensorineural hearing loss, often profound and occasionally progressive is relatively common (9, 73, 74). The prognosis for the silently infected newborn must also be guarded. Ten to 25 percent of these neonates may later develop sensorineural hearing deficits and 5–10% may suffer from various degrees of psychomotor disability (43, 75, 93). Because of the high incidence of congenital CMV, 0.5% to 2.5% of newborn populations, precisely defining the long-term outcome of the silent intrauterine infection is an important public health consideration (43, 111).

Infection in the neonatal period rarely results in clinical illness. A protracted pneumonitis syndrome has been associated with primary infection in this age group (139).

Postnatal infection as documented serologically becomes increasingly prevalent with advancing age. While HCMV has been implicated in the genesis of dysfunction in virtually every organ system, well-established clinical syndromes are few. A heterophil antibody-negative mononucleosis syndrome occurs spontaneously in adults (51, 61) and can develop following infection acquired by blood transfusion at any age (65, 87, 125). In contrast to the Epstein-Barr virus (EBV)-induced syndrome, tonsillopharyngitis, lymphadenopathy, and splenomegaly are usually absent. Individuals with immune suppression, whether iatrogenically or naturally induced, are subject to illness ranging from pneumonitis (most common), hepatitis, or fever with leukopenia, as isolated entities, to generalized disease often associated with a fatal outcome (1, 27, 104, 108). In immunosuppressed patients, the relative contributions of primary and recurrent infection in the production of disease remains to be clearly determined, although the former is seemingly more important at least in transplant recipients (11, 45). In contrast to the fetal disorder, injuries to the central nervous system and perceptual organs are uncommon with postnatal infection (82).

Incidence, period of infectivity, and mode of transmission. The incidence of HCMV infection is inversely related to socioeconomic status (64). In underdeveloped countries, virtually everyone has acquired the infection by young adulthood (64), and higher infection rates have been found in socially disadvantaged groups in developed nations (117). In this country, fetal infection occurs in as many as 2% of offspring of low-income mothers (111); rates among the infants of middle- and upper-income groups are significantly less (13, 43). On the average, congenital CMV occurs in 1% of newborn populations in developed nations. Acquisition in the newborn period can be as high as 10% in low-socioeconomic settings in this country (92). Prevalence studies from Japan and Finland demonstrated active infection in 60% and 34%, respectively, of 6-month-old infants of middle-income families (69, 83). The reasons for the higher rates seen in these populations relative to those observed in this country are unclear. Beyond early infancy there is a gradual increase in infection rates. In the United States between 50% and 90% of the adult population, depending on living standards, have antibody to HCMV (64). Active infection in adults, as determined by virus excretion in urine and genital secretions, is likewise prevalent varying from 2% to 20% in the adult female populations studied (13, 83, 92). The rate of virus shedding among adult males has not been as accurately defined. Two large-scale studies found the rates of urinary excretion in men to be less than 3% (52, 117). Excretion among adult females is usually due to recurrent rather than primary infection (83, 92).

A unique feature of HCMV infection is the long persistence of viral excretion, at least from the urinary tract. Congenitally and neonatally infected children shed virus from this site for years, (75, 112) and adults with CMV mononucleosis can excrete the virus for many months (61). Comparable periods of infectivity following inapparent infection at any age are probable although not well documented. Thus, persistent excretion and recurrent episodes of shedding from peripheral sites provide this virus with a unique ability to maintain itself in human populations. The duration of viremia following primary or recurrent infection is not well established; the frequency of infection following blood transfusion suggests that it may be prolonged. Efforts to document viremia among blood donors, however, have produced mostly negative results (20, 52, 79).

Transmission of infection from mother to fetus can occur not only as a consequence of primary maternal infection during pregnancy but also following a recurrent episode. In fact, in highly seroimmune pregnant populations, the latter event may be more common than the former (111). This observation raises serious questions about the potential efficacy of a vaccine designed to prevent fetal infection (84).

The exact sequence of events attending intrauterine transmission remains unclear. Blood-borne spread to the placenta and, ultimately, to the fetus is generally accepted. Whether local reactivation or reinfection in the genital tract of the mother with contiguous spread to the conceptus is also a possible route of transmission awaits clarification.

Transmission from mother to offspring at the time of birth via contact with infected maternal genital secretions is now reasonably well established (92). Infection may also be acquired by the neonate or young infant secondary to the ingestion of virus-containing breast milk (92). With known exposure in these two situations the attack rate approximates 50% (92). The possibility for nosocomial spread of this infection within nurseries or other units within the hospital is poorly defined.

Beyond the neonatal period, there is minimal information on the routes of natural transmission. Based on the frequent shedding of virus in oropharyngeal secretions of children and the high attack rates, it is reasonable to presume that respiratory spread is a common event in this age group and likely plays a role in adult infection as well. Direct contact with infected urine may also be an important mode of acquiring infection for individuals so exposed, i.e., young children and their adult caretakers. HCMV is frequently shed in genital secretions by adult females (83, 92) and to a lesser extent by adult males (66). In the latter group, high levels of virus and prolonged excretion are characteristic. These findings plus comparative infection rates among sexually promiscuous, celibate, and control female populations suggest that the infection may be sexually transmitted (18, 50).

Iatrogenic primary infection has been clearly shown to occur following blood transfusion, the risk of which is directly related to the amount transfused (87). It has been postulated that blood transfusion may also activate latent infection via an inapparent graft versus host reaction. Active infection as documented by virus excretion and/or rises in specific antibody titer commonly occurs in organ transplant patients and other immunosuppressed individuals. Among the former group, clear evidence establishing the role of the donor organ as a source of primary infection has been obtained (11, 45). Reactivation of latent infection secondary to debilitation of cell-mediated immunity (21) and/or the introduction of foreign antigens (blood, donor organs) is commonly observed in immunosuppressed patients. Whether exogenous reinfection plays a role in recurrent episodes observed in such patients or normal individuals remains a moot point at present. From the foregoing, it becomes obvious that a much clearer definition of the natural history of primary and recurrent HCMV infections is required in order to appropriately design chemotherapeutic and preventive programs. The antigenic heterogeneity, multiple sources and routes of transmission, and the peculiar host-virus relationship make this undertaking a very challenging one.

Pathology

Pathological assessments have been confined until recently to histopathologic searches for CMV inclusion-bearing cells in various organs. Such studies document the presence of virus in virtually every organ with the lungs, kidney, liver, intestine, and brain (neonates) being most prominently involved (70, 74, 77). Within organs, only a minority of cells appear to be involved. With the use of the fluorescent-antibody (FA) assay and the more sophisticated autoradiographic methods for detecting evidence of the viral genome (48), the infection is apparently much more widespread than indicated by classic staining techniques. Widespread involvement of the acoustical structures of the inner ear, including nerve tissue in cases of fatal congenital infection, was recently demonstrated by FA, thus providing a pathologic correlate of the sensorineural hearing loss seen in survivors with this infection (110). In the kindney, virus replication is apparently confined to the cells of the distal convoluted and collecting tubules (48).

While epithelial cells, especially in the kidneys, liver, lungs, pancreas and salivary glands, are prominently involved, similar changes may occur in endothelial and connective tissue cells. In the generalized disease of infancy, an associated focal or diffuse inflammatory cell infiltrate occurs; hepatitis is the rule. The brain may be extensively damaged, with focal necrosis and calcification most marked in the subependymal areas. In immunosuppressed patients, the lung is the major target organ and the inflammatory response is less marked (77).

The mechanism(s) by which HCMV induces pathology have not been precisely defined. Clearly, direct viral cytolysis is one such possibility. Direct injury to the vasculature with ischemic necrosis is rarely seen. Other possibilities include antibody-complement and antibody-lymphocyte mediated immune lysis of infected cells, T-lymphocyte cytotoxicity and injury attending deposition of circulating immune complexes. There is no direct evidence for involvement of any of these mechanisms; however, recently, immune complexes were demonstrated in the blood and glomeruli of congenitally infected infants, clearly suggesting a possible pathologic role for these moieties (113). In contrast to being harmful, normal T-lymphocyte responsiveness is likely a major prerequisite for the containment of this infection. This is suggested by experimental infection in animals (32, 114), as well as by the virulence of the infection in patients with suppression of cell-mediated immunity.

Oncogenic potential

Like its kindred viruses, herpes simplex (HSV) and Epstein-Barr (EBV), HCMV has been shown to have oncogenic potential. Both infected permissive and nonpermissive host cells are stimulated to increase DNA and RNA synthesis (95, 121)—a feature shared by other known oncogenic DNA viruses. Of more importance is the documentation that ultraviolet (UV)-irridated HCMV transformed hamster embryo fibroblasts and clones from these transformants proved oncogenic for weanling hamsters (2). More direct evidence suggesting that HCMV may be oncogenic for humans has recently been obtained. A clinical isolate recovered from prostate tissue of a 3-year-old boy induced transformation of human embryo fibroblasts. These transformants were oncogenic for weanling athymic nude mice producing poor differentiated tumors (34). The presence of a functioning HCMV genome in the transformed heterologous and homologous cells, as well as the tumor cells that they induced, was established by the detection of surface and intracellular HCMV-specific antigens by FA. Since the majority of the population becomes infected by HCMV in early life, proving an etiologic role for cancer in humans will be difficult.

Description and Nature of Cytomegalovirus

Size and morphology

Morphologically, the HCMV virion is typical of the other herpesviruses and is, therefore, quite similar to the virions of HSV, varicella-zoster virus V-Z, or EBV (106, 140). Following negative staining and electron microscopic analysis the virion is shown to consist of a 64-nm core enclosed by a 110-nm icosahedral capsid with 162 capsomeres (105, 140). Complete particles are surrounded by a double membrane envelope and measure approximately 180 nm in diameter. The typical core is comprised of aggregates of globular subunits, although a toroidal configuration has been observed in naked nucleocapsids in human tumor cells (39).

Electron microscopic (EM) studies of infected human fibroblasts (49, 105) demonstrate capsids with and without cores in skein-like nuclear inclusions. Acquisition of an envelope occurs by budding through the inner lamella of the nuclear membrane or through the membrane of cytoplasmic vacuoles. An additional viral structure, the dense body, consisting of a homogeneous electron-dense sphere enclosed in a double membrane identical to that of mature virions is also found in the cytoplasmic vacuoles from which it derives its membrane. These particles measure 250–500 nm in diameter.

Chemical composition

The genome of HCMV is DNA which is linear in configuration with a length ranging from 56 nm to 76 nm (35, 58, 98). There are apparently 2 species of DNA, a larger one with an approximate molecular weight of 150×10^6 daltons and a smaller one of 100×10^6 daltons (35, 58). The envelope of the virion contains essential lipid (94). Twenty-three to 33 structural proteins with molecular weights ranging from 11,000 to 290,000 have been detected (25, 60, 97, 118). Eight of these proteins are glycosylated and reside in the envelope (118). The dense bodies contain a qualitatively similar complement of polypeptides but lack DNA (25, 97).

Reaction to chemical and physical agents

HCMV is completely inactivated by exposure to 20% ether for 2 hr (94), to pH of less than 5, to 56 C for 30 min (137), or to UV light for 5 min (2). The addition of 5–10% serum to the diluent stabilizes the virus at 37 C but not at 4 C (130). Infectivity is better preserved at each temperature when the virus is suspended in distilled water or medium without $NaHCO_3$ (130). Strain variability relative to inactivation at 4 C has been observed.

CMV does not withstand freezing and thawing or storage at −20 to −50 C without stabilizers (137). The infectivity of cell-free virus is best preserved by storage in $NaHCO_3$ free diluent at −90 C in the presence of 35% sorbitol (129). Virus infected cells suspended in Eagle minimal essential medium (MEM) with 10–20% serum and 10% dimethylsulfoxide (DMSO) can be stored with minimal loss of infectivity indefinitely in liquid nitrogen (−190 C).

The growth of HCMV in permissive cells is inhibited by all DNA inhibitors, rifampicin (31), phosphonoacetic acid (46), and interferon (86). HCMV induces little or no interferon *in vitro* (38).

Antigenic characteristics

Following infection, antibodies of the IgG, IgM and IgA classes can be detected using a variety of serologic tests. Antigens responsible for the various antibodies have not been precisely defined. However, 2 complement-fixing (CF) antigens have been described, a soluble and a viral associated component (17, 59, 131). The soluble antigen contains at least 2 polypeptides with molecular weights of 66,000 and 140,000 daltons. The smaller moeity is glycosylated and hyperimmune animal serum prepared against it does not neutralize homologous virus (131). Soluble antigen is stable at 4 C and withstands repeated cycles of freezing and thawing but marked loss of potency occurs at 37 C or with boiling (59). The virus-associated CF antigen extracted by glycine buffer treatment of infected cells appears to derive its antigenicity primarily from nucleocapsids (17). Both antigens develop primarily after viral DNA replication and are mostly cell associated. Supernatant fluids from infected cell cultures contain minimal amounts of CF antigen.

Antigens responsible for neutralizing-antibody production are found in the envelopes of mature virions and dense bodies and are likely glycoproteins (118). Antiserum prepared against purified virion and dense-body membrane glycoproteins neutralize infectivity and react with cytoplasm and membranes of infected cells in indirect fluorescent-antibody (IFA) tests, yet elicit no fluorescence of the membranes of uninfected cells (118). Thus, it is doubtful that host-cell membrane antigens are incorporated into the virion envelope to any significant extent. Neither hemagglutinating nor hemabsorbing antigens are elaborated.

Previous data (5) using human serum suggested, and recent work confirmed, that HCMV possesses a broad antigenic mosaic. Examination of the DNA of 5 laboratory strains as well as 6 clinical isolates by DNA-DNA reassociation kinetics indicated that, while all shared at least 80% homology, none were identical (48). A similar spectrum of DNA content of the strains was found by restriction enzyme analysis using Echo RI and Hind III (48). No genetic grouping of strains was possible by these procedures. Hyperimmune animal serum prepared against these 11 strains likewise confirmed the antigenic heterogeneity when each was cross-reacted in the CF test (48). A few strains failed to elicit cross-reacting antibody suggesting the need to use a broadly reactive antigen, i.e., AD 169 strain, for diagnostic work (5, 48). One instance of complete homology between different strains was recently reported (111). These 2 strains were isolated from consecutive siblings with congenital CMV infection.

Biologic differences between strains have received little systematic evaluation. It is generally accepted that Davis and AD 169 laboratory strains cause distinctively different cytopathic effects.

Murine CMV and HCMV have no serologic cross-reactivity. A one-way cross-reaction between normal simian serum and certain HCMV strains has been observed in both the CF and neutralization (Nt) assays (78). Hyperimmune serum raised in simians and goats against both human and simian strains, however, reveal strict species specificity in the Nt test (41). Recently, cross-reactivity between immune human serum and simian CMV-infected human cells has been observed by the FA technique (120). Thus, human and simian strains share various degrees of antigenic similarity.

Host range

All attempts to infect animals with HCMV have failed. Likewise, productive infection of heterologous cell systems has not been achieved. Abortive infection occurs in a variety of nonhuman cells, including mouse, bovine, hamster, and guinea pig fibroblasts, as well as Vero cells (14, 133). Induction of late antigens and productive infection in infected mouse fibroblasts by 5-indo-2'-deoxyuridine (IUDR) treatment suggests that a functioning host-cell genome is required for suppression (14). Productive infection of human fibroblast cells is likewise enhanced by pretreatment with IUDR (96).

Successful *in vitro* propagation of CMV is in general limited to homologous fibroblast cells. Exceptions have been documented, the most notable of which is the growth of CMV from the Cercopithecus monkey in human fibroblasts (22). This affinity for fibroblastic cells *in vitro* is in contrast to the more frequently observed involvement of epithelial tissue in humans.

Growth in tissue culture

Cell system

Although limited growth of HCMV in homologous epithelial cells has been observed (76, 126, 128), the virus is most successfully isolated and propagated in homologous fibroblast cells. For diagnostic work, the tissue of origin of the fibroblast is apparently of little consequence; various tissues, including embryonic skin, muscle, lung, testis, foreskin, and myometrium, have been used successfully. Serially propagated diploid strains of embryonic fibroblasts (such as WI-38) can be purchased commercially. However, high passages of these cell lines may have too short a lifespan to be ideal for isolation of HCMV. A readily available tissue source is neonatal foreskin. In our hands, foreskin cells can be propagated for diagnostic use through the tenth and fifteenth passage after which sensitivity and cell longevity become unreliable.

Virus-cell interaction (cytopathic effect; fluorescence and electron microscopic analysis)

The virus-cell interaction varies depending on whether the virus strain is laboratory adapted or a recent clinical isolate. Fresh isolates must be serially passed *in vitro* in order to adapt the strains for extracellular virus production. The mechanism responsible for the change in replicative ability is unknown.

Laboratory adapted strains. In infected monolayers fixed with Bouin solution and stained with hematoxylin and eosin (53), cell enlargement and/ or rounding (strain dependent) is visualized within 6 hr after infection. By 24 hr, the nucleus is eccentrically placed with prominent nucleoli. An eosinophilic paranuclear inclusion develops and cell enlargement is more apparent. Between 48 and 72 hr following infection, an irregular skein-like basophilic nuclear inclusion appears. The cytoplasm stains more basophilic, and the eosinophilic paranuclear inclusion is more prominent. Occasionally, smaller and denser eosinophilic inclusions with distinct margins are observed in the cytoplasm. Multinucleated cells can be seen with the inclusion bearing nuclei arranged concentrically around the large eosinophilic inclusion. Cytopathology at the level of the individual cell is little influenced by the multiplicity of input; however, multi-nucleation, presumably occurring by cell fusion, is observed more frequently with large inocula of virus. Two prototype laboratory strains, Davis and AD 169, cause clear differences in cytopathic affect (CPE) (see Fig 13.1 and 13.2). The Davis strain causes early cell rounding, margination and reniform distortion of the nucleus, and the development of a single very prominent eosinophilic paranuclear inclusion. In contrast, AD 169 infected cells retain their fibroblastic shape. Nuclear morphology is likewise preserved except for margination and the paranuclear inclusions formed are less distinct and often biopolar. Nuclear inclusions produced by each strain tend to conform to the shape of the cell nucleus but are otherwise indistinguishable. In our experience, the great majority of clinical isolates are of the Davis type.

EM analysis (49, 105, 106) of virus replication reveals that virions and dense bodies enter the cell either by fusion of the envelope with the cell membrane or are uncoated following phagocytosis. Nucleocapsids can be visualized in the vicinity of the nuclear membrane within minutes after entry. The early eosinophilic paranuclear inclusion is composed of small vesicles, smooth endoplasmic reticulum, and mitochondria. Progeny virus in the form of nucleocapsids, with or without cores, appear in the nuclear inclusion between 48 and 72 hr after infection. Margination of nucleoli which appear to project into the inclusion is a prominent feature of this stage. Envelopment takes place either at the inner leaflet of the nuclear membrane or by budding into cytoplasmic vacuoles. Cytoplasmic envelopment of virions and dense bodies (which appear *de novo* in the cytoplasm) occurs primarily in the paranuclear eosinophilic inclusion. The smaller, randomly placed inclusion contains only virions and dense bodies surrounded by a limiting membrane. Exit of mature virions and dense bodies from the cell apparently takes place via ostia from the vacuoles and connecting microtubules.

According to sequential IFA analysis in our hands (Fig 13.3A–D), a homogeneous nuclear fluorescence appears within 1-3 hr after inoculation of HCMV in fibroblast cells. By 24 hr, aggregates of antigen appear in the nucleus, the cytoplasm stains diffusely, and a paranuclear inclusion is easily identified. Viral DNA replication at 48-72 hr after infection is accompanied by a prominent staining for the newly formed nuclear inclusion, as well as the perinuclear cytoplasmic inclusion. Pseudopodic extensions of the cytoplasm are frequently observed, and nuclear fluorescence in adjacent cells

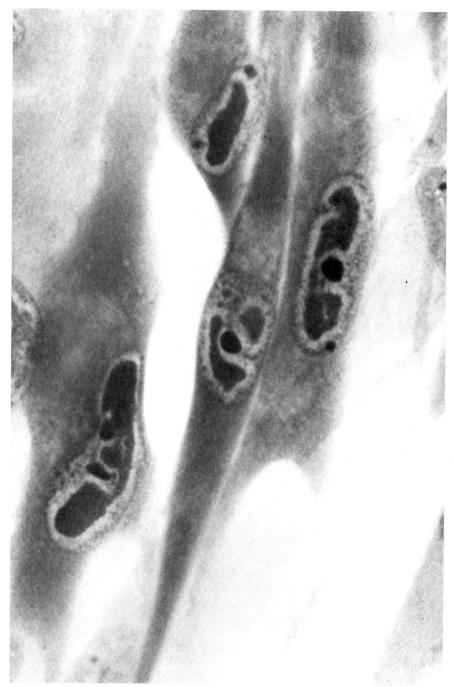

Figure 13.1—Cytopathic effect of the AD 169 strain of HCMV in human foreskin fibroblasts; focal lesion. Hematoxylin—eosin stain, 500X.

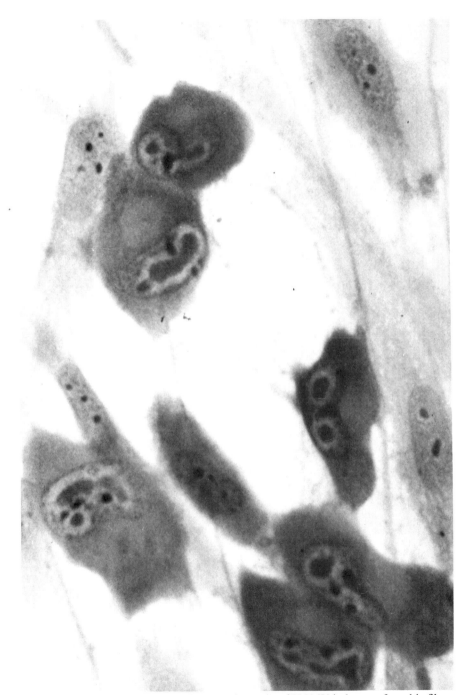

Figure 13.2—Cytopathic effect of the Davis strain of HCMV in human foreskin fibro-blasts; focal lesion. Hematoxylin—eosin stain, 500X.

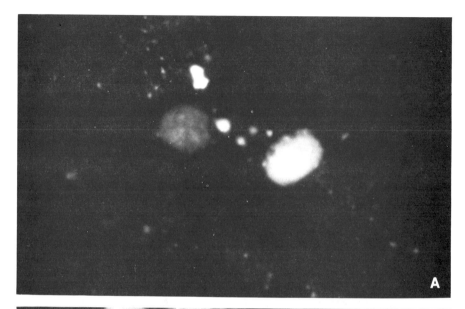

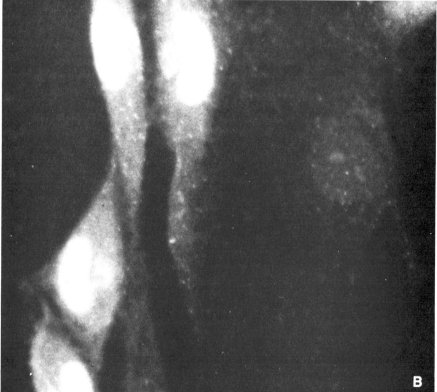

Figure 13.3 A and B—Development of HCMV antigens in infected monolayers of fibroblasts as detected by antihuman IgG; stain AD 169. A) 3 hr after infection, immune human serum; B) 24 hr after infection, immune human serum.

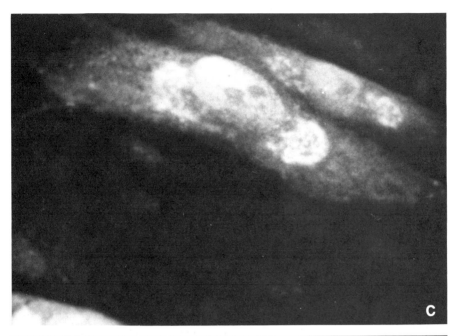

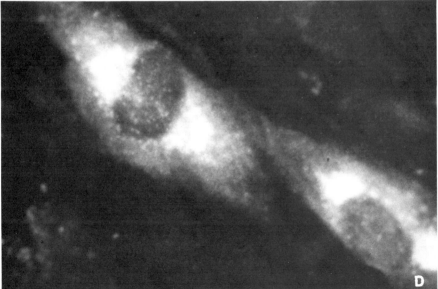

Figure 13.3 C and D—Development of HCMV antigens in infected monolayers of fibroblasts as detected by antihuman IgG immunofluoresence; strain AD 169. C) 72 hr after infection, immune human serum; D) 72 hr after infection, nonimmune human serum. Magnification 400X.

indicates extracellular spread of the infection. At approximately 24 hr after infection, a receptor for the Fc portion of IgG develops in the cytoplasm, (57, 138). Concomitant with viral DNA synthesis, these receptors appear as diffuse cytoplasmic fluorescence with discrete aggregates in the area of the perinuclear viral inclusion. Infection in the presence of DNA inhibitors prevents the synthesis of the perinuclear portion of this structure. Fc receptors are also synthesized on the surface of viable HCMV infected cells in a similar time sequence (138).

Clinical isolates. A light microscope and EM study of an unadapted, wild strain revealed cellular changes similar to those described above with several important exceptions (53, 54). Most cytoplasmic nucleocapsids had incomplete cores, and the paranuclear cytoplasmic inclusion was surrounded by lysosomes. In addition, early cell death from lysis supervened. The contribution of defective virion formation and lysosomal injury to the observed inability of fresh isolates to immediately adapt to extracellular virus production seems apparent but awaits definition.

Clinical specimens containing HCMV produce characteristic CPE within hours to weeks following inoculation depending on the amount of virus present. Initially, the CPE consists of small, round, or elongated foci of enlarged, refractile cells (Fig 13.4A). Most clinical isolates produce early and marked cell rounding. Often the affected cells have brownish refractile granules. Spread of infection in the monolayers is quite slow, involving adjacent cells first. Foci thus gradually enlarge (Fig 13.4B), often with central degeneration; satellite foci usually form, but rarely does the initial infection progress to involve the entire monolayer unless the inoculum was quite large (Fig 13.4C). This slowly developing process may last for several weeks to months. When large quantities of HCMV are in the inoculum, generalized cell rounding may appear within 24 hr.

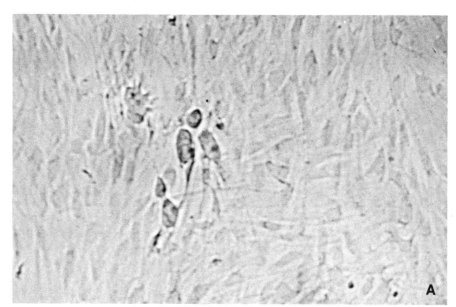

Figure 13.4A—Cytopathic effect of clinical isolates of HCMV in human foreskin fibroblasts, unstained preparation. A) Early focus, 5 days after inoculation.

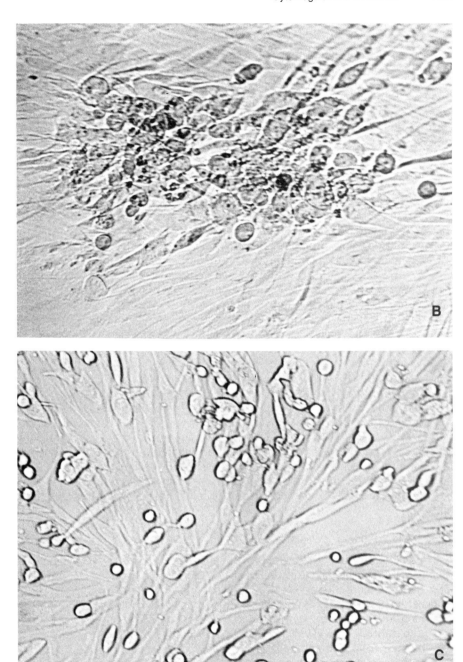

Figure 13.4 B and C—Cytopathic effect of clinical isolates of HCMV in human foreskin fibroblasts; unstained preparations. B) Advanced focus,
14 days after inoculation; C) High multiplicity of infection, 5
days after inoculation.

Virus propagation and storage

To assure continued survival of the strain, early passage of intact infected cells is recommended. This can be accomplished in two ways depending on the condition of the uninfected cells in the monolayers. Assuming good longevity for the monolayer, the simplest method is make a cell suspension and replate in fresh growth medium (MEM supplemented with 10% calf serum, glutamine 2 mM/ml and gentamicin 50 μg/ml). This provides for a substantial increase in infected to uninfected cell contact with subsequent cell-to-cell spread. In contrast, senescent monolayers should be dispersed and fed onto or co-cultivated with fresh, uninfected cells. Monodispersion is achieved by washing and flooding the cell monolayer with an equal mixture of 0.2% EDTA and 0.25% trypsin. The dispersing agent is removed and the monolayers incubated at 37 C for 5 min in the residual fluid. Immediately thereafter, medium is added and the individual cells replated according to one of the following procedures. For feeder cultures, the infected cell suspension in maintenance medium (MM) (medium No. 199 supplemented with 2-5% calf serum, glutamine 2 mM/ml and gentamicin 50 μg/ml) is allowed to settle onto washed preformed cell monolayers. Fresh MM is replaced after 2 hr in order to remove nonviable cells. Co-cultivation with an uninfected cell suspension is carried out in growth medium and the cell mixture is allowed to form a monolayer in an appropriate vessel over a 24-hr period at which time growth is replaced with MM. Ratios of infected to uninfected cells, as well as appropriate passage intervals, are best gauged by the degree of CPE and condition of the uninvolved cells in the monolayers.

Infectivity can be best preserved in early passages by storing viable, infected cells in liquid nitrogen at −190 C. Infected monolayers are dispersed and the cells resuspended in medium with 20% fetal calf serum and 10% DMSO in glass vials. Specimens are frozen at −20 C for 1 hr, placed at −70 C overnight, and transferred to liquid nitrogen the following day. Although infectivity can be maintained at −70 C for variable periods, storage at the lower temperatures is clearly superior. Virus cultivation from cryopreserved infected cells is carried out by feeder culture or co-cultivation techniques.

Preparation of cell-free virus stocks

For quantitative laboratory work, cell-free virus stocks are mandatory. Such stocks can be harvested from either the medium of infected monolayers, the infected cells per se, or a combination of the two. Earlier work (7) suggesting that intracellular virus is preferable has not been refuted, although numerous recent reports document the suitability of extracellular virus preparations. Stock-virus pools of unadapted strains must, of necessity, be obtained from infected cells.

Intracellular virus is harvested from monolayers, infected with as high a multiplicity as possible, showing extensive or preferably complete CPE on days 4-7 after inoculation; however, serial, high multiplicity passages may result in decreasing yields of infectivity due to the generation of defective interferring particles (30). Cells are dislodged mechanically by a rubber policeman or removed by EDTA-trypsin treatment, washed once, and resuspended in Eagle MEM free of $NaHCO_3$ (or in supernatant cell culture fluid) to the desired volume. The cell suspension is disrupted by a 30–60 sec exposure in a sonic oscillator at 10 Kc/sec, clarified by spinning at 500 × g for 10 min and aliquoted. Storage of this preparation at −70 C with a final concentration of 35% sorbitol (in water) has been shown to preserve infectivity for over a year (7). Inocula with sorbitol concentrations of this magnitude may be toxic to monolayers when used undiluted. Experience in our laboratory indicates that storage in 10% sorbitol is suitable for periods of up to 6 months.

Extracellular virus stocks are prepared simply by clarifying the cell culture fluid at 500 × g for 10 min and storing in the presence of sorbitol at −70 C. Sequential daily harvests of extracellular virus from the culture fluid with replacement of fresh MM can be obtained in this way.

Using these procedures, titers of 10^6 pfu/ml of stock virus are regularly obtained with intracellular virus preparations usually providing a higher yield.

Virus assay

The most commonly used procedures for titration of HCMV are the tube dilution method (7) and the plaque assay (16, 100). The second method is recommended for laboratories in which CO_2 incubators are available. The plaque assay is more sensitive, precise, and can be read at 8–14 days as compared to 21–28 days for the tube dilution technique. A 3-day FA cell assay (132) compares favorably with the plaque assay. Many of the technical details of these procedures are described in Laboratory Diagnosis, pages 420–433. Serial 10-fold dilutions of the virus pool are assayed for infectivity. Titers are determined by the enumeration of plaques and single fluorescing cells at the various dilutions in the plaque and fluorescing cell assays, respectively. In the tube dilution method, infectivity is expressed as the highest dilution of virus which produces CPE in 50% of the culture tubes ($TCID_{50}$).

Preparation of Hyperimmune Serum

Standard typing antiserum for HCMV is not yet readily available. Antiserum has been produced in variety of species, including rabbits, guinea pigs, goats, baboons, and monkeys by immunization with crude virus preparations; however, such serum uniformly contains anticellular antibodies which severely limit its utility for assays other than Nt. Crude virus antigens can be prepared as described in the preceeding section. Soluble CMV antigens prepared by alkaline extraction of infected cells produce antibody with less host-cell reactivity but fail to elicit Nt antibody (131). With the advent of methods for obtaining relatively large amounts of highly purified HCMV (28, 47, 97), potent antiserum essentially free of host-cell reactivity has been prepared in hamsters and guinea pigs. The antiserum can be used in a variety of serologic assays, including radioimmunoassay (RIA), IFA, CF, and Nt tests.

Different purification and immunization methods have been employed, but all share the basic elements of the following scheme. Confluent monolayers are infected at a high MOI and extracellular virus is harvested from the culture fluids at 4–10 days after infection. Following low-speed centrifugation to remove cell debris, the virus is pelleted at 50,000 × g for 1 hr, resuspended in 1/100 the original volume in Tris-buffered saline (TBS), pH 7.4, and homogenized on a Vortex mixer. Polyethylene glycol precipitation has been used successfully to accomplish this concentration step in lieu of high-speed centrifugation (28). The concentrated virus preparations are purified by density gradient centrifugation on 10–50% sucrose followed by isopycnic banding in cesium chloride (density 1.15 to 1.35 g/cm³). Purification by isopycnic potassium tartrate gradient centrifugation (20–50%) has also been reported (60). Bands from each density gradient separation are dialyzed against TBS and stored in this solution at −70 C. The centrifugation in sucrose results in a substantial loss in infectivity, while exposure to cesium chloride is less damaging to virion integrity (28, 47).

Animals are injected at 1–2 weekly intervals with antigen mixed with an equal volume of Freund complete adjuvant by one or more routes, i.e., intraperitoneally (ip), intramuscularly, or intradermally for a total of 4–6 injections. Each animal should receive 200 μg of viral protein; this is usually accomplished in small animals by the injection of 0.25 ml of antigen in multiple sites. Following this schedule, between 1.0–2.0 mg of viral protein is required for each animal to be immunized. Animals should be free of pre-existing HCMV antibody as determined by the most sensitive serologic assay available. Hyperimmunization may cause an increase in antibody levels to uninfected cells (28). This same study claims the superiority of the ip route of administration.

Antiserum prepared in this manner can be used to great advantage in the investigation of interstrain and interspecies differences in antigenic composition. From the diagnostic standpoint, antiserum can serve as an antigen probe in looking for HCMV in cellular specimens by the IFA technique, as well as providing a highly specific antibody source for the serologic identification of HCMV isolates. Until such an antiserum becomes routinely available, immune human serum free of antibody to HSV and V-Z, remains the reagent of choice for diagnostic assays.

Collection and Preparation of Specimens for Laboratory Diagnosis

Specimens for virus isolation

Isolation of virus is the most specific method to establish the diagnosis of HCMV infection whether congenitally or postnatally acquired. Virus can be recovered from several body fluids (urine, saliva, tears, milk, semen, stools, and vaginal or cervical secretions), and blood elements, as well as from various tissues obtained by biopsy or at autopsy. Although virus isolation proves productive HCMV infection, it does not necessarily confirm an etiologic relationship with an existing disease.

All samples submitted to the laboratory for virus isolation should be processed within a few hours after collection. Until processed, all specimens are maintained at 4 C (23, 71, 136). For shipment this is also the preferred temperature (23, 136). Swabbed specimens are obtained in collecting medium such as medium No. 199 with 100 μg/ml of gentamicin, 100 u/ml of mycostatin, and 1-2% calf serum (or 0.5% bovine serum albumin). Isotonic intravenous saline solutions containing 0.5% human serum albumin may be substituted if necessary. Conventional freezing (-20 C) of the clinical specimen, even for a few days is undesirable because of the known lability of HCMV to freezing (23, 71, 136).

Urine. Clean voided urine samples should be collected in sterile containers and treated as soon as possible with an antibiotic solution. We employ a solution containing 100 μg/ml of gentamicin and 100 u/ml of mycostatin. However, penicillin 500 u/ml, streptomycin 500 μg/ml and mycostatin are used by others. After incubation for 30 min at 4 C or room temperature, the samples are clarified by centrifugation at 500 $\times$ g for 15 min. Two-tenths milliliter of supernatant fluid is inoculated into each of a minimum of 2 culture tubes.

Saliva, tears, stools, and cervical or vaginal secretions. Sterile swabs immersed in collecting medium are used for sampling. To obtain specimens of saliva, the swab is rubbed over the buccal mucosa opposite the upper molars in the proximity of the Stenson ducts then over the floor of the mouth anterior to the tongue. For tears, the swab should be rubbed over the tarsal surface of the conjunctiva. A swab inserted 1-2 cm through the anal sphincter and swirled in place will provide an adequate sample for stool culture. To collect a sample of cervical secretions, visualization of the cervix uteri by means of speculum examination is a prerequisite. Secretions are obtained by swirling the cotton swab on the external os of the cervical canal. Vaginal secretions can also be collected during the speculum examination or by simply inserting the swab in the vagina until resistence is encountered and swirling it in place. The latter procedure has the advantage that it can be performed by the patient. After incubation for 30 min at 4 C or room temperature, the samples are clarified by centrifugation at 500 $\times$ g for 15 min. Two-tenths milliliter of supernatant fluid is inoculated into each of a minimum of 2 culture tubes.

Biopsy and autopsy specimens. Portions of each organ to be tested are collected with a seperate set of sterile instruments and placed in Petri dishes or vials containing collecting medium. Specimens should be processed immediately upon arrival in the laboratory. Storage at 4 C for 24 hr or freezing at -20 C reduces the recovery rate of CMV (71).

The tissue specimens can be processed by the following methods (see Chapter 3):

1. Feeder cultures — A 10% (w/v) suspension of the specimen in maintenance medium is prepared by trimming and finely mincing with sterile scissors. Two-tenths milliliter of this suspension is inoculated directly into established monolayer cultures. The preferred method is to disperse the cells by incubating the minced tissues in an equal mixture of 0.2% EDTA and 0.25% trypsin for 2-4 hr at 37 C with magnetic stirring. After centrifugation at 300 × g for 15 min, the cells are resuspended in MM (10% wt/vol). Two-tenths milliliter of the cell suspension is inoculated into several monolayer cultures. Potential toxicity can be minimized by changing the medium 4–24 hr after inoculation.

2. *Co-cultivation*—Cell suspensions from trypsinized tissues are mixed with equal amounts (1 × 10^5 cells/ml each) of freshly trypsinized human fibroblasts in growth medium. Cultures of combined cells are prepared in tubes (1 ml/tube), Petri dishes (5 ml/dish) or in flasks (10, 20, or 40 ml/flask).

Containers are incubated in a stationary position at 37 C. Depending on the growth rate of the cells, growth medium is replaced after 24–72 hr with MM. Secondary and tertiary cultures can be propagated in a similar manner following EDTA-trypsin dispersion of the established cell cultures in an effort to speed virus recovery (119). Further passages are unwarranted due to the low yield.

3. *Propagation of the specimens as cell cultures*—The *in vitro* cultivation of cells from biopsy specimens or tissues obtained at autopsy offers an advantage over the procedures for virus isolation from tissue suspension in that it allows for the detection of minute amounts of virus that may be present in the tissues. Tissues are minced and dispersed by trypsinization as described above. The resulting cells are suspended in growth medium at a concentration of 5 × 10^5 cells/ml. Cultures are prepared in tubes (1 ml/tube), Petri dishes (5 ml/dish), or flasks (10–40 ml/flask). Coverslip cultures in Leighton tubes or in Petri dishes can be made for histologic observation. Cultures are incubated at 37 C. Growth medium (containing 0.225% NaH-CO_3 when cultures are grown in CO_2) should be replaced every 3–5 days until the monolayers are well established. Thereafter, cultures are maintained in MM with twice weekly feedings and may be serially passed as described for the co-cultivation method. Since occasional specimens, particularly those obtained at autopsy grow poorly *in vitro*, it is advisable to always process samples by one or both of the above methods as well.

Milk and semen. These samples are diluted 10-fold in collecting medium to avoid toxicity and then incubated for 30 min at 4 C or room temperature (66, 92). After centrifugation at 500 × g for 10 min, 0.2 ml of supernatant fluid is inoculated into each of at least 4 monolayer cultures.

Peripheral blood leukocytes. Ten milliliters of blood collected in a syringe containing 0.1 ml of heparin (1000 u/ml) is allowed to settle in an upright position for 1–2 hr at room temperature (15). The leukocyte-rich plasma is expelled into a sterile tube through a 21-gauge needle bent at a 45° angle. This fraction contains most of the blood leukocytes, many platelets, and some erythrocytes (RBC). Attempts at isolation from the buffy coat free of autologous plasma is accomplished by first centrifuging the leukocyte-rich plasma at 400 × g for 15 min. The cell pellet is then resuspended and washed twice with MM. To more completely separate the blood elements, Ficoll-Hypaque gradient separation is employed (15). Ficoll-Hypaque is prepared by combining 2.4 parts of a 9% (wt/vol) solution of Ficoll (400,000 MV) in distilled water with 1 part of a 33.9% solution of Hypaque in distilled water (final density, 1.077). Forty milliliters of a 1:4 dilution of heparinized blood in phosphate-buffered saline (PBS), pH 7.4, is layered on top of a 10 ml Ficoll-

Hypaque gradient in polystyrene tubes followed by centrifugation at 400 × *g* for 40 min at room temperature. The mononuculear cells are then aspirated from the interface, washed with 50 ml of MM and spun at 400 × *g* for 10 min. The pelleted cells which consist of 70-80% lymphocytes and 20-30% monocytes and platelets are resuspended in *RPMI* 1640 medium. The RBC and granulocytes in the bottom of the tube are mixed with 4.5% Dextran (MW 5 × 10^5) dissolved in 0.9% NaCL and transferred to tubes with an appropriate diameter to make a cell column at least 40 mm high. The suspension is kept upright at 4 C for about 40 min to allow the RBC to settle to the bottom. Granulocytes and RBC are then harvested from the upper and lower phases, respectively, washed twice in PBS, and resuspended in MM. One × 10^6 cells are inoculated on performed monolayers or co-cultivated with 1 × 10^5 freshly dispersed fibroblasts.

Because of the frequent occurrence of toxicity in cultures inoculated with blood cell elements, it is recommended that 6-10 culture tubes be used for each of the separated components. If toxicity damages the monolayers during the 4- to 6-week period of incubation and observation, a fresh suspension of fibroblasts (1 × 10^5 cells/ml) can be added to repair the tissue culture (67).

Serum for antibody testing

Several serologic methods are now available for routine laboratory diagnosis. Of these, CF, Nt, indirect hemagglutination (IHA), and IFA are the most widely used. While single serum samples may be adequate to define past experience with HCMV, specimens collected immediately and at 2-, 4-, and 8-week intervals after onset, along with attempts at virus isolation, are required to establish the diagnosis of a primary infection.

A venous blood sample collected aseptically is allowed to clot in a sterile tube for 2 hr at room temperature. After clot retraction, preferably over night at 4 C, the serum is separated and stored at −20 C.

Specimens for exfoliative cytology

Cytomegalic inclusion-bearing cells have been found in the sediment smears of several body fluids and secretions, as well as in touch preparations of tissue sections. However, because of the low yield, exfoliative cytology is of limited diagnostic value (6, 24, 44, 72, 80, 103).

Cervix uteri. A cervical specimen obtained with a spatula is smeared on a glass slide which is immediately placed in 95% ethanol for fixation, and stained with hematoxylin and eosin or Papanicolaou stains (80).

Urine. The sediment of freshly obtained urine is mixed with an equal volume of 95% ethanol, filtered onto a 0.45 µm millipore filter, smeared, and stained as described immediately above (24, 72, 103). Diagnostic yield can be improved if the cells are sedimented on glass slides by means of centrifugation at 900 rpm in a cytocentrifuge (103). The smear is covered with 2 drops of Parlodion (1 g Parlodion mixed with 200 ml each of 95% ethanol and anhydrous ether). The slides are then fixed for 15 min in a solution of 1 part acetic acid and 9 parts of 95% ethanol and stained by the Papanicolaou technique.

Laboratory Diagnosis

Virus isolation in tissue culture

For isolation or propagation of HCMV in the laboratory, fibroblasts of human origin must be employed. Embryonic skin-muscle and lung or neonatal foreskin are suitable sources. The preparation and passage of the fibroblast cultures are carried out as described in Chapter 3. Cultures must be maintained in good condition for prolonged periods of time (4–6 weeks) because of the slow growth of fresh isolates of HCMV. To maintain the monolayers in this state, MM is replaced at least once a week. With serial passages, the cells may become less able to support the growth of the virus; therefore, low passage cell material is preferred. Since fresh medium often induces mytoses, microscopic observation of the cultures for CPE should be postponed for at least 24–48 hr in order to avoid a false-positive reading.

Growth and identification of isolates

Vital cell preparation. Inoculated cultures are examined once or twice a week for a minimum of 5 weeks for the appearance of CPE. This may first appear anywhere from 1 day to several weeks depending on the amount of virus contained in the inoculum. As shown in Figure 13.3, HCMV CPE is focal and progresses slowly; it can be easily distinguished from the cytopathology induced by HSV (81) and V-Z (88) even in the unstained preparations. Although the CPE induced by V-Z is characteristically focal and spreads slowly like HCMV, the individual foci are more delicate and the affected cells lack the typical brownish cytoplasmic granules (88).

Fixed and stained preparations. In stained preparations the cytopathology is pathognomonic of HCMV. The staining can be easily accomplished using coverslip or tissue culture slide preparations or directly in the original culture tubes by means of the collodion-staining technique described in Chapter 22 (56).

Growth characteristics as a means of identification. One of the most distinctive characteristics of HCMV is its slow growth in culture. HSV cytopathology appears much sooner following inoculation. In addition, the rapid production of large amounts of extracellular virus leads to involvement of the entire monolayer within 2–5 days (81). In contrast, fresh isolates of HCMV produce only cell-associated infection in early passages causing a slowly progressing, focal CPE. In human fibroblasts, V-Z infection is also primarily an intracellular process although low levels of extracellular virus can be detected in early passage (88). However, as previously mentioned the focal lesions induced by this virus can be distinguished morphologically from those of HCMV, and progression of the CPE is more rapid. More importantly, HSV and V-Z can be isolated and propagated in virtually all standard cell lines and epithelial cells of human and simian origin, respectively.

Plaque production. The plaques produced by HCMV can be distinguished from V-Z (88) and HSV (81); however, the methods previously described are of greater utility for this purpose. Both cell-free and cell-associated HCMV produce small plaques in fibroblasts under an overlay of methylcellulose, ionoagar, or agarose within 14 days of incubation. The plaques can be best enumerated and observed following methylene blue staining and the use of simple magnification (85).

Identification of CPE by indirect immunoperoxidase and immunofluorescence techniques. Both assays can be used to identify HCMV antigens in infected cells before cytopathology is evident by light microscope (36, 40, 132). Neither technique, however, has been adequately evaluated clinically and is not described in detail here. If utilized, care should be taken to assure the specificity of the antiserum with respect to HCMV.

Exfoliative cytology and histopathology

Light Microscopy. Cytologic techniques can be applied in an attempt to find characteristic intranuclear inclusions in specimens collected as previously described (see pages 416–419). Inclusion-bearing cells may be found in saliva, milk, cervical and trachael secretions, and in touch preparations from biopsy or necropsy tissues. Such cells are large (10–40μ), have scanty but distinct cytoplasm, and display a prominent central inclusion separated from the marginated chromatin by a clear zone (halo). The sensitivity of the standard cytologic techniques is low relative to virus isolation, irrespective of the type of specimen (70, 80). Only 50% of the urine samples from infants with symptomatic congenital CMV infection yield positive results (44). In addition, the presence of these cells in urine sediment is not pathognomonic of HCMV, since they may be found for short periods of time in the urine of patients suffering from a variety of viral infections (103).

Anticomplement immunofluorescence test (ACIF). This assay is a potentially useful diagnostic tool to detect HCMV infected cells because it is highly sensitive, specific, and relatively simple (48, 113). The test is based on the ability of specific antigen-antibody reactions to fix complement. Its superiority compared to other FA tests such as direct or indirect methods is due to the amplifying effect of the fluorescein isothiocyanate (FITC) conjugated anticomplement staining and its ability to detect both IgG and IgM classes of antibody-antigen reactions.

Exfoliated cells or thin sections (4 μm) of frozen tissue mounted on glass slides are air-dried and fixed for 10 min in chilled acetone (48, 113). Slides are first incubated with anti-HCMV (purified virus) hyperimmune serum or with a human serum containing a high titer of HCMV antibodies and preferably lacking antibodies to the other members of the herpesvirus family. Hyperimmune serum prepared against crude viral antigens can also be used following extensive absorption with normal fibroblasts in order to remove anticellular antibody. After incubation in a moist chamber for 1 hr at 37 C, followed by thorough washing in PBS, the preparations are incubated for 1 hr with a 1:10 dilution of fresh normal human serum lacking antibodies to HCMV and preferably to EB, V-Z, and HSV as the source of complement. Following washing in PBS, the slides are then incubated for 1 hr with FITC-conjugated goat antihuman C_3 at a dilution of 1:30. The specific fluorescence of HCMV antigens is distributed uniformly in the cytoplasm and nucleus of the infected cells. For correct intrepretation of this test, it is essential that identical specimens be tested with serum lacking HCMV antibodies, as well as with a heat-inactivated source of complement. The reliability of the assay to detect HCMV antigens depends on the specificity of the three reagents employed; to be certain of the presence of HCMV antigens the use of hyperimmune serum is required. There are no data to indicate that tissue-bound immune complexes may cause a false-positive result in this assay; however, this theoretical possibility must be considered.

Nucleic acid hybridization. The detection of HCMV genome in exfoliated cells, touch preparations, and tissue sections can be accomplished by nucleic acid hybridization techniques, the most well studied of these being the *in situ* complementary RNA-DNA cytohybridization assay (48). Specific radiolabeled viral complementary RNA or DNA are required as probes. These very sophisticated techniques are for investigational use only at present.

Electron microscopy. Various specimens can be examined with the electron microscope for the presence of HCMV but its morphologic similarity to the other herpesviruses precludes establishing a definitive diagnosis by this method (54, 105, 106).

Serologic diagnosis

CF and Nt tests have been available for several years. Both have been used with success for epidemiologic surveys and for diagnostic purposes. In recent years the serologic armamentarium for quantitating HCMV antibodies has been greatly increased. These newer assays include IFA, IHA, RIA, enzyme-linked immunosorbent assay (ELISA), and immune adherence hemagglutination (IAHA). The AD 169 strain of HCMV is recommended for routine diagnostic work because of its broad reactivity (5, 48). In certain circumstances, it may be advisable to employ an additional laboratory strain, ex. Davis, as well as homologous virus when available. Such an approach allows for a more comprehensive assessment of the patient's antigenic experience with HCMV.

Neutralization tests

Although the Nt assay is seldom used in diagnostic serology, it is the standard method against which other procedures are compared particularly for specificity. Several types of tests are currently available for quantitating neutralizing HCMV antibodies (4, 16, 85, 99).

Plaque reduction micro-Nt test. Human fibroblast cells are grown in 24-well plastic tissue culture trays. Fibroblasts are suspended in growth medium at a concentration of 1×10^5 cells/ml and each well is seeded with 1 ml of this cell suspension. Confluent monolayers are usually formed after 72 hr incubation at 37 C in a humidified atmosphere with 5% CO_2. Virus stocks are prepared as described on pages 414–415 and stored at -70 C. The titer of the stock to be employed in the test is predetermined by plaque assay.

For the Nt test, serum is inactivated at 56 C for 30 min prior to testing. Serial 2-fold dilutions of serum (0.2 ml) in MEM are mixed with equal volumes of virus suspended in the same diluent (approximately 400–800 pfu/0.2 ml) containing 10% guinea pig complement (4, 99). Ideally, the guinea pig complement should be pretested for viral inhibitory activity; however, in our experience using a 1:10 dilution of this reagent, nonspecific neutralization has not been observed. The controls consist of equal volumes of diluent and virus or nonimmune serum and virus. The latter is necessary when test serum is to be assayed at dilutions of ≤1:4. After a 60 min incubation at 37 C, 0.1 ml of the test and control mixtures are inoculated into duplicate wells from which medium has been removed. The inoculated cultures are incubated for 60 min at 37 C in a CO_2 incubator to allow for absorption of unneutralized virus. The inocula are then removed and cell sheets are washed once with MEM and overlaid with 1.5 ml of MEM containing 2% methylcellulose and 2–5% calf serum. After 10–14 days of incubation, the monolayers are fixed with 10% formalin and stained with 0.03% aqueous solution of methylene blue. Plaques are counted with the aid of an inverted microscope.

Serum Nt antibody titers are expressed as the highest serum dilution causing 60% plaque reduction as compared to the counts in control wells. Serum having a titer ≥1:2 are considered positive for Nt HCMV antibodies.

The Nt test can be completed more rapidly by using neutral red dye for plaque identification (99). This medium consists of MEM prepared without phenol red, supplemented with 0.1% bovine serum albumin, 0.1% yeastolate, and 0.5% ionogar #2 or agarose and buffered with 1.5 ml of 8.8% $NaHCO_3$/100 ml. After plates are incubated for 7 days, 0.25 ml of the above medium containing 7% of a 1:1000 stock solution of neutral red is added to each well and incubation is continued for an additional 24-hr period. Serum Nt antibody titers are expressed as described above.

Three-day fluorescent cell assay. This method compares favorably with the plaque assay and results can be obtained in 3 days (132). For this procedure, fibroblast monolayers are grown to confluency on tissue culture slides or coverslips. The Nt procedure and inoculation of the monolayers are identical to that described for the plaque Nt assay. Following absorption and subsequent washing, MM without methylcellulose is added. Between 72 and 96 hr after infection, the cultures are air-dried, fixed in acetone for 10 min at room temperature, and stained immediately or stored at −20 C. For staining, fixed monolayers are reacted for 1 hr at 37 C with a 1:10 dilution of pooled immune human serum or hyperimmune animal serum. After washing in PBS, the cell cultures are reacted with an appropriate fluorescein-conjugated antiglobulin for 1 hr at 37 C. Staining may also be carried out using the ACIF technique. Slides are mounted in glycerol/PBS (1:1) and fluorescent cells are counted at low power under a fluorescence microscope. The antibody titer is expressed as the highest serum dilution which reduces the number of fluorescent cells by 60%.

The tube Nt test. Neutralizing-antibodies can also be measured by the inhibition of CPE in tube cultures. However, this method is less precise and requires more time (21–28 days) for completion than the plaque reduction Nt test.

The mechanics of Nt are performed as described above. The indicator system comprises 3 tube cultures per virus-serum dilution and virus-diluent control. The serum titer is expressed as the highest serum dilution which completely inhibits CPE in all 3 cultures.

Complement fixation test

The CF test remains the most widely used routine serologic assay for quantitating HCMV antibodies (8, 17, 22, 63, 109, 112, 122, 134, 135).

Preparation of antigen. Monolayer cell cultures are infected at a MOI of approximately 1. When the cultures show 90–100% CPE (5–7 days), the infected cells are scraped into the medium and centrifuged at $600 \times g$ for 15 min. The supernatant fluid is removed. Intracellular antigen can be obtained by several methods (8, 17, 134); however, the most potent preparations are those obtained by glycine extraction (12, 17, 63). The infected cell pellet is resuspended to 5% of the original culture volume in 0.1 M glycine buffered saline (pH 9.5) and incubated with occasional shaking at 37 C for 6 hr (17). The suspension is then clarified by centrifugation at $600 \times g$ for 20 min. The supernatant fluid containing the CF antigen is stored at -70 C in 0.5 ml volumes. A control antigen from uninfected fibroblasts is similarly prepared and stored. Alternatively, antigen may be prepared by incubating disrupted (tissue grinder), infected cells in 0.5 M glycine-buffered saline, pH 8.5, at 4 C overnight (134).

Crude antigen is harvested by disrupting the resuspended cells (1/20 the original volume in Veronal-buffered saline, pH 7.2 or in Hanks balanced salt solution) by 3 cycles of freeze and thaw or by treatment for 2 min in a ultrasonic oscilator at 10 Kc/second (8, 42, 74). The potency and specificity of each batch of CF antigen must be determined by checkerboard titration against a known positive human serum pool employing both viral and control antigens. The antigen is preferably used unheated; however, if anticomplementary activity is present, it may be lessened without appreciable loss of antigenicity by heating at 56 C for 15 min.

Performance of the assay. The test is performed by the micromethod described in Chapter 1. Two units of antigen, 2 units of complement, and a 2% suspension of optimally sensitized sheep RBC (2 units of hemolysin) are used. Veronal buffer is used as diluent for all reagents, as well as a substitute for the antigen in the wells that serve as controls for anticomplementary activity of the serum. Prior to testing, all sera must be heat inactivated at 56 C for 30 min. Antibody titers are expressed as the highest dilution of serum giving 75% or more CF (3+ to 4+) as estimated by the size of the nonhemolyzed RBC button. In the absence of anticomplementary activity, positive reactions at serum dilutions of ≥1:8 indicate the presence of HCMV antibody. The anticomplementary activity encountered in approximately 10% of clinical specimens is a technical disadvantage of this assay (12, 112).

Indirect hemagglutination

The IHA method has proved highly sensitive and reproducible with the advantage that it can detect both IgG and IgM antibodies (10, 29).

Antigen preparation. The methods used to prepare the IHA antigen are identical to those described for obtaining the CF antigen (10, 29).

Performance of the assay. The IHA test is performed by a standard micromethod utilizing plastic plates. A 2.5% suspension of sheep RBC in PBS (pH 7.2) are tanned by mixing with an equal volume of a freshly made tannic acid solution (1:20,000 dilution in PBS) and incubating at 37 C for 10 min in a water bath. After centrifugation at $500 \times g$ for 10 min and 1 wash in PBS, the cells are resuspended in PBS to 2.5% and should be used within 2–4 hr. The sensitization of the tanned cells is accomplished by mixing in the following order: 4 volumes of PBS, 1 volume of the optimal dilution of antigen (determined by checkerboard titration, usually a 1:8 dilution) and 1 volume of 2.5% tanned RBC. After 30 min at room temperature, the cells are washed twice with rabbit serum diluent (normal rabbit serum—heat inactivated, absorbed with 50% sheep RBC at 4 C for 30 min and diluted 1:100 in PBS), and then adjusted to a 0.5% suspension in this diluent.

Test serum is diluted 1:8 in rabbit serum diluent, heat inactivated (56 C for 30 min), and absorbed with 0.025 ml of packed tanned RBC at 4 C for 30 min to remove nonspecific agglutinins. Two-fold dilutions (0.05 ml) are incubated with 0.05 ml of sensitized RBC for 2–4 hr at room temperature followed by incubation at 4 C until the cells settle. Antibody titers are expressed as the highest dilution of serum giving a 3+ to 4+ agglutination on a scale of 0 to 4+.

Serum exhibiting agglutination at a $\geq$1:8 dilution is considered positive in the absence of nonspecific agglutination of nonsensitized cells.

Immunofluorescence assays

FA procedures have become widely accepted for the measurement of specific HCMV antibodies. Several methods are currently available for this purpose (33, 44, 101, 112, 123, 124).

Indirect fluorescent-antibody assay to measure IgG antibodies against late HCMV induced antigens. The antigen for this assay consists of fixed, whole, infected cells obtained by inoculating monolayers with a high MOI of HCMV. Cells are harvested by EDTA—trypsinization when CPE involves 90–100% of the monolayer 5–7 days after infection (112). These cells are mixed in a 3:1 proportion with similarly prepared uninfected cells to provide an internal control. Approximately 2×10^4 cells are placed on each of 5-mm wells on preprinted slides, air-dried and then fixed for 10 min in cold acetone. These slides can be stored at -70 C for several months. Serial 2- or 4-fold dilutions of test serum in PBS are delivered by Pasteur pipette to each well. After incubation for 60 min at 37 C followed by thorough washing in PBS for 10 min, wells are similarly treated with fluorescein conjugated anti-human IgG. In order to reduce nonspecific staining, highly purified anti-serum to the Fc fragment of human IgG is recommended. The appropriate dilution of the conjugate depends on its protein concentration and F:P ratio and must be determined with known positive and negative control sera for each batch. Counterstaining is done by immersing the slides for 1 min in a 0.02% solution of Evans blue in PBS. Slides are mounted in glycerol/PBS (1:1) and observed under a fluorescence microscope for the presence of nuclear and diffuse cytoplasmic fluorescence. A titer of $\geq 1:16$ is considered positive. It is imperative to include positive and negative control sera in each run.

It is now well established that HCMV induces an Fc-IgG receptor in the cytoplasm of infected human fibroblasts. This receptor appears at 24–36 hr after infection and is seen as dim cytoplasmic and dense perinuclear staining, most prominently seen at 72–96 hr after infection. No receptor for IgA or IgM can be demonstrated by FA (57). The Fc-IgG receptor may result in a false-positive reading in the IFA assay (57, 120, 138). The variables that influence accurate assessment of specific staining are the use of conjugates of good quality, cells harvested on the fifth to seventh day after infection, and most importantly, careful observation of distribution of cellular fluorescence (112). For ease of interpretation, many observers restrict a positive reading to nuclear staining. At lower serum dilutions, however, bright whole cell fluorescence with prominent membrane staining is frequently observed with immune serum. One report indicates that simian CMV infection of human fibroblasts does not result in the production of an Fc receptor, whereas specific antibody detection in this preparation correlates well with that obtained using the homologous system (120).

Indirect fluorescent-antibody assay to measure IgG antibodies produced against early CMV-induced antigens. This assay is technically similar to the IFA test described above except in the preparation of the antigen (37, 112, 123). To obtain "early antigen," (EA) confluent monolayers of human fibroblasts are exposed to HCMV (MOI, ~1) for 1 hr at 37 C, then the inoculum is replaced by MM containing 20 μg/ml of cytosine arabinoside (ara-C) (112). After 72 hr of incubation cells are dispersed by EDTA-trypsin and fixed onto preprinted slides as described above.

The fluorescent staining in this assay is always restricted to the nucleus of the infected cells (Fig 13.5). A titer of $\geq 1:8$ indicates a positive result.

Anticomplement immunofluorescence test. The ACIF assay is specific and gives brighter staining than the IFA test by virtue of the amplifying effect of the activation of a large number of C_3 (B1c/B1a) molecules for each IgG duplet (33, 37, 48, 89, 113). The antigen is prepared as described for the IFA assay. Following heat inactivation, serial 2- or 4-fold dilutions of test serum in PBS are delivered by Pasteur pipette to each well on preprinted slides. After incubation for 60 min at 37 C followed by thorough washing in PBS, 1 drop of a 1:20 dilution of fresh normal human serum lacking antibodies to HCMV (as defined by IFA or Nt assays) and preferably to the other herpesviruses is placed on each well for 1 hr. After 1 wash in PBS, the binding of C_3 to the specific antigen-antibody complexes is assayed for with a 1:30 dilution of FITC-conjugated goat anti-human $C_3/C_3\mathbf{c}$ for 30 min. The optimum dilutions of the complement source and conjugate should be determined empirically by titration employing known immune and nonimmune control sera. Slides are then processed for fluorescence examination as in the IFA assay. The specific fluorescent staining with this assay is again restricted to the nuclei of the infected cells (Fig 13.6). This test offers the clear advantages of easy interpretation of the bright nuclear fluorescence and the lack of reaction with the Fc-IgG receptor. A titer of $\geq 1:8$ is considered as evidence of infection. When standardizing the reagents employed in this test, controls for specificity should include an antigen consisting of uninfected cells, the use of PBS instead of positive and negative control sera for background fluorescence, and the use of inactivated complement (48, 113). Subsequently, in each run, positive- and negative-control sera must be tested along with patient's serum. The ACIF test can also be used to quantitate antibody to the EA of HCMV (37).

Indirect fluorescent-antibody-IgM assay. The main purpose for the development of this assay was the detection of specific IgM antibodies to HCMV in neonates with suspected congenital infection (44, 75, 101, 102). Since IgM antibodies do not normally cross the placenta, their presence in serum obtained from the umbilical cord or during the early neonatal period indicates fetal production of antibody. Procedures that detect specific IgG antibodies are unable to distinguish fetal from maternal antibodies and hence cannot be used to distinguish active intrauterine infection.

For the purpose of diagnosis of congenital HCMV infection this assay has serious limitations. First, when compared to virus isolation for the detection of congenital infection, its sensitivity is no greater than 50% (75). Conversely, false-positive reactions can occur due to the presence of rheumatoid factor (anti-IgM-IgG antibodies) in the serum of neonates with HCMV or other congenital infections (90).

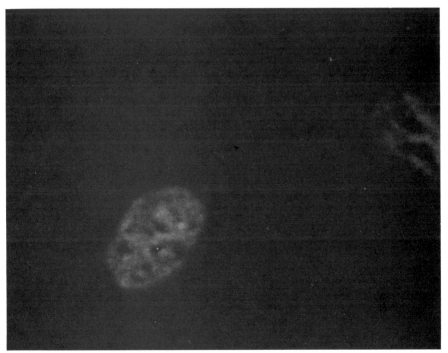

Figure 13.5—Early antigen detected in the nucleus of cytosine arabinoside treated, infected human foreskin fibroblasts by antihuman IgG immunofluorescence; strain AD 169, 400X.

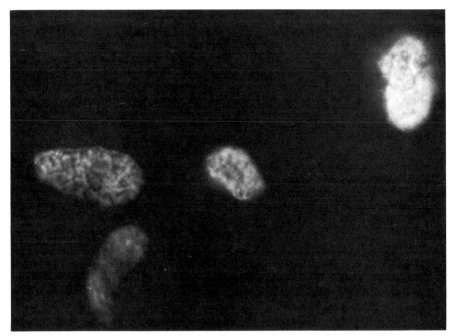

Figure 13.6—Late antigen detected in the nucleus of infected human foreskin fibroblasts by anticomplement immunofluorescence; strain AD 169 400X.

The antigen preparation and technical procedure for this assay are identical to those described for the IFA test except that the conjugate is an antihuman IgM antiserum (44, 75, 101, 102). A variation of this method is the
double indirect procedure which employs first a rabbit antihuman IgM
(heavy chain) antiserum followed by incubation with fluorescein-labeled
anti-rabbit IgG antiserum (102). A titer of ≥1:8 is considered evidence of
IgM-HCMV antibodies. The specificity of this assay is greatly dependent on
the purity of the conjugate. Contaminating anti-IgG antibody produces false-
positive results.

*Indirect fluorescent-antibody to measure antibodies to HCMV-induced
membrane antigens.* This assay can measure class-specific antibody directed against HCMV-induced antigens on the surface of viable infected cells.
Its clinical usefulness as a diagnostic procedure has not been adequately
assessed (124). A confounding feature of this procedure is the development
of an IgG receptor on the membranes of HCMV-infected cells (138), thus
making quantitation of specific IgG antibody difficult. According to the only
clinical study reported to date, however, it appears that IgM is the major
class of antibody reactive in this assay (124).

Other methods

Several of the newer serologic techniques are highly sensitive and permit detection of antibodies of different classes. However, since their clinical

applicability is yet to be adequately tested only a brief description of the technical details are presented here.

Radio immunoassay. An indirect solid-phase micro—RIA has been developed for the detection of class-specific IgM and IgG HCMV antibodies (28, 62). The HCMV antigen for this assay is prepared by glycine extraction of infected cells as described on page 424. The optimal concentration of antigen is defined for each batch with a known positive serum and ^{125}I-labeled goat anti-human IgG or IgM as described below. The appropriate concentration of antigen is then desiccated on the flat-bottom surface of the wells of microtiter plates and fixed with 10% formaldehyde (pH 7.4) at room temperature for 20 min. Twenty-five microliters of serial dilutions of serum in PBS are added to duplicate wells and incubated for 1 hr at 37 C for IgG determinations and 3 hr at a similar temperature to measure IgM antibodies. After rinsing several times in PBS, 0.025 ml of the radiolabeled antiserum is added to each well. Following incubation at 37 C for 1 hr, rinsing in PBS, and dehydration with 95% alcohol, the bottom of each well is clipped into the scintillation vials and counted in a gamma scintillation spectrometer. Serum titration curves are obtained by plotting the logarithm of specific radioactivity on the vertical axis and the serum dilution on the horizontal axis. The endpoint titer is defined as the dilution which gives twice the radioactivity of the background sample. HCMV and control antigens incubated with diluent and nonimmune human sera and subsequently with ^{125}I radiolabeled antiserum should be employed to define the level of background radioactivity. Preliminary results indicate that the RIA is a sensitive, specific and reproducible technique that has the advantage over some other serologic methods in that class antibody responses can be determined.

Immune adherence hemagglutination. This is a complement-mediated assay in which there is agglutination of indicator human RBC (type O, Rh positive) (19). The sensitivity of the IAHA is 4- to 16-fold greater than the CF test. The equipment, reagents and procedures used in the IAHA are basically the same as those employed in the CF test. Dithiothreitol is added to protect C_3 from C_3-inactivator. The assay is based on the fact that surface receptor sites of nonsensitized RBC bind to C_3 when it is activated by binding HCMV antigen-antibody complexes. Hemagglutination is evaluated on a 0 to 4+ scale and patterns of 3+ or 4+ are considered positive, provided nonspecific hemagglutination is not observed in the corresponding uninfected antigen control wells. Serum titers are expressed as the reciprocals of the highest serum dilution at which 3+ to 4+ hemagglutination occurs.

Enzyme-linked immunosorbent assay. Although enzyme-labeled antibodies have been utilized for several years for virus identification in cell cultures, their use for the measurement of specific HCMV antibodies has only recently been systematically evaluated (100, 127). ELISA appears to hold significant promise as a routine test in diagnostic virology because of its simplicity and ability to measure Ig class-specific antibodies. A preliminary report indicates that an indirect micromethod is satisfactory for the detection of antibodies to HCMV (127).

The test is performed in microplates to which viral antigen has been passively adsorbed. After incubation with dilutions of test serum followed by washing with PBS, the enzyme (alkaline phosphatase)-labeled anti-globulin (IgG or IgM) is added to the wells for an additional hour. After washing and drying, P-nitrophenyl phosphate is added as a substrate. As hydrolysis proceeds in each well, the substrate changes color and this can be quantitated spectrophotometrically at 400 nm. The absorbance is proportional to the rate of enzyme hydrolysis which is related to the amount of antiserum attached to the specific antigen-antibody complex formed on the plate. Since the antiserum concentration and the antigen are constant, the absorbance values can be related to the amount of antibodies present in the test serum. The antiserum can be linked to a variety of other enzymes including peroxidase, glucose oxidase, or B-galactoxidase yielding highly reactive and stable reagents. Standardization of the assay for the presence and amount of specific antibody is obtained by a procedure similar to that described for RIA.

Interpretation of serologic results

In order to define previous HCMV infection, an antibody determination on a single serum sample is usually adequate, provided this measurement is done by means of a sensitive serologic assay. This assessment can be made by any of the routine methods, perhaps with the exception of the CF test. A negative result with this assay cannot be equated with lack of previous HCMV exposure when crude antigen prepared by freeze-thaw disruption or sonication is employed (12, 17). With the use of the more potent glycine extracted antigen, however, the sensitivity of the CF assay closely approximates that of the IHA and IFA tests (10, 12, 52), although anti-complementary activity may occur (12). Thus, for seroepidemiologic studies, it is recommended that either the IFA, IHA, or ACIF tests be employed. Considering the practical advantages of the CF assay for many laboratories, this procedure may also be used for this purpose provided glycine-extracted antigen is available.

Primary HCMV infection is diagnosed by demonstrating the *de novo* appearance of antibody in convalescent-phase serum (seroconversion). The IFA, ACIF, IHA, or Nt test are reliable procedures for determining seroconversions. Longitudinal studies of blood donors (134), pregnant females, and infants with perinatal HCMV infections (112) indicate that CF-antibody titers may fluctuate between undetectable and low-positive (8–32) levels in otherwise seroimmune individuals; such reactions must be viewed as false seroconversions. This peculiar activity appears to be virtually eliminated when the more sensitive glycine extracted antigens are employed (10, 12). Comparative serologic studies done longitudinally in the various forms of HCMV infection would help resolve this matter by better defining whether each of these antibody moieties persist, which ones are boosted with recurrent HCMV infections, and what proportion of the infected population manifest these serologic phenomena.

Limited prospective follow-up studies of normal individuals with spontaneous mononucleosis (3, 51, 109), renal transplant recipients (3, 12, 110) and ''natal'' (112) HCMV infections indicate that IFA and IHA antibodies first appear within a few weeks after primary HCMV infection followed by

1–2 and 4-week delay, respectively, in CF- and Nt-antibody responses. Differential Ig class-specific HCMV antibody responses are currently not adequately described to be definitively useful in the diagnosis of primary infection (65, 68, 101, 102). Although IgM antibody has been found in the convalescent-phase serum of patients with primary infection (65, 68), it remains to be established whether this response is a transient one and, if so, is subject to reactivation with recurrent infection. Preliminary data suggest that this may be the case (102). Likewise, with recurrent HCMV infection in normal individuals differential serologic responses are not well delineated, but minimal or no changes in total or IgG antibody titer have been the rule (92). In contrast, recurrent infections following immunosuppression, organ transplantation, and multiple transfusions are frequently associated with rapid, variable rises in total or IgG antibody levels accompanied by virus shedding (12, 26, 45, 55, 87). Whether recurrences represent reinfection or reactivation cannot be determined serologically. However, based on epidemiologic evidence, it appears that reactivation of infection is more common.

Intrauterine infection is classically diagnosed by demonstrating persisting or rising total or IgG-antibody levels in serial serum samples collected beyond the time of expected disappearance of maternally derived antibody. Clearly, however, this diagnostic approach does not differentiate between HCMV infections acquired *in utero* from those acquired at or around the time of delivery (112).

In uninfected infants born to seropositive mothers, equivalent levels of IgG-HCMV antibodies due to placental transfer are detectable in umbilical cord serum. The latter disappear during the first year after delivery at variable rates, depending on the initial titer and the sensitivity of the testing system (112). When infection is acquired at or around the time of delivery, the mother is usually seropositive and excreting virus from different sites, most often cervix, urine, and breast (92). Indeed, we currently believe the mother is the most likely source of infection for the baby, via transmission from infected cervical secretions or breast milk (92). Pharyngeal shedding is another possible source, maternal and otherwise. Infection is then established in the neonate or young infant usually in the face of placentally transferred maternal antibodies. This situation confuses serial serologic diagnosis of congenitally acquired infection when using techniques that measure IgG antibodies. To emphasize this point the differential antibody responses of infants who acquire HCMV infection at or around delivery is summarized in Figure 13.7 (112). At birth, the level of antibodies in the umbilical cord serum are equivalent to the comparable titers in the mother's serum. On the average, IFA levels are the highest followed in order by IHA, Nt, IFA-EA, and CF (crude antigen). In the baby, levels of all antibody types decrease during the early weeks after delivery due to catabolism of maternal IgG antibody. In certain cases with low initial levels, they may even disappear, a phenomenon more often seen with CF antibody but occassionally with IFA-EA. Less significant decreases occur in the IFA antibody.

With the advent of virus excretion between 3 and 12 (average 5) weeks after birth, all antibody titers, except IFA, are significantly boosted (Fig

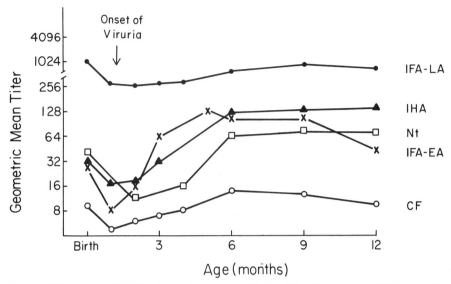

Figure 13.7—Group CF (○), IF (early antigen; X), Nt (□), IHA (▲), and IF (late antigen; ●) antibody responses among infants acquiring HCMV in the
immediate newborn period.

13.7). Nt, IFA, and IHA titers along with urinary virus excretion persist with
minimal waning at least for a year or more. IFA-EA antibody wanes more
rapidly, but low levels are most often maintained for at least 2 years. CF-
antibody titers appear to wane even more quickly and somewhat unpredict-
ably, at least when crude antigens are employed in the testing system. CF
antibody which rises more slowly than the others may fall to low (8–16) or
even undetectable levels and then fluctuate between 8 and 32 for reasons
that are presently unknown.

With congenital HCMV infection, virus initially acquired *in utero* continues to replicate productively for a number of years after birth whether the
infection is symptomatic or subclinical (75, 112). Fetal production and placental transfer of antibody apparently proceed under these circumstances
with the latter mechanism likely providing the bulk of antibody to the infected newborn. Thus, at birth, antibody levels in cord serum of congenitally
infected infants are equivalent to those in maternal serum, as with the uninfected baby born to a seropositive mother or those who acquire infection
during delivery or in the early postnatal period. Comparing antibody levels
between mother and baby at birth is therefore of no diagnostic value in des-
ignating the congenitally infected newborn.

After birth, the IFA- and CF-antibody levels generally follow the pattern shown in Figure 13.7 for infants with early postnatal infection. The cata-
bolic period of maternal antibody is slightly foreshortened with congenital
infection, likely as a result of ongoing production of antibody by the infant
who is already infected at birth. In symptomatic congenital infection, the CF

antibody is generally maintained at higher levels during the early weeks and months after birth but with subclinical infection the pattern of early waning and later fluctuation is much like that previously described for perinatal infections as shown in Figure 13.7. In contrast to the pattern observed with early postnatal infection, congenitally infected infants maintain relatively stable levels of IFA-EA antibody during the first 6 months of life. The IHA- and Nt-antibody responses have not been well contrasted between the two types of HCMV infection.

In symptomatic newborns showing stable levels of any type of IgG antibody from birth throughout the first 6 months of life there is strong presumptive evidence for intrauterine involvement by HCMV. In the absence of the clinical illness, the demonstration of stable IFA-EA-antibody levels from birth onward clearly indicates congenital acquisition of infection. However, if the initial serologic monitoring is delayed for over 2 months following delivery, it is nearly impossible to distinguish intrauterine from natal or early postnatal acquisition because of the similarity of the antibody responses associated with persistent virus replication in both conditions.

The serologic diagnosis of congenital HCMV infection could be best established by the detection of fetal IgM antibody in cord or early neonatal serum, thus, obviating the need for sequential monitoring for total or IgG antibody. The IFA-IgM procedure has been used with limited success both for diagnosis of symptomatic infants and in screening for subclinical infection (44, 75). The problems of low sensitivity (50% effectiveness with subclinical infection) and sepcificity need resolution. Clearly, rheumatoid factor (IgM antibody directed against maternal IgG) can give false-positive reactions in the IgM-IFA test and rheumatoid factor is produced in a fairly high percentage of patients with either subclinical or symptomatic congenital HCMV infections (90). However, the IFA-IgM test is better for screening for subclinical infection in newborns than is screening for nonspecific elevations of total IgM (75).

Because of all the complications of serologic diagnosis of congenital infection, virus isolation from urine in the first week of life remains the best way to prove intrauterine involvement. The virus in urine has a high enough titer and is sufficiently stable at 4 C so that shipment to virology laboratories should pose no problem. Proving intrauterine infection, especially in suspect infants, is of paramount importance because of associated developmental disabilities.

References

1. ABDALLAH PS, MARK JB, and MERIGAN TC: Diagnosis of cytomegalovirus pneumonia in compromised hosts. Am J Med 61:326–332, 1976
2. ALBRECHT T and RAPP F: Malignant transformation of hamster embryo fibroblasts following exposure to ultraviolet-irradiated human cytomegalovirus. Virology 55:53–61, 1973
3. ANDERSEN HK: Complement-fixing and virus-neutralizing antibodies in cytomegalovirus infection as measured against homologous and heterologous antigen. Acta Pathol Microbiol Scand 78:504–508, 1970
4. ANDERSEN HK: The influence of complement on cytomegalovirus neutralization by antibodies. Arch Gesamte Virusforsch 36:133–140, 1972

5. ANDERSEN HK: Studies of human cytomegalovirus strain variations by kinetic neutralization tests. Arch Gesamte Virusforsch 38:297–305, 1972

6. BENIRSCHKE K, MENDOZA GR, and BAZELEY PL: Placental and fetal manifestations of cytomegalovirus infection. Virchows Archiv [Cell Pathol] 16:121–139, 1974

7. BENYESH-MELNICK M, PROBSTMEYER F, McCOMBS R, BRUNSCHWIG JP, and VONKA V: Correlation between infectivity and physical virus particles in human cytomegalovirus. J Bacteriol 92:1555–1561, 1966

8. BENYESH-MELNICK M, VONKA V, PROBSTMEYER T, and WIMBERLY I: Human cytomegalovirus: properties of the complement-fixing antigen. J Immunol 96:261–267, 1966

9. BERENBERG W and NANKERVIS GA: Long-term follow-up cytomegalic inclusion disease of infancy. Pediatrics 46:403–410, 1970

10. BERNSTEIN MT and STEWART JA: Indirect hemagglutination test for detection of antibodies of cytomegalovirus. Appl Microbiol 21:84–89, 1971

11. BETTS RF, FREEMAN RB, DOUGLAS RG, and TALLEY TE: Clinical manifestations of renal allograft derived primary cytomegalovirus infection. Am J Dis Child 131:759–763, 1977

12. BETTS RF, GEORGE SD, RUNDELL BB, FREEMAN RB, and DOUGLAS RG JR: Comparative activity of immunofluorescent antibody and complement-fixing antibody in cytomegalovirus infection. J Clin Microbiol 4:151–156, 1976

13. BIRNBAUM G, LYNCH JI, and MARGILETH AM: Cytomegalovirus infections in newborn infants. J Pediatr 75:789–795, 1969

14. BOLDOGH I, GÖNCZÖL E, GÄRTNER L, VACZI L, MICHELSON S: Latent infection of mouse cells with human cytomegalovirus. Bull Cancer (Paris) 63:411–416, 1976

15. BOYUM A: Separation of leucocytes from blood and bone marrow. Scand J Clin Lab Invest 21:77–89, 1968

16. CHIBA S, STRIKER RL JR, and BENYESH-MELNICK M: Microculture plaque assay for human and simian cytomegalovirus. Appl Micro 23:780–783, 1972

17. CREMER NE, SCHMIDT NJ, JENSEN F, HOFFMAN M, OSHIRO LS, and LENNETTE EH: Complement-fixing antibody in human sera reactive with viral and soluble antigens of cytomegalovirus. J Clin Micro 1:262–267, 1975

18. DAVIS LE, STEWART JA, and GARVIN S: Cytomegalovirus infection: a seroepidemiologic comparison of nuns and women from a venereal disease clinic. Am J Epidemiol 102:327–330, 1975

19. DIENSTAG JL, CLINE WL, and PURCELL RH: Detection of cytomegalovirus antibody by immune adherence hemagglutination. Proc Soc Exp Biol Med 153:543–548, 1976

20. DIOSI P, MOLDOVAN E, and TOMESCU N: Latent cytomegalovirus infection in blood donors. Br Med J 4:660–662, 1969

21. DOWLING JN, SASLOW AR, ARMSTRONG JK, and HO M: Cytomegalovirus infection in patients receiving immunosuppressive therapy for rheumatologic disorders. J Infect Dis 133:399–408, 1976

22. DRESSMAN GR and BENYESH-MELNICK M: Spectrum of human cytomegalovirus complement-fixing antigens. J Immunol 99:1106–1114, 1967

23. FELDMAN RA: Cytomegalovirus in stored urine specimens. J Pediatr 73:611–614, 1968

24. FETTERMAN GH: A new laboratory aid in the clinical diagnosis of inclusion disease of infancy. Am J Clin Pathol 22:424–425, 1952

25. FIALA M, HONESS RW, HEINER DC, HEINE JW JR, MURNANE J, and WALLACE R: Cytomegalovirus proteins. I. Polypeptides of virus and dense bodies. J Virol 19:243–254, 1976

26. FIALA M, PAYNE JE, BERNE TV, MOORE TC, HENLE W, MONTGOMERIE JZ, CHATTERJEE SN, and GUZE LB: Epidemiology of cytomegalovirus infection after transplantation and immunosuppression. J Infect Dis 132:421–433, 1975

27. FINE RN, GRUSHKIN CM, ANAND S, LIBERMAN E, and WRIGHT HT JR: Cytomegalovirus in children post renal transplantation. Am J Dis Child 120:197–202, 1970

28. FORGHANI B, SCHMIDT NJ, and LENNETTE EH: Antisera to human cytomegalovirus produced in hamsters: reactivity in radioimmunoassay and other antibody assay systems. Infect Immun 14:1184–1190, 1976

29. FUCCILLO DA, MODER FL, TRAUB RG, HENSEN S, and SEVER JL: Micro indirect hemagglutination test for cytomegalovirus. Appl Microbiol 21:104–107, 1971

30. FURUKAWA T, JEAN JH, and PLOTKIN SA: Characteristics of defective human cytomegalovirus. Abstracts of Annual Meeting, Am Soc Microbiol, 1977, p 313
31. FURUKAWA T, TANAKA S, and PLOTKIN SA: Inhibition of human cytomegalovirus by rifampin. J Gen Virol 28:355-362, 1975
32. GARDNER MB, OFFICER JE, PARKER J, ESTES JD, and RONGEY RW: Induction of disseminated virulent cytomegalovirus infection by immunosuppression of naturally chronically infected wild mice. Infect Immun 10:966-969, 1974
33. GEDER L: Evidence for early nuclear antigens in cytomegalovirus-infected cells. J Gen Virol 32:315-319, 1976
34. GEDER L, KREIDER J, and RAPP F: Human cells transformed *in vitro* by human cytomegalovirus: tumorigenicity in athymic nude mice. J Natl Cancer Inst 58:1003-1009, 1977
35. GEELEN JLMC and VAN DER NOORDAA J: Characterization of human cytomegalovirus DNA: isolation and molecular weight. 3rd International Symposium on Oncogenesis and Herpesviruses, Program and Abstracts, Cambridge, Mass, July 25-29, 1977, p 44
36. GERNA G, VASQUEZ A, McCLOUD CJ, and CHAMBERS RW: The immunoperoxidase technique for rapid human cytomegalovirus identification. Arch Virol 50:311-321, 1976
37. GIRALDO G, BETH E, HAMMERLING U, TARRO G, and KOURILSKY, FM: Detection of early antigens in nuclei of cells infected with cytomegalovirus or herpes simplex virus type 1 and 2 by anti-complement immunofluorescence, and use of a blocking assay to demonstrate their specificity. Int J Cancer 19:107-116, 1977
38. GLASGOW LA, HANSHAW JB, MERIGAN TC, and PETRALLI JK: Interferon and cytomegalovirus *in vivo* and *in vitro*. Proc Soc Exp Biol Med 125:843-849, 1967
39. HAGUENAU F and MICHELSON-FISKE S: Cytomegalovirus: nucleocapsid assembly and core structure. Intervirology 5:293-299, 1975
40. HAHON N, SIMPSON J, and ECKERT HL: Assessment of virus infectivity by the immunofluorescent and immunoperoxidase techniques. J Clin Microbiol 1:324-329, 1975
41. HAINES HG, VON ESSEN R, and BENYESH-MELNICK M: Preparation of specific antisera to cytomegaloviruses in goats. Proc Soc Exp Biol Med 138:846-849, 1971
42. HANSHAW JB: Cytomegalovirus complement-fixing antibody in microcephaly. N Engl J Med 275:476-479, 1966
43. HANSHAW JB, SHEINER AP, MOXLEY AW, GAEV L, and ABEL V: CNS sequelae of congenital cytomegalovirus infection *In* Infections of the Fetus and Newborn Infant, Vol 3, Krugman S and Gershon AA (eds). Alan R Liss, New York, 1975, pp 47-54
44. HANSHAW JB, STEINFELD HJ, and WHITE CJ: Fluorescent-antibody test for cytomegalovirus macroglobulin. N Engl J Med 279:566-570, 1968
45. HO M, SUWANSIRIKUL S, DOWLING JN, YOUNGBLOOD LA, and ARMSTRONG JA: The transplanted kidney as a source of cytomegalovirus infection. N Engl J Med 293:1109-1112, 1975
46. HUANG ES: Human cytomegalovirus. IV. Specific inhibition of virus induced DNA polymerase activity and viral DNA replication by phosphonoacetic acid. J Virol 16:1560-1565, 1975
47. HUANG YT, HUANG ES, and PAGANO JS: Antisera to human cytomegalovirus prepared in the guinea pig: specific immunofluorescence and complement fixation tests. J Immunol 112:528-532, 1974
48. HUANG ES, KILPATRICK BA, HUANG YT, and PAGANO JS: Detection of human cytomegalovirus and analysis of strain variation. Yale J Biol Med 49:29-43, 1976
49. IWASAKI Y, FURUKAWA T, PLOTKIN S, and KOPROWSKI H: Ultrastructural study on the sequence of human cytomegalovirus infection in human diploid cells. Arch Gesamte Virusforsch 40:311-324, 1973
50. JORDAN MC, ROUSSEAU WE, NOBLE GR, STEWART JA, and CHIN TDY: Association of cervical cytomegalovirus with venereal disease. N Engl J Med 288:932-934, 1973
51. JORDAN MC, ROUSSEAU WE, STEWART JA, NOBLE GR, and CHIN TDY: Spontaneous cytomegalovirus mononucleosis. Ann Intern Med 79:153-160, 1973
52. KANE RC, ROUSSEAU WE, NOBLE GR, TEGTMEIER GE, WULFF H, HERNDON HB, CHIN TDY, and BAYER WL: Cytomegalovirus infection in a volunteer blood donor population. Infect Immun 11:719-723, 1975
53. KANICH RE, and CRAIGHEAD JE: Human cytomegalovirus infection of cultured fibroblasts. I. Cytopathologic effects induced by an adapted and a wild strain. Lab Invest 27:263-271, 1972

54. KANICH RE and CRAIGHEAD JE: Human cytomegalovirus infection of cultured fibroblasts II. Viral replicative sequence of a wild and an adapted strain. Lab Invest 27:273–282, 1972

55. KANTOR GL and JOHNSON BL: Cytomegalovirus infection associated with cardiopulmonary bypass. Arch Intern Med 125:488–492, 1970

56. KATZ SL and ENDERS JF: Measles virus In Diagnostic Procedures for Viral and Rickettsial Diseases, 4th edition, Lennette EH and Schmidt NJ (eds). Am Public Health Assoc, Inc, New York, 1969, pp 504–528

57. KELLER R, PEITCHEL R, GOLDMAN JN, and GOLDMAN M: An IgG-Fc receptor induced in cytomegalovirus-infected human fibroblasts. J Immunol 116:772–777, 1976

58. KILPATRICK BA and HUANG ES: Structural organization of human cytomegalovirus DNA. 3rd International Symposium on Oncogenesis and Herpesviruses, Program and Abstracts, Cambridge, Mass, July 25–29, 1977, p 45

59. KIM KS, MOON HM, SAPIENZA VJ, and CARP RI: Complement-fixing antigen of human cytomegalovirus. J Infect Dis 135:281–288, 1977

60. KIM KS, SAPIENZA VJ, CARP RI, and MOON HM: Analysis of structural polypeptides of purified human cytomegalovirus. J Virol 20:604–611, 1976

61. KLEMOLA E, VON ESSEN R, WAGER O, HALTIA K, KOIVUNIEMI A, and SALMI I: Cytomegalovirus mononucleosis in previous healthy individuals. Ann Intern Med 71:11–19, 1969

62. KNEZ V, STEWART JA, and ZIEGLER DW: Cytomegalovirus specific IgM and IgG response in humans studied by radioimmunoassay. J Immunol 117:2006–2013, 1976

63. KRECH VM, JUNG M, and SONNABEND WA: Study of complement fixing, immunofluorescent, and neutralizing antibodies in human cytomegalovirus infections. Z Immunitaetsforsch Immunobiol 141:411–429, 1971

64. LANG DJ: The epidemiology of cytomegalovirus infections: interpretation of recent observations In Infections of the Fetus and Newborn Infant, Vol 3, Krugman S and Gershon AA (eds). Alan R Liss, New York, 1975, pp 35–46

65. LANG DJ and HANSHAW JB: Cytomegalovirus infection and the postperfusion syndrome. N Engl J Med 280:1145–1149, 1969

66. LANG DJ and KEUMMER JF: Cytomegalovirus in semen: Observations in selected populations. J Infect Dis 132:472–473, 1975

67. LANG DJ and NOREN B: Cytomegalovirema following congenital infection. J Pediatr 73:812–819, 1968

68. LANGENHUYSEN MMAC: IgM levels, specific IgM antibodies and liver involvement in cytomegalovirus infection. Scand J Infect Dis 4:113–118, 1972

69. LEINIKKI P, HEINONEN K, and PATTAY O: Incidence of cytomegalovirus infections in early childhood. Scand J Infect Dis 4:1–5, 1972

70. MACASAET FF, HOLLEY KE, SMITH TF, and KEYS TF: Cytomegalovirus studies of autopsy tissue. I. Incidence of inclusion bodies and related pathologic data. Am J Clin Pathol 63:859–865, 1975

71. MACASAET FF, SMITH TF, and HOLLEY KE: Effect of storage on recovery of cytomegalovirus from necropsy tissue. J Clin Pathol 29:1077–1080, 1976

72. MARGILETH AM: The diagnosis and treatment of generalized cytomegalic inclusion disease of the newborn. Pediatrics 15:270–283, 1955

73. MCCRACKEN GH JR, SHINEFIELD HR, COBB K, RAUSEN AR, DISCHE R, and EICHENWALD HF: Congenital cytomegalic inclusion disease: a longitudinal study of 20 patients. Am J Dis Child 117:522–539, 1969

74. MEDEARIS DN JR: Observations concerning human cytomegalovirus infection and disease. Bull Johns Hopkins Hosp 114:181–211, 1964

75. MELISH ME and HANSHAW JB: Congenital cytomegalovirus infection: developmental progress of infants detected by routine screening. Am J Dis Child 126:190–194, 1973

76. MICHELSON-FISKE S, ARNOULT J, and FEBVRE H: Cytomegalovirus infection of human lung epithelial cells in vitro. Intervirology 5:354–363, 1975

77. MILLARD PR, HERBERTSON BM, NAGINGTON J, and EVANS DB: The morphological consequences and the significance of cytomegalovirus infection in renal transplant patients. Q J Med 167:585–596, 1973

78. MINAMISHIMA Y, GRAHAM BJ, and BENYESH-MELNICK M: Neutralizing antibodies to cytomegalovirus in normal simian and human sera. Infect Immun 4:368–373, 1971

79. MIRKOVIC R, WERCH J, SOUTH MA, and BENYESH-MELNICK M: Incidence of cyto-megaloviremia in blood-bank donors and infants with congenital cytomegalic in-clusion disease. Infect Immun 3:45-50, 1971

80. MORSE AR and COLEMAN DV: An evaluation of cytology in the diagnosis of herpes sim-plex virus infection and cytomegalovirus infection of the cervix uteri. J Obstet Gynae-col Br Commonw 81:393-398, 1974

81. NAHMIAS AJ and ROIZMAN B: Infection with herpes simplex viruses 1 and 2. N Engl J Med 289:667-674, 719-725, 781-789, 1973

82. NICHOLSON DH: Cytomegalovirus infection of the retina. Int Ophthalmol Clin 15:151-162, 1975

83. NUMAZAKI Y, YANO N, MORIZUKA T, TAKAI S, and ISHIDA N: Primary infection with human cytomegalovirus: virus isolation from healthy infants and pregnant women. Am J Epidemiol 91:410-417, 1970

84. PLOTKIN SA, FARQUHAR J, and HORNBERGER E: Clinical trials of immunization with the Towne 125 strain of human cytomegalovirus. J Infect Dis 134:470-475, 1976

85. PLUMMER G and BENYESH-MELNICK M: A plaque reduction neutralization test for human cytomegalovirus. Proc Soc Exp Biol Med 117:145-150, 1964

86. POSTIC D and DOWLING JN: Susceptibility of clinical isolates of cytomegalovirus to hu-man interferon. Antimicrob Agents Chemother 11(4):656-660, 1977

87. PRINCE AM, SZYMUNESS W, MILLIAN SJ, and DAVID DS: A serologic study of cyto-megalovirus infections associated with blood transfusions. N Engl J Med 294:1125-1131, 1971

88. RAPP F and BENYESH-MELNICK M: Plaque assay for measurement of cells infected with zoster virus. Science 141:433-434, 1963

89. REEDMAN BM, HILGERS J, HILGERS F, and KLEIN G: Immunofluorescence and anti-com-plement immunofluorescence absorption tests for quantitation of Epstein-Barr virus-associated antigens. Int J Cancer 15:566-571, 1975

90. REIMER CB, BLACK CM, PHILLIPS DJ, LOGAN LC, HUNTER EF, PENDER BJ, and MCGREW BE: The specificity of fetal IgM: antibody or anti-antibody? Ann NY Acad Sci 254:77-93, 1975

91. REYNOLDS DW, STAGNO S, and ALFORD CA: Recurrent cytomegalovirus (CMV) infec-tion in adult females. Pediatr Res Program Issue, APS/SPR 9:526, 1975

92. REYNOLDS DW, STAGNO S, HOSTY TS, TILLER M, and ALFORD CA JR: Maternal cyto-megalovirus excretion and perinatal infection. N Engl J Med 289:1-5, 1973

93. REYNOLDS DW, STAGNO S, STUBBS KG, DAHLE AJ, LIVINGSTON MM, SAXON SS, and ALFORD CA: Inapparent congenital cytomegalovirus infection with elevated cord IgM levels. N Engl J Med 290:291-296, 1974

94. ROWE WP, HARTLEY JW, WATERMAN S, TURNER HC, and HUEBNER RJ: Cytopathogenic agent resembling human salivary gland virus recovered from tissue cultures of human adenoids. Proc Soc Exp Biol Med 92:418-424, 1956

95. ST JOER SC, ALBRECHT TB, FUNK FD, and RAPP F: Stimulation of cellular DNA Syn-thesis by human cytomegalovirus. J Virol 13:353-362, 1974

96. ST JOER S and RAPP F: Cytomegalovirus replication in cells pretreated with 5-indo-2'-deoxyuridine. J Virol 11:986-990, 1973

97. SARVO I and ABADY I: The morphogenesis of human cytomegalovirus isolation and poly-peptide characterization of cytomegalovirus and dense bodies. Virology 66:464-473, 1975

98. SARVO I and FRIEDMAN A: Electron microscopy of human cytomegalovirus DNA. Arch Virol 50:343-347, 1976

99. SCHMIDT NJ, DENNIS J, and LENNETTE EH: Plaque reduction neutralization test for hu-man cytomegalovirus based upon enhanced uptake of neutral red by virus-infected cells. J Clin Microbiol 4:61-66, 1976

100. SCHMITZ H, DOERR HW, KAMPA D, and VOGT A: Solid-phase enzyme immunoassay for immunoglobulin M antibodies to CMV. J Clin Microbiol 5:629-634, 1977

101. SCHMITZ H and HAAS R: Determination of different cytomegalovirus immunoglobulins (IgG, IgA, IgM) by immunofluorescence. Arch Gesamte Virusforsch 37:131-140, 1972

102. SCHMITZ H, KAMPA D, DOERR HW, LUTHARDT T, HILLEMANNS HG, and WURTELE A: IgM antibodies to cytomegalovirus during pregnancy. Arch Virol 53:177-184, 1977

103. SCHUMANN GB, BERRING S, and HILL RB: Use of the cytocentrifuge for the detection of cytomegalovirus inclusions in the urine of renal allograft patients. Acta Cytol 21:168-172, 1977

104. SIMMONS RL, LOPEZ C, and BALFOUR H JR: Clinical correlations in renal transplant recipients. Ann Surg 180:623-632, 1974

105. SMITH JD and DE HARVEN E: Herpes simplex virus and human cytomegalovirus replication in WI-38 Cells. I. Sequence of viral replication. J Virol 12:919-930, 1973

106. SMITH JD and DE HARVEN E: Herpes simplex virus and human cytomegalovirus replication in WI-38 cells. II. An ultrastructural study of viral penetration. J Virol 14:945-956, 1974

107. SMITH MG: Propagation in tissue culture of a cytopathogenic virus from human salivary gland virus (SGV) disease. Proc Soc Exp Biol Med 92:424-430, 1956

108. SPENCER ES: Clinical aspects of cytomegalovirus infection in kidney graft recipients. Scand J Infect Dis 6:315-323, 1974

109. SPENCER ES and ANDERSEN HK: The development of immunofluorescent antibodies as compared with complement-fixing and virus-neutralizing antibodies in human cytomegalovirus infection. Scand J Infect Dis 4:109-112, 1972

110. STAGNO S, REYNOLDS DW, AMOS CS, DAHLE AJ, MCCOLLISTER FP, MOHINDRA I, ERMOCILLA R, and ALFORD CA: Auditory and visual defects resulting from symptomatic and subclinical congenital cytomegalovirus and toxoplasma infections. Pediatrics 59:669-678, 1977

111. STAGNO S, REYNOLDS DW, HUANG ES, THAMES S, SMITH RJ, and ALFORD CA: Congenital cytomegalovirus infection: Occurrence in an immune population. N Engl J Med 296:1254-1258, 1977

112. STAGNO S, REYNOLDS DW, TSIANTOS A, FUCCILLO DA, LONG W, and ALFORD CA: Comparative serial virologic and serologic studies of symptomatic and subclinical congenitally and natally acquired cytomegalovirus infections. J Infect Dis 132:568-577, 1975

113. STAGNO S, VOLANAKIS JE, REYNOLDS DW, STROUD R, and ALFORD CA: Immune complexes in congenital and natal cytomegalovirus infections of man. J Clin Invest 60:838-845, 1977

114. STARR S and ALLISON AC: Role of T lymphocytes in recovery from murine cytomegalovirus infection. Infect Immun 17:458-462, 1977

115. STARR JB, BART RD, and GOLD E: Inapparent congenital cytomegalovirus infection. N Engl J Med 282:1075-1077, 1970

116. STERN H: Isolation of cytomegalovirus and clinical manifestations of infection at different ages. Br Med J 1:665-669, 1968

117. STERN H and TUCKER SM: Prospective study of cytomegalovirus infection in pregnancy. Br Med J 2:268-270, 1973

118. STINSKI MF: Human cytomegalovirus: glycoproteins associated with virions and dense bodies. J Virol 19:594-609, 1976

119. STULBERG CS, ZUELZER WW, PAGE RH, TAYLOR PE, and BROUGH AJ: Cytomegalovirus infections with reference to isolation from lymph nodes and blood. Proc Soc Exp Biol Med 123:976-982, 1966

120. SWACK NS, MICHALSKI FJ, BAUMGARTEN A, and HSIUNG GD: Indirect fluorescent-antibody test for human cytomegalovirus infection in the absence of interfering immunoglobulin G receptors. Infect Immun 16:522-526, 1977

121. TANAKA S, FURUKAWA T, and PLOTKIN SA: Human cytomegalovirus stimulates host cell RNA synthesis. J Virol 15:297-304, 1975

122. TEGTMEIER GE: Antigenic activity of dense bodies from human cytomegalovirus-infected cells in the complement fixation test. Yale J Biol Med 49:69-70, 1976

123. THE TH, KLEIN G, and LANGEHUYSEN MMAC: Antibody reactions to virus-specific early antigens (EA) in patients with cytomegalovirus (CMV) infection. Clin Exp Immunol 16:1-12, 1974

124. THE TH and LANGENHUYSEN MMAC: Antibodies against membrane antigens of cytomegalovirus infected cells in sera of patients with a cytomegalovirus infection. Clin Exp Immunol 11:475-482, 1972

125. UMETSU M, CHIBA Y, HORINO K, CHIBA S, and NAKAO T: Cytomegalovirus—mononucleosis in a newborn infant. Arch Dis Child 50:396-398, 1975

126. VESTERINEN E, LEINIKKI P, and SAKSELA E: Cytopathogenicity of cytomegalovirus to human ecto—and endocervical epithlial cells *in vitro*. Acta Cytol 19:473–481, 1975

127. VOLLER A and BIDWELL DE: Enzyme-immunoassays for antibodies in measles, cytomegalovirus infections and after rubella vaccination. Br J Exp Path 57:243–247, 1976

128. VONKA V, ANISIMOV AE, and MACEK M: Replication of cytomegalovirus in human epitheloid diploid cell line. Arch Virol 52:283–296, 1976

129. VONKA V and BENYESH-MELNICK M: Interactions of human cytomegalovirus with human fibroblasts. J Bacteriol 91:213–220, 1966

130. VONKA V and BENYESH-MELNICK M: Thermoinactivation of human cytomegalovirus. J Bacteriol 91:221–226, 1966

131. WANER JL: Partial characterization of a soluble antigen preparation from cells infected with human cytomegalovirus: properties of antisera prepared to the antigen. J Immunol 114:1454–1457, 1975

132. WANER JL and BUDNICK JE: A three-day assay for human cytomegalovirus applicable to serum neutralization tests. Appl Microbiol 25:37–40, 1973

133. WANER JL and WELLER TH: Behavior of human cytomegaloviruses in cell cultures of bovine and simian origin. Proc Soc Exp Biol Med 145:379–384, 1974

134. WANER JL, WELLER TH, and KEVY SV: Patterns of cytomegaloviral complement-fixing antibody activity: a longitudinal study of blood donors. J Infect Dis 127:538–543, 1973

135. WELLER TH: The cytomegaloviruses: ubiquitous agents with protean clinical manifestations. N Engl J Med 285:203–214, 267–274, 1971

136. WELLER TH and HANSHAW JB: Virologic and clinical observations on cytomegalic inclusion disease. N Engl J Med 266:1233–1244, 1962

137. WELLER TH, MACAULEY JC, CRAIG JM, and WIRTH P: Isolation of intranuclear inclusion producing agents from infants with illnesses resembling cytomegalic inclusion disease. Proc Soc Exp Biol Med 94:4–12, 1957

138. WESTMORELAND D, ST JOER S, and RAPP F: The development by cytomegalovirus-infected cells of binding affinity for normal human immunoglobulin. J Immunol 116:1566–1570, 1976

139. WHITLEY RJ, BRASFIELD D, REYNOLDS DW, STAGNO S, TILLER RE, and ALFORD CA: Protracted pneumonitis in young infants associated with perinatally acquired cytomegaloviral infection. J Pediatr 89:16–22, 1976

140. WRIGHT HT JR, GOODHEART CR, and LIELAUSIS A: Human cytomegalovirus morphology by negative staining. Virology 23:419–424, 1964

CHAPTER 14

INFECTIOUS MONONUCLEOSIS AND EPSTEIN-BARR VIRUS-ASSOCIATED MALIGNANCIES

Werner Henle, Gertrude Henle, and Charles A. Horwitz

Introduction

The first description of infectious mononucleosis is usually credited to Filatov (29) and Pfeiffer (110) who in the late 1880s reported independently on a disease with fever, lymphadenopathy, and splenomegaly which occurred mainly in children and was designated Drüsenfieber or glandular fever by the second author. Because of the young age of most of the patients and the observation of epidemic episodes, it is doubtful that the disease conformed to what is now called infectious mononucleosis (IM), a term introduced in 1920 by Sprunt and Evans (125) who provided also the first definitive description of this disease. In 1932, Paul and Bunnell (107) reported that patients with IM develop high titers of antibodies to sheep erythrocytes (RBC). Demonstration of this heterophil antibody response by a later modified procedure to differentiate between Paul-Bunnell, Forssman, and other sheep RBC agglutinins, has become, and will remain, an important serologic diagnostic tool in IM. After a long search, the causative agent of IM was finally identified in 1968 by serendipity. G. Henle and her coworkers (46) observed that a laboratory technician, who previously had no antibodies to the Epstein-Barr virus (EBV), seroconverted when she developed IM. This "lead" has been amply confirmed subsequently in extensive studies with improved serologic techniques involving several EBV-related antigens and by other evidence so that the etiologic role of EBV in IM is now firmly established and generally accepted (26, 51, 95).

EBV, a member of the herpes group of viruses, was initially detected by electron microscopy in a small proportion of lymphoblastoid cells cultured from African Burkitt lymphoma (BL) by Epstein and his associates in 1964 (24). It has been considered ever since to be involved in the etiology of this tumor. Indeed, the virus transforms lymphocytes *in vitro* into permanently growing lymphoblasts, viral nucleic acid sequences are demonstrable in BL biopsies, and BL patients have high titers of antibodies to EBV-related antigens. Similarly strong evidence has linked EBV with another human malignancy; i.e., undifferentiated nasopharyngeal carcinoma

(NPC). The intimate association of EBV with these 2 malignancies has been discussed in several reviews (53, 76, 94, 137).

Clinical and laboratory features

General. IM is a self-limited lymphoproliferative disease which usually has a benign course but can occasionally be accompanied by severe, though rarely fatal complications. In its classic form, it presents with the triad of fever, sore throat, and extensive lymphadenopathy. Splenomegaly and hepatomegaly, accompanied by abnormal liver function tests, are frequent. White blood cell counts show a relative and absolute lymphocytosis with many atypical lymphocytes. The patients usually, but not always, develop a transient heterophil antibody response of the Paul-Bunnell type. These antibodies are dominantly of the IgM class and agglutinate sheep and horse RBCs and lyse bovine RBCs in the presence of complement. The uncomplicated disease usually runs its course within 1–4 weeks but occasionally may linger for several months.

White blood cell picture. Soon after onset, the leukocyte count may be normal or reveal a leukopenia due to a decrease in granulocytes. By the second or third week, the total count rises to between 10,000 and 20,000/mm^3, rarely higher. Blood smears characteristic for acute IM are found during the first or second week of illness. These show $\geq$50 mononuclear cells (lymphocytes and monocytes) with at least 10 atypical lymphocytes per 100 WBC. In most cases there are 60–80% mononuclear cells, >25 atypical lymphocytes per 100 WBC, and significant cellular pleomorphism. The blood smear abnormalities persist at least 2 weeks and on occasion up to several months (5). The morphologic findings are not specific for IM since they are encountered also in mononucleosis-like illnesses due to cytomegalovirus or toxoplasmosis. Significant numbers of reactive lymphocytes are also seen in active viral hepatitis, rubella, adenovirus infections, and a variety of other conditions (109, 135).

Liver function tests. The majority of IM patients show involvement of the liver as evident from abnormal liver function tests. Serum levels of gamma glutamyl transpeptidase (SGGT) or glutamic-oxalacetic transamidase (SGOT) are elevated in over 95% of the patients when serial specimens are tested. In 85% of the cases, the liver function profile shows peak bilirubin levels of <2.0ng in association with mild to moderate SGOT levels (<500mU/ml). In the 15% of patients with bilirubin levels above 2.0 ng, peak SGOT values are, as a rule, still <500mU/ml. The finding of an "anicteric" biochemical profile and mild to moderate levels of SGOT favors a diagnosis of IM over active viral hepatitis (32, 120). The cephalin flocculation or thymol turbidity tests also are positive in at least 85% of IM patients (26). Elevated levels of serum lactic dehydrogenase (LDH), while present in the vast majority of patients, are thought to originate from white blood cells rather than the liver (32).

Heterophil antibody responses. Several heterophil antibodies, which are mostly of the IgM class, arise transiently in IM. They include antibodies to sheep, horse, and beef RBCs, the Ii blood groups, IgG, *Proteus* OX$_{19}$, and others (6, 83). By far the most extensively studied heterophil antibodies are the agglutinins for native sheep and horse RBCs and the hemolysins for beef RBCs. These reactions are probably different expressions of the same antibody molecules (86). The agglutinins for sheep and horse RBCs are not absorbed by Forssman antigen (guinea pig kidney), but are removed by absorption with beef RBCs (13, 14). These heterophil antibodies of the Paul-Bunnell-Davidsohn (PBD) type are, with very rare exceptions, specific for IM (10, 15), but it is presently unknown why they arise. They are usually already detectable during the first week of illness but occasionally appear later. A variable proportion of IM patients, depending on their ages, fail to show PBD antibody responses. The heterophil antibodies may persist at gradually diminishing titers for many months after onset of IM.

Complications. These may accompany or follow classical signs of IM or, on occasion, they may be the only presenting features with or without subsequent clinical evidence of IM and with or without heterophil antibody responses. Complications involving the central nervous system include the Guillain-Barré syndrome, Bell's palsy, transverse myelitis, meningoencephalitis, and cerebellar ataxia. Other complications are pneumonitis, nephritis, rupture of the spleen, myo- or pericarditis, acquired hemolytic anemia, thrombocytopenic purpura, agranulocytosis, and others. Overwhelming fatal infections have been described in young males of 2 families suggesting a sex-linked immunogenetic defect in handling of the disease (4, 114).

Differential diagnosis. In heterophil antibody-negative IM-like illnesses, infections by cytomegalovirus (CMV), *Toxoplasma gondii*, adenovirus, and several other viruses can be the cause. In cases with central nervous system involvement, prominent hepatitis, pneumonitis, myo- or pericarditis, or other complications, numerous pertinent viruses must be considered. Detection of heterophil antibodies of the PBD type or EBV-related serologic patterns indicative of primary EBV infections tend to implicate this virus in the conditions under study. Occasionally, lymphoproliferative malignancies are considered in the differential diagnosis but rarely by experienced hematologists.

Epidemiology

The mode of transmission of IM has not been clearly established although intimate salivary contact, having led to the eponym of "kissing disease", appears to be the most frequent route (68). Salivary contamination of eating and drinking vessels and airborne dissemination of EBV also may be implicated (37, 68).

The incubation period of IM has been estimated to be 4–7 weeks, but there are few solid data. In colleges, the incidence of IM among contacts of cases is generally no greater than in the rest of the students (39, 122). The source and date of exposure can rarely be identified because a third or more primary EBV infections remain silent (27, 39, 101, 122, 129) and healthy individuals long after primary infections may sporadically excrete virus into the oropharynx (36, 97).

The period of infectivity probably begins before onset of illness and persists for weeks or months, based on detection of virus in oropharyngeal excretions (36, 97). In fact, the virus persists regularly in the lymphoreticular system as evident from the establishment of EBV-positive lymphoblast lines from peripheral leukocytes at moderate frequency and nearly uniformly from lymph node cells (19, 104). These carriers excrete virus sporadically into the oropharynx. About 15% of carriers selected randomly, at given times excrete virus, and the rate of excretion is enhanced in immuno-suppressed patients (126). Such excretors undoubtedly can transmit EBV to susceptible individuals. These observations account for the usual failure to identify the source of infection and to observe chains of overt IM cases.

Based on antibody surveys, primary EBV infections occur, as a rule, in early childhood under conditions of crowding or poor hygiene (42, 75). In this age range, they are thought either to remain silent or to cause such mild illnesses that IM is not a diagnostic consideration. Thus, IM is essentially unknown in developing nations in which practically all children seroconvert before 2-5 years of age. In economically advanced countries, especially among the affluent segments of their populations, primary EBV infections are often delayed until adolescence or later (43), when they frequently lead to the development of classical IM. The ratio between overt cases of IM and silent infections among college students was found to range between 2:1 and 1:2 (27, 39, 101, 122, 129). The preferential occurrence of IM in adolescents and young adults does not preclude occasional cases of IM in individuals over 50 years of age (69) nor the detection of characteristic cases of the disease among children (38). It is presently unknown, however, what percentage of primary EBV infections in childhood is accompanied by typical signs of IM, by mild, noncharacteristic illness, or by no signs of disease. It is also unknown, at what frequency primary EBV infections in childhood induce heterophil antibody responses.

Pathology and pathogenesis

The outstanding features of IM are the extensive hyperplasia of the lymphoreticular tissues, leading to lymphadenopathy, hepatosplenomegaly, and lymphoid hyperplasia in the naso- and oropharynx. The lymph nodes usually retain their follicular appearance. However, the sinuses are partially effaced or distended by macrophages, atypical lymphocytes, and pyroninophilic immunoblasts. Variable numbers of plasma cells, focal necrosis, and occasional Reed-Sternberg cells are also seen (21). Focal and perivascular infiltration of mononuclear cells, many being atypical, may be noted in almost every organ. A patchy pleomorphic mononuclear cell infiltrate is noted not only in the portal tracts and lobular sinosoids of the liver but also around parenchymal cells. Ill-defined, noncaseating granulomas are often seen in bone marrow biopsies.

The pathogenesis of IM has not been elucidated beyond speculative suggestions (7, 47, 92). At present, only lymphocytes with B cell characteristics are known to be susceptible to infection by EBV (73), although it is suspected that another, highly permissive type of cell might be the initial target of the virus, since B lymphocytes can hardly be considered permissive for the virus. EBV can transform B lymphocytes *in vitro* into lymphoblasts with permanent growth potential which henceforth carry viral genomes in a largely repressed state, usually leading only to expression of virus-related antigens in the nucleus and cell membranes. Only few of these cells replicate virus particles. Such transformation might also occur *in vivo* and thus contribute to the lymphoproliferation. The altered cells would be expected to become targets for T cells and the resulting interaction could account for part of the histopathology and symptomatology of IM (47, 121, 128). The atypical lymphocytes, having T-cell characteristics (106, 123, 130), might represent activated effector cells.

The Epstein-Barr Virus

Physical properties

Based upon size, shape, and chemical composition, EBV belongs to the herpes group of viruses. It has a DNA core surrounded by 162 capsomeres arranged in an icosahedral array, and this nucleocapsid is enclosed in an envelope derived from host-cell membranes.

Biological properties

The virus, apparently being limited in its replication to lymphoid cells with B-cell characteristics, can be maintained at present in the laboratory only in continuous lymphoblastoid cell lines (LCL) derived from Burkitt lymphoma or peripheral lymphocytes of IM patients or viral carriers. These LCL are divided into producer and nonproducer cultures, depending on whether a generally small proportion of the cells (<0.1% to at most 10%) or none of the cells synthesizes virus. All cells of producer and nonproducer lines carry EBV genomes as detected by nucleic acid hybridization techniques (105, 138) and by the expression of the EBV-associated nuclear antigen (EBNA) (115). It is very rare to obtain LCL with B-cell characteristics in the absence of the virus.

EBV preparations can be divided into "lytic" and "transforming" populations according to their dominant properties (99). Some LCL shed mainly lytic virus which induces in cells from nonproducer cultures a usually abortive, yet fatal, cycle of viral replication; i.e., EBV-related early antigens (EA) are synthesized but not viral-capsid antigen (VCA), and thus there is no production of virus particles (VP) (48, 60). However, at high-input multiplicities of infection, some of the cells produce VCA as well as VP. Virus populations, derived from other producer lines, the oropharynx of IM patients, or viral carriers, do not induce abortive infections in nonproducer cells but, unlike lytic virus preparations, they transform peripheral or cord blood lymphocytes *in vitro* into permanently growing, EBNA-positive LCL which, again, may be producers or nonproducers (20, 35, 54, 96, 112). No cells other than B lymphocytes have been found to date, although they well may exist, which are susceptible to infection or transformation by EBV.

Virus-related antigens

Because of the limited growth of virus in LCL, the differentiation of virus-specific antigens and the development of tests for the corresponding antibodies depended largely on immunofluorescence (FA). By such techniques it was shown, first of all, that EBV is antigenically distinct from the 3 known groups of human herpesviruses (Herpes simplex virus, CMV, and Varicella-zoster virus) as well as from any of the numerous animal herpesviruses that were tested (41). Furthermore, at least 4 different groups of EBV-related antigens have now been differentiated with the aid of selected human sera in LCL *per se* or after various manipulations (Table 14.1).

TABLE 14.1—EBV-RELATED ANTIGEN-ANTIBODY SYSTEMS

ANTIGEN	LYMPHOBLAST LINE	FIXATION		ANTIBODY DETERMINATION	
		ACE-TONE	METH-ANOL	METHOD	POSITIVE SERUM
VCA—Viral capsid antigen	Producer (cell smears)	+ or	+	Indirect immuno-fluorescence	All viral carriers
MA—Cell membrane antigen E-MA (Early) L-MA (Late)	Producer or abortively infected non-producer (suspensions)			Blocking or direct immuno-fluorescence	Most viral carriers
EA—Early antigens	Abortively infected non-producer (cell smears)			Indirect immuno-fluorescence	
D (Diffuse)		+ or	+		Mainly IM and NPC patients
R (Restricted)		+	−		Mainly BL patients
EBNA—EBV Nuclear antigen	Non-producer (cell smears)	+ and	+	Anti-C′ immuno-fluorescence	All viral carriers
S—Soluble antigen	Non-producer (cell extracts)			Complement fixation	Most viral carriers
VP—Enveloped virus particles	Producer (media or centrifugal concentrates)			Neutraliza-tion (prevention of abortive infection or of transformation)	All viral carriers

EBV-capsid antigen (VCA). This antigen is present in all virus-producing cells and was the first to be identified by indirect immunofluorescence (41) in acetone-fixed smears from producer LCL. Sera from all individuals who have experienced primary EBV infections in the past (virus carriers) react with VCA in the IgG test at titers ranging from 1:10 to 1:160, rarely higher. The percentages of virus-producing cells in given LCL match the percentages of immunofluorescent cells (41, 79). Thin sections prepared from individually selected fluorescent cells were shown to contain numerous VP, but these are not present in similarly prepared nonfluorescent cells (22, 139). Non-enveloped nucleocapsids extracted and concentrated from cells of producer LCL are coated and partly agglutinated when exposed to FA-positive but not FA-negative serum as shown by negative contrast electronmicroscopy (63, 93). Thus, the antibodies detected are clearly directed against viral nucleocapsids, and smears from producer LCL serve to detect VCA-specific IgG, IgM, or IgA antibodies by indirect immunofluorescence (IFA).

EBV-determined cell membrane antigens (MA). These antigens are detectable by FA or IFA with suspended live cells (79). They are divided into early and late MA, depending on whether or not viral DNA replication precedes their synthesis (25, 124). Antibodies to MA components are present in most sera from virus carriers. To avoid interaction of membrane-reactive antibodies unrelated to EBV, a blocking test has been devised to measure EBV-specific antibodies to MA; i.e., the cells are first exposed to the test serum and then to fluorescein isothiocyanate (FITC)-conjugated antibodies to MA from a donor without detectable iso- or other nonspecific antibodies (78). If the test serum contains anti-MA, it specifically blocks staining by the conjugate. The complexities of these techniques have prevented their wide application to serologic diagnosis and serologic surveys.

EBV-induced early antigens (EA). These antigens are present in every virus-producing (VCA-positive) cell, but they often are the only product in cells from nonproducer LCL after superinfection by lytic virus at moderate input multiplicities (48, 60). Antibodies to EA are rarely present in serum from healthy virus carriers; they are found occasionally at only low titers ($\leq$1:20) among those donors who maintain relatively high anti-VCA IgG antibody titers ($\geq$1:160). In contrast, antibodies to EA are observed frequently in serum from patients with EBV-associated diseases, often at substantial titers. They are therefore to a considerable extent disease-related, including some patients who experience reactivations of latent persistent EBV infections due to immunosuppressive diseases or therapy.

EA is a complex of at least 2 distinct components which are differentiated by the morphology of the immunofluorescent staining and by resistance to methanol fixation (48). One, called D, causes diffuse staining of the nucleus and cytoplasm of abortively EBV-superinfected cells and is resistant to methanol. The other component, called R, is restricted to a mass in the cytoplasm and is denatured by methanol. No method has been found to denature D without also affecting R. Antibodies to D arise transiently in about 85% of IM patients (58, 59), reach high titers in NPC with advancing tumor burden (62), and may appear in some BL patients, especially in the terminal stage (56). High titers of antibodies to R are virtually limited to BL (56). Reactivation of the persistent EBV infection may call forth in some instances either anti-D or anti-R (52). The early antigens are therefore of considerable serologic diagnostic importance.

EBV-associated nuclear antigen (EBNA). This antigen is detectable only by the sensitive anticomplement FA technique (115). It is present in every EBV-transformed cell, whether from producer or nonproducer lines. It is also found in the vast majority of cells from nearly all African and a proportion of nonAfrican BL biopsies (74, 116), as well as in the undifferentiated carcinoma cells in touch imprints from NPC biopsies (72), attesting to the intimate association of EBV with these 2 malignancies. Efforts to detect EBNA-positive cells in any other human tumor have thus far failed. Antibodies to EBNA are titrated on cell smears from nonproducer lines, using serum from anti-VCA negative donors as source of C'. Practically every anti-VCA-positive serum contains anti-EBNA, except serum from patients in the early acute phase of IM (47) or patients with severe immunologic defects or immunosuppressive diseases. In healthy carriers of EBV, the anti-EBNA titers usually range from 1:10 to 1:160.

Complement-fixing antigens.

1. Concentrated virus suspension—Such preparations have been used as CF antigen (34) which presumably measures antibodies to MA, as well as to VCA, depending on the relative representation of enveloped and nonenveloped VP. Because of the mixture of antigens and difficulties in obtaining sufficient quantities of virus particles, this test has not found wide application.

2. Soluble complement-fixing antigen (S)—Soon after the discovery of EBV, a soluble CF antigen was extracted from cells of producer lines, but it was not immediately recognized as EBV-related since it was found also in nonproducer LCL which had not yet been shown to contain viral genomes (1). It was found, however, that only anti-VCA positive serum reacted with this antigen, thus associating it with EBV (113). Although S preparations from nonproducer LCL are likely to contain some MA components, their main constituent appears to be EBNA. The titers of anti-S and anti-EBNA in given sera are closely similar (81).

Neutralization of EBV. Superinfection of nonproducer LCL by lytic EBV and establishment of LCL from cord blood leukocytes after exposure to transforming EBV have provided means to detect and titrate EBV neutralizing (Nt) antibodies. In the first system, neutralization (Nt) of the virus is ascertained by absence of EA synthesis in the exposed cells (108) or by their survival as determined by colony formation (118). In the second system, Nt of the virus becomes apparent by failure to establish LCL (96, 98), by reduced incorporation of ^{3}H-thymidine into exposed cells (117), or by non-emergence of EBNA-positive lymphoblasts (2, 88). These various techniques have yielded similar results in comparative Nt tests (16). There is some evidence that Nt antibodies are identical with antibodies to some of the MA components, probably late MA (16, 108), since these antigens are present in the viral envelope as well as on cell membranes (124). Nt antibodies are, with rare exceptions, present in anti-VCA-positive serum (64, 119). Nt tests have not been employed for serologic diagnosis because of their complexity and the time required for obtaining results.

Other serologic techniques. Efforts are being made to develop other sensitive serologic techniques for determination of antibodies to specific EBV-related antigens, such as radioimmune assays (RIA), enzyme-linked immunosorbent assays (ELISA), immune adherence tests (IA), etc. Such tests will require a high degree of purification of various EBV-related antigens to permit differential determination of the antibody spectra and titers as needed for the EBV-specific serologic diagnosis of IM. While the immunofluorescence techniques appear to be cumbersome and few diagnostic laboratories are prepared to perform them, they have the advantage of built-in controls in that only the appropriate numbers of cells must be stained (the others serving as controls) and the morphology of the fluorescent pattern has to conform with that of the antigen under test.

Antibody Responses in EBV-Associated Diseases

Infectious mononucleosis

General pattern. Figure 14.1 presents schematically the serologic responses and virologic observations in the course of IM. Serum obtained by chance or by design in prospective studies of IM well in advance of primary infections is uniformly devoid of all antibodies to EBV-related antigens (39, 46, 66, 102, 122, 129). In the acute phase, both IgM and IgG antibodies to VCA have usually reached peak titers by the time the patient comes to a physician's attention, so that ≥4-fold increases in antibody titer in subsequent sera are observed in not more than 20% of the patients (58). The IgM antibodies subsequently disappear within 4 or more weeks, whereas the IgG antibodies decline merely to lower but persistent levels. Since the lower range of peak IgG titers in IM may overlap with the upper range of titers in healthy virus carriers, only very high levels of VCA-specific IgG ($\geqq 1{:}320$) would be of some significance. About 85% of the patients show an early, transient anti-D response which does not necessarily reflect the severity of illness (58, 59). Also Nt antibodies, which seem to parallel anti-MA responses (not shown), arise early and then persist presumably for life (64, 77, 98, 119). In contrast to the early appearance of the above mentioned antibodies, those to EBNA and the probably identical S antigen appear, with few exceptions, only weeks or even months after onset of illness (47, 131) but then remain persistently detectable.

This differential appearance of the 2 groups of antibodies suggests that the corresponding antigens become available for antibody stimulation at different times and under different sets of circumstances. VCA, late MA, EA, and VP are products of lytically infected cells and thus are released from degenerating cells early during the incubation period. EBNA and S might be derived mainly later from EBV genome-carrying lymphoid cells after their destruction by T-cell action. EBNA-positive large lymphocytes have been observed among the circulating B-cell population of IM patients (80), and

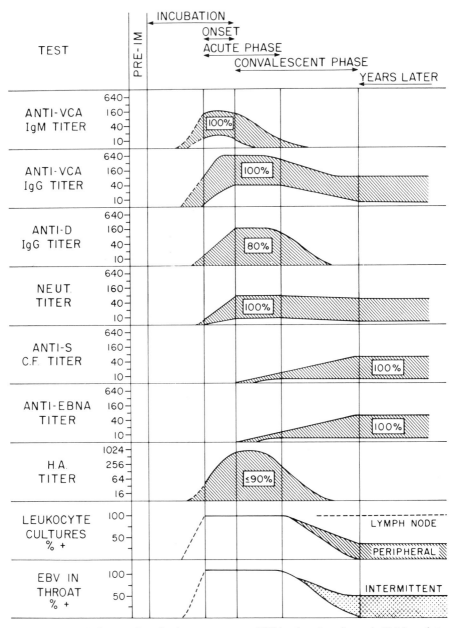

Figure 14.1.—Scheme of antibody responses to EBV-related antigens in IM (reprinted with permission of Stratton Intercontinental Book Corp.).

cells attacking specifically EBV-transformed cells *in vitro* have been separated from the T-cell fraction of peripheral lymphocytes obtained during the acute phase of the disease but not later (121, 128).

Implications of the serologic data. The data presented in Figure 14.1 have 3 implications regarding immunity to IM, the serologic diagnosis of primary EBV infections, and the persistence of some of the antibodies.

1. Determination of immunity—Absence of VCA-specific IgG antibodies denotes susceptibility, and their presence indicates immunity to IM. While anti-VCA does not neutralize EBV, serum containing anti-VCA almost invariably also has Nt antibodies. The anti-VCA test thus serves as a dependable indicator of the immune status.

2. Specific serologic diagnosis of primary EBV infections—These can often be identified serologically by testing of a single acute-phase serum; i.e., by demonstration of high titers of IgM and IgG antibodies to VCA, the presence of anti-D, and the absence of anti-EBNA. Second and later sera are needed only for confirmation or for the few patients with delayed antibody responses. The specific serologic diagnosis is thus established by (i) early presence and later disappearance of IgM antibodies to VCA; (ii) very high or, occasionally, still rising VCA-specific IgG antibody titers and their later decline to lower persistent levels; (iii) a transient anti-D response; and (iv) the early absence and later emergence of antibodies to EBNA or to S antigen. Of these test procedures, the anti-EA test is not essential, although helpful at times, but the other three are needed for accurate interpretation of results.

3. Latent persistent carrier state—The apparently life-long persistence of VCA-specific IgG, EBNA-specific, and Nt antibodies is explained by the persistent virus-carrier state which regularly becomes established in the course of primary EBV infections. EBNA-positive LCL can be established with considerable frequency from peripheral leukocytes and nearly uniformly from lymph nodes of healthy donors with antibody to VCA (104), and such donors, furthermore, may sporadically excrete EBV into the oropharynx (36, 97). For these reasons, the establishment of LCL or the demonstration of EBV in oropharyngeal secretions are, as a rule, of little diagnostic significance.

Need for EBV-specific serodiagnosis. EBV-specific serologic diagnostic tests are not required in classical cases of IM since the heterophil antibody response, as determined by the Paul-Bunnell-Davidsohn (PBD) technique, is practically specific for the disease. However, rapid slide tests performed with commercially available test kits (Monospot®, and others) may on occasion yield false-positive results. Furthermore, HA responses fail to develop in some patients with otherwise typical IM, especially in the pediatric age range. The absence of PBD antibodies was considered in the past by some clinicians to be incompatible with a diagnosis of IM. A proportion of such cases can now be shown clearly to be EBV-associated on the basis of specific serologic diagnostic tests (38, 71, 82, 103). The majority of heterophil antibody-negative IM-like illnesses are, however, caused by CMV (71, 82, 132) and others by *Toxoplasma gondii*, adenoviruses, or other viruses. EBV-specific serologic diagnostic tests are needed also for patients presenting with unusual manifestations of primary EBV infections with few or no other signs of typical IM.

EBV-associated malignancies

Detection of EBNA in tumor cells. As mentioned earlier, EBV-nucleic-acid sequences and EBNA-positive tumor cells are demonstrable in biopsies from most African and a proportion of nonAfrican BL, as well as in all undifferentiated NPC patients but not from patients with other malignancies (72, 74, 90, 116, 136, 140). While tests for EBV-DNA sequences are not readily available, tests for EBNA-positive cells are relatively simple. Merely by shaking minced BL biopsies in culture medium, sufficient cells are dispersed from the tissue for preparation of cell smears and EBNA staining. With freshly cut surfaces from NPC biopsies, touch preparations are made on coverslips to deposit small fragments of tissue (72). After drying and fixation, the preparations are stained for EBNA. To date, only undifferentiated carcinomas of the nasopharynx, but no other carcinomas or tumors of the head and neck region, have shown foci of EBNA-positive cells (67). These techniques may be useful, therefore, in the diagnosis of EBV-associated malignancies.

Antibody patterns of tumor patients. Patients with BL or NPC often have high titers of VCA-specific IgG antibodies which are to a considerable extent related to the total tumor burden (45, 49, 56, 57). Antibody levels to MA components are also elevated as compared to those of controls (17, 18). The majority of patients also show antibodies to EA, often at high titers, which in NPC are dominantly directed against D (48, 62), and in BL are often solely against R (48, 56). These differential responses are presently unexplained. VCA-specific IgM antibodies are not found in BL or NPC, but rheumatoid factor may mimic positive tests. An outstanding feature of NPC patients before treatment is the nearly uniform presence of serum IgA antibodies to VCA and, frequently, also to D; these often occur at substantial titers which at times may match those of IgG antibodies (44). VCA-specific IgA antibodies are noted only at low titers ($\leq$1:20) in no more than 30% of BL patients, transiently in about 40% of IM cases, and in less than 2% of controls or patients with other diseases who are among those who maintain relatively high VCA-specific IgG titers. In NCP anti-EBNA titers are usually also elevated, whereas in BL they may range from barely detectable to very high titers, thus extending the range of control titers at both ends of the scale.

The spectrum and titers of EBV-related antibodies are characteristic in advanced cases of BL or NPC and thus serve to support the diagnosis or to suggest it in problematic cases. The EBV-related serology appears to be more significant in monitoring of BL or NPC patients, since it provides some information on the effectiveness of therapy and thus the prognosis of the patients (56, 61, 62). When no antibodies to R are detectable or the anti-R titers decline steadily following chemotherapy, BL patients have a good prospect of becoming long-term survivors. However, when the anti-R (or anti-D) titers remain elevated or emerge and increase to high levels, the patients face one or more relapses, even after several years of complete remission, which ultimately terminate fatally (56). In NPC patients who respond only transiently to radiation therapy, antibodies of the IgG or IgA classes remain elevated or show substantial increases in titers with progression of the disease (61). In contrast, patients responding well to therapy show slow, steady declines in the antibody titers so that, depending on their initial concentrations, D-specific IgA and IgG and VCA-specific IgA antibodies gradually reach low or nondetectable levels. However, some of these patients may show arrest of the downward trend or reversal to a renewed broadening of the antibody spectrum and increasing titers. Such increases in the spectrum and titers of antibodies often become evident months before clinical recognition of renewed tumor activity or metastases (61). The EBV-related serology thus may serve to forewarn of imminent relapses or metastases.

Diseases not associated with EBV

Elevated VCA-specific IgG antibody titers, as compared to those of appropriate controls, are noted among patients with a variety of malignant or nonmalignant diseases; e.g., Hodgkin disease, other lymphomas, leukemias, various carcinomas, systemic lupus erythematosus, sarcoidosis, rheumatoid arthritis, etc. (52). In some of these cases, anti-EA, either anti-D or anti-R, may also be detectable, usually at low, but occasionally high titers for anti-D. In each disease category, a variable proportion of the patients, depending on the age ranges affected, have no antibodies to EBV so that a causal role of the virus in these diseases seems unlikely. Since all the conditions mentioned have immunosuppressive effects or require immunosuppressive therapy, activation of persistent EBV infections appears to be the most likely reason for the elevated antibody titers. Because of these observations caution is required in the interpretation of serologic diagnostic tests on patients of these types. Positive tests for VCA-specific IgM antibodies, noted in some cases of Hodgkin disease or other lymphomas, are caused by rheumatoid factor (unpublished). Also, very low anti-EBNA titers may be noted. It is unfortunate that serologic diagnostic tests may fail to provide clarification in cases in which a lymphoproliferative neoplasm and IM are considered in the differential diagnosis. However, an anti-EBNA titer of $\geq 1:20$ would tend to exclude a diagnosis of current IM.

Serologic Diagnostic Procedures

Only serologic diagnostic tests are at present useful for identification of primary EBV infections. These are divided into EBV-specific and heterophil-antibody determinations.

EBV-specific serologic diagnostic tests

Lymphoblast cultures required for the test procedures

Maintenance. The LCL are maintained in most laboratories on medium RPMI-1640 supplemented with 10% fetal calf serum (FCS), preferably heat-inactivated, and antibiotics. With 2% FSC, cultures usually do not survive.

Since some batches of FCS reduce the cellular growth rate, it is recommended to pretest lots and select those yielding optimal replication. Satisfactory batches can be stored for many months at -20 C. The cultures are usually incubated in stoppered glass or plastic flasks at 37 C but lower temperatures (32 C) may increase the numbers of virus-producing cells (see below). The cells do not attach to the surface of the vessels but settle to the bottom. Stock cultures are usually fed once a week, either by removing and replenishing part of the medium or by sedimentation of counted cells by low-speed centrifugation and resuspension in fresh medium to obtain in both instances about $2\text{-}3 \times 10^5$ viable cells/ml based on trypan blue exclusion. The cell numbers increase within 4 days to 8×10^5 to 2×10^6 cells, depending on the line, and then remain stationary. The limited feeding schedule prevents the continuous logarithmic growth which tends to gradually reduce the number of virus-producing cells. Even under the conditions described, a decline in VCA-positive cells may become apparent after a prolonged series of passages. For this reason, cells from all LCL are preserved in a liquid nitrogen freezer and revived when indicated. This precaution also serves to replace cultures which may be lost due to microbial contamination.

Types of LCL required.

1. Producer LCL provide VCA-positive cells for detection of the corresponding IgG, IgA, or IgM antibodies. It is desirable that the cultures contain between 5–15% VCA-positive cells to have sufficient numbers per microscopic field for rapid reading of results. Producer lines rarely show that many positive cells. The EB3 (24) and the HR-1 subline of P3J cultures (65), both of BL origin, are most commonly used. Before preparation of cell smears, the EB3 line is kept for 48 hr on an arginine-deprived medium (Eagle basic medium without arginine) which increases VCA-positive cells 5- to 10-fold (50). HR-1 cultures are kept at 32 C either continuously or at least for 5 days before making smears to obtain the desired numbers of VCA-positive cells.

2. Non-producer LCL are needed for the anti-EBNA and the anti-EA tests. The Raji line of BL origin (23) is commonly employed, although several others may be used. These cells contain EBNA, and smears from stock cultures are used to measure the corresponding antibodies. For the anti-EA test, Raji cells are either superinfected with EBV, which has been separated and concentrated from spent HR-1 culture medium (48, 60), or they are exposed to 20–50 μg of IUDR or BUDR/ml of medium for 1–3 days followed by further incubation in drug-free medium for 3–5 days (33, 40, 127) which derepresses the indigenous viral genome and usually leads to synthesis of only EA in a proportion of the cells. With the first method, the percentage of EA-positive cells can be adjusted readily to the desired 10%, whereas induction by IUDR is less reproducible and, furthermore, affects the quality of the smears, since the cells are often aggregated and do not flatten out.

Virus for superinfection is sedimented from HR-1 culture media (e.g., 1L) by centrifugation at about 50,000 g for 30 min and resuspended in 1 or 2 ml of fresh medium to affect a 500- to 1000-fold concentration. The virus concentrates are dispensed in small volumes (0.2–0.5 ml) and stored at -70 C or in a liquid nitrogen freezer. For titration of the virus, lots of 10^7

viable Raji cells are sedimented, resuspended in one of several serial 10-fold dilutions of virus, and incubated on a mechanical shaker at 37 C for 1 hr. Thereafter, sufficient medium is added to yield 5×10^5 cells/ml, and the cultures are further incubated for 48 hr when the maximal number of EA-positive cells is reached. For preparation of cell smears, the dilution of virus is adjusted according to the results of the titration to yield about 10% EA positive cells. The negative cells in the preparation serve as controls.

3. EBV-free LCL are required as EBNA-negative controls for the anti-EBNA test to detect the possible presence of antibodies to nuclear antigens unrelated to EBV. The MOLT-4 line (100), which has T-cell characteristics and was derived from a leukemic patient, can be used for this purpose.

Preparation of cell smears

After cell counts are made on the various untreated or treated cultures, the cells are sedimented at low speed in pointed centrifuge tubes, and the supernatant fluids are discarded (or, in the case of HR-1 cultures, saved for preparation of viral concentrates). The sedimented cells are resuspended in the remaining fluid, and a small amount of medium is added, sufficient to yield about 3×10^5 cells per drop as delivered by a finely drawn-out Pasteur pipette.

Smears are prepared either in the wells of teflon-coated microscope slides (8/slide) or on 6×30-mm coverslips. Since leakage of EBNA or D antigen from Raji cells during drying has been a continuing problem, the coverslip preparations seem to be preferable because they usually contain some satisfactory areas, even when leakage of the antigens has occurred. Six of these coverslips are each fixed by paper tape to microscope slides so that the long ends extend freely at right angles from the slides (Figure 14.2). A small drop of the cell suspension is placed on each of the 6 coverslips and spread over the surface with the drawn-out end of the Pasteur pipette. The smears are rapidly dried by an electric fan at room temperature and, in the case of Raji cells for EBNA tests, also under an infrared light, yielding a temperature of about 50 C at the coverslip level. After the smears appear to be dry, they are kept at room temperature for 1–2 hr before fixation. The slides are placed in trays of staining jars with the protruding coverslips hanging downward. The level of fixative in the staining jars is adjusted to avoid contact with the paper tape.

The fixative for VCA-positive cell smears (EB3 or HR-1) is usually acetone, although methanol can be used. EA-positive cell smears (EBV-super-infected or IUDR-induced Raji cells) are fixed either in acetone (D+R+ cells) or in methanol (D+R− cells). Both types of fixed smears are used in parallel to confirm the interpretation of the results based on the morphology of the immunofluorescent staining. For EBNA-positive cells, fixation with a precooled (−20 C) mixture of equal parts of acetone and methanol appears to be optimal. Fixation periods ranging from 3 to 10 minutes are satisfactory for all types of smears. The fixed smears are stored in covered containers at −20 C until used. Removal of needed slides from the freezer should be rapid so that the remaining slides do not attract much moisture from the air, since hydration and repeated freezing and thawing affects the integrity of the

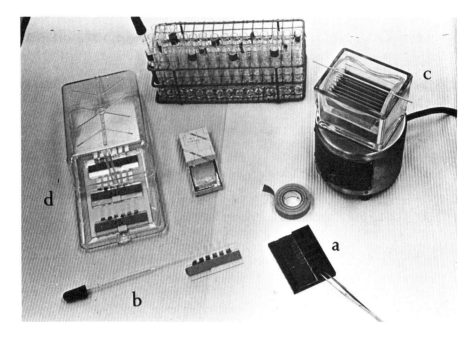

Figure 14.2.—Equipment used for preparation of cell smears and immunofluorescent staining.
    Six coverslips (6- × 30-mm) are lined up over a microscope slide
in a plastic mold (a) and attached to the slide by tape. Drops of cell
suspension are spread simultaneously over the 6 coverslips by the
drawn-out tip of a Pasteur pipette (b). After drying, the smears are
fixed, and after the staining procedure they are washed in a staining
jar (c) without or with magnetic stirring. After application of test reagents, the preparations are incubated as shown in a plastic container
(d) serving as a moist chamber. For further details see text.

smears. Before use, heavy (colored) nail polish is applied to the base of the
coverslips at the juncture with the slide to serve as a barrier. The test-serum
number and dilutions are written in insoluble ink on the tape. Each coverslip
thus remains identified throughout the staining procedure.

    Several commercial companies now sell cell smears in wells of teflon-
coated microscope slides. If they prove to be satisfactory, much labor can be
saved by diagnostic laboratories.

Serum collection and dilution

    No special precautions are needed for the collection of serum. It can be
sent to the laboratory without refrigeration as long as it is handled aseptically. It can be used for IF tests fresh or after inactivation at 56 C for 30 min.

    Serum is diluted in a veronal-buffered saline solution containing Ca^{++}
and Mg^{++} so that the same dilutions can be used for all test procedures.
While 2-fold serum dilution steps would be preferable, in order to permit

large-scale screening of serum, 4-fold dilutions are made changing pipettes for each dilution, beginning at 1:10 or 1:40, depending on anticipated results. In this manner, most endpoints are reached within 3 dilution steps. If not, higher or lower dilutions are tested subsequently. For the serologic diagnosis of IM, a 1:2 dilution is included for the anti-EBNA test.

Specific immunofluorescence tests

Since the basic procedures are described in Chapter 4, only those technical details are mentioned here which apply to the EBV-specific tests.

Indirect immunofluorescence.

1. Determination of the working dilution of FITC-conjugated antibodies to human immune globulins—For this purpose, a standard human serum with known IgG, IgM, or IgA antibodies to VCA is titrated in 2-fold steps on appropriate cell smears against serial 2-fold dilutions of conjugate, starting at 1:10. The antibody titers remain constant over several conjugate dilutions, although the intensity of staining gradually fades. At the endpoint of conjugate reactivity (1 unit), the antibody titers decline. Eight units of conjugate are employed in the test, usually corresponding to dilutions of 1:20 to 1:40 with good products such as the anti-IgG and anti-IgA conjugates from Hyland Laboratories, Costa Mesa, California, and other companies. Commercial anti-IgM conjugates are, however, often unsuitable for determination of VCA-specific IgM antibodies, but those produced by Dakopatts/AS, Copenhagen, Denmark, have been uniformly satisfactory for this purpose.

2. Determination of VCA-specific IgG or IgA antibodies—For this test, EB3 or HR-1 cell smears are first overlayered with 2 drops of test-serum dilution sufficient to cover the smear and incubated in a moist chamber for 45 min at 37 C. After rinsing with PBS, the smears are treated with FITC-conjugated antibodies to either human IgG (γ chain-specific) or to human IgA (α chain-specific) and again incubated for 45 min at 37 C. Known anti-VCA positive and negative sera serve as controls. The smears are then washed in staining jars on a magnetic stirrer twice with PBS for 5 min, rinsed finally with distilled water, and permitted to dry. The coverslips are then broken off at the base and, with forceps, mounted face down on microscope slides with elvanol-glycerol medium, 3 per slide; i.e., the 3 serial 4-fold dilutions of a given serum. The mounting medium permits storage of the preparations at 4 C for many months so that the slides can be read when convenient or rechecked months later.

3. Determination of VCA-specific IgM antibodies—For this test, HR-1 cell smears are required since a proportion of EB3 cells produces IgM. VCA-positive cells in advanced stages of degeneration are optimal to permit access of the large IgM molecules to the intracellular antigen. Therefore HR-1 cell smears are made 5 or more days after the last feeding from cultures kept at 32 C. To increase penetration of the antibodies to the intracellular antigenic sites, the incubation of the serum charge is prolonged to 3 hr at 37 C. Known VCA-specific IgM positive and negative sera are included in each test. The remainder of the procedures are conducted as for the VCA-specific IgG or IgA antibody tests, using FITC-conjugated antibodies to human IgM (μ-chain-specific). Tests for rheumatoid factor, an IgM antibody to the Fc regions of IgG, are needed to exclude its intervention in cases where clinical and laboratory data do not support a primary EBV infection (103).

4. *Determination of EA-specific IgG or IgA antibodies* —EBV-super-infected (or IUDR induced) Raji cell smears, fixed either in acetone (D+R+) or in methanol (D+R−), are used in parallel. All other procedures correspond to those described for the VCA-specific IgG or IgA test, except that known anti-D positive, anti-R positive, and anti-EA negative sera serve as controls. If immunofluorescence is obtained with acetone-fixed but not with methanol-fixed smears, the antibodies are directed solely against the R component. If acetone- and methanol-fixed smears yield equal titers, the antibodies are dominantly directed against D. Any anti-R reactions of lower titers that might also be present in such sera cannot be discerned in the presence of brilliant D fluorescence. If acetone-fixed smears yield a higher antibody titer than methanol-fixed smears, anti-R is the dominant antibody, its titer being revealed by the acetone-fixed smears and the anti-D titer by the methanol-fixed smears. Unfortunately, EBV-superinfected Raji cells are unsuitable for measuring EA-specific IgM antibodies since the conjugate alone gives considerable background staining.

Anti-C′ immunofluorescence determination of antibodies to EBNA. For this procedure, smears of Raji cells from stock cultures or cells from other nonproducer LCL are used. The smears are successively overlayed with test-serum dilution, human serum from a donor negative for VCA antibodies as source of C′, and FITC-conjugated antibodies to human $\beta_1 C/\beta_1 A$ globulins, each for 45 min at 37 C, rinsing after the first and second charges. The final (third) washing and rinsing in distilled water as well as the mounting of the coverslips follows the procedures described for the indirect FA tests. For determination of the working dilution of C′, cell smears are overlayed successively with a standard human anti-EBNA positive serum diluted 1:10 or 1:20, one of serial 2-fold dilutions of C′ beginning at 1:10 and the anti-human $\beta_1 C/\beta_1 A$ conjugate. Four times the last effective amount of C′, usually corresponding to dilutions between 1:20 and 1:40, is used for the test. The working dilution of the conjugate is determined by titration using serial 2-fold dilutions of a standard anti-EBNA positive serum and 4 units of C′. Mixing of the serum dilution and C′ to reduce the number of steps in this procedure is not acceptable because the C′ activity may be reduced or abolished by anticomplementary sera leading to false-negative or prozone reactions (55). Known anti-EBNA-positive- and -negative sera as well as EBNA-negative cell smears (e.g., MOLT-4 cells) serve as controls, the last to exclude false-positive results due to nonspecific antinuclear factors.

Evaluation of immunofluorescence tests

The required microscopic equipment, illumination, and filters for FA procedures are described in Chapter 4. While with dark-field illumination the immunofluorescent cells can easily be seen at low magnification (10X objective), the glycerol required on the dark-field condenser needs to be removed from the underside of the slides if they are to be kept. For this reason, incident illumination is now prefered, but it requires examination of the slides at higher magnification (40X objective). Under these conditions, weak staining may still be detectable with serum dilutions which are judged negative at lower magnification under dark-field illumination, increasing the antibody titers by a factor of about 2.

When the proportion of VCA- or EA-reactive cells is of the order of 10% based upon brilliant staining by low dilutions of a positive serum, the percentage of weakly stained cells at the endpoint dilution of this serum may possibly be reduced to 3%, because the cells do not contain equal amounts of antigen or the antibodies may be unevenly distributed. An occasional, brightly stained, degenerating cell at or beyond the antibody endpoint has to be disregarded because of nonspecific attachment of IgG and/or the anti-IgG conjugate.

With the 4-fold dilution scale, the highest serum dilution yielding immunofluorescence is taken as the endpoint if the staining is weak. However, if the immunofluorescence elicited by this dilution is still moderately strong, the endpoint is considered to be 2-fold higher. While this interpolation requires a subjective grading, the titers so determined have been well reproducible in simultaneous multiple titrations of given sera or on repetition of tests at different times.

In the anti-C' IF test for antibodies to EBNA, nearly all of the cells show nuclear fluorescence decreasing in intensity up to the endpoint, at least in satisfactory portions of the smears. However, at the endpoint and higher dilutions of the test sera, staining of C' receptors at the cell surface becomes increasingly evident. These reactions are easily differentiated from specific nuclear staining. C' receptors are not detectable in the presence of strong EBNA staining because C' evidently binds preferentially to antigen-antibody complexes. Nuclear staining due to nonspecific antinuclear factors as detected with control smears of EBNA-negative cells is often distinct from typical EBNA fluorescence but in some instances may mimic it closely.

Heterophil antibody tests

A variety of techniques have been developed for determination of heterophil antibody responses, using sheep, horse, or beef erythrocytes (RBC). Some require treatment of the RBC or adsorption of the sera. Most are performed in test tubes, but rapid slide tests have been developed and the reagents are commercially available so that tests can be performed in a physician's office.

Tests with native sheep erythrocytes

The presumptive test. This tube test measures titers of agglutinins for sheep RBCs as originally described by Paul and Bunnell (107). Davidsohn and others had earlier noted similar, at times substantial, reactivities in serum from patients with several other conditions, including serum sickness, leukemias, viral hepatitis, etc., and generally low titers in serum from some healthy individuals (8). Until 1968 this test, referred to as the Paul-Bunnel test, was considered as the screening test of choice for heterophil-antibody-positive IM.

Test procedure: 0.1 ml of heat-inactivated serum (56 C for 30 min) is added to 0.4 ml of 0.85% NaCl in the first of 12 10- × 75-mm test tubes. 0.25 ml of 0.85% NaCl is then added to the other tubes (#2-12) and 2-fold dilutions are made by transferring 0.25 ml from the first tube to the second and so on; 0.25 ml is discarded from the final tube. To each tube (#1-12) 0.1 ml of a 2% suspension of sheep RBCs is added. The final dilution in the first tube is 1:5 before adding the cell suspension and 1:7 after adding the sheep cell suspension. Dilutions in subsequent tubes are 1:14, 1:28, 1:56, etc. up to 1:14,336. The tubes are shaken and incubated at room temperature for 2 hr. The settled RBCs are resuspended by agitation and read for macroscopic agglutination. Positive sera often show agglutination after 15–30 min; however, negative results (<1:7) should be reported only after 2 hr of incubation (83).

Interpretation: Titers ≧ 1:224 are usually considered as positive for IM. Such levels are occasionally encountered, however, in other conditions such as serum sickness or following blood transfusions (13). Titers of <1:7 to 1:112 are seen in healthy individuals, many patients with diseases other than IM and, also in at least 20% of patients with IM, especially early in the disease (12, 13). A positive presumptive test at any level needs to be followed by a differential absorption test (see below) in all cases where clinical and hematologic findings suggest IM.

The differential absorption test. This tube test, commonly referred to as the Paul-Bunnel-Davidsohn (PBD) test, measures sheep RBC agglutinins before and after absorption of the test serum with Forssman antigen, usually guinea pig kidney (GPK) suspensions, and beef RBCs, respectively, both in 0.8% NaCl (9, 14). The anti-sheep agglutinins of IM (i.e., IM-specific heterophil antibodies) are not absorbed by GPK suspensions but are removed by beef RBCs. In contrast, the anti-sheep agglutinins in non-IM diseases and healthy controls are absorbed by GPK suspensions but not by beef RBCs.

Absorption of serum: 0.2 ml of inactivated serum is added to separate 1.0 ml volumes of absorbing reagents, usually 20% suspensions of GPK and boiled beef RBCs. The 2 mixtures are incubated at room temperature with frequent shaking for 10 min. They are then centrifuged, and the clear supernatant fluids representing GPK- and beef cell-absorbed serum samples are used for the test. Since the initial absorbing suspensions are 20% solid, only 0.8 ml is used to dilute the serum. Thus, the supernatant serum after absorption represents a 1:5 dilution. The GPK or beef RBC suspensions are available from several commercial sources, including Difco Laboratories, Detroit, Michigan. A 20% suspension of horse kidney can be substituted for the GPK preparation.

Test procedure: The set-up of the differential test is the same as for the presumptive test, except that 0.25 ml of absorbed serum, without further dilution, is added to the first tube (containing no saline) and to the second tube (with 0.25 ml of saline). Serial dilutions are then carried out from the second tube to the third and so on, and 0.1 ml volumes of a 2% sheep RBC suspension are then added to each tube resulting in final dilutions of 1:7, 1:14, 1:28, etc. up to 1:14,336 in the twelfth tube. The test is then incubated for 2 hr as in the presumptive test, after which they are read macroscopically for agglutination and interpreted against the baseline titer from the presumptive test (13, 83).

Interpretation: Positive reactions are recorded only if the differential absorption pattern is typical for IM; i.e., the GPK-absorbed anti-sheep agglutinins should decrease by no more than 3 tubes in titer, while beef cell-absorbed agglutinins should be almost completely removed or show a drop in titer of at least 4 tubes compared to the baseline titers in the presumptive test. If the presumptive titer is less than 1:56, any incomplete removal by GPK and complete removal by beef RBCs is considered as a positive test (13).

Comment: The PBD test is the best documented reference test available for IM. Since its original description in 1935, this confirmatory test has been found to be highly specific for IM (3, 15). In over 30 years of study, Davidsohn has encountered false-positives in only 2 cases, one a patient with Hodgkin disease and the other a patient with rheumatoid arthritis (10). False-positive reactions have also been reported in isolated patients with lymphosarcoma, diabetes, tularemia, progressive polyarthritis, the myelo-proliferative syndrome, and in a few patients receiving antithymocyte serum (10, 70, 111). Bender concluded that there was no satisfactory evidence that a positive PBD test could be caused by any condition other than IM (5). Thus, in patients with clinical signs and hematologic features of IM, a positive test establishes the diagnosis.

The sensitivity of the PBD test depends in part on the time after onset when the test is done and the criteria utilized for clinical diagnosis. Peak titers are encountered during the second and third weeks of illness. The test is qualitative rather than quantitative, and its main purpose is to separate heterophil antibodies of the IM type from Forssman antibodies. It should not be used to follow the clinical course of illness, as there is a poor correlation between the titer of GPK-absorbed anti-sheep agglutinins and either the stage and severity of illness or the numbers of atypical lymphocytes (5, 30). While the majority of patients are positive on initial specimens, a few patients turn positive 2–4 weeks after onset, usually after blood smears have already suggested a diagnosis of IM.

The differential test with horse erythrocytes

This tube test, referred to as the *Lee-Davidsohn Test*, measures titers of agglutinins for horse RBCs after differential absorption of the serum. In 1968, Lee and Davidsohn reaffirmed the greater sensitivity of horse over sheep RBCs in the detection of heterophil antibodies and reported cases of heterophil-antibody-positive IM that by standard sheep cell methods (PBD test) would have been considered negative or inconclusive (85). The test is specific and has increased sensitivity over that of the PBD test. The criterion for a positive test is simplified, and baseline unabsorbed anti-horse agglutinin titers are not needed (87).

Test procedure: Absorption of serum and the antibody titrations are performed exactly as in the PBD test; however, a 2% suspension of horse RBCs replace sheep cells as the indicator antigen for heterophil antibodies.

Interpretation: If the GPK-absorbed agglutinin titer exceeds the beef RBC-absorbed titer, the test is interpreted as positive. If the beef cell-absorbed titer is equal or greater than the GPK-absorbed titer, the test is interpreted as negative for heterophil-positive IM.

Comment: Initial studies with horse RBCs by Lee and Davidsohn suggested that specificity was retained if differential absorption was included as part of their sensitive tube test system (87). They then established the potential usefulness of this test in the *early* diagnosis of IM and recommended its use when agglutinin titers obtained with sheep RBCs were ≦1:28 and the clinical and hematologic findings suggested IM (83). These observations were confirmed by Nikoskelainen et al, who suggested that all clinical cases resembling IM be tested with horse RBCs when the classic PBD test was negative (103).

Over the past 6 years, one of the authors (CAH) utilized the Lee-Davidsohn test and confirmed the increased sensitivity of horse RBCs for detection of heterophil antibodies as compared to the PBD reaction. Also the specificity was confirmed by negative test results in greater than 99% of over 2000 patients without acute heterophil-positive IM. During this interval, 14 individuals were encountered who gave positive-heterophil-antibody reactions but did not fulfill minimal hematologic criteria for IM and generally had no or minimal signs of this disease (70). Four of these 14 patients showed EBV-specific serologic evidence of current or recent primary EBV infections. The other 10 patients had stable EBV-related antibody patterns indicative of past primary infections, leaving the heterophil-antibody reactions unexplained. However, the Lee-Davidsohn test permits detection of IM-specific heterophil antibodies for longer periods of time than does the PBD tests; i.e., for many months or even years following acute IM. Positive differential absorption tests were recorded for at least 12 months in 25% of 95 serially studied patients and in several cases for up to 30 months (28, 70). Due to its sensitivity and specificity, the horse RBC system appears to be optimal for detection of a maximal number of heterophil-antibody-positive cases of IM, and the Lee-Davidsohn test thus should replace the PBD test, as recommended also by Evans et al (28).

The ox cell hemolysin test

This test detects hemolysins for beef RBCs that occur in high titer in serum from patients with IM (11, 89, 91).

Test procedure: Heat-inactivated serum (56 C for 30 min) is diluted in 2-fold steps from 1:20, to 1:10,240 in buffered saline, using 1 ml volumes, and 0.5 ml of a 1.1% beef RBC suspension is added to each tube. After incubation for 10 min at room temperature, 0.5 ml of diluted (1:40) guinea pig complement is added to each tube and, after mixing, the test is incubated for 30 min at 37 C. Known positive and negative sera serve as controls. The highest test serum dilution yielding a degree of hemolysis greater than that of the 50% hemolysis standard is recorded as the titer (11, 83).

Interpretation: Positive results are reported with titers of 1:40 or above.

Comment: With a cut-off level for positive and negative results at a serum dilution of 1:40, false positives are uncommon (11). They occasionally occur in patients who have received blood group substances or transfusions, but the test is generally considered to be as specific and sensitive for IM as the PBD test (13). In contrast to differential absorption tests, this test is usually negative (<1:40) by 6–9 months after onset (28). Because of its specificity and relative sensitivity, this test serves as a valuable reference test for IM. It can also be automated and thus is particularly useful for epidemiologic surveys.

Tests with enzyme-treated sheep erythrocytes

Wöllner discovered that the IM-specific antigen, but not the Forssman antigen, on sheep RBCs is destroyed by various plant enzymes, including papain. He devised 2 enzyme tests (I and II) using both native and papain-treated sheep RBCs (133, 134).

Enzyme Test I. Inactivated normal and IM sera are tested against both papain-treated and untreated sheep RBCs. Normal serum has higher titers with papain-treated cells than with native cells, whereas the situation is reversed with IM serum. This test is severely limited by a significant number (30%) of false-negative test results in IM.

Enzyme Test II. The patient's serum is absorbed with papain-treated sheep RBCs and then compared with untreated serum. Results are interpreted as in the PBD test. In IM, the agglutinin titer of the absorbed serum titrated against untreated cells is always 4 or more tubes higher than the titer with papain-treated cells. In illnesses other than heterophil-antibody-positive IM, papain-treated cells completely absorb the sheep agglutinins or the absorbed sera yield higher titers with treated than with untreated cells.

Comment: The enzyme test II gives results that parallel the PBD test (11). Despite excellent specificity for IM, this test offers no particular advantages over the PBD test, and the lability of papain solutions significantly limits the usefulness of this test.

Rapid slide tests

Most of the 1- to 2-min rapid slide tests for IM utilize *fine* suspensions of GPK and beef RBC stromas for rapid differential absorption and *horse* RBCs for sensitive detection of heterophil antibodies (31, 84). A drop of serum is first mixed on the slide with the absorbent and then with the horse RBC antigen. An IM-specific reaction is revealed when rapid agglutination is observed with the untreated and GPK-absorbed serum samples but not with the beef stroma-absorbed preparation. Because of their sensitivity, simplicity, and convenience the slide tests have replaced the presumptive test in many laboratories as the screening test of choice for IM. The tests should be sensitive enough so that a negative result implies the absence of significant titers of IM-specific heterophil antibodies. As with all tests for IM, results must always be correlated with hematological and clinical findings.

It has been the experience of one of the authors (CAH) with one of the commercially available rapid slide test kits (Monospot®, Ortho-Diagnostics) that false-negative reactions are uncommon (<1.0%), whereas false-positive agglutination occurs with about 3% of serum samples. The incidence of false-positive or false-negative results depends in part on the sensitivity of the reagents provided by the rapid slide test kits (31). In general, sensitive rapid tests should detect GPK-absorbed agglutinins against horse RBCs of titers ≧1:56–1:112, while less sensitive commercially available tests may require titers of 1:224–1:448 before positive slide reactions are recorded. The preservative used for the horse RBCs by different companies may affect the sensitivity of the test; formalinized RBCs being least sensitive, thus yielding more false-negative results than RBCs preserved by other means. The descriptions and instructions inserted into the test kit packages should be consulted to determine the advantages and limitations of particular products. Deviation from the recommended technical performances of the tests may produce incorrect results.

A practical approach to the diagnosis of IM.

The following have proved to be suitable for the serologic diagnosis of IM.

1. When positive results are obtained in a rapid slide test with serum from an acutely ill patient whose blood smears show significant numbers of atypical lymphocytes, the diagnosis of IM is established. Reference tube

tests, while providing confirmation, are not essential, as the antibody titers do not correlate in individual cases with the severity of illness or the prognosis (30).

2. When a positive rapid slide test is recorded but blood smears do not suggest IM, the reference differential absorption tube test, using horse RBCs (Lee-Davidsohn test), should be performed to differentiate between a false-positive screening test result and IM-specific heterophil antibodies. If the Lee-Davidsohn test indicates that the beef cell-absorbed agglutinin titer is greater than the GPK-absorbed titer, the result of the rapid test was falsely positive. When an IM-specific pattern of heterophil antibodies is found (GPK-absorbed titer > beef RBC-absorbed titer) the patient should be questioned regarding illnesses resembling IM that might have occurred during the preceding months or year. EBV-specific serologic diagnostic tests may then be indicated for final clarification.

3. If the rapid slide test is negative but blood smears strongly suggest IM, the Lee-Davidsohn test is performed to determine whether the patient developed no or only low titers of IM-specific heterophil antibodies. Follow-up serum specimens should be requested to exclude a late evolution of IM-type heterophil agglutinins. In such cases, EBV-specific and other serologic diagnostic tests are required to differentiate between heterophil antibody-negative EBV-induced IM and IM-like illnesses due to CMV, *Toxoplasma gondii,* adenovirus, or other viruses.

References

1. ARMSTRONG D, HENLE G, and HENLE W: Complement fixation tests with cell lines derived from Burkitt's lymphoma and acute leukemias. J Bacteriol 91:1257–1262, 1966
2. AYA T and OSATO T: Early events in transformation of human cord leukocytes by Epstein-Barr virus: induction of DNA synthesis and virus-associated nuclear antigen. Int J Cancer 13:341–347, 1974.
3. BAILEY GH and RAFFEL S: Hemolytic antibodies for sheep and ox erythrocytes in infectious mononucleosis. J Clin Invest 14:228–244, 1935.
4. BAR R, DeLOR CL, CLAUSEN KP, HURTUBISE P, HENLE W, and HEWETSON J: Fatal infectious mononucleosis in a family. N Engl J Med 290:363–367, 1974.
5. BENDER CE: Interpretation of hematologic and serologic findings in the diagnosis of infectious mononucleosis. Ann Intern Med 49:852–865, 1958
6. CARTER RL: Antibody formation in infectious mononucleosis. II. Other 19S antibodies and false-positive serology. Br J Haematol 12:268–275, 1966
7. CARTER RL: Infectious mononucleosis: model for self limiting lymphoproliferation. Lancet 1:846–849, 1975
8. DAVIDSOHN I: Heterophile antibodies in serum sickness. J Immunol 16:259–273, 1929
9. DAVIDSOHN I: Serologic diagnosis of infectious mononucleosis. J Am Med Assoc 108:289–295, 1937
10. DAVIDSOHN I and LEE CL: The laboratory in the diagnosis of infectious mononucleosis. Med Clin North Am 46:225–244, 1962
11. DAVIDSOHN I and LEE CL: Serologic diagnosis of infectious mononucleosis. A comparative study of five tests. Am J Clin Pathol 41:115–125, 1964
12. DAVIDSOHN I and LEE CL: The clinical serology of infectious mononucleosis. *In* Infectious Mononucleosis, Carter RL and Penman HG (eds), Oxford, Blackwell Scientific Publications, 1969, pp 177–200
13. DAVIDSOHN I and NELSON DA: The Blood. *In* Todd-Sanford's Clinical Diagnosis by Laboratory Methods, 14th edition, Davidsohn I and Henry JB (eds), Philadelphia, W.B. Saunders Co., 1969, Chap 5

14. DAVIDSOHN I, STERN K, and KASHIWAGI C: The differential test for infectious mononucleosis. Am J Clin Pathol 21:1101–1113, 1951

15. DAVIDSOHN I and WALKER PH: The nature of the heterophilic antibodies in infectious mononucleosis. Am J Clin Pathol 5:455–465, 1935

16. DE SCHRYVER A, KLEIN G, HEWETSON J, ROCCHI G, HENLE W, HENLE G, and POPE J: Comparison of EBV neutralization tests based on abortive infection or transformation of lymphoid cells and their relation to membrane reactive antibodies (anti-MA). Int J Cancer 13:353–362, 1974

17. DE SCHRYVER A, FRIBERG S, JR, KLEIN G, HENLE W, HENLE G, DE-THE G, CLIFFORD P, and HO HC: Epstein-Barr virus (EBV)-associated antibody patterns in carcinoma of the post-nasal space. Clin Exp Immunol 5:443–459, 1969

18. DE SCHRYVER A, KLEIN G, HENLE W, CAMERON H, SANTESSON L, and CLIFFORD P: EB-virus associated serology in malignant disease: Antibody levels to viral capsid antigens (VCA), membrane antigens (MA) and early antigens (EA) in patients with various neoplastic conditions. Int J Cancer 9:353–364, 1972

19. DIEHL V, HENLE G, HENLE W, and KOHN G: Demonstration of a herpes group virus in cultures of peripheral leukocytes from patients with infectious mononucleosis. J Virol 2:663–669, 1968

20. DIEHL V, HENLE G, HENLE W, and KOHN G: Effect of a herpes group virus (EBV) on growth of peripheral leukocyte cultures. In Vitro 4:92–99, 1969

21. DORFMAN RF and WARNKE R: Lymphadenopathy simulating the malignant lymphomas. Human Pathol 5:519, 1974

22. EPSTEIN MA and ACHONG BG: Specific immunofluorescence test for the herpes-type EB virus of Burkitt lymphoblasts, authenticated by electron microscopy. J Nat Cancer Inst 40:593–607, 1968

23. EPSTEIN MA, ACHONG BG, BARR YM, ZAJAC B, HENLE G, and HENLE W: Morphological and virological investigations on cultured Burkitt tumor lymphoblasts (Strain Raji). J Nat Cancer Inst 37:547–559, 1966

24. EPSTEIN MA, BARR YM, and ACHONG BG: Studies with Burkitt's lymphoma. Wistar Inst Sympos Monogr 4:69–82, 1965

25. ERNBERG I, KLEIN G, KOURILSKY FM, and SILVESTRE D: Differentiation between early and late membrane antigen on human lymphoblastoid cell lines infected with Epstein-Barr virus. I. Immunofluorescence. J Nat Cancer Inst 53:61–65, 1974

26. EVANS AS: Infectious mononucleosis. *In* Textbook of Hematology, Williams I, Beutler E, Erslev AJ, and Rundles RW (eds), New York, McGraw-Hill, 1972, pp 843–853

27. EVANS AS, NIEDERMAN JC, and McCOLLUM RW: Seroepidemiologic studies of infectious mononucleosis with EB virus. N Engl J Med 279:1121–1127, 1968

28. EVANS AS, NIEDERMAN JC, CENABRE LC, WEST B, and RICHARDS VA: A prospective evaluation of heterophile and Epstein-Barr virus-specific IgM antibody titers in clinical and subclinical infectious mononucleosis: specificity and sensitivity of the tests and persistence of antibody. J Infect Dis 132:546–553, 1975

29. FILATOV NF: Lektsii ob Ostrykh Infektsionnykh Boleznyakh u Detey. Vol. 1, pp 13–14 Lang, Moscow, 1885

30. FINCH SC: Laboratory findings in infectious mononucleosis. *In* Infectious Mononucleosis, Carter RL and Penman HG (eds), Oxford, Blackwell, 1969, pp 47–62

31. GALLOWAY E: Comparison of three slide tests for infectious mononucleosis with Davidsohn's presumptive and differential heterophil test. Can J Med Technol 31:197–206, 1969

32. GELB D, WEST M, and ZIMMERMAN HJ: Serum enzymes in disease. IX. Analysis of factors responsible for elevated values in infectious mononucleosis. Am J Med 33:249–261, 1962

33. GERBER P: Activation of Epstein-Barr virus by bromodeoxyuridine in "virus-free" human cells. Proc Nat Acad Sci USA 69:83–85, 1972

34. GERBER P and DEAL DR: Epstein-Barr virus-induced viral and soluble complement-fixing antigens in Burkitt's lymphoma cell cultures. Proc Soc Exp Biol Med 134:748–751, 1970

35. GERBER P, WHANG-PENG J, and MONROE JH: Transformation and chromosome changes induced by Epstein-Barr virus in normal human leukocyte cultures. Proc Nat Acad Sci USA 63:740–747, 1969

36. GERBER P, NONOYAMA M, LUCAS S, PERLIN E, and GOLDSTEIN LI: Oral excretion of Epstein-Barr virus by healthy subjects and patients with infectious mononucleosis. Lancet 2:988–989, 1972

37. GINSBURG CM, HENLE G, and HENLE W: An outbreak of infectious mononucleosis among the personnel of an outpatient clinic. Am J Epidemiol 104:571–575, 1976

38. GINSBURG CM, HENLE W, HENLE G, and HORWITZ CA: Infectious mononucleosis in children: evaluation of the Epstein-Barr virus-specific serology. J Am Med Assoc 237:781–785, 1977

39. HALLEE TJ, EVANS AS, and NIEDERMAN JC: Infectious mononucleosis at the United States Military Academy. A Prospective study of a single class over 4 years. Yale J Biol Med 3:182–192, 1974

40. HAMPAR B, DERGE JG, MARTOS LM, and WALKER JL: Synthesis of Epstein-Barr virus after activation of the viral genome in a "virus-negative" human lymphoblastoid cell (Raji) made resistant to 5-bromodeoxyuridine. Proc Nat Acad Sci USA 69:78–82, 1972

41. HENLE G and HENLE W: Immunofluorescence in cells derived from Burkitt's lymphoma. J Bacteriol 91:1248–1256, 1966

42. HENLE G and HENLE W: Immunofluorescence, interference and complement fixation techniques in the detection of the herpes-type virus in Burkitt tumor cell lines. Cancer Res 27:2442–2446, 1967

43. HENLE G and HENLE W: Observations on childhood infections with the Epstein-Barr virus. J Infect Dis 121:303–310, 1970

44. HENLE G and HENLE W: Epstein-Barr virus-specific IgA serum antibodies as an outstanding feature of nasopharyngeal carcinoma. Int J Cancer 17:1–7, 1976

45. HENLE G, HENLE W, CLIFFORD P, DIEHL V, KAFUKO GW, KIRYA BG, KLEIN G, MORROW RH, MUNUBE GMR, PIKE MC, TUKEI PM, and ZIEGLER JL: Antibodies to EB virus in Burkitt's lymphoma and control groups. J Nat Cancer Inst 43:1147–1157, 1969

46. HENLE G, HENLE W, and DIEHL V: Relation of Burkitt tumor associated herpes-type virus to infectious mononucleosis. Proc Nat Acad Sci USA 59:94–101, 1968

47. HENLE G, HENLE W, and HORWITZ CA: Antibodies to Epstein-Barr virus-associated nuclear antigen in infectious mononucleosis. J Infect Dis 130:231–239, 1974

48. HENLE G, HENLE W, and KLEIN G: Demonstration of two distinct components in the early antigen complex of Epstein-Barr virus infected cells. Int J Cancer 8:272–282, 1971

49. HENLE G, HENLE W, KLEIN G, GUNVEN P, CLIFFORD P, MORROW RH, and ZIEGLER JL: Antibodies to early Epstein-Barr virus-induced antigens in Burkitt's lymphoma. J Nat Cancer Inst 46:861–871, 1971

50. HENLE W and HENLE G: Effect of arginine-deficient media on the herpes-type virus associated with cultured Burkitt tumor cells. J Virol 2:182–191, 1968

51. HENLE W and HENLE G: Epstein-Barr virus: The cause of infectious mononucleosis. In Oncogenesis and Herpesviruses, Biggs IM, de Thé G, and Payne LN (eds), IARC Sci Publ No. 2, Lyon, 1972, pp 269–274

52. HENLE W and HENLE G: Epstein-Barr Virus (EBV)-Related Serology in Hodgkin's Disease. Natl Cancer Inst Mono. No. 36, Kaplan HS (ed), 1973, pp 79–84

53. HENLE W and HENLE G: Epstein-Barr virus and human malignancies. Cancer 34:1368–1374, 1974

54. HENLE W, DIEHL V, KOHN G, ZUR HAUSEN H, and HENLE G: Herpes-type virus and chromosome marker in normal leukocytes after growth with irradiated Burkitt cells. Science 157:1064–1065, 1967

55. HENLE W, GUERRA A, and HENLE G: False-negative and prozone reactions in tests for antibodies to Epstein-Barr virus-associated nuclear antigen. Int J Cancer 13:751–754, 1974

56. HENLE W, HENLE G, GUNVÉN P, KLEIN G, CLIFFORD P, and SINGH S: Patterns of antibodies to Epstein-Barr virus-induced early antigens in Burkitt's lymphoma. Comparison of dying patients with long-term survivors. J Nat Cancer Inst 50:1163–1173, 1973

57. HENLE W, HENLE G, HO HC, BURTIN P, CACHIN Y, CLIFFORD P, DE-SCHRYVER A, DE-THÉ G, DIEHL V, and KLEIN G: Antibodies to Epstein-Barr virus in nasopharyngeal

carcinoma, other head and neck neoplasms and control groups. J Nat Cancer Inst 44:225–231, 1970

58. HENLE W, HENLE G, and HORWITZ CA: Epstein-Barr virus-specific diagnostic tests in infectious mononucleosis. Human Pathol 5:551–565, 1974

59. HENLE W, HENLE G, NIEDERMAN JC, KLEMOLA E, and HALTIA K: Antibodies to early antigens induced by Epstein-Barr virus in infectious mononucleosis. J Infect Dis 124:58–67, 1971

60. HENLE W, HENLE G, ZAJAC B, PEARSON G, WAUBKE R, and SCRIBA M: Differential reactivity of human sera with EBV-induced "early antigens". Science 169:188–190, 1970

61. HENLE W, HO HC, HENLE G, CHAU JCW, and KWAN HC: Nasopharyngeal carcinoma: Significance of changes in Epstein-Barr virus-related antibody patterns following therapy. Int J Cancer 20:663–672, 1977

62. HENLE W, HO HC, HENLE G, and KWAN HC: Antibodies to Epstein-Barr virus-related antigens in nasopharyngeal carcinoma. Comparison of active cases and long term survivors. J Nat Cancer Inst 51:361–369, 1973

63. HENLE W, HUMMELER K, and HENLE G: Antibody coating and agglutination of virus particles separated from the EB3 line of Burkitt lymphoma cells. J Bacteriol 92:269–271, 1966

64. HEWETSON JF, ROCCHI G, HENLE, W, and HENLE G: Neutralizing antibodies against Epstein-Barr virus in healthy populations and patients with infectious mononucleosis. J Infect Dis 128:283–289, 1973

65. HINUMA Y, KOHN M, YAMAGUCHI J, WUDARSKI DJ, BLAKESEE JR, JR, and GRACE JT, JR Immunofluorescence and herpes-type virus particles in the P3HR-1 Burkitt lymphoma cell line. J Virol 1:1045–1051, 1967

66. HIRSHAUT Y, CHRISTENSON WN, and PERLMUTTER JC: Prospective study of herpes-like virus role in infectious mononucleosis. Clin Res 19:459–463, 1971

67. HO HC, HUANG DP, HENLE W, HENLE G, and CHAU JCW: Study of biopsies from nasopharyngeal and other carcinomas of the head and neck for Epstein-Barr virus-associated nuclear antigen. In preparation.

68. HOAGLAND RJ: The transmission of infectious mononucleosis. Am J Med Sci 229:262–272, 1955

69. HORWITZ CA, HENLE W, HENLE G, SEGAL M, ARNOLD T, LEWIS FB, ZANICK D, and WARD PCJ: Clinical and laboratory evaluation of elderly patients with heterophil-antibody positive infectious mononucleosis—report of seven patients, ages 40–78. Am J Med 61:333–339, 1976

70. HORWITZ C, HENLE W, HENLE G, POLESKY H, WEXLER H, and WARD PCJ: The specificity of heterophil antibodies and healthy donors with no or minimal signs of infectious mononucleosis. Blood 47:91–98, 1976

71. HORWITZ CA, HENLE W, HENLE G, POLESKY H, BALFOUR HH JR, SIEM RA, BORKEN S, and WARD PCJ: Heterophil-negative infectious mononucleosis and mononucleosis-like illnesses: laboratory confirmation of 43 cases. Am J Med 63:947–957, 1977

72. HUANG DP, HO JHC, HENLE W, and HENLE G: Demonstration of EBV-associated nuclear antigens in NPC cells from fresh biopsies. Int J Cancer 14:580–588, 1974

73. JONDAL M, and KLEIN G: Surface markers on human B and T lymphocytes. II. Presence of Epstein-Barr virus receptors on B lymphocytes. J Exp Med 138:1365–1378, 1973

74. JUDSON SC, HENLE W, and HENLE G: A cluster of Epstein-Barr virus-associated American Burkitt's lymphoma. N Engl J Med 297:464–468, 1977

75. KAFUKO GW, DAY NE, HENDERSON BE, HENLE G, HENLE W, KIRYA G, MUNUBE G, MORROW RH, PIKE MC, SMITH PG, TUKEI P, and WILLIAMS EH: Epstein-Barr virus antibody levels in children from the West Nile District of Uganda: Report of a field study. Lancet 1:706–709, 1972

76. KLEIN G: The Epstein-Barr virus and neoplasia. N Engl J Med 293:1353–1356, 1975

77. KLEIN G, PEARSON G, HENLE G, HENLE W, DIEHL V, and NIEDERMAN JC: Relation between Epstein-Barr viral and cell membrane immunofluorescence in Burkitt tumor cells. II. Comparison of cells and sera from patients with Burkitt's lymphoma and infectious mononucleosis. J Exp Med 128:1021–1030, 1968

78. KLEIN G, PEARSON G, HENLE G, HENLE W, GOLDSTEIN G, and CLIFFORD P: Relation between Epstein-Barr viral and cell membrane immunofluorescence in Burkitt tumor cells. III. Comparison of blocking and direct membrane immunofluorescence and anti-EBV reactivities of different sera. J Exp Med 129:697–705, 1969

79. KLEIN G, PEARSON G, NADKARNI JS, NADKARNI, JJ, KLEIN E, HENLE G, HENLE W, and CLIFFORD P: Relation between Epstein-Barr viral and cell membrane immunofluorescence of Burkitt tumor cells. I. Dependence of cell membrane immunofluorescence on presence of EB virus. J Exp Med 128:1011–1020, 1968

80. KLEIN G, SVEDMYR E, JONDAL M, and PERSSON PO: EBV-determined nuclear antigen (EBNA)-positive cells in the peripheral blood of infectious mononucleosis patients. Int J Cancer 17:21–26, 1976

81. KLEIN G, and VONKA V: Relationship between the Epstein-Barr virus (EBV) determined complement-fixing antigen and the nuclear antigen (EBNA) detected by anti-complement fluorescence. J Natl Cancer Inst 53:1645–1646, 1971

82. KLEMOLA E, VON ESSEN R, HENLE G, and HENLE W: Infectious mononucleosis-like disease with negative heterophil agglutination test. Clinical features in relation to Epstein-Barr virus and cytomegalovirus antibodies. J Infect Dis 121:608–614, 1970

83. LEE CL, and DAVIDSOHN I: Serologic test for infectious mononucleosis. Chicago, American Society of Clinical Pathologists Commission on Continuing Education, 1972

84. LEE CL, DAVIDSOHN I, and PANCZYSZYN O: Horse agglutinins in infectious mononucleosis. II. The spot test. Am J Clin Pathol 49:12–18, 1968

85. LEE CL, DAVIDSOHN I, and SLABY R: Horse agglutinins in infectious mononucleosis. Am J Clin Pathol 49:3–11, 1968

86. LEE CL, TAKAHASKI T, and DAVIDSOHN I: Sheep erythrocyte agglutinins and beef erythrocyte hemolysins in infectious mononucleosis serum. J Immunol 91:783–790, 1963

87. Lee CL, Zandrew F, and DAVIDSOHN I: Horse agglutinins in infectious mononucleosis. III. Criterion for differential diagnosis. J Clin Pathol 21:631–634, 1968

88. LEIBOLD W, FLANAGAN TD, MENENEZ J, and KLEIN G: Induction of Epstein-Barr virus (EBV)-associated nuclear antigen (EBNA) during *in vitro* transformation of human lymphoid cells. J Natl Cancer Inst 54:65–68, 1975

89. LEYTON GB: Ox-cell hemolysins in human serum. J Clin Pathol 5:324–328, 1952

90. LINDAHL T, KLEIN G, REEDMAN BM, JOHANSSON B, and SINGH S: Relationship between Epstein-Barr virus (EBV) DNA and the EBV-determined nuclear antigen (EBNA) in Burkitt lymphoma biopsies and other lymphoproliferative malignancies. Int J Cancer 13:764–772, 1974

91. MASON JK: An ox cell hemolysin test for the diagnosis of infectious mononucleosis. J Hyg 49:471–481, 1951

92. MANGI RJ, NIEDERMAN JC, KELLEHER JE JR, DWYER JM, EVANS AS, and KANTOR FS: Depression of cell mediated immunity during acute infectious mononucleosis. N Engl J Med 291:1149–1153, 1974

93. MAYYASI SA, SCHIDLOVSKY G, BULFONE LM, and BUSCHECK FT: The coating reaction of the herpes-type virus isolated from malignant tissues with an antibody present in sera. Cancer Res 27:2020–2024, 1967

94. MILLER G: Oncogenicity of Epstein-Barr virus. J Infect Dis 130:187–205, 1974

95. MILLER G: Epstein-Barr herpesvirus and infectious mononucleosis. Progr Med Virol 20:84–112, 1975

96. MILLER G, LISCO H, KOHN HI, and STITT D: Establishment of cell lines from normal adult human blood leukocytes by exposure to Epstein-Barr virus and neutralization by human sera with Epstein-Barr virus antibody. Proc Soc Exp Biol Med 137:1459–1465, 1971

97. MILLER G, NIEDERMAN JC, and ANDREWS L: Prolonged oropharyngeal excretion of EB virus following infectious mononucleosis. N Engl J Med 137:140–147, 1973

98. MILLER G, NIEDERMAN JC, and STITT DL: Infectious mononucleosis: appearance of neutralizing antibody to Epstein-Barr virus measured by inhibition of formation of lymphoblastoid cell lines. J Infect Dis 125:403–406, 1972

99. MILLER G, ROBINSON J, HESTON L, and LIPMAN M: Differences between laboratory strains of Epstein-Barr virus based on immortalization, abortive infection and interference. Proc Nat Acad Sci USA 71:4006–4010, 1974

100. MINOWADA J, OHNUMA T, and MOORE GE: Rosette-forming human lymphoid cell lines. I. Establishment and evidence for origin of thymus-derived lymphocytes. J Nat Cancer Inst 49:891–895, 1972

101. NIEDERMAN JC, EVANS AS, SUBRAMANYAN MS, and MCCOLLUM RW: Prevalence incidence and persistence of EB virus antibody in young adults. N Engl J Med 282:361–365, 1970

102. Niederman JC, McCollum RW, Henle G, and HENLE W: Infectious mononucleosis. J Am Med Assoc 203:139–143, 1968

103. NIKOSKELAINEN J, LEIKOLA J, and KLEMOLA E: IgM antibodies specific for Epstein-Barr virus in infectious mononucleosis without heterophil antibodies. Br Med J 72–75, 1974

104. NILSSON K, KLEIN G, HENLE W, and HENLE G: The establishment of lymphoblastoid lines from adult and foetal human lymphoid tissue and its dependence on EBV. Int J Cancer 8:443–450, 1971

105. NONOYAMA M and PAGANO JS: Detection of Epstein-Barr viral genome in non-productive cells. Nature 233:103–106, 1971

106. PATTENGALE PK, SMITH RW, and PERLIN E: Atypical lymphocytes in acute infectious mononucleosis, identification by multiple T and B lymphocyte markers. N Engl J Med 291:1145–1148, 1974

107. PAUL JR and BUNNELL WW: The presence of heterophile antibodies in infectious mononucleosis. Am J Med Sci 183:80–104, 1932

108. PEARSON G, DEWEY F, KLEIN G, HENLE G, and HENLE W: Relation between neutralization of Epstein-Barr virus and antibodies to cell membrane antigens induced by the virus. J Nat Cancer Inst. 45:989–995, 1970

109. PEJME J: Infectious mononucleosis. A clinical and haematological study of patients and contacts and a comparison with healthy subjects. Acta Med Scand (suppl) 413:34 1964

110. PFEIFFER E: Drüsenfieber. Z Kinderheilk 29:257–264, 1889

111. PIROFSKY B, RAMIREZ-MATEOS JC, and AUGUST A: "Foreign serum" heterophile antibodies in patients receiving antithymocyte antisera. Blood 42:385–393, 1973

112. POPE JH, HORNE MK, and SCOTT W: Identification of the filtrable leukocyte-transforming factor of QIMR-WIL cells as herpes-like virus. Int J Cancer 4:255–260, 1969

113. POPE JH, HORNE MK, and WETTERS EJ: Significance of a complement-fixing antigen associated with herpes-like virus and detected in the Raji cell line. Nature 222:166–167, 1969

114. PURTILO DT, CASSEL CK, YANG JPS, HARPER R, STEPHENSON SR, LANDING BH, and VAWTER GF: X-linked recessive progressive combined variable immunodeficiency (Duncan's disease). Lancet 1:935–941, 1975

115. REEDMAN BM and KLEIN G: Cellular localization of an Epstein-Barr virus (EBV)-associated complement-fixing antigen in producer and non-producer lymphoblastoid cell lines. Int J Cancer 11:499–520, 1973

116. REEDMAN BM, KLEIN G, POPE JH, WALTERS MK, HILGERS J, SINGH S, and JOHANSSON B: Epstein-Barr virus-associated complement-fixing antigen and nuclear antigen in Burkitt's lymphoma biopsies. Int J Cancer 13:755–763, 1974

117. ROBINSON J and MILLER G: Assay for Epstein-Barr virus based on stimulation of DNA synthesis in mixed leukocytes from umbilical cord blood. J Virol 15:1065–1072, 1975

118. ROCCHI G and HEWETSON JF: A practical and quantitative micro test for determination of neutralizing antibodies against Epstein-Barr virus. J Gen Virol 18:385–391, 1973

119. ROCCHI G, HEWETSON J, and HENLE W: Specific neutralizing antibodies in Epstein-Barr virus associated diseases. Int J Cancer 11:637–647, 1973

120. ROSALKI SB, JONES TG, and VERNEY AF: Transaminase and liver function study in infectious mononucleosis. Br Med J 1:929–932, 1960

121. ROYSTON I, SULLIVAN JL, PERLMAN PO, and PERLIN E: Cell-mediated immunity to Epstein-Barr virus-transformed lymphoblastoid cells in acute infectious mononucleosis. N Engl J Med 293:1159–1163, 1975

122. SAWYER RN, EVANS AS, NIEDERMAN JC, and MCCOLLUM RW: Prospective studies of a group of Yale University freshmen. I. Occurrence of infectious mononucleosis. J Infect Dis 123:263–270, 1971

123. SHELDON PJ, PAPAMICHAEL M, HEMSTED EH, and HOLBOROW EJ: Thymic origin of atypical lymphoid cells in infectious mononucleosis. Lancet 1:1153–1155, 1973

124. SILVESTRE D, KOURILSKY FM, KLEIN G, YATA Y, NEUPORT-SAUTES C, and LEVY JP: Relationship between EBV-associated membrane antigen on Burkitt lymphoma cells

and the viral envelope, demonstrated by immunoferritin labeling. Int J Cancer 8:222–233, 1971

125. SPRUNT TP and EVANS FA: Mononuclear leucocytosis in reaction to acute infection ("infectious mononucleosis"). Bull Johns Hopkins Hosp 31:410–417, 1920

126. STRAUCH B, ANDREWS L, SIEGEL N, and MILLER G: Oropharyngeal excretion of Epstein-Barr virus by renal transplant recipients and other patients treated with immuno-suppressive drugs. Lancet 1:234–237, 1974

127. SUGAWARA K, MIZUNO F, and OSATO T: Induction of Epstein-Barr virus-related membrane antigens by 5-iododeoxyuridine in non-producer human lymphoblastoid cells. Nature 246:70–72, 1973

128. SVEDMYR E and JONDAL M: Cytotoxic effector cells specific for B cell lines transformed by Epstein-Barr virus are present within patients with infectious mononucleosis. Proc Nat Acad Sci USA 72:1622–1626, 1975

129. UNIVERSITY HEALTH PHYSICIANS and P.H.L.S. LABORATORIES JOINT INVESTIGATION: Infectious mononucleosis and its relation to EB virus antibody. Br Med J 4:643–646, 1971

130. VIROLAINEN M, ANDERSSON LC, LALLA M, and VAN ESSEN R: T-lymphocyte proliferation in mononucleosis. Clin Immunol Immunopath 2:114–120, 1973

131. VONKA V, VLCKOVA I, ZAVADOVA H, KOUBA K, LAZONSKA Y, and DUBEN J: Antibodies to EB virus capsid antigen and soluble antigen of lymphoblastoid cells in infectious mononucleosis. Int J Cancer 9:529–535, 1972

132. WAHREN B, ESPMARK A, and WALDÉN G: Serologic studies on cytomegalovirus infection in relation to infectious mononucleosis and similar conditions. Scand J Infect Dis 1:145–151, 1969

133. WÖLLNER D: Über die serologische Diagnose der infektiösen Mononukleose nach Paul-Bunnell mit nativen und fermentierten Hammelerythrozyten. Z Immunitaetsforsch 112:290–308, 1955

134. WÖLLNER D: Differenzierungsmethoden zur serologischen Diagnose der infektiösen Mononukleose. I. Die Differential-agglutination mit nativen und papainisierten Hammelerythrozyten nach Absorption mit Meerschweinchennierenzellen und papainisiertem Hammelblut. Z Immunitaetsforsch 113:301–318, 1956

135. WOOD TA and FRENKEL EP: The atypical lymphocyte: Am J Med 42:923–936, 1967

136. ZIEGLER JL, ANDERSSON M, KLEIN G, and HENLE W: Detection of Epstein-Barr virus DNA in American Burkitt's lymphoma. Int J Cancer 17:701–706, 1976

137. ZUR HAUSEN H: Oncogenic Herpesviruses. Biochim Biophys Acta 417:25–35, 1975

138. ZUR HAUSEN H and SCHULTE-HOLTHAUSEN H: Presence of EB virus nucleic acid homology in a "virus-free" line of Burkitt tumor cells. Nature 227:245–248, 1970

139. ZUR HAUSEN H, HENLE W, HUMMELER K, DIEHL V, and HENLE G: Comparative study of cultured Burkitt tumor cells by immunofluorescence, autoradiography and electron microscopy. J Virol 1:830–837, 1967

140. ZUR HAUSEN H, SCHULTE-HOLTHAUSEN H, KLEIN G, HENLE W, HENLE G, CLIFFORD P, and SANTESSON L: EB-virus DNA in biopsies of Burkitt tumors and anaplastic carcinomas of the nasopharynx. Nature 228:1056–1058, 1970

CHAPTER 15

ENTEROVIRUSES

Joseph L. Melnick, Herbert A. Wenner,
and C. Alan Phillips

Introduction

The enterovirus group was established in 1957 (17) in order to bring together the polioviruses, the group A and B coxsackieviruses, and the echoviruses. All are inhabitants of the human alimentary tract; as a group they are associated with a variety of clinical syndromes, but their most severe expression is in diseases involving the central nervous system (CNS) of man. Poliovirus, the oldest member of the group, was identified in 1908 by Landsteiner and Popper (70), group A coxsackievirus in 1948 by Dalldorf and Sickles (26), and group B coxsackievirus in 1949 by Melnick et al (96). The refinement of tissue culture methods and the expansion of their use into the field of virology in the 1950s led to the isolation of large numbers of hitherto unknown viruses that are not pathogenic for laboratory animals. It early became apparent that these agents could be isolated from healthy children (39, 49, 110), as well as from patients with the aseptic meningitis syndrome (82, 116), and that multiple types exist (82, 110). As more investigators entered the field, more and more of these new agents became recognized. Because their relationship to human disease was unknown, and because they failed to produce illness in laboratory animals, including infant mice, they were called "orphan" viruses or human enteric viruses, a name later changed to enteric cytopathogenic human orphan viruses or ECHO viruses. A cooperative study by Melnick, Sabin, and Hammon on the prototype strains then available resulted in the differentiation of 13 antigenically distinct viruses (15). The enteroviruses have been classed as one of the major subdivisions of the picornaviruses (56). In the recently proposed Latinized taxonomy, enteroviruses are classified as the genus *Enterovirus*, one of the four genera of the family, *Picornaviridae* (20, 87). Currently, over 70 human enterovirus types have been recognized; additional antigenically distinct strains are under study as possible new prototypes.

Clinical aspects of infection

Clinical syndromes. Most enteroviral infections, even with the more virulent members of the group, cause few or no clinical symptoms. However, several discrete clinical syndromes may occur, ranging through severe paralysis, aseptic meningitis, herpangina, pleurodynia, myocarditis, skin rash, coryza, and a variety of other manifestations. Different enteroviruses, as well as nonenteric viruses, may produce some of the same clinical syndromes. On the other hand the same enterovirus may cause different syndromes under different circumstances. A summary of the major clinical manifestations associated with human enteroviruses appears in Table 15.1. Descriptive aspects of many of these syndromes are found in several treatises. For fuller discussion of certain of the topics, especially as related to clinical, epidemiologic, pathologic, immunologic, and prophylactic aspects, the reader is referred to *Viral Infections of Humans: Epidemiology and Control*, Evans AS (ed), Plenum, 1976, p 163-207, and also to Papers and Discussions presented at the 1st-5th International Congresses on Poliomyelitis.

The listing of clinical syndromes in the table is not complete; enteroviruses have been found in patients with cerebellar ataxia, ocular disturbances, lymphadenopathy with fever, etc. Several nonpolio enteroviruses (e.g., coxsackievirus type A7, echovirus types 2, 4 and others) may cause spinal paralysis; in most instances, paralysis is incomplete and reversible.

Mode of transmission. Enteroviruses can be spread by respiratory droplets, by fecal contamination (fingers, table utensils, foodstuffs, milk), and by flies and cockroaches, which in nature become contaminated with human feces and can act as mechanical carriers. Enteroviruses are regularly found in sewage, even after treatment (86, 162).

TABLE 15.1—CLINICAL SYNDROMES ASSOCIATED WITH INFECTIONS BY ENTEROVIRUSES

Polioviruses, types 1–3
    Paralysis (complete to slight muscle weakness)
    Aseptic meningitis
    Undifferentiated febrile illness, particularly during the summer
Coxsackieviruses, group A, types 1–24*
    Herpangina (types 2, 3, 4, 5, 6, 8, 10)
      Acute lymphatic or nodular pharyngitis (type 10)
    Aseptic meningitis (types 2, 4, 7, 9, 10)
    Paralysis (infrequently) (types 7, 9)
    Exanthem (types 4, 5, 6, 9, 16)
    A "hand-foot-and-mouth" disease (types 5, 10, 16)
    Pneumonitis of infants (types 9, 16)
    "Common cold" (types 21, 24)
    Hepatitis (types 4, 9)
    Infantile diarrhea (types 18, 20, 21, 22, 24)
    Acute hemorrhagic conjunctivitis (type 24)
Coxsackieviruses, group B, types 1–6
    Pleurodynia (types 1–5)
    Aseptic meningitis (types 1–6)
    Paralysis (infrequently) (types 2–5)
    Severe systemic infection in infants, meningoencephalitis and myocarditis (types 1–5)
    Pericarditis, myocarditis (types 1–5)
    Upper respiratory illness and pneumonia (types 4, 5)
    Rash (type 5)
    Hepatitis (type 5)
    Undifferentiated febrile illness (types 1–6)

Incubation period. The incubation period between implantation of virus and clinical expression of the disease varies widely, ranging from 2 to 35 days.

Period of infectivity. The high communicability of enteroviruses has been amply documented. Intrafamilial spread commonly occurs. Overall attack rates range from 10% to 20% and may exceed 50% in young children, since all susceptible members of the family are usually infected. Epidemiologic data indicate that communicability is greatest during the early phase of infection, when virus may be recovered in highest concentration from body fluids and excreta. Virus is present in the blood, oropharynx, and feces several days before onset of symptoms (in cases of apparent illness). Most enteroviruses are still being shed in feces 2–4 weeks later; at this time virus usually cannot be recovered from the cerebrospinal fluid (CSF) or oropharynx, and certainly not from blood.

Pathogenesis. The portal of entry of enteroviruses is believed to be the alimentary tract. The susceptibility of humans to these viruses may be enhanced during pregnancy and during the administration of corticosteroids. After initial and continuing multiplication, probably in lymphoid tissue of the pharynx and gut, viremia may occur and in turn lead to further virus proliferation in the cells of the reticuloendothelial system, and finally to involvement of the target organs (spinal cord and brain, meninges, myocardium, skin). The virus is excreted in the stools for several weeks and is present in the pharynx 1–2 weeks postinfection in individuals having either

TABLE 15.1—CLINICAL SYNDROMES ASSOCIATED WITH INFECTIONS BY ENTEROVIRUSES *(cont.)*

Echoviruses, types 1–34**

Aseptic meningitis (all serotypes except 12, 24, 26, 29, 32, 33, 34)

Paralysis (types 2, 4, 6, 9, 11, 30; possibly 1, 7, 13, 14, 16, 18, 31)

Encephalitis, ataxia, or Guillain-Barré syndrome (types 2, 6, 9, 19; possibly types 3, 4, 7, 11, 14, 18, 22)

Exanthem (types 2, 4, 6, 9, 11, 16, 18; possibly 1, 3, 5, 7, 12, 14, 19, 20)

Respiratory disease (types 4, 9, 11, 20, 25; probably 1, 2, 3, 6, 7, 8, 16, 19, 22)

Others: Diarrhea (different types have been recovered; a consistent association has not been established)

Epidemic myalgia (types 1, 6, 9)

Pericarditis and myocarditis (types 1, 6, 9, 19)

Hepatic disturbances (types 4, 9)

Enterovirus, types 68–71†

Pneumonia and bronchiolitis (type 68)

Acute hemorrhagic conjunctivitis (type 70)

Aseptic meningitis (type 71)

Meningoencephalitis (type 71)

Hand-foot-and-mouth disease (type 71)

*Coxsackievirus A23 was never formally accepted as a new type, since it was found to be identical with the previously described echovirus 9.

**Echovirus type 10 was excluded from the group, it is a larger RNA virus with 92 capsomeres; Type 28 was reclassified as rhinovirus type 1; Type 34 is related to coxsackievirus A24 as a prime strain.

†Since 1969, new enterovirus types have been assigned enterovirus type numbers rather than being subclassified as coxsackieviruses or echoviruses. The vernacular names of the previously identified enteroviruses have been retained.

clinical or subclinical infection. Individuals infected with live poliovaccine excrete the virus abundantly in the stools.

Two or more enteroviruses may propagate simultaneously in the alimentary tract (107), but under many circumstances multiplication of one virus may interfere with growth of the heterologous type. Interference with the growth ("take") of live poliovaccine by other concurrent enterovirus infections is now well established. The nature of the so-called local or cellular immunity, which is manifested by protection against intestinal reinfection after recovery from the natural infection or after immunization with the live vaccine, has not been satisfactorily elucidated. Locally produced antibodies, or perhaps interferon, are more likely to be responsible than are nonhumoral factors.

Enteroviruses have been isolated from feces, pharyngeal washings, CSF, heart, blood (buffy coat as well as whole blood), CNS, urine, and lesions of skin or mucous membrane. Enterovirus 70 has been isolated most often from conjunctival swabs.

Immunology. The natural history of infection by enteroviruses often militates against consistent demonstration of significant antibody responses. During the earliest stages, the infection is often localized, and virus has not penetrated into the more vulnerable organs (for example, CNS). Quite often, such extension occurs later, and concurrent with or soon after onset of neurologic signs, neutralizing (Nt) antibodies have already attained maximal levels (73, 100). However, there is considerable variability in antibody responses for the enteroviruses (14). The choice of laboratory diagnostic methods is of some importance. For example, rises in complement fixing (CF) antibody titer may be revealed much less consistently when inactivated rather than fully infectious viral antigens are used.

Nt, CF, flocculating, and precipitating antibodies develop after natural infections from enteroviruses or vaccination with live polioviruses. Hemagglutination-inhibiting (HAI) antibodies also occur, but they can be detected only for those enteroviruses that possess a demonstrable hemagglutinin. Nt antibodies are generally type-specific, appear soon after infection, and persist for many years. However, infection with one type may also give rise to a low level of transient Nt antibodies to certain other serotypes; this has also been found to occur after infection with oral poliovaccine. CF antibodies appear within 10 to 20 days after infection, reach a peak between 1 and 3 months, decline in a few months, and then persist at a low level for 2 or more years. After immunization with the killed poliovaccine, the CF antibody response is variable and appears to depend on previous natural infection. These antibodies acquired from poliovirus and coxsackievirus infections may be less enduring and often are demonstrable for only a few months. But for echovirus types 6 and 16, CF antibodies, after early decline, have persisted for several years (13, 103).

During infection, antibodies to the denatured viral antigen appear before antibodies to the native antigen, and subsequently the levels of antibodies to the denatured antigen are first to fall. Type-specific CF antibodies are formed only after the first infection, usually in the very young; subsequent infection with any other type induces antibodies against the heatstable, group-specific antigen.

HAI antibodies appear at about the same time as, or even slightly earlier than, CF antibodies (within 21 days after onset of infection), decline less rapidly, and for most enteroviruses, generally endure longer. Nonspecific inhibitors for hemagglutinins of enteroviruses may be present in many human sera.

Epidemiology. Enteroviruses are found in persons living in all parts of the world. They are ubiquitous in tropical and semitropical zones. They may spread rapidly in silent or overt epidemics, particularly in temperate climates, where they are encountered more commonly during the late summer and early fall. Because of their antigenic inexperience, children are the prime targets of enterovirus infections and thus serve as the main vehicle for the spread of the virus; the rate of infection among them may exceed 50% in warmer lands where unsanitary and poor socioeconomic conditions prevail. In all populations, natural immunity is acquired with increasing age. The poorer the sanitary conditions, the earlier the age at which infection first occurs and immunity develops. Children living under poor hygienic circumstances are infected early in life, so that over 90% may be immune to the prevailing enteroviruses by the age of 5 years. As personal and community hygiene improves, spread of enteroviruses becomes limited, and increasing numbers of individuals reach adult life without having been infected and immunized. In some isolated Eskimo communities, the whole population has lacked antibodies. The shift in the highest age-specific incidence of poliomyelitis from preschool children to schoolchildren and young adults, which took place in the 1940s in many parts of the globe, has been attributed to improvement in sanitary conditions. Since the introduction of poliomyelitis vaccines, the few cases of polio that occur are in the nonimmunized groups.

Pathology

Enteroviruses may leave pathologic evidence of cell injury, often in newborn and older infants and in young children. Intrauterine transfer of group B coxsackieviruses is recognized. It is not clear whether the viruses have a teratogenic effect on the fetus. Older children and adults may develop disease (herpangina, pleurodynia, paralytic poliomyelitis, etc.) which is often severe and sometimes fatal.

As a rule, persons with fatal cases of poliomyelitis show severe neural damage. Histologically, inflammatory lesions are most abundant in the anterior horns of the spinal cord, various centers of the hindbrain, and rarely in the forebrain, except in motor and premotor areas. There is lymphatic hyperplasia; myocarditis is not uncommon.

Some coxsackieviruses, notably A7 and occasionally others (e.g., B5), may elicit corresponding cellular pathology (137). Group B coxsackieviruses in newborn infants cause a severe generalized disease. Characteristic pathologic changes consist of focal necrosis accompanied by infiltration of lymphocytes and polymorphonuclear leukocytes. Lesions are most pronounced in the heart, but are also present in the brain, spinal cord, liver, kidney, and adrenals (32,65). Muscle fibers of the myocardium show necrosis and peripheral inflammatory responses. Early lesions consist of focal necrosis with pyknosis and karyorrhexis of myocardial nuclei, with polymorphonuclear cells in interstices; late lesions show profound myocardial injury with mononuclear cells and histiocytes predominating among injured myofibrils. Group B coxsackieviruses may involve both white and gray matter of the CNS, producing features of meningoencephalomyelitis. In infants there is an apparent predilection of the disease for the brain stem, especially the inferior olivary nuclei. Anterior horns of the spinal cord are not involved as constantly, and seldom so severely, as in poliomyelitis.

Biopsied muscle from pleurodynia patients yielding group B coxsackieviruses has shown severe inflammatory infiltration or degeneration of muscle fibers, or both. Pancreatic lesions have been observed in the newborn; these consist of parenchymal infiltrates of polymorphonuclear cells, necrobiosis of acinar tissue, and destruction of islet cells. The testes show nonspecific subacute inflammation. Biopsied muscles of polymyositis patients have shown coxsackievirus aggregates at the site of muscle damage (Fig 15.1) (35).

Deaths caused by echoviruses are uncommon; hence, knowledge of pathologic changes is fragmentary. Among infants who unexpectedly die, echoviruses (notably type 7) as well as other enteroviruses have been recovered from parenchymal tissue. Interstitial pneumonitis has been found in these infants, as well as in older individuals (e.g., echovirus 20), but the etiologic relationship requires further definition. Interstitial myocarditis has been reported for types 3 and 22. Clinical evidence indicates various degrees of involvement of the CNS, including at least transient injury to motor neurones (by echovirus 6, among others) (76). Bulbospinal paralysis has been associated with types 2, 4, and 11. In at least one instance (echovirus 2 infection), sections of the CNS showed typical distribution and character of lesions ordinarily associated with poliovirus. In another, similar lesions considered to be caused by echovirus 9 were probably related to type 2 poliovirus, which was also recovered from the CNS tissues. Thus, it appears that some echoviruses can simulate the pathologic picture of poliomyelitis (25, 138, 139).

Description and Nature of the Enteroviruses

Common characteristics

Enteroviruses comprise at present a group of over 70 members. They are composed of a single-strand ribonucleic acid (RNA) core enclosed in a protein coat (capsid). The protein coat of the mature extracellular virus carries the antigenic specificity and provides the protective shell for the RNA, which is the virus genetic material and serves as the essential infectious component. Agents within this group possess the following properties (16):

1. Particle size is 20–30 nm in diameter. Cubic symmetry of the icosahedral type has been suggested as the structural form of some of these viruses, but only a few have been studied in detail (80).

2. Evidence for an RNA core includes susceptibility of infectious nucleic acid to ribonuclease and resistance to deoxyribonuclease, red staining with acridine orange, and failure of 5-fluorodeoxyuridine to prevent virus synthesis. The nucleic acid core comprises 20–30% of the particle. The mo-

lecular weight of nucleic acid in the virion is 2.5–2.8 × 10⁶ daltons. Infectious RNA has been extracted from representative serotypes of polioviruses, coxsackieviruses, and echoviruses. Because it is freed of the surface protein antigen, such RNA cannot be neutralized by viral antiserum.

3. Resistance to ether, due to lack of essential lipids, is demonstrated by retention of full infectivity after treatment with 20% ethyl ether for 18 hr at 4 C.

4. Cationic stabilization to thermal inactivation is shown by protection of enteroviruses from thermal inactivation (50 C for 1 hr) by 1M $MgCl_2$.

Reactions to chemical and physical agents

Enteroviruses are resistant to all known antibiotics and chemotherapeutic agents. Laboratory disinfectants, such as 70% alcohol, 5% lysol, or 1% quaternary ammonium compounds (Roccal), are ineffective. The viruses are insensitive to ether, deoxycholate, and various detergents, which destroy other viruses (arboviruses, myxoviruses, etc.). Enteroviruses are insusceptible to exposure to acid (pH 3–5), a procedure which partially inactivates rhinoviruses (146). However, virulent and attenuated polioviruses also have marked differences in their sensitivity to acids (153). Treatment with 0.3% formaldehyde, 0.1 N HCl, or free residual chlorine at a level of 0.3–0.5 ppm causes rapid inactivation, but the presence of extraneous organic matter protects the virus from inactivation (145). Thus, caution must be exercised before carrying over laboratory findings on the chlorination of enteroviruses, often in purified form, to chlorination under natural conditions. Enteroviruses are inhibited from propagating in cell cultures by 2-(α-hydroxybenzyl)-benzimidazole (HBB), with the exception of group A coxsackieviruses 7, 11, 13, 16, and 18 and echoviruses 22 and 23 (144). Guanidine is also a potent inhibitor of poliovirus (and other enterovirus) synthesis in cell cultures (22, 115). However, virus progeny grown in the presence of guanidine become resistant to the drug (89).

Exposure of these viruses to a temperature of 50 C destroys them rapidly. However, in the presence of molar magnesium and other divalent cations, virtually no detectable inactivation occurs in 1 hr at 50 C (151). In late harvests, virus is thermostabilized by cystine, which is present in most nutrient media (157). Enteroviruses are stable at freezing temperatures for many years, remain active for weeks at refrigerator temperatures (4 C), and for days at room temperature. Their inactivation at all temperatures is inhibited by $MgCl_2$. Molar NaCl, on the other hand, protects enterovirus activity at 50 C but markedly increases the rate of inactivation at 37 C (151, 152).

Enteroviruses are rapidly inactivated by ultraviolet (UV) light and usually by drying, unless special conditions are observed (8, 44, 60). Vital dyes (neutral red, acridine orange, proflavine) when incorporated into the structure of these viruses render them readily susceptible to visible light (21, 120).

Classification

The International Committee on Nomenclature of Viruses, now the International Committee on Taxonomy of Viruses, recommended that viruses

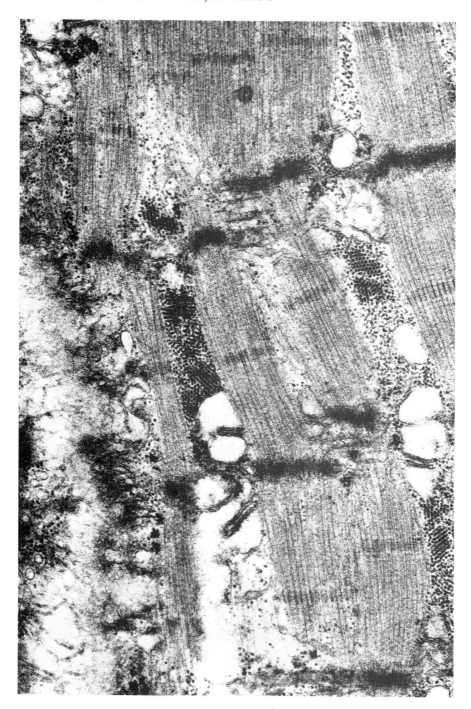

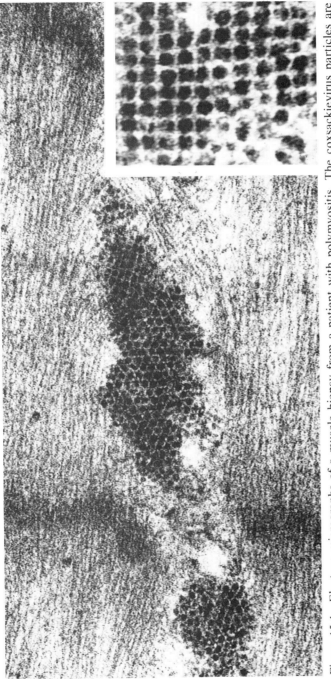

Figure 15.1.—Electron micrographs of a muscle biopsy from a patient with polymyositis. The coxsackievirus particles are localized within muscle cells. Facing page: 55,000X. This page: 100,000X. Inset: The individual particles within an array have a center-to-center distance of 23 nm. 245,000X. (*Source:* Ref 35).

TABLE 15.2—POLIOVIRUSES

TYPE	PROTOTYPE STRAIN	GEOGRAPHIC ORIGIN	ILLNESS IN PERSON YIELDING PROTOTYPE VIRUS	INVESTIGATOR(S)
1	Brunhilde	Maryland	Paralytic polio*	Howe and Bodian
2	Lansing	Michigan	Fatal paralytic polio**	Armstrong
3	Leon	California	Fatal paralytic polio**	Kessel

*Virus recovered from feces.
**Virus recovered from spinal cord.

be classified into major groups on the basis of common biochemical and biophysical properties. In keeping with this recommendation, an international study group charged with the classification of enteroviruses and related agents created the picornavirus group, made up of the small, ether-insensitive RNA viruses (20, 87, 56). Within this group the following biological subgroups are recognized:

I. Picornaviruses of human origin
  A. Enteroviruses
    1. Polioviruses, types 1–3
    2. Coxsackieviruses of group A, types 1–24*
    3. Coxsackieviruses of group B, types 1–6
    4. Echoviruses, types 1–34**
    5. Enteroviruses, types 68–71
  B. Rhinoviruses (over 100 types)
II. Picornaviruses of lower animals
  A. Enteroviruses (monkeys, pigs, cows, mice)
  B. Rhinoviruses (horses)
  C. Aphthoviruses (foot-and-mouth disease viruses)
  D. Encephalomyocarditis virus (rats)

The first subgroup had been previously brought together as the enteroviruses (17). Strains belonging to all types have been isolated from the lower as well as the upper alimentary tract of human beings. The strains listed in Tables 15.2–6 have been approved as prototypes (17, 97, 106), and the World Health Organization (WHO) International Reference Centre and Regional Enterovirus Laboratories have accepted them as international standards (169). The prototype strains are deposited in the American Type Culture Collection, Rockville, MD 20852, and in the WHO Virus Laboratories; from both of these sources, they are available for worldwide distribution to suitably equipped virus laboratories. For information on obtaining reference enteroviruses and antisera against them, the investigator should contact the

---

*Type 23 was never formally accepted as a new type, as it was found to be identical with the previously described echovirus 9.

**Type 10 echovirus (reovirus) was removed from the group, as it is a larger RNA virus with 92 capsomeres; Type 28 is now recognized as rhinovirus type 1; Type 34 is related to coxsackievirus A24 as a prime strain.

TABLE 15.3—COXSACKIEVIRUSES GROUP A*

TYPE	PROTOTYPE STRAIN	GEOGRAPHIC ORIGIN	ILLNESS IN PERSON YIELDING PROTOTYPE VIRUS**	INVESTIGATOR
1	Tompkins	Coxsackie, NY	Poliomyelitis†	Dalldorf
2	Fleetwood	Delaware	Poliomyelitis†	Dalldorf
3	Olson	New York	Aseptic meningitis	Dalldorf
4	High Point	North Carolina	(Sewage of polio community)	Melnick
5	Swartz	New York	Poliomyelitis	Dalldorf
6	Gdula	New York	Aseptic meningitis	Dalldorf
7	Parker	New York	Aseptic meningitis	Dalldorf
8	Donovan	New York	Poliomyelitis	Dalldorf
9	Bozek	New York	Aseptic meningitis	Dalldorf
10	Kowalik	New York	Aseptic meningitis	Dalldorf
11	Belgium-1	Belgium	Epidemic myalgia	Curnen
12	Texas-12	Texas	(Flies in polio community)	Melnick
13	Flores	Mexico	None	Sickles
14	G-14	South Africa	None	Gear
15	G-9	South Africa	None	Gear
16	G-10	South Africa	None	Gear
17	G-12	South Africa	None	Gear
18	G-13	South Africa	None	Gear
19	NIH-8663	Japan	Guillain-Barré syndrome	Huebner
20	IH-35	New York	Infectious hepatitis	Sickles
21	Kuykendall; Coe	California	Poliomyelitis† Mild respiratory disease‡	Lennette
22	Chulman	New York	Vomiting and diarrhea	Sickles
24	Joseph	South Africa	None	Gear

*Cross-reactivity has been observed between A3 and 8, A11 and 15, A13 and 18.

**All isolates were from stools, except for prototypes of A4 and A12, which were isolated from sewage and flies, as indicated. Numerous strains of each of these types were isolated from stools also.

†When coxsackieviruses have been isolated from patients with paralytic poliomyelitis, the patients have often been found to have a dual infection, the poliovirus presumably being responsible for the paralytic illness.

‡The Coe virus was isolated from throat washings.

Research Resources Branch, National Institute of Allergy and Infectious Diseases, Bethesda, MD 20014, USA; or the WHO Collaborating Centre for Virus Reference and Research, Department of Virology, Baylor College of Medicine, Houston, TX 77030, USA.

The members of the second subgroup, the rhinoviruses (146), differ from the enteroviruses in several properties: a) Whereas the cytopathic enteroviruses are readily isolated in primary cultures of human and monkey kidney (MK) cells and certain strains may be isolated directly in continuous human heteroploid lines (such as HeLa or HEp-2), rhinoviruses are more readily isolated in embryonic human kidney or human diploid cell strains (lung fibroblasts) than in MK cells—in fact, many strains can only be recov-

TABLE 15.4—COXSACKIEVIRUSES GROUP B

TYPE	PROTOTYPE STRAIN	GEOGRAPHIC ORIGIN	ILLNESS IN PERSON YIELDING PROTOTYPE VIRUS*	INVESTIGATOR
1	Conn-5	Connecticut	Aseptic meningitis	Melnick
2	Ohio-1	Ohio	Summer grippe	Melnick
3	Nancy	Connecticut	Minor febrile illness	Melnick
4	JVB	New York	Chest and abdominal pain	Sickles
5	Faulkner	Kentucky	Mild paralytic disease with residual atrophy	Steigman
6	Schmitt	Philippine Islands	None	Hammon

*All isolates were from stools.

ered in cells of human origin. b) Rhinoviruses are isolated from the nose and throat rather than from the feces because they cannot withstand the acidic pH levels of the gastrointestinal tract. c) Their growth is favored when cultures are rolled at 33 C, whereas enteroviruses grow readily in stationary cultures at 36–37 C. d) Unlike the enteroviruses, rhinoviruses are unstable at pH 3–5, decreasing about 2 $\log_{10}$ units of infectious titer when exposed to this degree of acidity for 1–3 hr. They have been recovered from patients with colds, croup, bronchiolitis, and bronchopneumonia. Echovirus-28 seems to have been the first rhinovirus recovered (101), and it has been reclassified as rhinovirus type 1.

Antigenic characteristics

Poliovirus types 1 and 2 share common antigens. Intratypic strain differences are known for all three poliovirus serotypes, and pronounced intratypic variation has been encountered among both coxsackie- and echoviruses. Four such variants are known for A20 coxsackieviruses (6).

With some enteroviruses antigenic variation results in the appearance of prime strains (85). The prime strain is poorly neutralized by antiserum to the originally characterized (prototype) strain, but it induces the production of antibody which neutralizes the prime strain and the prototype strain equally well. Prime strains have been found for coxsackievirus A24 and for echovirus types 1, 4, 5, 6, 8, 11, and 30; they probably exist for many more enterovirus types (36). The prime strains, however, share CF and precipitin antigens with their prototypes; tests for these antigens using prototype antiserum can readily be performed for typing prime strains.

Another problem has been the difficulty of neutralizing certain strains. For example, the prototype echovirus 4 strain (Pesascek) is poorly neutralized by homologous antiserum. The Du Toit strain is much more sensitive and is preferred for the Nt test (170). The poor neutralization of the Pesascek strain was shown to be due to aggregation of virus particles; virus in nonneutralizable aggregates was found to constitute up to 30% of untreated Pesascek stock preparations, but only 0.1% of Du Toit. With monodispersed virus obtained by filtration through Millipore membranes of appropriate porosity, efficient neutralization of Pesascek strain can be achieved (158).

TABLE 15.5—ECHOVIRUSES*

TYPE	PROTOTYPE STRAIN	GEOGRAPHIC ORIGIN	ILLNESS IN PERSON YIELDING PROTOTYPE VIRUS**	INVESTIGATOR(S)
1	Farouk	Egypt	None	Melnick
2	Cornelis	Connecticut	Aseptic meningitis	Melnick
3	Morrisey	Connecticut	Aseptic meningitis	Melnick
4	Pesascek	Connecticut	Aseptic meningitis	Melnick
5	Noyce	Maine	Aseptic meningitis	Melnick
6	D'Amori	Rhode Island	Aseptic meningitis	Melnick
6'	Cox	Ohio	None	Ramos-Alvarez, Sabin
6"	Burgess	Connecticut	Aseptic meningitis	Melnick
7	Wallace	Ohio	None	Ramos-Alvarez, Sabin
8	Bryson	Ohio	None	Ramos-Alvarez, Sabin
9	Hill	Ohio	None	Ramos-Alvarez, Sabin
11	Gregory	Ohio	None	Ramos-Alvarez, Sabin
12	Travis	Philippine Islands	None	Hammon, Ludwig
13	Del Carmen	Philippine Islands	None	Hammon, Ludwig
14	Tow	Rhode Island	Aseptic meningitis	Melnick
15	CH 96-51	West Virginia	None	Ormsbee, Melnick
16	Harrington	Massachusetts	Aseptic meningitis	Kibrick, Enders
17	CHHE-29	Mexico City	None	Ramos-Alvarez, Sabin
18	Metcalf	Ohio	Diarrhea	Ramos-Alvarez, Sabin
19	Burke	Ohio	Diarrhea	Ramos-Alvarez, Sabin
20	JV-1	Washington, DC	Fever	Rosen
21	Farina	Massachusetts	Aseptic meningitis	Enders, Kibrick
22	Harris	Ohio	Diarrhea	Sabin
23	Williamson	Ohio	Diarrhea	Sabin
24	DeCamp	Ohio	Diarrhea	Sabin
25	JV-4	Washington, DC	Diarrhea	Rosen
26	Coronel	Philippine Islands	None	Hammon
27	Bacon	Philippine Islands	None	Hammon
29	JV-10	Washington, DC	None	Rosen
30	Bastianni	New York	Aseptic meningitis	Plager, Duncan, Lennette
31	Caldwell	Kansas	Aseptic meningitis	Wenner, Lennette, von Magnus
32	PR-10	Puerto Rico	Aseptic meningitis	Branche
33	Toluca-3	Mexico	None	Rosen, Kern
34	DN-19†	Texas	Infantile diarrhea	Melnick

*Types 1 and 8 share antigens, type 1 having the broader spectrum.

**All isolates were from stools.

†DN-19 antiserum partially neutralizes coxsackievirus A24, but A24 antiserum does not neutralize DN-19 virus, although it reacts with the virus in complement-fixation and gel-diffusion tests. Thus, DN-19 should be considered a prime strain of coxsackievirus A24, rather than as a distinct echovirus.

TABLE 15.6—NEW ENTEROVIRUS TYPES

TYPE	PROTOTYPE STRAIN	GEOGRAPHIC ORIGIN	ILLNESS IN PERSON YIELDING PROTOTYPE VIRUS	INVESTIGATORS
68	Fermon	California	Lower respiratory illness*	Schieble, Lennette
69	Toluca-1	Mexico	None**	Rosen, Schmidt
70	J670/71	Japan and Singapore	Acute hemorrhagic conjunctivitis†	Kono, Yin-Murphy, Melnick
71	BrCr	California	Aseptic meningitis‡	Schmidt, Lennette

*Prototype isolated from throat swabs.

**Prototype isolated from rectal swab.

†Prototype recovered from conjunctival swabs.

‡Prototype recovered from stool; strains have also been isolated from brains of fatal encephalitis cases.

A number of cross-relationships exist between several enteroviruses; for example, coxsackieviruses A3 and A8, A11 and A15, A13 and A18, echoviruses 1 and 8, 12 and 29, 6 and 30, and polioviruses 1 and 2 to a minor degree. Previously reported relationships between echoviruses 1 and 12 appear to have been due to contamination of an echovirus 12 stock by type 1 virus (43).

Poliovirus preparations contain two antigens detectable in precipitin and CF tests. They are called native (D) and denatured (C) antigens. The native antigen is associated with the intact virion and is present to a high degree in fully infectious preparations, but it may be converted to the denatured antigen associated with empty capsids by heating at 56 C, alkaline pH, and phenol or UV irradiation. During infection, antibodies to the denatured antigen appear before antibodies to the native antigen, and subsequently the levels of antibodies to the denatured antigen are first to fall. Type-specific CF antibodies are formed only after the first infection, usually in the very young; subsequent infection with any other type induces antibodies against the heat-stable, group-specific antigen.

Type-specific precipitating and flocculating antibodies usually appear concurrently with Nt antibodies in infected individuals. They can be detected in tubes (regular or capillary) or by the agar gel-diffusion technique.

Two precipitating antigens have been differentiated for A9, B1, B3, and B5 coxsackieviruses, both by density gradient and gel-diffusion separation. The "group" precipitating antigen is identical with the "group" CF antigen, which appears to be responsible for the heterotypic reactivity of some human sera. The other—the "specific" precipitating antigen—also fixes complement with homotypic monkey antiserum, but not with human serum. Heating at 56 C for 30 min activates the CF capacity of the latter antigens with homotypic and heterotypic human sera.

A number of the enteroviruses agglutinate erythrocytes (RBC) (34, 117). Strains of group A coxsackieviruses 20, 21, and 24, group B coxsackieviruses 1, 3, 5 and 6, and echoviruses 3, 6, 7, 11, 12, 13, 19, 20, 21, 24, 25, 29, 30, and 33 agglutinate human group O cells; coxsackievirus A7 agglutinates those chicken RBC agglutinable with vaccinia virus. For some serotypes, only a few hemagglutinating strains have been found, while for others (e.g., echovirus 11) almost all strains have this property. The hemagglutinins are associated with the infectious virus particles because both are sedimented together by ultracentrifugation and are also adsorbed together by RBC during hemagglutination. Some enteroviruses agglutinate human RBC to the same titer at 4 C and at 37 C and at pH extremes from 5.8 to 7.4, while others vary under these conditions. Coxsackie A7 hemagglutinin derived from infected mouse tissue, although particulate, has been differentiated from the infectious particle (168). Factors affecting hemagglutination by enteroviruses are agglutinability of RBC, thermolability of agglutinins, pH, and temperature of incubation. While the data available at present suggest that most strains of a given enterovirus type either do or do not hemagglutinate, exceptions have been found in sufficient number to rule out definitive identification based on hemagglutination, although this property is useful for initial screening of new isolates. Titers of hemagglutinin observed with enteroviruses may be as high as 1:2048.

Pathogenicity for animals

Rhesus (*Macaca mulatta*) and cynomolgus (*Macaca irus*) monkeys, as well as other species (i.e., *Cercopithecus aethiops,* the African green or grivet monkey) can be readily infected with polioviruses by the intraspinal (the most sensitive), intracerebral, and intranasal routes. Furthermore, certain poliovirus strains may infect monkeys on intradermal or intramuscular (im) injection; cynomolgus monkeys have been infected with some strains by way of the gastrointestinal tract. Feeding poliovirus can cause infection of chimpanzees and cynomolgus monkeys, with prolonged excretion of virus in the stools, viremia, and the development of serum antibodies. Naturally acquired infection, and even paralysis, has occurred in captive primates, particularly in chimpanzees. The use of monkeys in the polio laboratory is described by Paul and Melnick (108). With the introduction of tissue culture procedures, the monkey is no longer required as a diagnostic test animal.

By and large, laboratory rodents are resistant to freshly isolated polioviruses, although strains belonging to all three types have been adapted to cotton rats and to both suckling and adult mice. These animals usually develop flaccid paralysis when inoculated intracerebrally or intraspinally.

Newborn mice are the animals in which coxsackieviruses were first isolated, and their differentiation into groups A and B is based upon the pathologic lesions produced in this test animal. Group A viruses cause generalized myositis accompanied by a flaccid type of paralysis. Group B viruses cause focal myositis and typical lesions in the interscapular fat pad and brain. Myocarditis, endocarditis, hepatitis, and necrosis of acinar tissue of the pancreas may also be produced. Suckling hamsters develop similar pathologic changes. Both group A and B viruses induce lesions in the bones of mice simulating neoplastic growth (79).

Coxsackievirus A7 inoculated intracerebrally in rhesus monkeys produces flaccid paralysis and severe neuronal lesions. On the basis of studies with strains isolated from paralytic cases, Soviet investigators believe that

A7 resembles polioviruses and that consideration should be given to its being classified as poliovirus type 4 (147). A14 virus causes similar CNS lesions in both rhesus monkeys and adult mice, but on subsequent passage in newborn mice, the same virus causes only myositis (24). In chimpanzees, coxsackieviruses produce inapparent infections characterized by heterotypic anamnestic responses (67, 91) similar to those occurring in humans.

None of the prototype strains of the echoviruses produce overt disease in laboratory animals. However, intracerebral and intraspinal inoculation of monkeys with some strains has caused neuronal destruction associated with fever, viremia, and occasionally muscle weakness or paralysis. Similar neuronal lesions have been produced by im inoculation (164). Oral, im, or intracutaneous administration of some echoviruses to chimpanzees produces an inapparent infection with excretion of virus in the throat and feces and development of serum antibodies (57). Some strains of echovirus 9, after passage in tissue cultures, produce a widespread, coxsackievirus-type of myositis in newborn mice. The pathogenicity of these viruses for laboratory animals is summarized in Table 15.7, but individual variations occur within types.

Growth in tissue cultures

The enteroviruses are divided into subgroups depending upon their capacity to grow and produce characteristic cellular damage in different *in vitro* and *in vivo* test systems. The main properties dividing the enteroviruses are shown in Table 15.7, but the footnotes to the table and the discussion which follows illustrate in part the variations which may be expected in strains within a single antigenic type. There is ample evidence that host range is not a good criterion for dividing the enteroviruses into subgroups, inasmuch as there are many strain differences within a single type (16, 72).

In general, enteroviruses grow best in primate epithelial cells. Thus, all three types of polioviruses grow well in cultures of MK, HeLa, and human amnion cells. All group B coxsackieviruses grow readily in MK—rhesus (*M. mulatta*), African green monkey (*C. aethiops*), and patas monkey (*Erythrocebus patas*)—as well as in a variety of human cell lines (HeLa, amnion, etc.). Coxsackieviruses B3, 4, and 5 have also been grown in kidney cell cultures of hamsters, pigs, lambs, and mice (72). Of the group A coxsackieviruses, A7 and A9 grow readily in MK cells. Coxsackievirus A21 grows best on primary isolation in HeLa, HEp-2, KB, and primary or diploid human embryonic kidney cell cultures. A7, A9, A11, A13, A15, A16, A18, A20, and A24 also can be isolated directly in primate cell cultures. Most group A viruses have been adapted to grow in human amnion cells (165); A2 and A4 have been propagated also in chick embryo cell cultures (134), and A9 in hamster kidney cells (72).

RD cells, derived from a human rhabdomyosarcoma, support replication of a number of group A coxsackieviruses, including types A5 and A6, which previously had been propagable only in suckling mice (125). A number of the group A coxsackievirus types that replicated in RD cells had higher titers in this cell line than in other cell culture systems. In tests on a limited number of clinical specimens, RD cells were slightly less sensitive

TABLE 15.7—ENTEROVIRUSES: GROWTH IN MONKEY KIDNEY AND HUMAN CELL CULTURES
AND PATHOGENICITY FOR ANIMALS

| | MONKEY | | PATHOGENICITY | |
VIRUS	KIDNEY CELLS	HUMAN CELLS	MICE	MONKEYS
Poliovirus	+	+	0*	+**
Coxsackievirus A	0†	0‡	+†	0‖
Coxsackievirus B	+	+	+†	0‖
Echovirus	+#	0‡	0¶	0‖
Enterovirus 68-71	±	+	±	0§

*Some strains of each type have been adapted to mice.

**Attenuated strains used for oral vaccine produce mild localized lesions when introduced intraspinally and almost no lesions when inoculated intracerebrally.

†Coxsackie A7, A9, and B strains grow readily in monkey kidney cells; some strains grow poorly in mice and fail to produce disease in these animals.

‡Some strains grow preferentially in, or have been adapted to human cell cultures. Coxsackie viruses A11, 13, 15, 16, 18, 20 and 21 may be isolated directly in human cells.

‖Coxsackie A7 produces a severe polioencephalomyelitis in monkeys; other coxsackie- and echovirus strains produce *mild* lesions in the CNS that resemble mild poliomyelitis.

#Echovirus type 21 is cytopathogenic for human epithelial cells but not for monkey kidney cells.

¶Whereas the prototype and other strains of echovirus 9 are not pathogenic for mice, a number of other strains, especially after passage in monkey kidney cells, produce paralysis in mice (severe coxsackievirus type of myositis).

§Enterovirus 70 may produce lesions in the CNS.

than suckling mice for isolation of group A coxsackieviruses, but they did permit the recovery of certain virus types which previously could be isolated only in suckling mice. Group B coxsackieviruses replicated poorly or not at all in RD cells.

Echoviruses (with the exception of type 21) grow readily in primary MK cells and almost always produce characteristic cytopathic effects (CPE); most of these viruses will grow in human cells, such as primary amnion, thyroid, and kidney cells. They also grow in WI-38 cells, although generally such cell culture lines are less sensitive than primary cultures, especially for isolation purposes. Diploid lines of human fetal kidney (126) and the BGM line of African green monkey (23) have also been recommended. However, sensitivity for isolation of echoviruses may vary with the passage level of the cells.

The growth of enteroviruses in cultured cells is generaly associated with a characteristic CPE (2, 59, 111). Infected cells round up, show shrinkage and marked nuclear pyknosis, become refractile, eventually degenerate, and fall off the glass surface (Figs 15.2-4). In stained preparations (Fig 15.5 and 15.6), enterovirus CPE is manifested by the appearance of an eosinophilic mass, increasing in size in the cell center and displacing the shrinking nucleus and the marginal basophilic "hyaline" cytoplasm to the cell periphery. Figures 15.2-6 illustrate poliovirus and echovirus CPE in MK cell monolayers. The enterovirus type of CPE is not produced in cell cultures by the EMC-Mengto group or by the reoviruses (formerly classified as echovirus 10) (2, 112).

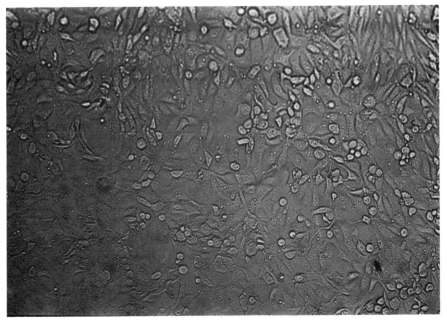

Figure 15.2—Monkey kidney culture infected with poliovirus, showing cytopathic effect (CPE) in approximately 25% of cells. Infected cells have assumed the round shape. The CPE score is 1+.

Electron microscopic studies of ultrathin sections of enterovirus-infected cell cultures or tissues show cytoplasmic arrays or crystals of dense spherical particles, each approximately 17–28 nm in diameter (59, 105, 113, 140) (Fig 15.1). The cytologic changes caused by echoviruses 22 and 23, although resembling those of other enteroviruses at an early stage, involve distinct nuclear manifestations at later stages (132). The nucleolus disintegrates. Chromatin granules tend to aggregate at the nuclear membrane with the intranuclear structures fading and leaving an empty-appearing nucleus. Furthermore, when stained with acridine orange, infected cells show abnormal staining characteristics.

Under agar overlay, plaques are formed by various members of the enterovirus group in cultures of susceptible cells (54). Agar often inhibits plaque formation, and neutral red may reduce the plaque count (photodynamic effect). However, if proper precautions are taken, with suitable agar (Difco agar, ionagar, agarose, diethyl-aminoethyl dextran, 25 mM MgCl$_2$, etc.) and filtered (rather than autoclaved) neutral red, plaques may be obtained with all echoviruses (159, 160).

Polioviruses produce circular plaques with clear centers and sharp boundaries. Plaques of group B coxsackieviruses are round, resembling those of poliovirus, except that they may have rather diffuse boundaries and their appearance may be delayed. Coxsackievirus A9 on MK cells produces similar plaques with less clear centers (due to the presence of healthy cells) and fuzzy boundaries. Many of the group A coxsackieviruses propagable in

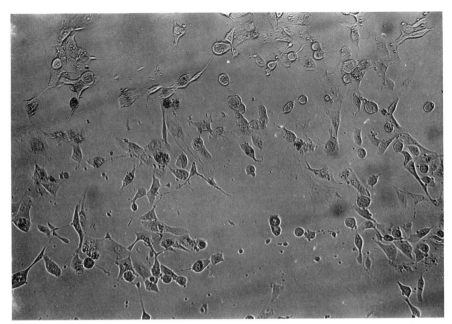

Figure 15.3—Culture infected with poliovirus, showing more advanced stage of CPE, 4+, that is, almost 100% of the cells are infected.

human amnion cells form plaques of quite variable morphology. The number and size of plaques produced by most strains of enteroviruses are increased by the incorporation of 25 mM of MgCl2 in agar overlay (160). Plaque morphology and differential susceptibility of cell cultures to the enteroviruses have been utilized for preliminary presumptive identification (52–55).

Preparation of Enteroviral Typing Antisera

Type-specific antisera against enteroviruses are produced in a variety of experimental animals. Some of the most practical and satisfactory procedures are outlined below. To obtain *reference* enteroviruses and antisera against them, contact the Research Resources Branch, National Institute of Allergy and Infectious Diseases, Bethesda, MD 20014, USA; or the WHO Collaborating Centre for Virus Reference and Research, Department of Virology, Baylor College of Medicine, Houston, TX 77030, USA.

Monkey antiserum (64, 119)

Monkeys previously tested to show the absence of demonstrable antibodies against enteroviruses are used for the preparation of high-titer type-specific antiserum. The antigen consists of either infected tissue culture fluid or infected mouse tissue. It is mixed with an equal amount of adjuvant (1

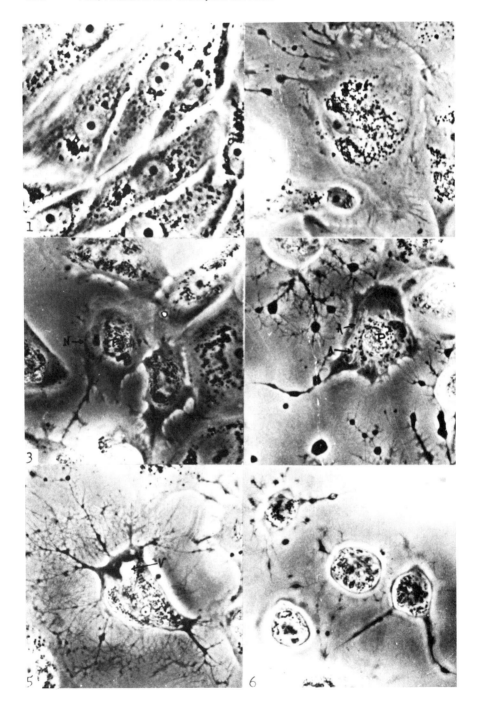

part Arlacel A and 9 parts standard mineral oil like Bayol F). The ingredients are emulsified by expressing them back and forth between 2 syringes connected to a Swinney filter with a fine wire screen. Stable emulsions are characterized by their retention of droplet form when dropped on water. Spreading of the droplet calls for additional mixing.

The emulsion is injected in 2-ml amounts into the calf muscle of each leg 4 times at 2-week intervals. The monkeys are exsanguinated 2 weeks after the last injection. The Nt titers against 100 mean tissue culture infectious doses ($TCID_{50}$) of homologous virus usually range between 1:1000 and 1:10,000, while those against 100 $TCID_{50}$ of heterologous viruses are almost always $\leq 1:16$. These sera have not always been found satisfactory for CF testing; nonspecific CF reactions are encountered, presumably from some common nonviral protein in the immunizing antigen and the CF antigen preparations. The most suitable method is to immunize monkeys with virus grown in monkey cells without serum; this avoids the production of antibodies to foreign host proteins.

Rabbit and guinea pig antiserum

Potent antiserum has been prepared by the following procedures (102). With use of undiluted tissue culture fluid as antigen, each rabbit is injected im at 4 sites on day 1 with 10 ml of a virus-adjuvant mixture, plus 1 ml of tissue culture fluid intravenously (iv) on days 1, 7, 14, 21, and 30; 10 ml of virus-adjuvant are also given im on day 21. Bleedings are generally begun about day 37, and the rabbits are given a booster dose (0.5 ml iv) and bled on alternate weeks thereafter. Thus, each rabbit receives a minimum of 15 ml of tissue culture fluid, the exact amount depending on the life span of the rabbit.

Enterovirus antiserum has been prepared in guinea pigs by immunizing the animals with fluorocarbon-treated virus (37). In this way, antiserum without host CF antibodies may be produced. Each animal is immunized 3 times with 1 ml of antigen at intervals of 3–4 weeks, and is bled 1 week after

Figure 15.4—Micrographs of living cells as seen in the phase-contrast microscope. Normal and poliovirus-infected monkey kidney epithelial cells in culture. (1) Normal monolayers, uninfected. (2) Cell in early phase of infection with type 1 poliovirus. (3) Cells from the same culture at a slightly more advanced stage. Cells are beginning to pull away from each other. (4) Another field of the culture at a more advanced stage. In the cell at the center of the field, the outlines of the nucleus are obscured by the paranuclear mass. Clear, filamentous areas are seen in the cytoplasm (A). (5) Culture at a slightly more advanced stage. The cell has begun to round up, and large clear vacuoles (V) are seen in the upper left of the cytoplasm. The nucleus is masked by the cytoplasmic paranuclear mass (P). (6) Last stages of cytopathic degeneration induced by poliovirus. (*Source:* Ref 111)

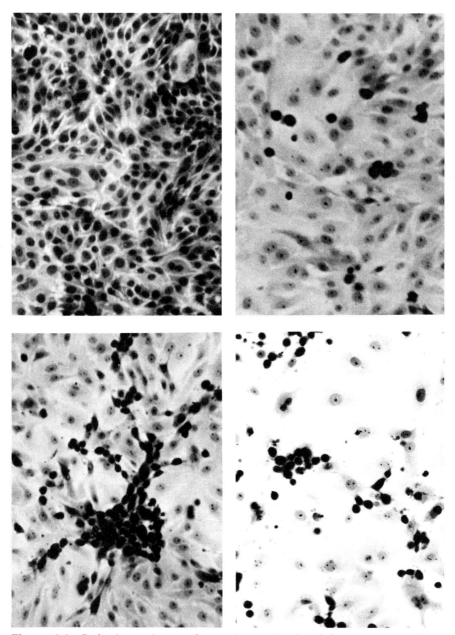

Figure 15.5—Stained monolayers of normal and echovirus-infected monkey kidney
epithelial cells shown at low power. (Upper left) normal uninfected culture 6 days old. (Upper right) culture infected with echovirus 1 shown
24 hr after inoculation. Rounded infected cells are scattered throughout
the field. (Lower left) 66 hr after inoculation. Infected cells are seen as
foci of rounded, densely staining cells. (Lower right) 90 hr after inoculation. Many infected cells have sloughed off the glass; most remaining are rounded because of viral infection.

the last injection. The first and second injections are given subcutaneously, the last intracerebrally or intraperitoneally (ip).

Mouse and hamster antiserum and ascitic fluid (18, 27)

These animals are used for the preparation of antisera against coxsackieviruses that grow only in suckling mice. Aqueous extracts (10% infected muscle) are inoculated ip in 4 increasing doses at weekly intervals. A suitable course for mice is 0.5, 1.0, 1.5, and 2.0 ml; for hamsters, 1.0, 1.5, 2.0, and 3.0 ml. Animals are bled 7-10 days after the last inoculation.

Ascitic fluid is a satisfactory alternative to serum from immune mice for use in CF tests with group A coxsackieviruses and several other enteroviruses. Large quantities of fluid can be obtained from a small number of mice. Immune ascitic fluids are usually equal in potency, are just as specific, and have less anticomplementary activity than immune sera.

Adult mice are inoculated with use of the schedule described above. Two days after the last virus dose (2 ml), each mouse receives 0.1 ml of Sarcoma 180 cell suspension by ip injection. Ascitic fluid is harvested 10-12 days later, at which time the mice are exsanguinated for antiserum (31).

Antiserum from Horses and Other Large Domestic Animals (41, 42, 90)

For preparing large amounts of antisera, horses, cows, sheep, goats, and pigs have been found to yield potent antisera against the enteroviruses, with the highest titers found in the horse (1:1000–1:20,000 except for echovirus 4, which yields low titers as it does in monkeys). Antigens are prepared as follows (99):

1. One part of 4 M $MgCl_2$ is added to 3 parts of virus (undiluted tissue culture harvest) to preserve infectivity of the virus. (Adventitious simian agents may be eliminated from viral seeds by heating virus at 50 C for 1 hr in the presence of 1 M $MgCl_2$.)

2. $AlCl_3$ is added to the virus-Mg mixture to give a final concentration of 25 mM. This is accomplished by adding 1 ml of 2 M $AlCl_3 \cdot 6 H_2O$ to 79 ml of the virus-Mg mixture.

3. To the virus-Mg-Al mixture, Na_2CO_3 is added to give a final concentration of approximately 50 mM. This is done by adding 2 ml of 2.5 M Na_2CO_3 to the 80 ml of the virus-Mg-Al mixture. A precipitate is formed by this addition.

4. The virus suspension is placed on a magnetic stirrer and mixed gently to prevent foaming until the suspension is homogeneous. It is allowed to stand at room temperature for 15-30 min, and is then centrifuged at 3000 rpm for 20 min. or at 5000 rpm for 10 min. The supernatant fluid is decanted and discarded, as it contains less than 1% of the virus.

5. The sediment is reconstituted in saline solution at 10% of original volume, that is, to make 8 ml in the example cited. This sediment contains more than 99% of the virus.

6. If higher concentration of virus is desired, the suspension can be centrifuged at 4000-5000 rpm for 15 min. The sediment is more tightly packed and can be suspended in 3-10% of the original volume.

A schedule that has produced Nt antiserum titers of about 1:2000–1:20,000 against 100 $TCID_{50}$ of virus is as follows:

1. Horses are inoculated im with three 20-ml doses of concentrated antigen at intervals of 4 weeks.

2. Multiple large bleedings are taken 2, 4, 6, and 8 weeks after the third dose, and a booster antigen dose (20 ml) is administered 20-26 weeks after the first dose of antigen.

3. The animals may then be exsanguinated 2 weeks after the booster dose or held and bled frequently thereafter if this is preferred. At least 25 liters of potent antiserum can be obtained from 2 animals. The availability of such serum has led to the preparation of large amounts of combined pools to facilitate typing isolates.

Collection and Preparation of Specimens for Laboratory Diagnosis

Precautions

Laboratory-acquired infections are not uncommon among persons working with enteroviruses. The various kinds of risks in the laboratory are discussed in Chapter 2, and little more can be said here except that disability

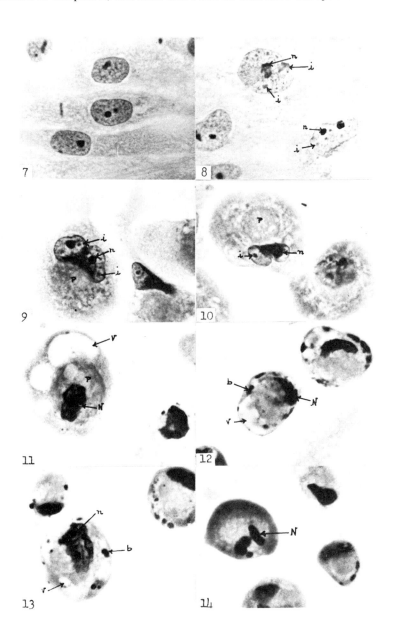

and death have occurred in laboratory workers from poliovirus infections; such possibilities attend other enteroviruses. Since personnel in enterovirus laboratories may be exposed to wild-type polioviruses, they should be immunized against them.

Collection of specimens

Enteroviruses have been recovered from the following specimens obtained during the clinically apparent infection: feces (or rectal swabs), pharyngeal washings (or throat swabs), CSF, blood, vesicle fluids, conjunctival swabs, and urine; during inapparent infection they have been isolated from fecal and pharyngeal samples. The importance of proper collection of the appropriate specimens (body tissues, feces, pharyngeal washings, blood, vesicle fluid, or CSF) at the right time, during the earliest days of illness or immediately after death, cannot be overemphasized; a summary of specimens and their handling is given in Table 15.8. An unsatisfactory specimen does not warrant the waste of a good test.

As soon as specimens are obtained, they are taken or shipped to the laboratory (see Table 15.8 for conditions of shipment). At the laboratory they are recorded and examined to make sure they are suitable for use in tests (that is, still frozen, with no leakage, etc.); they are processed for testing (for example, serum separated from whole blood) and then tested. Specimens that cannot be tested at once can be stored at -20 C (which is satisfactory for enteroviruses) or preferably at -70 C to preserve infectivity of other viruses which may be present. Serum is stored without preservative at 4 C, or it may be frozen. Repeated freezing and thawing ($>4X$) may adversely affect both viruses and antibodies.

Whenever possible, blood should be obtained after overnight fasting. Collect blood (10–20 ml) in sterile dry tubes as early as possible after onset of illness, and again in the third or fourth week, during convalescence. A third sample obtained around the sixth to eighth week is often helpful. Care should be taken to avoid hemolysis both at the time of collection from the

Figure 15.6—Normal and poliovirus-infected monkey kidney cells, fixed and stained with hematoxylin and eosin. (7) Uninoculated culture. (8) After inoculation with poliovirus type 3. Cell at upper center has lost most of its nuclear chromatin; the nucleus contains 2 acidophilic inclusions (i). Lower cell has lost most of its chromatin, has several intranuclear inclusions (i) clearly differentiated from nucleolus (n). The 2 nuclei at left appear unaltered. (9) Cells showing more advanced degeneration; distorted nucleus contains several inclusion bodies and 2 nucleoli. (10) Cells at a more advanced stage. Cell at left center shows well-defined cytoplasmic eosinophilic mass (P); nucleolus (n) can be distinguished in distorted nucleus, which also contains an acidophilic inclusion body (i). (11) Cells in last stages of virus degeneration; characteristic vacuoles (V) in periphery of cytoplasm. (12) and (13) Cells showing basophilic cytoplasmic granules (b); nucleolus (n) still visible in wrinkled nucleus. (14) Late stage. Nucleus (N) already fragmenting. (*Source:* Ref 111)

TABLE 15.8—KINDS OF SAMPLES; WAYS OF OBTAINING AND PREPARING THEM FOR DIAGNOSTIC STUDIES

| SPECIMEN | COLLECTION OF SPECIMENS | | | | PREPARATION OF SPECIMENS | | | |
| | AMOUNT | MEDIUM* | CONTAINER** | SHIPMENT† | STORAGE IN LABORATORY | EXTRACTIONS, IF ANY | | ANTIBIOTICS ADDED |
						PRIMARY	REFINED	
Fecal:								
Stool	4–8 g (≥ 1 tsp)	None	Screw-cap jar	Freeze	–20 C	10% wet wt. in BSS at 2000 rpm/20 min	10,000 rpm/1 hr	§
Rectal swab	≥ 2 swabs	BSS	Tube	Freeze	–20 C	Twirl swabs in medium	10,000 rpm/1 hr	§
Pharyngeal:								
Gargle	10–15 ml	BSS	Tube	Freeze	–20 C	None	10,000 rpm/1 hr	§
Swab	≥ 2 swabs	BSS	Tube	Freeze	–20 C	Twirl swabs in medium.	None	§
Blood:								
Whole	≥ 10 ml	None	Tube	Do not Freeze	Clot	Triturate clot at 2000 rpm/20 min	Rarely	None
Serum	5–10 ml	None	Tube	Freeze	–20 C	None	Rarely	None
Cerebrospinal fluid	≥ 3 ml	None	Tube	Freeze	–70 C	None	Rarely	None
Miscellaneous:								
Vesicle fluid	0.2 ml	BSS	Tube	Freeze	–70 C	None (as a rule)	Rarely	Rarely
Pericardial fluid / Ascitic fluid	≥ 1 ml	None	Tube	Freeze	–70 C	None (as a rule)	Rarely	Rarely
Urine	10 ml	None	Tube	Freeze	–20 C	None	Rarely	§
Autopsy:								
Blood	Samples	None	Sterile containers and tubes	Freeze	–70 C	None (as a rule)	Rarely	Rarely
Cerebrospinal fluid	Samples							
Central nervous system	Samples					Tissues ground to 10–20% suspension in medium, clarified by low-speed centrifugation		
Effusion fluid, visceral organs, etc.	ca 3 g or ≥ 3 ml							

* BSS—Balanced salt solutions (Hanks, Earle), or Melnick medium A or B, or bacteriologic broth are used.

** Tubes of heavy glass with screwcaps and rubber gaskets preferred. These may be placed in sealable plastic bags to further decrease the chance for spillage.

† By fastest transportation, preferably on dry ice. If wet ice is used, specimens must be in watertight containers.

§ Elective, according to laboratory preference.

patient and in the laboratory. The clot from acute-phase blood may be used for virus isolation studies (viremia).

Specimens obtained at postmortem may be helpful in establishing a laboratory diagnosis, but only if properly taken. The likelihood of recovering viruses from tissues obtained at necropsy depends on the time interval between onset of fatal illness and death. The longer this interval, the less the chance of recovering viruses. The pathologist may, after histologic studies, be able to guide virus studies; often he cannot. Information on the clinical features of illness is helpful. Any one of three conditions—illness of short duration, signs of possible virus origin, and compatible histologic lesions (10)—warrants institution of viral studies.

Improved histologic techniques, including histochemical and immunochemical labeling (11), are sometimes valuable adjuncts to virus studies. In addition to general-purpose fixatives (neutral buffered formalin, Zenker and Carnoy fluids), special fixatives (sucrose-formalin, acetone, etc.) may be required for prospective cytologic studies and fluorescence microscopy.

Feces. A 4- to 8-g specimen is desirable. Small plastic ointment boxes or small wide-mouth jars are useful as containers. The specimens are kept frozen or at least cold until tested.

Rectal swabs. If a stool specimen cannot be obtained, a rectal swab is often a useful substitute. However, the chances of isolating virus from a swab may be 50% less than from a fecal specimen. To obtain best results, a moist sterile swab is inserted well into the rectum, and the mucosa rubbed until fecal material adheres to the swab; it is then placed in a test tube containing 1–2 ml of Hanks or Earle balanced salt solution (BSS). It is important that the specimen be tested promptly or kept frozen until used.

Pharyngeal (or nasopharyngeal) washings. Various types of irrigating fluid, such as sterile distilled water, broth, or salt solutions, may be used to obtain nasopharyngeal washings from patients or suspected carriers of the virus. The fluid is introduced into the patient's mouth, either from a drinking glass or through a large glass syringe without attached needle. With the head retracted, the patient is requested to gargle the material, which is then collected in a sterile drinking glass or small basin. The procedure is repeated over a period of at least 3 min; the amount of washing fluid is kept under 20 ml. Isotonic solutions are tolerated better than others for nasopharyngeal washings. Nasal swabs may be used; suitable cotton applicators are available commercially. The swab should be inserted so as to pass just posteriorly to the turbinates.

Throat swabs. Material is obtained by rubbing the oropharynx vigorously with 2 sterile cotton swabs. The samples should include material from the posterior pharynx, the tonsils, and the faucial pillars. The swabs are transferred immediately to a test tube containing 1–2 ml of BSS. The specimens should be tested promptly or kept frozen.

Ocular samples. Material is obtained by gently rubbing the surface of the eye with 2 sterile cotton swabs or by gentle conjunctival scraping. The swabs or scrapings are transferred to a test tube containing 1–2 ml of BSS. If not tested at once, they should be held frozen until tested.

Spinal fluid. Spinal fluid is collected under aseptic conditions, placed in a sterile test tube, and either tested immediately or preserved frozen.

Vesicle fluid. The area containing the lesions is cleansed with ether or acetone. Aspiration into a tuberculin syringe fitted with a 26-gauge needle has occasionally provided an adequate sample. Another method consists of rupturing the vesicles and absorbing the escaping fluid on cotton swabs. At the same time the vesicle base is gently rubbed with the swab. Aspirated fluids are dispensed in 1 ml of diluent, after which the syringe barrel is rinsed with the diluent. Swabs are also deposited in tubes containing 1 ml of diluent.

Urine. A clean, voided, midstream sample (10 ml) is collected directly into a sterile test tube. It should be tested immediately, or if this is not feasible, the sample should be stored frozen.

Autopsy specimens. Enteroviruses, particularly the polioviruses, are isolated from human autopsy material such as spinal cord, medulla, and pons, or from intestinal contents and intestinal wall. Other materials, such as heart muscle and lymph nodes, etc., may also be taken. Autopsy material should be collected as soon as possible after death. Whenever possible, the virologist should attend the autopsy. Several sets of sterile instruments must be available. Tissues are collected in a planned order so that contamination from gastrointestinal contents is avoided. Organs outside the body cavities (e.g., CNS, parotid, and lymph nodes) should be obtained before the cavities are opened. Tissues from the thorax should be obtained before those in the peritoneum, and those in the peritoneum before the intestines are removed. Each tissue is removed with a separate set of sterile instruments, and after removal, each is placed in a suitable sterile container such as a 1-oz heavy glass vial with a screw cap.

Serum. Two blood samples are required for antibody tests. The first (acute phase) is collected at the onset of illness or as soon as possible thereafter; the second (convalescent phase) is collected 2–3 weeks later. Each time, a fasting specimen (10 ml) of venous blood should be obtained in a sterile test tube. The blood is allowed to clot at room temperature for 2 hr, and the serum separated under aseptic conditions. If this is not practicable, the blood is refrigerated as soon as possible after collection, and the serum removed within the next 24 hr. Sterile glassware is used throughout. Serum is centrifuged, if necessary, to remove traces of RBC, and is kept in the refrigerator. If there is to be a delay of more than a few days before the tests can be performed, the serum is frozen.

Sewage. For surveillance of enteroviruses present in a community, particularly during epidemics of enteroviral disease, monitoring of sewage, stream water, etc., is often desirable. Detection is made more practicable by methods recently developed for concentration of viruses from large volumes of fluid (9, 148, 162).

Storage and shipment of specimens

Material awaiting testing or shipment may be held for short periods at refrigerator temperature; for longer storage, it should be frozen. Ordinary glass test tubes may break when frozen if they contain excess amounts of fluid. Therefore, fluid specimens are placed in special containers, such as plastic tubes or thick-walled glass containers. They are then frozen in a deep-freeze box, in the freezing compartment of a refrigerator, or in a specially constructed insulated box containing dry ice (CO_2) that can maintain a temperature as low as -70 C. Enteroviruses, unlike certain other viruses, do not require temperatures below -20 C for their preservation. Multiple freezing and thawing of specimens, which may inactivate the virus, should be avoided.

For shipping, frozen material is packed in an insulated box containing dry ice and preferably sent by air. Serum for serologic tests should be properly packed and sent by air, but refrigeration is not required.

Preparation of materials for inoculation

Feces and rectal swabs. A 10% or 20% fecal suspension is made in a cold, sterile salt solution in a tightly stoppered tube or flask containing glass beads. After vigorous shaking to emulsify the feces, the specimen is allowed to settle in the cold. For preparing inoculum from rectal swabs, the fluid is thoroughly expressed from the swab. The fluid must be slightly alkaline (pH 7.5) to elute virus from the cotton swab.

The eluate of the swab, or the supernatant fluid of the stool specimen, is then poured into a centrifuge tube and clarified at 2500 rpm for about 10 min. The supernatant fluid is removed, antibiotic solution is added to give a final concentration per ml of 1000 units of penicillin and 1000 μg of streptomycin (or some other suitable antibiotic mixture), and the sample is held at room temperature for 1 hr. The specimen is then centrifuged in the cold at speeds from 3000 (for 1 hr) to 10,000 rpm (for 20 min), depending on the availability of equipment. If the supernatant fluid is not readily removed from the sediment, a second spinning may be necessary. The supernatant fluid is inoculated immediately or kept frozen until used.

1. Concentration of virus by ultracentrifugation (81, 109)—The virus contained in fecal suspensions can be concentrated and separated from much extraneous material by use of the ultracentrifuge. A larger amount of fecal suspension is prepared by low-speed spinning as above, and 10–100 ml, depending upon the availability and degree of concentration desired, are spun in the ultracentrifuge for 60–90 min at 106,000 $\times g$. The supernatant fluid is discarded, and the virus-containing sediment taken up in 1–3 ml of tissue culture maintenance medium. This suspension is prepared for inoculation by centrifugation for 30 min at 1500 rpm (or 20 min at 18,000 rpm) to remove debris in the sediment, and antibiotics are added as above. While this method is more sensitive and valuable for special studies, its use is not mandatory; therefore an ultracentrifuge is not considered essential equipment for the usual enterovirus laboratory.

2. Other methods of concentration—Recently described methods include the adsorption of viruses to aluminum hydroxide salts (148) or to collodion membranes (162), from which the adsorbed viruses are then eluted (48). Under these conditions, the viruses are recovered in concentrated form from sewage or fecal extracts. Not only is the virus concentrated, but it is also freed from toxins that are often present in sewage and feces.

3. Freon treatment (50)—Virus bound to an inhibitor may be released by Freon-113 (trifluorotrichloroethane), which destroys the inhibitor and so permits detection of the virus. A chilled stool suspension is treated with an equal volume of Freon, and then the mixture, while still cold, is homogenized in a high-speed mixer. The material is centrifuged, antibiotics are added, and the material is ready for inoculation.

Pharyngeal washings and throat swabs. The fluid is thoroughly expressed from the swab, as above, and the swab discarded. Pharyngeal washings and swab extracts are then processed by centrifugation and treated with antibiotics as described in the preceding sections.

Spinal fluid. This material, if properly collected, may be used as it is received. If blood cells are present, they may be separated by light centrifugation. Spinal fluids suspected of being bacterially contaminated are treated with antibiotics and prepared for inoculation as described above.

Blood. Enteroviruses have been recovered from serum early in infection. Virus in the serum may be bound to the first antibody that develops (94). Thus, the opportunities for its detection are increased if the virus-binding antibody is destroyed (94, 78). The following technique has been used successfully (94).

A portion (0.5 ml) of each serum sample is placed in each of three 100-× 13-mm tubes. To each tube is added 0.25 ml of acid buffer-gelatin-Tris, as described by Mandel (78), and 0.2 ml of 0.3 N HCl, both of which are prewarmed to 37 C. This brings the pH of the serum to 2.5, where it is maintained at room temperature for 2 hr. The serum is then returned to pH 7 by addition of 0.45 ml of alkaline buffer-gelatin-Tris (78) and 0.2 ml of 0.3 N NaOH to each tube. Next, 0.3 ml of each sample is inoculated onto each of 5 monkey or human kidney tube cultures from which maintenance medium has been drained. The tubes are covered by aluminum foil and incubated at 37 C for 2-3 hr in a stationary rack. The monolayers are then rinsed gently twice with 1 ml of maintenance medium, and 1 ml of fresh maintenance medium is added to each tube. Tubes are stoppered, reincubated at 37 C for 1 week, and then observed at least every other day for CPE. Positive tubes are harvested and stored frozen as soon as 50% of the cells show CPE, and the virus is identified.

Controls on the sensitivity of this acid-dissociation procedure are carried out with a known enterovirus that is tested against a standardized antiserum. The virus is titrated and portions containing 100 $TCID_{50}$/ml are combined with equal volumes of the homotypic antiserum. The mixtures are incubated at 37 C for 6 hr and then placed at 4 C overnight. Samples of 0.5 ml each of a control virus-antibody system are included in each test. Recovery of over 50% of the control virus from its neutralized mixture indicates proper functioning of the test.

Vesicle fluid. For obtaining inoculum from swabs, cotton pledgets are removed from the applicators and placed in the barrel of a 5-ml syringe; 1 ml of phosphate-buffered saline (pH 7.5) is added to the barrel, and the plunger is inserted into place. The fluid is thoroughly expressed from the pledget into the original swab tube by applying adequate pressure to the plunger. Antibiotics (adequate amounts of penicillin and streptomycin, depending on the degree of contamination) are added to the specimen and mixed. After light centrifugation in the cold, the supernatant fluid is either inoculated immediately or stored frozen until used.

Urine. Antibiotics are added, and the specimen is inoculated without further treatment.

Autopsy specimens. Weighed fragments (1–2 g are usually sufficient) are placed in a sterile mortar containing a small amount of sterile abrasive (alundum or sand); the specimen is then ground with enough sterile BSS—not more than 2 ml at first—to make it into a fairly thick paste. Grinding is usually done for at least 5 min, during which time cold, sterile salt solution is slowly added to make a 20% suspension. This suspension is transferred to a centrifuge tube and spun at 2000 rpm for 5–10 min, and the supernatant fluid is removed. The supernatant fluid is either inoculated immediately or kept frozen until used. It is advisable to make from 10 to 15 ml of suspension so that some of the material may be kept frozen for possible future use. Before inoculation, antibiotics are added to the suspension to yield a final concentration of 1000 units of penicillin and 1000 μg of streptomycin per ml. Neomycin and bacitracin are also used by some laboratories.

Serum for antibody. There is little loss of specific virus-neutralizing capacity, or of other antibodies (e.g., HAI, CF, etc.) in serum stored at 4 C or −20 C. Lyophilized immune sera retain Nt, HAI, and CF titers for years. Repeated freezing and thawing of serum, however, is not recommended; antibody losses may occur when this procedure is followed. Ordinarily, preservatives are not added to serum, except in some instances for the HAI test.

Specimens for microscopic examination

The cytopathology observed in tissues obtained after death may become more meaningful in association with recovery of virus from the target organ. Lesions characteristically associated with some enteroviruses (poliovirus being the prototype) may be found in brain or spinal cord specimens taken at autopsy; tissue changes found in parenchymal organs (e.g., myocardium, liver, etc.) or in cells of the alimentary tract are not, as a rule, specific for enteroviruses.

Few specific histopathologic effects have been observed in tissues collected antemortem. The histologic changes in dermal lesions associated with some of the enteroviruses have not been described, at least to our knowledge.

In practice, enterovirus particles (electron microscopy) or cellular damage (light and electron microscopy) are not visible in clinical specimens directly, but only in infected cell cultures or laboratory animals or (as indicated above) in selected tissues after death. Fluorescence microscopy, however, has been applied directly to autopsy specimens (12) and to clinical specimens, particularly CSF cellular deposits and leukocytes obtained in the

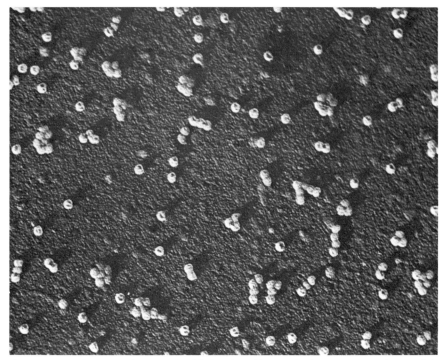

Figure 15.7—Electron micrograph of field of purified poliovirus prepared for particle counting. Negatively charged virus particles are sedimented at high speed directly upon positively charged grids which were prepared by coating collodion-covered grids with a thin layer of aluminum. Grids with poliovirus are shadowed with chromium and examined in the electron microscope. By counting the number of particles per field, the number of particles per ml of the original virus suspension can be calculated. 90,000X. (*Source:* Smith KO and Melnick JL in J Immunol 89:279, 1962)

early phases of illness, to reveal specific viral antigens (136, 143). Thus far the method has not been applied successfully to cells of the alimentary tract nor to cellular debris from dermal vesicles.

Laboratory Diagnosis

Direct examination of specimens

Electron microscopy. Virus particles 18–25 nm in diameter may be observed directly and enumerated quantitatively by electron microscopy, provided their concentration is $\geq 10^7$/ml. By counting representative fields in which the particles have been sedimented, it is possible to arrive at the concentration of virus/ml of suspension. Figures 15.7 and 15.8 illustrate fields

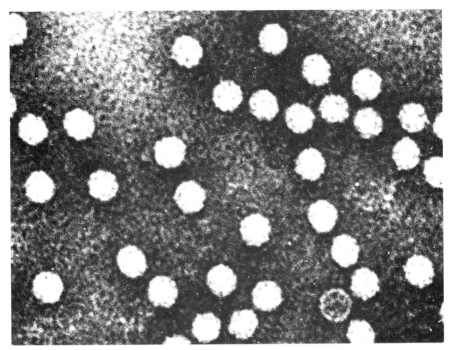

Figure 15.8—Poliovirus prepared for high-resolution electron microscopy to show fine structure of the poliovirus. An empty viral capsid is shown in the lower right corner. Negatively stained with phosphotungstic acid. 286,000X. (*Source:* Unpublished electron micrograph, Department of Virology, Baylor College of Medicine, Houston, TX)

of poliovirus prepared for particle counting. The method is applicable to other enteroviruses for obtaining directly the concentration of virus particles in a suspension, and for determining whether viruses from 2 different groups are present (e.g., enterovirus and adenovirus). Specific antibody will produce agglutination of the virions.

Immunofluorescence microscopy. This procedure is becoming increasingly useful in the virus diagnostic laboratory but has not been used extensively in typing enteroviruses directly in clinical specimens. However, the method seems promising (143).

Up to the present, immunofluorescence (FA) methods for enteroviruses have been used chiefly for typing isolates by labeling of infected cell cultures. Antisera conjugated with fluorescein isothiocyanate are effective reagents for typing enteroviruses (45, 133).

Globulins are precipitated from monkey antiserum by 50% saturation with ammonium sulfate and labeled with fluorescein isothiocyanate. This compound is added in a powdered form with stirring to globulin solutions (at pH 9) in an ice-bath. Conjugates are absorbed twice with monkey liver powder and once with a suspension of MK cells before use.

The virus is grown in tube cultures or in Leighton tubes containing cover slips. With regular tubes when 1+ to 2+ CPE is present, maintenance medium is removed, and cells are dispersed with 0.02% versene and are then centrifuged at 2000 rpm for 5 min. Smears of sedimented cells are prepared on slides, air dried, and fixed in acetone at room temperature for 10 min. Leighton tube coverslips, when 1+ to 2+ CPE is present, are removed, dried, and fixed similarly. Slides and coverslips are stained immediately or stored at −20 C until stained. In the direct method of FA staining, conjugates, either undiluted or diluted 1:2 with buffered saline solution, are added to infected cell preparations and examined in the microscope (114).

The FA technique has been applied directly to CSF cells (136, 143) and leukocytes of human patients (136) and to human myocardial tissues (12). Such tests must be rigidly controlled to assure the specificity of the reaction.

Isolation of viral agents

Isolation in animals

Monkeys, once the mainstay of the poliovirus laboratory, have been entirely replaced now by tissue cultures—except for use in neurovirulence testing. The care and inoculation of monkeys and the description of experimental poliomyelitis in these animals can be found in reference 108.

Enteroviruses are now isolated in tissue cultures or in newborn mice, but neither test system can be relied upon to recover all enteroviruses. The three polioviruses, most of the group B coxsackieviruses, coxsackievirus A9 (and A7 and A16 to a lesser degree), and most echoviruses (except type 21) grow readily in MK cultures and produce typical CPE.

While many of the prototype strains of coxsackievirus group A (and all of group B) were adapted by serial passage to various tissue culture systems (71, 167), most group A viruses can be isolated from clinical specimens only by the inoculation of newborn mice; specimens that fail to produce CPE in cultures therefore should be passaged in newborn mice. Some strains multiply in mice but insufficiently to produce lesions in primary passage, and they are easily missed. However, in addition to the types readily isolated in MK cultures (see above), types A11, 13, 15, 18, 20, 21, and 24 grow well in human cell cultures.

Coxsackievirus groups A and B, in suckling mice

As indicated above, newborn mice (or hamsters) are essential hosts for the propagation of certain enteroviruses in the laboratory, particularly for group A coxsackieviruses. Mice should preferably be no more than 1 day old. Each sample may be inoculated by a single route into 3 litters of mice; routes and dosages used are subcutaneous, 0.03 ml; ip, 0.05 ml; and intracerebral, 0.02 ml. If supplies are limited, a single litter may be inoculated by multiple routes. Mice are examined and scored daily for 14 days.

Features of group A infection. Preferably, mice should be less than 24 hr and not more than 72 hr old at the time of inoculation. After a variable incubation period (1–9 days), mice become less active; a progressive flaccid paralysis sets in. Encephalitis signs are absent. After onset of paralysis, breathing is weak and shallow, and mice die within 12–48 hr. Some viruses produce characteristic foot drop of front limbs with later onset of stiffness, flexion deformities, and generalized paralysis.

Histologic studies reveal widespread lesions of the voluntary muscles. Lesions consist of edema, waxy degeneration, and coagulation necrosis, depending upon the phase of infection; sarcolemma sheaths are collapsed; interstitial cellular exudates develop; there is a variable degree of infiltration by inflammatory cells. Severely damaged muscles such as paraspinal, pelvic, and limb muscles, show considerable wasting and apparent increase in cellularity. Other muscles (masseter, diaphragm, etc.) are less extensively or barely (tongue) involved. Group A strains almost always induce muscle lesions without injury to CNS, fat tissue, or other tissue. Focal inflammatory lesions have been seen in CNS tissues after infection with groups A7, A14, and A16 viruses.

Features of group B infection. Mice should be inoculated within 24–48 hr after birth. Older mice are more resistant; even in younger mice primary infections are sometimes less easily revealed for group B than for group A viruses. Several passages may be required before typical signs of infection develop in these animals.

Illness is characterized by weakness, tremors, generalized muscular spasm, or spastic paralysis. Dyspnea and cyanosis may develop prior to death, which often occurs within 48 hr. Some mice may survive several days longer, and some may remain alive, showing only stunting and transient incoordination.

Encephalomalacia with cyst formation occurs, particularly after intracerebral inoculation; interscapular fat pads (as well as others) become swollen, mucoid, and grayish white, with visible focal opacities. None of the white linear streaks seen in skeletal muscles of group A-infected mice are found (seen best in mice surviving a week or more).

Histologic studies reveal encephalitis with widespread necrosis of neurones; in the cord, lesions chiefly involve the gray matter. Panniculitis is characterized by the death of young fat cells, leading to necrosis with subsequent healing, regeneration, and calcium deposition. Acinar cells of the pancreas degenerate; islets of Langerhans and ducts are spared. Other lesions may include interstitial myocarditis and hepatitis. Only focal myositis has been encountered.

Weanling mice develop pancreatitis, which may be detected with trypan blue (51) (0.5 ml of 5% solution, delivered ip). By the fourth day lesions in the pancreas usually stain blue.

Problems encountered. Anatomical findings indicative of both group A and group B infections in mice suggest the presence of two (or more) viruses in the inoculum. More than one type of coxsackievirus, or multiple enteroviruses, are known to occur in the same isolate (5, 18, 92). Possibly of equal importance is the report that when two coxsackievirus strains are present in the inoculum one may interfere with the growth of the other (163). (Enteroviral interference with oral poliovaccine "takes" is well known.)

Other difficulties may arise in working with suckling mice. These animals have their own infectious diseases, which may intrude overtly or covertly during searches for coxsackieviruses. Some of these, as well as other viruses (of human origin), may multiply in mice and thereby provide stocks containing unrecognized mixtures of viruses.

Differences in susceptibility between litters are known (141); these may be related to factors transmitted to suckling mice in the colostrum (7). When many tests are performed, litters should be pooled, and infant mice distributed randomly to foster mothers. However, the advantages gained by this precaution are sometimes offset by cross-infections with indigenous microorganisms, cannibalism, or failure of mice to thrive.

Virus harvest. Mice that develop paralysis, tremors or spasms are sacrificed. Tissues for virus studies are collected as follows: Wet the dead mouse with 70% alcohol; secure it, belly down, to a sterile board. Use sterilized instruments to remove first the brain, and then the legs (or the entire skinned, eviscerated torso). These tissues, made into 20% suspensions with BSS, constitute the materials for further passage for differentiation and identification. Store each at −20 C. For histologic studies slit the abdominal wall, and open the cranium of one whole skinned mouse inoculated by each route. Transfer to Bouin or other suitable fixative. For passage in mice, the ip or subcutaneous route may be used.

Isolation in tissue cultures

The ideal cell culture system of universal application in the recovery of all enteroviruses has yet to be found. At present there are some strains which fail to elicit CPE in any cell culture system. Human enteroviruses, except those requiring newborn mice for their propagation, are usually isolated in primary MK cell cultures (poliovirus, certain of the A coxsackieviruses, all of the B coxsackieviruses and echoviruses except type 21). Primary human amnion (28) and human fetal kidney and lung (19, 46, 121, 124, 126, 171) may also be used if available, especially for the new enterovirus types 68–71 and for some group A coxsackieviruses. Continuous epithelial cell lines (such as HeLa) have not proved to be as sensitive for isolation of viruses, although MK-grown virus can be adapted to HeLa cells. BGM cells have also been useful for enterovirus isolation (23, 29). The general procedures for the preparation of cell cultures are given in Chapter 3. Some special aspects of tissue culture procedures concerning the enteroviruses are described below.

Preparation of kidney cell cultures. The following modifications, when used with trypsin solution (149), have consistently produced the largest yields of cells; the entire time for trypsinization is about 60–80 min.

Kidneys are obtained aseptically from exsanguinated monkeys and the capsules removed. The entire kidneys (without removing the pelvis) are placed in an appropriate glass tube and minced with uterine scissors into 5- to 7-mm pieces. The minced tissue is then transferred to a trypsinization flask, processed, and grown as described in Chapter 3. It appears that the swirling action created by the presence of fibrous tissue of the pelvis increases the cell yields. This procedure consistently yields 10^8 cells/g of kidney.

Tissue culture tubes. Inexpensive lime glass tubes may be used (156). Since the tubes are disposable, rewashing and resterilizing of glassware are avoided. New glass is less liable to strain than reheated glass; consequently, the breakage of old tubes during stoppering, which constitutes a considerable laboratory hazard, is eliminated. During the outgrowth of cells, about 100 tubes are incubated unstoppered in a box with a neoprene gasket, which eliminates a tedious stoppering process (150).

Growth and maintenance media for MK cell cultures. The following 2 media have been used for several years for the isolation and typing of enteroviruses with highly satisfactory results. The growth medium contains only 2% calf serum; the serum-free maintenance medium keeps the cells for the usual length of time required for the isolation and typing of enteroviruses (about 10 days).

Growth Medium (M-H) (Melnick Medium A)

Hanks BSS containing 0.002% phenol red	86.7	ml
5% lactalbumin hydrolysate in Hanks BSS without bicarbonate and phenol red	10.0	ml
Calf serum	2.0	ml
7.5% NaHCO$_3$	0.3	ml
Antibiotic solution containing 10,000 units of penicillin and 10,000 μg of streptomycin per ml or 25 μg of gentamycin per ml	1.0	ml

Maintenance Medium (M-E) (Melnick Medium B)

Earle BSS containing 0.002% phenol red	86.0	ml
5% lactalbumin hydrolysate in Hanks BSS without bicarbonate and phenol red	10.0	ml
7.5% NaHCO$_3$	3.0	ml
Antibiotic solution (same as in growth medium)	1.0	ml

The addition of 1.0 ml of autoclaved skim milk (10% powdered milk in distilled water) to the maintenance medium is recommended for longer maintenance of cells in a serum-free medium.

Incorporation of 25 mM MgCl$_2$ into maintenance medium enhances the multiplication of polioviruses as manifested in earlier CPE (154), and it produces larger plaques with most of the enteroviruses tested (160). It also increases the rate of poliovirus isolations from clinical specimens, although certain echoviruses are inhibited by the high concentration of magnesium ions.

Isolation procedures. The clinical sample, prepared as described above, is inoculated in 0.2-ml amounts into each of 3 or 4 primary MK or human fetal diploid kidney tube cultures containing 1 ml of maintenance medium and incubated in an almost horizontal position at 36–37 C. (In some laboratories the chances of isolating an enterovirus have been found to be improved if the culture tube is first drained of medium, the inoculum added— up to 1 ml per culture—and virus adsorption allowed to take place for 2–3 hr at 36–37 C. The inoculum is then removed, 1 ml of maintenance medium is added, and the cultures are incubated at 36–37 C. Cultures showing early ($\sim$18 hr) degeneration, which is probably due to the toxicity of the inoculum, are subpassaged.) The addition of a second cell line such as WI-38 increases the chances of isolating a virus. Microscopic readings for CPE are performed at least every other day. Uninoculated cultures derived from the same cell suspension are included as cell controls, and they must remain negative if the test is to be considered valid. CPE is characterized by cellular disorganization consisting of separation, swelling, increased refractivity, lysis, and detachment from the glass wall (Figs 15.2-6). Cultures showing degeneration of about 50% of the cell sheet are harvested and stored at -20 C.

Specimens harvested before the seventh day are titrated and typed as described below. For all the specimens harvested after the seventh day, an additional passage is made in an attempt to raise the titer before the virus is typed.

Identification of isolates

As noted earlier, a rough guide to grouping of isolates can be obtained by their pathogenetic expression in monkey and human cell cultures or in suckling mice. Not all agents recovered from feces and oropharynx are enteroviruses. Others that might be recovered from the feces are reoviruses and adenoviruses. In addition, the following might be isolated from the oropharynx: rhinoviruses, measles, mumps, rubella, herpes simplex, and cytomegaloviruses. Many of these agents produce distinctive CPE, which at once differentiates them from enteroviruses. Several evoke fatal encephalitis in newborn mice.

While the isolation of an enterovirus is simple and relatively rapid, its identification may be slow, expensive, and sometimes tedious. The decision to identify isolates depends on a number of factors; the most important, in our opinion, are those relating to clinical reference and community guidance.

The cytopathic changes, rapidity of development of CPE, and nature of lysis often provide clues to the type of virus. The cytopathic changes for enteroviruses are shown in Figures 15.2-6. In addition, nuclear "ballooning" or "bubbling" is a feature found with echovirus types 22 and 23 (132). The staining patterns of enteroviruses in infected cells are usually helpful only in indicating absence of other viruses that produce characteristic cytoplasmic or nuclear inclusion bodies. Enteroviruses are identified by specific serologic responses in Nt, HI, CF, FA, or precipitin tests, or other antigen-antibody reactions. All such tests hinge on the availability of high-titer type-specific antiserum.

Homogeneity of virus stocks. Several enteroviruses may be found in feces, sewage, and flies. In the laboratory, several serotypes may be inadvertently mixed while infected fluid overlays or mouse carcasses are being combined into single virus pools. Such mixtures, in later studies, provide inconsistent serologic responses. Mixtures are seldom recognized at the time of isolation or during serial passage. Some difficulties may be avoided by using the purification steps noted below. Unfortunately these procedures unduly hinder work in a busy diagnostic laboratory. A practical scheme would be to set aside strains which give uncertain serologic responses for later study as possible mixtures, variants within types, or potential new serotypes.

Two methods can be used for obtaining "purified" stocks: purification by terminal dilution and plaque purification. With the former the single culture showing CPE at the end of the dilution series (4 cultures per 10-fold dilution) in a titration is used to form a stock. The positive culture at the end of the third titration is used to form the virus pool. The method is applicable also to viruses propagable in newborn mice.

In the plaque purification method, with use of dilutions estimated to yield <10 plaques per culture, a single plaque is picked, and the progeny is grown on cell monolayers under fluid overlay. This procedure is repeated 2 more times. The third passage plaque is used to form the virus stock.

Other problems relate to the presence in cultures of adventitious agents such as simian viruses in MK cells and mycoplasma in continuous cell lines (such as HeLa or KB). Viruses indigenous to the species providing cells for culture are not readily eliminated.

Nt tests with mouse isolates. Tests in mice are carried out only when the isolated virus fails to propagate in tissue culture. The virus preparation, consisting of infected mouse torso suspension, is titrated in suckling mice to establish its 50% lethal dose (LD_{50}) titer. Approximately 100 LD_{50} of virus are mixed with equal amounts of type-specific serum, either singly or in pools as described below. The mixtures are incubated at 37 C for 2 hr, and 0.05 ml is inoculated into each of 8 suckling mice. With each series of Nt tests, control titrations of virus diluted with sterile saline solution are included. Some variation (0.4 log) in the calculated dose of 100 LD_{50} used in the Nt test is permissible; thus tests in which controls show that 40–250 LD_{50} were used need not be repeated. If serum pools are used, a confirmatory test is made using proper dilutions of the indicated homotypic antiserum.

Nt tests with tissue culture isolates. Several methods are available, but the use of a constant amount of virus (100 $TCID_{50}$) mixed with serial dilutions of serum is recommended. These are assayed by using cells grown in tubes or microtiter plates, with CPE or pH change as the index, or in cell monolayers under agar (bottles or vertical tube cultures (161)), with plaque formation or reduction as the index. Suitable tests for a suspected enterovirus are outlined below.

1. Inhibition of CPE in tube cultures—Add 0.3 ml of tissue culture fluid containing an estimated 100 $TCID_{50}$ of virus/ml to each of 3 tubes containing 0.3 ml of antisera for polioviruses 1, 2, and 3, respectively. Each serum sample is diluted so that 20 antibody units are present (i.e., 20 times that necessary to neutralize 100 $TCID_{50}$). The incubation period for the virus-serum mixtures is 2 hr at 37 C. Two MK cultures are inoculated with 0.2 ml of each virus-serum mixture. The unknown virus is titrated in the test to determine the number of virus $TCID_{50}$ actually present in the test. Inoculated cultures are incubated at 36–37 C and observed daily. Results are usually apparent on day 3 or 4, and the final readings are made on day 6 or 7. To enhance the appearance of CPE due to polioviruses, 25 mM $MgCl_2$ may be added to the maintenance medium (154).

2. Micromethod in plates—The micro Nt tests described in Chapter 3 provide other methods for identification of virus isolates. The techniques have been adapted to Nt tests using monolayer cell cultures with CPE as the index (69, 131, 142). There is considerable saving of antiserum, stock virus, tissue culture, and tissue culture reagents. A comparison of results obtained by macro- and micromethods showed 97% agreement (69).

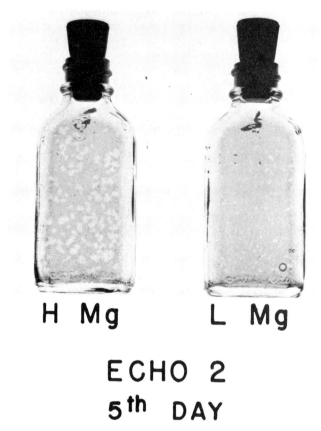

H Mg   L Mg

ECHO 2
5th DAY

Figure 15.9—Growth of echovirus 2 on monkey kidney cells in bottle cultures under agar, in media containing high (at left, 25 mM) and low (at right, 1 mM) MgCl$_2$ concentrations, 5 days after seeding. For echovirus 2 to form plaques, the agar overlay should be made with Bacto-agar; when Noble agar was used in the overlay, plaques did not develop in the low-magnesium cultures.

3. Plaque technique for enteroviruses—The advantages of using the plaque technique in assaying virus infectivity, in purifying viruses, and in carrying out plaque-reduction Nt tests with sera of low neutralizing titers are discussed in Chapter 3. Several modifications (160) in the plaquing technique used for enteroviruses have improved the results considerably so that plaques are now readily produced with enterovirus types previously regarded as difficult to plaque (Fig 15.9). Furthermore, with these modifications most enteroviruses grow faster and produce larger plaques. Counts of poliovirus plaques are possible at 24 hr, and the final readings are made at 48 hr. The modifications involve the incorporation of 25 mM MgCl$_2$ into the agar overlay, the use of Difco Bacto-agar (Noble agar inhibits plaque formation of certain enteroviruses and reoviruses), and filtration of materials (particularly the neutral red solution) through membrane filters rather than asbestos pads. The agar overlay medium is prepared as follows:

Bacto-agar (Difco) . . . .   3.0 g
Distilled water . . . .   163.0 ml

Sterilize at 15 lb for 15 min, cool to 45 C, and add:

10X Earle salt solution (containing antibiotics)* . . . .   20.0 ml
7.5% NaHCO₃* . . . .   10.8 ml
Neutral red (1:1000)* . . . .   3.0 ml
10% skim milk† . . . .   1.0 ml
50% MgCl₂ · 6 H₂O . . . .   2.0 ml
     The temperature of the agar overlay should not be above 44 C when added to the cell cultures. Before adding to the agar medium, centrifuge lightly and use the supernatant fluid only.
*Sterilized by membrane filtration.
†Dry skim milk reconstituted in distilled water and autoclaved at 10 lb for 10 min.

A rapid plaque method has been described that uses vertical tube culture for titration of viruses and measurement of Nt antibodies (161).

General comment on Nt tests for virus identification. Many isolates are not neutralized by poliovirus antiserum; therefore enteroviruses are typed by using antiserum pools according to a combination pattern so designed that each serum specimen is included in more than 1 pool (77, 123). It is possible to test a virus isolate against 42 serotypes using only 8 pools of sera in a single test (see below). (This method has been modified by Schmidt et al (123) so that each serum specimen is incorporated into 2 "intersecting serum" pools. By this method a virus isolate may be screened against 16 serotypes using 8 serum pools, or against 25 serotypes using 10 serum pools.)

In order to keep the number of serum samples in a pool to reasonable limits, 2 intersecting schemata can be used. The first schema would include those viruses which grow readily in tissue culture. The second would include the group A coxsackieviruses which do not grow in tissue culture. Reacting a new isolate against the group A coxsackievirus pools is recommended because some coxsackievirus A isolates are known to grow in cell cultures even more readily than they grow in mice. The possibility that such cytopathogenic strains are present is thus taken into account.

Strains that are not neutralized by immune sera to known enterovirus types are purified by three serial plaque passages or, if they do not produce plaques, by three terminal dilution passages. The purified virus is retested against the serum pools to eliminate the possibility that a mixture of viruses was present in the original isolate. If the strain is still not shown to be related to any of the known viruses and has the properties of an enterovirus (including stability at pH 3–5, which distinguishes enteroviruses from the acid-labile rhinoviruses), it should be filtered to remove the persistent fraction (158). If the monodispersed filtrate still is not neutralized by known antisera, then antiserum against the isolate should be prepared for further characterization of the strain and for further testing against the known enteroviruses.

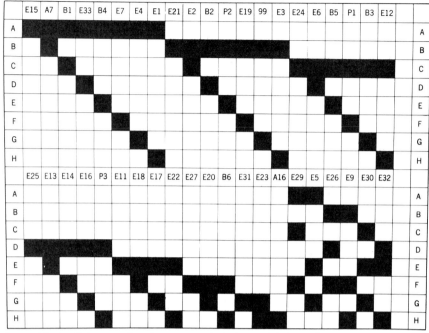

Figure 15.10—Schema of antiserum pools (77). Multiple antisera are incorporated into different pools; a virus isolate can be specifically typed by its pattern of neutralization in tests against the pools. With the antiserum combinations shown, new isolates of 42 enteroviruses can be identified in tests against only 8 pools.

Preparation and use of combination pools for typing isolates (77). To avoid the almost prohibitive time and expense that would be required for typing a new enterovirus isolate by individual tests against the entire battery of enteroviral antisera, isolates are often typed by using antiserum pools. These pools are prepared according to a combination so designed that an isolate can be screened for identity against as many as 42 sera using only 8 pools in a single test. In the test 100 TCID$_{50}$ of virus are set up with each serum pool, as in carrying out a conventional Nt test. Figure 15.10 shows the schema for 8 combination antiserum pools, A-H, which can be used to identify 42 enterovirus serotypes in the Nt tests.

Steps in preparation of pools:

1. High-titer antiserum is used (from a large stock made in horses).

2. Serum titers should be known. If the titer is not available, a titration should be done using 100 plaque-forming units (pfu) or 100 TCID$_{50}$ of the prototype virus against serial dilutions of serum. The serum titers are expressed per 0.1 ml, as the dilution that contains 1 antibody unit.

3. The dilution of serum containing 50 antibody units per 0.1 ml is then calculated (Table 15.9), and a determination can be made of the amount of undiluted serum required to incorporate 20 antibody units in a 1-liter pool.

TABLE 15.9—SERA FOR POOLS*

SERUM	TITER PER 0.1 ML (RECIPROCAL OF DILUTION THAT CONTAINS 1 ANTIBODY UNIT)	RECIPROCAL OF DILUTION CONTAINING 50 ANTIBODY UNITS PER 0.1 ML	AMOUNT OF UNDILUTED SERUM REQUIRED FOR EACH 1-LITER POOL (ML)	POOL ASSIGNMENT(S)
Polio 1	8,000	400	2.50	C, F
Polio 2	19,000	950	1.05	B, E
Polio 3	16,000	800	1.25	D, H
Coxs. A7	9,200	460	2.18	A, B
Coxs. A9	8,000	400	2.50	B, G
Coxs. A16	1,500	75	13.33	H
Coxs. B1	38,000	1,900	0.52	A, C
Coxs. B2	22,000	1,100	0.90	B, D
Coxs. B3	4,000	200	5.00	C, G
Coxs. B4	20,000	1,000	1.00	A, E
Coxs. B5	22,000	1,100	0.90	C, E
Coxs. B6	32,000	1,600	0.62	F, H
Echo 1	11,000	550	1.80	A, H
Echo 2	35,000	1,750	0.56	B, C
Echo 3	4,700	235	4.20	B, H
Echo 4	6,000	300	3.30	A, G
Echo 5	13,000	650	1.53	A, E, G
Echo 6	8,000	400	2.50	C, D
Echo 7	15,000	750	1.33	A, F
Echo 9	7,500	375	2.66	B, F, H
Echo 11	2,000	100	10.00	E
Echo 12	26,000	1,300	0.76	C, H
Echo 13	17,000	850	1.18	D, E
Echo 14	7,300	365	2.73	D, F
Echo 15	2,000	100	10.00	A
Echo 16	12,500	625	1.58	D, G
Echo 17	5,000	250	4.00	E, G
Echo 18	15,000	750	1.33	E, F
Echo 19	35,000	1,750	0.58	B, F
Echo 20	13,000	650	1.50	F, G
Echo 21	2,000	100	10.00	B
Echo 22	13,200	660	1.51	E, H
Echo 23	16,000	800	1.25	G, H
Echo 24	3,400	170	5.90	C
Echo 25	2,000	100	10.00	D
Echo 26	19,000	950	1.05	B, D, F
Echo 27	2,000	100	10.00	F
Echo 29	8,000	400	2.50	A, C, F
Echo 30	5,500	275	3.63	C, E, G
Echo 31	9,600	480	2.08	G
Echo 32	16,000	800	1.25	D, E, H
Echo 33	8,000	400	2.50	A, D

* All sera prepared in horses (41, 42, 90).

TABLE 15.10—SERUM CONSTITUENTS INCLUDED IN EACH POOL

POOL	CONSTITUENT SERA
A	CA7, CB1, CB4, E1, E4, E5, E7, E15, E29, E33
B	P2, CA7, CA9, CB2, E2, E3, E9, E19, E21, E26
C	P1, CB1, CB3, CB5, E2, E6, E12, E24, E29, E30
D	P3, CB2, E6, E13, E14, E16, E25, E26, E32, E33
E	P2, CB4, CB5, E5, E11, E13, E17, E18, E22, E30, E32
F	P1, CB6, E7, E14, E18, E19, E20, E26, E27, E29
G	CA9, CB3, E4, E5, E16, E17, E20, E23, E30, E31
H	P3, CA16, CB6, E1, E3, E9, E12, E22, E23, E32

Example: For poliovirus type 1, 1:8000 is the original titer. A titer of 1:160 = 50 antibody units per 0.1 ml, and for preparing 1 liter of a pool containing 50 antibody units per 0.1 ml, 6.25 ml of undiluted serum will be required. Several types of undiluted sera in predetermined quantities are distributed into each pool, in accordance with the schema outlined.

4. After calculations have been made on each serum sample, a schema is developed to incorporate the sera into the pools in such a way that there is a mixture of low- and high-titer antisera in each pool, in order to have about the same amount of serum protein in each pool. The pool assignment(s) for each serotype are shown in the right-hand column of Table 15.9.

5. A list of the serum constituents of each pool is shown in Table 15.10. In order to obtain 1-liter pools, the required amount of each constituent serum, undiluted, is added to the appropriate pool, and the remainder of the 1-liter volume is made up with Melnick medium B.

Example: Pool C contains various quantities of the following sera: P1, CB1, CB3, CB5, E2, E6, E12, E24, E29, and E30. The total volume of undiluted sera will be 24.77 ml. To this are added 975.23 ml of Melnick medium B to make 1 liter, the total volume of the pool.

6. Completed pools should be distributed in small volumes (about 10 ml) that can be readily available as working stocks for use in Nt tests.

7. The code for interpreting results on the basis of the schema described (Fig. 15.10) is shown in Table 15.11.

Explanatory notes:

One-Class Neutralization: In this class, each serotype is added to a single pool, and only that pool will neutralize a virus of this type.

Two-Class Neutralization: In this class, each serum is present in 2 different pools. Example: Poliovirus 3 antiserum is included in pools D and H, and type 3 poliovirus isolates will be neutralized by these 2 pools.

Three-Class Neutralization: In this class, each serum is present in 3 different pools. Example: If the virus under test is echovirus 29, it will be neutralized by pools A, C, and F.

8. Combination pools J-P of equine antiserum are also available for identification of 19 group A coxsackieviruses. Their preparation, test procedures, and availability are described in a recent publication (95).

Hemagglutination-inhibition tests. (Note: This section was prepared essentially by Leon Rosen, Pacific Research Section, National Institute of Allergy and Infectious Diseases, Honolulu, HI.) Although only about one-third of the presently recognized enteroviruses are known to hemagglutinate, the relative simplicity of the HAI technique makes this procedure attractive as the first step in attempting to identify an enterovirus. The enterovirus serotypes for which hemagglutination has been demonstrated are listed in Table 15.12 (34, 61, 68, 117). It should be noted that not all strains

TABLE 15.11—CODE FOR READING RESULTS

IF NEUTRALIZED BY POOL(S):	VIRUS IS:	IF NEUTRALIZED BY POOL(S):	VIRUS IS:
A	E15	CD	E6
B	E21	CE	CB5
C	E24	CF	P1
D	E25	CG	CB3
E	E11	CH	E12
F	E27	DE	E13
G	E31	DF	E14
H	CA16	DG	E16
AB	CA7	DH	P3
AC	CB1	EF	E18
AD	E33	EG	E17
AE	CB4	EH	E22
AF	E7		
AG	E4	FG	E20
AH	E1	FH	CB6
BC	E2	GH	E23
BD	CB2		
BE	P2	ACF	E29
BF	E19	AEG	E5
BG	CA9	BDF	E26
BH	E3	BFH	E9
		CEG	E30
		DEH	E32

of the serotypes listed in the table hemagglutinate. Furthermore, hemagglutination may be quite variable from one tissue culture passage to the next, and this variation limits usefulness of the HAI technique for routine identification purposes. For some serotypes (e.g., coxsackievirus B3) only a few hemagglutinating strains have been found, while for others (e.g., echovirus 11) practically all strains have this property. In addition to the viruses listed in Table 15.12, a number of other hemagglutinating enteroviruses are known (among them strains with the properties of the coxsackieviruses in group A) that are probably antigenically distinct from all presently recognized serotypes but that have not as yet been completely characterized. All the viruses in Table 15.12 agglutinate human RBC with the exception of coxsackievirus A7, which agglutinates those chicken RBC agglutinable by vaccinia virus. Other factors known to influence hemagglutination by enteroviruses include temperature, pH, and the age of the RBC donor.

1. Preparation of antigens—Enteroviruses to be tested for hemagglutination should be grown in either MK or human kidney tissue cultures maintained on medium No. 199. Although in some instances it has been demonstrated that enteroviruses propagated in other types of tissue culture or in suckling mice will hemagglutinate, the data available are not sufficient to permit recommendation of these alternative methods for routine use. Similarly, sufficient experience has not as yet been gained to permit routine use of other maintenance media. If possible, the maintenance medium used on

TABLE 15.12—ENTEROVIRUSES KNOWN TO HEMAGGLUTINATE

Coxsackievirus A7	Echovirus 3	Echovirus 21
Coxsackievirus A20	Echovirus 6	Echovirus 24
Coxsackievirus A21	Echovirus 7	Echovirus 25
Coxsackievirus A24	Echovirus 11	Echovirus 29
Coxsackievirus B1	Echovirus 12	Echovirus 30
Coxsackievirus B3	Echovirus 13	Echovirus 33
Coxsackievirus B5	Echovirus 19	Enterovirus 68
Coxsackievirus B6	Echovirus 20	

the infected tissue cultures should be free of serum. If serum is necessary, it is recommended that chicken serum be used, as this variety is less apt to agglutinate human RBC than sera of most of the commonly used mammalian species. Supernatant fluid from infected tube or bottle cultures is tested after the tissue sheets have been completely destroyed by the virus and after the cultures have been frozen and thawed once. It is difficult to anticipate the quantity of infected supernatant fluid required to complete the identification process, since this is largely dependent on the titer of hemagglutinin obtained, which varies widely. Consequently, it is recommended that only a small quantity of supernatant fluid (1 ml) be prepared for the initial screening procedure to determine whether or not hemagglutination can be demonstrated, and that, if necessary, a further passage be made to provide sufficient material for the definitive typing. For coxsackievirus A21, hemagglutinin titers have been higher when infected cells have been harvested together with the culture fluids.

2. *Erythrocytes*—Human type O RBC are collected, stored, and standardized exactly as described for work with reoviruses in Chapter 17. Erythrocytes from newborn infants (collected from the umbilical cord after it has been tied) are the most sensitive to agglutination by enteroviruses, but cells from adult donors are suitable for most serotypes.

3. *Hemagglutinin titration*—Four sets of serial 2-fold dilutions of tissue culture fluid are prepared in 12- × 75-mm test tubes with hemispherical bottoms or in Linbro or Cooke "U" plates for the microtiter system. The dilutions should range from 1:8 to 1:4096, and each tube or well should contain 0.4 or 0.05 ml (0.025 virus + 0.025 diluent), respectively. Two sets of dilutions are prepared in 0.01 M phosphate-buffered 0.85% NaCl at a pH of approximately 5.8, and another 2 sets are prepared in 0.01 M phosphate-buffered 0.85% NaCl at a pH of approximately 7.4. The standard RBC suspension, prepared in the same diluents, is then added (0.2 ml to each tube or 0.05 ml to each well). The tubes or plates are shaken, and the RBC allowed to settle at either 4 C or 37 C (i.e., 1 set of the pH 5.8 dilutions and 1 set of the pH 7.4 dilutions at 4 C, the others at 37 C). The highest dilution of tissue culture fluid which shows a 1+ pattern of sedimentation is taken as the endpoint, and this tube or well is considered to contain 1 unit of hemagglutinin. If a large number of strains is to be tested for hemagglutination, it is more efficient to screen the fluids at a single dilution of 1:8 at each pH and temper-

ature specified and then titrate only those found positive. Some enteroviruses agglutinate human RBC to the same titer at 4 C and at 37 C and at both pH extremes; others do not. While the presently available data suggest that most strains within a given serotype behave consistently in this respect, exceptions have been found in sufficient number to rule out definitive identification based on these characteristics. Titers of hemagglutinin observed with enteroviruses range from 1:8 to 1:2048, depending on serotype and other conditions mentioned above.

4. *Preparation and standardization of typing antiserum*—Generally, antiserum suitable for HAI typing procedures can be prepared by any method suitable for serum to be used in Nt tests. (In the case of those picornaviruses that produce CPE in human kidney but not in MK cultures, difficulty has been encountered in preparing high-titer antiserum suitable for either the HAI or tissue culture Nt procedures.) As a typical example of the HAI titers that can be obtained, the NIH reference monkey serum for echovirus type 7 has a homologous HAI titer of 1:10,240 and heterologous HAI titers of <1:40 against all the hemagglutinating enteroviruses with which it has been tested. Of course, lower homologous HAI titers are usually obtained when rabbits are immunized by shorter procedures, but these titers are almost always sufficiently high for routine typing purposes. Antiserum is considered suitable for HAI typing purposes if its homologous titer is at least 1:160 and any heterologous titers are at least 8-fold lower. It is usually quite easy to prepare sera with titers much higher than these minimal requirements. In some instances (e.g., echovirus type 20) it is necessary to use a nonprototype antigen to determine the titer of an antiserum because the prototype strain does not hemagglutinate.

Before use in the HAI tests, typing antisera are adsorbed with kaolin and human RBC exactly as described for work with the reoviruses (see Chapter 17). The sera are not inactivated. HAI tests are set up and are interpreted as described for the reoviruses, except that phosphate-buffered saline solution and an RBC sedimentation temperature of either 4 C or 37 C are employed to correspond with the optimal conditions observed in titration of the particular hemagglutinin to be used.

5. *HAI typing procedure*—To identify hemagglutinating enterovirus isolates, 4 units of hemagglutinin are set up against single dilutions of typing antisera known to contain at least 8 antibody units. Isolates are routinely tested against antisera of each of the enteroviruses known to hemagglutinate, except that those isolates that produce CPE in rhesus kidney are not ordinarily run against antisera of serotypes that do not, and vice versa. The pH and temperature conditions found most suitable in the antigen titration are usually employed in the HAI tests. An isolate is considered typed if it is completely inhibited by one of the typing antisera and not by any of the others. As a confirmatory procedure, the typing antiserum may be titrated to its end point against the isolate.

6. *Interpretation*—If an enterovirus isolate hemagglutinates but is not inhibited by any of the standard typing antisera, one of the following factors may be responsible: The isolate is a "prime" strain of a serotype known to hemagglutinate and the typing serum is not sufficiently "broad" to pick this

up; the isolate is a hemagglutinating strain of a recognized enterovirus serotype for which hemagglutination has not been demonstrated previously; the
isolate is a hemagglutinating strain of a previously unrecognized enterovirus
serotype; or the isolate is a mixture of two hemagglutinating enteroviruses.

With regard to prime strains, the only solution to this difficulty, as in the
Nt procedures, is to use the broadest available strain to prepare the standard
typing antiserum. In the case of a hemagglutinating strain of a recognized
serotype not previously known to have this property, this can usually be
determined by setting up the hemagglutinin against high-titer Nt antisera of
these serotypes. All the problems enumerated above can be further investigated by preparing an antiserum against the isolate in question and testing
this serum against known hemagglutinating antigens.

In practice, it has been found possible to identify, by HAI procedures,
between 30% and 40% of random groups of enterovirus isolates cytopathic
for MK cultures. The difficulty encountered with the enteroviruses not cytopathic for MK, and with coxsackievirus A7, renders HAI unsuitable at the
present time for identification of these viruses.

Complement-fixation tests. Although at present not all enteroviruses
can be identified by the CF technique, this test is of considerable practical
value in the identification of many enteroviruses (18, 33). However, it fails
to indicate prime relationships among strains which might have epidemiologic significance. Enteroviruses producing rapid and complete CPE in MK cell
cultures and those group A coxsackieviruses that grow to high titers in newborn mice are most readily identified by the CF procedure. On the other
hand, enteroviruses that produce a slowly progressive CPE in MK cell cultures, produce CPE only in human cell cultures, and grow to relatively low
titers in suckling mice are not satisfactorily identified by the CF procedure.
The principal difficulties encountered with the CF typing procedure are the
inability to produce a sufficiently potent CF antigen from some isolates by
simple techniques, the anticomplementary effect of some antigens, occasional nonspecific fixation of obscure origin, and the inability to produce
satisfactory antiserum for certain enterovirus serotypes.

It is usually relatively easy to prepare typing serum for those prototype
viruses that can be propagated in MK cultures or in newborn mice. Viruses
grown in these systems can be used to immunize monkeys and adult mice,
respectively. These animals, unlike humans, almost always respond with the
production of type-specific CF antibody. No completely satisfactory system
has as yet been found for producing type-specific CF sera for isolates that
must be grown in human cultures.

1. Preparation of antigens—Antigens may be prepared from isolates
which grow in MK cultures by inoculating an appropriate number of such
tube cultures containing 1 ml of Melnick medium B: lactalbumin enzymatic
hydrolysate, 0.5%, plus inactivated (56 C for 30 min) calf serum, 2%, and
Earle BSS, 97.5%. In some laboratories, HeLa cell cultures yield more potent CF antigens than do MK cell cultures. It is desirable that tubes be inoculated with a dilution of seed virus such that a complete degeneration of
the tissue culture will take place rapidly, but not before 48 hr post-
inoculation. After complete degeneration of cells has taken place, the cul-

tures are frozen and thawed once, and the uncentrifuged pooled fluids are used as antigen. Antigens for isolates which are comparatively slow-growing in the presence of calf serum should be prepared in cultures maintained on medium No. 199 alone, or on Melnick medium B without calf serum.

Antigens may be prepared from isolates which grow only in newborn mice (and produce gross lesions typical of coxsackieviruses of group A) by the following technique: Litters of 2- to 4-day-old mice are inoculated ip with 0.04 ml of virus diluted (usually 10^{-2} or 10^{-3}) so as to produce typical signs of disease in most of the mice on the second or third day after inoculation. When a majority of the mice are paralyzed, all living mice are killed and stored at -20 C until used for the preparation of antigen. Mice found dead are discarded. In preparing the antigen, the mice are thawed, and the head, tail, feet, viscera and skin removed. The torso and limbs are then homogenized intermittently in a Waring Blendor for a total of 3 min, with 10 ml of sterile 0.85% NaCl as a diluent for each mouse. The suspension is centrifuged at 1500 rpm for 10 min, the supernatant fluid is transferred to a separatory funnel, and 4 ml of diethyl ether are added for each 10 ml of suspension. The mixture is shaken vigorously for several minutes and then held overnight at 4 C. The following morning the aqueous phase is withdrawn, and the residual ether removed from this material by water vacuum. The suspension is stored at -20 C.

2. Preparation and standardization of typing sera—Satisfactory antiserum may be prepared in monkeys or in adult mice, with use of schedules given in this chapter. Most of the rhesus sera prepared at the University of Kansas under the auspices of the Committee on Enteroviruses have also been found satisfactory for CF typing (63, 166). For CF typing the sera must be of high titer and must be used at dilutions beyond the point at which they show any nonspecific activity. For most coxsackie- and several echoviruses, immune ascitic fluids prepared in mice yield high-titer and specific CF antibody.

The antisera are tested insofar as possible with prototype homologous and heterologous antigens to establish their specificity. These antigens can be prepared as described above or by more refined techniques. It is desirable to use 4 antigen units in these tests, but it is frequently not possible to achieve high titers. A serum is considered satisfactory if its specific titer is at least 8-fold higher than any dilution which is anticomplementary or which shows nonspecific fixation. The minimal satisfactory homologous titer is considered to be 1:32. Much higher titers than this are often obtained with rhesus sera. Some heterotypic CF titers have been observed in rhesus and mouse sera, and these usually correspond to antigenic relationships also observed in Nt tests. Such heterotypic reactions must be taken into consideration in interpreting typing tests.

3. Technique of the CF test—Procedures utilized in the CF test are described in Chapter 1.

4. Typing procedure—To identify an isolate, its antigen is tested against serum (containing 4 or more antibody units) of each of those enterovirus serotypes known to have the same general characteristics; that is, isolates that produce CPE in MK are tested against antisera of serotypes that produce CPE in this tissue culture, and isolates that produce lesions typical of coxsackieviruses of group A in mice are tested against coxsackievirus A antiserum, etc.

In practice, tissue culture antigens are tested undiluted and may be run in duplicate, heated (56 C for 30 min) and unheated. Heating usually lowers the titer of the antigen but often eliminates anticomplementary activity. This may make possible a satisfactory test if the unheated antigen is anticomplementary. Mouse antigens are usually tested at dilutions of 1:2 and 1:4. Both dilutions should be tested for anticomplementary effect. Sometimes with a weak antigen only the 1:2 dilution will react. With others, a satisfactory result may be obtained with the 1:4 dilution if the lower dilution is anticomplementary.

In a satisfactory test the antigen reacts with only one antiserum type, unless such related serotypes as echovirus types 1 and 8 are involved. In many instances 4+ fixation is not observed with the single antiserum that reacts. However, lesser degrees of fixation with one antiserum—and no reaction at all with the others—usually indicate a successful typing. At the present state of knowledge, all CF typing of critical importance should be confirmed by Nt tests. Examples of mouse isolates reacting with 2 sera are known, and this has led to the recognition and separation of two virus types from the single isolates (18).

If no fixation occurs, one may be dealing with an insufficiency of antigen or with a serotype not represented among the sera used. Unfortunately, there is no way at present to distinguish between these possibilities. If the antigen is anticomplementary, the test is unsatisfactory. This happens most often with those viruses that grow slowly in MK cultures, necessitating the maintenance of the tissue cultures for long periods of time. Occasionally, it may be observed that an antigen prepared in MK cultures causes fixation with more than one type of serum in the absence of demonstrable anticomplementary activity. The explanation for this phenomenon is not known. It may represent a reaction of latent viruses in the MK cultures with corresponding antibodies in the monkey serum, or it may be the result of borderline anticomplementary effect of the antigen added to a similar effect of some sera.

Despite the many limitations of the CF typing technique, it has proved very valuable in practice where many enterovirus isolates have to be identified. In one longitudinal study of enteroviral infections in children, it was possible by this technique to identify approximately 90% of those isolates producing CPE in MK cultures.

Fluorescent antibody-antigen techniques. The procedures thus far found useful for identifying enterovirus serotypes have been discussed in "Direct Examination of Specimens" in this chapter.

Precipitin methods. Methods were first developed for polioviruses and coxsackieviruses A9 and B. Partially purified and concentrated (high-speed centrifugation) suspensions of polioviruses grown in tissue culture produce direct flocculation or precipitation when mixed with rabbit or human immune serum under proper conditions. The techniques used to demonstrate this phenomenon are the macro tube test (135), the microflocculation test (128, 135), and an agar gel-diffusion method which has proved useful for revealing antigenic relationships between heterologous enteroviruses (129).

Viral antigen preparations are concentrated (200- to 400-fold or to $\geq 10^7$ $TCID_{50}$ per 0.1 ml) by ultracentrifugation. Clean microscope slides (1×3 inch) are coated on 1 side with about 3 ml of 0.8% Ionagar No. 2 (Consolidated Laboratories, Inc) in 0.15 M NaCl. Wells (5 mm diameter for antigens in the center and 3–4 mm diameter for antisera around the central well) are cut with an agar gel cutter. Viral antigens (undiluted, or at 1:2 dilutions), 0.4 ml each and 0.015 ml of each serum are added to the proper wells. The precipitin reaction is monitored during an 18- to 24-hr incubation period at 37 C in a humid chamber. The prepared slides are inspected periodically using dark-field illumination. Usually, no staining is required for photographic recording of the observed precipitin reactions.

Flow Chart of Procedures for Isolation and Identification of Enteroviruses

For viruses which cannot be typed by the procedures outlined in Figure 15.11 determine thermostability in the presence of M $MgCl_2$, an important property of enteroviruses, and perform an acid lability test for a rhinovirus. Separate mixtures of two or more viruses by plaque purification and then obtain "pure" culture and retype. Strains that remain untypable may be prime serotypes, or new serotypes, or aggregated virus populations. Monodispersed stocks should be obtained by ultrafiltration (158) and the procedure should be repeated.

Serologic diagnosis

After enteroviral infection, Nt, CF, and HAI antibodies, among others, may be found in convalescent-phase serum. Diagnosis of an individual patient's illness on the basis of serology alone would require too large a battery of tests against known enteroviruses unless the choice of serotypes for testing can be narrowed by a strongly suggestive clinical picture frequently associated with specific enteroviral serotypes, isolation of a known enterovirus from the patient, and/or presence of a community outbreak of infections with a known enterovirus serotype. Of the available techniques for measurement, tests for these three antibody responses (Nt, CF, and HAI) have had sufficient trial for detailed description.

Tests for determination of antibodies are carried out either for clinical diagnosis or for epidemiologic studies. In acute cases, antibodies may already be present at the time the patient is admitted to the hospital. For epidemiologic studies a single blood sample from each person in the study suffices. Careful attention to selection of the persons to be sampled is essential to obtain valid results. For a discussion of serologic surveys, including the selection and size of samples, see Immunological and Haematological Surveys, Report of a Study Group. WHO Tech Rep Series No. 181, 1959. For clinical diagnostic purposes 2 samples of serum are required, one obtained as soon as possible after the onset of illness, and another 2–3 weeks later. The relationship of antibodies to infection is indicated when a significant quantitative increase is detected in the second sample (75, 122). A 4-fold or

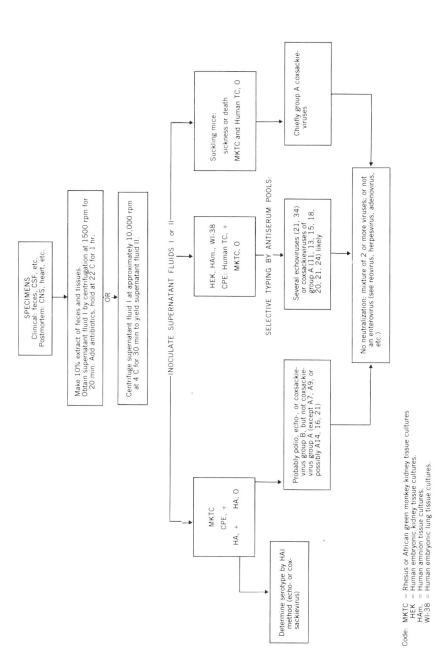

Figure 15.11—Flow chart of procedures for isolation and identification of enteroviruses.

TABLE 15.13—TISSUE CULTURE NEUTRALIZATION TEST WITH PAIRED SERA OF PATIENT INFECTED WITH TYPE 1 POLIOVIRUS

POLIO-VIRUS*	SERUM (DAY AFTER ONSET)	CELLULAR DEGENERATION (CPE) AT SERUM DILUTION														50% SERUM TITER	
		1:2			1:10			1:50			1:250			1:1250			LOG	ANTILOG
Type 1	1	0	0	0	+	+	+	+	+	+	+	+	+	+	+	+	0.7	5
	20	0	0	0	0	0	0	0	0	0	0	0	+	+	+	+	2.5	320
Type 2	1	0	0	0	+	+	+	+	+	+	+	+	+	+	+	+	0.7	5
	20	0	0	0	0	0	0	0	+	+	+	+	+	+	+	+	1.5	32
Type 3	1	+	+	+	+	+	+	+	+	+	+	+	+	+	+	+	0	0
	20	+	+	+	+	+	+	+	+	+	+	+	+	+	+	+	0	0
None:	1	0	0	0														
	20	0	0	0														

*100 TCID$_{50}$ of each virus used in the test.

greater rise in antibody titer is considered significant in serologic tests conducted in vitro, and neutralization of 2 logs$_{10}$ of virus is considered significant in the test done in animals.

Neutralization tests

Tissue culture systems. The principles and general procedure for this are discussed in previous sections and need not be repeated here. Other procedures, such as the metabolic-inhibition test, are described in Chapter 3. The following procedures in monolayer tube cultures are those recommended by the Committee on the Enteroviruses (17).

Cytopathic endpoint tests. Tests are carried out in MK cultures grown in Melnick medium A and, before use, changed to Melnick medium B or to medium No. 199. Virus and serum dilutions are made with Melnick medium B. Virus in 0.5-ml amounts, calculated to contain 100 TCID$_{50}$ per 0.1 ml, is added to 0.5 ml of each serum dilution and mixed. After incubation for 2 hr at 37 C, 0.2 ml of the mixture is added to each of 4 MK tubes. When the virus-serum mixtures have been inoculated, control virus (a challenge dose containing the calculated 100 TCID$_{50}$ per 0.1 ml) is diluted 10, 100, and 1000 times, and 0.1 ml of each dilution is inoculated into each of 4 cultures. The cultures are incubated at 37 C; results are recorded 3-4 and 7-8 days later. The earlier readings are made to detect any initial neutralization that is followed by breakthrough of virus, since partial neutralization may indicate antigenic relatives. At the time of the last reading, the control titration indicates the amount of virus which was present in the challenge dose; this should be approximately 100 TCID$_{50}$. Serum titer should be calculated for the 50% endpoint per 0.1 ml against the challenge dose of virus. A typical protocol using paired sera of a patient infected with poliovirus type 1 is presented in Table 15.13.

Plaque reduction tests. Some enterovirus strains are difficult to neutralize in tube cultures (e.g., the prototype Pesascek strain of echovirus 4) unless monodispersed virus stock is prepared by ultrafiltration (158). Other strains of the same type (e.g., the DuToit strain of echovirus 4) that have fewer nonneutralizable aggregates may be used in the tube Nt test (1, 170). A plaque-reduction Nt test (57, 160) detects antibodies even with aggregated virus stocks because the test does not require neutralization of over 99% of the stock. A description of a satisfactory plaque-reduction test for enteroviruses follows.

Plaque reduction tests for Nt antibody are carried out in MK cultures grown in Melnick medium A with 2% calf serum and washed once before use with either saline or Melnick medium B without serum. Twofold serum dilutions are mixed with an estimated 100 pfu of virus per 0.1 ml. Equal volumes of diluted serum and virus in saline solution or Melnick medium B are employed. The mixture is incubated for 1 hr at 37 C, and 0.2 ml of each mixture is inoculated into each of 2 drained bottle cultures. After an adsorption period of 2 hr at 37 C, the monolayers are covered with agar. The overlay contains 1.5% Bacto agar, 0.1% skim milk, 1:60,000 (filtered, not autoclaved) neutral red, and 0.225% sodium bicarbonate in final concentrations in Earle salt solution. For each milliliter of overlay, 100 units of penicillin and 100 μg of streptomycin are included. The bottles are left about 1 hr at room temperature for solidification of the overlay and then are inverted and incubated at 37 C. The plaque counts of both bottles at each serum dilution are compared with the number of plaques in the control bottles without serum. A 90% reduction in plaque count is taken as the lower limit of significant neutralization, and the highest dilution of serum which gives such neutralization is considered as the titer of the serum.

Microneutralization test. The microtiter technique provides a convenient method for quantitative tests of large numbers of sera. In these virus-serum Nt tests, tissue culture cell suspensions are propagated and maintained in Linbro or Cooke U or flat-bottom wells in plastic plates; antibody titer endpoints are determined on the basis of CPE. Readings are made with an inverted microscope. The basic features of the technique are described in Chapter 3; here human acute- and convalescent-phase sera are diluted by loop, and virus dosage is added by dropper pipette. Controls include 1:4 serum dilution to detect toxicity, cell controls in dilution media, and virus titration. The vertical tube test (161) also can be used for rapid measurement of antibody, in this case by the index of plaque inhibition.

Mouse Nt test. This is the test for antibodies against coxsackieviruses that have not been adapted to tissue culture (3, 4, 27, 93). The same principles apply and virus-serum mixtures are set up in the same way as just described, except that the original virus concentration is 100 LD_{50} per 0.02 ml. The inoculation dose is 0.04 ml ip into each of 8 newborn mice randomly distributed in mixed litters.

Mice are observed daily for 10–14 days. Those missing, cannibalized, or found dead within 48 hr are recorded as nonspecific deaths and are not scored. After 48 hr, signs of disease, as well as deaths, should be recorded. The virus controls must develop disease in the allotted period if the test is to be considered valid.

The complement-fixation test

CF was once fairly widely employed for the diagnosis of poliovirus infections. It has also been used for the diagnosis of other enteroviral infections, but to a lesser extent because of the great number of heterotypic crossings that have been observed, which render the test of little value for type-specific diagnosis (38, 66).

Hemagglutination-inhibition test

Almost all individuals experiencing naturally acquired infections with enteroviruses known to hemagglutinate respond with the development of significant titers of HAI antibodies against the homologous virus. Such individuals may also respond to a varying degree with significant HAI antibody rises to heterologous enterovirus serotypes. Moreover, individuals infected with nonhemagglutinating serotypes may also develop HAI antibodies against heterologous hemagglutinating enteroviruses. Thus the HAI procedure is of little value for type-specific diagnosis if the infecting virus is not known. On the other hand, it can be quite useful in the detailed investigation of an outbreak known to be caused by an enterovirus serotype that does hemagglutinate. Persons infected with one of the serotypes listed in Table 15.12 develop HAI antibodies even though their homologous isolates may not have the property of hemagglutination. HAI antibodies usually appear within 21 days after onset of infection and can usually be detected for at least 6 months thereafter. Since these antibodies are very common in human sera, it is essential that paired sera be employed for diagnostic purposes. A ≥4-fold rise in titer is considered a positive result.

HAI tests are carried out by essentially the same procedures as those used to type isolates. The test antigens are prepared from the prototype strain, or if the prototype does not hemagglutinate, from another suitable strain. All sera are adsorbed either with kaolin or with filtrate from cultures of a psychrophilic *Pseudomonas* sp. Many human sera contain nonspecific inhibitors for hemagglutinins of group B coxsackieviruses and very likely other hemagglutinating enteroviruses. Kaolin is not always effective in removing such inhibitors, whereas pseudomonas filtrate is highly effective (130). Kaolin carries the additional risk of removing or reducing the specific enteroviral serum antibodies. HAI antibody responses with properly treated sera correlate very closely with Nt antibody responses to group B coxsackieviruses (130), but low levels of HAI antibodies in the absence of corresponding Nt antibody have been encountered in some echovirus infections (13).

Optimal conditions of pH and temperature for each hemagglutinating antigen must be determined. Paired sera are always run in the same test and are usually titrated in 2-fold dilutions from 1:10 through 1:320 against 4 units of antigen.

Passive-hemagglutination test

As noted above, no serologic screening test has proved useful in most laboratories for detecting the presence of enteroviral disease. A passive hemagglutination test using paired sera has been developed and has been used over a 6-year period to successfully detect epidemic coxsackievirus B5 disease and smaller outbreaks of echovirus 9 and echovirus 6 disease well before virus isolations and associated clinical syndromes make the diagnosis evident (30, 47). Because of cross-reactivity among the enteroviruses, the test is not useful for determining the specific enterovirus serotype causing disease. It has, however, proved useful as a screening test for detecting rises in enteroviral antibody, and its lack of specificity is more than offset by its simplicity and the fact that results may be obtained on the day that the test is performed. This test for detecting enteroviral disease must await more widespread trial in other laboratories before it can be recommended as a routine diagnostic procedure. A $\geq$4-fold rise in titer is considered a positive result.

To perform this test, 1 volume (0.1 ml) of washed guinea pig or human group O RBC is mixed with 1 volume of viral antigen (usually echovirus 11) and 1 volume of a 1:20 dilution of 0.0375 M stock solution of chromic chloride ($CrCl_3$-6 H_2O). The cells, antigen, and $CrCl_3$-6 H_2O are prepared in PO_4-free, 0.15 M saline. The stock solution of $CrCl_3$-6 H_2O is 1% in distilled water and is kept in a brown, light-proof bottle at 5 C. The mixture of cells, antigen, and chromium is allowed to react for 5 min at room temperature and is then washed 4 times in phosphate-buffered saline (PBS) with use of 30-sec periods of centrifugation. The washed cells are reconstituted as 0.1% suspension in PBS containing 0.1% bovine serum albumin.

Microtiter plates (V type) are used. A diluent containing PBS, Tween (1:20,000), and polyvinyl pyrrolidone (2.5 mg/dl) is added to each well, and an equal volume of the serum under study is added to the first well of the microtiter trays and serially diluted with a microtiter loop. Control tests are done in the last 2 wells of each row for all experiments: these include antigen-coated cells without test serum, and noncoated RBC with test serum. All test wells then receive an equal volume of the 0.1% suspension of virus-coated RBC. The titration plates are covered with a clear tape to minimize evaporation and are left at room temperature for 1 hr. They are then spun for 1 min at 1000 rpm in a centrifuge equipped with special carriers for microtiter trays. The clear tape is removed and the plates are inclined at a 60° angle on an illuminated platform for 20 min. Cells that remain as a button at the bottom of a well signify a positive reaction, and smooth running patterns of RBC denote a negative reaction.

Association of Enteroviruses with Disease

In order that a virus be clearly established as the etiologic agent of the patient's disease, it is not always sufficient that a virus be isolated and that specific antibodies be found to develop. Since no evidence can be sought to show that the recovered virus produces the same disease in susceptible humans, caution must be exercised in interpretation of laboratory findings. Inapparent infections are common, and dual, triple, and quadruple enteroviral infections have been recorded (107). Some of the enteroviruses (polioviruses; coxsackieviruses A7, A9, A16, A21, and A24; echovirus types 4, 6, 9, 11, 16, 30, and enteroviruses 70 and 71) are associated periodically with epidemic outbreaks and are known to be pathogens, but they, as well as others, have been recovered also from persons without any malaise or with only minor complaints.

Associations based on serologic data alone are particularly deserving of critical scrutiny. Mention has been made of some cross-reactions obtained with immune sera from animals; cross-reactions are even more pronounced with human sera. The majority of these cross-reactions have been obtained by CF, some by HAI, and a few by Nt. A few examples may be cited. Ditypic and tritypic antibody responses to inactivated antigens occur in poliomyelitis (83, 127). Antibodies neutralizing type 2 poliovirus have appeared for a brief period during type 1 infections (118). Infections with several group A coxsackieviruses engender antibodies to other group A viruses (3) and also to group B viruses (66); similarly group B infections are occasionally attended by antibody rises against other group B viruses (75) and against some group A coxsackieviruses (66), echoviruses, and polioviruses (13). Conversely, some echoviruses may call forth antibodies against group B coxsackieviruses and polioviruses. Antibodies against echovirus types 6 and 9 have followed echovirus type 4 infections; rises to echovirus 16 have been noted after infection with echoviruses types 6, 9, and 20 (40, 62, 74, 104, 122).

Thus, the isolation of an enterovirus from the alimentary tract, even with subsequent ≥4-fold rise in antibodies, may have no relationship to the patient's illness. On the other hand, the consistent recovery of an enterovirus from similar illnesses and from asymptomatic familial associates, in conjunction with homotypic seroconversion, provide strong evidence of an etiologic relationship.

Recovery of an enterovirus from body fluids (CSF, blood, etc.) or from tissues of CNS, heart muscle, etc.; the disclosure of compatible anatomic lesions; and the demonstration of viral antigen within affected cells also constitute convincing evidence that the virus recovered is related to the patient's disease. Recovery of a single serotype from patients with similar clinical features during an outbreak, particularly when reinforced by data noted above, relates the serotype to the disease. While a single experience of this sort may not be absolute proof of the relationship, it is about all that can be obtained in most clinical and laboratory settings. Confirmation of the epidemiologic and laboratory findings in other areas and in different years is desired for final proof of causal relationship.

References

1. BARRON AL and KARZON DT: Characteristics of ECHO 4 virus (Shropshire) isolated during epidemic aseptic meningitis. J Immunol 87:608–615, 1961
2. BARSKI G. The significance of *in vitro* cellular lesions for classification of enteroviruses. Virology 18:152–154, 1962
3. BEEMAN EA and HUEBNER RJ: Evaluation of serological methods for demonstrating antibody responses to group A coxsackie (herpangina) viruses. J Immunol 68:663–672, 1952
4. BEEMAN EA, HUEBNER RJ and COLE RM: Studies of coxsackie viruses. Laboratory aspects of group A viruses. Am J Hyg 55:83–107, 1952
5. BEEMAN EA, PARROTT RH, and COLE RM: Simultaneous occurrence of two immunological types of group A ''coxsackie'' virus in a case of herpangina. Proc Soc Exp Biol Med 78:295–298, 1951
6. BEHBEHANI AM, LEE LH and MELNICK, JL: Identification of Thai C-18 virus as a member of the coxsackievirus A20 subgroup. Proc Soc Exp Biol Med 116:661–662, 1964

7. BEHBEHANI AM, SULKIN SE, and WALLIS C: Factors influencing susceptibility of mice to coxsackie virus infection. J Infect Dis 110:147–154, 1962
8. BENYESH M, POLLARD EC, OPTON EM, BLACK FL, BELLAMY WD, and MELNICK JL: Size and structure of echo, poliomyelitis, and measles virus determined by ionizing radiation and ultrafiltration. Virology 5:256–274, 1958
9. BERG G, BODILY HL, LENNETTE EH, MELNICK JL, and METCALF TG (eds): Viruses in Water. American Public Health Association, Washington, 1976
10. BODIAN D: The virus, the nerve cell, and paralysis. A study of experimental poliomyelitis in the spinal cord. Bull Johns Hopkins Hosp 83:1–106, 1948
11. BUCKLEY SM: Visualization of poliomyelitis virus by fluorescent antibody. Arch Gesamte Virusforsch 6:388–400, 1956
12. BURCH GE, SUN S, CHU K, SOHAL RA, and COLCOLOUGH HL: Interstitial and coxsackievirus B myocarditis in infants and children. J Am Med Assoc 203:1–8, 1968
13. BUSSELL RH, KARZON DT, BARRON AL, and HALL FT: Hemagglutination-inhibiting, complement-fixing and neutralizing antibody responses in ECHO 6 infection, including studies on heterotypic responses. J Immunol 88:47–54, 1962
14. CHIN TDY, LEHAN PH, RUBIN H, and WENNER HA: Epidemic infection with coxsackie virus, group B type 5. II. Virus excretion and neutralizing antibody response. Am J Hyg 67:321–330, 1958
15. COMMITTEE ON THE ECHO VIRUSES: Enteric cytopathogenic human orphan (ECHO) viruses. Science 122:1187–1188, 1955
16. COMMITTEE ON ENTEROVIRUSES: Classification of human enteroviruses. Virology 16:501–504, 1962
17. COMMITTEE ON THE ENTEROVIRUSES, NFIP: The enteroviruses. Am J Public Health 47:1556–1566, 1957
18. CONTRERAS G, BARNETT VH, and MELNICK JL: Identification of coxsackie viruses by immunological methods and their classification into 16 antigenically distinct types. J Immunol 69:395–414, 1952
19. COONEY MK: Relative efficiency of cell cultures for detection of viruses. Health Lab Sci 10:294–302, 1973
20. COOPER PD, MELNICK JL ET AL: Picornaviridae: second report. Intervirology 10:165–180, 1978
21. CROWTHER D and MELNICK JL: The incorporation of neutral red and acridine orange into developing poliovirus particles making them photosensitive. Virology 14:11–21, 1961
22. CROWTHER D and MELNICK JL: Studies of the inhibitory action of guanidine on poliovirus multiplication in cell cultures. Virology 15:65–74, 1961
23. DAHLING DR, BERG G, and BERMAN D: BGM, a continuous cell line more sensitive than primary rhesus and African green kidney cells for the recovery of viruses from water. Health Lab Sci 11:275–282, 1974
24. DALLDORF G: Neuropathogenicity of group A coxsackie viruses. J Exp Med 106:69–76, 1957
25. DALLDORF G: The enteroviruses and paralytic disease. In Virus Infections of Infancy and Childhood. Symposium of the Section on Microbiology, The New York Academy of Medicine, Hoeber-Harper, 1960, pp 125–144
26. DALLDORF G and SICKLES GM: An unidentified, filtrable agent isolated from the feces of children with paralysis. Science 108:61–62, 1948
27. DALLDORF G and SICKLES GM, The coxsackie viruses, In Diagnostic Procedures for Virus and Rickettsial Diseases, 2nd edition, American Public Health Association, New York, 1956, pp 153–168
28. DUNNEBACKE TH and ZITCER EM: Preparation and cultivation of primary human amnion cells. Cancer Res 17:1043–1046, 1957
29. FARRAH SR, GOYAL SM, GERBA CP, WALLIS C, and MELNICK JL: Concentration of enteroviruses from estuarine water. Appl Environ Microbiol 33:1192–1196, 1977
30. FAULK WP, VYAS GN, PHILLIPS CA, FUDENBERG HH, and CHISM K: A passive hemagglutination test for antirhinovirus antibodies. Nature New Biol 231:101–104, 1971
31. GAMBLE DR and KINSLEY ML: The routine typing of coxsackie viruses by complement fixation. Mon Bull Min of Health Public Health Lab Serv 22:6–14, 1963
32. GEAR JHS: Coxsackie virus infections of the newborn. Prog Med Virol 1:106–121, 1958

33. GNESH GM, PLAGER H, and DECHER W: Enterovirus typing by complement fixation. Proc Soc Exp Biol Med 115:898–900, 1964
34. GOLDFIELD MS, SRIHONGSE S, and FOX JP: Hemagglutinins associated with certain human enteric viruses. Proc Soc Exp Biol Med 96:788–791, 1957
35. GYORKEY F, CABRAL GA, GYORKEY PK, URIBE-BOTERO G, DREESMAN GR, and MELNICK JL: Coxsackievirus aggregates in muscle cells of a polymyositis patient. Intervirology 10:69–77, 1978
36. HAGIWARA A, TAGAYA I, and YONEYAMA T: Epidemic of hand, foot and mouth disease associated with enterovirus 71 infection. Intervirology 9:60–63, 1978
37. HALONEN P and HUEBNER RJ: ECHO and poliomyelitis virus antisera prepared in guinea pigs with fluorocarbon-treated cell culture antigens. Proc Soc Exp Biol Med 105:46–49, 1960
38. HALONEN P, ROSEN L, and HUEBNER RJ: Homologous and heterologous complement fixing antibody in persons infected with ECHO, coxsackie, and poliomyelitis viruses. Proc Soc Exp Biol Med 101:236–241, 1959
39. HAMMON WMcD, LUDWIG EH, SATHER G, and YOHN DS: Comparative studies on patterns of family infections with polioviruses and ECHO virus type 1 on an American military base in the Philippines. Am J Public Health 47:802–811, 1957
40. HAMMON WMcD, YOHN DS, LUDWIG EH, PAVIA RA, SATHER GE, and McCLOSKEY LW: A study of certain nonpoliomyelitis and poliomyelitis enterovirus infections: clinical and serologic associations. J Am Med Assoc 167:727–735, 1958
41. HAMPIL B and MELNICK JL: WHO collaborative studies on enterovirus reference antisera: second report. Bull WHO 38:577–593, 1968
42. HAMPIL B, MELNICK JL, WALLIS C, BROWN RW, BRAYE, ET, and ADAMS RR JR: Preparation of antiserum to enteroviruses in large animals. J Immunol 95:895–908, 1965
43. HARA M, KOMATSU T, SASAKI M, and TAGAYA I: On the lack of serological relationship of echovirus types 1 and 12. Proc Soc Exp Biol Med 128:683–687, 1968
44. HARPER GJ: Airborne micro-organisms: survival tests with four viruses. J Hyg 59:479–486, 1961
45. HATCH MH, KALTER SS, and AJELLO GW: Identification of poliovirus isolates with fluorescent antibody. Proc Soc Exp Biol Med 107:1–4, 1961
46. HATCH MH and MARCHETTI GE: Isolation of echoviruses with human embryonic lung fibroblast cells. Appl Microbiol 22:736–737, 1971
47. HAWLEY HB, MORIN DP, GERAGHTY MB, TOMKOW J, and PHILLIPS CA: Coxsackievirus B epidemic at a boy's summer camp: isolation of virus from swimming water. J Am Med Assoc 226:33–36, 1973
48. HENDERSON M, WALLIS C, and MELNICK JL: Concentration and purification of enteroviruses by membrane chromatography. Appl Environ Microbiol 32:689–693, 1976
49. HONIG EI, MELNICK JL, ISACSON P, PARR R, MYERS IL, and WALTON M: An endemiological study of enteric virus infections. Poliomyelitis, coxsackie, and orphan (ECHO) viruses isolated from normal children in two socio-economic groups, J Exp Med 103:247–262, 1956
50. HOWE HA: Detection of poliovirus in feces of chimpanzees during late convalescence by means of Freon 113. Proc Soc Exp Biol Med 110:110–113, 1962
51. HOWES DW: Intravital staining in titrations of group B coxsackie viruses in weaned mice. Nature 173:270–271, 1954
52. HSIUNG GD: Further studies on characterization and grouping of ECHO viruses. Ann NY Acad Sci 101:413–422, 1962
53. HSIUNG GD and MELNICK JL: Comparative susceptibility of kidney cells from different monkey species to enteric viruses (poliomyelitis, coxsackie, and ECHO groups). J Immunol 78:137–146, 1957
54. HSIUNG GD and MELNICK JL: Morphologic characteristics of plaques produced on monkey kidney monolayer cultures by enteric viruses (poliomyelitis, coxsackie and ECHO groups). J Immunol 78:128–136, 1957
55. HSIUNG GD and MELNICK JL: Orphan viruses of man and animals. Ann NY Acad Sci 70:342–360, 1958
56. INTERNATIONAL ENTEROVIRUS STUDY GROUP: Picornavirus group. Virology 19:114–116, 1963

57. ITOH H and MELNICK JL: The infection of chimpanzees with ECHO viruses. J Exp Med 106:677–688, 1957
58. JAMISON RM and MAYOR HD: Comparative study of seven picornaviruses of man. J Bacteriol 91:1971–1976, 1966
59. JAMISON RM, MAYOR HD, and MELNICK JL: Studies on ECHO 4 virus (picornavirus group) and its intracellular development. Exp Molec Pathol 2:188–202, 1963
60. JENSEN MM: Inactivation of airborne viruses by ultraviolet radiation. Appl Microbiol 12:418–420, 1964
61. JOHNSON KM and LANG DJ: Separation of hemagglutinating and non-hemagglutinating variants of coxsackie A-21 virus. Proc Soc Exp Biol Med 110:653–657, 1962
62. JOHNSSON T, BÖTTIGER M, and LÖFDAHL A: An outbreak of aseptic meningitis with a rubella-like rash probably caused by ECHO virus type 4. Arch Gesamte Virusforsch 8:306–317, 1958
63. KAMITSUKA PS, LOU TY, FABIYI A,and WENNER HA:Preparation and standardization of coxsackievirus reference antisera. I. For twenty-four group A viruses. Am J Epidemiol 81:283–306, 1965
64. KAMITSUKA PS, SOERGEL ME, and WENNER HA: Production and standardization of ECHO reference antisera. I. For 25 prototypic ECHO viruses. Am J Hyg 74:7–25, 1961
65. KIBRICK S and BENIRSCHKE K: Severe generalized disease (encephalohepatomyocarditis) occurring in the newborn period and due to infection with coxsackie virus, group B: evidence of intrauterine infection with this agent. Pediatrics 22:857–875, 1958
66. KRAFT LM and MELNICK JL: Complement fixation tests with homologous and heterologous types of coxsackie virus in man. J Immunol 68:297–310, 1952
67. KRAFT LM and MELNICK JL: Quantitative studies of the virus-host relationship in chimpanzees after inapparent infection with coxsackie viruses. II. The development of complement-fixing antibodies. J Exp Med 97:401–414, 1953
68. LAHELLE O: Capacity of certain Echo virus 6 strains to cause hemagglutination. Virology 5:110–119, 1958
69. LAMB GA, PLEXICO K, GLEZEN WP, and CHIN TDY: Use of micro technique for serum neutralization and virus identification. Public Health Rep 80:463–466, 1965
70. LANDSTEINER K and POPPER E: Übertragung der Poliomyelitis acuta auf Affen. Z Immunitätsforsch 2:377–390, 1909
71. LEHMANN-GRUBE F and SYVERTON JT: Pathogenicity for suckling mice of coxsackie viruses adapted to human amnion cells. J Exp Med 113:811–829, 1961
72. LENAHAN MF and WENNER HA: Propagation of entero- and other viruses in renal cells obtained from non-primate hosts. J Infect Dis 107:203–212, 1960
73. LENNETTE EH and SCHMIDT NJ: Studies on the development and persistence of complement-fixing and neutralizing antibodies in human poliomyelitis. Am J Hyg 65:210–238, 1957
74. LENNETTE EH, SCHMIDT NJ, and MAGOFFIN RL: Observations on the complement-fixing antibody response to poliovirus in patients with certain coxsackie and ECHO virus infections. J Immunol 86:552–560, 1961
75. LENNETTE EH, SHINOMOTO TT, SCHMIDT NJ, and MAGOFFIN RL: Observations on the neutralizing antibody response to group B coxsackie viruses in patients with central nervous system disease. J Immunol 86:257–266, 1961
76. LEPOW ML, COYNE N, THOMPSON LB, CARVER DH, and ROBBINS FC: A clinical, epidemiologic, and laboratory investigation of aseptic meningitis during the four-year period, 1955–1958. II. The clinical disease and its sequelae. N Engl J Med 266:1188–1193, 1962
77. LIM KA and BENYESH-MELNICK M: Typing of viruses by combinations of antiserum pools. Application to typing of enteroviruses (coxsackie and ECHO). J Immunol 84:309–317, 1960
78. MANDEL B: Reversibility of the reaction between poliovirus and neutralizing antibody of rabbit origin. Virology 14:316–328, 1961
79. MARKOWA J and MAREK A: Experimental bone tumors caused by common viruses. Nature 213:831–833, 1967
80. MAYOR HD: Picornavirus symmetry. Virology 22:156–160, 1964

81. MELNICK JL: The ultracentrifuge as an aid in the detection of poliomyelitis virus. J Exp Med 77:195-204, 1943

82. MELNICK JL: Application of tissue culture methods to epidemiological studies of poliomyelitis. Am J Public Health 44:571-580, 1954

83. MELNICK JL: Antigenic crossings within poliovirus types. Proc Soc Exp Biol Med 89:131-133, 1955

84. MELNICK JL: Tissue culture methods for the cultivation of poliomyelitis and other viruses In Diagnostic Procedures for Virus and Rickettsial Diseases, 2nd edition, American Public Health Association, New York, 1956, pp 97-151

85. MELNICK JL: ECHO viruses In Cellular Biology, Nucleic Acids, and Viruses. Spec Publ NY Acad Sci 5:365-381, 1957

86. MELNICK JL: Water as a reservoir of virus in nature and means for control In Viruses and Environment: Proceedings of the Third International Conference on Comparative Virology, 1978, in press.

87. MELNICK JL ET AL.: Picornaviridae. Intervirology 4:303-316, 1974

88. MELNICK JL and Ågren K: Poliomyelitis and coxsackie viruses isolated from normal infants in Egypt. Proc Soc Exp Biol Med 81:621-624, 1952

89. MELNICK JL, CROWTHER D, and BARRERA-ORO J: Rapid development of drug-resistant mutants of poliovirus. Science 134:557, 1961

90. MELNICK JL, and HAMPIL B: WHO collaborative studies on enterovirus reference antisera. Bull WHO 33:761-772, 1965

91. MELNICK JL and KAPLAN AS: Quantitative studies of the virus-host relationship in chimpanzees after inapparent infection with coxsackie viruses. I. The virus carrier state and the development of neutralizing antibodies. J Exp Med 97:367-400, 1953

92. MELNICK JL, KAPLAN AS, ZABIN E, CONTRERAS G, and LARKUM NW: An epidemic of paralytic poliomyelitis characterized by dual infections with poliomyelitis and coxsackie viruses. J Exp Med 94:471-492, 1951

93. MELNICK JL and LEDINKO N: Immunological reactions of the coxsackie viruses. I. The neutralization test: technic and application. J Exp Med 92:463-482, 1950

94. MELNICK JL, PROCTOR RO, OCAMPO AR, DIWAN AR, and BEN-PORATH E: Free and bound virus in serum after administration of oral poliovirus vaccine. Am J Epidemiol 84:329-342, 1966

95. MELNICK JL, SCHMIDT NJ, HAMPIL B, and HO HH: Lyophilized combination pools of enterovirus equine antisera: preparation and test procedures for the identification of field strains of 19 group A coxsackievirus serotypes. Intervirology 8:172-181, 1977

96. MELNICK JL, SHAW EW, and CURNEN EC: A virus from patients diagnosed as non-paralytic poliomyelitis or aseptic meningitis. Proc Soc Exp Biol Med 71:344-349, 1949

97. MELNICK JL, TAGAYA I, and VON MAGNUS H: Enteroviruses 69, 70, and 71. Intervirology 4:369-370, 1974

98. MELNICK JL, WENNER HA, and ROSEN L: The enteroviruses In Diagnostic Procedures for Viral and Rickettsial Diseases, 3rd edition, Lennette EH and Schmidt NJ (eds), American Public Health Association, Inc. New York, 1964, pp 194-242

99. MIDULLA M, WALLIS C, and MELNICK JL: Enterovirus immunizing antigens in the form of cation-stabilized and concentrated virus preparations. J Immunol 95:9-12, 1965

100. MILLER CA and WENNER HA: Antibody responses to naturally occurring poliomyelitis infections in children. I. Neutralizing antibodies against the prototype and patient's own viruses. Pediatrics 14:573-586, 1954

101. MOGABGAB WJ: 2060 virus (ECHO 28) in KB cell cultures. Characteristics, complement-fixation and antigenic relationships to some other respiroviruses. Am J Hyg 76:15-26, 1962

102. NATIONAL FOUNDATION FOR INFANTILE PARALYSIS, INC, COMMITTEE ON ECHO VIRUSES; and MICROBIOLOGICAL ASSOCIATES, INC, Bethesda, Maryland: Statement Concerning the Use of ECHO and Coxsackie Virus Antisera, 1957

103. NEVA FA and MALONE MF: Persistence of antibodies to ECHO-16 viruses following Boston exanthem disease. Proc Soc Exp Biol Med 102:233-235, 1959

104. NEVA FA and MALONE MF: Specific and cross reactions by complement fixation with Boston exanthem disease virus (ECHO-16). J Immunol 83:645-652, 1959

105. Nuñez-Montiel O, Weibel J, and Vitelli-Flores J: Electron microscopic study of the cytopathology of ECHO virus infection in cultivated cells. J Biophys Biochem Cytol 11:457-467, 1961
106. Panel for Picornaviruses: Classification of nine new types. Science 141:153-154, 1963
107. Parks WP, Queiroga LT, and Melnick JL: Studies of infantile diarrhea in Karachi, Pakistan. II. Multiple virus isolations from rectal swabs. Am J Epidemiol 85:469-478, 1967
108. Paul JR and Melnick JL: Poliomyelitis In Diagnostic Procedures for Virus and Rickettsial Diseases, 2nd edition, American Public Health Association, New York, 1956, pp 53-90
109. Peizer LR, Mandel B, and Weissman D: An improved method for rapid laboratory diagnosis of poliomyelitis. Proc Soc Exp Biol Med 106:772-776, 1961
110. Ramos-Alvarez M and Sabin AB: Characteristics of poliomyelitis and other enteric viruses recovered in tissue culture from healthy American children. Proc Soc Exp Biol Med 87:655-661, 1954
111. Reissig M, Howes DW, and Melnick JL: Sequence of morphological changes in epithelial cell cultures infected with poliovirus. J Exp Med 104:289-304, 1956
112. Rhim JS, Jordan LE, and Mayor HD: Cytochemical, fluorescent-antibody and electron microscopic studies on the growth of reovirus (ECHO 10) in tissue culture. Virology 17:342-355, 1962
113. Rifkind RA, Godman GC, Howe C, Morgan C, and Rose HM: ECHO 9 virus in tissue culture observed by light and electron microscopy. Virology 12:331-334, 1960
114. Riggs JL and Brown GC: Application of direct and indirect immunofluorescence for identification of enteroviruses and titrating their antibodies. Proc Soc Exp Biol Med 110:833-837, 1962
115. Rightsel WA, Dice JR, McAlpine RJ, Timm EA, McLean IW Jr, Dixon GJ, and Schabel FM: The antiviral effect of guanidine. Science 134:558-559, 1961
116. Robbins FC, Enders JF, Weller TH, and Florentino GL: Studies on the cultivation of poliomyelitis viruses in tissue culture. V. The direct isolation and serologic identification of virus strains in tissue culture from patients with nonparalytic and paralytic poliomyelitis. Am J Hyg 54:286-293, 1951
117. Rosen L and Kern JK: Hemagglutination and hemagglutination-inhibition with coxsackie B viruses. Proc Soc Exp Biol Med 107:626-628, 1961
118. Sabin AB: Transitory appearance of type 2 neutralizing antibody in patients infected with type 1 poliomyelitis virus. J Exp Med 96:99-106, 1952
119. Salk JE, Lewis LJ, Youngner JS, and Bennett BL: The use of adjuvants to facilitate studies on the immunological classification of poliomyelitis viruses. Am J Hyg 54:157-173, 1951
120. Schaffer FL: Binding of proflavine by and photoinactivation of poliovirus propagated in the presence of the dye. Virology 18:412-425, 1962
121. Schmidt NJ: Tissue culture in the laboratory diagnosis of viral infections. Am J Clin Pathol 57:820-828, 1972
122. Schmidt NJ, Dennis J, Hagens SJ, and Lennette EH: Studies on the antibody responses of patients infected with ECHO viruses. Am J Hyg 75:168-182, 1962
123. Schmidt NJ, Guenther RW, and Lennette EH: Typing of ECHO virus isolates by immune serum pools. The "Intersecting Serum Scheme." J Immunol 87:623-626, 1961
124. Schmidt NJ, Ho HH, and Lennette EH: Comparative sensitivity of human fetal diploid kidney cell strains and monkey kidney cell cultures for isolation of certain human viruses. Am J Clin Pathol 43:297-301, 1965
125. Schmidt NJ, Ho HH, and Lennette EH: Propagation and isolation of group A coxsackieviruses in RD cells. J Clin Microbiol 2:183-185, 1975
126. Schmidt NJ, Ho HH, and Lennette EH: Comparative sensitivity of the BGM cell line for isolation of enteric viruses. Health Lab Sci 13:115-117, 1976
127. Schmidt NJ and Lennette EH: Modification of the homotypic specificity of poliomyelitis complement-fixing antigens by heat. J Exp Med 104:99-120, 1956

128. SCHMIDT NJ and LENNETTE EH: A microflocculation test for poliomyelitis with observations on the flocculating antibody response in human poliomyelitis. Am J Hyg 70:51-65, 1959

129. SCHMIDT NJ, LENNETTE EH, and DENNIS J: Gel double diffusion studies with group B and group A, type 9, coxsackieviruses. III. Antigen-antibody absorption tests. J Immunol 94:482-491, 1965

130. SCHMIDT NJ, LENNETTE, EH, and DENNIS J: Hemagglutination-inhibiting antibody responses in human infections with group B coxsackieviruses. J Immunol 96:311-318, 1966

131. SCHMIDT NJ, LENNETTE EH, and HANAHOE EH: A micro method for performing parainfluenza virus neutralization tests. Proc Soc Exp Biol Med 122:1062-1067, 1966

132. SHAVER DN, BARRON AL, and KARZON DT: Distinctive cytopathology of ECHO viruses types 22 and 23. Proc Soc Exp Biol Med 106:648-652, 1961

133. SHAW ED, NEWTON A, POWELL AW, and FRIDAY CJ: Fluorescent antigen-antibody reactions in coxsackie and ECHO enteroviruses. Virology 15:208-210, 1961

134. SHAW M; Cultivation of coxsackie virus in embryonated eggs and in chick tissue cultures. Proc Soc Exp Biol Med 79:718-720, 1952

135. SMITH W: Direct virus antibody flocculation reactions. Prog Med Virol 1:280-304, 1958

136. SOMMERVILLE RG: Rapid diagnosis of viral infections by immunofluorescent staining of viral antigens in leucocytes and macrophages. Prog Med Virol 10:398-414, 1968

137. STEIGMAN AJ: Viruses in search of disease. Discussion: Part I. Ann NY Acad Sci 67:249-250, 1957

138. STEIGMAN AJ: Poliomyelitic properties of certain non-polio viruses: enteroviruses and Heine-Medin disease. J Mt Sinai Hosp 25:391-404, 1958

139. STEIGMAN AJ and LIPTON MM: Fatal bulbospinal paralytic poliomyelitis due to ECHO 11 virus. J Am Med Assoc 174:178-179, 1960

140. STUART DC JR and FOGH J: Electron microscopic demonstration of intracellular poliovirus crystals. Exp Cell Res 18:378-381, 1959

141. SULKIN SE, SCHWAB M, and WALLIS HC: Isolation of coxsackie viruses. Litter differences among suckling mice. Proc Soc Exp Biol Med 77:354-356, 1951

142. SULLIVAN EJ and ROSENBAUM MJ: Methods for preparing tissue culture in disposable microplates and their use in virology. Am J Epidemiol 85:424-437, 1967

143. TABER LH, MIRKOVIC RR, ADAM V, ELLIS SS, YOW MD, and MELNICK JL: Rapid diagnosis of enterovirus meningitis by immunofluorescent staining of CSF leukocytes. Intervirology 1:127-134, 1973

144. TAMM I and EGGERS HJ; Differences in the selective virus-inhibitory action of 2-(α-hydroxybenzyl)-benzimidazole and guanidine-HC1. Virology 18:439-447, 1962

145. TRASK JD, MELNICK JL, and WENNER HA: Chlorination of human, monkey-adapted and mouse strains of poliomyelitis virus. Am J Hyg 41:30-40, 1945

146. TYRRELL DAJ and CHANOCK RM: Rhinoviruses. A description. Science 141:152-153, 1963

147. VOROSHILOVA MK and CHUMAKOV MP: Poliomyelitis-like properties of AB-IV coxsackie A7 group of viruses. Prog Med Virol 2:106-170, 1959

148. WALLIS C, HOMMA A, and MELNICK JL: A portable virus concentrator for testing water in the field. Water Res 6:1249-1256, 1972

149. WALLIS C, LEWIS RT, and MELNICK JL: Preparation of kidney cell cultures. Texas Rep Biol Med 19:194-197, 1961

150. WALLIS C and MELNICK JL: A rapid method for production of replicate monkey kidney tissue cultures in unstoppered tubes. Texas Rep Biol Med 18:670-673, 1960

151. WALLIS C and MELNICK JL: Stabilization of poliovirus by cations. Texas Rep Biol Med 19:683-700, 1961

152. WALLIS C and MELNICK JL: Cationic stabilization—a new property of enteroviruses. Virology 16:504-505, 1962

153. WALLIS C and MELNICK JL: Effect of organic and inorganic acids on poliovirus at 50°C. Proc Soc Exp Biol Med. 111:305-308, 1962

154. WALLIS C and MELNICK JL: Magnesium chloride enhancement of cell susceptibility to poliovirus. Virology 16:122-132, 1962

155. WALLIS C and MELNICK JL: Suppression of adventitious agents in monkey kidney cultures. Texas Rep Biol Med 20:465–475, 1962
156. WALLIS C and MELNICK JL: A disposable, constricted tissue culture tube. Proc Soc Exp Biol Med 112:344–346, 1963
157. WALLIS C and MELNICK JL: Thermosensitivity of poliovirus. J Bacteriol 86:499–504, 1963
158. WALLIS C and MELNICK JL: Virus aggregation as the cause of the non-neutralizable persistent fraction. J Virol 1:478–488, 1967
159. WALLIS C and MELNICK JL: Mechanism of enhancement of virus plaques by cationic polymers. J Virol 2:267–274, 1968
160. WALLIS C, MELNICK JL, and BIANCHI M: Factors influencing enterovirus and reovirus growth and plaque formation. Texas Rep Biol Med 20:693–702, 1962
161. WALLIS C, PARKS W, SAKURADA N, and MELNICK JL: A rapid plaque method using vertical tube cultures for titration of viruses and neutralizing antibodies. Bull WHO 33:795–801, 1965
162. WALLIS C, STAGG CH, FARRAH SR, and MELNICK JL: Problems related to the concentration of viruses from large volumes of wastewater In Virus Aspects of Applying Municipal Wastes to Land, University of Florida Press, Gainesville, 1976 pp 37–44
163. WEIGAND H: Interference between coxsackie viruses in mice. Proc Soc Exp Biol Med 101:103–106, 1959
164. WENNER HA: The ECHO viruses. Ann NY Acad Sci 101:398–412, 1962
165. WENNER HA: Problems in working with enteroviruses. Ann NY Acad Sci 101:343–356, 1962
166. WENNER HA, BEHBEHANI AM, and KAMITSUKA PS: Preparation and standardization of coxsackievirus reference antisera. II. For six group B viruses. Am J Epidemiol 82:27–39, 1965
167. WENNER HA and LENAHAN MF: Propagation of group A coxsackie viruses in tissue cultures. II. Some interactions between virus and mammalian cells. Yale J Biol Med 34:421–438, 1961/2
168. WILLIAMSON JD and GRIST NR: Studies on the hemagglutinin present in coxsackie A7 virus-infected suckling mouse tissue. J Gen Microbiol 41:283–291, 1965
169. WORLD HEALTH ORGANIZATION: The Work of WHO Virus Reference Centres and the Services They Provide. WHO, Geneva, 1968, pp 49–52
170. YOHN DS and HAMMON WMcD: ECHO-4 viruses: improved methods and strain selection for identification and serodiagnosis. Proc Soc Exp Biol Med 105:55–60, 1960
171. ZDRAŽILEK J: Sensitivity of human diploid embryonic lung cells for isolation of echoviruses from sewage. J Hyg Epid Microbiol Immunol 18:2–8, 1974

CHAPTER 16

RHINOVIRUSES

Vincent V. Hamparian

Introduction

The rhinoviruses constitute the largest subgroup of the *Picornaviridae* family. Although they share some properties with the enterovirus subgroup, they can be easily differentiated by their lability at low pH. In addition, the rhinoviruses are recognized as the single most important cause of mild upper respiratory illnesses in adults and, in contrast to enteroviruses, they are not found in the gut of infected individuals.

The rhinoviruses are a relatively recent addition to our collection of defined human viruses. The first definitive isolation of a rhinovirus from patients with common colds was accomplished in the middle 1950s, and between 1960 and 1962 six additional serotypes were isolated. These early isolates were recovered in either primary rhesus monkey kidney (MK) or human embryonic kidney (HEK) cultures. The environmental conditions needed for growth and production of cytopathic effects (CPE) were different from those of most other viruses. Cell cultures were maintained on a medium with a lower pH than usual and were incubated at 33 C instead of 37 C. In addition, incubation of tube cultures on a slowly turning roller drum appeared to be helpful for development of CPE. Generally, the infectivity titers obtained with these methods were relatively low (compared with those for most enteroviruses) and variability in the sensitivity of different batches of primary cells added to the difficulties of working with these viruses. Under these circumstances, the accumulation of new knowledge was relatively slow, and the recruitment of new investigators into the rhinovirus field was delayed.

The development of human diploid cell strains (HDCS) was an important advance in our ability to work with rhinoviruses. Such cells generally have proven to be sensitive and reproducible host-cell systems for the routine isolation and propagation of rhinoviruses and have provided much of the impetus for the rapid increase in our knowledge of these agents. The adaptation of rhinoviruses to growth in stable cell lines provided a second excellent host-cell system, one in which rhinoviruses could be easily and reproducibly plaqued and in which they could be propagated to high titers. With the avail-

535

ability of better host-cell systems and the belief that rhinoviruses were new and important pathogens of humans, our knowledge of rhinoviruses increased rapidly.

Since the purpose of this chapter is to present a compendium of diagnostic information, the reader is referred to other publications for a detailed consideration of the history of rhinoviruses (1, 3, 61, 66, 76, 101, 192, 205, 213).

Clinical aspects

Rhinoviruses are recognized as the single most important cause of mild upper respiratory illness (common colds) in adults and may well be responsible for the majority of all acute respiratory infections in humans (54, 76, 81, 86, 93, 144, 149, 164, 175). Although there is no question that rhinoviruses primarily cause upper respiratory illnesses in children and adults, their importance in the etiology of lower respiratory illnesses, particularly in children, remains unsettled (29, 45, 54, 58, 76, 93, 101, 149, 188, 189, 220). Recently, evidence has been accumulating on the importance of rhinoviruses in acute exacerbations of chronic bronchitis (48, 134, 138-141, 187, 189). For a comprehensive review of clinical aspects, the reader is referred to the recent publications by Dick and Chesney (33) and Gwaltney (61).

Evidence for the physical mechanisms by which rhinoviruses are transmitted from person to person comes from volunteer studies. Rhinovirus type 2 produced illness in volunteers when administered in nasal drops or by nasal and conjunctival swabs, whereas throat swabs were ineffective (11). Airborne transmission of rhinoviruses by droplets also occurred but required about a 20-fold greater amount of virus than did intranasal inoculation (28). In addition, oral contact between infected and susceptible volunteers and putting virus into the mouth were inefficient means of spreading infection (61). Quantitation of rhinovirus in the respiratory secretions of individuals with natural infections indicated that the amount of virus in pharyngeal secretions was 10- to 100-fold less than in nasal mucus (82). Virus was not always present in saliva and usually could not be recovered from coughs and sneezes; however, self-inoculation of the nose and eye with contaminated fingers transmitted infection. The concept of self-inoculation with infected hands was supported by the finding of rhinovirus on the fingers of 16 of 38 infected volunteers and on 6 of 40 objects they had handled (170). Transmission to susceptible volunteers and recovery of virus from hands were directly related to the presence of peak titers of virus in nasal secretions (30). In a recent volunteer study (68), it was found that transmission of infection by the hand route was significantly more efficient than exposure to either large- or small-particle aerosols. Because of these findings, it has been suggested that relatively simple control measures such as frequent hand washing might be successful in reducing person-to-person transmission of rhinoviruses (30, 68).

The uncomplicated, natural illness is characterized most commonly by rhinorrhea, nasal obstruction, mild pharyngitis, and cough. Fever and systemic complaints are infrequent. Symptomatology peaks on the second and third days of illness and usually lasts for about 7 days (64). Studies in volunteers indicate that the onset of illness is usually between 2 and 4 days after infection and closely correlates with the time of peak virus shedding. Excretion of small amounts of virus may continue for as long as 3 weeks after onset (40). Studies involving intensive surveillance of families for rhinovirus infections have shown that rhinoviruses can be recovered from 14% of specimens obtained 3-4 days before onset and from about 30% of specimens obtained 2 days before onset (109).

Certain aspects of the epidemiology of rhinovirus infections are unusual. Longitudinal studies indicate that a multiplicity of serotypes may be present and causing disease in a limited geographic locale. Most serotypes appear and disappear randomly, while a few serotypes may remain endemic. However, outbreaks of disease may also occur where only 10-15 serotypes account for over 50% of the illnesses. Long-term studies indicate that viruses isolated in earlier studies are slowly being replaced by "newer" serotypes. These findings could indicate either that the number of serotypes existing in nature is extremely high or that some form of antigenic variation is occurring. Since the details of the epidemiology of rhinovirus infections are beyond the scope of this chapter, the interested reader is directed to the epidemiologic studies by Fox et al (54), Monto and Cavallaro (150), and Gwaltney et al (65), to the editorial by Fox (53), and to the excellent reviews by Hamre (76), Gwaltney (61), and Dick and Chesney (33), which contain comprehensive sections on epidemiology.

Pathology

Knowledge of the specific pathology produced during rhinovirus infection is limited. Nasal biopsies obtained from infected volunteers and examined histologically did not show changes that could be associated consistently with either infection or illness (41). Studies involving infection of human nasal polyps in organ culture also have not been helpful. When stained and examined histologically, infected and uninfected polyps could not be distinguished. No changes that could represent viral foci of infection were seen (69).

Description and Nature of Rhinoviruses

Common characteristics

Human rhinoviruses are classified as a genus within the family *Picornaviridae* (154, 197, 218). They share the properties of a single-strand ribonucleic acid (RNA) genome, small size (about 28 nm in diameter), naked icosahedral capsid, buoyant density in CsCl ranging between 1.38 and 1.41 g/cm^3, lability at low pH, ether and chloroform stability, and capsid assembly in the cytoplasm. Base analyses of RNA of human rhinovirus types 2, 4, and 14 indicate a higher content of adenylic acid than is present in other picornaviruses (130, 154). However, more rhinoviruses need to be tested to determine if a high adenylic acid content is a characteristic that can differentiate rhinoviruses from other picornaviruses. Thus, except for the well-established properties of higher density and lability at low pH, characteristics of rhinoviruses closely resemble those of other picornaviruses.

Size and shape

The size of rhinovirus particles has been determined by filtration, thin-section electron microscopy (EM), and observation of negatively stained particles. Most of the early determinations on size were obtained by filtration. Even with differences in materials and methods, the relatively crude filtration methods indicated that rhinoviruses were small, ranging between 17 and 30 nm in diameter (37, 38, 72, 100). Thin-section EM reveals intracellular crystals of virus particles with center-to-center spacing of 25–28 nm and diameters between 17 and 28 nm (5, 50, 72, 107). Reports of size determination by negative staining are more plentiful and give virion diameters of 20–27 nm (14, 59, 102, 113, 126, 128, 131, 165). The hexagonal shape of rhinovirus virions indicates that they possess icosahedral symmetry and are constructed in a manner similar to that of other picornaviruses (178).

Chemical composition

Human rhinovirus virions contain about 30% RNA. The size of the RNA in types 1A and 2 is about 2.5×10^6 daltons, similar to that of other picornaviruses (7, 128, 135, 153, 185). The capsid of rhinovirus 1A appears to contain 60 copies of each of 4 distinct polypeptides, VP1, VP2, VP3, and VP4. These 4 polypeptides are formed by cleavage of a common precursor VP0 (9, 113, 133, 193). No uncleaved precursor (VP0) has been found in highly purified preparations of rhinovirus type 2; this indicates that it has no important role in virion structure (119). The molecular weights of the 4 structural polypeptides of rhinovirus type 1A (VP1-4) have been determined by sodium dodecyl sulfate (SDS)-polyacrylamide gel electrophoresis as 35,000, 30,000, 25,000 and 8000, respectively (9, 135).

Density

Buoyant density of picornaviruses in CsCl is a property that can be used to differentiate subgroups of the *Picornaviridae* (154, 177). The buoyant densities of human and bovine rhinoviruses generally fall between 1.385 and 1.405 g/cm³. These values are higher than those reported for caliciviruses (1.36–1.38 g/cm³) and enteroviruses and cardioviruses (1.34 g/cm³) and lower than those reported for foot-and-mouth disease virus (1.43 g/cm³) and equine rhinovirus (1.44 g/cm³). In contrast to the acid-stable picornaviruses, buoyant-density values for rhinoviruses generally have not been consistent. Values in CsCl have ranged from 1.38 to 1.41 g/cm³, and 2 different densities have been reported for type 14 (192). These discrepancies apparently are due to a variety of factors, including methodology and the physical state of preparations used for buoyant-density determinations. The buoyant-density values for acid-labile picornaviruses are affected by pH, the kind of anion present, and the length of centrifugation time. Thus, the density values for human rhinovirus type 4 increased from 1.40 g/cm^3 at pH 7.1 to 1.42 at pH 9.0 and from 1.36 g/cm^3 in $CsSO_4$ to 1.40 in CsCl (177). Furthermore, a proportion of virus particles in preparations of rhinovirus type 14 have been found sequestered in a fibrous, proteinaceous material. Such preparations yield bands at 2 positions in CsCl gradients with average density values of 1.409 and 1.386 g/cm^3, with the lower-density band containing the sequestered particles. The attachment of virus to the fibrous material can be reversed either by treatment with proteases or by a second isopycnic centrifugation resulting in recovery of most of the infectious virus at a density of about 1.41 g/cm^3 (57). Until more information is available about the buoyant densities of rhinoviruses, comparisons of values may be valid only when 2 viruses are cosedimented (192). With this technique, the density of rhinovirus type 2 is significantly greater than that of type 14 (113).

Sedimentation

The sedimentation coefficients of rhinovirus types 2 and 14 have been determined in sucrose as 150 S (113). This value was obtained by cosedimenting the individual rhinoviruses with poliovirus type 2 and assuming a sedimentation coefficient of 156 S for poliovirus (179). Prior to sedimentation analysis, rhinoviruses prepared in CsCl had to be dialyzed or dialyzed and stored at 4 C for 1 week to preclude anomalous high results apparently caused by CsCl reversibly bound to the virions (136).

Effect of physical and chemical agents

Lipid solvents and detergents. Rhinoviruses and other picornaviruses are not affected by lipid solvents such as ethanol, fluorocarbon, ether, or chloroform. Surface active agents such as sodium deoxycholate, Nonidet P40, and SDS do not appear to affect human rhinoviruses (192). However, SDS does inactivate a bovine rhinovirus (98), has been reported to interfere with plaque formation by human rhinovirus type 2, and appears to stabilize it against inactivation by low pH or heat (122). Since information on the effects of detergents on rhinoviruses is still limited, no generalizations can be made.

Proteases. Trypsin destroys the infectivity of some rhinoviruses (111). Human rhinovirus types 1B, 13, 15, 16, 17, 32, and 33 are inactivated when exposed to 5 mg/ml of trypsin for 1 hr at 37 C. Types 3, 4, 5, 6, and 14 are resistant, and type 2 is "partially" sensitive. Recently, purified type 2 has been found to be resistant to trypsin exposure (192). However, it has been stated that proteolytic enzymes can inactivate rhinovirus receptor sites on host cells (10). Thus, the possibility that residual trypsin in virus-enzyme reaction mixtures or virion-associated trypsin could inhibit viral absorption can not be excluded. Such an occurrence could be interpreted as sensitivity to trypsin.

Heat. Early studies with rhinovirus type 1A indicated that this virus was stable after 2 cycles of freezing (-70 C) and thawing (37 C) or after 1 week at 4 C. Below 39 C, rhinoviruses appear to be less stable than polioviruses; loss of infectivity appears to be due to inactivation of RNA and not to changes in the capsid protein (36).

At 50 C or 56 C rhinoviruses, like polioviruses, are inactivated and converted into empty capsids with C-type serologic reactivity (95, 122, 123, 128). However, human rhinoviruses appear to be less labile than enteroviruses at 50 C (38, 110, 130). Enteroviruses are completely stabilized in the presence of 1 M $MgCl_2$ when exposed to 50 C for 1 hr (Melnick JL, see page 477), whereas some rhinoviruses are partially stabilized and others are not (37, 38). It is likely that some rhinoviruses can be differentiated from enteroviruses on the basis of heat lability in the presence of a bivalent cation such as Mg^{++}. However, since the results with rhinoviruses are variable, this kind of test does not provide a simple, routine procedure for differentiating all rhinoviruses from enteroviruses.

Because of differences in procedures for inactivation, it is often difficult to compare experiments done in different laboratories. In addition, some virus preparations tested have contained animal serum while others have been highly purified. More pertinent to viral diagnosis, no comprehensive, quantitative studies have been done on the stability of rhinoviruses present in clinical specimens.

pH. Rhinoviruses are inactivated below pH 6. This property of rhinoviruses is still the simplest means of differentiating them from enteroviruses. The amount of inactivation and the effect on the integrity and serologic reactivity of the virion is a function of pH, time, and temperature (38, 94, 96, 98, 113, 123, 174). Variability in results of pH inactivation studies in different laboratories probably is due to differences in purity of the preparations tested and the methods employed. At pH 3 inactivation appears to be very rapid, requiring less than 10 sec for human rhinovirus type 14 (96). In addition, exposure to pH 3 appears to cause complete dissolution of rhinovirus virions (96, 174). The products of mild acidification (pH 5) formed from 4 rhinoviruses include A particles that sediment at 135 S and lack VP4, and B particles that lack both VP4 and RNA and sediment at 80 S (113, 156). The production of A and B particles results in significant loss of D-reactive (neutralizing) antigen (123). The type of buffer used also may affect the inactivation of rhinoviruses. For example, bovine rhinovirus strain RS 3x is partially inactivated by neutral McIlvaine buffer (98). Although human rhinoviruses do not appear to be affected by this buffer, this observation emphasizes that screening tests for pH lability should be performed with the same buffer at both low and neutral pH.

Ultraviolet irradiation (UV). The kinetics of UV inactivation of rhinovirus types 17 and 40 were determined in one study and compared with those for inactivation of poliovirus type 2 (Hughes JH, Mitchell M, and Hamparian VV, unpublished data). Prior to testing the viruses were partially purified by fluorocarbon extraction. Inactivation curves were plotted with use of the best-fit line as determined by the least-squares method. The inactivation rates of the 3 viruses were similar. Half-life times for rhinovirus types 17 and 40 were approximately 3 and 5 sec, respectively. For poliovirus type 2 the half-life was approximately 4.5 sec. After 90 sec of exposure, no infectious virus could be detected in any of the preparations. Even after 13 min of UV inactivation, all virus preparations were still capable of eliciting neutralizing-antibody responses in guinea pigs.

Other agents. After exposure to 2 M urea for 1 hr at 22 C, rhinovirus type 2 is partially degraded (123). B particles free from RNA and soluble RNA are produced. The effect of urea on enteroviruses may be similar since treatment of poliovirus with 4 M urea produces empty capsids, probably analagous to the B particles produced by rhinoviruses (27).

There are some data indicating that hydrogen peroxide can inactivate rhinoviruses (137). Approximately 100 mean tissue culture infectious doses ($TCID_{50}$) of human rhinovirus types 1A, 1B, and 7 were exposed to H_2O_2 at concentrations of 3%, 1.5%, 0.75%, and 0.375% for various periods of time. The time required for inactivation of all 3 serotypes by 3% H_2O_2 was 6–8 minutes. This time increased with decreasing concentrations of H_2O_2, and approximately 60 min was required for inactivation with 0.75% H_2O_2.

A wide variety of substances with diverse chemical structures are known to inhibit rhinovirus replication *in vitro*. These include guanidine, substituted guanidines, 2-(α-hydroxybenzyl) benzimidazole (HBB), substituted HBB compounds, triazinoindoles, isoquinolines, zinc, ascorbic acid, interferon, and a variety of interferon inducers. Thus far, no antiviral substances that might be useful in the laboratory diagnosis of rhinovirus infections have been described.

For recent information on antiviral substances with activity against rhinoviruses, the reader can consult some other publications (10, 33, 61). For a comprehensive review of rhinovirus structure and replication, the reader is referred to the excellent review by Butterworth et al (10).

Antigenic composition

Number of immunotypes

A collaborative program involving many laboratories and sponsored by the National Institutes of Allergy and Infectious Diseases and the World Health Organization has led to a numbering system for 89 rhinoviruses and 1 subtype. The details of the development of the numbering system and the basis for regarding a virus as a distinct prototype have been reported (16, 17, 101, 103, 104). Table 16.1 presents the numbering system according to prototype strain and the original descriptive reference. This numbering system is the result of phases 1 and 2 of the collaborative program. A third phase has now been completed, and 22 additional rhinoviruses that are serologically distinct from types 1A–89 have been identified (71). If all of these viruses eventually are designated as new serotypes, the numbering system would be extended to 111.

One of the major questions still unresolved concerns the total number of serotypes existing in nature. The accumulating evidence suggests the existence of many rhinoviruses that are untypable with sera for the 89 numbered

TABLE 16.1—Rhinovirus Numbering System

Rhinovirus Number	Prototype Strain	Original Reference
1A	Echo-28	159, 160, 168
1B	B632	202
2	HGP	202
3	FEB	202
4	16/60	202
5	Norman	202
6	Thompson	202
7	68-CV 11	72
8	MRH-CV 12	72
9	211-CV 13	72
10	204-CV 14	72
11	1-CV 15	72
12	181-CV 16	72
13	353	99, 100
14	1059	99, 100
15	1734	99, 100
16	11757	99, 100
17	33342	99, 100
18	5986-CV 17	110
19	6072-CV 18	110
20	15-CV 19	110
21	47-CV 21	110
22	127-CV 22	110
23	5124-CV 24	110
24	5146-CV 25	110
25	5426-CV 26	110
26	5660-CV 27	110
27	5870-CV 28	110
28	6101-CV 29	110
29	5582-CV 30	110
30	106F	21, 78
31	140F	21, 78
32	363	217
33	1200	217
34	137-3	77, 78
35	164A	77, 78
36	342H	77
37	151-1	77, 78
38	CH 79	66, 67
39	209	151
40	1794	151
41	56110	151
42	56822	151
43	58750	151
44	71560	151
45	Baylor 1	162
46	Baylor 2	162
47	Baylor 3	162

TABLE 16.1—Rhinovirus Numbering System (*continued*)

Rhinovirus Number	Prototype Strain	Original Reference
48	1505	106
49	8213	106
50	A2 No. 58	142, 103
51	F01-4081	117, 103
52	F01-3772	117, 103
53	F01-3928	117, 103
54	F01-3774	117, 103
55	WIS 315E	32
56	CH82	66
57	CH47	66
58	21-CV 20	110
59	611-CV 35	73
60	2268-CV 37	73
61	6669-CV 39	73
62	1963M-CV 40	73
63	6360-CV 41	73
64	6258-CV 44	73
65	425-CV 47	73
66	1983 CV 48	73
67	1857-CV 51	73
68	F02-2317-Wood	181
69	F02-2513-Mitchinson	181
70	F02-2547-Treganza	181
71	SF365	65
72	K2207	142, 104
73	107E	77, 78
74	328A	75, 104
75	328F	78
76	H00062	78
77	130-63	189
78	2030-65	188
79	101-1	77, 78
80	277G	75, 104
81	483F2	75, 104
82	03647	75, 104
83	Baylor 7	164
84	432D	78
85	50-525-CV-54	124
86	121564-Johnson	180, 104
87	F02-3607-Corn	180, 104
88	CVD-01-0165-Dambrauskas	180, 104
89	41467-Gallo	180, 104

types and the 22 phase-3 viruses. In a longitudinal epidemiologic study covering the years 1966–1971, a total of 6.2% of 81 rhinovirus isolates from 1966–67 could not be typed with antiserum for types 1–89, 11.8% of 127 isolates from 1968–69 were untypable, and 37.3% of 59 isolates from 1970–71 could not be typed with 112 different rhinovirus sera (Monto AS, personal communication). As part of a fourth and final phase of the collaborative rhinovirus program, 108 viruses untypable with serum for the 89 numbered viruses were tested against the 22 phase-3 sera. Most of these viruses were isolated in the late 1960s and early 1970s. Sixty-eight (63%) of the 108 viruses could not be typed (71). Since antisera for these 68 viruses are not available, the number of different serotypes present among these strains could not be determined. It is theoretically possible that all of these viruses are identical. However, the large number of viruses involved and the fact that they were isolated in 6 different laboratories, most of which are geographically widely separated, argues against this possibility. Judging from past experience, it would not be surprising if 30–50% of these viruses were new serotypes.

The possibility also can not be excluded that rhinoviruses are undergoing continuous and relatively rapid antigenic change and that this process might be contributing to the very large number of serotypes that seem to exist (146). Two different studies have shown that antigenic differences between strains of the same type isolated several years apart were great enough to interfere with their typing (182, 195). In addition, as mentioned above, the indication that many recent isolates tend to be untypable argues against the existence of a finite number of serotypes. Continuous long-term epidemiologic studies and appropriate sera for antigenic analysis are needed to clarify this situation.

Description of various antigens

Complement-fixing (CF) antigen. Attempts to use CF antigens for serologic diagnosis of rhinovirus infection have been unsuccessful. A CF antigen for type 1A prepared in KB cells was used to demonstrate CF antibody increases in paired sera from individuals with respiratory illnesses. However, since antibody increases to various enteroviruses also were observed, the specificity of this antigen was questionable (143). A CF antigen prepared with rhinovirus type 2 was tested against sera from individuals of various ages. CF antibody was present at birth, decreased in frequency and titer during the first decade of life, and then increased rapidly and was retained into old age. There was no correlation between CF and serum neutralizing (Nt) antibodies (15). In tests with sera from very young children, CF antibody rises could be demonstrated in a proportion of paired sera with antigen for the serotype recovered from the clinical specimen. These reactions were specific but could only be demonstrated with serum relatively free of CF antibody for enteroviruses and rhinoviruses (Author, unpublished data). These results suggest that as individuals experience repeated rhinovirus (picornavirus) infections, group-reactive antibody for C-type antigens are produced and may mask specific reactions. Studies on the CF activity of native rhinovirus type 1A antigens prepared in CsCl gradients showed the presence of 2 peaks of activity; one was associated with the virion and had a density of 1.41 g/cm^3, and the other had a lower density (1.30 g/cm^2). Both antigens fixed complement with homotypic antisera. With similar preparations of rhinovirus type 2, it was shown that only the less-dense fraction would fix complement with type 1A antiserum, suggesting the presence of an heterotypic antigen (31). More recently, it has been demonstrated that treatment of type 2 virus at pH 5, at 56 C, or in 2 M urea converts particles with Nt or D determinants to 2 types of subviral particles, both with C antigenicity. Untreated or native antigens generally have yielded type-specific reactions when tested with homotypic animal sera. In CF tests using treated antigens, types 1A and 2 have been shown to share a common C-type antigen (123). Similar C- and D-type antigens have been demonstrated for enteroviruses (55, 184). It is apparent from the above discussion that the CF test is not practical for serologic diagnosis of rhinovirus infections.

Immunodiffusion (ID) antigens. Antigens for use in gel double-diffusion experiments have been prepared for some rhinoviruses. At least 2 antigens reactive in ID tests appear to be present in native rhinovirus preparations. In one investigation a single precipitin line was formed when antigens prepared from 2 plaque mutants of virus type 34 were diffused against homotypic animal sera (20). Highly purified preparations of type 1A, 2, and 14 produced only single lines of precipitation with homotypic sera prepared in rabbits. However, in another study mild acid treatment of type 2 virus yielded an ID antigen able to react with type 1A antiserum (123). Similar reactions were obtained with type 2 virions after heating or treatment with 2 M urea. The results of CF tests were similar to those obtained by ID. In a different study, single precipitin lines also were formed when hyperimmune guinea pig sera were tested with native ID antigens for virus types 2, 14, 34, and 36. The reactions were highly specific. However, 2 precipitin lines were observed when these antigens were diffused against human sera containing homologous Nt antibody (94). To confirm that human serum with Nt antibody would yield 2 ID lines, antigen for virus type 2 was used to examine 21 human sera. Nine sera with Nt titers $\geq$1:8 yielded 2 precipitin lines. Sera with no detectable Nt antibody yielded 1 line. Lines formed in the presence of Nt antibody were highly specific and always appeared closest to the serum well. When a human serum specimen was diffused against echovirus type 4, poliovirus type 2, coxsackievirus type B5, and rhinovirus type 2 antigens, the precipitin lines merged, indicating a pattern of identity (94). These results suggest that rhinoviruses probably share a common group antigen with enteroviruses. The results of ID experiments with rhinoviruses are similar to those reported for other human picornaviruses (184).

It appears that the ID test probably can be used to screen human sera for the presence of Nt antibody for rhinoviruses. The test has not been used in attempts to demonstrate antibody increases in paired sera.

Hemagglutinating (HA) antigen. Among serotypes 1–55, several rhinoviruses have been found to agglutinate sheep erythrocytes. These include types 3–6, 15, 20, 23, 29, 35, 37, 47, and 50–54 (191). Since some serotypes tested were of low titer, no conclusions can be drawn about their ability to cause hemagglutination (HA).

Some of the conditions for HA were studied. It was found that HA titers were highest at pH 8 and 9. High titers were obtained at both 4 C and room temperature. No HA occurred at 37 C, and cells agglutinated at 4 C disaggregated when placed at 37 C. Addition of magnesium, potassium, phosphate, or calcium ions did not affect the reaction. Human group O, chick, goose, horse, and rhesus and African green monkey erythrocytes were not agglutinated by rhinovirus type 5. Guinea pig, hamster, dog, and rabbit cells were agglutinated but were 500-fold less sensitive than were sheep cells. Erythrocyte receptors for rhinovirus type 5 were destroyed by crude filtrate of *Vibrio cholerae* but not by exposure to trypsin.

The property of HA appears to be associated with the infectious particle. The HA antigen is not affected by chloroform but is abolished by treatment at pH 4, heating at 56 C, and exposure to 8 M urea. In CsCl gradients 97% of the HA activity bands with the infectious particle at a density of 1.40 g/cm^3. In sucrose gradients the infectivity and 80% of the HA activity band with a sedimentation coefficient of 150 S.

Specific inhibition of HA was obtained with hyperimmune animal serum, and paired sera from volunteers infected with rhinovirus type 3 or 4 showed increases in titers specific for the infecting virus (191).

The relationship between hemagglutination-inhibiting (HAI) antibody and infection has been studied in paired sera from volunteers infected with rhinovirus types 3 and 4 (171). There was good correlation between HAI and serum neutralization (Nt) tests. High levels of serum HAI antibody were associated with protection, but low serum titers did not always imply susceptibility. HAI activity also was demonstrable in concentrated nasal washings and appeared to be related to protection. Following infection, increases in serum HAI antibody appeared to be specific for the infecting virus. These results indicate that the HAI test may provide an alternative method for detecting specific antibody for certain rhinoviruses. More work is needed to determine how useful the HAI test is for diagnosis of rhinovirus infections. Whether HA is a general property of rhinoviruses or is limited to certain strains remains to be determined.

Pathogenicity for animals

The human rhinoviruses have a very limited animal-host spectrum. Anthropoid apes such as the chimpanzee and gibbon are the only animals known to be susceptible (34). All rhinoviruses tested appear to be highly infectious for the chimpanzee, and virus excretion patterns resemble those seen in humans. Nevertheless, natural infections in chimpanzees are rare, and only one such outbreak has been reported (34). No clinically apparent disease has occurred in either experimentally or naturally infected animals.

There is no evidence for replication of rhinoviruses in a variety of other laboratory animals: no evidence of infection was produced in rhesus monkeys after intracerebral and intraspinal inoculation with virus type 1A (157); in suckling mice inoculated intracerebrally, intraperitoneally (ip) or subcutaneously; in guinea pigs inoculated ip or intramuscularly (im); in adult mice inoculated intranasally or ip; or in rabbits inoculated by the intradermal or intracorneal routes (72, 100, 157). Furthermore, rhinoviruses did not replicate in embryonated chicken eggs when inoculated by the yolk sac, amniotic, or allantoic routes (72).

A number of agents resembling human rhinoviruses in certain properties have been isolated from some naturally infected animals, including horses (39, 167) and cattle (6, 97, 115, 127, 147, 173, 176, 219). However, the so-called equine rhinoviruses have some biological and physicochemical properties that differ significantly from those of human rhinoviruses (154, 155). The degree of relationship between bovine and human rhinoviruses has not been fully established. There appear to be at least 2 bovine rhinovirus serotypes (116). The reported biologic and physicochemical properties of some bovine rhinoviruses closely resemble those of most human rhinoviruses (98, 115, 147, 173, 176). Similar biologic properties include improved CPE and replication at 33 C, improved CPE when cultures are rolled, the need for careful control of medium pH within the range 6.8–7.0, and a limited host-cell range. All of the above biological properties were determined in primary bovine cell culture systems. Common physicochemical properties include RNA genome, size, lability at low pH, resistance to lipid solvents, variable sensitivity to trypsin, and variability to heat inactivation in the presence of $MgCl_2$. Additional information about virion structure and replication of bovine rhinoviruses is needed to fully clarify their relatedness to human rhinoviruses.

Growth in cell cultures

The host-cell and tissue culture spectrum of rhinoviruses is limited to cells derived from humans and monkeys. Rhinoviruses have been propagated in primary HEK and primary MK cultures, HDCS, and human heteroploid cell lines. Occasionally, secondary cultures of MK and HEK have been used. In addition, organ cultures of human embryonic trachea, turbinates, and nasal septum have been used to grow some strains that could not be isolated in conventional cell cultures.

The details of early attempts to grow rhinoviruses, the basis for using certain unusual growth conditions, and the results of numerous host-cell-spectrum studies have been described by Kapikian in the fourth edition of this publication (101). Because of the importance of this information, Kapikian's sections on growth in tissue and organ cultures and on the comparative sensitivity of various cell culture systems for primary isolation have been modified and updated and are presented below.

Rhinovirus type 1A strains 2060 and JH were first isolated in primary rhesus MK cell cultures; stationary cultures were used for 2060, and rolled cultures for JH virus. Both viruses grew slowly, and most of the strains required a blind passage before they produced any CPE in the MK cells (160, 168); even after 12 passages of rhinovirus type 1A (2060) in MK cultures, complete destruction of cells occurred only after 10–14 days (160). CPE was also produced in monkey testis and HEK but not in HeLa, KB, chick embryo, human conjunctiva, or monkey cornea cultures (160). It was later found that second passage MK cultures supported the growth of rhinovirus type 1A (JH and 2060) more consistently than did primary MK cultures; in the former cultures CPE appeared earlier and involved more of the cell sheet (145, 169). Rolling of infected MK culture tubes increased the virus yield and enhanced the CPE (89, 145, 168, 169). The use of "islands of cells" usually appearing about 4 days after planting of cultures also facilitated the interpretation of CPE (89). Infectivity titers of rhinovirus type 1A (2060) were highest in neutral or slightly acid maintenance medium (158); 10- to 100-fold reduction in infectivity occurred at pH 7.6–7.8 when compared with infectivity at pH 7.0–7.2. It was therefore recommended that for optimal growth the pH should be maintained between 6.8 and 7.2 (145, 158). With these and other modifications, rhinovirus type 1A (2060 and JH) could be propagated satisfactorily.

Rhinovirus types 2 (HGP) and 3 (FEB) could be propagated in rolled HEK cultures without showing CPE; virus growth was measured by virus-interference tests and by production of illness in volunteers inoculated with tissue cultures harvests (87, 211). It was felt that virus grew more efficiently in cultures incubated at 33 C than at 36 C (211). When the pH of the maintenance medium was reduced to about 7, rhinovirus type 2 (HGP) produced CPE in HEK, primary and secondary rhesus MK, and secondary cyno-mologous MK cultures incubated at 33 C; optimal virus growth occurred in roller tubes maintained at 33 C in medium containing 0.3% sodium bicarbonate (216). Secondary rhesus MK cultures (cells in patches rather than in continuous sheets) were more sensitive than primary cultures. Environmental conditions for facilitating the growth of rhinovirus type 2 were similar to those for rhinovirus type 1A except for the important additional requirement of incubation at 33 C.

Rhinovirus type 2 (HGP) produced CPE in both HEK and MK cultures, whereas strain FEB (type 3) produced CPE only in rolled HEK cultures (216). It was found later that 8 of 25 patients with common colds had shed viruses that grew in rolled tissue cultures maintained in low bicarbonate medium at 33 C; these agents did not produce CPE in stationary tube cultures incubated at 37 C and maintained with standard medium (88).

Later, other strains were found which grew only in HEK cells and were designated "H" strains, while those which grew in both human and monkey cells were designated "M" strains (207). However, this property may be related to the amount of virus inoculated into the MK culture (42). Rhinovirus types 13, 14, and 15 originally described as "H" strains, produced CPE in primary MK tissue cultures if 10^4 $TCID_{50}$ or more were inoculated, while rhinovirus type 17, also described as an "H" strain, required $10^{5.2}$ $TCID_{50}$. In another study, of 4 strains of rhinovirus type 33 originally described as "H" strains, only 2 could be adapted to MK cultures (166). The ability to replicate in MK cultures, although occasionally helpful for grouping strains, is variable and is not commonly used for this purpose.

Rhinovirus types 7–12 were isolated from patients with common colds in a HDCS of human fetal kidney (WI-10) and a HDCS of human fetal lung (WI-26). The CPE was easy to recognize; the cultures were rolled in medium with a more conventional pH (7.2–7.4) at 33 C (72). The availability of sensitive HDCS cultures in almost unlimited quantities provided a great impetus to rhinovirus research and facilitated the isolation of many additional serotypes (80).

In early studies comparing the sensitivity of primary HEK and 2 HDCS of human embryonic lung (HEL), BW and WI-38, for isolation of rhinovirus types 3 and 4 from volunteers' nasal washings, it was found that rhinovirus type 4 could be isolated with equal efficiency in all 3 cultures; however, for isolation of rhinovirus type 3, HEK was the most sensitive, BW intermediate, and WI-38 insensitive (199). The D.C. virus, now classified as rhinovirus type 9 (18), was cultivated successfully in 1962 producing CPE on initial passage into HDCS WI-26 and HEL-110; it did not produce CPE in HEK cells. Growth was optimal when cultures were rolled at 33 C and maintained in a medium at pH 7.2 (210). It did not produce CPE when incubated at 36 C with the other conditions remaining optimal, and it grew poorly both in roller tubes at 33 C in a medium at pH 7.6 and in stationary tubes at 33 C in a medium with pH at 7.2 (210). It is noteworthy that the virus could be isolated in only 4 of 11 HDCS derived from different HEL, although it could be adapted to grow in 10 of the 11 and in HEK after primary isolation (209). In further studies the sensitivity of HDCS WI-26 to rhinovirus type 2 varied significantly, and primary cultures of HEK derived from different embryos had a variable sensitivity over at least as wide a range as the diploid cells (8). A comparison of the relative sensitivity of primary cultures of HEK and HEL showed that the primary HEL cells were much less sensitive than the HEK; however, with subculture the sensitivity of the lung cells increased, although usually it was less than that of the HEK cells. The reasons for the resistance of the first passage cells and the varying sensitivity of different lots of tissue from the same fetus and of different lots from different fetuses are not understood. Different lots of HDCS did not vary in sensitivity to poliovirus, but did to one rhinovirus studied (8).

The relative sensitivity of primary HEK and HDCS WI-26 or WI-38 was studied in several laboratories during epidemiologic surveys. In 1 study of students with upper respiratory infections, 82 rhinoviruses were isolated over 3 periods: 52 (63%) were recovered in WI-38, 53 (65%) in HEK, and 52 (63%) in human aorta cultures, another HDCS. However, 24 (29%) were recovered in HEK alone, 9 (11%) in WI-38 alone, and 10 (12%) in human aorta cultures alone. In addition, the relative sensitivity of the cell lines changed during the study, with the ratio of isolations in WI-38 to those in HEK varying from 11:1 to 1:18 to 1.9:1 during the 3 phases of the study (163). In another study of upper respiratory illnesses among students, approximately 12% of 281 specimens inoculated in HDCS WI-26 or WI-38, 4% of 175 inoculated into HEK, and 2% of 263 inoculated in secondary MK cultures yielded rhinoviruses (67).

A lack of superiority of either HDCS WI-38 or HEK and evidence of fluctuating sensitivity of these cultures at different times was demonstrated in a large study of nose and throat swabs from 1578 patients with acute respiratory infections in which 92 rhinoviruses were isolated as follows: 32 (35%) were isolated only in HEK, 43 (47%) only in WI-38, and 17 (18%) in both cell cultures (83). The sensitivity of the 2 systems varied during the study: during the first 18 months, 24 rhinoviruses were isolated in HEK and 10 in WI-38, while in the last 22 months of the study twice as many (50 vs 25) rhinoviruses were isolated in WI-38 as in HEK cultures. Since only 1 tube of each culture had been used in the above study, 6 original specimens that had yielded a rhinovirus only in HEK and 6 that had yielded a rhinovirus only in WI-38 cultures were diluted 3-fold (1:1, 1:3, 1:9) and inoculated into 3 tubes each of both HEK and WI-38 cultures. In all cases CPE was observed only in the tissue from which the virus had been originally isolated. It was noteworthy that the 1:9 dilution was positive in 3 of the 6 specimens positive only in HEK and 3 of the 6 specimens positive only in WI-38, and at the same time the undiluted specimen was negative in the opposite culture, revealing a remarkable difference in sensitivity between these 2 cell systems (83). In a more recent study of respiratory illness, of 30 viruses isolated only in human cell cultures, 22 were detected in HEK and only 17 in WI-38 (86). Of 15 viruses recovered in MK cells, 6 were detected in MK only, and 9 in both MK and WI-38 cells.

It is apparent that different lots of HDCS will vary in sensitivity to rhinoviruses, as will cultures of HEK derived from different embryos; the reasons for the varying sensitivity are unknown. Therefore, it would be good practice for diagnostic laboratories to perform sensitivity studies at certain intervals by titrating a standardized seed virus into new lots of HDCS.

The cell culture systems used for the original isolation of the 89 numbered rhinoviruses plus one subtype, the 22 distinct phase-3 viruses, and the 68 untypable phase-4 strains were determined from the records of the collaborative rhinovirus program (see Antigenic Composition above). Of these 180 rhinoviruses, 2 were isolated in MK cells, 28 in HEK cultures, 146 in various HDCS (primarily WI-26 and WI-38), and 4 in more than one cell type. No comparisons for efficacy of isolation can be made since in most cases the various cell culture systems were not used simultaneously. However, these results suggest that because of their availability and relatively consistent susceptibility to rhinoviruses, HDCS are used for most epidemiologic studies.

Rhinoviruses have been adapted to grow in human heteroploid cell lines such as HEp-2, KB, HeLa, and L132 cells (88, 99, 100, 110, 143, 186, 190, 200). A study of factors affecting growth of type 2 virus in suspension cultures of L132 cells showed that freshly trypsinized cells absorbed little if any virus (190). This finding was interpreted as being due to tryptic destruction of viral receptor sites, which required some time to regenerate. In addition, it was found that type 2 virus produced optimal yields at pH 7.7, supporting earlier findings that low pH was not necessary for rhinovirus replication in all cell culture systems (100, 110). Growth of rhinoviruses in HeLa cells has been used for the typing of rhinovirus serotypes (17). The first 55 numbered rhinoviruses were readily adapted to a sensitive line of HeLa cells from HDCS WI-26 or WI-38 harvests and yielded consistently higher infectivity titers in the HeLa cells (16). All 55 types grown in HeLa cells were passaged easily into HDCS WI-38 and demonstrated CPE for 3 consecutive passages, while in contrast only 9 of 55 serotypes produced CPE in HEp-2 cells for 3 consecutive passages. Rhinovirus types 56-89 also were readily adapted to the same HeLa cell line from inocula prepared in HDCS (104). Further, over 350 rhinovirus strains (representing over 100 serotypes) submitted to the collaborative program have been adapted to grow with relative ease in these HeLa cells (Author, unpublished data). HeLa cells also have been used to plaque rhinovirus types 1A-55 (19, 50). The HeLa cells used in these studies have been referred to as M (Merck) HeLa, HeLa M, (24, 52, 192, 194), rhino-HeLa (113), H-HeLa (135) and HeLa "R" (118). All of these cell lines are from the same source—a horse serum line obtained originally from Microbiological Associates, Bethesda, MD (16, 73, 110). To avoid confusion and because these cells have been referred to most often as either M HeLa or HeLa M, the author suggests that the designation HeLa M be retained. This HeLa line is contaminated with *Mycoplasma orale* (Somerson NL, personal communication).

HeLa M cells maintained on medium with 30 mm $MgCl_2$ were compared with rhinovirus-sensitive HDCS for susceptibility to various inocula containing rhinoviruses (194). Four of 7 samples of organ culture fluids produced CPE in both HeLa and HDCS cultures. Of 10 nasal washings tested, 4 produced CPE in both HeLa and HDCS cultures, 1 sample produced CPE in HeLa cultures only, and one in HDCS cultures only. CPE was produced in HeLa M cells inoculated with 70 rhinoviruses passaged only in HDCS. The 70 inocula represented at least 30 distinct serotypes (194). HeLa M cells maintained in the presence of 30 mm $MgCl_2$ also have been used for isolation of rhinoviruses from clinical specimens. HeLa M and WI-38 cells were inoculated in parallel with nasal washings from volunteers infected with 4 different rhinovirus serotypes, 1A, 2, 9, 43. Of 198 specimens tested, 86 isolations were obtained in WI-38 and 132 in HeLa M (196). The use of fetal bovine serum in the medium reduced the sensitivity of WI-38 cells but not of the HeLa cells.

In another study HeLa M and a HDCS (HEL) known to be as sensitive to rhinoviruses as WI-38 were compared for the isolation of rhinoviruses from patients with respiratory disease (118). Over a 4-year period, 526 rhinoviruses were isolated from 117 patients, 32% in both cell types, 59% in HeLa only, and 9% in HEL only. No typing was done, and the agents isolated were regarded as rhinoviruses on the basis of failure to produce CPE in monkey cells unless the virus was an M strain and showed characteristic CPE and lability at acid pH. The initial CPE occurring in HeLa cells was sometimes less characteristic of rhinovirus infection than that seen in HEL cells, but once initiated it always went to completion. In HEL cells the initial foci of CPE often disappeared within a few days. Whether the higher isolation rate in HeLa was due to a prevalence of serotypes more easily isolated in these cells was not determined. Known virus-positive specimens were used to compare a HDCS [fetal trachea (FT)] and the HeLa M line for ability to reisolate rhinoviruses (24). A total of 112 (83.5%) rhinovirus strains representing 22 different serotypes were reisolated in FT cultures, while only 71 isolates (52.6%) were recovered in HeLa M cultures after up to 4 blind passages in medium with 30 mm $MgCl_2$. Twenty-eight isolates were obtained in HeLa cells without $MgCl_2$. Rhinovirus CPE was not observed at first passage and required 1–2 blind passages. However, the isolation attempts in HeLa probably were not conducted under optimal conditions. After only 2 days of incubation on a roller drum, HeLa cultures began spontaneously degenerating, and to prevent this, medium was changed and incubation was continued in stationary racks. The poor condition of the HeLa cells during the first 48 hr following inoculation and incubation in a stationary position instead of on roller drums could have adversely affected the recovery of rhinoviruses in these cells. Probably the most interesting finding in this study was the demonstration of dual rhinovirus infections. Two different rhinoviruses were isolated from each of 5 clinical specimens. The FT cells yielded the serotype originally recovered, but a second rhinovirus type was isolated in HeLa M cells. The second strains isolated in HeLa were two of type 3, two of type 42, and one of type 48. These results suggest that some rhinovirus strains may be isolated more readily in HeLa cells.

Growth in organ cultures

Human embryonic organ culture (OC) of fragments of nasal septum, turbinates, and trachea were found to support the growth of rhinovirus type 2, an M strain and an H strain as well (91). The ciliary activity of the cultures was unaffected by rhinovirus type 2 infection but was destroyed in cultures infected with echovirus 11. Rhinovirus type 2 grew to higher titers for a longer period of time in the nasal OC; it did not grow in either human esophageal or palatal OC or rhesus monkey nasal and tracheal OC (91).

Because agents from many patients with common-cold–like illnesses, were not recoverable in conventional tissue cultures, even though washings from these patients produced colds when administered to volunteers, OC were used in an attempt to cultivate such fastidious agents (92). Nasal washings obtained from a patient with an upper respiratory infection were inoculated into OC of human embryonic nasal epithelium; the fifth day after inoculation the ciliary activity stopped. The agent (HS) could be passaged serially to additional nasal OC in which it caused the cessation of ciliary action the day after inoculation. The HS virus grew in human embryonic tracheal and esophageal OC as well, but in titration studies the nasal OC was somewhat more sensitive than the tracheal OC, and the tracheal OC was considerably more sensitive than the esophageal. The HS virus did not grow in 4 strains of human diploid lung fibroblasts, primary HEK, human amnion, MK, or HeLa cells; it passed a 50-nm filter, was ether stable and acid labile, and grew better at 33 C than at 37 C and at neutral pH than in an alkaline medium (92). The HS virus was found to be antigenically distinct from 41 rhinoviruses in 1-way or reciprocal Nt tests and was capable of inducing colds in volunteers (90). Two other viruses resembling rhinoviruses (MT, FT) were isolated from nasal washings of patients with common colds in human embryonic tracheal OC (inducing a reduction in ciliary activity) but could not be isolated on first passage in any conventional tissue culture system. However, the OC harvests grew in a HDCS (HEL) but not in MK or HEK cultures (208). More recently a modified method of organ culture has been described (206) and used to isolate 11 rhinoviruses undetectable in conventional cell culture systems (212). The major changes included the use of Eagle medium in place of No. 199 and incubation of cultures in an atmosphere of 5% CO_2. Since the original and modified methods were not tested together, it is not known if the modified method is better for rhinovirus isolations from clinical specimens. In another study the OC, HEK, and WI-38 systems were compared for the isolation of rhinoviruses from specimens obtained from military recruits with respiratory illness (86). Of 62 presumptive rhinoviruses isolated, 17 could be recovered in OC only, indicating that the use of OC of ciliated epithelium is advantageous when rhinovirus isolations are attempted. It appears that there are various grades of fastidiousness of known rhinoviruses, including those (such as rhinovirus type 2) cultivable in both conventional cell cultures and OC, those (such as MT) that do not initially grow in conventional cultures but after passage in OC are cultivable in cell cultures, and those (such as HS) that cannot be cultivated in conventional cultures, even after passage in OC.

It is possible that the variability in the sensitivity of cell cultures to rhinoviruses can be explained to some extent on the basis of the quality and quantity of specific rhinovirus receptor sites on host-cell membranes. Rhinoviruses, like other picornaviruses, require specific receptor sites for attachment to HeLa cells and can be grouped into receptor families. It has been suggested that the grouping of serotypes into receptor families may be related to H and M host-range characteristics (120, 121). The attachment is temperature dependent, and the rate of attachment depends upon the serotype. It also has been stated that rhinovirus receptors are sensitive to proteolytic enzymes, which suggests the possibility that trypsinization may alter host-cell receptors (120, 121). Perhaps the methods used for preparation of OC and primary cell cultures and for subcultivation of cell strains and cell lines might affect rhinovirus receptor sites, thus influencing the sensitivity of host cell systems. It would be of interest to study cell systems with varying susceptibility to rhinoviruses to determine the status of receptor sites during sensitive and insensitive periods.

It is clear from the foregoing discussion that no conclusions can be drawn as to the single best cell culture system for isolation of rhinoviruses. It appears that the greatest number of isolations are obtained when a range of culture systems are used. Ideally, these would include OC, a sensitive HDCS, primary HEK, and a rhinovirus-sensitive line of heteroploid cells. Because of our cumulative experience with HDCS, and because of their availability and wide susceptibility to rhinoviruses, such culture systems are used for routine isolation of rhinoviruses by most viral diagnostic laboratories.

Preparation of Immune Serum

A variety of animals have been used to prepare rhinovirus antisera. These include guinea pigs, rabbits, dogs, goats, calves, monkeys, baboons, and degus—a south American rodent. In early studies antigens used for immunization usually were of low potency, and rigorous immunization procedures were sometimes required to prepare usable antisera. Consequently, many sera used for antigenic analysis were of low titer and were occasionally cytotoxic. With improved methods for growing rhinoviruses (16, 22, 204) high-titer immunogens can be prepared routinely in HeLa M cells (22), and immune animal sera with titers in the thousands can be produced with as few as 2 injections (94). Although a variety of immunization schedules, dosages, antigens (both concentrated and unconcentrated), and adjuvants have been used to prepare immune sera, comparative studies demonstrating the superiority of any one procedure have not been done (21, 22, 72, 94, 100, 151, 161, 181, 183). However, a study was done defining the minimal dose of infectious virus needed to elicit an immune response in rabbits receiving a course of 6 injections (22). The minimal infectious dose needed to elicit high levels of antibody to rhinovirus type 1A was 1.4×10^7 plaque-forming units (pfu)/ml; type 2 required 10^8 pfu/ml. Although satisfactory antibody titers were obtained with other rhinovirus immunogens with titers between 2.3×10^5 and 2.6×10^6 pfu/ml, uniformly successful production of potent antisera required immunogens with titers of at least 10^7 pfu/ml. In another study the South American hystricomorph *Octodon degus* (degu) was compared with guinea pigs as a source of antiserum (161). The degu is a rodent with 2 distinct thymus glands, one of which retains its size and structural integrity throughout life. With use of the same antigen pool and identical methods (2 inoculations 6 weeks apart) antisera for each of 6 rhinovirus serotypes were prepared simultaneously in guinea pigs and degus. The infectivity titers of the pools were between 3.5 and 5.5 $TCID_{50}$/ml. With 3 of the serotypes, the titers achieved were either comparable in both animals or somewhat higher in the degu. For the other 3 serotypes, the titers obtained were clearly higher in the degu. The immunogen with the lowest titer ($10^{3.5}$ $TCID_{50}$/ml) elicited poor responses in guinea pigs but produced sera with titers of over 1:1000 in the degu (161). Exemplary methods for preparing immune sera in guinea pigs and rabbits follow.

Preparation in guinea pigs

Antigen pools with minimal titers of $10^{6.0}$ $TCID_{50}$/ml are treated once with fluorocarbon (freon 113, E.I. DuPont, Wilmington, Delaware); 2 parts virus and 1 part fluorocarbon are blended at maximal speed for 3 1-min intervals in a Sorvall Omni-mixer submerged in an ice bath. Equal parts of Freon and antigen can be used if host cell debris has not been removed or if the serum concentration in the antigen preparation is 5% or higher. The mixture is centrifuged at $1000 \times g$ for 10 min, and the supernatant fluid containing the virus is removed and emulsified with an equal volume of Freund incomplete adjuvant until droplets of the emulsion are nondispersible in water. If many antisera are to be made, a Mulsi-Churn Reciprocator (Mulsi Jet Inc., Elmhurst, Illinois) or similar instrument can be used for efficient and easy production of emulsions. Animals (400–600 g) are inoculated intramuscularly (im) with 2–3 ml of emulsion (1–1.5 ml into the thigh of each hind leg). One month later, the animals are inoculated ip with 3–5 ml of aqueous antigen and exsanguinated a week later while under carbon dioxide anesthesia. Modifications of this method include using antigen-adjuvant emulsion for the second im injection and Freund complete adjuvant instead of the incomplete.

Preparation in rabbits

Fluorocarbon treated antigen pools with minimal titers of 10^7 pfu/ml are emulsified with Freund incomplete adjuvant, and 1 ml of emulsion is injected into each of 4 im sites. Twenty-one days later, each rabbit is injected by the intravenous (iv) route with 0.1 ml of aqueous antigen. Three days later, a series of iv injections of 0.2, 0.3, and 0.4 ml are initiated and given at 3- to 4-day intervals. Seven days later, a final iv injection of 1 ml is given, and the rabbits are bled 1 week later. With this schedule many rabbits may have peak antibody levels after the fourth iv injection, but a fifth iv injection may be needed before all rabbits develop high antibody levels.

Specificity of animal antisera

In recent years the more consistent availability of potent immune animal serum for studies of antigenic relationships has resulted in the description of extensive cross-relationships between rhinovirus serotypes (25, 183). In addition, heterotypic immunization of rabbits has led to the detection of previously unsuspected relationships (26). In some cases it has been possible to remove heterotypic Nt activity from immune serum by absorption with human liver powder (17, 183). These results have been interpreted as being due to the removal of anticellular antibodies produced during the course of immunization. In other studies, however, where the kinetics of heterotypic Nt reactions have been determined, the reactions have been shown to proceed at a constant rate, indicating that anti-host cell antibody is not involved in heterotypic Nt (23, 25). In addition, it has been shown that even a single injection of rabbits with a potent antigen can elicit heterotypic Nt antibody responses (26).

In a recent review current knowledge of cross-relations among rhinoviruses was summarized (53). The data were obtained from published reports of Nt antibody responses in animals and in humans. Among 47 different serotypes, tests with a variety of immune animal sera demonstrated about 31 reciprocal and 53 one-way relationships (53). Among 22 distinct but unnumbered phase-3 viruses in the collaborative rhinovirus program (see Antigenic Composition above), 3 phase-3 viruses were found to be related to 3 other phase-3 strains, and 11 phase-3 viruses cross-reacted with various numbered rhinoviruses (70). It is clear from this discussion that a) many rhinovirus immune sera can contain heterotypic antibody and must be standardized carefully prior to use for typing purposes and b) immune sera with heterotypic antibody should be examined by Nt kinetics or be absorbed appropriately to help determine the specificity of the heterotypic reaction. Perhaps antibody directed against host cell rhinovirus receptor sites is present in some immune sera and may play a role in blocking rhinovirus infection. In such circumstances absorption of immune sera with certain absorbents, e.g., freshly trypsinized HeLa cells, could be ineffective if receptors are not present on the cell surface. The use of purified antigens and immunization schedules involving only 2-3 injections of animals should be helpful in reducing the amount of host-cell antibodies formed during the production of immune sera.

Collection and Preparation of Specimens for Laboratory Diagnosis

Precautions

Clinical materials should be handled with precautions normally used for respiratory secretions.

Preparations for virus isolation

Source of specimen. Nasopharyngeal wash specimens are superior to nasal or pharyngeal swabs for isolation. This was demonstrated when volunteers were inoculated with rhinovirus types 13, 15, or 16 and these methods of collection were compared. Among 13 antibody-free volunteers, 76% of the nasopharyngeal washings, 36% of nasal swabs, and 35% of pharyngeal swabs were positive during the first 7 days after inoculation (12). The collecting fluid was veal infusion broth containing 0.5% bovine albumin.

Nasopharyngeal washings may be obtained as follows. With the patient in a sitting position and with the head tilted slightly backward, 5–10 ml of normal saline solution without antibiotics is instilled into 1 nostril. After 5–10 sec, the patient expels the fluid into a beaker or glass. The procedure is repeated for the other nostril.

If nasopharyngeal washings cannot be obtained, nasal swabs are preferred over pharyngeal swabs and saliva specimens. In a study of naturally occurring rhinovirus infections in adults, rhinovirus isolations were made from 35 of the 176 illnesses: 30 (86%) from nasal swabs, 21 (60%) from pharyngeal swabs, and 17 (49%) from saliva. Fourteen (40%) of the 35 isolates were recovered from a single source only; 10 (71%) were from nasal swabs, 3 from pharyngeal swabs, and 1 from the saliva (63). In a study involving children, comparison of nasal and pharyngeal cotton-swab specimens demonstrated that of 19 virus-positive children, 9 (47%) isolations were made from the nose alone, 2 (11%) from the pharynx alone, and 8 (42%) from both nose and pharynx (81). The collecting medium in these studies was beef heart infusion broth containing 1% bovine serum albumin. Thus, it appears that if nasopharyngeal washings cannot be taken, nasal swabs are preferable to pharyngeal swabs, and using both kinds of swabs is probably better than using either alone. Attempts to isolate rhinoviruses from anal swabs have been consistently unsuccessful (4, 13, 125), as have attempts to recover rhinoviruses from conjunctival swabs (11).

Importance of collecting specimens early in the course of illness. As generally recognized for most viral infections, clinical specimens obtained soon after onset of illness are more likely to yield viruses than those obtained later. In one report serial specimens from patients with rhinovirus-positive illnesses yielded the highest rate of isolations on the initial day of illness and the first 3 days after onset. The isolation rate remained relatively high up to 8 days after onset of symptoms (76). In a study in which different patients were sampled at various times after onset of symptoms, the isolation rate remained relatively constant from 0 to 5 days after onset. The recovery rate was much lower from samples obtained on days 6 and 7 after onset (63). In another study the isolation rate did not vary significantly during the first 5 days of illness (152).

Importance of inoculating specimens directly into cell cultures. Ideally, specimens should be inoculated soon after collection without freezing and thawing. In a study in which specimens initially were inoculated directly into cell cultures, an attempt was made to reisolate rhinoviruses from the known positive specimens (in veal infusion broth with 0.5% bovine albumin) after

6-8 months of storage at -60 C. Only 24 (61%) of 39 previously positive specimens yielded isolates, and fewer H strains than M strains yielded isolates again (4). Specimens originally inoculated after a freeze-thaw cycle and positive for rhinoviruses were examined again after up to 13 months of storage at -60 C in the above medium or in medium No. 199 with 0.5% gelatin. Of 171 previously positive specimens, 140 (81%) yielded an isolate again with more M than H strains being recovered (4). In another study using veal infusion broth containing 0.5% bovine albumin as collecting medium for swab specimens, 19 rhinovirus strains were recovered from fresh specimens, and 16 were reisolated after 6 months or more of storage at -30 C (152). In a different study involving the influence of storage on isolation of rhinoviruses from fresh (unfrozen) specimens, no differences in isolation rates were obtained when specimens were inoculated after 30 min, 1.5 hr, or 3.5 hr of storage on wet ice (85).

Serologic diagnosis

Acute- and convalescent-phase serum specimens must be tested simultaneously to demonstrate a significant increase in antibody titer. A single serum specimen is of no value since it is well established that rhinovirus antibody may persist for years at relatively high levels (61, 74, 201). The acute-phase blood specimen should be obtained within 3-4 days after onset of illness, and a convalescent-phase serum specimen about 3 weeks after onset. The clot should be allowed to retract at room temperature for 1-3 hr or overnight at 4 C. Serum can be separated from whole blood by centrifugation and either drawn off with a pipette or carefully decanted. If a centrifuge is not available, a Pasteur pipette or a syringe and needle can be used to draw off the serum without disturbing the clot. Serum can be stored at -20 C or even at 4 C for a short time. Since serum Nt tests must be done in cell cultures, serum specimens should be handled under aseptic conditions.

Laboratory Diagnosis

Direct examination of material

The only reports of direct examination of clinical specimens for diagnosis of rhinovirus infections have been on the use of immunofluorescence (FA). Indirect FA (IFA) tests with specific immune rabbit or goat sera were used in attempts to detect rhinovirus type 1B antigen in cells of nasopharyngeal epithelium from 48 patients with acute respiratory disease or pneumonia (44). Specific cytoplasmic fluorescence was observed in cells from 5 patients, and rhinoviruses were isolated from 3 of these patients. In addition, 50 patients with acute conjunctivitis and trachoma with conjunctivitis were examined. Specific cytoplasmic fluorescence was observed in conjunctival scrapings from 4 (8%) of these patients (44). In a more recent study, nasopharyngeal smears from 238 patients with respiratory disease were examined by IFA for antigens to rhinovirus types 1B, 7, 17, and 48.

Of these patients 183 were examined for type 1B infections, 220 for type 17, 86 for type 7, and 123 for type 48. Immune rabbit sera diluted to contain 32–64 units of Nt antibody were used for each virus type. Rhinovirus infections were detected in 24 of these patients by this method (43). However, the correlation between virus isolation and positive FA results was generally poor. Of 14 clinical specimens positive by FA, rhinoviruses were isolated from only five, and one of the isolates did not correspond to the serotype detected by FA. Because of the large number of rhinovirus serotypes and the difficulties of working with large numbers of monovalent sera, the FA method is presently impractical for the direct examination of clinical material on a routine basis.

Virus isolation

Isolation in animals. The chimpanzee and the gibbon are the only animals known that can be infected with rhinoviruses. Rhinoviruses have not been propagated in embryonated chicken eggs.

Isolation in cell cultures. HEK and HDCS, such as WI-26 or WI-38 have been used most widely for isolation of rhinoviruses from clinical specimens. Also, recent results with HeLa M cells indicate that this heteroploid cell line may be useful for this purpose. Rhesus MK cultures, which were important in the isolation of rhinovirus type 1A, are not used routinely for isolation of rhinoviruses since most rhinoviruses cannot be cultivated in this cell system from clinical specimens. The results of some exemplary studies comparing the relative sensitivities of different cell culture systems for primary isolation of rhinoviruses have been discussed above under Growth in Cell Cultures.

Isolation in HDCS. WI-26 and WI-38 has been used most often for the recovery of rhinoviruses, and both appear to be equally sensitive although, as mentioned above, variations occur at unpredictable intervals necessitating monitoring of sensitivity. These cell strains were originally derived from HEL tissue (80) and can be carried in serial culture by established procedures (see Chapter 3). In our laboratory, the growth medium consists of Eagle minimal essential medium (MEM) in Earle balanced salt solution (BSS), supplemented with 10% fetal bovine serum, 0.09% $NaHCO_3$, pencillin (100 units/ml), and streptomycin (100 μg/ml). The maintenance medium consists of Eagle MEM in Earle BSS containing 2% fetal bovine serum, penicillin 100 units/ml and mycostatin (50 units/ml), chlortetracycline 50 and streptomycin (100 μg/ml); it also contains 0.006 M Tris (hydroxymethyl) aminomethane (tris) buffer and 0.09% $NaHCO_3$, which gives an initial pH of 7.2–7.4. Additional $NaHCO_3$ can be added in place of Tris buffer and Eagle basal medium (BME) can be substituted for MEM. The specimen to be studied is inoculated in 0.2-ml amounts into each of 2 tubes of WI-26 or WI-38 cultures; the tubes are incubated at 32–34 C on drums rotating at one-third rpm.

Studies with a few rhinoviruses indicated that in WI-26 cultures these viruses grew as well at 37 C in stationary tube cultures with medium containing 0.22% $NaHCO_3$ (with pH above the neutral range) as at 33 C in rolling tubes with medium containing 0.06% $NaHCO_3$ (with a pH around neutrality). In contrast, these viruses did not grow as well under the former conditions in HEK cultures (100). However, these studies were not done with original specimens inoculated into WI-26 cultures for the first time. Others found that incubating cultures at 33 C under conditions of motion with maintenance medium at about pH 7.2 was necessary for the propagation of some rhinoviruses in HDCS derived from HEL (21, 66, 210). Rotation of HDCS cultures at temperatures of 32–34 C in medium at about pH 7.2 is recommended because under such conditions rhinoviruses have been recovered successfully from clinical specimens. In addition, there are no statistical data available on the effectiveness of various incubation conditions for isolation of rhinoviruses in HDCSs from original specimens.

On initial isolation the CPE generally appears within the first week of inoculation and frequently by the second day; however, isolates also may be recovered during the second week and rarely during the third week after inoculation. Thus, cultures can be observed for approximately 3 weeks. CPE may be recognized early when a few of the cells in the monolayer appear rounded or oval and become refractile, forming a "focus." A single focus or several foci may be present when the CPE is first seen. Gradually, these foci spread throughout the entire monolayer, blending into one another, until eventually the cells are lysed, leaving a granular debris. Occasionally, the CPE does not progress and may be manifested by only a few foci, even after 2–3 weeks; passage of harvests of such tubes may increase the CPE. Rarely, a few foci may appear and then disappear several days later. It may be worthwhile to passage cultures as soon as CPE has stopped progressing since further incubation might only serve to inactivate the virus. The CPE in HDCS cultures is easily seen since any foci of round cells stand out very clearly in fibroblast cultures, which normally contain very few round cells when the monolayers are confluent.

Isolation in primary HEK cultures. A method for growing primary HEK cultures (87) is described in Chapter 3. A method for growing HEK cultures used for isolation of rhinoviruses has been described as follows (207, 211):

> 1. Growth medium consists of 5–10% calf serum plus 0.5% lactalbumin hydrolysate in Hanks BSS containing 0.03% sodium bicarbonate, penicillin (100 units/ml), streptomycin (100 μg/ml), and mycostatin (20 units/ml). Maintenance medium is 2% unheated calf serum and 0.25% lactalbumin hydrolysate in Hanks BSS containing 0.03% sodium bicarbonate, penicillin (100 units/ml), streptomycin (100 μg/ml), and mycostatin (20 units/ml). The pH of both growth and maintenance media is about 7.0–7.2.
>
> 2. The clinical specimen (0.2 ml) is inoculated into each of 2 HEK tubes, which are incubated at 33 C on a roller drum. Incubation at 33 C on a roller drum, in medium with lower than usual bicarbonate concentration (with a pH about 7), is necessary for successful propagation of rhinoviruses in primary HEK cells (207, 216).

The CPE produced by clinical specimens varies from marked CPE originating 3–4 days after inoculation and destroying the entire monolayer within 1 week to 1 or 2 foci per tube appearing during the first 2 weeks after inoculation and occasionally regressing a few days later. The CPE generally begins with foci of degeneration consisting of a few cells in which the cytoplasm becomes refractile or looks like ground glass (216). Later the cytoplasm becomes irregular in outline, with long branching processes; eventually the cells become rounded and fall off the glass.

No comparative information is available on the importance of the ingredients in growth and maintenance media for primary isolation of rhinoviruses in HEK cultures. Recently, the use of lactalbumin hydrolysate and calf serum in cell culture media has declined. Most commercial houses supplying HEK cultures use a growth medium consisting of BME or MEM in Hanks BSS supplemented with fetal bovine serum to a final concentration of 10%; antibiotics such as penicillin (100 units/ml) and streptomycin (100 μg/ml) are added, and the pH is adjusted to about 7.0-7.2 by adding NaHCO$_3$ to 0.035%. It is not known if the absence of lactalbumin hydrolysate and the use of fetal bovine serum in place of calf serum in HEK media will affect the sensitivity of these cells for isolation of rhinoviruses.

Isolation in continuous cell lines. The only continuous cell line successfully used for recovery of rhinoviruses from clinical specimens is the HeLa M line (see Growth in Cell Cultures, page 547). Experience with the use of HeLa M cells for primary isolation of rhinoviruses is very limited (24, 118, 196). Additional longitudinal studies comparing the sensitivity of HeLa M with HDCS and HEK cultures for isolation of rhinoviruses need to be done. Various kinds of media have been used for growth and maintenance of this cell line during rhinovirus recovery attempts. One study employed Eagle medium (the kind was unspecified) with 5% calf serum for growth. For maintenance the medium was supplemented with 30 mM MgCl$_2$, and fetal bovine serum at a final concentration of 2% was substituted for calf serum (118). No other details or information about medium ingredients were given. In another study HeLa M cells were grown in BME containing 10% filtered ox serum, 0.10% NaHCO$_3$, penicillin (100 units/ml), streptomycin (100 μg/ml), and achromycin (22.5 units/ml). The cells were maintained in a similar medium with ox serum reduced to 2% and supplemented with 30 mM MgCl$_2$ and tryptose phosphate broth to a final concentration of 5% (196). Cultures were trypsinized weekly, and tubes or bottles were implanted with 10^5 cells/ml. In still a different study, the growth medium was Eagle MEM with 10% fetal bovine serum. Maintenance medium was MEM with 1% fetal bovine serum and 30 mM MgCl$_2$ (24).

In our laboratory HeLa M cells have been used almost exclusively for working with over 350 rhinovirus strains (at least 100 different serotypes). The cells have not been used for virus isolations, and except for plaque assays, medium has not been supplemented with MgCl$_2$. The details of the techniques used for handling these cells and for adapting HDCS-propagated rhinoviruses to grow in them have been reported (16). It is likely that with the addition of MgCl$_2$ to the maintenance medium the general methodology described would be appropriate for isolation of rhinoviruses from clinical specimens. Therefore, a description of the methods used to adapt rhinoviruses to growth in HeLa M cells follows:

1. The HeLa cells are grown in a medium consisting of Eagle MEM in Earle BSS, with 10% uninactivated fetal calf serum, 0.15% sodium bicarbonate, penicillin (100 units/ml), streptomycin (100 μg/ml), chlortetracycline (40 μg/ml). Roller tube cultures are prepared by inoculating 70,000-100,000 cells/ml and are used after 2-4 days incubation.

2. The maintenance medium is the same as the growth medium except that 2% fetal calf serum is used and the sodium bicarbonate level is raised to 0.30% and Tris buffer is added to a final concentration of 0.001 M.

3. For adapting rhinoviruses to HeLa cells, 0.3 ml of undiluted virus is added to HeLa tube cultures 2-3 days after planting (before the cell monolayer is fully confluent) and is incubated at 33 C on a roller drum.

4. The cultures are harvested within 3-5 days after inoculation when CPE is complete or has stopped progressing, and the harvests are passed to fresh tubes as described above until CPE is complete within 4 days after inoculation.

Isolation in organ culture. Human embryonic nasal and tracheal OC are capable of supporting the growth of certain rhinoviruses which cannot be propagated in any known tissue culture system (84, 92, 208, 209). OC would undoubtedly increase the number of rhinoviruses isolated and should be used if available; in addition, OC would permit the isolation of coronaviruses of human origin since with one exception (229E) all of these viruses were originally isolated in OC and could not be adapted to tissue cultures (79, 105, 132, 208). Methods of preparing human embryonic tracheal or nasal OC have been described as follows (91, 215):

1. The trachea and nasal epithelium are cut into 1- to 3-mm square pieces. Sharp knives are used and the ciliated surface is never touched.

2. Four to 6 tissue fragments are placed on the bottom of a 60 × 15-mm plastic Petri dish where it has been scratched with a scalpel blade to facilitate adherence.

3. Medium No. 199 is added until level with or slightly above the fragment tops. The medium contains penicillin (100 units/ml), streptomycin (100 μg/ml), mycostatin (50 units/ml), and $NaHCO_3$ (0.35 g/liter), and the pH remains at 7.0-7.2 during the next 24 hr. The medium is replaced daily.

4. Each dish is incubated in a humidified plastic box at 33 C. Although not done in these studies, it is possible that incubation on a rocker platform might facilitate isolation of rhinoviruses.

5. The ciliary activity is observed through a dissecting microscope with reflected light. The cultures are inoculated with fresh specimens by dropping about 0.4 ml of the specimen over the tissue fragments. Each culture is observed for ciliary activity daily, and every day or every other day, the fluid is harvested and replaced with new maintenance medium.

6. Pooled harvested fluids from the organ cultures are passaged to other organ cultures or to cell cultures.

Identification of isolates and of serotypes. Hyperimmune sera are not available from commercial sources for any of the rhinovirus serotypes. Seed viruses and hyperimmune sera have been prepared for the 89 numbered serotypes under the auspices of the Research Resources Branch of the National Institute of Allergy and Infectious Diseases. These reference grade reagents have been released under contract to the American Type Culture Collection, Rockville, MD, for distribution, and small quantities of these reagents can be obtained from this source. Thus, typing of rhinovirus isolates remains essentially a research problem unless a laboratory is willing to take the considerable time and expense required to prepare and standardize its own hyperimmune sera. However, even in the absence of hyperimmune sera, certain characteristics of rhinoviruses can be used to place an isolate into the rhinovirus subgroup of picornaviruses. The properties an agent should possess to be grouped as a rhinovirus are as follows:

1. Ability to produce CPE, generally resembling that produced by enteroviruses, in HDCS (such as WI-26 or WI-38), in primary HEK cultures, or in HeLa cells.

2. Stability on exposure to lipid solvents such as chloroform or ether. A procedure for determining ether sensitivity has been described (2):

One part of diethyl ether is mixed with 4 parts of a suspension of the unknown virus, and the mixture is incubated in a sealed container at 4 C for approximately 18-24 hr. The ether is removed by transferring the specimen to an uncovered Petri dish and swirling it at room temperature in a fume hood for about 10 min. The ether also may be eliminated by bubbling nitrogen gas through the mixture for 5 min. The infectivity titer of the virus is determined in appropriate cell cultures. An equal volume of the unknown virus is handled in an identical manner, except that diethyl ether is not used. A known ether-sensitive virus, such as herpes simplex, and an ether-resistant virus, such as an enterovirus, should be included as controls and handled in a similar manner as the unknown virus. The infectivity titers of the viruses with and without ether treatment are compared. No significant loss in infectivity should occur with ether-resistant viruses.

A procedure for determining chloroform sensitivity has been described (49). A slightly modified version follows:

A mixture of 0.1 ml of analytical reagent-grade chloroform, and 1 ml of cell culture fluid containing virus is shaken either by hand or by mechanical mixer for approximately 10 min at room temperature. Immediately after shaking, the mixture is centrifuged at about 1000 x g for 5 min. The clear, upper aqueous phase is removed and used to determine the infectivity titer of the virus in appropriate cell cultures. An equal volume of unknown virus is handled in an identical manner but without chloroform. A known chloroform-sensitive virus such as herpes simplex, and a chloroform-resistant virus such as an enterovirus, are included as controls. The infectivity titers of the viruses are compared with and without chloroform treatment.

3. Complete or almost complete inactivation on treatment at pH 3 distinguishes the rhinoviruses from the enteroviruses, the latter being acid resistant. Procedures for this test have been described (37, 110). One method follows:

Virus is diluted 1:10 in Eagle MEM prepared without bicarbonate, pH about 2.7, and in Eagle MEM without bicarbonate but buffered with 0.01 M tris to pH 7; both mixtures are incubated for 3 hr at room temperature. A known acid-labile virus, such as rhinovirus type 1A, and an acid-stable virus, such as one of the enteroviruses, are treated in a similar way. Infectivity titrations are determined in appropriate cell cultures. Infrequently, high-titer preparations may not be completely inactivated at pH 3, and in such cases a 100-fold or greater reduction in titer would be interpreted as acid lability. Citrate-phosphate buffer at pH 3 and pH 7 can be used in place of MEM. In this buffer system rhinovirus type 14 is completely inactivated at pH 3 within 10 sec (96).

4. Small size (15–30 nm) as determined by filtration through nitrocellulose or polycarbonate membranes or by electron microscopy.

5. RNA genome as determined by lack of inhibition by DNA inhibitors such as 5-fluorodeoxyuridine (110) or by extraction of the intact RNA from the virion (35, 56, 110, 112, 153, 185). Characteristics 1, 2, and 3 above are sufficient for presumptive identification of an isolate as a rhinovirus.

If antisera are available, an isolate can be typed by a conventional Nt test in tube cultures as follows:

Equal volumes of unknown virus diluted to contain 10–1,000 TCID$_{50}$ (the test virus dose, [TVD]) and specific antiserum diluted to contain at least 20 antibody units are mixed and incubated with occasional shaking for 2 hr at room temperature. The diluent can consist of Hanks or Earle BSS containing an added protein such as gelatin (0.5%) or fetal bovine serum (2%) to help protect against inactivation of the TVD. In addition, equal volumes of TVD and diluent are mixed and incubated simultaneously. This is to determine the actual amount of virus used in the test. The serum-virus mixture is inoculated in 0.2-ml amounts into each of 2 cell-culture tubes; 10-fold dilutions of the TVD-diluent mixture are inoculated similarly. The cultures are examined at 2- to 3-day intervals for approximately 1 week. If CPE is present in tubes inoculated with serum-virus mixtures and the amount of TVD in the test is not overwhelming, the virus has not been typed. However, if there is no CPE, it cannot be assumed that the virus has been typed unless the TVD contains at least 10 $TCID_{50}$ and the antiserum is known to be free of heterologous cross-reactivity.

As discussed above some hyperimmune animal sera have demonstrated heterotypic reactions emphasizing the need for all sera to be standardized prior to use for routine typing purposes. Because such cross-reactions occur and additive effects of pooled sera may further complicate results, the use of intersecting or combinatorial pools of hyperimmune sera is not recommended unless such pools have been carefully standardized with known rhinovirus serotypes. Intersecting and combinatorial pools of guinea pig, rabbit, bovine, and goat hyperimmune sera have been used for typing rhinoviruses (60, 73, 108, 183).

Serologic diagnosis

Neutralization test

This is the only test system available on a routine basis for the serologic diagnosis of rhinovirus infections. A variety of methods for conducting Nt tests have been reported. These include a microplaque reduction test (203), a conventional plaque reduction (PR) test (51), micro-Nt tests (60, 95, 114, 148), the conventional tube endpoint Nt test (201, 203), and a micro-metabolic inhibition test (194).

The intensity of the serum Nt-antibody response following a rhinovirus infection appears to vary with the infecting serotype. In general, individuals infected with M strains develop $\geq$ 4-fold rises and higher titers more often than individuals infected with H strains (or what appears to be H strains when titers are low).

In one study, 14 individuals infected with M strains (6 children and 8 adults) developed $\geq$4-fold rises in titer, with median titers of <1:8 in acute-phase and of >1:128 in convalescent-phase sera, while only 8 of 19 (9 children and 10 adults) infected with H strains developed $\geq$4-fold increases in titers, with median titers of <1:8 in acute-phase and of 1:8 in convalescent-phase sera (201). Similar results were obtained in another study in which 11 of 12 M-strain positive and only 8 of 15 H-strain positive individuals developed $\geq$4-fold titer increases (67). In studies of only a few rhinovirus types, M-strain antibody persisted for long periods while H-strain antibody was found to wane (198). In studies with rhinovirus types 1A-55 on the prevalence of neutralizing antibodies in sera from 148 normal individuals, antibodies were present for all of the serotypes. However, serotypes with high antibody prevalence tended to be M strains, and those with low antibody prevalence tended to be H strains (61).

The microplaque reduction Nt test is more sensitive than the conventional endpoint tube Nt test when 15–20 microplaques and 100 $TCID_{50}$ of virus, respectively, are used (203). However, when 3–10 $TCID_{50}$ of virus is used, the sensitivity of the conventional tube Nt test compares favorably with that of the microplaque method. If the virus dosage in the conventional test is increased to 100–320 $TCID_{50}$, titers obtained in human sera are reduced or become undetectable (201). The microplaque reduction test is not in routine use, probably because it is too laborious, requiring the use of a microscope to count foci of CPE (microplaques) in replicate tube cultures.

The conventional 50% PR test and the conventional tube Nt method were used in one study to determine Nt antibody titers in sera from volunteers infected with rhinovirus type 2 and from students from whom rhinovirus type 1A was isolated. An estimated 40–100 pfu were used in the PR tests. The number of $TCID_{50}$ employed in the tube Nt tests was not stated (51). A combination of both single and paired sera from 10 individuals were tested by both methods. Most of the PR titers were significantly higher than the corresponding tube Nt titers. In addition, the PR test detected antibody in 4 acute-phase sera which were negative by the tube Nt assay. The conventional PR test is preferable to the micro–PR test because it can be easily read without the aid of a microscope. However, more experience is needed with this test before it can be used routinely.

Micro-neutralization test

A variety of micro-Nt tests have been described for identification of rhinovirus serotypes and detection of antibody. These include techniques in which WI-38 cells are added to serum-virus mixtures in either 6-mm glass precipitin tubes (60) or in disposable "V" microtiter plates (Cooke Engineering Co., Alexandria, Virginia) (114), in which HeLa M cells are added to serum-virus mixtures in flatbottom plastic microplates (148), or in which serum-virus mixtures are added to HeLa M cells planted 24 hr earlier in Microtest II tissue culture plates (Falcon Plastics, Oxnard, California) (95). A micro-Nt method in which HeLa M cells are added to serum-virus mixtures present in plastic microplates and which can be read with the unaided eye has been described as follows (148):

1. Tests are done in sterile flat-bottom plastic microplates.

2. The diluent (which also serves as medium) consists of Eagle MEM in Earle salts containing 7.5% calf serum inactivated at 56 C for 30 min, penicillin (100 units/ml), and streptomycin (100 μg/ml). Diluent is added to the wells in 0.025-ml amounts, and the unknown serum already at 1:2 is serially diluted in duplicate wells with microloops calibrated to contain 0.025 ml.

3. The test virus in 0.025 ml amounts is added to the residual 0.025 ml of diluted serum in each well. (The viruses have been previously diluted to contain 32–100 $TCID_{50}$/0.025 ml.)

4. The plates are covered loosely and placed in a CO_2 incubator at 33 C for 1 hr. Subsequently, 10,000–12,000 HeLa M cells contained in 0.1 ml are added to each well. Finally, 0.05 ml of diluent is added to each well. Serum and cell controls and a titration of the test virus dose are included in each test.

5. Plates are covered loosely and placed in a CO_2 incubator at 33 C for 6 days. After incubation, the medium is removed, and 1 drop of a crystal violet solution is added to each plate. This solution is prepared by dissolving 7.5 g of crystal violet in 50 ml of 70% ethyl alcohol and adding 250 ml of formalin and enough distilled water to bring the volume to 1 liter.

6. Cells are stained for 5–10 min, washed 3 times with distilled water, and allowed to dry overnight.

7. The preserved and stained cell sheet can be visualized best at this time, and endpoints can be read macroscopically with the unaided eye. A scoring system of 1–4 is used in recording CPE based on the amount of cell sheet destroyed. A well is considered virus positive if it is scored as 3 or more.

The conventional tube neutralization test

This is the most commonly used test system for detecting rhinovirus antibody in serum specimens.

1. Serial 4-fold dilutions (1:2, 1:8, 1:32, 1:128) of the patient's acute- and convalescent-phase sera (inactivated at 56 C for 30 min) are prepared in diluent consisting of Hanks BSS with 0.5% gelatin.

2. An equal volume of virus diluted to contain 6–20 $TCID_{50}$/0.2 ml (the TVD) is mixed with each serum dilution and incubated at room temperature for 2 hr. The TVD is also mixed with an equal volume of diluent and incubated at room temperature for 2 hr; this is for the simultaneous titration of the TVD. The cell-culture tubes subsequently inoculated should contain 3–10 $TCID_{50}$/0.2 ml since the TVD is diluted 2-fold in serum or the diluent.

3. Serial 10-fold dilutions of the TVD are made; 0.2 ml of each dilution is inoculated into each of 4 tubes containing about 1.5 ml of the maintenance medium. The serum-virus dilutions (0.2-ml amounts) are inoculated into each of 2 tube-cultures. If the test is large, requiring several hours for completion, a virus titration should be performed at the start of the inoculation (initial virus titration) and at its conclusion (final virus titration).

4. Cell cultures are incubated at 32–34 C on a roller apparatus turning at 12–20 revolutions/hr and are examined microscopically at 2- to 3-day intervals for about 1 week; serum Nt endpoints are calculated according to the method of Reed and Muench (172). If 3–32 $TCID_{50}$ of test virus is present in the simultaneous titration, the test should be satisfactory. A $\geq$ 4-fold rise in Nt antibody titer is considered significant. Roller-tube cultures of HDCSs, HeLa, HEK, or MK cells (for M strains) can be used.

One report describes the failure to correctly identify an unknown rhinovirus because of viral aggregation (62). This problem was encountered with a single passage level of a strain (SF1684) of type 2. When the sixth passage level of this strain prepared in WI-38 cells was used in tests with homologous hyperimmune guinea pig sera, the Nt titers obtained were 32- to 64-fold lower than those obtained with other passage levels of the same strain. Treatment of this passage level with 1% sodium deoxycholate, with 0.01% trypsin, or by filtration disaggregated the virions and restored full susceptibility to Nt. Thus, the possibility of viral aggregation must be considered when Nt failure or an unexpectedly low homologous serum titer is encountered.

Metabolic inhibition test

A micro-metabolic inhibition test has been shown to be as sensitive as conventional endpoint Nt tests and the micro-PR test. Significant antibody increases were demonstrated by each of these 3 tests in 10 of 13 paired sera from volunteers inoculated with rhinovirus type 2 and in 2 of 5 paired sera from volunteers inoculated with rhinovirus type 43 (194). The technique has been described as follows:

1. Rigid disposable plastic microtiter plates are used with microtiter loops and droppers, each delivering 0.025 ml.

2. Serial dilutions of serum (inactivated at 56 C for 30 min) are made in Medium No. 199 containing ox serum at a final concentration of 5%, 0.17% $NaHCO_3$, 30 mM $MgCl_2$, 0.3% glucose, and an additional 2 ml of a 0.1% phenol red solution per 98 ml of medium.

3. About 100 $TCID_{50}$ of virus in 0.025 ml are added to each serum dilution, and the serum-virus mixtures are incubated at 36 C for 1 hr; 15,000 HeLa M cells in 0.1 ml of BME with 5% ox serum, 0.11% $NaHCO_3$, 30 mM $MgCl_2$ and 0.3% glucose solution are added to each well.

4. The plate is sealed with transparent tape and incubated at 33 C for 7 days; the tape is removed, and the plate is covered with sterile aluminum foil and held at 36 C for 2 hr. After the 2-hr period, the color of the medium in all cups should have changed from yellow or orange to red. The plate is then resealed and incubated for 1 or 2 days before reading. This technique is also used for typing isolates; however, there is somewhat more nonspecific Nt in the microtest than in the tube test (194).

Hemaggregation-inhibition test

This test is based on the fact that trypsin-treated human erythrocytes suspended in buffered glucose at pH 5 aggregate and rapidly sediment in a photometer tube. Such aggregation can be inhibited by certain viruses, including rhinoviruses, and this inhibition can be prevented by homologous antiserum (46, 47, 214). Rhinovirus types 1B, 2, 3, 4, 5, and 6 were tested, and hemaggregation-inhibition was observed with all 6 types. In different preparations there were up to 100-fold differences in the ratio between infectivity and hemaggregation-inhibition titers (47). The 6 rhinoviruses were also used in tests with hyperimmune animal serum and with human serum. Although heterologous reactions did occur with animal sera, the homologous anti-hemaggregation-inhibition titers were higher. There was no correlation between homologous anti-hemaggregation-inhibition titers and those obtained in Nt tests. Also, cross-reactions occurred between rhinovirus serotypes 2 and 4 for which there is no evidence by Nt tests. With human serum, the correlation between presence of Nt antibody and significant anti-hemaggregation-inhibition titers was good. When paired sera from adults infected with or vaccinated against rhinovirus types 1A, 1B, or 2 were tested, the correlation between both rising Nt and rising anti-hemaggregation-inhibition titers was poor. More experience with this test is needed before its usefulness in rhinovirus serology can be determined.

Hemagglutination-inhibition test (HAI)

This procedure has the potential of becoming a useful adjunct to the serum Nt test for the serologic diagnosis of rhinovirus infections. It has been described as follows (171):

1. HA antigens are prepared in HeLa M cells grown in 80-oz roller bottles maintained in Eagle medium with 2% bovine serum, 5% tryptose phosphate broth, and 30 mM $MgCl_2$.

2. Bottle cultures are inoculated with enough virus to produce almost complete CPE after 18–24 hr at 33 C.

3. Cells remaining on the glass are shaken off into the medium, and the cells and cellular debris are sedimented at 2000 rpm for 10 min. The supernatant fluid is discarded, and the cell sediment is suspended in PBS to 5% of the volume of the original medium.

4. The suspension is frozen and thawed twice and clarified by low-speed centrifugation. The supernatant fluid, with an infectivity titer of $10^{7.5}$–$10^{8.0}$ $TCID_{50}$ per ml, constitutes the HA antigen. Titers of antigens prepared in this manner are between 1:32 and 1:128.

5. For the HAI test serum samples are absorbed for 3–18 hr at 4 C with about one-third their volume consisting of washed and packed sheep erythrocytes. After clarification at 4 C, the serum is removed and inactivated at 56 C for 30 min.

6. The HAI test is done in microtiter plates (IS-MVC-96, Cooke Engineering) by using 4 units of antigen. Serum-antigen mixtures are incubated for 1 hr at room temperature before addition of a 0.5% suspension of sheep erythrocytes.

7. The test is read after settling overnight at 4 C. The diluent used for resuspending the sheep erythrocytes (the diluent for serum is not described) consists of 50% CF-test

buffer (Oxoid Ltd.), 50% glucose (4.5%) in deionized water, and 0.5% gelatin, adjusted to pH 8.5 with 0.1 M HEPES buffer (191).

References

1. ANDREWS CH: *In* The Common Cold, Norton, New York, 1965
2. ANDREWES CH and HORSTMANN DM: The susceptibility of viruses to ethyl ether. J Gen Microbiol 3:290-297, 1949
3. ANDREWES CH and TYRRELL DAJ: Rhinoviruses *In* Viral and Rickettsial Infections of Man, 4th edition, Horsfall FL Jr and Tamm I (eds), JB Lippincott, Philadelphia, 1965, pp 546-548
4. BLOOM HH, FORSYTH BE, JOHNSON KM, and CHANOCK RM: Relationship of rhinovirus infection to mild upper respiratory disease. I. Results of a survey in young adults and children. J Am Med Assoc 186:38-45, 1963
5. BLOUGH HA, TIFFANY JM, GORDON G, and FIALA M: The effect of magnesium on the intracellular crystallization of rhinovirus. Virology 38:694-712, 1969
6. BÖGEL K and BÖHM H: Ein rhinovirus des rindes. Zentralbl Bakteriol Parasitenkd Infektionskr Hyg Abt 1 187:2-14, 1962
7. BROWN F, NEWMAN JFE, and STOTT EJ: Molecular weight of rhinovirus ribonucleic acid. J Gen Virol 8:145-148, 1970
8. BROWN PK and TYRRELL DAJ: Experiments on the sensitivity of strains of human fibroblasts to infection with rhinoviruses. Br J Exp Pathol 45:571-578, 1964
9. BUTTERWORTH BE: A comparison of virus-specific polypeptides of encephalomyocarditis virus, human rhinovirus-1A and poliovirus. Virology 56:439-453, 1973
10. BUTTERWORTH BE, GRUNERT RR, KORANT BD, LONBERG-HOLM K, and YIN FH: Replication of rhinoviruses: brief review. Arch Virol 51:169-189, 1976
11. BYNOE ML, HOBSON D, HORNER J, KIPPS A, SCHILD GC, and TYRRELL DAJ: Inoculation of human volunteers with a strain of virus isolated from a common cold. Lancet 1:1194-1196, 1961
12. CATE TR, COUCH RB, and JOHNSON KM: Studies with rhinoviruses in volunteers: production of illness, effect of naturally acquired antibody, and demonstration of a protective effect not associated with serum antibody. J Clin Invest 43:56-67, 1964
13. CATE TR, DOUGLAS RG JR, JOHNSON KM, COUCH RB, and KNIGHT V: Studies on the inability of rhinovirus to survive and replicate in the intestinal tract of volunteers. Proc Soc Exp Biol Med 124:1290-1295, 1967
14. CHAPPLE PJ and HARRIS J: Biophysical studies of a rhinovirus. ultracentrifugation and electron microscopy. Nature 209:790-792, 1966
15. CHAPPLE PJ, HEAD B, and TYRRELL DAJ: A complement fixing antigen from an M rhinovirus. Arch Gesamte Virusforsch 21:123-126, 1967
16. CONANT RM and HAMPARIAN VV: Rhinoviruses: basis for a numbering system. I. HeLa cells for propagation and serologic procedures. J Immunol 100:107-113, 1968
17. CONANT RM and HAMPARIAN VV: Rhinoviruses: basis for a numbering system. II. Serologic characterization of prototype strains. J Immunol 100:114-119, 1968
18. CONANT RM, HAMPARIAN VV, STOTT EJ, and TYRRELL DAJ: Identification of rhinovirus strain DC. Nature 217:1264, 1968
19. CONANT RM, SOMERSON NL, and HAMPARIAN VV: Plaque formation by rhinoviruses. Proc Soc Exp Biol Med 128:51-56, 1968
20. CONANT RM, THOMAS DC, and HAMPARIAN VV: Properties of rhinovirus plaque mutants. Proc Soc Exp Biol Med 134:677-682, 1970
21. CONNELLY AP JR and HAMRE D: Virologic studies on acute respiratory disease in young adults. II. Characteristics and serologic studies of three new rhinoviruses. J Lab Clin Med 63:30-43, 1964
22. COONEY MK and KENNY GE: Immunogenicity of rhinoviruses. Proc Soc Exp Biol Med 133:645-650, 1970
23. COONEY MK and KENNY GE: Reciprocal neutralizing cross-reactions between rhinovirus types 9 and 32. J Immunol 105:531-533, 1970

24. COONEY MK and KENNY GE: Demonstration of dual rhinovirus infection in humans by isolation of different serotypes in human heteroploid (HeLa) and human diploid fibroblast cell cultures. J Clin Microbiol 5:202–207, 1977

25. COONEY MK, KENNY GE, TAM R, and FOX JP: Cross relationships among 37 rhinoviruses demonstrated by virus neutralization with potent monotypic rabbit antisera. Infect Immun 7:335–340, 1973

26. COONEY MK, WISE JA, KENNY GE, and FOX JP: Broad antigenic relationships among rhinovirus serotypes revealed by cross-immunization of rabbits with different serotypes. J Immunol 114:635–639, 1975

27. COOPER PD: Studies on the structure and function of the poliovirion: effect of concentrated urea solutions. Virology 16:485–495, 1962

28. COUCH RB, CATE TR, DOUGLAS RG JR, GERONE PJ, and KNIGHT V: Effect of route of inoculation on experimental respiratory viral disease in volunteers and evidence for airborne transmission. Bacteriol Rev 30:517–529, 1966

29. CRAIGHEAD JE, MEIER M, and COOLEY MH: Pulmonary infection due to rhinovirus type 13. N Engl J Med 281:1403–1404, 1969

30. D'ALESSIO DJ, PETERSON JA, DICK CR, and DICK EC: Transmission of experimental rhinovirus colds in volunteer married couples. J Infect Dis 133:28–36, 1976

31. DANS PE, FORSYTH BR, and CHANOCK RM: Density of infectious virus and complement-fixing antigens of two rhinovirus strains. J Bacteriol 91:1605–1611, 1966

32. DICK EC, BLUMER CR, and EVANS AS: Epidemiology of infections with rhinovirus types 43 and 55 in a group of University of Wisconsin student families. Am J Epidemiol 86:386–400, 1967

33. DICK EC and CHESNEY PJ: Rhinoviruses In Pediatric Infectious Diseases, Feigin RD and Cherry JD (eds), Saunders, 1977

34. DICK EC and DICK CR: Natural and experimental infections of nonhuman primates with respiratory viruses. Lab Anim Sci 24:177–181, 1974

35. DIMMOCK NJ: Biophysical studies of a rhinovirus. Extraction and assay of infectious ribonucleic acid. Nature 209:792–794, 1966

36. DIMMOCK NJ: Differences between the termal inactivation of picornaviruses at "high" and "low" temperatures. Virology 31:338–353, 1967

37. DIMMOCK NJ and TYRRELL DAJ: Physicochemical properties of some viruses isolated from common colds (rhinoviruses). Lancet 2:536–537, 1962

38. DIMMOCK NJ and TYRRELL DAJ: Some physico-chemical properties of rhinoviruses. Br J Exp Pathol 45:271–280, 1964

39. DITCHFIELD J and MACPHERSON LW: The properties and classification of two new rhinoviruses recovered from horses in Toronto, Canada. Cornell Vet 55:181–189, 1965

40. DOUGLAS RG JR: Pathogenesis of rhinovirus common colds in human volunteers. Ann Otol Rhinol Laryngol 79:563–571, 1970

41. DOUGLAS RG JR, ALFORD BR, and COUCH RB: Atraumatic nasal biopsy for studies of respiratory virus infection in volunteers. Antimicrob Agents Chemother 8:340–343, 1968

42. DOUGLAS RG JR, CATE TR, and COUCH RB: Growth and cytopathic effect of H type rhinoviruses in monkey kidney tissue culture. Proc Soc Exp Biol Med 123:238–241, 1966

43. DREIZIN RS, BOROVKOVA NM, PONOMAREVA TI, VIKHNOVICH EM, KHEINITIS AA, and LEICHINSKAYA TV: Diagnosis of rhinovirus-infections by virological and immuno-fluorescent methods. Acta Virol 19:413–418, 1975

44. DREIZIN RS, VIKHNOVICH EM, BOROVKOVA NM, and PONOMAREVA TI: The use of indirect fluorescent antibody technique in studies on the reproduction of rhinoviruses and for the detection of rhinoviral antigen in materials from patients with acute respiratory diseases and conjunctivitides. Acta Virol 15:520, 1971

45. DREIZIN RS, VIKHNOVICH EM, BOROVKOVA NM, PONOMAREVA TI, GEINE GV, PYLAEVA EY, KLIMANSKAYA EV, RODOV, MN, KHEINITIS AA, and ZUBANOVA GN: Human rhinoviruses circulating in Moscow. Vop Virusol 75:592–597, 1975

46. DRESCHER J and SCHRADER K: Titration of poliovirus and influenza virus by means of the hemaggregation test. Am J Hyg 79:218–235, 1964

47. DRESCHER J and TYRRELL DAJ: The titration of rhinoviruses and of antibodies against them by means of the photometric hemaggregation-inhibition test. Am J Epidemiol 89:98–109, 1969

48. EADIE MB, STOTT EJ, and GRIST NR: Virological studies in chronic bronchitis. Br Med J 2:671-673, 1966
49. FELDMAN HA and WANG SS: Sensitivity of various viruses to chloroform. Proc Soc Exp Biol Med 106:736-738, 1961
50. FIALA M: Plaque formation by 55 rhinovirus serotypes. Appl Microbiol 16:1445-1450, 1968
51. FIALA M: A study of the neutralization of rhinoviruses by means of a plaque-reduction test. J Immunol 103:107-113, 1969
52. FIALA M and KENNY GE: Enhancement of rhinovirus plaque formation in human heteroploid cell cultures by magnesium and calcium. J Bacteriol 92:1710-1715, 1966
53. FOX JP: Reviews and commentary—is a rhinovirus vaccine possible? Am J Epidemiol 103:345-354, 1976
54. FOX JP, COONEY MK, and HALL CE: The Seattle virus watch. V. Epidemiologic observations of rhinovirus infections, 1965-1969 in families with young children. Am J Epidemiol 101:122-143, 1975
55. FROMMHAGEN LH: The separation and physicochemical properties of the C and D antigens of coxsackievirus. J Immunol 95:818-822, 1965
56. GAUNTT CJ: Synthesis of ribonucleic acids in KB cells infected with rhinovirus type 14. J Gen Virol 21:253-267, 1973
57. GAUNTT CJ, GRIFFITH MM, SUACK JR, UPSON RH, and CARLSON EC: Properties and origins of infectious rhinovirus type 14 particles of different buoyant densities. J Virol 16:1265-1272, 1975
58. GEORGE RB and MOGABGAB WJ: Atypical pneumonia in young men with rhinovirus infections. Ann Intern Med 71:1073-1078, 1969
59. GERIN JL, RICHTER WR, FENTERS JD, and HOLPER JC: Use of zonal ultracentrifuge systems for biophysical studies of rhinoviruses. J Virol 2:937-943, 1968
60. GWALTNEY JM JR: Micro-neutralization test for identification of rhinovirus serotypes. Proc Soc Exp Biol Med 122:1137-1141, 1966
61. GWALTNEY JM JR: Rhinoviruses In Viral Infections of Humans, Evans AS (ed), Plenum, New York, 1976
62. GWALTNEY JM JR and CALHOUN AM: Viral aggregation resulting in the failure to correctly identify an unknown rhinovirus. Appl Microbiol 20:390-392, 1970
63. GWALTNEY JM JR, HENDLEY JO, SIMON G, and JORDAN WS JR: Rhinovirus infections in an industrial population. I. The occurrence of illness. N Engl J Med 275:1261-1268, 1966
64. GWALTNEY JM JR, HENDLEY JO, SIMON G, and JORDAN WS JR: Rhinovirus infections in an industrial population. II. Characteristics of illness and antibody response. J Am Med Assoc 202:494-500, 1967
65. GWALTNEY JM JR, HENDLEY JO, SIMON G, and JORDAN WS JR: Rhinovirus infections in an industrial population. III. Number and prevalence of serotypes. Am J Epidemiol 87:158-166, 1968
66. GWALTNEY JM JR and JORDAN WS JR: Rhinoviruses and respiratory disease. Bacteriol Rev 28:409-422, 1964
67. GWALTNEY JM JR and JORDAN WS JR: Rhinoviruses and respiratory illnesses in university students. Am Rev Resp Dis 93:362-371, 1966
68. GWALTNEY JM JR, MOSKALSKI PB, and HENDLEY JO: Hand-to-hand transmission of rhinovirus colds. Ann Intern Med 88:463-467, 1978
69. HAMORY BH, HENDLEY JO, and GWALTNEY JM JR: Rhinovirus growth in nasal polyp organ culture. Proc Soc Exp Biol Med 155:577-582, 1977
70. HAMPARIAN VV and HUGHES JH: Rhinovirus Reference Laboratory, Annual Contract Report to the National Institute of Allergy and Infectious Diseases, April 1, 1971-March 31, 1972
71. HAMPARIAN VV and HUGHES JH: Rhinovirus Reference Laboratory, Final Contract Report to the National Institute of Allergy and Infectious Diseases, September 1, 1973 to May 31, 1974
72. HAMPARIAN VV, KETLER A, and HILLEMAN MR: Recovery of new viruses (coryzavirus) from cases of common cold in human adults. Proc Soc Exp Biol Med 108:444-453, 1961
73. HAMPARIAN VV, LEAGUS MB, and HILLEMAN MR: Additional rhinovirus serotypes. Proc Soc Exp Biol Med 116:976-984, 1964

74. HAMPARIAN VV, LEAGUS MB, HILLEMAN MR, and STOKES J JR: Epidemiologic investigations of rhinovirus infections. Proc Soc Exp Biol Med 117:469-476, 1964

75. HAMRE D: (Virus submitted by).

76. HAMRE D: Rhinoviruses *In* Monographs in Virology, Melnick JL (ed), S Karger, AG, Basel, Switzerland, 1968

77. HAMRE D, CONNELLY AP JR, and PROCKNOW JJ: Virologic studies of acute respiratory disease in young adults. III. Some biologic and serologic characteristics of seventeen rhinovirus serotypes isolated October, 1960 to June, 1961. J Lab Clin Med 64:450-460, 1964

78. HAMRE D, CONNELLY AP JR, and PROCKNOW JJ: Virologic studies of acute respiratory disease in young adults. IV. Virus isolations during four years of surveillance. Am J Epidemiol 83:238-249, 1966

79. HAMRE D and PROCKNOW JJ: A new virus isolated from the human respiratory tract. Proc Soc Exp Biol Med 121:190-193, 1966

80. HAYFLICK L and MOOREHEAD PS: The serial cultivation of human diploid cell strains. Exp Cell Res 25:585-621, 1961

81. HENDLEY JO, GWALTNEY JM JR, and JORDAN WS JR: Rhinovirus infections in an industrial population. IV. Infections within families of employees during two fall peaks of respiratory illness. Am J Epidemiol 89:184-196, 1969

82. HENDLEY JO, WENZEL RP, and GWALTNEY JM JR: Transmission of rhinovirus colds by self-inoculation. N Engl J Med 288:1361-1364, 1973

83. HIGGINS PG: The isolation of viruses from acute respiratory infections. IV. A comparative study of the use of cultures of human embryo kidney and human embryo diploid fibroblasts (WI-38). Mon Bull Min Health Public Health Lab Serv 25:223-229, 1966

84. HIGGINS PG: The isolation of viruses from acute respiratory infections. V. The use of organ cultures of human embryonic nasal and tracheal ciliated epithelium. Mon Bull Min Health Public Health Lab Serv 25:283-288, 1966

85. HIGGINS PG, ELLIS EM, and BOSTON DG: The isolation of viruses from acute respiratory infections. III. Some factors influencing the isolation of viruses from cases studied during 1962-64. Mon Bull Min Health Public Health Lab Serv 25:5-17, 1966

86. HIGGINS PG, ELLIS EM, and WOOLLEY DA: Viruses associated with acute respiratory infections in royal air force personnel. J Hyg 68:647-654, 1970

87. HITCHCOCK G and TYRRELL DAJ: Some virus isolations from common colds. II. Virus interference in tissue cultures. Lancet 1:237-239, 1960

88. HOBSON D and SCHILD GC: Virological studies in natural common colds in Sheffield in 1960. Br Med J 2:1414-1418, 1960

89. HOLPER JC, MILLER LF, CRAWFORD Y, SYLVESTER JC, and MARQUIS GS JR: Further studies on multiplication, serology and antigenicity of 2060 and JH viruses. J Infect Dis 107:395-401, 1960

90. HOORN B, BYNOE ML, CHAPPLE PJ, and TYRRELL DAJ: Inoculation of a novel type of rhinovirus (HS) to human volunteers. Arch Gesamte Virusforsch 18:226-230, 1966

91. HOORN B and TYRRELL DAJ: On the growth of certain "newer" respiratory viruses in organ cultures. Br J Exp Pathol 46:109-118, 1965

92. HOORN B and TYRRELL DAJ: A new virus cultivated only in organ cultures of human ciliated epithelium. Arch Gesamte Virusforsch 18:210-225, 1966

93. HORN ME, BRAIN E, and GREGG I: Respiratory viral infection in childhood. A survey in general practice, Roehampton 1967-1972. J Hyg 74:157-168, 1975

94. HUGHES JH, CHEMA S, LIN N, CONANT RM, and HAMPARIAN VV: Acid lability of rhinoviruses: loss of C and D antigenicity after treatment at pH 3.0. J Immunol 112:919-925, 1974

95. HUGHES JH, GNAU JM, HILTY MD, CHEMA S, OTTOLENGHI AC, and HAMPARIAN VV: Picornaviruses: rapid differentiation and identification by immune electromicroscopy and immunodiffusion. J Med Microbiol 10:203-212, 1977

96. HUGHES JH, THOMAS DC, and HAMPARIAN VV: Acid lability of rhinovirus type 14: effect of pH, time and temperature. Proc Soc Exp Biol Med 144:555-560, 1973

97. IDE PR and DARYBSHIRE JH: Rhinoviruses of bovine origin. Br Vet J 125:7-8, 1969

98. IDE PR and DARBYSHIRE JH: Studies with a rhinovirus of bovine origin. II. Some physical and chemical properties of strain RS 3x. Arch Gesamte Virusforsch 36:177-188, 1972

99. JOHNSON KM, BLOOM HH, CHANOCK RM, MUFSON MA, and KNIGHT V: Acute respiratory diseases of viral etiology. VI. The newer enteroviruses. Am J Public Health 52:933–940, 1962

100. Johnson KM and ROSEN L: Characteristics of five newly recognized enteroviruses recovered from the human oropharynx. Am J Hyg 77:15–25, 1963

101. KAPIKIAN AZ: Rhinoviruses *In* Diagnostic Procedures for Viral and Rickettsial Diseases 4th edition, Lennette EH and Schmidt NJ (eds), Am Public Health Assoc, Inc, New York, 1969

102. KAPIKIAN AZ, ALMEIDA JD, and STOTT EJ: Immune electron microscopy of rhinoviruses. J Virol 10:142–146, 1972

103. KAPIKIAN AZ, CONANT RM, HAMPARIAN VV, CHANOCK RM, CHAPPLE PJ, DICK EC, FENTERS JD, GWALTNEY JM JR, HAMRE D, HOLPER JC, JORDAN WS JR, LENNETTE EJ, MELNICK JL, MOGABGAB WJ, MUFSON MA, PHILLIPS CA, SCHIEBLE JH, and TYRRELL DAJ: Rhinoviruses: a numbering system. Nature 213:761–762, 1967

104. KAPIKIAN AZ, CONANT RM, HAMPARIAN VV, CHANOCK RM, DICK EC, GWALTNEY JM JR, HAMRE D, JORDAN WS JR, KENNY GE, LENNETTE EH, MELNICK JL, MOGABGAB WJ, PHILLIPS CA, SCHIEBLE JH, STOTT EJ, and TYRRELL DAJ: A collaborative report: rhinoviruses—extension of the numbering system. Virology 43:524–526, 1971

105. KAPIKIAN AZ, JAMES HD JR, KELLY SJ, DEES JH, TURNER HC, MCINTOSH K, KIM HW, PARROTT RH, VINCENT MM, and CHANOCK RM: Isolation from man of "avian infectious bronchitis virus-like" viruses (coronaviruses) similar to 229E virus, with some epidemiological observations. J Infect Dis 119:282–290, 1969

106. KAPIKIAN AZ, MUFSON MA, JAMES HD JR, KALICA AR, BLOOM HH, and CHANOCK RM: Characterization of two newly recognized rhinovirus serotypes of human origin. Proc Soc Exp Biol Med 122:1155–1162, 1966

107. KAWANA R and MATSUMOTO I: Electron microscopic study of rhinovirus replication in human fetal lung cells. Jpn J Microbiol 15:207–217, 1971

108. KENNY GE, COONEY MK, and THOMPSON DJ: Analysis of serum pooling schemes for identification of large numbers of viruses. Am J Epidemiol 91:439–445, 1970

109. KETLER A, HALL CE, FOX JP, ELVEBACK L, and COONEY MK: The virus watch program: a continuing surveillance of viral infections in metropolitan New York families. VIII. Rhinovirus infections: observations of virus excretion, intrafamilial spread and clinical response. Am J Epidemiol 90:244–254, 1969

110. KETLER A, HAMPARIAN VV, and HILLEMAN MR: Characterization and classification of ECHO 28-rhinovirus-coryzavirus agents. Proc Soc Exp Biol Med 110:821–831, 1962

111. KISCH AL, WEBB PA, and JOHNSON KM: Further properties of five newly recognized picornaviruses (rhinoviruses). Am J Hyg 79:125–133, 1964

112. KOLIAS SI and DIMMOCK NJ: Replication of rhinovirus RNA. J Gen Virol 20:1–15, 1973

113. KORANT BD, LONBERG-HOLM K, NOBLE J, and STASNY JT: Naturally occurring and artificially produced components of three rhinoviruses. Virology 48:71–86, 1972

114. KRIEL RL, WULFF H, and CHIN TDY: Microneutralization test for determination of rhinovirus and coxsackievirus A antibody in human diploid cells. Appl Microbiol 17:611–613, 1969

115. KUROGI H, INABA Y, GOTO Y, TAKAHASHI A, SATO K, OMORI T and MATUMOTO M: Isolation of rhinovirus from cattle in outbreaks of acute respiratory disease. Arch Gesamte Virusforsch 44:215–226, 1974

116. KUROGI H, INABA Y, TAKAHASHI E, SATO K, GOTO Y, and OMORI T: Serological differentiation of bovine rhinoviruses. Nat Inst Anim Health Q 15:201–202, 1975

117. LENNETTE EH and SCHIEBLE JH: (Virus submitted by).

118. LEWIS FA and KENNETT ML: Comparison of rhinovirus-sensitive HeLa cells and human embryo fibroblasts for isolation of rhinoviruses from patients with respiratory disease. J Clin Microbiol 3:528–532, 1976

119. LONBERG-HOLM K and BUTTERWORTH BE: Investigation of the structure of polio- and human rhinovirions through the use of selective chemical reactivity. Virology 71:207–216, 1976

120. LONBERG-HOLM K, CROWELL RL, and PHILIPSON L: Unrelated animal viruses share receptors. Nature 259:679–681, 1976

121. LONBERG-HOLM K and KORANT BD: Early interaction of rhinoviruses with host cells. J Virol 9:29-40, 1972

122. LONBERG-HOLM K and NOBLE-HARVEY J: Comparison of *in vitro* and cell-mediated alteration of a human rhinovirus and its inhibition by sodium dodecyl sulfate. J Virol 12:819-826, 1973

123. LONBERG-HOLM K and YIN FH: Antigenic determinants of infective and inactivated human rhinovirus type 2. J Virol 12:114-123, 1973

124. MASCOLI CC, LEAGUS MB, HILLEMAN MR, WEIBEL RE, and STOKES J JR: Rhinovirus infection in nursery and kindergarten children. new rhinovirus serotype 54. Proc Soc Exp Biol Med 124:845-850, 1967

125. MASCOLI CC, LEAGUS MB, WEIBEL RE, STOKES J JR, REINHART H, and HILLEMAN MR: Attempt at immunization by oral feeding of live rhinoviruses in enteric-coated capsules. Proc Soc Exp Biol Med 121:1264-1268, 1966

126. MAYOR HD: Picornavirus symmetry. Virology 22:156-160, 1964

127. MAYR A, WIZIGMANN G, WIZIGMANN I, and SCHLIESSER T: Untersuchungen über Infektiöse Kälbererkrankungen während der Neugeborenen-phase. Zentralbl Veterinaermed Beih 12:1-12, 1965

128. MCGREGOR S and MAYOR HD: Biophysical studies on rhinovirus and poliovirus. I. Morphology of viral ribonucleoprotein. J Virol 2:149-154, 1968

129. MCGREGOR S and MAYOR HD: Biophysical and biochemical studies on rhinovirus and poliovirus. II. Chemical and hydrodynamic analysis of the rhinovirion. J Virol 7:41-46, 1971

130. MCGREGOR S and MAYOR HD: Internal components released from rhinovirus and poliovirus by heat. J Gen Virol 10:203-207, 1971

131. MCGREGOR S, PHILLIPS CA, and MAYOR HD: Purification and biophysical properties of rhinoviruses. Proc Soc Exp Biol Med 122:118-121, 1966

132. MCINTOSH K, DEES JH, BECKER WB, KAPIKIAN AZ, and CHANOCK RM: Recovery in tracheal organ cultures of novel viruses from patients with respiratory disease. Proc Natl Acad Sci USA 57:933-940, 1967

133. MCLEAN C and RUECKERT RR: Picornaviral gene order: comparison of a rhinovirus with a cardiovirus. J Virol 11:341-344, 1973

134. MCNAMARA MJ, PHILLIPS IA, and WILLIAMS OB: Viral and *Mycoplasma pneumoniae* infections in exacerbations of chronic lung disease. Am Rev Resp Dis 100:19-24, 1969

135. MEDAPPA KC, MCLEAN C, and RUECKERT RR: On the structure of rhinovirus-1A. Virology 44:259-270, 1971

136. MEDAPPA KC and RUECKERT RR: Binding of cesium ions to human rhinovirus-14. Abstr Annu Meet Am Soc Microbiol, Abstr 207, 1974

137. MENTEL R and SCHMIDT J: Investigations on rhinovirus inactivation by hydrogen peroxide. Acta Virol 17:351-354, 1973

138. MINOR TE, BAKER JW, DICK EC, DEMEO AN, OUELLETTE JJ, COHEN M, and REED CE: Greater frequency of viral respiratory infections in asthmatic children as compared with their nonasthmatic siblings. J Pediatr 85:472-477, 1974

139. MINOR TE, DICK EC, BAKER JW, OUELLETTE JJ, COHEN M, and REED CE: Rhinovirus and influenza type A infections as precipitants of asthma. Am Rev Resp Dis 113:149-153, 1976

140. MINOR TE, DICK EC, DEMEO AN, OUELLETTE JJ, COHEN M, and REED CE: Viruses as precipitants of asthmatic attacks in children. J Am Med Assoc 227:292-298, 1974

141. MINOR TE, DICK EC, PETERSON JA, and DOCHERTY DE: Failure of naturally acquired rhinovirus infections to produce temporal immunity to heterologous serotypes. Infect Immun 10:1192-1193, 1974

142. MOGABGAB WJ: (Virus submitted by).

143. MOGABGAB WJ: 2060 virus (ECHO 28) in KB cell cultures. Characteristics, complement-fixation and antigenic relationships to some other respiroviruses. Am J Hyg 76:15-26, 1962

144. MOGABGAB WJ: Acute respiratory illnesses in university (1962-1966), military and industrial (1962-1963) populations. Am Rev Resp Dis 98:359-379, 1968

145. MOGABGAB WJ and HOLMES B: 2060 and JH viruses in secondary monkey kidney cultures. J Infect Dis 108:59-62, 1961

146. MOGABGAB WJ, HOLMES BJ, and POLLACK B: Antigenic relationships of common rhinovirus types from disabling upper respiratory illnesses. Dev Biol Stand 28:400–411, 1975

147. MOHANTY SB and LILLIE MG: Isolation of a bovine rhinovirus. Proc Soc Exp Biol Med 128:850–852, 1968

148. MONTO AS and BRYAN ER: Microneutralization test for detection of rhinovirus antibodies. Proc Soc Exp Biol Med 145:690–694, 1974

149. MONTO AS and CAVALLARO JJ: The Tecumseh study of respiratory illness. II. Patterns of occurrence of infection with respiratory pathogens, 1965-1969. Am J Epidemiol 94:280–289, 1971

150. MONTO AS and CAVALLARO JJ: The Tecumseh study of respiratory illness. IV. Prevalence of rhinovirus serotypes, 1966-1969. Am J Epidemiol 96:352–360, 1972

151. MUFSON MA, KAWANA R, JAMES HD JR, GAULD LW, BLOOM HH, and CHANOCK RM: A description of six new rhinoviruses of human origin. Am J Epidemiol 81:32–43, 1965

152. MUFSON MA, WEBB PA, KENNEDY H, GILL V, and CHANOCK RM: Etiology of upper-respiratory-tract illnesses among civilian adults. J Am Med Assoc 195:1–7, 1966

153. NAIR CN and LONBERG-HOLM KK: Infectivity and sedimentation of rhinovirus ribonucleic acid. J Virol 7:278–280, 1971

154. NEWMAN JFE, ROWLANDS DJ, and BROWN F: A physico-chemical sub-grouping of the mammalian picornaviruses. J Gen Virol 18:171–180, 1973

155. NEWMAN JFE, ROWLANDS DJ, BROWN F, GOODRIDGE D, BURROWS R, and STECK F: Physicochemical characterization of two serologically unrelated equine rhinoviruses. Intervirology 8:145–154, 1977

156. NOBLE J and LONBERG-HOLM K: Interactions of components of human rhinovirus type 2 with HeLa cells. Virology 51:270–278, 1973

157. PELON W: Classification of the '2060' virus as ECHO 28 and further study of its properties. Am J Hyg 73:36–54, 1961

158. PELON W and MOGABGAB WJ: Further studies on 2060 virus. Proc Soc Exp Biol Med 102:392–395, 1959

159. PELON W, MOGABGAB WJ, PHILLIPS IA, and PIERCE WE: Cytopathogenic agent isolated from recruits with mild respiratory illnesses. Bacteriol Proc 1956, p 67

160. PELON W, MOGABGAB WJ, PHILLIPS IA, and PIERCE WE: A cytopathogenic agent isolated from naval recruits with mild respiratory illnesses. Proc Soc Exp Biol Med 94:262–267, 1957

161. PHILLIPS CA and BORAKER DK: Preparation of rhinovirus antisera in the South American hystricomorph rodent, *Octodon degus*. Proc Soc Exp Biol Med 148:208–210, 1975

162. PHILLIPS CA, MELNICK JL, and GRIM CA: Characterization of three new rhinovirus serotypes. Proc Soc Exp Biol Med 119:798–801, 1965

163. PHILLIPS CA, MELNICK JL, and GRIM CA: Human aorta cells for isolation and propagation of rhinoviruses. Proc Soc Exp Biol Med 119:843–845, 1965

164. PHILLIPS CA, MELNICK JL, and GRIM CA: Rhinovirus infections in a student population: isolation of five new serotypes. Am J Epidemiol 87:447–456, 1968

165. PHILLIPS CA, MELNICK JL, and SULLIVAN L: Characterization of four new rhinovirus serotypes. Proc Soc Exp Biol Med 134:933–935, 1970

166. PHILLIPS CA, RIGGS S, MELNICK JL, and GRIM CA: Rhinoviruses associated with common colds in a student population. J Am Med Assoc 192:277–280, 1965

167. PLUMMER G: An equine respiratory enterovirus some biological and physical properties. Arch Gesamte Virusforsch 12:694–700, 1963

168. PRICE WH: Isolation of a new virus associated with respiratory clinical disease in humans. Proc Natl Acad Sci USA 42:892–896, 1956

169. PRICE WH, EMERSON H, IBLER I, LaCHAINE R, and TERRELL A: Studies of the JH and 2060 viruses and their relationship to mild upper respiratory disease in humans. Am J Hyg 69:224–249, 1959

170. REED SE: An investigation of the possible transmission of rhinovirus colds through indirect contact. J Hyg 75:249–258, 1975

171. REED SE and HALL TS: Hemagglutination-inhibition test in rhinovirus infections of volunteers. Infect Immunity 8:1–3, 1973

172. REED LJ and MUENCH H: A simple method of estimating fifty per cent endpoints. Am J Hyg 27:493–497, 1938

173. REED SE, TYRRELL DAJ, BETTS AO, and WATT RG: Studies on a rhinovirus (EC11) derived from a calf. I. Isolation in calf tracheal organ cultures and characterization of the virus. J Comp Path 81:33-41, 1971

174. REEVES JD and MAYOR HD: The effects of hydrogen ions on the morphology and infectivity of rhinovirions. Arch Gesamte Virusforsch 40:325-333, 1973

175. ROSENBAUM MJ, DEBERRY P, SULLIVAN EJ, PIERCE WE, MUELLER RE, and PECKINPAUGH RO: Epidemiology of the common cold in military recruits with emphasis on infections by rhinovirus types 1A, 2, and two unclassified rhinoviruses. Am J Epidemiol 93:183-193, 1971

176. ROSENQUIST BD: Rhinoviruses: isolation from cattle with acute respiratory disease. Am J Vet Res 32:685-688, 1971

177. ROWLANDS DJ, SANGAR DV, and BROWN F: Buoyant density of picornaviruses in cesium salts. J Gen Virol 13:141-152, 1971

178. RUECKERT RR: Picornaviral architecture In Comparative Virology, Academic Press, New York, 1971, pp 225-306

179. SCHAFFER RL and SCHWERDT CE: Purification and properties of poliovirus. Advan Virus Res 6:159-204, 1959

180. SCHIEBLE JH and LENNETTE EH: (Virus submitted by).

181. SCHIEBLE JH, LENNETTE EH, and FOX VL: Rhinoviruses: the isolation and characterization of three new serologic types. Proc Soc Exp Biol Med 127:324-328, 1968

182. SCHIEBLE JH, LENNETTE EH, and FOX VL: Antigenic variation of rhinovirus type 22. Proc Soc Exp Biol Med 133:329-333, 1970

183. SCHIEBLE JH, FOX VL, LESTER F, LENNETTE EH: Rhinoviruses: an antigenic study of the prototype virus strains. Proc Soc Exp Biol Med 147:541-545, 1974

184. SCHMIDT NJ, DENNIS J, FROMMHAGEN LH, and LENNETTE EH: Serologic reactivity of certain antigens obtained by fractionation of coxsackie viruses in cesium chloride density gradients. J Immunol 90:654-662, 1963

185. SETHI SK and SCHWERDT CE: Studies on the biosynthesis and characterization of rhinovirus ribonucleic acid. Virology 48:221-229, 1972

186. SHARMA R and WERNER GH: Studies on the 2060 JH viruses. I. Biological characteristics of the agents. Arch Gesamte Virusforsch 12:42-57, 1962

187. STENHOUSE AC: Rhinovirus infection in acute exacerbations of chronic bronchitis: a controlled prospective study. Br Med J 3:461-463, 1967

188. STOTT EJ, EADIE MB, and GRIST NR: Rhinovirus infections of children in hospital; isolation of three possibly new rhinovirus serotypes. Am J Epidemiol 90:45-52, 1969

189. STOTT EJ, GRIST NR, and EADIE MB: Rhinovirus infections in chronic bronchitis: isolation of eight possibly new rhinovirus serotypes. J Med Microbiol 1:109-118, 1968

190. STOTT EJ and HEATH GF: Factors affecting the growth of rhinovirus 2 in suspension cultures of L132 cells. J Gen Virol 6:15-24, 1970

191. STOTT EJ and KILLINGTON RA: Hemagglutination by rhinoviruses. Lancet 2:1369-1370, 1972

192. STOTT EJ and KILLINGTON RA: Rhinoviruses. Annu Rev Microbiol 26:503-524, 1972

193. STOTT EJ and KILLINGTON RA: The polypeptides of three rhinoviruses. J Gen Virol 18:65-68, 1973

194. STOTT EJ and TYRRELL DAJ: Some improved techniques for the study of rhinoviruses using HeLa cells. Arch Gesamte Virusforsch 23:236-244, 1968

195. STOTT EJ and WALKER M: Antigenic variation among strains of rhinovirus type 51. Nature 224:1311-1312, 1969

196. STRIZOVA V, BROWN PK, HEAD B, and REED SE: The advantages of HeLa cells for isolation of rhinoviruses. J Med Microbiol 7:433-438, 1974

197. STUDY GROUP OF PICORNAVIRIDAE: Intervirology 4:303-316, 1974

198. TAYLOR-ROBINSON D: Laboratory and volunteer studies on some viruses isolated from common colds (rhinoviruses). Am Rev Resp Dis 88:262-268, 1963

199. TAYLOR-ROBINSON D and BYNOE ML: Inoculation of volunteers with H rhinoviruses. Br Med J 1:540-544, 1964

200. TAYLOR-ROBINSON D, HUCKER R, and TYRRELL DAJ: Studies on the pathogenicity for tissue cultures of some viruses isolated from common colds. Br J Exp Pathol 43:189-193, 1962

201. TAYLOR-ROBINSON D, JOHNSON KM, BLOOM HH, PARROTT RH, MUFSON MA, and CHANOCK RM: Rhinovirus neutralizing antibody responses and their measurement. Am J Hyg 78:285–292, 1963
202. TAYLOR-ROBINSON D and TYRRELL DAJ: Serotypes of viruses (rhinoviruses) isolated from common colds. Lancet 1:452–454, 1962
203. TAYLOR-ROBINSON D and TYRRELL DAJ: Serological studies on some viruses isolated from common colds (rhinoviruses). Br J Exp Pathol 43:264–275, 1962
204. THOMAS DC, CONANT RM, and HAMPARIAN VV: Rhinovirus replication in suspension cultures of HeLa cells. Proc Soc Exp Biol Med 133:62–65, 1970
205. TYRRELL DAJ: Rhinoviruses In Monographs in Virology 2, von Herausgegeben, Gard S, Hallauer C, Meyer KF (eds), Springer, New York, 1968
206. TYRRELL DAJ and BLAMIRE CJ: Improvements in a method of growing respiratory viruses in organ cultures. Br J Exp Pathol 48:217–227, 1967
207. TYRRELL DAJ and BYNOE ML: Some further virus isolations from common colds. Br Med J 1:393–397, 1961
208. TYRRELL DAJ and BYNOE ML: Cultivation of a novel type of common-cold virus in organ cultures. Br Med J 1:1467–1470, 1965
209. TYRRELL DAJ and BYNOE ML: Cultivation of viruses from a high proportion of patients with colds. Lancet 1:76–77, 1966
210. TYRRELL DAJ, BYNOE ML, BUCKLAND FE, and HAYFLICK L: The cultivation in human-embryo cells of a virus (DC) causing colds in man. Lancet 2:320–322, 1962
211. TYRRELL DAJ, BYNOE ML, HITCHCOCK G, PEREIRA HG, and ANDREWES CH: Some virus isolations from common colds. I. Experiments employing human volunteers. Lancet 1:235–237, 1960
212. TYRRELL DAJ, BYNOE ML, and HOORN B: Cultivation of "difficult" viruses from patients with common colds. Br Med J 1:606–610, 1968
213. TYRRELL DAJ and CHANOCK RM: Rhinoviruses: a description. Science 141:152–153, 1963
214. TYRRELL DAJ, HEAD B, and DIMIC D: The titration of tuberculin, nucleic acids, acids and viruses by means of haemaggregation inhibition, using a "pattern" test. Br J Exp Pathol 48:513–521, 1967
215. TYRRELL DAJ and HOORN B: The growth of some myxoviruses in organ cultures. Br J Exp Pathol 46:514–518, 1967
216. TYRRELL DAJ and PARSONS R: Some virus isolations from common colds. III. Cytopathic effects in tissue cultures. Lancet 1:239–242, 1960
217. WEBB PA, JOHNSON KM, and MUFSON MA: A description of two newly-recognized rhinoviruses of human origin. Proc Soc Exp Biol Med 116:845–852, 1964
218. WILDY P: Classification and nomenclature of viruses In Monographs in Virology, Melnick JL (ed), Karger, Basel, 1971
219. WIZIGMANN G and SCHIEFER B: Isolierung von Rhinoviren bei Kalbern and Untersuchungen uber die Bedeutung dieser Viren fur die Entstehung von Kalbererkrankungen. Zentralbl Veterinaermed Beih 13:37–50, 1966
220. WULFF H, NOBLE GR, MAYNARD JE, FELTZ ET, POLAND JD, and CHIN TDY: An outbreak of respiratory infection in children associated with rhinovirus types 16 and 29. Am J Epidemiol 90:304–311, 1969

CHAPTER 17

REOVIRUSES

Leon Rosen

Introduction

The genus *Reovirus* is only one of several genera now included in the family *Reoviridae* (5) which, as presently constituted, also includes at least 2 other viruses affecting humans, namely, Colorado tick fever virus in the genus *Orbivirus* and the infantile gastroenteritis agent (commonly referred to as a rotavirus) not yet assigned to a genus. While reoviruses are known to replicate only in vertebrates, the family *Reoviridae* includes viruses pathogenic for plants (e.g., rice dwarf virus), others pathogenic for arthropods (e.g., cytoplamsic polyhedrosis virus of the silkworm moth), and viruses which multiply both in vertebrates and arthropods and both in plants and arthropods. This chapter deals only with reoviruses (*sensu stricto*) known to infect humans.

Serologic studies have shown that reovirus infection in humans is very common throughout the world. Moreover, reoviruses apparently identical to those recovered from humans have been isolated from an exceptionally wide variety of mammals, including wild and laboratory mice, dogs, cats, cattle, sheep, swine, horses, *Macaca* and *Cercopithecus* monkeys, and chimpanzees. Hemagglutination-inhibition (HAI) or neutralizing antibodies to reoviruses are prevalent in practically every mammalian species that has been examined. Reoviruses also have been recovered from chickens and other birds but they differ from mammalian strains.

Since reoviruses of humans and lower animals are most frequently found in the feces, it is logical to suspect that the fecal-oral route is the primary means of transmission. Transmission to or from the respiratory tract may occur, but evidence to this effect is lacking. No well-established seasonal patterns of infection have been observed, and outbreaks among humans in institutions have occurred in summer, fall, and winter. There is no good evidence that transmission occurs by arthropod vectors or by the transplacental route under natural conditions.

Reoviruses have been isolated from patients with fever, exanthems, upper and lower tract respiratory disease, gastrointestinal disease (including steatorrhea), central nervous system disease, and hepatitis, but their importance as etiologic agents of such illnesses, some of which were fatal (8, 12, 24), is still unclear. Similarly, reoviruses (mainly type 3) have

577

been isolated from tumor tissue of many patients with Burkitt tumor, but no convincing evidence has as yet been found that the association is of etiologic significance (2). Apparently, most reovirus infections are associated with either mild or no clinical manifestations.

Reoviruses have been studied more intensively by molecular biologists than by those concerned with human and animal disease. This stems from the fact that they were the first animal viruses shown to have a double-stranded RNA genome. Later this genome was shown to be segmented. The most recent general review of reoviruses covers literature to the end of 1966 (16). More current reviews are available on the molecular biology of reoviruses (21, 22).

Description and Nature of Reoviruses

Reoviruses are approximately 75 nm in diameter and have an isometric double capsid with icosahedral symmetry. They have no envelope, resist lipid solvents, are acid-stable, and contain a genome of 10 segments of doublestranded RNA with a total molecular weight of 15×10^6 daltons. Virions also contain an RNA-dependent RNA polymerase. Virus is synthesized in and matures in the cytoplasm of cells with the formation of inclusions containing virus particles in crystalline array.

Reoviruses from humans and most from lower mammals can be grouped into three serotypes designated types 1, 2, and 3 (14). Insofar as they have been tested, strains of the same serotype from various species are indistinguishable from each other (15). Two additional serotypes have been reported from cattle in Japan (13), and a virus sharing some attributes both of mammalian and of avian reoviruses has been recovered from a bat in Australia (6). With one possible exception, reoviruses isolated from birds are serologically distinct from the mammalian types.

Mice, rats, hamsters, and other laboratory animals have been used to study the pathogenesis of reovirus infection (9–11, 23), but intact animals usually are not used for virus isolation. A possible source of error when mice are used for any purpose is the presence of pre-existing reovirus infection in most colonies of laboratory mice.

Mammalian reoviruses replicate and produce cytopathic effects (CPE) in a remarkably wide variety of cell cultures—including cultures derived from domestic animals, as well as those of primate origin. The type of cell culture most widely used for recovery of reoviruses is *Macaca mulatta* (rhesus) monkey kidney cells. In addition, KB cells, HeLa cells, human fibroblasts, stable human amnion lines, primary human kidney, primary *Cercopithecus* kidney, BS-C-1 cells, and L cells, among others, have been used in experimental studies.

Preparation of Immune Serum

Type-specific immune serum can be prepared in guinea pigs, rabbits, chickens, and geese (1, 3, 14). Since the serum of mammals frequently contains HAI antibodies against one or more reovirus serotypes, pre-immunization serum should be tested against antigens of each of the three serotypes before animals are used for immune serum production.

Guinea pigs are immunized by instilling 0.1 ml of undiluted infected cell culture fluid into each nostril of an anesthetized animal. The virus content of the fluid is not critical, since reoviruses multiply in guinea pigs after intranasal inoculation. (Infected guinea pigs can transmit their infection to animals housed in the same cage.) Animals should be exsanguinated as soon as a trial bleeding indicates that a sufficiently high titer of homotypic HAI antibody ($\leq$1:160) has appeared (usually 2–3 weeks after inoculation). The final serum also must be tested to determine whether the animal has responded with a type-specific reaction. Some animals develop heterotypic antibodies. An immune serum is considered satisfactory if it has a homotypic HAI titer $\geq$1:160 and heterotypic titers <1:10. The preimmunization serum of each animal yielding a satisfactory immune serum should be preserved for reference purposes, i.e., for use in the event that equivocal results are obtained in typing an isolate with the post-immunization serum. Considerable antigenic variation has been noted among strains of type 2, and it may be necessary to prepare several immune sera for this serotype with different strains.

Chickens can be immunized by a series of 3 intramuscular inoculations of 1 ml of undiluted cell culture fluid given 1 week apart, followed by exsanguination 1 week after the last inoculation. Geese can be immunized by an initial inoculation of 10 ml of cell culture fluid intraperitoneally and 5 ml intravenously, followed by 5 ml intraperitoneally on day 15, 5 ml intravenously on day 27, 2 ml intramuscularly on day 40, and exsanguination on day 50. Domestic fowl apparently do not transmit mammalian reoviruses to one another and can be housed in the same cage. Most mammalian species will respond with heterotypic antibodies when immunized with repeated parenteral inoculations of a single reovirus serotype.

Satisfactory immune serum also can be obtained by careful selection of serum from humans or animals with naturally acquired antibodies. Individual sera are tested against antigens of each of the three serotypes until some are found which have the desired homotypic titers and do not have heterotypic titers.

Collection and Preparation of Specimens

Most reoviruses recovered in both natural and experimental infections of humans have been obtained from fecal specimens, either from stools or from rectal swabs. Isolates have also been reported from throat swabs, nasal secretions, urine, blood, cerebrospinal fluid, and various organs obtained at autopsy. Although virus excretion has been observed to continue for several weeks in some human infections, it is suggested that specimens be obtained as early as possible in the course of illness and, if possible, on several successive days.

Reoviruses can be recovered from either spontaneously passed feces or from rectal swab specimens. To collect a rectal swab specimen, a dry cotton-tipped applicator stick is inserted at least 2 inches into the anal orifice, rotated, and then withdrawn, preferably with some fecal material adhering to the cotton. Immediately after collection, the swab is swirled vigorously in 3 ml Hanks balanced salt solution (BSS) containing 500 units of penicillin and 500 μg of streptomycin/ml, until a slightly turbid solution is obtained. Before the swab is discarded, as much fluid as possible is expressed from the cotton by pressing it against the inside wall of the container above the fluid line. If spontaneously passed feces are available, the same type of suspension is prepared by selecting a small amount of feces from a moist part of the specimen with a cotton-tipped applicator stick.

The fecal suspension is stored frozen at as low a temperature as is available. If it is to be used immediately, it is frozen and thawed once. To eliminate as many bacteria as possible, the suspension is centrifuged at approximately 2000 $\times$ g at 4 C for 30 min before use in a virus isolation procedure. The supernatant fluid, withdrawn carefully with a capillary pipette, is used as the inoculum.

Throat and nasal swabs are collected and processed by methods similar to those used for fecal specimens. Tissues removed aseptically by biopsy or at autopsy are triturated in Hanks BSS, and the supernatant fluid used as an inoculum. Reoviruses have been recovered from tissue fragments maintained in explant or Maitland-type cultures when the same specimens failed to yield the virus by direct inoculation of cell cultures (2).

Laboratory Diagnosis

Virus isolation

Host systems. Primary *Macaca* kidney cell cultures are satisfactory for routine isolation, but primary human kidney should be used in critical work when it is desired that the possibility of latent reovirus infection in the cells themselves be excluded. Reovirus type 1 has been recovered frequently from uninoculated simian kidney cell cultures maintained for long periods of time. However, pre-existing reovirus infection has not been encountered when *Macaca* kidney cells have been used as described below, nor has reovirus been recovered from uninoculated human kidney cell cultures, even when the latter have been maintained for long periods of time.

Conditions of incubation. Tube cultures of primary kidney cells are used when a confluent monolayer of cells has appeared. It is important that the cultures be washed free from serum before use, since it is likely that any mammalian serum present in the growth medium contains antibodies to one or more reovirus serotypes. Washing is accomplished by replacing the growth medium with 3 successive changes of 1 ml of Hanks BSS containing 100 units of penicillin and 100 μg of streptomycin/ml. After the last change, 1 ml of medium No. 199 or other suitable serum-free medium with the same concentration of antibiotics may be added as a maintenance medium.

The specimen is then inoculated into 1 or more culture tubes in 0.1 ml amounts. Tubes are incubated at 36–37 C and are observed microscopically every 2 or 3 days for 21 days. At the end of this time interval, 0.1 ml of the supernatant fluid of each tube is passed to a fresh culture tube which has been prepared in the same manner as the original tube. The passage tubes are incubated and observed for 7 days. Maintenance fluid is not changed on either the original or the passage tube, and the isolation tubes are ordinarily kept for 21 days, even though the cell sheet may have degenerated before then. However, if it appears from microscopic examination that cell degeneration is due to bacterial or fungal contamination, the isolation attempt is considered unsatisfactory.

Recognition of infection. Reoviruses usually can be distinguished from other viruses that are encountered in human fecal specimens by the nature of their CPE in unstained *Macaca* kidney cultures. The cells become granular and do not slough off the glass as readily as do cells affected by most enteroviruses. Often they remain fastened to the glass by a single process and flutter in the medium as the tube is agitated during microscopic examination. The typical effect is often confused by inexperienced personnel with nonspecific cellular degeneration. Doubtful cases can be resolved by additional cell culture passages and one can gain experience by observing the effect of various dilutions of a known reovirus in *Macaca* kidney cultures of good quality.

Reoviruses also can be recognized by the cytoplasmic inclusions visible by conventional microscopy in stained preparations of infected cell cultures and by their intra- or extracellular morphology when examined by electron microscopy.

Identification of isolates

Reoviruses usually are identified as to serotype by HAI techniques. All isolates so far described have the property of agglutinating human erythrocytes (RBC), although this phenomenon is sometimes difficult to demonstrate with strains of type 3. Isolates are tested for the presence and titer of hemagglutinin as follows.

Titration of hemagglutinin. Human type O RBC are collected in Alsever solution, by addition of 10–20 ml of blood to 50 ml of the solution. The cells are then washed 3 times in dextrose-gelatin-Veronal (DGV) solution and can be stored as a 10% suspension in this solution for at least 1 week. If the RBC are to be used within 24 hr after collection, they can be washed and stored temporarily in 0.85% NaCl.

To minimize variation in the number of RBC employed in titrations of hemagglutinin and in HAI tests, the concentration of cells is standardized by means of a spectrophotometer. The standard value is determined by allowing 0.2 ml amounts of various concentrations of human RBC in 0.85% NaCl to settle at room temperature in test tubes (12-mm $\times$ 75-mm) with hemispherical bottoms. The lowest concentration of cells producing a solid button of cells after complete sedimentation is chosen as the standard. The optical density of this test preparation is determined at a wave-length of 490 nm on a spectrophotometer, and thereafter all RBC suspensions are made up to this value. A simpler, but less satisfactory, technique is to prepare a 0.75% suspension of RBC in 0.85% NaCl based on the packed-cell volume.

Supernatant fluid from infected tube cultures is tested for hemagglutination after the cell sheets have been completely destroyed by the virus and after the cultures have been frozen and thawed once. Fluid from 2 or more culture tubes is usually pooled (before testing) so that there is enough hemagglutinin to complete the identification procedure. Serial 2-fold dilutions of the fluid are prepared in 0.85% NaCl in 12-mm × 75-mm test tubes. Dilutions should range between 1:2 and 1:1024, and each tube should contain 0.4 ml. The standard RBC suspension is then added in 0.2 ml amounts. The tubes are shaken and the RBC are allowed to settle at room temperature. The highest dilution of cell culture fluid which shows a 1+ pattern of sedimentation (4) is taken as the endpoint, and this tube is considered to contain 1 unit of hemagglutinin.

It is usually possible to demonstrate agglutination of human RBC by strains of reovirus types 1 and 2 in any passage fluid from *Macaca* kidney cultures. Strains of type 3 sometimes have low titers or give negative results when first tested. Thus far, it has always been possible to obtain titers of hemagglutinin sufficiently high (20 units per ml) for purposes of identification for all strains of type 3 by testing additional passage levels. Hemagglutinin titers of type 3 strains are not necessarily increased with continued cell culture passage. Rather, it appears, for reasons unknown, that the multiplication of virus in one lot of cell cultures simply results in the production of a higher titer of hemagglutinin than does multiplication in another, grossly similar, lot of cultures.

Hemagglutination-inhibition test. The HAI test for typing isolates is carried out as follows. The typing serum is adsorbed with kaolin by mixing a 1:5 dilution of serum in 0.85% NaCl with an equal volume of a 25% suspension of acid-washed kaolin in 0.85% NaCl (25 g of kaolin + 100 ml of saline solution) and allowing the mixture to stand for 20 min at room temperature. The mixture is then centrifuged briefly to sediment the kaolin, and supernatant fluid is considered a 1:10 dilution of serum. After this treatment, the serum is adsorbed with human type O RBC to remove any agglutinins for this type of cell which might be present. This is done by adding 0.1 ml of a 50% suspension of RBC to each 1.0 ml of the 1:10 dilution of serum and allowing the mixture to stand for 1 hr at approximately 4 C. The supernatant fluid is then withdrawn and is ready for use. The serum is not inactivated.

It is known that kaolin removes some antibody from serum, and alternative methods of removing nonspecific serum inhibitors have been proposed. However, the other methods are more complicated, and it has not been demonstrated that they offer any advantages from a practical point of view.

The HAI test is set up by adding 0.2 ml amounts of hemagglutinin diluted in 0.85% NaCl to contain 20 units/ml (4 units/0.2 ml) to 0.2 ml of serial 2-fold dilutions of serum in 0.85% NaCl. Each serum is used from a dilution of 1:10 to, or beyond, its endpoint. The mixtures are shaken briefly and are then allowed to stand for 1 hr at room temperature before the addition of 0.2

ml amounts of standard RBC suspension. The RBC are allowed to settle at room temperature, and the titer of a serum is taken as that dilution which completely inhibits agglutination. The lowest dilution of each serum used is tested for the presence of RBC agglutinins by substituting 0.2 ml of saline solution for the antigen. An antigen titration is also included in the test.

There is also available a simple micromethod for conducting the HAI test; a detailed procedure has been published by Schmidt (20).

An isolate is considered typed if it is inhibited at a titer of at least 1:40 by one of the typing antisera, and not at a dilution of 1:10 by the others. Because of the antigenic heterogeneity of type 2 strains (7), it may sometimes be necessary to prepare an antiserum against the isolated strain to demonstrate a relationship to this serotype.

Serologic diagnosis

Most diagnostic serology of reovirus infections has been done with the HAI test. Not only is this procedure simpler in general than either the neutralization (Nt) test or the complement fixation (CF) test, but the latter two procedures are also less satisfactory for diagnostic purposes in reovirus infections for the following reasons. In the Nt test, a relatively large amount of test virus is required to obtain a CPE before the cell cultures degenerate spontaneously. Consequently, small amounts of antibody are difficult to detect. In the CF test, it is difficult or impossible to detect CF antibodies in the convalescent-phase serum of many infected individuals. In other words, both tests are less sensitive than the HAI test. When CF antibodies are present, they apparently are group-specific rather than type-specific.

It has been possible to demonstrate a 4-fold rise in homologous HAI antibody in practically all natural or experimental reovirus infections which have been observed in humans. Individuals infected with reovirus type 3 almost invariably show only a homotypic HAI response, whereas those infected with types 1 or 2 often develop heterotypic antibody also (17–19). The heterotypic titers are usually, but not always, lower than the homotypic titers.

HAI antibodies are present 21 days after the experimental infection of humans, but may appear earlier. Ordinarily they can be detected for at least 1 year after natural infection, and they probably persist for much longer periods of time. Since reovirus antibodies are very common in human serum, it is essential that paired sera be employed for diagnostic purposes. A 4-fold rise in titer is considered a positive result.

HAI tests are carried out by a technique similar to that already described for typing reovirus isolates. The test antigens are prepared with representative strains or with homotypic strains in the manner described previously. All sera are adsorbed with kaolin, but it is usually not necessary to adsorb human serum with human type O RBC.

Paired sera are always run in the same test and are usually titrated in 2-fold dilutions from 1:10 through 1:320 against 4 units of hemagglutinin of each of the three serotypes. Because of the antigenic heterogeneity of type 2 strains, it may be necessary to use more than one antigen of this type. If available, an antigen prepared from a strain isolated from the patient would be the most satisfactory in type 2 infections. This procedure has not been found necessary for types 1 and 3.

References

1. BEHBEHANI AM, FOSTER LC, and WENNER HA: Preparation of typespecific antisera to reoviruses. Appl Microbiol 14:1051-1053, 1966
2. BELL TM: Viruses associated with Burkitt's tumor. Prog Med Virol 9:1-34, 1967
3. BRUGGEMAN CAMVA and VERSTEEG J: Studies on reovirus-antigens. I. Preparation of reovirus-specific immune serum in the rabbit by means of active immunization through the scarified skin. Arch Gesamte Virusforsch 42:371-377, 1973
4. CHANOCK RM and SABIN AB: The hemagglutinin of St. Louis encephalitis virus. I. Recovery of stable hemagglutinin from the brains of infected mice. J Immunol 70:271-285, 1953
5. FENNER F: Classification and nomenclature of viruses. Intervirology 7:1-115, 1976
6. GARD GP and MARSHALL ID: Nelson Bay virus. A novel reovirus. Arch Gesamte Virusforsch 43:34-42, 1973
7. HARTLEY JW, ROWE WP, and AUSTIN JB: Subtype differentiation of reovirus type 2 strains by hemagglutination-inhibition with mouse antisera. Virology 16:94-96, 1962
8. JOSKE RA, KEALL DD, LEAK PJ, STANLEY NF, and WALTERS MNI: Hepatitis-encephalitis in humans with reovirus infection. Arch Intern Med 113:811-816, 1964
9. KILHAM L and MARGOLIS G: Hydrocephalus in hamsters, ferrets, rats, and mice following inoculations with reovirus type I. I. Virologic studies. Lab Invest 21:183-188, 1969
10. KILHAM L and MARGOLIS G: Pathogenesis of intrauterine infections in rats due to reovirus type 3. I. Virologic studies. Lab Invest 28:597-604, 1973
11. KILHAM L and MARGOLIS G: Congenital infections due to reovirus type 3 in hamsters. Teratology 9:51-64, 1974
12. KRAINER L and ARONSON BE: Disseminated encephalomyelitis in the human with recovery of hepatoencephalitis virus (HEV); pathologic and virologic report. J Neuropathol Exp Neurol 18:339-342, 1959
13. KUROGI H, INABA Y, TAKAHASHI E, SATO K, GOTO Y, OMORI T, and MATUMOTO M: New serotypes of reoviruses isolated from cattle. Brief report. Arch Gesamte Virusforsch 45:157-160, 1974
14. ROSEN L: Serologic grouping of reoviruses by hemagglutination-inhibition. Am J Hyg 71:242-249, 1960
15. ROSEN L: Reoviruses in animals other than man. Ann NY Acad Sci 101:461-465, 1962
16. ROSEN L: Reoviruses In Virology Monographs 1, Springer-Verlag, Vienna-New York, 1968, pp 73-107
17. ROSEN L, EVANS HE, and SPICKARD A: Reovirus infections in human volunteers. Am J Hyg 77:29-37, 1963
18. ROSEN L, HOVIS JF, MASTROTA FM, BELL JA, and HUEBNER RJ: Observations on a newly recognized virus (Abney) of the reovirus family. Am J Hyg 71:258-265, 1960
19. ROSEN L, HOVIS JF, MASTROTA FM, BELL JA, and HUEBNER RJ: An outbreak of infection with a type 1 reovirus among children in an institution. Am J Hyg 71:266-274, 1960
20. SCHMIDT NJ: Antibody assays for enteroviruses and reoviruses In Manual of Clinical Immunology, Rose NR and Friedman H (eds), Am Soc Microbiol, Washington DC, 1976
21. SHATKIN AJ: Viruses with segmented ribonucleic acid genomes: multiplication of influenza versus reovirus. Bacteriol Rev 35:250-266, 1971
22. SILVERSTEIN SC, CHRISTMAN JK, and ACS G: The reovirus replicative cycle. Annu Rev Biochem 45:375-408, 1976
23. STANLEY NF: The reovirus murine models. Prog Med Virol 18:257-272, 1974
24. TILLOTSON JR and LERNER AM: Reovirus type 3 associated with fatal pneumonia. N Engl J Med 276:1060-1063, 1967

CHAPTER 18

INFLUENZA VIRUSES

Walter A. Dowdle, Alan P. Kendal, and Gary R. Noble

Introduction

Influenza is an acute infectious respiratory disease of humans caused by influenza virus types A and B. The disease usually occurs in epidemic form with abrupt onset and rapid spread over a geographic region. The extent may range from small focal outbreaks to worldwide epidemics or pandemics. A third influenza virus, type C, causes a mild common cold-like or subclinical illness (33, 77), and epidemics have not been documented. On epidemiologic grounds, at least 10 global influenza epidemics (pandemics) have occurred during the past 200 years. The first type A virus from humans was isolated in 1933 (75), and the first type B, in 1940 (23). Serologic evidence suggests that the pandemics near the turn of the century and in 1918 were also caused by type A viruses (11, 25, 51). In temperate zones influenza epidemics of either type occur mainly from late fall until spring, but in tropical areas the season of prevalence is less well defined. Influenza outbreaks occur somewhere in the world most of the year, alternating between the Northern and Southern Hemispheres.

Epidemics of influenza A viruses are a veterinary, as well as a public health, problem. Type A strains are found in horses, pigs, and many species of birds, both wild and domestic. Types B and C virus have been isolated only from humans. Unpredictable antigenic mutability of influenza A and B viruses and the theoretical possibility that type A viruses may emerge in some form from animal reservoirs have made laboratory surveillance of these viruses an important component of early warning and defense against epidemic influenza.

For further information on influenza and influenza viruses, two recent monographs (38, 76) and an earlier historical review are available (30).

Clinical

Influenza is transmitted through inhalation of virus-containing droplets expelled from the respiratory tract of symptomatic or asymptomatic individuals. Crowding and environmental conditions during winter may enhance transmission. The incubation period is dose dependent and may vary from 1 to 4 days, but it is usually about 2 days. Influenza virus multiplies in the ciliated columnar epithelium of the upper and lower respiratory tract, causing cell necrosis and sloughing. The greatest period of viral shedding occurs from 1 day before to 3–4 days after the onset of illness. Reduced quantities of virus may be shed for 1 week or more.

Influenza infections may cause no recognized illness in up to half of the individuals infected, but in the remainder it may produce symptoms ranging from a minor respiratory illness to fatal viral pneumonia. Malaise, fever, and a mild sore throat or dry cough are typical during the first 2–4 days of illness. A systemic febrile respiratory disease affecting family members of all ages should suggest influenza A or B infection.

Acute influenza virus pneumonia may rapidly lead to alveolar fluid accumulation, hypoxia, and death. Bacterial pneumonia may follow influenza infection, particularly in the elderly and in those with compromised function of the lungs, heart, kidney, or endocrine system. A number of non-respiratory complications may rarely occur: polyneuritis, encephalopathy, and inflammation of cardiac and skeletal muscles. Reye syndrome, characterized by noninflammatory encephalopathy, fatty infiltration of abdominal viscera, and elevated serum transaminase and ammonia concentrations may occur after influenza B infection (8) and, less commonly, after influenza A infections (65). Additional references to clinical manifestations of influenza may also be found in Dowdle et al (19).

Pathology

In uncomplicated influenza, patchy desquamation may occur in the ciliated columnar epithelium of the respiratory tract. In influenza pneumonia, virus is found in the epithelial cells of the distal bronchioles and alveoli, which may be lined with a hyaline membrane; the air spaces are filled with fluid, erythrocytes (RBC), and leukocytes. Submucosal capillaries and lymphatics may become distended, with accumulation of interstitial fluid and lymphocytes (54).

Description and Nature of the Agents

Common characteristics

Influenza viruses contain a segmented single-strand RNA genome, enclosed within a viral modified host-cell membrane. The virion RNA has been shown to contain 8 segments (60, 63): the largest 3 RNA segments contain the genetic code for the polypeptides (P_1, P_2, and P_3), believed to be required for virus-specific RNA-dependent RNA polymerase activity; the 3 intermediate-sized segments of the viral genome contain the code for hemagglutinin, nucleoprotein (NP), and neuraminidase (NA) polypeptides; and the 2 smallest RNA segments contain the code for an internal structural virion protein (M protein) and a nonstructural (NS) polypeptide found only in virus-infected cells (12). Influenza B viruses probably resemble influenza A in these general properties. Precise information is lacking about the total number of genes in influenza C viruses or their coding assignments. Although influenza C contains hemagglutination (HA) and receptor-destroying activities, these do not appear to have the chemical specificity for sialic acid-containing substrates demonstrated for influenza A and B (34).

Size and shape

All influenza viruses are pleomorphic. Virions are generally spherical, with an approximate diameter of 100 nm, or filamentous, with a total length of several microns. The greatest degree of pleomorphism and aggregation is usually found with newly isolated viruses grown in eggs. Surface projections about 8–10 nm long and spaced at 8-nm intervals may usually be observed in influenza viruses examined by negative-staining techniques. Influenza C viruses may, in addition, possess a reticular structure on the surface, although this may not be reliably observed on newly isolated virions (50). The available evidence suggests that influenza A and B nucleocapsids may be packaged as a large coil about 50 nm in diameter and of variable length (1).

Chemical composition

Virions are composed of about 70–75% protein, 20–24% lipid, 5% carbohydrate, and 1% RNA (24). Carbohydrate and lipids are largely host specified, but sialic acid is absent in influenza A and B viruses because of the activity of NA (40).

Resistance to inactivation

Influenza virus infectivity may be destroyed by heating to 56 C, treatment with lipid solvents, acid, formaldehyde, beta-propiolactone, or irradiation with ultraviolet light. Infectivity is lost on repeated freezing and thawing or storage in standard −20 C freezers. Infectious virus can be preserved by lyophilization with 0.5% gelatin and maintenance at 4 C or by freezing of liquid suspensions to −60 C or colder in the presence of at least 1% protein stabilizer.

Classification

The family *Orthomyxoviridae* contains the genus *Influenzavirus* (which includes influenza types A and B) and a probable genus (with no approved name) for influenza C. The World Health Organization (WHO) provides rules for nomenclature (80) and periodically updates them on the basis of new information. Influenza virus nomenclature is based on antigenic type and epidemiologic information, including host of origin and place and year of isolation. For influenza A viruses, an antigenic description follows the strain designation and indicates the antigenic character of the hemagglutinin and NA subtypes. For example, prototype strains for the 4 human hemagglutinin subtypes are A/Puerto Rico/8/34(H0N1), A/Fort Monmouth/1/47(H1N1), A/Singapore/1/57(H2N2), and A/Hong Kong/1/68(H3N2). An additional 11 different hemagglutinin subtypes and 7 different NA subtypes are recognized among type A viruses isolated from horses, pigs, and birds. These are designated by host of origin, such as A/equine/Prague/1/56(Heq1Neq1) and A/tern/South Africa/61(Hav1Nav2). Certain hemagglutinin and NA subtypes are shared by strains isolated from different species. Each hemagglutinin and NA subtype may encompass strains exhibiting a considerable degree of antigenic heterogeneity. For example, A/Hong Kong/8/68 and A/Victoria/3/75 cross-react by immunodiffusion and are both considered as H3N2 strains, yet they may be readily differentiated by hemagglutination-inhibition (HAI) and neuraminidase-inhibition (NI) tests. Thus, the provision for full names for each strain permits the designation of selected strains as representative of antigenic groupings within a subtype.

Antigenic composition

Type-specific antigens. The NP (31) or "soluble" antigen of influenza viruses is type-specific for influenza A, B, or C viruses (59). The M (membrane or matrix) protein associated with the inner structure of virion envelopes is also type-specific (68).

Strain-specific antigens. Antigenic variation in influenza viruses occurs primarily in the surface antigens of virions, originally designated the "V" antigen (30). This variation is mediated by multiple determinants in the hemagglutinin and NA, which are independent antigens (72, 75). The degree of variation in influenza B strains is less than that in influenza A strains, and antigenic variation in influenza C viruses has been studied for only a few isolates (59). Abrupt change in the antigenic composition of influenza A viruses is called "antigenic shift," and in the case of the hemagglutinin, is usually associated with worldwide epidemics, such as in 1957 with the Asian (H2) and in 1968 with the Hong Kong (H3) viruses. More gradual changes in the antigens within a subgroup are described as "antigenic drift," which may or may not be associated with epidemics. The 4 main subgroups of hemagglutinins, described above for human influenza A isolates, do not necessarily represent antigenic shifts. Some antigenic determinants are shared by Hsw1, H0, and H1 strains, which can be recognized by cross-reactivity in HAI tests and immunologic priming studies (10, 14). H2 and H3 strains each appear to represent more distinct antigenic subgroups with less evidence of shared determinants (72). The 2 main subgroups of NA antigens (N1 and N2) of human influenza A isolates are not antigenically related (78).

Viruses possessing Hsw1N1 antigens (swine influenza virus) are believed, for seroepidemiologic reasons, to have infected humans from about 1918 to 1930 (9, 35); they have also been shown to have caused occasional infections in humans, but with limited transmission, in 1974, 1975, and 1976 (18, 28). The initial source of the recent Hsw1N1 viruses that have infected humans is believed to be infected pigs. Other animal influenza viruses are known to exist with hemagglutinin and/or NA antigens related to those of human strains. Even though contemporary influenza B strains diverge considerably from the prototype strain (B/Lee/40), strains from intermediate years cross-react with earlier and later isolates. All influenza C viruses isolated thus far cross-react to a considerable extent in HAI tests.

Other antigens. Influenza viruses grown in eggs contain host carbohydrate antigens (29). In some circumstances, antibodies to egg host antigens can result in cross-reactivity between unrelated strains. The nonstructural protein synthesized in influenza-infected cells and the viral RNA polymerase have not been studied for type or strain specificity.

Host range in animals

The developing chick embryo is the simplest and most widely used animal host system for the growth of influenza viruses. Ferrets are useful for some experimental purposes because they can be readily infected by intranasal instillation of clinical material (75) or laboratory-grown virus. The illness produced in ferrets by influenza A viruses is typical of the human disease. Influenza types B and C can also infect ferrets, but in contrast to types A and B, influenza C virus has not been recovered from lungs, only from nasal turbinates.

Influenza A and B viruses initially replicate poorly in mice, but on sequential passage with use of mouse lung suspensions at 2- to 3-day intervals, adapted viruses are selected that cause severe lung lesions and death. Influenza C virus has not been adapted to growth in mouse lung. Hamsters and guinea pigs are also susceptible to experimental infection with adapted strains of influenza.

Influenza A (but not types B or C) viruses in nature may also have as their normal host avian, equine, or porcine species (59). Several investigators (4) have observed naturally occurring infection of swine with human H3N2 influenza strains (43), and evidence has been recently obtained that viruses similar to human H3N2 strains may on occasion infect various animals, including primates, cows, and chickens.

As more studies of the antigenic relationships between influenza viruses are done, more cross-reactions are found between isolates from different species, suggesting that viruses in different ecologic systems may independently evolve antigens having common structures, or that mixed infections of an animal can occur with two viruses that result in the production of a virus deriving host-range genes from one parent and genes specifying hemagglutinin and/or NA antigens from the other parent.

Growth in tissue culture

Influenza A and B viruses have been propagated in primary chick embryo fibroblasts, in kidney or lung cells from embryonic chickens, and in human tissue, hamster kidney, porcine kidney, and calf kidney cells, but the most widely used cells for isolation purposes are primary rhesus monkey kidney (PRMK) cells. Recent studies have shown that the host range of influenza viruses may be increased by growing the viruses in the presence of a suitable concentration of a proteolytic enzyme, usually trypsin (3, 39, 41, 44).

In this way, many influenza viruses have been grown in primary chick embryo fibroblast cells, as well as in two cell lines, MDBK and MDCK, all of which cells are refractory to replication of most influenza strains in the absence of proteolytic enzymes. The possibility of using this technique for the isolation of viruses from clinical specimens needs to be further evaluated.

Preparation of Immune Serum for Identification of Viruses

Strain-specific antiserum

Strain-specific antiserum for use in the HAI test in the diagnostic laboratory can be prepared in chickens by iv inoculation of 5 ml of allantoic fluid containing a minimum of 160 HA units (HAU)/ml (57). Animals are exsanguinated 9–10 days later. Antibody titers of ≥ 160 against the homologous antigens are desirable (57).

For more definitive characterization of antigenic relationships, strain-specific antiserum produced in ferrets is recommended. Ferrets are infected by intranasal instillation of 1 ml of allantoic or amniotic fluid containing at least 10^4 infectious virus particles. Animals are bled 14 days after being immunized. Ferrets are highly susceptible to infection with influenza A and influenza B viruses and must be kept isolated during immunization. Pre-immunization serum should also be tested to rule out natural infection. Both of the above procedures have the advantage that antibodies will not be produced to host (egg) components as may occur if goats or rabbits are immunized.

Type-specific antiserum

Antiserum for use in the complement fixation (CF) test can be prepared in guinea pigs. Animals should be bled before immunization, and the serum tested to determine absence of antibody to the parainfluenza viruses. The animals under light ether anesthesia are then inoculated intranasally with 0.5 ml of allantoic fluid containing 10^5–10^6 infectious virus particles (EID_{50}). Generally, the initial antibody-evoking strain is chosen from prototype strains least likely to be encountered in typing unknown human viruses, i.e., a strain dissimilar from contemporary strains of influenza and B/Lee/40 for type B. Five weeks later the low concentration of type-specific antibody is boosted by simultaneous intraabdominal injection of 1 ml of purified NP antigen and im injection of 2.5 ml of an emulsion containing equal quantities of concentrated antigen and Freund complete adjuvant. The NP antigen is prepared by ether treatment of the intact virus, which releases the internal antigen (46), or by isoelectric precipitation from tissue culture harvests (64). The choice of a strain for production of the NP antigen is not critical since most hemagglutinin and NA antigens should have been removed by RBC adsorption in the process of purifying the NP antigen. Goats are exsanguinated 7–10 days after the booster injection. Antibody titers should be determined by block titration (61) with soluble type A and B antigens (see section below) of known titer, with controls prepared in the same manner.

Matrix protein antiserum for typing viruses by the immunodiffusion test is prepared by injecting rabbits or goats with purified M antigen from an influenza A or B strain. Goats are initially injected in both thighs and the tail with 1000 μg of M protein mixed with Freund complete adjuvant. Thirty days later, 300 μg of aqueous antigen is given iv, and an equal amount of antigen mixed with adjuvant is injected into the thigh. The animal may be bled 7 days later (57). Purified M protein can be prepared by electrophoresis of detergent-disrupted virus on cellulose acetate membrane (68).

Collection and Preparation of Specimens for Laboratory Diagnosis

Precautions

No special precautions are required for collecting respiratory specimens from patients, although health personnel may benefit from influenza immunization.

Virus isolation. Best results are obtained when cultures are taken within the first 3 days of illness. A swab culture of the throat and nasal passage is the most practical method of collecting the specimen for influenza virus isolation, although larger quantities of virus and higher isolation rates are obtained from nasal washings. The specimens are obtained as follows. The pharynx is vigorously swabbed with a cotton-tipped applicator, the secretions are eluted from the cotton, and the applicator stick is broken off in a vial of transport medium. A wire nasopharyngeal swab is passed into the nostril parallel with the palate and gently rotated; the secretions are then eluted from the swab in the same vial of transport medium containing the throat swab. A suitable transport medium is approximately 5 ml of either tryptose phosphate broth (pH 7.0-7.2) or veal infusion broth, each containing 0.5% gelatin. Nasal washes are collected by instilling 5 ml of saline alternately in each nostril while the patient sits with head tipped back and closes the airway by beginning to say "car."

Specimens should be transported to the laboratory on wet ice and maintained at 4 C before being inoculated into eggs or tissue culture (5). If they cannot be inoculated within 3-4 days, specimens should be rapidly frozen to −70 C soon after being collected and maintained in a mechanical freezer or on dry ice. Vials should be tightly sealed to prevent entry of CO_2, which might inactivate the virus. Before the embryonated eggs or tissue cultures are inoculated, a 10X solution of antibiotics is added to the vials to yield a final concentration of 800 units of penicillin and 400 μg of streptomycin sulfate per ml. Before the nasal washes are inoculated, specimens are agitated and then centrifuged at 4 C for 15 min at 1500 × g to remove particulate debris and bacteria.

Postmortem specimens from the respiratory tract should be obtained as soon after death as possible to avoid loss of virus viability and excessive bacterial growth. Swab cultures, secretions, or blocks of tissue 1 cm^3 should be collected aseptically from areas of the respiratory tract lined with ciliated epithelium. In patients with acute fatal viral pneumonia, involved portions of the peripheral lung should also be collected. In patients who died of Reye syndrome, virus isolation may be attempted from muscle and other involved organs, although better isolation rates are obtained from the respiratory tract early in the illness (48, 58).

Serologic diagnosis. An acute-phase serum specimen should be collected within 7 days after onset of illness, and a convalescent-phase serum specimen should be collected between the fourteenth and twenty-first days after the onset of illness. From 1 to 5 ml of serum should be removed aseptically from clotted blood and placed in a tightly closed screw-cap vial, and both early and late serum specimens sent together to the laboratory. Serum specimens may be stored frozen below -20 C or unfrozen at 4 C. Shipping serum frozen on dry ice reduces leakage and the risk of bacterial growth. When long-distance shipping without refrigeration is required, sodium azide may be added to a final concentration of 0.1% to prevent bacterial growth.

Light microscopy. Examination of tissue specimens by light microscopy provides no virus-specific diagnostic information. A needle biopsy of the liver may be useful in establishing a diagnosis of Reye syndrome, but the changes observed by light microscopy do not establish a specific viral etiology.

Electron microscopy. The demonstration of influenza virus in respiratory secretions by electron microscopy (EM) has been reported (32), although other respiratory viruses are more commonly detected by EM in cells of the respiratory tract (13).

Immunofluorescence examination. Secretions containing respiratory epithelial cells may be aspirated from the nasopharynx through the nose with a fine plastic catheter connected to a mucus trap and a suction machine. Cells are sedimented by centrifugation at 1500 rpm for 10 min at 4 C and suspended in phosphate-buffered saline (PBS) by gentle pipetting. Visible mucus is removed, and the cells are again sedimented by centrifugation. The cells are resuspended and placed on chemically clean glass slides, allowed to dry, and fixed in acetone at 4 C for 10 min.

If a suction machine is not available, cells may be obtained with pharyngeal and nasal swabs. The pharynx is swabbed vigorously until the patient coughs or gags, and with a second swab the nasal mucosa is rubbed thoroughly; both swabs are broken off and placed in a single vial of transport medium. Cells are removed from the cotton by pipetting the transport medium over the swabs, the cell suspension is centrifuged, and smears are prepared as above. Tracheal and bronchial secretions obtained at autopsy may be similarly processed. Frozen sections of lung tissue may also be examined by immunofluorescent staining. Immunofluorescence techniques have been described in detail by Gardner and McQuillan (27).

Laboratory Diagnosis

Direct examination of clinical material

Fluorescent-antibody (FA) staining of respiratory epithelial cells, first demonstrated by Liu (49), is the only method of direct examination to gain general acceptance for documenting influenza infection. The examination of intact cells that are free of mucus and present in sufficient numbers has shown a high correlation between FA staining and virus isolation (37). Discrete, specific staining is visible in the cytoplasm or the nucleus, depending on the stage of viral infection in each cell. Nonspecific staining may occur in degenerating cells collected late in the illness or in specimens allowed to deteriorate after collection. Failure to obtain bright fluorescence may also result from the use of antiserum prepared against the surface proteins of strains that are antigenically distinct from new pandemic strains. Conversely, the use of antiserum raised against the internal NP or M proteins common to either influenza A or B will not distinguish the appearance of antigenically novel strains. The use of rapid methods of influenza diagnosis for hospitalized patients may allow infected patients to be segregated from high-risk patients or newborn nurseries, thus potentially decreasing nosocomial infections (26).

Virus isolation

In general, influenza A viruses are reliably isolated in eggs and usually can be isolated in PRMK cells (see schema). In some instances, swine influenza-like viruses that infect humans may also be isolated in PRMK cells (74). PRMK cells often are better than eggs for growth of influenza B viruses. The ability of different isolates of types A and B influenza to grow in the egg or PRMK cells is variable, emphasizing the advisability of using both host systems when maximal isolation rates are required. Influenza C viruses have been isolated only in eggs.

Embryonated eggs. Embryonated white-leghorn eggs, incubated for 10–11 days, are optimal for isolation of influenza A and B viruses. Eggs 7–8 days old (which may be incubated for 5 rather than 2–3 days after infection) may be best for isolation of influenza C viruses, but in many instances influenza C viruses have been isolated under conditions similar to those used for influenza A and B strains. Eggs are candled to verify the presence of a live embryo.

To inject the sample, a syringe with a 23-gauge 1.5-inch needle is used. The needle is gently pushed through a hole in the air-sac end of the shell into the allantoic cavity and then, with a short, stabbing motion, is inserted into the amniotic sac. If the needle is correctly inserted, it will be capable of moving the embryo. Between 0.1 and 0.2 ml of specimen is inoculated. As the needle is withdrawn from the amnion, a further 0.1–0.2 ml of specimen is inoculated into the allantoic cavity. The hole in the shell may be sealed with a rapidly drying glue, collodion, or molten wax. Usually, three eggs are inoculated per specimen, and the eggs are incubated at 33–34 C for 2–3 days (virus may sometimes be detected within 1 day).

In harvesting fluids, eggs are chilled (overnight at 4 C, or for 30 min at −20 C and then for several hr at 4 C) to minimize bleeding. After the area over the air sac is swabbed with 70% alcohol, the egg shell is cracked by tapping with sterile forceps, and sufficient shell is pulled away to open the allantoic cavity. Allantoic fluid is harvested with a 10-ml syringe and a wide needle with a blunted end; 0.5 ml is dispensed into an open tube for HA testing; the remainder is dispensed into a capped tube for later use. Amniotic fluids can be harvested with a 3-ml syringe and a 20- to 23-gauge needle; occasionally, the amniotic sac may have to be washed with saline to recover virus, since the volume of amniotic fluid may shrink if viral growth has occurred. Because of the small volume of amniotic fluid usually obtained, fluid from different eggs may be pooled, and an appropriately sized sample of the pool or a dilution of the pool tested for HA in tubes (0.25–0.5 ml) or on microtiter plates (0.05 ml).

To detect hemagglutinins, add an equal volume of 0.5% chicken RBC to the allantoic or amniotic fluids in tubes or on microtiter plates, mix well, and allow cells to settle. Because of its ability to elute, influenza C virus might not be detected if specimens are incubated at room temperature rather than at 4 C, or if guinea pig RBC are used instead of chicken RBC. Human "O" cells or guinea pig cells at a concentration of 0.4% are otherwise suitable for detection of influenza viruses, and guinea pig cells may be more sensitive than chicken cells for detection of hemagglutinin from newly isolated viruses. If no hemagglutinin is detected, a pool containing an equal volume of the amniotic and allantoic fluids of each egg is reinoculated as above. A third blind passage is rarely warranted but may be useful for some strains.

Once influenza A and B viruses have been isolated in eggs, they then grow in the allantoic cavity, but influenza C strains must be passaged continually in the amnion. Use of a control-positive influenza virus (e.g., a laboratory-adapted strain) to verify the susceptibility of the eggs to influenza is not recommended since it introduces a risk of contaminating clinical specimens. Unusual isolates of influenza virus (e.g., those isolated outside of the normal influenza season or those with different antigenic or growth characteristics from current strains) should be authenticated if possible by reisolation and by serologic confirmation of infection of the patient.

Tissue culture. Because serum components may keep many influenza viruses from replicating, PRMK cells should be washed at least twice with Hanks balanced salt solution (BSS) and maintained with serum-free medium before being infected. Two tubes should be inoculated with the antibiotic-treated specimen (0.3 ml/tube, if available) and incubated at 33 C. The use of a roller drum will increase the rate of viral replication. Cytopathic effect (CPE) is usually produced by influenza B isolates and, less predictably, influenza A isolates within the first week. Possible presence of influenza viruses is evidenced either by production of hemagglutinin in the medium or by the ability of the cells to cause hemadsorption (HAd) (73), usually before CPE can be detected. Thus, if CPE becomes pronounced, medium from one or both tubes should be harvested and titrated for HA activity with 0.4% guinea pig RBC at 4 C. Alternately, in the absence of CPE by 7 days, fluid should be removed from one inoculated tube, and the cells tested for HAd. This is done by adding 1 ml of Hanks BSS and 0.2 ml of fresh 0.4% guinea pig RBC and leaving the solution over the PRMK cells for 30 min at room temperature. Inspections for HAd are made at 10-min and 30-min intervals. (Several uninoculated tubes should be tested for HAd in parallel as a control for adventitious viruses in the cells and for nonspecific adsorption of the RBC.) If HAd is observed, the fluid from the tested tube should be combined with fluids recovered from the other tube after the cells have been subjected to a single freeze-thaw cycle. The pooled fluids should be tested for hemagglutinin titer, and if the titer is sufficient (≥ 16), the virus may then be identified with the HAI test. However, should the pooled fluid from the PRMK tubes have only a low HA activity or should HAd not be detected, then a second passage is made by inoculating fresh PRMK cells with 0.2 ml/tube of the pooled medium from the first passage.

Identification of the isolates

Methods available. Physical and chemical methods, such as 1- or 2-dimensional electrophoretic or chromatographic comparisons of the nucleic acids and proteins (or their partial digests), and/or nucleic acid hybridization techniques might be used in the future to characterize influenza isolates, and some studies along these lines have been undertaken (45, 56, 71). Until now, however, these procedures have been used primarily for determining the genetic relatedness of strains determined to be of interest by serologic procedures, which remain the most practical means of diagnosing influenza infections and characterizing isolates.

All serologic methods for identification of influenza viruses are in one or the other of two categories: those based on reactions of components that are type-specific (NP and/or M protein) and those based on components that are strain-specific (hemagglutinin and NA). Methods in the later category provide more precise identification of the virus. Tests specific for NA are not recommended for routine diagnostic purposes. Tests available for detecting type-specific components include CF, double immunodiffusion (DID) (16, 69), and labeled-antibody methods such as FA. A strain-specific test, such as HAI, should be considered first, however, since one of the main purposes of isolating influenza viruses is to identify the strain responsible for an outbreak or epidemic. The HAI test has the advantage of accuracy of antigen control, thus permitting reproducible comparisons between isolates and known reference strains. Possible disadvantages of the HAI test are the requirement for an antigen with reasonable levels of HA activity and the need to destroy nonspecific HA inhibitors present in many animal reference sera.

Alternatives to HAI are HAd-inhibition (HAdI) (73), neutralization (Nt), hemagglutinin-specific single radial hemolysin (SRH) (21, 66, 70), DID (67), CF, or labeled-antibody tests. With the HAdI test, the drawback is that there is no way to control the amount of antigen, and therefore valid comparisons between the isolate and a reference strain cannot be made. Furthermore, excess antigen present on the cells or antigenic variation of an isolate may result in little or no inhibition of HAd. The Nt test requires an effort that is not normally warranted. Its primary advantage is that specimens with low concentrations of virus can be used. It is usually simpler, however, to repassage virus or to concentrate specimens with low levels of virus by centrifugation to obtain sufficient concentrations for use in HAI tests. In the HAI, HAdI, and Nt tests, non-antibody serum components may cause nonspecific inhibition (42).

Methods of treatment of serum are described in detail later in this chapter. Methods must be appropriate in respect to source of serum and viral sensitivity. In general, chicken or goat serum contains few inhibitors of influenza hemagglutinin and may be successfully treated with receptor-destroying enzyme (RDE). Horse serum contains gamma inhibitors which are highly reactive with H2 and H3 strains of influenza A virus and must be inactivated with potassium periodate. Treatment of rabbit or ferret serum with RDE or periodate is dictated by the sensitivity of the influenza strain to be tested. Accordingly, serum from these animals is not recommended for routine diagnostic purposes; neither is guinea pig serum, which contains inhibitors to H2 and H3 strains that can normally be removed only by adsorption with kaolin.

The SRH test is not affected by non-antibody inhibitors of HA, but it requires relatively large amounts of antigen. A major drawback to the strain-specific CF or DID tests is the need for either purified hemagglutinins as antigen or reference serum known to be specific for the HA antigen. Otherwise the tests may measure reactions due to NA, NP, and/or M protein, which would compromise the ability of the tests to differentiate between virus strains.

In the HAI test, antiserum to a new variant often reacts well with an earlier reference strain, although antiserum to the reference strain may consistently react poorly with the new isolate. The simultaneous recovery of isolates with this property from geographically distinct outbreaks may be a valuable indication of antigenic drift. The ability of serum to discriminate between variants of the same antigenic subtype is clearly of prime importance. In general, serum from singly infected animals (e.g., ferrets) is more strain-specific than serum from animals immunized by stimulation with a nonreplicating antigen, as when serum is produced in chickens, rabbits, or goats. In addition, hyperimmune serum produced with nonreplicating whole virus may contain high concentrations of NA antibodies, which may, with some strains, cause apparent cross-reactions in the HAI tests that can mask antigenic variation between strains (39, 72). This problem can be avoided by the use of serum prepared against antigenic hybrid viruses containing the hemagglutinin of interest, but an irrelevant NA. Because of these potential problems, WHO has established a network of influenza laboratories to assure broad sampling and definitive characterization of influenza variants. Representative strains isolated each year and potentially unusual strains are sent to the international influenza center in either Atlanta or London for comparative studies.

Occasionally, a newly isolated agent, suspected of being an influenza type A or B virus, does not react at all in HAI tests with antiserum to current strains (including swine influenza). In such cases, the agent might (1) not be an influenza A or B virus, (2) represent a strain exhibiting a major antigenic divergence from the reference strain, or (3) be an example of an isolate with low avidity for antibody. If the agent is clearly not influenza C, a type-specific test (see below) should be used to determine whether it is an influenza A or B virus before further attempts are made to identify the strain. EM examination of infected allantoic fluid or PRMK-cell harvests, by pseudoreplica technique, may also be helpful in demonstrating the presence of typical influenza viruses.

Methods of choice

Hemagglutination inhibition test. Either egg fluids or PRMK-cell harvests are titrated in duplicate 2-fold serial dilution in 0.5-ml volumes of PBS. This is done in 10- × 75-mm tubes or in specially designed clear plastic plates (57). One-half milliliter of chicken RBC (0.5%) is added to each dilution in the first series, and 0.5 ml of guinea pig RBC (0.4%) is added to each dilution in the second series; then the mixtures are shaken and incubated at room temperature until the cells have settled. A control containing diluent, but not virus, is included for each RBC suspension. The titration may also be done by using microplates and 0.05-ml volumes of antigen dilution and RBC, particularly if it is desirable to conserve antigen or only small volumes of antigen are available which may have a low titer (e.g., tissue-culture fluids). The titration done in microplates may, however, be somewhat less reproducible than that done with the larger volumes because of the error that can occur when serial dilutions are done with loops. An HAU is defined as the reciprocal of the highest dilution of virus causing complete agglutination when reacted with an equal volume of appropriately diluted RBC. If influenza C is suspected, prechilled reagents should be used in the titration and the chicken RBC should settle in the cold.

The HAI test to identify the isolate is done by using the RBC indicator system that gives the highest virus titers, 4 HAU of virus, and serum that has been appropriately treated to inactivate non-antibody inhibitors of HA. Each isolate should be tested with antiserum to current influenza type A and B strains, with homologous reference antigens used as internal controls. The isolate should be inhibited only by antiserum to one virus type, and, likewise, each control antigen should be inhibited only by its homologous antiserum. If both reference sera inhibit the isolate, even though the sera are specific for their control antigens, residual non-antibody inhibitors of HA are probably present, or the hemagglutinin of the isolate may not be of influenzal origin. In this event, the hemagglutinin could be caused by other myxoviruses or a bacterial contaminant.

Differences in HAI titers of ≥4-fold between an isolate and its control antigen of the same type (A or B), when reacted with reference serum, provide a preliminary indication that the isolate may be an antigenic variant. But newly isolated influenza viruses can have a low avidity for antibody; therefore, they must be further examined by preparing homologous antiserum and performing a reciprocal HAI test. Reaction of this antiserum with antigens of the reference strain at a titer equal to or less than that with the isolate provides more substantial evidence of antigenic variation. Antigenic characterization of a variant may be complicated by the asymmetric nature of its relationship with a reference strain or by the variable degrees of strain specificity exhibited by serum from animals immunized in different ways.

Hemadsorption inhibition test. This test is usually done on second viral passage to obtain a sufficient number of cell cultures to accommodate the desired number of test serum samples. A minimum of three tubes of infected cells are required: two for current type A and B strain-specific reference antiserum and one for a positive HAd control. Infected and control PRMK-cell cultures are washed twice with Hanks BSS. Then 0.8 ml of a 2.5% dilution of serum in Hanks BSS is added to the infected cells and to several tubes of control cells from the same batch. Before being used, the serum must be treated appropriately, usually with RDE, to inactivate nonantibody inhibitors of HA and adsorbed with guinea pig RBC to remove agglutinins. The entire cell sheet is covered by the diluted serum solution, and cultures are incubated for 30 min at room temperature. Then 0.2 ml of 0.4% guinea pig RBC is added to each tube and reacted for a further 30 min at room temperature, and the cultures are examined under a microscope for residual HAd. Isolates are identified by the serum that prevents HAd although, as noted above, strains cannot be positively identified.

Neutralization test. The Nt test permits a direct assay for Nt antibody; the HAI test, an indirect assay. In practice, the results of the two tests are similar; however, for research studies or for special circumstances, a Nt test for differentiating virus strains may be desired. The test may be performed as follows: viruses are diluted in 10-fold series; 0.1 ml per dilution is inoculated into 4–5 tubes of susceptible tissue culture. Infectivity titers are calculated according to the method of Reed and Muench (62) and are based on the presence of HAd in tissue culture after 7 days. Virus suspensions diluted to contain 100 $TCID_{50}$ are mixed with equal volumes of heat-inactivated (56 C for 30 min) antiserum or with a normal serum control from the same species and incubated at room temperature for 1 hr. Serum-virus mixtures (0.2 ml) are inoculated in triplicate into tissue-culture tubes. Because the presence of NA antibody may inhibit release and spread of unneutralized virus from infected foci (17), it is desirable to replace the cell-culture medium with fresh medium 1 hr after inoculation and incubation at 35 C. The reciprocal of the highest dilution of serum inhibiting HAd in 2 or more of the triplicate tubes after 7 days at 35 C is considered to be the titer. Neutralization of virus by normal serum controls suggests susceptibility of test strains to serum inhibitors that may be removed by appropriate serum treatment. However, sometimes influenza virus antibodies, resulting from cross-infections or contact with infected handlers, may be found in preimmune ferret serum.

Type-specific complement-fixation test. Isolates which are suspected of being influenza viruses but cannot be identified by HAI may be typed with the CF test and NP antigens. Test antigens of the isolates are prepared from infected chorioallantoic membranes or by ether treatment of virus (47). Increasing dilutions of antigen are tested against three dilutions of type A and type B antiserum that encompass the known titers.

Type-specific double-immunodiffusion test. Reference antiserum to isolated M protein of influenza A and B viruses is used in this alternative to the type-specific CF test (16). NP antiserum can also be used. Either PRMK-cell or egg fluids are suitable as sources of antigen, preferably with hemagglutinin titers of ≥32, although satisfactory results have been obtained in some cases with lower concentrations. For antigen preparation, approximately 5–10 ml of cold fluid is acidified by adding 1 N HCl (0.03 ml of 1 N HCl/ml of allantoic fluid) to give a final pH of about 4.0 when tested with pH paper. After a 60-min reaction in the cold, precipitated virus is recovered by centrifugation at 1000 × *g* for 10 min, and the supernatant fluid is removed by decantation and drainage. The virus-containing precipitates are suspended in glycine buffer, pH 9.0, containing 10% of the detergent sodium lauryl sarcosinate (Sarkosyl NL-97, Geigy Industrial Chemicals, Ardsley, NY 10502). Ten microliters of buffer are used for each 1 ml of original virus fluid. Preparations of unknown antigens, control antigens prepared with known influenza A and B isolates, uninfected egg or PRMK-cell fluids, and reference serum are dispensed into wells of an Ouchterlony plate (Meloy Industries, Springfield, VA) according to the pattern shown in Figure 18.1 (in which the unknown is a type B influenza virus). All control reactions of reference serum with homologous antigen must be positive, and neither reference serum should react with the negative control antigen. The isolate may not react if it is not an influenza A or B isolate, or if it *is* an influenza A or B isolate but is not present in sufficient concentration (i.e., initial hemagglutinin titer <32).

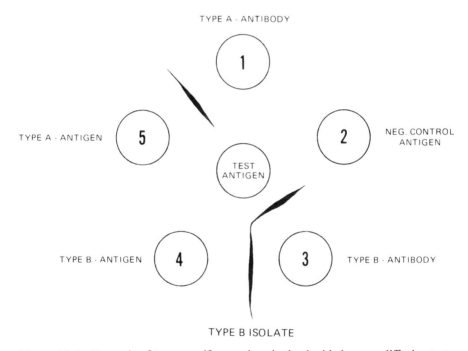

Figure 18.1—Example of type-specific reactions in the double immunodiffusion test.

Neuraminidase-inhibition test. Because of its relative complexity, this test is usually done only with epidemiologically important viruses, or viruses of special significance. WHO has described details of an NI-test procedure, which encompasses features developed by several investigators (4). Antigen dosage is standardized by reacting dilutions of virus with an equal volume of the high-molecular-weight fetuin substrate at 34–37 C for about 15 hr. In many cases, egg fluids or cell-culture harvests can be used as antigens without being purified or concentrated. Tests with shorter reaction times are less sensitive, and proportionately more antigen is needed. Antigen may, however, be concentrated by high-speed centrifugation and resuspended in one-tenth its original volume so that rapid NI tests can be performed with fluids or harvests containing new isolates in low concentration (36). The amount of sialic acid released from the substrate by the action of the virus enzyme is determined by a colorimetric reaction (2, 79). A viral dilution is then selected which will liberate about 20 μg of sialic acid, which corresponds to an optical density reading (A_{549}) of about 0.8–1.0 when measured with a 1-cm path length cell.

The antigenic characteristics of the NA are determined by reacting samples of the appropriately diluted antigen for 1 hr at 34 C with each of a series of 3.2-fold or 4-fold dilutions of reference antiserum. Fetuin substrate is added, and residual enzyme activity is determined after 15 hr. Control reference antigens are tested in parallel. The NI titer of a serum sample is defined as the reciprocal of the dilution which inhibits 50% of the activity of the standard amount of antigen. This titer is usually determined by graphical or mathematical interpolation of results from serum dilutions that inhibit the enzyme >50% and <50%, respectively. With practice, within-test error should be less than about ±1.5-fold, so that when a reference serum is tested against its control homologous antigen and the unknown antigen, 3-fold differences in serum titer can be considered significant. Cross-reactions between antigens of different subgroups have not been detected, but differences in titer of >100-fold with samples of a single serum tested against different antigens within a subgroup are not uncommon. Asymmetric differences may exist between strains within the same subgroup and can only be detected by performing reciprocal tests. In some instances, antibodies to hemagglutinin may, by steric hindrance, block the activity of NA and give low-level false-positive results (20). Therefore, reference antiserum for characterization of the NA antigen should be prepared either with isolated NA or with antigenic hybrid viruses containing a hemagglutinin of a different subgroup from that of the viruses to be examined. NA in different strains may sometimes vary in thermostability, and the enzyme reaction may have to be performed at a temperature as low as 25 C to prevent thermal inactivation of the virus. Alternately, it may be advantageous to stabilize the enzyme by adding normal serum and/or calcium. With troublesome enzymes, individual parameters should be varied so that the conditions giving optimal results can be found.

Serologic diagnosis

Since most persons experience their first influenza infection before school age and may have one or more infections each decade of life, the presence of serum antibody to influenza is not necessarily evidence of recent infection. Serologic diagnosis requires demonstration of a significant increase in antibody titer between the acute-phase serum collected at onset of disease and the convalescent-phase serum collected 2–3 weeks later. A serologic diagnosis of influenza may be made on the basis of a significant antibody rise to any of the four virion antigens, M protein, NP, NA, and hemagglutinin; however, tests for antibody to each antigen are not equally sensitive, and rises in antibody titers are not observed with the same frequency for each antigen. The internal M and NP antigens, unlike the virion surface NA and hemagglutinin antigens, are type specific and antigenically stable; therefore, one of these antigens, in theory, could detect infection with any influenza virus of that type. Preliminary studies by SRD tests have shown that rises in serum antibody to the M antigen of influenza A viruses occur infrequently and only after severe influenza infection (53). In contrast, antibody increases to the NP antigen occur frequently, and tests for this antibody have proven to be useful diagnostic tools. Antibody to the NP antigen may be detected by SRD or CF tests. The SRD test is highly sensitive (53), but the requirement for large amounts of antigen makes the test prohibitive for most diagnostic laboratories. CF is the most frequently used test for measuring serum antibody to the NP antigen. The NP antigen for the CF test is available commercially. The CF test has the additional advantage of being widely used for the serologic diagnosis of other respiratory-disease agents. Influenza antigens can therefore be included in a set of antigens for testing serum from a person with undifferentiated viral respiratory disease.

Antibody to the two virion surface antigens, hemagglutinin and NA, may be assayed by a number of different tests. Among these are the HAI, CF, SRD, SRH, and Nt tests for hemagglutinin antibody and the NI and SRD tests for NA antibody. The HAI and NI tests are the most widely used, in that order. Serologic diagnosis of influenza by HAI tests for antibodies to the hemagglutinin antigen is far simpler than by NI tests for antibody to the NA antigen. Further, the NA antigen is probably less effective in stimulating antibodies in the infected host. The CF and HAI tests are both effective, but the results of the two tests do not always agree. The relative effectiveness of each test depends upon a number of variables, such as the age and previous antigenic experience of the individual, the appropriateness of the strain used in the HAI test, and the interval between collection of the acute-phase and convalescent-phase serum samples. When influenza is suspected, serum found to be negative by one test may be reexamined by the other test for maximal diagnostic efficiency. Serologic techniques will not detect 100% of infections, however, even when more than one test is used. A small proportion of subjects may be ill and may shed virus but may fail to respond with detectable increase in antibody.

The requirement for destroying nonspecific inhibitors before the serum is examined in the HAI test should not be considered a serious disadvantage. The mechanics of serum treatment are simple, and the risk of antibody loss is slight with most procedures. Failure to treat serum or to destroy inhibitors can, particularly in the presence of NA antibody, produce false-positive HAI reactions. Serum treatment can be avoided to some extent by selecting inhibitor-resistant test strains, but some such strains may also have reduced susceptibility to antibody.

The CF test with crude allantoic fluid harvests used as antigens detects antibody to strain-specific virion surface antigens. Not surprisingly, results with this test are often similar to those obtained by HAI. The number of

THROAT AND/OR NASAL SPECIMEN

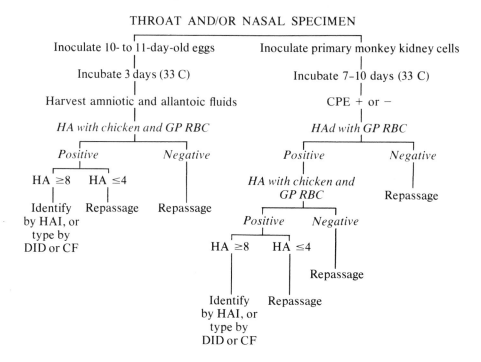

Figure 18.2—Schema for isolation of influenza viruses. CF=complement fixation test, DID=double immunodiffusion test, GP=guinea pig, HA=hemagglutination test, HAd=hemadsorption test, HAI=hemagglutination-inhibition test, RBC=erythrocytes.

serologic diagnostic rises appears to be similar or slightly less by strain-specific CF than by HAI; but more importantly, this CF test does not discriminate between antibody to the different virion antigens that may be contained in the crude allantoic fluid harvests. The CF test with unpurified antigens should be clearly distinguished from the type-specific test with purified NP antigen previously described and the strain-specific test Lief (46) described.

The SRD test appears to be about as sensitive for serologic diagnosis as the HAI test, although the SRD test is capable of detecting antibodies with specificity that might not react in the HAI test. A major disadvantage of the SRD test is the requirement for purified virus concentrates.

SRH results appear to resemble closely those obtained by the HAI test for serologic diagnosis of influenza A or B infections (21). The SRH test is simple to perform, and some may find it more useful than HAI for their purposes.

The Nt test, because of its laborious and complex nature, only rarely and in very special circumstances is used for serologic diagnosis of influenza. In general, results of Nt tests performed in embryonated eggs, with the allantoic membranes on eggshell bits (22), or with monkey kidney tissue culture parallel HAI test results. True neutralization of virus infectivity is specific for antibody to the hemagglutinin antigen. Under certain conditions, however, the presence of NA antibody throughout the viral replication cycle may repress spread of the virus and cause apparent neutralization (17, 39).

In tests for hemagglutinin antibody, where whole virions are used as antigens, antibody to the NA may also react. Under such circumstances (and provided that in the HAI test all serum inhibitors are destroyed) antibody to the NA usually does not interfere with demonstration of antibody rises to the hemagglutinin antigens. Therefore, for serologic diagnostic purposes standard virus preparations may be used.

Complement-fixation test

NP antigens and control serum for type A and type B influenza viruses are available from commercial sources, or they may be prepared in the laboratory. Antigens are prepared by inoculating the virus into 10- to 11-day-old embryonated eggs by the intra-allantoic route and then incubating the eggs for 48 hr at 35 C. The eggs are then chilled overnight, and the chorioallantoic membranes are removed and washed in sterile 0.1M PBS, pH 7.2. The membranes are ground in a mortar with sterile alundum (or homogenized) and suspended in 1 ml of PBS per membrane. After centrifugation at $250 \times g$ (about 1000 rpm) for 15 min, the supernatant fluid containing NP antigen and hemagglutinating particle is withdrawn. Hemagglutinin is absorbed by mixing 1 ml of packed chicken RBC with 15 ml of chilled supernatant fluid; the mixture is then centrifuged. The absorption procedure is carried out in the cold and is repeated until the supernatant fluid fails to agglutinate chicken RBC. The resulting hemagglutinin-free fluid is titrated for use as NP antigen in the CF test.

NP antigens of type A and B, together with control material similarly prepared from uninoculated eggs, are used to measure antibody in acute-and convalescent-phase sera. Antiserum for control of antigen reactivity and specificity is the type-specific antiserum described in the section on the identification of isolates (page 595). The procedure for performance of the CF test is described in Chapter 1. Modifications of the test may also be used (61).

Hemagglutination-inhibition test

Antigens for use in the HAI test are commercially available, or they may be prepared in the laboratory. Antigens for this test are allantoic fluids from eggs infected with strains which have been well adapted to growth in this host. Such fluids normally give satisfactory hemagglutinin titers with chicken RBC.

Hemagglutinin titration. The following procedure is described for the use of microtiter equipment. Beginning with a 1:10 dilution of the virus in 0.01M PBS, pH 7.2, make 2-fold serial dilutions, in duplicate, in 0.05-ml volumes. Add 0.05 ml of chicken or guinea pig RBC to each well in the series. Include 1 well for each RBC suspension as a cell control (diluent plus RBC). Mix and incubate at room temperature until the cells settle. Consider the highest dilution of virus causing agglutination as the titration endpoint; that dilution contains 1 HAU/0.05 ml, and its reciprocal value is the antigen titer.

Preparation of test antigen. The HAI test is done with a test antigen preparation that contains 4 HAU in 0.025 ml. The proper dilution of virus to be used in the HAI test is determined by dividing its hemagglutinin titer (determined as above) by 8. For example, if the hemagglutinin titer is 160, then a 1:20 dilution would contain 8 HAU in 0.05 ml, or 4 HAU in 0.025 ml.

To assure accuracy in determining HAI reactions, each antigen should be retitrated after being diluted to confirm that it contains 8 HAU/0.05 ml. Prepare a row of 6 wells, each containing 0.05 ml of diluent. Add 0.05 ml of the working dilution of virus (8 HAU) to the first well and make the 2-fold dilution series through 5 wells. To the sixth well, add 0.05 ml of diluent in place of virus, to serve as the cell control. Add 0.05 ml of the appropriate RBC suspension to all wells, and after mixing, allow the contents to settle. The cell control and the last 2 wells should show compact buttons of normal settling. Agglutination in the first 3 wells of the series indicates that the working dilution contains 8 HAU of virus per 0.05 ml, as required for the HAI test. The viral concentration of the working dilution should be adjusted, if necessary, by adding PBS or virus as appropriate. Whenever the working antigen dilution is adjusted, its hemagglutinin titer should be confirmed by retitration as described above.

Serum treatment. Non-antibody factors which inhibit influenza virus agglutination may be present in serum from a wide variety of animals. Inhibitors in human and chicken sera, which otherwise react with many influenza strains, can be successfully removed by treatment with the RDE of *Vibrio cholerae* (6, 57). RDE preparations consisting of crude bacterial filtrates are satisfactory for serum treatment. Such preparations may actually be more useful than the purified NA since they contain proteolytic enzymes as well. RDE treatment is performed as follows: add 4 volumes of RDE (100 units/ml) to each volume of serum. Incubate the mixture overnight in a water bath at 37 C. Add 5 volumes of 1.5% sodium citrate, and incubate the mixture at 56 C for 30 min to yield a final 1:10 dilution of treated serum.

Successful destruction of inhibitors in other than human and chicken sera varies with the virus to be tested. Treatment with potassium periodate, a combination of trypsin/periodate, or kaolin (7) may be required. Periodate treatment is performed as follows: add 0.3 ml M/90 potassium periodate to 0.1 ml of serum previously heated to 56 C for 30 min, mix well, and incubate for 15 min at room temperature. Add 0.6 ml of 0.6% glycerol in saline to neutralize excess periodate, and bring final volume of serum dilution up to 1:10. For the combination trypsin/periodate treatment, crystalline trypsin (e.g., Difco 1:250) is dissolved in 0.1M PBS, pH 8.2, at a concentration of 8 mg/ml. To 1 volume of serum, one-half volume of the trypsin solution is added, and the mixture is immediately placed in a 56 C water bath for 30 min. After it cools to room temperature, treat the serum with periodate as above, using 0.15 ml of trypsin-treated serum and only 0.55 ml of glycerol saline to achieve a final 1:10 serum dilution.

Guinea pig serum may require adsorption of inhibitors with kaolin. To verify the success of treatment with serum from different species, normal serum must be tested in parallel with immune serum against the isolates. In some instances treatment of serum with periodate or trypsin/periodate may increase nonspecific inhibitor activity. If chicken cells are used in HAI tests, adsorption to remove nonspecific agglutinins is usually unnecessary and should be done only if agglutination occurs with controls prepared by substituting PBS for virus. Should guinea pig or human O cells be used, non-specific agglutination of RBC may be avoided by adsorbing the treated serum at a ratio of 0.1 ml of 50% RBC to 1 ml of the 1:10-diluted serum. Allow adsorption to proceed for 1 hr at 4 C, and then remove RBC by centrifugation.

Performance of the hemagglutination-inhibition test. Prepare 2-fold dilutions of treated reference antiserum from 1:10 through 1:2560 in 0.025-ml volumes. Add 0.025 ml of the test virus suspension containing 4 HAU to each well. To test for RBC agglutinins in the serum, prepare a control containing 0.025 ml of diluent instead of antigen, mixed with 0.025 ml of the 1:10 dilution of serum. Also prepare cell controls (PBS only) and antigen controls (PBS and antigen) for each test; shake tray and incubate for 30 min at room temperature.

Add 0.05 ml of RBC to each well, shake, and incubate at room temperature until the cell control shows the button of normal settling. The HAI titer is the reciprocal of the highest dilution of serum which completely inhibits agglutination. The normal compacting of RBC in the presence of a high concentration of serum protein (low serum dilutions) should not be mistaken for inhibition. Complete inhibition can best be judged by tilting the plates, thus causing nonagglutinated cells to stream freely.

Interpretation of test. A $\geq$4-fold increase in antibody titer between an acute- and a convalescent-phase serum specimen is considered indicative of infection with type A or type B influenza virus. The strain of virus used as antigen does not necessarily identify the strain of virus causing disease. Anamnestic responses conditioned by prior experience with influenza virus antigens are frequent, and antibody responses to an earlier antigen may be greater than to the current infecting virus. Anamnestic responses are usually confined to broad antigenic groups such as H0/H1 strains and H2/H3 strains. Occasionally, however, rises to Hsw1, H0, or H1 antigens may occur after infections with H3 strains.

Presumptive serologic diagnosis

Through the use of the unpaired-serum technique, a suspected outbreak of influenza can usually be confirmed within 24 hr. The technique is based on the assumption that, by the time an influenza outbreak is recognized, cases have already been occurring in the community for 2 weeks or more. Serum specimens are collected from 10 or more patients who are in the acute stage of the disease and from the same number of age-matched cohorts who experienced the same symptoms 10 or more days earlier. All serum specimens are tested simultaneously for influenza A and B hemagglutinin or NP antibody titers. If the epidemic was caused by influenza, the geometric mean antibody titer for type A or B should be significantly higher (by Student's t test) in the latter group than in the former (52, 55).

If the difference in antibody titer is ≥4-fold, the difference may be considered significant without resorting to statistical analysis. A diagnosis made on this basis should then be confirmed by conventional methods of viral isolation, usually requiring several days, and diagnosis with paired sera.

References

1. ALMEIDA JD and WATERSON AP: Two morphological aspects of influenza virus *In* The Biology of Large RNA Viruses, Barry RD and Mah BWJ, (eds), Academic Press, London, 1970, pp 27–51

2. AMINOFF D: Methods for the quantitative estimation of N-acetyl-neuraminic acid and their application to hydroysates of sialomucoids. Biochem J 81:384–392, 1961

3. APPLEYARD G and MABER HB: Plaque formation by influenza viruses in the presence of trypsin. J Gen Virol 25:351–358, 1974

4. AYMARD-HENRY M, COLEMAN MT, DOWDLE WR, LAVER WG, SCHILD GC, and WEBSTER RG: Influenzavirus neuraminidase and neuraminidase-inhibition test procedures. Bull WHO 48:199–202, 1973

5. BAXTER BD, COUCH RB, GREENBERG SB, AND KASEL JA: Maintenance of viability and comparison of identification methods for influenza and other respiratory viruses of humans. J Clin Microbiol 6:19–22, 1977

6. BURNET FM and STONE JD: The receptor-destroying enzyme of V(ibrio) cholerae. Aust J Exp Biol Med Sci 25:227–233, 1947

7. CLARKE DH and CASALS J: Techniques for hemagglutination and hemagglutination-inhibition with arthropod-borne viruses. Am J Trop Med Hyg 7:561–573, 1958

8. COREY L, RUBIN RJ, HATTWICK MAW, NOBLE GR, and CASSIDY E: A nationwide outbreak of Reye's syndrome. Its epidemiologic relationship to influenza B. Am J Med 61:615–625, 1976

9. DAVENPORT FM, HENNESSY AV, and FRANCIS T JR: Epidemiologic and immunologic significance of age distribution of antibody to antigen variants of influenza virus. J Exp Med 98:641–656, 1953

10. DAVENPORT FM, HENNESSY AV, and FRANCIS T JR: Influence of primary antigenic experience upon the development of a broad immunity to influenza. Trans Assoc Am Phys 70:81–90, 1957

11. DAVENPORT FM, MINUSE E, HENNESSY AV, and FRANCIS T: Interpretation of antibody patterns of man. WHO Bull 41:453–460, 1969

12. DIMMOCK NJ: New virus-specific antigens in cells infected with influenza virus. Virology 39:224–234, 1969

13. DOANE FW, ANDERSON N, ZBITNEW A, and RHODES AJ: Application of electron microscopy to the diagnosis of viral infections. Can Med Assoc J 100:1043–1049, 1969

14. DOWDLE WR, COLEMAN MT, HALL EC, and KNEZ V: Properties of the Hong Kong influenza virus, 2. Antigenic relationship of the Hong Kong virus hemagglutinin to that of other influenza A viruses. Bull WHO 41:419–424, 1969

15. DOWDLE WR, DOWNIE JC, and LAVER WG: Inhibition of virus release by antibodies to surface antigens of influenza viruses. J Virol 13:269–275, 1974

16. DOWDLE WR, GALPHIN JC, COLEMAN MT, and SCHILD GC: A simple double immunodiffusion test for typing influenza viruses. Bull WHO 51:213–218, 1974

17. DOWDLE WR, LAVER WG, GALPHIN JC, and DOWNIE JC: Antigenic relationships among influenza virus A neuraminidase (N2) antigens by immunodiffusion and postinfection netralization tests. J Clin Microbiol 3:233–238, 1976

18. DOWDLE WR and HATTWICK MW: Swine influenza virus infections in humans. J Infect Dis Supplement 136:S386–S389, 1977

19. DOWDLE WR, NOBLE GR, and KENDAL AP: Orthomyxovirus—influenza: comparative diagnosis unifying concept *In* Comparative Diagnosis of Viral Diseases, Kurstak E (ed), Academic Press, New York, San Francisco, London, 1977, pp 447–501

20. EASTERDAY BC, LAVER WG, PEREIRA HG, and SCHILD GC: Antigenic composition of recombinant virus strains produced from human and avian influenza A viruses. J Gen Virol 5:83-91, 1969

21. FARROHI KH, FARROHI FK, NOBLE GR, KAYE HS, and KENDAL AP: Evaluation of the single radial hemolysis test for measuring hemagglutinin- and neuraminidase-specific antibodies to H3N2 influenza strains and antibodies to influenza B. J Clin Microbiol 5:353-360, 1977

22. FAZEKAS DE ST. GROTH S and WHITE DO: Comparison of the infectivity of influenza viruses in two host systems: the allantois of intact eggs and surviving allantois-on-shell. J Hyg 56:535-546, 1958

23. FRANCIS T: A new type of virus from epidemic influenza. Science 91:405-408, 1940

24. FROMMHAGEN LH, KNIGHT CA, and FREEMAN NK: The ribonucleic acid, lipid and polysaccharide constituents of influenza preparations. Virology 8:176-197, 1959

25. FUKUMI H: Interpretation of influenza antibody patterns in man: existence and significance of Hong Kong antibody in old people prior to the Hong Kong influenza epidemic. WHO Bull 41:469-473, 1969

26. GARDNER PS, COURT SDM, BROCKLEBANK JT, DOWNHAM MAPS, and WEIGHTHAM D: Virus cross-infection in paediatric wards. Br Med J 2:571-575, 1973

27. GARDNER PS and McQUILLIN J: Rapid Virus Diagnosis: Application of Immunofluorescence. Butterworth & Company, Ltd., Great Britain, 1974

28. GOLDFIELD M, BARTLEY JD, PIZZUTI W, BLACK HC, ALTMAN R, and HALPERIN WE: Influenza in New Jersey in 1976: isolations of A/New Jersey/76 at Fort Dix. J Infect Dis, 136:S347-S355, 1977

29. HARBOE A: The influenza virus haemagglutination inhibition by antibody to host material. Acta Path Microbiol Scand 57:317-330, 1963

30. HOYLE L: The Influenza Viruses. Virology Monographs, 4, Springer-Verlag, New York, 1968, pp 243-254

31. HOYLE L, JOLLES B, and MITCHELL RG: The incorporation of radioactive phosphorus in the influenza virus, and its distribution in serologically active virus fractions. J Hyg (London) 52:119-127, 1954

32. JONCAS JH, BERTHIAUME L, WILLIAMS R, BEAUDRY P, and PAVILANIS V: Diagnosis of viral respiratory infections by electron microscopy. Lancet 1:956-959, 1969

33. JOOSTING ACC, HEAD B, BYNOE ML, and TYRRELL DAJ: Production of common colds in human volunteers by influenza C virus. Br Med J 4:153-154, 1968

34. KENDAL AP: A comparison of "influenza C" with prototype myxoviruses: receptor-destroying activity (neuraminidase) and structural polypeptides. Virology 65:87-99, 1975

35. KENDAL AP, MINUSE E, MAASSAB HF, HENNESSY AV, and DAVENPORT FM: Influenza neuraminidase antibody patterns of man. Am J Epidemiol 98:96-103, 1973

36. KENDAL AP, GOLDFIELD M, NOBLE GR, and DOWDLE WR: Identification and preliminary antigenic analysis during an influenza outbreak at Fort Dix, New Jersey. J Infect Dis, 136:S381-S385, 1977

37. KERR AA, DOWNHAM MAPS, McQUILLAN J, and GARDNER PS: Gastric 'flu: influenza B causing abdominal symptoms in children. Lancet 1:291-295, 1975

38. KILBOURNE ED (ed): The Influenza Viruses and Influenza. Academic Press, New York, San Francisco, London, 1975

39. KILBOURNE ED, LAVER WG, SCHULMAN JL, and WEBSTER RG: Antiviral activity of antiserum specific for an influenza virus neuraminidase. J Virol 2:281-288, 1968

40. KLENK HD, COMPANS RW, and CHOPPIN PW: An electron microscopic study of the presence or absence of neuraminic acid in enveloped viruses. Virology 42:1158-1162, 1970

41. KLENK HD, ROTT R, ORLICH M, and BLODOM J: Activation of influenza A viruses by trypsin treatment. Virology 68:426-439, 1975

42. KRIZANOVA O and RATHOVA V: Serum inhibitors of myxoviruses. Curr Top Microbiol Immunol 47:125-151, 1969

43. KUNDIN WD and EASTERDAY BC: Hong Kong influenza infection in swine: experimental and field observations. Bull WHO 47:489-491, 1972

44. LAZAROWITZ SG and CHOPPIN PW: Enhancement of the infectivity of influenza A and B viruses by proteolytic cleavage of the hemagglutinin polypeptide. Virology 68:440-454, 1975

45. LAVER WG and WEBSTER RG: Studies on the origin of pandemic influenza. II. Peptide maps of the light and heavy polypeptide chains from the haemagglutinin subunit of A2 influenza viruses isolated before and after the appearance of Hong Kong influenza. Virology 48:445-455, 1972

46. LIEF FS: Antigenic analysis of influenza viruses by complement fixation. VII. Further studies on production of pure anti-S serum and on specificity of type A S antigens. J Immunol 90:172-177, 1963

47. LIEF FS and HENLE W: Methods and procedures for use of complement-fixation technique in type- and strain-specific diagnosis of influenza. Bull WHO 20:411-420, 1959

48. LINNEMANN CC JR, SHEA L, KAUFFMAN CA, SCHIFF GM, PARTIN JC, and SCHUBERT WK: Association of Reye's syndrome with viral infection. Lancet 2: 179-182, 1974

49. LIU C: Rapid diagnosis of human influenza infection from nasal smears by means of fluorescein-labeled antibody. Proc Soc Exp Biol Med 92:883-887, 1956

50. MARTIN ML, PALMER EL, and KENDAL AP: Lack of characteristic hexagonal surface structure on a newly isolated influenza C virus. J Clin Microbiol 6:84-86, 1977

51. MASUREL N and MARINE WM: Recycling of Asian and Hong Kong influenza virus A hemagglutinins in man. Am J Epidemiol 97:44-49, 1973

52. MILSTONE JH, LINDBERG RB, BAYLISS BM, DeCOURSEY E, and BECK ME: Influenza B epidemic in the Pacific area. Mil Surg 99:777, 1946

53. MOSTOW SR, SCHILD GC, DOWDLE WR, and WOOD RJ: Application of the single radial diffusion test for assay of antibody to influenza type A viruses. J Clin Microbiol 2:531-540, 1975

54. MULDER J and HERS JFPh: Influenza. Wolters-Noorhoff nv Groningen, Publishers, The Netherlands, 1972

55. National Communicable Disease Center. Influenza-Respiratory Disease Surveillance Report, No. 84. Public Health Service, US Department of Health, Education, and Welfare, Atlanta, Ga., 1968

56. PALESE P and SCHULMAN JL: Mapping of the influenza virus genome: identification of the hemagglutinin and the neuraminidase genes. Proc Nat Acad Sci USA, 73:2142-2146, 1976

57. PALMER DF, COLEMAN MT, DOWDLE WR, and SCHILD GC: Advanced Laboratory Techniques for Influenza Diagnosis. Public Health Service, US Department of Health, Education, and Welfare, Center for Disease Control, Atlanta, GA, 1975

58. PARTIN JC, SCHUBERT WK, PARTIN JS, JACOBS R, and SAALFELD K: Isolation of influenza virus from liver and muscle biopsy specimens from a surviving case of Reye's syndrome. Lancet 2:599-603, 1976

59. PEREIRA HG: Influenza antigenic spectrum. Progr Med Virol 11:46-79 (Karger, Basel), 1969

60. PONS MW: A reexamination of influenza single- and double-stranded RNAs by gel electrophoresis. Virology 69:789-792, 1976

61. Public Health Monograph No. 74: Standardized Diagnostic Complement Fixation Method and Adaptation to Micro Test. Public Health Service, US Department of Health, Education, and Welfare, Center for Disease Control, Atlanta, GA, 1965

62. REED LJ and MUENCH H: A simple method of estimating 50% end points. Am J Hyg 27:493-497, 1938

63. RITCHEY MB, PALESE P, and SCHULMAN JL: Mapping of the influenza virus genome. III. Identification of genes coding for nucleoprotein, membrane protein and nonstructural protein. J Virol 20:307-313, 1976

64. ROTT R, WATERSON AP, and REDA IM: Characterization of "soluble" antigens derived from cells infected with Sendai and Newcastle disease viruses. Virology 21:663-665, 1963

65. RUBEN FL and MICHAELS RH: Reye's syndrome with associated influenza A and B virus infection. J Am Med Assoc 234:410-412, 1975

66. RUSSELL SM, McCAHON D, and BEARE AS: A single radial haemolysis technique for the measurement of influenza antibody. J Gen Virol 27:1-10, 1975

67. SCHILD GC: Studies with antibody to the purified haemagglutinin of an influenza AO virus. J Gen Virol 9:191-200, 1970

68. SCHILD GC: Evidence for a new type-specific structural antigen of the influenza virus particle. J Gen Virol 15:99-103, 1972

69. SCHILD GC and PEREIRA HG: Characterization of the ribonucleoprotein and neuraminidase of influenza A viruses by immunodiffusion. J Gen Virol 4:355–363, 1969

70. SCHILD GC, PEREIRA MS, and CHAKRAVERTY P: Single-radial-haemolysis: a new method for the assay of antibody to influenza haemagglutinin. Applications for diagnosis and seroepidemiologic surveillance of influenza. Bull WHO 52:43–50, 1975

71. SCHOLTISSEK C, ROHDE W, HARRIS E, and ROTT R: Correlation between base sequence homology of RNA segment 4 and antigenicity of the hemagglutinin of influenza viruses. Virology 79:330–337, 1977

72. SCHULMAN JL and KILBOURNE ED: Independent variation in nature of hemagglutinin and neuraminidase antigens of influenza virus. Distinctiveness of hemagglutinin antigen of Hong Kong/68 virus. Proc Nat Acad Sci USA 63:326–333, 1969

73. SHELOKOV A, VOGEL JE, and CHI L: Haemadsorption (adsorption-haemagglutination) test for viral agents in tissue culture with special reference to influenza. Proc Soc Exp Biol Med 97:802–809, 1958

74. SMITH TF, BURGERT EO, DOWDLE WR, NOBLE GR, CAMPBELL RJ, and VAN SCOY RE: Isolation of swine influenza virus from autopsy lung tissue of man. N Engl J Med 294:708–710, 1976

75. SMITH W, ANDREWES CH, and LAIDLAW PO: A virus obtained from influenza patients. Lancet 2:66–68, 1933

76. STUART-HARRIS CH and SCHILD GC: Influenza: The Viruses and the Disease. Edward Arnold, Ltd., London, 1976

77. TAYLOR RM: A further note on 1233 (influenza C) virus. Arch Gesamte Virusforsch 4:485–500, 1951

78. TUMOVA B and SCHILD GC: Antigenic relationships between type A influenzaviruses of human, porcine, equine, and avian origin. Bull WHO 47:453–460, 1972

79. WARREN L: The thiobarbituric acid assay of sialic acids. J Biol Chem 234:1971–1975, 1959

80. WHO Study Group: A revised system of nomenclature for influenza viruses. Bull WHO 45:119–124, 1971

CHAPTER 19

PARAINFLUENZA VIRUSES

Robert M. Chanock

Introduction

The parainfluenza viruses are important respiratory tract pathogens that are medium sized (150-200 nm), RNA containing, ether-sensitive members of the paramyxovirus group. Although the initial strain (Sendai virus, a murine agent) was isolated from the laboratory mouse, the types which infect man were recognized with the application of tissue culture and hemadsorption techniques (3, 8, 11, 42).

Parainfluenza viruses share many properties with influenza viruses, but they are different from these agents in several respects. Parainfluenza viruses have a larger ribonucleoprotein-containing inner helix (18 nm vs. 9 nm for the influenza viruses) and, unlike influenza viruses, are capable of fusing cells and hemolyzing certain types of erythrocytes (RBC) (20, 67-69). The parainfluenza viruses have common antigens which are not shared by the influenza viruses. The viruses of mumps and Newcastle disease (NDV) share the foregoing properties, including antigenic relationships, with the parainfluenza viruses (19, 25, 42, 63).

Four distinct serologic types have been recovered from humans. Strains of parainfluenza viruses related to the human types but, antigenically separable from them, have also been isolated from a number of animal species (Table 19.1).

Epidemiology

Types 1-4 parainfluenza viruses have a wide geographic distribution. The first 3 types have been identified in most areas when appropriate tissue culture and hemadsorption techniques were applied to the study of childhood respiratory tract diseases. Thus far, type 4 viruses, which are more difficult to recover in tissue culture, have been isolated in fewer areas, but, serologic studies suggest that they are also relatively ubiquitous.

Each of the 4 parainfluenza virus types can cause acute respiratory tract disease in humans. This etiologic relationship is indicated by two observations. First, each of the virus types has been recovered significantly more often from patients with respiratory diseases than from individuals free of such illness (7, 9, 11-13, 30, 34, 42-44, 47, 52, 65). Second, types 1, 2, 3, and 4A viruses each have produced upper respiratory tract infections and illness when administered to adult volunteers.

The parainfluenza viruses are exceeded only by respiratory syncytial virus (RSV) as important causes of lower respiratory tract disease in young children, and they commonly reinfect older children and adults to produce upper respiratory tract disease (12, 34).

There is considerable diversity in both epidemiologic and clinical manifestations of infections due to the parainfluenza viruses. Parainfluenza virus type 1 is the principal cause of croup (laryngotracheobronchitis) in children, and parainfluenza type 3 virus is second only to RSV as a cause of pneumonia and bronchiolitis in infants less than 6 months of age. Parainfluenza virus type 2 resembles type 1 virus in clinical manifestations, but serious illness occurs less frequently; infections with type 4 parainfluenza virus are detected infrequently, and associated illnesses are usually mild.

The parainfluenza viruses are most important as respiratory tract pathogens during infancy and childhood. In this age group, type 1, 2, and 3 viruses cause a spectrum of effects which ranges from inapparent infection to life-threatening lower respiratory tract disease. Studies in different parts of the world indicate that type 1, 2, and 3 viruses are associated with approximately 40% of severe croup (acute laryngotracheobronchitis) (13, 43, 44, 47, 52, 65). Type 1 virus is the most important of the parainfluenza viruses in the croup syndrome. In addition to croup, type 1, type 2, and type 3 viruses are also responsibile for smaller but appreciable percentages of other acute respiratory tract diseases of infancy and early childhood.

Parainfluenza infection generally occurs very early in life. Sixty percent of children are infected with parainfluenza type 3 virus by 2 years of age, and approximately 80% are infected by 4 years of age (12). Infection with type 1 or type 2 virus generally occurs somewhat later, but a majority of children are infected with type 2 virus by 4 years of age, and over 75% are infected with type 1 virus by 5 years of age. Infections with type 3 virus occur often in the first months of life while infants still possess circulating antibody derived from their mothers. In contrast, in young infants maternally derived anti-

TABLE 19.1.—ANTIGENIC TYPES AND NATURAL HOSTS OF PARAINFLUENZA VIRUSES

VIRUS TYPE	STRAINS WHICH INFECT HUMANS (SYNONYM)	RELATED BUT ANTIGENICALLY DISTINCT STRAINS WHICH INFECT OTHER HOSTS	
		STRAIN (SYNONYM)	HOST
1	Hemadsorption type 2 (HA-2)	Sendai, or hemagglutinating virus of Japan (HVJ)*	Mouse, pig
2	Croup-associated (CA)	Simian virus 5 (SV5)†	Monkey, dog
		Simian virus 41 (SV41)	Monkey
3	Hemadsorption type 1 (HA-1)	Shipping fever (SF4)	Cow
4	M_{25}		

*Human infections have been reported, but authenticity of those claims has been questioned (30).

†Two isolations from humans have been reported, DA and WB viruses (39, 45). SV5 is antigenically identical with SA virus; origin of latter (human? hamster?) is unknown.

body appears to prevent both infection and severe disease with either type 1 or type 2 virus (34). Severe illness caused by type 1 or type 2 virus is rather rare under 4 months of age. After 4 months of age there is a rise in the number of cases of croup and other lower respiratory tract diseases caused by type 1 and type 2 viruses. This high incidence continues until approximately 6 years of age. After a child reaches school-age there is a much lower incidence of lower respiratory tract disease caused by type 1 and type 2 parainfluenza viruses, and the occurrence of lower respiratory tract illness in individuals infected with either virus during adolescence or adult life is distinctly unusual, although this does occur on occasion.

From 1957 to 1961, type 1 virus appeared to be endemic; infection occurred sporadically and without a definite seasonal pattern (34). Beginning in 1962, a different pattern developed in which sharp outbreaks of type 1 virus occurred every 2 years in the autumn of even-number years, and this pattern has continued to the present time. When the virus is epidemic, there is generally a marked increase in the incidence of croup in the pediatric population.

Type 2 virus is nearly as ubiquitous as type 1 virus, and infection occurs in outbreaks which are most prominent in the fall of odd-number years, the years in which type 1 virus is absent from the population (34). Type 3 virus invariably has exhibited an endemic pattern, with infection occurring in all seasons of the year. Small outbreaks have been noted, but there has been no predictable periodicity in their occurrence.

The parainfluenza viruses are particularly troublesome as causes of infection in the hospital. Children who are admitted to the hospital for non-respiratory tract illness are often infected during their hospital stay, and this is often associated with the development of serious lower respiratory tract disease (51).

Clinical aspects

Mode of transmission. Transmission of parainfluenza viruses is by direct person-to-person contact or large droplet spread. The viruses do not persist long in the environment, however. The high rate of infection early in life, coupled with the frequency of reinfection, suggests that the virus spreads readily from person to person. Reinfected individuals appear to be infectious, and a relatively low inoculum is able to produce infection. The type 3 virus appears to be most efficient in its ability to spread from person to person. Type 3 virus generally infects all susceptible individuals in a semi-closed population, such as a nursery (12). Such outbreaks generally involve all susceptible individuals within a short period of time. In contrast, the type 1 and type 2 viruses appear to be less effective in this regard, infecting between 40–70% of susceptible individuals in semiclosed populations (12). There is no evidence that infection is transmitted from humans to animals or vice versa.

Pathogenesis. Initially, in parainfluenza virus infection the mucous membranes of the nose and throat are involved. Paranasal and eustachian tube obstruction may also occur. In many patients the inflammatory process descends into the lower respiratory tract and produces limited changes in the bronchi. If more extensive changes occur in the lower tract, there is a tendency for type 1 and type 2 infections to involve the larynx, resulting in the croup syndrome; there may also be extensive involvement of the trachea and bronchi, with accumulation of inspissated mucus resulting in additional obstruction of the airway. When type 3 virus produces severe disease, there is a tendency for extension to occur into the lungs and small bronchi, and bronchopneumonia develops.

Approximately 80% of infants and children undergoing initial infection with type 3 virus develop a febrile illness, and in one-third of primary type 3 infections there is involvement of the lower respiratory tract resulting in either pneumonia or bronchitis (9, 11). One-half of initial type 1 virus infections and two-thirds of initial type 2 infections produce a febrile illness (12). Lower respiratory tract involvement also occurs commonly during primary type 1 infection; about 25% of primary infections produce bronchitis or pneumonia. Severe acute laryngotracheobronchitis (croup), although the most dramatic manifestation of initial parainfluenza virus infection, is not the rule and is noted in only 2–3% of primary type 1 or type 2 infections (34).

Severe respiratory tract disease caused by type 1, 2, or 3 parainfluenza virus generally occurs in the first 3–5 years of life. This finding suggests that primary infection confers upon the host a relative resistance to subsequent severe parainfluenza virus illness.

Reinfection of adults, as well as of children, with parainfluenza virus has been recognized on a number of occasions, particularly with type 3 virus. Although the frequency of reinfection is not known, it is probable that many individuals have repeated experience with type 3 virus. In a series of outbreaks of type 3 infection in a nursery population, it was observed that 17% of the children infected during one outbreak were reinfected during subsequent outbreaks, although the interval between outbreaks was not more than 9 months (12). Illness usually occurs less often and is less severe during reinfection than during primary infection.

In one study of type 3 virus infection in infants and young children, presence of serum neutralizing antibodies correlated with resistance to infection and illness (12). However, resistance associated with serum neutralizing antibody was not complete but only partial. One-third of infants and children with high serum-antibody levels became infected. Although reinfection occurred, an effect of antibody was indicated by the shorter period of virus shedding in contrast to the pattern observed during primary infection. Moderate levels of serum antibody were not associated with complete protection against febrile illness, since such illnesses occurred approximately 40% as often as during first infection.

Studies with the type 1 and type 2 viruses indicate that immunity to infection and to disease appears to be mediated through local respiratory tract secretory antibody, while antibody in serum plays a lesser role in resistance (59). Similar information has not been obtained as yet for the type 3 virus.

Incubation period. In experimental infection of adult volunteers, the interval between administration of type 1, 2, or 3 virus and onset of upper respiratory tract symptoms ranged from 3–6 days (12). The incubation period in pediatrics infections has not been defined; however, information is available concerning the interval between exposure to type 3 virus and the subsequent initial shedding of this virus. In several institutional outbreaks of infection this interval was 2–4 days (12).

Period of infectivity. The interval during which an individual infected with a parainfluenza virus can infect another person is not known. However, long range epidemiologic studies indicate that type 3 virus can be recovered for 3–10 days (median of 8 days) from the oropharynx during initial infection, whereas during reinfection virus is detected for a shorter interval (9).

Symptoms and signs. In children, the most common type of illness consists of rhinitis, paryngitis, and bronchitis, usually with fever. The most common initial symptoms are cough and fever. There may be some croupiness to the cough, but respiratory distress is not present. Approximately three-fourths of such ill children have temperatures above 100 F; fever usually lasts 2–3 days. Coarse breath sounds, rhonchi, erythema of the pharyngeal mucous membranes, and rhinitis are the characteristic physical findings. Cervical adenopathy is uncommon.

Cough and fever are the most common symptoms of infants and children with bronchopneumonia or croup. Approximately two-thirds of such patients exhibit respiratory distress. In the croup syndrome this takes the form of inspiratory stridor, inspiratory retractions of the sternum and the rib cage, and a variable degree of respiratory obstruction. Inspiratory wheezes are commonly heard on auscultation. Individuals with bronchopneumonia commonly exhibit dyspnea, and fine rales or ronchi can be heard by auscultation. In some patients, a combined bronchopneumonia-croup illness may occur. On X-ray examination, patients with bronchopneumonia usually exhibit a diffuse or localized peribronchiolar infiltrative process which may involve any portion or portions of the lung fields.

Complications. The most severe complications are associated with laryngeal obstruction, which on occasion can be fatal.

Pathology

The pathologic changes produced by parainfluenza viruses in humans have not been adequately described.

Description and Nature of the Agents

Common characteristics

The parainfluenza viruses share a number of properties which are also common to other paramyxoviruses, such as mumps and measles viruses. These properties include compound helical symmetry, helical ribonucleoprotein inner component, lipoprotein outer envelope which is studded with periodic glycoprotein projections, and maturation of the virion at the host cell membrane.

Size, shape, and chemical composition

The parainfluenza viruses are extremely pleomorphic and vary in size from 150-250 nm, with occasional large particles in the range of 800-1000 nm. A single ribonucleoprotein helix with a diameter of approximately 18 nm and a length of approximately 1 μ is present inside the virion (15, 16, 67-69). This structure contains the unsegmented RNA viral genome. The molecular weight of paramyxoviruses RNA is estimated to be 6 × 10⁶ (15, 18). Its sedimentation coefficient is 50-57 S when measured in a sucrose gradient. There is general agreement that the parainfluenza virion contains at least 5 proteins. In order of decreasing molecular weight these are: 1) the P protein with a molecular weight of 69,000; 2) HN glycoprotein, molecular weight 67-74,000; 3) F glycoprotein, molecular weight 65,000; 4) NP protein, molecular weight 56-61,000 and 5) M protein, molecular weight 38-41,000 (15). The HN and F glycoproteins are located on the surface of the virion attached to the viral envelope. The HN glycoprotein has both hemagglutinating and neuraminidase activites, while the F protein is responsible for initiation of infection (presumably brought about by focal lysis of the host cell membrane) and cell fusion. The F glycoprotein is not active until it is cleaved by a host cell protease (15, 56). Following this reaction, the complex containing the cleavage products (F1 and F2) is able to bring about fusion between the viral and cell membranes. The viral membrane consists of a lipid bilayer beneath which is the M protein. Within this envelope is the helical ribonucleoprotein that contains the NP protein and the viral RNA. Also associated with ribonucleoprotein is the P protein that may be involved in the synthesis of RNA complementary to the viral genome.

Resistance

Parainfluenza viruses are relatively unstable at temperatures of 37 C and above. The rate of inactivation is markedly influenced by the composition of the suspending medium; serum proteins tend to protect these viruses from heat inactivation. Each of the 4 virus types can be stored without loss of infectivity for several years at −60 C if 0.5% bovine albumin or 5% chicken serum is incorporated in the suspending medium. The parainfluenza viruses are rapidly inactivated at pH 3 (35). Infectivity is also completely destroyed by exposure to 20% ether for 18 hr at 4 C, indicating that lipid is essential for the integrity of the virion.

Classification

The parainfluenza viruses are members of the paramyxovirus group (15, 67). The basis for their differentiation from the myxoviruses is their wider inner helical component (18 nm vs. 9 nm).

Antigenic composition

Immunotypes

Thus far, 4 immunotypes have been recognized among the parainfluenza viruses that infect humans (19, 42). The first 3 appear to be both antigenically stable and homogeneous, i.e., each of these types contains only one serotype (12, 19, 60). Prime strains of type 2 virus exist and may create confusion unless serum against such strains are used for virus identification by hemagglutination inhibition (HAI) or tissue culture neutralization (Nt) tests (50). The type 4 serotype contains two subtypes which are designated subtype A and subtype B (7). These subtypes are closely related but can be distinguished by appropriate serologic techniques. The parainfluenza viruses share related antigens. Despite antigenic relatedness, these viruses can be differentiated easily by complement fixation (CF), HAI, or tissue culture NT using post-infection guinea pig serum. Homotypic serum titers of 1:80–1:2560 are obtained when CF tests are performed with virus suspensions or "soluble" nonhemagglutinating antigens, whereas heterotypic titers are usually less than 1:10 (19, 60, 63). Comparable specificity is observed in HAI or Nt tests. The two subtypes of type 4 parainfluenza virus cannot be distinguished by CF but can be differentiated by Nt or hemadsorption-inhibition (HAdI) tests (7).

Strains of parainfluenza virus related to type 1, 2, or 3 virus have been recovered from a number of animal species. Sendai virus, recovered from mice and pigs, is related to but distinct from the type 1 virus of humans (19). Similarly, the SV5 and SV41 agents of simian origin are related to human type 2 virus, while the shipping fever virus of cows (SF4) is related to the type 3 virus of humans (1, 10, 60).

When human and animal subtypes within a type are tested by CF with guinea pig immune serum, relationships of a reciprocal or nonreciprocal nature are observed. Thus, the human and the bovine parainfluenza 3 subtypes exhibit a reciprocal relationship in which homologous serum titers are 4- to 8-fold higher than the heterologous titers (1). Human and murine parainfluenza 1 subtypes exhibit a nonreciprocal relationship in which antiserum for the latter virus exhibits broad reactivity, while antiserum for the human subtype reacts in a more specific fashion (19, 60). Parainfluenza 2 subtypes also display a nonreciprocal relationship in which antiserum for the simian subtypes exhibits broad reactivity (10, 60).

Antigens

Soluble. Soluble, nonhemagglutinating, specific CF antigens have been prepared from types 1, 2, and 3 viruses by ether treatment and subsequent RBC adsorption of hemagglutinins (19). The soluble, nonhemagglutinating antigen of type 1 (muris) virus is associated with the inner helical component of the virion, and it is probable that similar antigens of the other parainfluenza viruses are of the same nature (55). Parainfluenza viruses do not share a common soluble CF antigen (19).

Viral. Specific antigens are present on the envelope of the parainfluenza viruses. Thus, parainfluenza types 1, 2, 3, and 4 viruses react in a specific manner when tested with the appropriate antiserum by Nt, HAdI, or HAI tests (7, 19, 42). Specific antigenic activity has been demonstrated for the hemagglutinating subunits of type 1 (muris) parainfluenza virus released from the virion by ether disruption; such subunits are located at the surface since they are composed of envelope material and its projections and since they hemagglutinate and exhibit neuraminidase activity (54).

Hemagglutinin. Parainfluenza viruses agglutinate certain fowl and mammalian RBC. Except for type 4 virus, moderate to high levels of hemagglutinins are produced in infected tissue cultures. At 4 C, type 1 and type 2 viruses produce higher hemagglutination (HA) titers with chicken than with guinea pig RBC. However, maximal titers with all types are obtained when tests are performed with guinea pig RBC at 37 C; an increase in HA titers occurs when virus-guinea pig RBC mixtures originally sedimented at 4 C are resuspended and permitted to sediment at 37 C (20, 36). This patterns of reaction is also characteristic of NDV and mumps virus, but does not occur with the influenza viruses. After virus preparations have been subjected to sonic oscillation at 20 kc for 10 min, the HA titer of types 1-3 viruses at 4 C equals that obtained at 37 C (36). This suggests that originally a considerable proportion of the hemagglutinin exists in an aggregated form and that disaggregation occurs when the hemagglutinin is in contact with the RBC at 37 C (36). The use of such "aggregated" hemagglutinin results in a 4- to 16-fold lower HAI titer than that obtained with a sonically treated preparation of virus (37). With high-titer preparations of type 1 and 3 virus, a negative zone in the lower dilutions is commonly observed at 37 C. A similar pattern is exhibited by SV41 strain of type 2 virus.

Hemagglutinating subunits consisting of envelope material, and its spikelike projections are released from parainfluenza type 1 virus when it is treated with ether. Such subunits are unstable in ether, but they are stabilized in the presence of Tween 20 or 80 (38). Tween-ether treatment of type 2 virus produces a marked increase in HA titer, presumably by releasing hemagglutinating subunits from the liproprotein outer envelope (41).

Irreversible binding of virus antigen to RBC occurs when type 2 (simiae) virus is incubated at 37 C with chicken RBC (39). RBC to which this virus has adsorbed agglutinate fresh RBC and are agglutinated when exposed to high dilutions of serum containing antibody for type 2 (simiae) virus. It is likely that this effect is due to fusion of the viral envelope with the cell membrane brought about by the F glycoprotein (15).

Pathogenicity for animals

Some strains of types 1, 2, and 3 viruses will replicate in the embryonated chicken egg, others will not (8, 11, 24, 40). To date, eggs appear to be less sensitive to infection with naturally occurring virus than are monkey kidney cells; with the exception of the murine subtype of type 1 (Sendai virus) and 3 strains of type 2 virus from humans, isolation of a parainfluenza virus in embryonated eggs has not been reported (66).

Types 1, 2, and 3 viruses multiply slowly after inoculation into the amniotic cavity of 7- to 8-day-old embryonated eggs; to obtain maximal titers, incubation at 34-36 C for 5-7 days is required. Type 3 virus grows only in the amniotic cavity, whereas one strain of type 2 and several strains of type 1 virus have been adapted to the allantoic cavity of the egg (24, 40). Amniotic (types 1, 2, and 3) and allantoic (types 1 and 2) fluids from embryos infected with well-adapted egg strains contain hemagglutinins for guinea pig or chicken RBC, or both. Most strains of type 2 virus, however, multiply only in the amniotic cavity, and the amount of virus produced is insufficient to cause agglutination of RBC.

Types 1-4 viruses infect guinea pigs without producing overt disease. Hamsters are sensitive to intranasal inoculation of type 1, 2, or 3 virus; 1 $TCID_{50}$ is sufficient to infect this animal (21, 22). The hamster also undergoes a silent infection without obvious signs of illness.

Growth in tissue culture

Primary monkey kidney tissue culture is a sensitive and satisfactory system for recovery of all 4 types of virus. Rhesus and vervet monkey kidney cultures are equally sensitive for isolation of types 1, 2, and 3 virus strains. However, for recovery of type 4 virus, rhesus cultures are considerably more sensitive than vervet cells (7). In a limited number of tests, human embryonic kidney cell cultures have also proven satisfactory for recovery of types 1, 2, and 3 viruses (64). Isolation of type 1, 2, or 3 virus in diploid human fibroblasts is possible, but in quantitative tests this tissue was found to be much less sensitive than monkey renal cells. Serially propagated heteroploid human cell lines (HEp-2, HeLa, or KB) support the growth of naturally occurring types 1, 2, and 3 viruses, but they are less sensitive for virus recovery than are primary human or monkey renal cell cultures. This is particularly true for type 1 strains (30).

Preparation of Immune Serum

Antigenic characterization of parainfluenza viruses is best accomplished with immune serum prepared by intranasal infection of guinea pigs. Care must be taken to use guinea pigs which are free of antibodies for the parainfluenza and mumps viruses (19). Such seronegative guinea pigs are given 0.2 ml of undiluted virus suspension intranasally under light ether anesthesia and then kept in isolation to prevent subsequent infection with myxoviruses and other paramyxoviruses. The animals are bled after 21-28 days, and a serum pool is prepared incorporating material from those guinea pigs with the highest antibody levels. Such serum exhibits specificity when tested by CF. Homologous serum titers ranging from 1:80 to 1:2560 are obtained with viral particle or soluble antigens, whereas heterotypic antigens fail to fix complement with a 1:10 dilution of serum (19, 63).

The serum is also specific by Nt and HAI tests. A varying proportion of guinea pigs develop low-level heterotypic HAI antibody responses, but these reactions do not pose any difficulty in strain identification.

Rabbit immune serum, produced by multiple intravenous inoculations, reacts specifically in CF, Nt, HAdI, and HAI tests, but the frequency, extent, and titer of heterotypic responses are generally greater than those found with guinea pig serum. Three biweekly intravenous inoculations of undiluted type 2 or 3 virus-infected tissue culture or egg fluid generally stimulate HAI antibody titers of 1:160-1:640. Satisfactory type 1 serum is more difficult to prepare in rabbits and may require multiple inoculations over a 4- to 6-month period.

Hyperimmune horse serum reacts in a specific manner in the HAdI test, and for this reason such serum is useful for identification of isolates. Equine antiserum is not useful for CF studies since it is broadly reactive when tested by this technique (29).

Collection of Specimens for Laboratory Diagnosis

Virus isolation

All parainfluenza types are readily recovered from the oropharynx. Specimens may be obtained by rubbing a cotton swab vigorously across the posterior pharyngeal wall or, in older individuals, by nasal wash or gargle. The pharyngeal swab is immersed in 2–5 ml of collecting fluid (see below) and agitated, after which the fluid is expressed from the swab; the swab is discarded. It is particularly important that specimens for virus isolation be taken as soon after onset of symptoms as possible. During initial infection, type 3 virus is shed from the pharynx for a minimum of 1 day and for an average of 6 days after onset of illness (9). During reinfection, type 3 virus is shed for an even shorter period than during the first infection. Isolates are rarely obtained from fecal specimens.

The viruses are relatively unstable in balanced salt solution and require a protein protective substance for stabilization. The addition of 0.5% gelatin or bovine albumin meets this need. Optimal results are obtained with veal infusion broth with 0.5% bovine albumin, or Hanks balanced salt solution (BSS) with 0.5% gelatin. Ideally, specimens should be tested fresh without prior freezing. If this is not possible, the throat swab or gargle fluid should be frozen rapidly and stored at − 60 C or lower, either in glass sealed ampules in a CO_2 chest or in screwcap ampules in a mechanical freezer.

Serologic diagnosis

An acute-phase serum specimen should be collected as early in the course of illness as possible, preferably before the fifth day. A convalescent-phase specimen should be taken 2–3 weeks later. Serum, separated from clotted blood, is stored in the frozen state until all specimens from the patient can be tested simultaneously.

Microscopy

Nasopharyngeal secretions, collected by aspiration, can be tested for the presence of characteristic paramyxovirus particles by electron microscopy (28). Secretions are suitable for such study even after storage at −20 C for 1–5 months.

Laboratory Diagnosis

Direct examination of clinical material

Electron microscopy. A small drop of nasopharyngeal secretion is placed on a drop of water resting on a waxed surface. A Formvar-carbon-coated copper grid is then touched briefly to the drop. A drop of 2% potassium phosphotungstate (pH 7) is then added to the grid. After removing excess fluid with filter paper, the grid is air-dried and is then examined with an electron microscope. This technique permits direct examination of type 1 parainfluenza virus particles in secretions from patients with croup (28). Since parainfluenza viruses cannot be differentiated from one another by electron microscopic examination, it is not possible to determine the serotype of the infecting virus by the phosphotungstate negative staining method.

In one study, the secretions from patients with croup which yielded type 1 virus in tissue cultures, and in which typical paramyxovirus particles were visible by electron microscopy, contained sufficient viral antigen to agglutinate human type O RBC and to permit identification by HAI test (26).

Immunofluorescence. Nasopharyngeal secretions are collected by gentle suction, emulsified in 0.5 ml of saline, and centrifuged at 1000 rpm for 10 min. The sediment is resuspended in phosphate-buffered saline (PBS) and recentrifuged (31–33). The resulting pellet is suspended in a few drops of saline and distributed to several areas on each of 2 slides. The slides are allowed to air dry. Slides are fixed in acetone for 10 min at 4 C. One of the spots containing fixed nasopharyngeal material is overlaid with type 1 parainfluenza virus immune rabbit serum, another spot with type 2 antiserum, and a third spot with type 3 antiserum. The slides are incubated at 37 C for 30 min in a moist chamber and then rinsed for 30 min in 3 changes of PBS. Fluorescein-conjugated anti-rabbit globulin is then added, and the slides are incubated again for 30 min at 37 C. This is followed by a 30 min rinse in 3 changes of PBS and a final wash for 2 min in distilled water. The slides are then viewed by UV microscopy. Exfoliated cells infected with parainfluenza virus exhibit cytoplasmic staining. Staining reactions are completely type specific and the indirect immunofluorescence technique appears to be as efficient as isolation of virus in tissue culture for diagnosis of parainfluenza virus infection (33).

Success of this technique is dependent upon the use of rabbit parainfluenza antiserum which is absorbed with human heteroploid cells (i.e., HeLa or HEp-2 cells) in order to remove reactivity against human tissue. Rabbit antiserum is prepared by immunization of animals with virus grown in the embryonated egg (Sendai, murine type 1 virus) or continuous LLC-MK-2 monkey cells (human type 2 or type 3 virus).

Virus isolation

Embryonated eggs. Naturally occurring strains of parainfluenza viruses grow poorly, or not at all, in embryonated hen's egg. Thus far, only three parainfluenza strains, all type 2, have been recovered in eggs (66).

Tissue culture. Rhesus monkey kidney cell cultures are the preferred system for recovery of parainfluenza viruses. Vervet monkey kidney and human embryonic kidney cell cultures are also suitable for recovery of types 1, 2, and 3 viruses but are considerably less sensitive for isolation of type 4 strains.

Tissue cultures are washed 3 times with BSS to reduce the quantity of residual serum from the growth medium. Monkey kidney and human embryonic kidney cells are maintained with medium No. 199 or a mixture of equal volumes of medium No. 199 and Eagle basal medium. The use of monkey kidney cells for the recovery of parainfluenza viruses has the serious disadvantage that a simian paramyxovirus (SV5) occurs frequently in such cultures. This agent has all the biologic properties of a parainfluenza virus and is antigenically distinct from the four human types except for a one-way relationship with type 2 virus demonstrable by CF with postinfection guinea pig serum (10). SV5 contamination of rhesus kidney cell cultures in the United States usually has a seasonal distribution, occurring from October to March. The extent of contamination of different lots of cultures may vary from 0.5–100% of all tubes. It is sometimes possible to control the simian parainfluenza contamination by adding 0.2% hyperimmune rabbit serum to both the growth and maintenance media of monkey kidney cell cultures (10). In this concentration, the serum does not inhibit types 1–4 viruses. Unfortunately, this concentration of rabbit serum may inhibit avid strains of influenza A virus.

Tissue cultures are incubated either stationary or in a roller drum. Rotation in a roller drum increases the sensitivity of cultures to type 4 parainfluenza viruses but not to the other serotypes (7). Recommended incubation temperature is from 33–36 C.

Type 1 virus rarely produces sufficient cell destruction during the isolation passage in monkey tissue culture cells to permit recognition. After several further passages, type 1 virus produces only a minimal rounding and destruction of tissue culture cells. Type 4 virus resembles type 1 and cannot be recognized by morphologic changes in the host cells. During the isolation passage, type 3 virus produces a minimal cytopathic effect (CPE) in monkey kidney cells, generally insufficient to permit recognition of the agent in inoculated cultures; however, after serial cultivation in monkey kidney cells, CPE is extensive. Type 3 virus induces infected cells to separate from the sheet; they assume an elongated fusiform shape and then fragment. Type 2 is the only virus of the group which can easily be recognized by its CPE, namely, by the formation of dark, granular, irregular syncytia. Affected areas assume a "Swiss cheese" appearance when the syncytia retract and fall away from the cell sheet (3, 8, 23). Both type 2 and 3 viruses produce syncytial CPE in serially propagated heteroploid human cell lines (HeLa, KB and HEp-2) (46).

All four parainfluenza viruses produce intracytoplasmic eosinophilic inclusions in monkey kidney cells (5, 42). These inclusions are particularly striking when infected cultures are fixed in Bouin solution and stained with hematoxylin and eosin.

Cultures infected with types 1-4 parainfluenza viruses are capable of hemadsorbing guinea pig RBC. This property is fundamental to the recognition of naturally occurring strains of types 1, 3, and 4 viruses (11, 42). In addition, hemadsorption is more sensitive than CPE for detection of type 2 strains (43).

Guinea pig or human RBC are employed at a concentration of 0.4%; 0.2 ml of such a suspension prepared in isotonic saline solution is added to a culture tube containing 1.0-1.5 ml of fluid medium. After addition of RBC, the cultures are incubated horizontally for 30 min at 4 C. Cultures infected with parainfluenza viruses give a hemadsorption reaction with guinea pig RBC at this temperature, with the exception of type 4 virus which requires an incubation temperature of 25-37 C for maximal patterns. For this reason, the cultures, if negative, are reincubated at 25 C for 30 min and reexamined. Temperatures above 25 C cause a reversal of positive patterns in cultures infected with types 1 and 3 viruses. Tests are read microscopically at 60-100X magnification. Before examination, the culture tube is gently rocked several times on the long axis to wash off any RBC which may have settled onto the cells without actually adsorbing to the monolayer.

Tissue cultures inoculated with clinical specimens are tested for hemadsorption after a 5-day incubation period and, subsequently, at the tenth to thirteenth day, and on the twentieth day. After each test for hemadsorption, the medium containing the added guinea pig RBC is withdrawn and replaced with fresh medium. It is important to remove most of the RBC since prolonged incubation of cultures containing large numbers of RBC may result in a confusing, nonspecific hemadsorption.

The quantity of free virus in the fluid medium of cultures infected with clinical specimens is usually insufficient to interfere with the hemadsorption reaction. However, during experimental laboratory studies, large quantities of free virus are often found in the medium 3-5 days after inoculation with 10^4 to 10^6 $TCID_{50}$ of virus. When RBC are added to such cultures, large free-floating aggregates of agglutinated RBC are formed with the result that few RBC are available for hemadsorption. This difficulty can be avoided by washing such cultures several times with BSS before the addition of RBC. In evaluating tissue cultures inoculated with clinical specimens, it is important to search for agglutinated RBC and, if such masses are found, the washing procedure should be carried out.

The majority of types 1 and 3 viruses recovered from children are detected by the fifth day after inoculation of tissue cultures (10). Types 2 and 4 isolates often require a longer interval of incubation before hemadsorption occurs (10, 43). CPE with type 2 virus generally appears several days after the occurrence of hemadsorption. When specimens from adults are tested, the quantity of parainfluenza virus present is commonly smaller than that found in specimens from infants or children (10). In such instances, the time required for occurrence of hemadsorption is generally 10 days or longer.

Identification of isolates. Tissue culture fluids from cultures which exhibit either hemadsorption or CPE are inoculated undiluted or at a dilution of 1:10 into fresh cultures or monkey or human kidney cells. After 2 days of incubation, one of the inoculated cultures is tested for hemadsorption. If 50% or more of the cell sheet shows hemadsorption, typing is attempted with specific immune serum, employing the HAdI technique. If negative, the cultures are reincubated and tested daily until hemadsorption is detected, at which time typing is performed. Types 1 and 3 viruses usually require 2 days of incubation before typing, while types 2 and 4 viruses usually require 3-6 days.

Rabbit, chicken, or guinea pig serum for parainfluenza types 1, 2, 3, and 4, mumps, SV5, and influenza types A, B, and C are used for typing. The serum is treated with an equal volume of receptor-destroying enzyme (RDE) overnight at 36 C, inactivated at 56 C for 30 min, and then diluted 1:10 in physiologic saline solution. The second passage cultures are washed twice with BSS; 0.6 ml of this solution and 0.2 ml of RDE-treated typing serum at a dilution of 1:10 are added; the cultures are incubated for 20-30 min at room temperature; 0.2 ml of guinea pig RBC suspension is added, and the cultures are reincubated at 4 C for 30 min and then examined for the occurrence and extent of hemadsorption. If hemadsorption is greater at 25 C or 37 C, as occurs with type 4 strains, incubation is performed at either of these temperatures. Isolates are identified by the serum that prevents hemadsorption. Generally, a serum must have an HAI titer of 1:160-1:320 before it will effectively prevent hemadsorption when used at a dilution of 1:10.

Isolates can also be identified by CF, HAI, or Nt in tissue culture. With many strains of type 4 virus, CF or Nt represents the method of choice since these viruses are extremely sensitive to hemadsorption inhibitors present in rabbit and chicken sera.

Serologic diagnosis

Antibody response

The serologic response of humans to parainfluenza infection is generally less specific than that exhibited by infected animals (guinea pigs or hamsters). In part, this appears to result from prior experience with other members of the parainfluenza group and with mumps virus. It is unusual to find individuals after the first year of life without antibody to at least one of the parainfluenza viruses (17, 52).

Heterotypic CF and HAI type 3 antibody responses occur commonly following type 1 infection during childhood (11, 14). Initial infection with type 3 virus generally occurs earlier than with type 1, and it is probable that prior sensitization to type 3 antigens accounts for the occurrence of heterotypic responses to type 1 virus. Type 3 heterotypic responses also occur frequently after type 2 infection during childhood. Adults infected with one of the parainfluenza viruses often develop heterotypic responses, most likely reflecting their extensive prior experience with members of this group.

Individuals infected with type 1, 2, or 3 virus not uncommonly develop an antibody response to related parainfluenza viruses from other species (Sendai, SV5, and SF4) (1, 11, 12). These responses, as well as heterotypic responses for the human strains, occur in an unpredictable fashion. The antigenic relation of mumps virus to the parainfluenza viruses is indicated by the frequent occurrence of heterotypic responses to the latter agents after mumps infection (8, 25, 42). Similarly, an antibody rise to mumps virus can occur after parainfluenza infection. The antigenic breadth of such heterotypic parainfluenza responses in adults has been described on a number of occasions (12).

It is clear that etiologic diagnosis by serologic means is hampered by the great frequency and irregularity of heterotypic responses. A specific diagnosis can best be made by virus isolation. The paired serum specimens can be examined by three serologic methods—CF, HAI, and Nt. Both specimens of a serum pair should always be assayed in the same test.

Complement fixation test

Antigens. Satisfactory antigens for virus types 1–4 can be prepared from infected monkey kidney cell cultures. Fluid and cells from types 1–3 infected cultures are harvested after 5–6 days of incubation and treated for 10 min in a sonicator at 0 C. Treated suspensions are clarified at 2000 rpm for 15 min and stored in the frozen state. Type 4 cultures are harvested after 6–10 days of incubation, and the viral antigens are concentrated 10 × by centrifugation at 30,000 rpm for 2 hr in a 30 rotor of the model L Spinco centrifuge and then stored in the frozen state. Antigens for types 2 and 3 viruses can also be prepared from infected KB or HeLa cell cultures; infected cultures are incubated for 5–6 days at 35 C before the cells and fluids are harvested. Amniotic fluid from eggs infected with type 1, 2, or 3 virus, or the allantoic fluid from type 1 or 2 infected eggs, can also be used as an antigen. Seven-day-old eggs are inoculated by the appropriate route and incubated at 35 C for 6–7 days. Although individual attempts may fail, it is generally possible to prepare material containing 4–8 units of antigen for each of the viruses.

Reference serum. Reference serum for standardization and certification of CF antigens is prepared by infecting guinea pigs by the intranasal route.

Special modifications of test. The CF test is performed essentially as described in Chapter 1. The guinea pig serum used as the source of complement should be free of paramyxovirus antibody. An excess of antigen— 4–8 units—is used since responses in infants and small children are often missed in tests utilizing 2 antigen units. For this reason, it is also desirable to standardize antigens to be used in tests with human serum with a serum obtained from a young child recently convalescent from parainfluenza virus infection. Antigens for each of the parainfluenza types are included in CF tests performed with serum from patients with respiratory disease.

Interpretation of test. A ≥4-fold rise in CF-antibody titer constitutes evidence of parainfluenza infection. A specific serologic diagnosis of the infecting parainfluenza virus cannot be made with certainty because of the frequent occurrence of heterotypic CF responses (14). A rise in antibody to only one type of virus does not guarantee specificity, since heterotypic rises can occur in the absence of a homotypic response. Caution in interpretation of serologic findings is also indicated because of the antigenic relation of mumps virus to the parainfluenza viruses; infection with the former agent is commonly associated with a rise in antibody to the latter agents, especially among adults (25, 42). For the reasons just described, it is clear that identification of the infecting virus can best be established by virus isolation.

The CF test is a moderatly sensitive procedure for diagnosis of parainfluenza infection among children with respiratory disease severe enough to require hospital care. This technique is also sensitive for the diagnosis of inapparent or mild type 3 virus infections in children, whereas the CF-antibody response after such infections with type 1 virus in the same age group is poor. Approximately one-third to one-half of reinfections with type 1 or 3 virus in adult life are accompanied by a CF-antibody response.

Hemagglutination-inhibiton test

Preparation of antigens. These can be prepared by the same method described for CF antigens. It is difficult to prepare type 4 hemagglutinin antigen with sufficient potency for use in the HAI test. The sensitivity of the HAI technique can be enhanced by using type 2 virus which has been treated with 0.125% Tween 80 and 33% ether (41). Similarly, antigens which have been sonically treated at 20 kc for 10 min show a 4- to 16-fold increase in HAI titer over that obtained with untreated hemagglutinins (37).

Treatment of serum. Human and rabbit sera contain nonspecific inhibitors for types 1, 2, and 3 hemagglutinins (8, 17, 26, 61). Not all virus preparations are sensitive to such inhibitors. Strains which have been passaged only a few times in tissue culture may be more sensitive than well-adapted strains (62).

Inhibitors can be effectively reduced in titer by treating the serum with RDE. Equal volumes of undiluted RDE and serum are incubated overnight at 37 C, and the mixture is then heated at 56 C for 30 min. For satisfactory removal of inhibitor from serum, the RDE preparation should have a titer of $\geq$1:128 when tested with parainfluenza type 3 virus by the following modified method of Burnet and Stone (6).

Serial 2-fold dilutions of RDE are made in 0.5 ml volumes of calcium acetate saline solution buffer, pH 6.2 (2); 0.5 ml of 0.4% guinea pig RBC is added to each tube; the mixture is incubated for 30 min at 37 C; the fluid is then withdrawn by capillary pipette and 1 ml of parainfluenza type 3 hemagglutinin (8 units) is then added to each tube. The RBC are resuspended and allowed to sediment at room temperature. The titer of RDE is the highest dilution which renders the RBC refractory to hemagglutination.

Standard serum. Reference serum is prepared in guinea pigs or rabbits as described above.

Procedure for test. The type of RBC used, the temperature of sedimentation, and the time of incubation of serum and virus before addition of RBC, all influence the inhibitory titer of the serum. Highest inhibitory levels are obtained when the test conditions include the RBC and temperature of sedimentation which produce the highest hemagglutination titer. Preincubation of serum-virus mixtures for 1 hr at room temperature is also required for maximal inhibitory titer (26, 27).

RDE-treated serum is diluted in a microtiter plate in serial 2-fold steps in isotonic saline solution; 0.025 ml of hemagglutinin diluted to contain 4 units is then added to the cups containing the serum dilutions. The titer of the virus preparation is determined by titration on the day of the test. The serum control cup containing the lowest serum dilution tested, usually 1:10, should receive 0.025 ml of saline solution. The serum-virus mixtures are shaken and then held at room temperature (20–25 C) for 1 hr. Guinea pig or human RBC (0.05 ml of 0.4% suspension) are added to each cup and the plate is shaken. The RBC are permitted to sediment at room temperature or at 37 C. The test is read when the RBC in the serum control cups have settled to a button, usually after 30–60 min. The inhibitory titer is the highest dilution of serum which completely or almost completely inhibits hemagglutination.

A simultaneous titration of the virus is performed to demonstrate that 4 units were used in the test. It is advisable to include a standard reference serum (either human or animal) for each virus tested as an additional check for specificity and test sensitivity. Some sera contain agglutinins for guinea pig RBC; these agglutinins may be removed by prior absorption for 1 hr at 4 C with such cells at a final concentration of 5%.

Interpretation of test. A 4-fold or greater rise in HAI antibody constitutes evidence of parainfluenza infection. As in the CF test, heterotypic responses often preclude definitive serologic diagnosis of the infecting virus by HAI test.

The HAI test is moderately sensitive for serologic diagnosis of mild, as well as severe, parainfluenza type 1 or 3 infection during childhood. Approximately 50% of adults reinfected with type 1 or 3 virus show a rise in HAI-antibody titer. Experience with the HAI test in type 2 infections is limited, but it appears that most infected children and adults respond with an increase in such antibody.

Virus neutralization test

Antigens. Pools of infectious virus are prepared in monkey kidney tissue culture cells (types 1–4) or in continuous cell line cultures (type 2 and type 3). Infected monkey kidney cell culture fluids are harvested after 3–4 days of incubation for types 1, 2, and 3 viruses and after 5 days for type 4 virus. Continuous cell line cultures (KB, HeLa, or Hep-2) infected with type 2 or 3 virus are harvested after 3 days of incubation. It is important to add a stabilizer to the monkey kidney culture harvests; 0.5% bovine albumin or 5% chicken serum is suitable for this purpose. The infected tissue culture fluid is centrifuged at 2000 rpm for 10 min. and the supernatant fluid is stored at −60 C in 1 ml volumes in sealed glass ampules in a CO_2 chest or in screw-cap tubes in a mechanical freezer.

Pools prepared in this manner have a titer of 10^6 to 10^7 $TCID_{50}$/ml except for type 4 virus which usually has a titer of 10^5 $TCID_{50}$/ml. Titrations are performed by inoculating each of a series of decimal dilutions of virus prepared in BSS with 0.5% gelatin into 3–4 monkey kidney cell cultures. After 3 days (types 1, 2 and 3) or 5 days (type 4) of incubation, the cultures are washed 3 times with 1 ml BSS; then 1 ml 0.1% guinea pig RBC suspension in BSS is added to each tube. After incubation in the horizontal position for 30 min at 4 C (types 1, 2, 3) or at 25 C (type 4), the cultures are examined microscopically for evidence of hemadsorption. The titer is calculated according to the Reed-Muench method (53).

Treatment of serum. Serum is heated at 56 C for 30 min except when being tested for type 2 antibody. Heating serum from children with type 2 infection reduces the level of neutralizing activity (8, 23).

Standard serum. Reference serum is prepared as described in the sections above on CF and HAI techniques.

Procedure for the test. Two-fold or 4-fold dilutions of serum are incubated for 1 hr at room temperature with an equal volume of virus diluted to contain 100 $TCID_{50}/0.1$ ml. For parainfluenza type 1 Nt tests, 10 $TCID_{50}/$ 0.1 ml are used because antibody responses occurring in infants and young children are often not detected with the larger dose of virus (14). Dilution of the virus to the estimated 10 or 100 $TCID_{50}$ is made in BSS with 0.5% gelatin. After incubation at room temperature for 1 hr, 0.2 ml of the serum-virus mixture is inoculated into 2-3 monkey kidney cell cultures. A simultaneous titration of the diluted virus suspension is performed to determine the actual quantity of virus used in the test. After incubation at 33-35 C for 3 days (for types 1-3) or for 5 days (type 4), the test is read using inhibition of hemadsorption as the antibody endpoint. As in the reading of infectivity titrations, the cultures are washed 3 times with BSS, and 1 ml of a 0.1% guinea pig RBC suspension is added to each tube. After incubation at either 4 C (types 1, 2 and 3) or at 25 C (type 4), the cultures are examined microscopically for the occurrence of hemadsorption. Complete inhibition of hemadsorption is taken to represent neutralization. The serum endpoint is estimated by the method of Reed and Muench (53).

Assay of neutralizing antibody can also be performed in microtiter plates (57, 58). In the microtiter plate modification, serial 2-fold dilutions of serum are performed in duplicate in 0.025 ml volumes of BSS with 0.5% gelatin utilizing transfer loops and microplates. An equal volume of medium containing 8-32 $TCID_{50}$ of parainfluenza virus is then added to each cup, and the mixtures are incubated for 1 hr at room temperature. Approximately 8000-10,000 second passage rhesus monkey kidney cells are then added to each cup; the cups are filled with tissue culture medium (Eagle) supplemented with 2% agamma calf serum, 0.2% SV5 rabbit antiserum, 250 units/ ml penicillin, and 250 μg/ml streptomycin. The plates are covered with a loose sheet of plastic and incubated at 37 C in a humidified 5% CO_2-air atmosphere, or sealed with tape and incubated in a conventional 37 C incubator. After 3 days, the fluid medium is removed, the cell sheets are washed in saline solution, and overlaid with a suspension of 0.1% guinea pig RBC in physiologic saline solution. After incubation at 4 C for 30 min the microplates are examined with a light-microscope for the presence of hemadsorption. The Nt titer of serum is calculated from the highest dilution which produces $\geq$ 50% reduction of hemadsorption when compared with that produced by virus in the absence of serum.

Serum titer endpoints can also be determined by the hemagglutination reaction after addition of 0.025 ml of 1% guinea pig RBC suspension to each cup (70).

Interpretation of test. A ≥ 4-fold rise in neutralizing antibody constitutes evidence of parainfluenza infection. As in the CF and HAI tests, heterotypic neutralizing antibody responses often preclude definitive serologic diagnosis of the infecting type by this technique.

The Nt test is moderately sensitive for the serologic diagnosis of infection with types 1-4 infections acquired during infancy or childhood. This technique is less sensitive for detecting infection in adults, since many older individuals possess moderate levels of neutralizing antibody as a result of prior parainfluenza virus experience.

Enzyme-linked immunosorbent assay

Preliminary data have been presented that this technique can be used for the detection of antibody to type 1 parainfluenza virus (4). In a preliminary test, the enzyme-linked immunosorbent assay (ELISA) was found to be more sensitive than CF for measurement of type 1 serum antibodies. Solid-phase coupled antigen was prepared by infecting a monolayer of African green monkey kidney cells. After thorough washing, infected tissue was fixed with acetone and stored at −70 C until used in the ELISA test. Serum was allowed to react with antigens present in the fixed tissue. After thorough washing, an anti-IgG serum conjugated with peroxidase was added, and the amount of enzyme bound to the tube determined by adding specific substrate (σ dianisidine hydrochloride). The intensity of the color which developed as a result of peroxidase activity was measured by colorimeter (4).

References

1. ABINANTI FR, CHANOCK RM, COOK MK, WONG D, and WARFIELD M: Relationship of human and bovine strains of myxovirus parainfluenza 3. Proc Soc Exp Biol Med 106:466-469, 1961

2. ADA GL and STONE JD: Electrophoretic studies of virus-red cell interaction: mobility gradient of cells treated with viruses of the influenza group and the receptor-destroying enzyme of *V. cholerae*. Br J Exp Pathol 31:263-274, 1950

3. BEALE AJ, McLEOD DL, STACKIW W, and RHODES AJ: Isolation of cytopathogenic agents from the respiratory tract in acute laryngotracheobronchitis. Br Med J 1:302-303, 1958

4. BISHAI FR and GALLI R: ELISA, a viral diagnostic method. Lancet 1:696-697, 1977

5. BRANDT CD: Cytopathic action of myxoviruses on cultivated mammalian cells. Virology 14:1-10, 1961

6. BURNET FM and STONE JD: Receptor-destroying enzyme of *V(ibrio) cholerae*. Aust J Exp Med Sci 25:227-233, 1947

7. CANCHOLA J, VARGOSKO AJ, KIM HW, PARROTT RH, CHRISTMAN E, JEFFRIES B, and CHANOCK RM: Antigenic variation among newly isolated strains of parainfluenza type 4 virus. Am J Hyg 79:357-364, 1964

8. CHANOCK RM: Association of a new type of cytopathogenic myxovirus with infantile croup. J Exp Med 104:555-576, 1956

9. CHANOCK RM, BELL JA, and PARROTT RH: Natural history of parainfluenza infection. *In* Perspectives in Virology, Pollard, M (ed), Burgess, Minneapolis, 1961, pp 126-138

10. CHANOCK RM, JOHNSON KM, COOK MK, WONG DC, and VARGOSKO AJ: The hemadsorption technique, with special reference to the problem of naturally occurring simian parainfluenza virus. Am Rev Resp Dis 83:125-129, 1961
11. CHANOCK RM, PARROTT RH, COOK MK, ANDREWS BE, BELL JA, REICHELDERFER T, KAPIKIAN AZ, MASTROTA FM, and HUEBNER RJ: Newly recognized myxoviruses from children with respiratory disease. N Engl J Med 258:207-213, 1958
12. CHANOCK RM, PARROTT RH, JOHNSON KM, KAPIKIAN AZ, and BELL JA: Myxoviruses: parainfluenza. Am Rev Resp Dis 88:152-166, 1963
13. CHANOCK RM, VARGOSKO AJ, LUCKEY A, COOKE MK, KAPIKIAN AZ, REICHELDERFER T, and PARROTT RH: Association of hemadsorption viruses with respiratory illness in childhood. J Am Med Assoc 169:548-55, 1959
14. CHANOCK RM, WONG D, HUEBNER RJ, and BELL JA: Serologic response of individuals infected with parainfluenza viruses. Am J Public Health 50:1858-1865, 1960
15. CHOPPIN PW and COMPANS RW: Reproduction of paramyxoviruses. In Comprehensive Virology, 4, Fraenkel-Conrat H and Wagner RR (eds) Plenum Press, New York, 1975, pp 95-178
16. CHOPPIN PW and STOECKENIUS W: The morphology of SV5 virus. Virology 23:195-202, 1964
17. CLARKE SKR and SAYNOR R: Hemagglutination-inhibition tests against CA virus. Arch Gesamte Virusforsch 9:288-294, 1959
18. COMPANS RW and CHOPPIN PW: Isolation and properties of the helical nucleocapsid of the parainfluenza virus SV5. Proc Nat Acad Sci USA 57:949-956, 1967
19. COOK MK, ANDREWS BE, FOX HH, TURNER HC, JAMES WD, and CHANOCK RM: Antigenic relationships among the "newer" myxoviruses (parainfluenza). Am J Hyg 69:250-264, 1963
20. COOK MK and CHANOCK RM: Unpublished data
21. COOK MK and CHANOCK RM: In vivo antigenic studies of parainfluenza viruses. Am J Hyg 77:150-159, 1963
22. CRAIGHEAD JE, COOK MK, and CHANOCK RM: Infection of hamsters with parainfluenza 3 virus. Proc Soc Exp Biol Med 104:301-304, 1960
23. CRAMBLETT HG: Isolation of a cytopathogenic agent resembling the CA virus from an infant with croup. Pediatrics 22:56-59, 1958
24. DeMEIO JL: Adaptation of parainfluenza 2 (croup-associated) virus to the embryonated hen's egg. J Bacteriol 85:943-944, 1963
25. DeMEIO JL and WALKER DL: Demonstration of antigenic relationship between mumps virus and hemagglutinating virus of Japan. J Immunol 78:465-471, 1957
26. DICK EC and MOGABGAB WJ: Characteristics of parainfluenza 1 (HA2) virus. II. Hemagglutination, hemagglutination-inhibition and neutralization. Am J Hyg 73:273-281, 1961
27. DICK EC and MOGABGAB WJ: Characteristics of parainfluenza I (HA2) virus. III. Antigenic relationships, growth, interaction and erythrocytes and physical properties. J Bacteriol 83:561-571, 1962
28. DOANE FW, ANDERSON N, CHATIYANONDA K, BANNATYNE RM, McLEAN DM and GHODES AJ: Rapid laboratory diagnosis of paramyxovirus infections by electron microscopy. Lancet 2:751-753, 1967
29. DOWDLE W and ROBINSON RQ: Unpublished data
30. FUKUMI H, NISHIKAWA F, SUGIYAMA T, YAMAGUCHI Y, NANBA J, NATSUURA T, and OIKAWA R: An epidemic due to HA2 virus in an elementary school in Tokyo, Japan. J Med Sci Biol 12:307-317, 1959
31. GARDNER PS, McQUILLIN J, and McGUCKIN R: The late detection of respiratory syncytial virus in cells of respiratory tract by immunofluorescence. J Hyg 68:575-580, 1970
32. GARDNER PS and McQUILLIN J: Application of immunofluorescent antibody technique in rapid diagnosis of respiratory syncytial virus infection. Br Med J 3:340-343, 1968
33. GARDNER PS, McQUILLIN J, McGUCKIN R, and DITCHBURN RK: Observations on clinical and immunofluorescent diagnosis of parainfluenza virus infections. Br Med J 2:7-12, 1971
34. Glezen WP, Loda FA, and DENNY FW: The parainfluenza virus. In Viral Infections of Humans, Epidemiology and Control, Evans AS (ed), Plenum Medical Book Company, New York, 1976, pp 337-349

35. HAMPARIAN VV, HILLEMAN MR, and KETLER A: Contributions to characterization and classification of animal viruses. Proc Soc Exp Biol Med 112:1040-1050, 1963

36. HERMODSSON S: Effect of ultrasonic vibration on the hemagglutinating activity of some parainfluenza viruses. Nature 188:1214, 1960

37. HERMODSSON S, DINTER Z and BAKOS K: Studies on variants of a bovine strain of parainfluenza 3 virus 2. Hemagglutinating activity. Acta Pathol Microbiol Scand 51:75-80, 1961

38. HOSAKA T, HOSOKAWA Y and FUKAI K: A new device for preparing subunits of myxovirus. Biken J 2:367-370, 1959

39. HSIUNG GD, ISACSON P and McCOLLUM RW: Studies of myxovirus isolated from human blood. I. Isolation and properties. J Immunol 88:284-290, 1962

40. JENSEN KE, PEELER BE and DULWORTH WG: Immunization against parainfluenza infections. Antigenicity of egg adapted types 1 and 3. J Immunol 89:216-226, 1962

41. JOHN TJ and FULGINITI VA: Parainfluenza 2 virus: increase in hemagglutinin titer on treatment with tween-80 and ether. Proc Soc Exp Biol Med 121:109-111, 1966

42. JOHNSON KM, CHANOCK RM, COOK MK and HUEBNER RJ: Studies of a new human hemadsorption virus. I. Isolation properties and characterization. Am J Hyg 71:81-92, 1960

43. KIM HW, VARGOSKO AJ, CHANOCK RM and PARROTT RH: Parainfluenza 2 (CA) virus: etiologic association with croup. Pediatrics 28:614-621, 1961

44. LEWIS FA, LEHMANN NE and FERRIS AA: The hemadsorption viruses in laryngo-tracheobronchitis. Med J Aust 48:929-932, 1961

45. LIEBHABER H, KRUGMAN S, McGREGOR D, and GILES JP: Studies of a myxovirus recovered from patients with infectious hepatitis. I. Isolation and characterization. J Exp Med 122:1135-1150, 1965

46. MARSTON RQ and VAUGHAN ER: Parainfluenza 3—Assay and growth in tissue culture. Proc Soc Exp Biol Med 104:56-60, 1960

47. McLEAN DM, BACH RD, LARKE RPB and McNAUGHTON GA: Myxoviruses associated with acute laryngotracheobronchitis in Toronto, 1962-63. Can Med Assoc J 89:1257-1259, 1963

48. McQUILLIN J and GARDNER PS: Rapid diagnosis of respiratory syncytial virus infection by immunofluorescent antibody techniques. Br Med J 1:602-605, 1968

49. McQUILLIN J, GARDNER PS and STURDY PA: The use of cough/nasal swabs in the rapid diagnosis of respiratory syncytial virus infection by the fluorescent antibody technique. J Hyg 68: 283-292, 1970

50. NUMAZAKI Y, SHIGETA S, YANO N, TAKAI S and ISHIDA N: A varient of parainfluenza type 2 virus. Proc Soc Exp Biol Med 127:992-996, 1968

51. MUFSON MA, MOCEGA HE and KRAUSE HE: Acquisitic of parainfluenza 3 virus infection by hospitalized children I. Frequencies, rates and temporal data. J Infect Dis 128:141-147, 1973

52. PARROTT RH, VARGOSKO AJ, KIM HW, BELL JA and CHANOCK RM: Acute respiratory diseases of viral etiology III. Myxoviruses: parainfluenza. Am J Public Health 52:907-917, 1962

53. REED LJ and MUENCH H: A simple method of estimating fifty percent endpoints. Am J Hyg 27:493-497, 1938

54. ROTT R: Antigenicity of Newcastle disease virus. In Newcastle Disease Virus. An Evolving Pathogen. Hanson RP (ed), Univ Wis Press, Madison, 1964, pp 133-146

55. ROTT R, WATERSON AP and REDA IM: Characterization of "Soluble antigens" derived from cells infected with Sendai and Newcastle disease viruses. Virology 21:663-665, 1963

56. SCHEID A and CHOPPIN PW: Identification of biological activities of paramyxovirus glycoproteins. Activation of cell fusion, hemolysis and infectivity by proteolytic cleavage of an inactivate precursor protein of Sendai virus. Virology 57:475-490, 1974

57. SCHMIDT NJ, LENNETTE EH, and HANAHOE MF: A micro-method for performing parainfluenza virus neutralization tests. Proc Soc Exp Biol Med 122:1062-1067, 1966

58. SMITH CB, CANCHOLA J, and CHANOCK RM: A micro-method for assay of neutralizing antibodies against parainfluenza virus types 1 and 3. Proc Soc Exp Biol Med 124:4-7, 1967

59. SMITH CB, PURCELL RH, BELLANTI JA and CHANOCK RM: Protective effect of antibody to parainfluenza type I virus. N Engl J Med 275:1145-1152, 1966
60. SPURRIER ER and ROBINSON RQ: Antigenic relationships among human and animal strains of parainfluenza viruses. Health Lab Sci 2:203-207, 1965
61. SUTTON RNP: Respiratory viruses in a residential nursery. J Hyg 60:51-67, 1962
62. VAN DER VEEN J: Personal communication
63. VAN DER VEEN J and SONDERKAMP HJA: Secondary antibody response of guinea pigs to parainfluenza and mumps viruses. Arch Gesamte Virusforsch 15:721-734, 1965
64. VARGOSKO AJ: Unpublished data
65. VARGOSKO AJ, CHANOCK RM, HUEBNER RJ, LUCKEY AH, KIM HW, CUMMING C, and PARROTT RH: Association of type 2 hemadsorption (parainfluenza i) virus and Asian influenza A virus with infectious croup. N Engl J Med 261:1-9, 1959
66. VON EULER L, KANTOR FS, and HSIUNG GD: Studies of parainfluenza viruses. I. Clinical, pathological and virological observations. Yale J Biol Med 35:523-533, 1963
67. WATERSON AP: Two kinds of myxovirus. Nature 193:1163-1164, 1962
68. WATERSON AP and HURRELL JMW: The fine structure of the parainfluenza viruses (brief report). Arch Gesamte Virusforsch 12:138-142, 1962
69. WATERSON AP, JENSEN KE, TYRRELL DAJ, and HORNE RW: The structure of parainfluenza 3 virus. Virology 14:374-378, 1961
70. WULFF H, SOEKEN J, POLAND JE, and CHIN TDY: A new microneutralization test for antibody determination and typing of parainfluenza and influenza viruses. Proc Soc Exp Biol Med 125:1045-1049, 1967

CHAPTER 20

MUMPS VIRUS

Hope E. Hopps and Paul D. Parkman

Introduction

Mumps virus is a member of the paramyxovirus subgroup which encompasses the parainfluenza viruses and Newcastle disease virus (35). The virus has a single-strand RNA-containing nucleoprotein core and an outer membrane which contains both a hemagglutinin and a neuraminidase. Mumps virus, found only in humans, can produce either clinically apparent or inapparent infections.

History

Mumps as a disease was probably first described in the fifth century B.C. by Hippocrates. By 1790, orchitis was recognized as a complication, but it was not until the twentieth century that meningoencephalitis was definitely associated with mumps infection. In 1934, the etiologic agent was identified as a virus by Johnson and Goodpasture (58).

Clinical aspects

Mumps is transmitted from one individual to another by saliva containing the virus. Transmission may occur by direct transfer, by air-suspended droplets, or by fomites recently contaminated with saliva. Although the pathogenesis of mumps infection is not yet precisely understood, the evidence available supports the following concept: virus first multiplies in an unknown site, presumably in the upper respiratory tract; invasion of the blood stream then occurs and infection of the salivary glands and other organs is thus established. In most instances 18 days elapse between the time of exposure and the first detectable enlargement of the salivary glands; the incubation period may range, however, from 14 to 24 days. The period of communicability, as determined by the isolation of virus from the saliva in naturally occurring mumps and in experimentally induced infections, can extend from 7 days before salivary gland involvement until 9 days thereafter (33, 39, 50, 72). The usual period of communicability, however, is probably shorter, lasting from a few days before to a few days after onset of parotitis. The virus can be present in saliva of cases of inapparent infection

633

and of cases of orchitis or meningitis in which enlargement of the salivary gland is absent (50, 63). Presumably, it is from such sources that cases of mumps infection can arise for which no known source of exposure can be determined. Mumps virus is also excreted in the urine for as long as 14 days after onset of illness (84, 85).

Uncomplicated infection of the salivary glands is manifested by enlargement of one or more of these organs—most often the parotids. The swelling in most cases reaches a maximum after 48 hours, and a gland usually remains enlarged from 7 to 10 days. Fever of short duration and of moderate degree can be present; sometimes the rise in temperature may be negligible or absent.

The two most common complications, orchitis (seen in about 20% of mature males) and meningoencephalitis (occurring in an incidence from 0.5–10% in different studies), often develop between the second and tenth day after the onset of parotitis. These conditions can also appear either before or at the same time the salivary glands become enlarged. Moreover, they can be the only presenting signs.

Ovaritis occurs in about 5% of adult females with mumps. Other complications, such as pancreatitis, thyroiditis, neuritis of various nerves (facial, trigeminal, optic, and auditory), involvement of the eye (conjunctivitis, keratitis, iritis, and retinitis), and of the inner ear are encountered more rarely. In addition to causing pancreatitis, there have been reports suggesting that diabetes mellitus can occasionally be a complication of mumps, although the association is at present inconclusive (82). While some investigators have suggested that intrauterine mumps infection can occur and lead to endocardial fibroelastosis (1, 79), more recent reports have failed to provide evidence for this route of infection (19, 76).

For obvious reasons, the pathologic changes in the salivary glands or other organs which can be affected have not been studied extensively. On the basis of the information available, however, they are not sufficiently characteristic to be of diagnostic value, even were it practicable to obtain tissues for routine examination.

The typical case of mumps is readily recognized, particularly during epidemic periods, and rarely requires laboratory confirmation. Specific diagnostic tests are needed mainly for establishing the etiology of complications, such as meningoencephalitis or orchitis, in the absence of salivary gland involvement. In cases presenting only involvement of the central nervous system, additional tests for viruses other than mumps must be performed.

Description and Nature of the Agent

Mumps virus has an RNA-containing nucleoprotein core, encased in a lipid-containing outer membrane which has surface projections. The outer surface of the virus has hemagglutinin and neuraminidase activity (35). An RNA-dependent RNA polymerase has been shown in mumps virus grown in embryonated eggs (5). The virus has the ability to hemolyze erythrocytes paramyxoviruses. Johnson and Goodpasture (58) demonstrated that virus from monkey parotid glands passes readily through Berkefeld N and V filters. Subsequent publications on filtration through gradocol membranes, analytical centrifugation, and electron microscopy have reported particle sizes ranging from 85μ to >300 μ diameter (16, 52). Electron micrographs obtained by negative contrast staining with phosphotungstic acid showed that the virus is composed of an internal helical structure enclosed in an outer envelope (54). The internal component, a ribonucleoprotein, is identical with the soluble (S) complement-fixing (CF) antigen (49). The outer envelope of the virus contains the viral (V) antigen and the hemagglutinating activity of the agent, first demonstrated by Levens and Enders (71).

Analysis of virus purified by density gradient ultracentrifugation using polyacrylamide gel electrophoresis revealed the presence of 6 polypeptides ranging in size from 40,000 to 64,000 daltons. There are only 2 glycoproteins; the larger one appears to be the site of hemagglutinating and neuraminidase activity (57).

The infectivity of the virus is inactivated by exposure to 0.1% formalin, ultraviolet irradiation, or treatment with ether without necessarily destroying its hemagglutinating activity and CF antigens. The virus is relatively stable; its infectivity is little changed on storage at 4 C for several days, at -20 C for weeks, and at -50 to -70 C for many months. The stability may be improved by addition of proteins, such as 1% bovine albumin, 0.5% gelatin, or 2% serum of various species if proven to be free of inhibitors (16).

Preparation of Immune Serum

For positive and negative control sera employed in various serologic tests, most laboratories have been using selected sera from individuals without past experience with mumps virus, or early acute-phase sera and sera taken 2 weeks or later after onset of disease. Consequently, few efforts have been made to produce immune serum in animals. No difficulties are encountered in inducing good antibody responses in rhesus monkeys, rabbits, guinea pigs, hamsters, and ferrets.

Antibody responses in guinea pigs have been studied to the greatest extent (56). A single dose of 10^3 EID_{50} administered intranasally yielded good antibody titers to the S-antigen within 2-3 weeks, whereas antibodies to the V-antigen arose later or not at all. An intraperitoneal injection of 10^7 EID_{50} elicited high titers of both types of antibodies within 2-3 weeks, whereas the same dose of ultraviolet-inactivated virus yielded essentially only antibodies to V-antigen. The observation that live, but not inactivated, virus yields anti-S suggests that a subclinical infection is induced in guinea pigs. The use of guinea pigs and a single dose of virus is advantageous because the resulting serum is generally free of anticomplementary and nonspecific reactivity.

Collection and Preparation of Specimens for Laboratory Diagnosis

Precautions

Mumps virus has been categorized in Class 2 by the US Public Health Service *Ad Hoc* Committee on the Safe Shipment and Handling of Etiologic Agents. Agents in this category are of ordinary potential hazard, i.e., they can produce disease from accidental inoculation but are contained by ordinary laboratory techniques (83). As with all potentially pathogenic organisms, correct and careful laboratory techniques, including effective decontamination and sterilization procedures, are indicated. If a worker is known to be susceptible, precautions should be taken to avoid the introduction of infected materials into the oral cavity or respiratory tract, since a laboratory infection has occurred by inadvertent contamination of the mouth with infected monkey salivary gland (28). If desired, susceptible persons can be vaccinated. A live attenuated mumps virus vaccine gives excellent protection (13, 34).

Virus isolation specimens

Mumps virus is readily recovered from the saliva of patients on the first and second day of disease, and occasionally later. Mumps virus has rather frequently been isolated from the spinal fluid of patients with meningoencephalitis within 6 days after onset (51, 63). It is also often excreted in the urine for as long as 14 days after appearance of symptoms (84, 85). Generally, it is desirable to collect specimens as early in the disease as possible. Virus has been isolated on some occasions also from blood (62), milk (64), the parotid gland, and other tissues (89). Stools and buffy-coat leukocytes are generally negative (84).

In young patients, saliva is collected by a suitable suction device (50) or by swabbing, especially of the area around the orifices of the Stenson duct. The swabs are placed immediately into tubes containing 1–3 ml of a suitable medium such as Hanks balanced salt solution (BSS) with a protein stabilizer and antibiotics; virus isolation from swabs is only slightly less successful than from saliva samples (84). Spinal fluid is obtained in the usual manner. For urine specimens, preferably the first voided morning urine is collected in a sterile container. All materials are immediately placed on ice where they may be kept for a few hours prior to inoculation. For longer storage, specimens should be maintained at -70 C or in liquid nitrogen. Freezing of the specimens diminishes the infectivity of the virus (45, 84). However, this adverse effect can be counteracted by the addition to the specimens of an equal volume of protein solutions such as 1% bovine albumin.

Penicillin (500 units/ml) and streptomycin (1000 μg/ml) are added to bacterially contaminated specimens before inoculation. For saliva, an equal volume of sterile infusion broth is added, and the mixture is then centrifuged. The addition of broth may aid in the deposition of bacteria by reducing viscosity. Concentration of the virus by high-speed centrifugation markedly increases the success of isolation from urine specimens (85). Approximately 15 ml of urine is clarified by centrifugation at 4 C for 10 min at 1500 rpm. The supernatant fluid is then spun at 40,000 rpm for 90 min in a Spinco Model-L centrifuge. The pellet, resuspended in one-tenth volume of Hanks BSS serves as inoculum. Spinal fluid is used directly as the inoculum.

Specimens for serologic diagnosis

Although virus isolation is the most certain means for establishing the laboratory diagnosis, serologic methods are also useful and easier technically. Between 5 and 10 ml of blood is obtained and allowed to clot; the serum is removed under sterile conditions with precautions to prevent hemolysis. The serum can be stored in tightly stoppered containers at 4 C for up to 4 weeks; after this period the antibody concentration in human serum may decline significantly. For this reason it is best to store serum at -10 to -15 C, at which temperature the antibody levels remain constant for years (30). Known positive and negative human sera to be used as controls in CF tests are stored in small volumes in the manner described to avoid frequent freezing and thawing, which also tends to reduce antibody titers. If the specimen will be in transit for more than 1 day, serum rather than clotted blood should be shipped to the laboratory.

Although strong presumptive evidence of infection by mumps virus can be obtained for a considerable proportion of patients from a single early serum specimen by using V- and S-antigens separately in the CF test (47, 49), it is essential for a final diagnosis to obtain at least 2 specimens of blood at an appropriate interval to demonstrate the development or increase of specific antibodies. Accordingly, a blood specimen is drawn as early as possible after the onset of symptoms, and another 7–14 days later. If no antibody is demonstrated in the second specimen, a third is obtained on the twenty-first day, by which time antibodies regularly are found.

Specimens for microscopic examination

Infected cell culture preparations can be examined for typical acidophilic intracytoplasmic inclusions, using coverslip cultures fixed in Bouin fluid and stained with hematoxylin and eosin (7, 41). For immunofluorescence microscopy, coverslips are washed in phosphate-buffered saline (pH 7.2), dipped in distilled water to remove salts, fixed in acetone at 22 C for 10–18 min, and air dried. Conjugate is prepared by ammonium sulfate fractionation of mumps antiserum produced in immunized guinea pigs. The globulin-rich fraction is conjugated with fluorescein isothiocyanate by using standard methods (69). Electron microscopic observations are most readily made on preparations purified and concentrated by differential centrifugation (54). Negative staining techniques employing collodion and carbon-coated 300-mesh copper grids and 1% sodium phosphotungstate are most commonly used.

Laboratory Diagnosis

Clinical pathology

Blood. In many patients with mumps uncomplicated by secondary bacterial infection, the total white cell count may be moderately elevated, but in others it is within normal limits and in some it may be depressed. The differential count frequently, but not invariably, may show an absolute or relative increase in lymphocytes from the first to the fourteenth day of the disease; the white cell count is of little importance in the diagnosis of infection due to mumps virus.

Spinal fluid. In mumps meningoencephalitis, the white cell counts of the spinal fluid can range from the normal 8–10 cells/mm³ to more than 2000 cells/mm³. For most patients, the differential count reveals 90–100% lymphocytes at some time during the illness (59, 63, 68). The proportion of lymphocytes can be lower in specimens taken early in the disease (68). In this connection, it should be recalled that in clinically uncomplicated parotitis an increase in the white cells in the spinal fluid has often been observed. Total counts entirely comparable with those encountered in frank meningoencephalitis have been recorded (4).

Serum amylase. The serum amylase regularly increases in mumps parotitis (3, 15, 90 ,91). An increase in this enzyme does not necessarily indicate pancreatic involvement (88). The maximum level is attained during the first week; thereafter, it declines until normal levels are commonly reached by the fourth week. The determination of serum amylase can be of assistance in the differentiation of mumps from other conditions that produce salivary gland enlargement or in the retrospective recognition of cases in patients in whom the swelling has subsided at the time of examination.

Virus isolation in animals

The early literature on transmission of mumps virus to monkeys, dogs, cats, and rabbits has been adequately reviewed (29). Small rodents, either newborn (65, 67) or adult (12, 38), are susceptible to various extents. For primary isolation of virus from patients, none of these species is of particular value because the chick-embryo and cell-culture techniques are more convenient for this purpose.

Virus isolation in embryonated eggs

Amniotic inoculation. For primary isolation of the virus in chick embryos, inoculation into the amniotic sac constitutes the route of choice. Yolk-sac inoculation can also be used for primary isolation but offers no advantage; in fact, the highest yields of hemagglutinin are found in the amniotic fluid.

Embryos at 7 to 8 days of development are used. The eggs are candled, the position of the embryonic eye is located, and a small hole is drilled into the shell over the air space at a distance of about 2 cm from the eye of the embryo. After disinfecting the area with tincture of iodine or 75% alcohol, the egg is placed in an almost horizontal position over the candling light.

With a $1^1/_2$ inch, 25-gauge hypodermic needle, the inoculation is made through the opening in the shell with a swift thrust toward the embryo. A lively movement of the latter indicates that the amniotic sac has been penetrated. After injecting 0.1–0.2 ml of inoculum and removing the needle, the opening is sealed with nail polish. Six to eight embryos are inoculated in this manner. Since the inoculum is administered "blindly", it can sometimes fail to enter the amniotic cavity. Some workers prefer injecting under direct vision (49, 72). An opening 1 cm in diameter is cut into the shell over the air sac toward the side where the embryo is located. With a pair of pointed forceps, a small sliver of the shell membrane is removed from the underlying chorioallantoic membrane (CAM). With appropriate illumination, the embryo can now be seen within the amnion through the bared part of the CAM, and the inoculum is injected into the amnion under observation. The hole in the shell is closed with cellophane tape. The eggs are then incubated for 5–7 days at 35–37 C.

Before harvest, the eggs are chilled in the refrigerator for several hours or in the freezer for 20–30 min to prevent bleeding during collection of the materials. The shell over the sac is disinfected and cut away with scissors. The allantoic fluid is withdrawn by pipette or decanted, depending whether it is wanted for the test. In early passages, the allantoic fluid usually contains little virus. The amniotic sac is then grasped with a pair of forceps, pulled upward and entered with a capillary pipette. The yield of amniotic fluid from infected embryos 13–14 days of age varies considerably; the average volume obtained is from 0.25 to 0.5 ml. Larger yields are derived from 11- to 12-day-old embryos.

Once the amniotic fluid has been removed, the tear is widened with a Pasteur pipette, and the embryo is dislodged from the cavity; the amniotic membrane is pulled out with the forceps, tearing it away from its points of attachment. This procedure often fails to secure the total sac; thus, some workers prefer to deposit the contents of the eggs into Petri dishes, holding the CAM against the shell by pressure with the forceps. The amnion is then stripped from the embryo and carefully teased away from the surface of the yolk sac, which it may cover to some extent. The weight of individual membranes is small, varying from 0.2 g to 0.5 g. The tissues are washed in about 10 ml of physiologic salt solution and their wet weight is determined. A 20% suspension is made by grinding the material in a mortar with sterile alundum and saline solution or in other appropriate types of grinders. Larger numbers of membranes can be emulsified in a blender. After centrifugation at about 1500 rpm for 10 min, the supernatant fluid is used for testing.

Tests for bacterial sterility are done immediately on each pool of material. All harvests are stored in the refrigerator overnight, but for longer storage, it is best to store the materials at -70 C or in liquid nitrogen.

Procedures for passage and adaptation of the virus

Further amniotic passages. The virus appears to multiply most regularly at first in the amniotic cavity as indicated by detectable and sometimes high concentrations of CF antigen in the membrane suspensions and by the presence of hemagglutinins in the amniotic fluid. Negative tests do not necessarily imply absence of virus. Indeed, virus frequently may not be detectable in the originally inoculated eggs. Before a negative result is recorded, second and third passages of pooled amniotic fluid or mixtures of amniotic fluid and membrane suspensions must be carried out by the technique described.

After serial passages by the amniotic route, the strains may become adapted to growth in the allantoic cavity. Occasionally, this can occur after 1 or 2 amniotic transfers; however, in other instances it may require a long series of amniotic passages and with certain strains, adaptation to the allantoic sac is not possible (16). Strains adapted to the allantoic sac are used for production of CF and HAI diagnostic reagents.

Allantoic sac inoculation. Embryos at 7 to 9 days of development are candled and the position of the embryo eye is marked. A small hole is drilled into the shell a little to one side of the mark. Through this aperture the sac is entered with a 1.3 cm (.5″), 26-gauge needle; the position of the needle is almost parallel to the shell when the injection is made; the volume of inoculum is 0.1 ml. At this stage of embryonic development, the allantoic sac is still relatively small and backflow of fluid after inoculation can present a problem, especially when inocula of >0.1 ml are used. To avoid this, a hole is cut into the shell over the air space and, by inserting a 2.58-cm (1″), 22-gauge needle, the injection is made just under the allantoic membrane facing the air space. After sealing the opening, the eggs are incubated at 35–37 C for various periods of time, depending upon the dose of virus inoculated. Maximal yields of virus may be reached within 5 days after large doses, whereas 7 days may be required with minimal infectious doses.

Before harvest, the eggs are chilled, and the allantoic fluid is withdrawn by pipette as described above. Volumes of 6–10 ml per egg may be obtained from 12- to 14-day-old embryos. The contents of the eggs are then decanted with care to retain the allantoic membrane within the shell. The membrane at this stage adheres to the shell and it is essential to separate its attachment to the embryo before the weight of the latter pulls it loose. The membrane is then washed *in situ* with saline solution before it is removed with forceps, and prepared into a suspension as described above on page 637.

Other routes. Although mumps virus does replicate in chick embryos inoculated into the yolk sac (43) and onto the CAM (6), these techniques have found little practical application and are not described here.

Indications of infection

Mortality and pathology. Death of the embryo is a variable criterion depending upon the strain of virus and the batches of embryos employed; therefore, it is not a reliable index of infection. There are no gross or microscopic pathologic lesions in the embryonic tissues, whether collected from dead or live embryos, that can be specifically associated with the effect of the virus.

Demonstration of a specific hemagglutinin. The detection of hemagglutinating activity in materials from inoculated embryos can be regarded as the most convenient and reliable index of infection (20), but its absence in fluids from initially inoculated or first passage eggs does not necessarily indicate that infection has failed to occur, since virus yields on the order of 10^6 infectious units of virus per ml are required for hemagglutination (HA) to occur. The presence and concentration of hemagglutinin is determined by the technique described below. Its specificity can be determined by showing that hemagglutinin is inhibited by specific antiserum (see below). Nonspecific HA in low titer, especially when tested with guinea pig erythrocytes (RBC), is observed on occasion with normal amniotic fluid (21).

The determination of specific CF antigens. The CF technique was the first to be employed as an index of infection in the embryo (43). It is possibly somewhat more sensitive at the first egg passage than the HA test, because it can yield positive results with CAM suspensions when the amniotic fluid may as yet be free of detectable hemagglutinins. Appropriate methods are described below. However, on account of its simplicity, HA has largely superseded the CF test.

Propagation in tissue culture. Mumps virus propagates in a variety of cell cultures. Virus in clinical specimens or virus which has undergone only a few passages in the chick embryo propagates well in simian cells (e.g., rhesus, cynomolgus, and *Cercopithecus* monkey kidney), continuous human cell lines (e.g., HeLa) or primary cultures (e.g., human amnion, human embryonic kidney). These virus strains produce cytopathic effects (CPE) and hemadsorption (HAd) and can be serially passaged (7, 10, 23, 26, 41, 45, 84, 85). Strains adapted to the allantoic cavity of the chick embryo also caused CPE in these cell cultures but, as a rule, cannot be maintained in them by serial transfers (6, 46). The chick-embryo-adapted virus, on the other hand, multiplies readily in cultures of chick embryo cells in contrast to the freshly isolated virus (8, 41). Primary human or simian renal cells appear to be the most sensitive for primary virus isolation. Mumps virus CPE is evidenced by cellular degeneration with or without accompanying syncytium formation. Syncytia have been described both with freshly isolated human strains and with virus at various stages of chick embryo adaptation (45, 46, 84); the cell membranes appear to dissolve, adjacent cells fuse, and the nuclei of the fused cells tend to aggregate (46). Infected cells contain acidophilic cytoplasmic inclusions (8, 41) and exhibit the phenomenon of HAd (81).

Primary isolation procedures

Early studies using HeLa and monkey renal cells showed them to be sensitive and more rapid for virus isolation than the chick embryo. Of the 2 cell types employed, monkey kidney cells proved to be more susceptible than HeLa cells (45, 84). Primary rhesus monkey kidney cells have been most commonly used for mumps virus isolation. Considerable experience in several laboratories suggests that primary cynomolgus cultures provide a satisfactory substitute for rhesus kidney cells. Primary *Cercopithecus* cultures have been used less widely but also appear to be satisfactory. Primary human embryo kidney cell cultures have also been used (23). No studies have been reported comparing frequency of isolation in serially passaged monkey cells such as BS-C-1, Vero, or DBS-FRhL-2 with primary cultures. The general impression, however, is that these cultures are less sensitive for virus isolation. WI-38 human fibroblasts have been shown to yield fewer isolates than primary rhesus cultures.

Primary rhesus, cynomolgus, or *Cercopithecus* monkey renal cell cultures are prepared as described in Chapter 3. After the cells have become confluent, the medium is removed, the cultures are inoculated with 0.1–0.2 ml of specimen of virus preparation, and the cultures are then maintained in a medium containing equal parts of medium No. 199 and Eagle minimal essential medium (MEM) without added serum and 100 units of penicillin and 100 μg of streptomycin per ml. Other conventional media can also be used. General experience suggests that fetal bovine serum does not contain inhibitors for mumps virus growth; if other types of sera (e.g., calf or horse serum) are used it is prudent to pretest for inhibitors of mumps virus replication.

HeLa cell tube cultures are prepared as described in Chapter 3. At the time of or just before the cell sheets become confluent, usually after 3–4 days at 37 C, the medium is removed, the cultures are inoculated as described above, and then refed with a medium containing Eagle MEM, 2% fetal bovine serum, and antibiotics.

The inoculated cultures are incubated at 36–37 C, and are examined daily for the appearance of CPE. The maintenance medium should be replaced as necessary to maintain the cells in good condition. Whether or not CPE is noted within 6–7 days, HAd tests should be carried out to confirm that the cytopathology is due to a hemadsorbing virus and to detect possible minimal degrees of infection. As a rule, additional passages are required to obtain enough materials for identification of the isolate. Negative first-passage cultures should be passaged once more to make certain that virus is not present.

Hemadsorption (HAd) test. The yield of virus in the cell culture medium is generally too small to be detected by the HA test, although some success has been recorded (84). Infected cells do, however, adsorb RBC due to the incorporation of viral hemagglutinin into the cell membrane (17, 81).

The HAd test is carried out as follows:

The medium need not be removed from the cultures, although some investigators prefer to wash the cell sheets with Hanks BSS before the test. A sterile suspension of 0.4% chicken or guinea pig RBC is prepared and added in 0.2 ml volumes to the tubes. Uninoculated cultures of the same batch are treated in the same manner for control purposes, especially when monkey renal cells are used, to exclude the possibility that an indigenous infection with a hemadsorbing virus such as SV-5 is present. The tubes are incubated in a near to horizontal position at room temperature for 3–5 min or at 4 C for 20–30 min. The tubes are then turned to permit the unattached RBC to float off, and the cell sheet is examined microscopically at low magnification (100–150X) for cell-attached clusters of RBC. Most striking results are seen when extensive lesions are present. A definite, though lesser, degree of hemadsorption may be noted in infected cultures even before the development of detectable CPE. After the test, the cultures are washed and refed for further incubation or used for additional passages so long as sterile RBC suspensions are employed.

Identification of the isolate

Hemadsorption inhibition (HAdI). The medium is removed from 4 infected cultures, and the cell sheets are washed once. Two of the tubes receive 0.8 ml of appropriately diluted antimumps serum, and the others receive normal serum or BSS. After incubation at room temperature or at 37 C (preferred by some workers) for 15–60 min in a nearly horizontal position, 0.2 ml of the RBC suspension is added to these tubes, as well as to the uninoculated control cultures. The cell sheets are inspected for HAd as described in the preceding section. Absence of HAd in tubes treated with antimumps serum indicates presence of mumps virus.

Neutralization (Nt) test. Material from infected cultures, clarified by centrifugation at 1500 rpm for 10 min and diluted to contain an estimated 10–50 $TCID_{50}$ of virus, is mixed with appropriately diluted antimumps- or antibody-negative reference serum. After 30–60 min at 37 C, portions of these mixtures are inoculated into several cultures each, these cultures are incubated at 36–37 C, and observed daily for the appearance of lesions. Suppression or significant reduction of CPE in the test culture, as compared to the controls, permits identification of the agent. HAd tests carried out as described above can also be used for evaluation of the results.

Immunofluorescence staining. The most rapid identification of mumps virus isolates from cell cultures can be accomplished by immunofluorescence staining (69), and conjugates are now available from commercial sources.

Serologic diagnosis

A serologic diagnosis of mumps virus infection can be made by testing for CF, HAI, or Nt antibodies. The CF and HAI procedures are of approximately equal sensitivity (27). The standard Nt test is generally slightly more sensitive in detecting antibodies than is the HAI test (14, 61). This difference is of particular importance in assessing antibody responses to vaccination when antibody titers are lower than those following natural mumps virus infection (34). Mumps virus shares antigenic relationships with other viruses of the paramyxovirus group as evidenced by serologic cross-reactions in each of these tests on serum from infected humans and animals (22, 55, 70, 87). Thus, serologic results must be interpreted in the light of the available clinical and epidemiologic information. It is conceivable that such cross-reactions might account for some of the occasional instances in which individuals with serologic evidence of immunity have subsequently developed mumps. The frequency with which cross-reactions are observed increases with increasing age and experience with the antigens of this virus group through natural infection (70).

Complement-fixation test

The CF test has proved to be practical for the diagnosis of mumps infections. By parallel use of the V-antigen and S-antigen, it is often possible to arrive at a presumptive diagnosis by testing an early specimen (47). S-antibodies frequently arise before V-antibodies, but the latter persist for longer periods of time. Thus, elevated S-antibody titers, accompanied by low or no levels of V-antibody are noted only in the first few days of illness. Whether this pattern is found or not, a second blood specimen must be taken 10–14 days later to confirm or establish the diagnosis by demonstration of rise in antibody levels. For the determination of immunity status, only V-antigen is required, since S-antibodies usually disappear within a few months. It should be noted that a negative test, especially in the older age groups, does not necessarily imply susceptibility, since 20–30% of the individuals in these groups may give a positive history. Furthermore, a few individuals with positive reactions (1–2%) can, upon subsequent exposure, develop mumps (48, 74). The CF test is not sufficiently sensitive to be used reliably for the detection of antibodies induced by mumps vaccine.

Preparation and standardization of reagents. The V- and S-antigens are derived most conveniently from infected allantoic fluids and membranes, respectively, although potent preparations can also be prepared from amniotic fluids and membranes. Chick embryos are infected with allantoic-sac-adapted virus, and the fluid and membrane are harvested as described above. On day 5–6 after inoculation, the allantoic fluids usually reveal only V-antigen activity. The V-antigen is located in the envelope of the virus particles, which covers the internal S-antigen so that it is inaccessible to homologous antibody. The virus particles may break down on storage, thereby exposing some S-antigen. The allantoic fluids are dialyzed against 20 volumes of 0.01 M phosphate-buffered saline solution (PBS), pH 7, to remove most of the urates which may precipitate on prolonged storage. This procedure is necessary as a preliminary step for efficient inactivation of the virus by ultraviolet light, should this be desired (47). The V-antigen is separated from the allantoic fluid by centrifugation at 20,000 rpm for 30 min and resuspended in BSS.

For S-antigen, a 20% suspension of the membranes is prepared and centrifuged at 20,000 rpm for 30 min to sediment most of the virus particles. The virus also can be removed by adsorption onto chicken RBC. Neither of these techniques affects the S-antigen titer of the supernatant fluid. It is recommended that 30% sucrose be added to the final preparation as a stabilizer. In this manner, the antigen can be kept at 4 C for weeks and in the frozen or lyophilized state, for years. The sucrose, after dilution in the test procedure, does not interfere with the CF reaction.

Control antigens are prepared in the same manner from uninfected embryos of the same batch. Merthiolate 1:10,000 is added to all antigens as a preservative.

The antigens are standardized in "box" or "checkerboard" titrations against appropriate human convalescent-phase sera or guinea pig immune sera. Increasing dilutions of antigen (undiluted through 1:64) are tested against the respective sera in suitable dilutions (e.g., 1:8 through 2 dilutions beyond the serum endpoint, which may be as high as 1:2048). The highest dilution of antigen which gives the highest serum titer (3+ to 4+ fixation) represents the optimal dose. Twice this amount is used in the test to guard against day-to-day variations in the sensitivity of the hemolytic system. It should be noted that the optimal dose determined with guinea pig serum is generally half that observed with human serum. If guinea pig serum is employed for standardization, 4 optimal doses of antigen are required for testing of human serum.

Serum is heated at 56 C for 30 min or at 60 C for 20 min. If a serum is found to be anticomplementary, heating for a second time at 60 C for 20 min often will remove this property without affecting the antibody level. If reactions with host control antigens are noted, absorption of the serum with sheep RBC (1 part of serum plus 1 part of 10% suspension, held 20 min at room temperature and then centrifuged) may serve to decrease this reactivity.

There are no special considerations as far as diluents and the hemolytic system are concerned. Both the complement and the antisheep hemolysin should be standardized in box or checkerboard titrations.

Procedure for the CF test. Any standard technique is satisfactory if reagents are well standardized and utilized at near optimal reactivities. An example of a suitable CF procedure is given in Chapter 1. Two-fold dilutions of the test sera are made in triplicate or quintuplicate, depending whether one or both of the specific antigens and the corresponding controls are to be employed. The range of dilutions may vary with the aim of the tests. For diagnostic purposes, a range from 1:8 to 1:512 is usually sufficient. For determination of immunity, an initial dilution of 1:2 is desirable, and the series need not exceed 1:32, since higher antibody levels are usually seen only in convalescent-phase serum. One row each receives optimally diluted V-antigen, S-antigen, normal allantoic fluid, normal membrane suspension, or saline solution, respectively. The test is then done using the chosen standard procedure and appropriate controls.

Interpretation of the CF test. The endpoint is taken as the reciprocal of the highest serum dilution causing a $\geq 3+$ fixation of complement. In tests of a single acute-phase serum, the presence of antibodies to the S-antigen, but not to the V-antigen, is highly suggestive of recent infection. A 4-fold increase in antibody titers or reproducible evidence of a change in serologic status from seronegative to seropositive in acute- and convalescent-phase sera is presumptive evidence of mumps infection (see general remarks above).

Hemagglutination-inhibition test (HAI)

The application of the HAI test is generally the same as that for the CF test. The HAI test has the advantage of being technically simpler and less expensive to perform than the other antibody tests. The disadvantages of the test are related to the difficulty in interpreting the meaning of low levels of HAI activity in serum which might be present as a result of difficulty in removing nonspecific inhibitors or as a result of cross-reacting antibodies to other paramyxoviruses (55, 78). Unlike the CF procedure, the HAI does not permit the early presumptive diagnosis provided with CF by the differential use of S- and V-antigens. On the other hand, the hemagglutinating activity and its inhibition by specific immune sera serve more readily than does the CF test to recognize infection of the chick embryo and to identify the isolated virus.

Preparation of antigen. Antigens for the HAI test are most conveniently prepared using allantoic fluids of infected chick embryos (see above) clarified by centrifugation at 1500 rpm for 10 min. Treatment of such antigens with Tween 80 and ether has been shown to increase the HA titer 2- to 4-fold and to improve the sensitivity of the HAI test slightly (14). For this purpose, allantoic fluids from infected eggs are sedimented by centrifugation (18,000 rpm in a No. 21 rotor of the Model-L Spinco centrifuge). The virus pellet is resuspended to one-tenth initial volume in PBS (pH 7.2). Tween 80 in a 1% solution is added slowly to a concentration of 0.1% and agitated using a magnetic stirrer for 5 min and then a half volume of anesthetic ether added. After 5 hr of stirring at room temperature, the aqueous phase is recovered and the residual ether is removed under vacuum. The HA activity remains constant at 4 C for at least 6 months.

Procedure for the HAI test. The same general procedures used for influenza virus are applicable. The test can be performed in glass tubes, plastic plates, or in a microtiter system. While the volume of the reagents employed in different laboratories can vary, and with it the initial concentration of RBC required, the final percentage of RBC in the test should be between 0.25 and 0.50. The following technique can serve as a guide.

Antigen titrations are performed by preparing serial 2-fold dilutions of the test material in 0.85% sodium chloride solution using 0.4 ml volumes and 10-× 100-mm test tubes. Thrice washed adult chicken RBC in 1% suspension are then added, 0.2 ml per tube. After thoroughly shaking the tubes, the test is held at room temperature or at 4 C for 45–60 min, and the degree of agglutination is read according to the pattern formed at the bottom of the tube. If guinea pig RBC are used, 60–90 min are required for their settling. In the absence of agglutination, the RBC settle out in a small firm button, 2–3 mm in diameter. Strong agglutination (+) causes the cells to form a shield of RBC covering the bottom of the tube. Partial agglutination (±) shows a small central button surrounded by a halo of a partial shield. The highest dilution of virus preparation giving + agglutination is taken to contain 1 HA unit (HAU) in 0.4 ml.

Serum to be HAI tested is inactivated at 56 C for 30 min and treated for removal of nonspecific inhibitors. For this purpose adsorption with acid washed kaolin (20), inactivation by treatment with the receptor destroying enzyme RDE of *V. cholera* (11), or periodate (48) can be used. The procedure for periodate treatment is as follows:

To 0.5 ml of serum is added 0.15 ml of 0.1 M $NaIO_4$. After incubation at 37 C for 30 min, 0.15 ml of 40% solution of glucose is added, and the volume is increased to 1 ml with saline solution, effecting a total serum dilution of 1:2. This treatment does not decrease high titers of specific antibodies, but it does reduce the inhibition in many low-titer sera. For the HAI test, serial 2-fold dilutions of serum are prepared in saline solution. To 0.2 ml of each serum dilution is added 0.2 ml of virus preparation diluted to contain 4 HAU (corresponding to 8 HAU in 0.4 ml). After incubation of the test for 1 hr at room temperature or at 37 C, 0.2 ml of 1% suspension of chicken RBC is added to each tube. After shaking the tubes, the RBC are held to settle for 60–90 min at 4 C or at room temperature; the results are read by the patterns as described above. The antihemagglutinin titer is expressed as the reciprocal of the highest serum dilution which completely prevents HA. The following controls are needed: (a) 0.2 ml of lowest serum dilution and 0.2 ml saline solution to show that the serum *per se* does not agglutinate the RBC; (b) 0.2 ml of the diluted virus suspension and 0.2 ml saline solution, as well as 3 further serial 2-fold dilutions of the virus to determine the exact units of hemagglutinin employed in the test; and (c) positive and negative human or animal reference sera in an appropriate range of dilutions to ascertain the specificity and the sensitivity of the test.

The clearest readings are obtained at about the time when the RBC have just settled. With a delay in reading, the positive patterns may be less well defined, because cells can slide toward the center of the well, resulting in partial or even negative agglutination patterns. If the serum is of high titer, no difficulties are encountered in reading of the results. With low-titer serum, the pattern observed often is atypical, in that a broad, flat button may be seen with irregular edges. This pattern may be caused by relatively high serum concentrations and inhibitors of HA. To ascertain whether or not HA has occurred, the test tubes are tilted; nonagglutinated RBC will stream toward the low side of the tube, whereas agglutinated cells will retain the pattern.

Interpretation of the test. A ≥4-fold rise in antihemagglutinin titer in a convalescent-phase serum, as compared to the titer of an acute-phase specimen, is taken as evidence of infection by mumps virus. If the first specimen is taken within 4 days after onset, a significant increase in this antibody can be demonstrated in nearly all cases; if taken between 4 and 8 days, an increase cannot always be detected, since maximal antibody levels may already have been attained. In the latter case, CF tests using the V-antigen may still demonstrate a diagnostically significant ≥4-fold rise in antibodies, since such antibodies reach their peak later in convalescence.

Virus neutralization test

Of the procedures available, the Nt test appears to be the most sensitive and specific. Demonstration of Nt antibodies in serum affords the best evidence of the immune status of an individual. Likewise, the development of Nt antibodies after vaccination provides the most accurate information as to the success of immunization.

Nt tests have been performed in suckling mice (66), embryonated hens' eggs (40, 73), and in a variety of types of cell cultures (14, 25, 31, 32, 42, 46, 60, 75). The cell culture tests are currently used most commonly and are the most sensitive and specific of the methods for detection of mumps antibodies. Serum, previously treated with periodate for HAI tests should not be used in Nt tests because formalin produced by the interaction between periodate and glucose can inactivate the mumps virus in the serum-virus mixtures.

In the embryonated egg. The technique described by Gotlieb et al (40) is as follows:

A pool of mumps-virus-infected allantoic fluid is prepared and stored in small volumes at -70 C or in liquid nitrogen. The virus is titrated under the same conditions as employed in the actual test (see below) to determine the dilution providing the appropriate number of infectious doses. The serum is inactivated at 56 C for 30 min or at 60 C for 20 min. Serial 2-fold dilutions of serum are made in 0.8 ml volumes using sterile saline as diluent. To these are added equal volumes of virus suspension, diluted to provide 1000–10,000 ID_{50} per egg. The serum-virus mixtures are incubated at 37 C for 1 hr or at 4 C for 18 hr, whichever is more convenient. Each mixture is then inoculated in 0.2 ml volumes into the allantoic cavity of 8-day-old chick embryos, using 6 eggs per dilution. After incubation of the eggs at 36–37 C for 6–7 days, individual allantoic fluids are harvested and tested for the presence of hemagglutinin as described above. In such tests, a standard known-positive serum is included, and the diluted test virus preparation is titrated in 3–4 further serial 10-fold dilutions to which equal volumes of saline solution are added to make up for the omitted serum. The results of the Nt test are evaluated on the basis of the presence or absence of HA in individual eggs at various serum dilutions and the 50% endpoint of serum Nt is calculated by the probit method (36).

Slight variations in the virus concentration used will not significantly influence the serum titers, since a 1000-fold increase in virus reduces the serum titer only 10-fold (40). Treatment of the individual allantoic fluids with periodate as described above for serum can assist in detecting small yields of virus which at the time of harvest are masked by inhibitors normally present in allantoic fluid.

In suckling mice and hamsters. Kilham et al (66) have described a direct Nt test in suckling mice using mouse or hamster brain passage virus. Their results were comparable to those obtained in parallel tests in eggs. To the inactivated serum dilutions, equal volumes of virus are added to provide the equivalent of 100 LD_{50} per suckling mouse or hamster. After 30 min of incubation at room temperature, groups of 8 randomly selected 1-day-old Swiss mice are each inoculated intracerebrally with one of the mixtures. Symptoms of encephalitis appear on the ninth day, and death is taken as the basis for calculation of 50% endpoints; animals are held for 3 weeks before the test is terminated.

In tissue culture. Nt tests in tissue cultures, grown in glass vessels or in microtiter plates, are the most advantageous. Nt is assessed by prevention of CPE in cultures with fluid media (25, 46, 60, 75), by reduction in the numbers of plaques in agar overlaid monolayers (32), or by inhibition of HAd (14, 42). The plaque test is technically the most demanding of the Nt procedures. It has advantages in that its greater sensitivity allows a more accurate assessment of response to mumps vaccination and of mumps immunity. Guinea pig complement has been used to enhance mumps neutralizing-antibody titers in tests performed in eggs (40, 73) and cell cultures (80). Since unheated guinea pig serum by itself has been shown to inhibit mumps virus replication, considerable caution is necessary to avoid misinterpretation of such results. Of more promise is the development of a highly sensitive plaque reduction Nt test based on the potentiation of the virus antibody complexes by heterologous anti-immunoglobulins (80). The general technique for detection of Nt antibodies in cell cultures grown in roller tubes is as follows:

Serial 2-fold dilutions of inactivated serum are mixed with equal volumes of virus diluted to the desired concentration determined by preliminary titration. Both serum and virus may be diluted in Hanks BSS. After incubation of the serum virus mixtures for 1 hr at 37 C or for 18 hr at 4 C, 2–4 cultures of HeLa cells, chick embryo fibroblasts, or the Vero line of continuous *Cercopithecus* monkey kidney cells are each inoculated with 0.2 ml of a given serum-virus mixture and incubated at 32 or 37 C (14). As controls, a standard antimumps serum is always included. The virus dilution employed is titrated in 1.0 log steps to ascertain the exact dose used in the test. With a dose in the order of 10 $TCID_{50}$, the most sensitive test is obtained.

The test is read usually after 4–7 days of incubation and the results are recorded in terms of (a) the percentage of cells showing cytolysis or degeneration, i.e., $\pm$ = minimal lesions; + to + + + + = from 25% to 100% of the cells affected; serum dilutions preventing destruction of about half of the cells (+ +) are taken as the endpoint or (b) reduction in HAd.

The results do not seem to differ significantly whichever of the following strains is used: an early amniotic strain (third to sixth passage) which produces infectious progeny and can be maintained by serial passage in HeLa cells (25, 45); an allantoic-sac-adapted strain which cannot be passed serially in HeLa cultures (46); or a strain which has been isolated in cell cultures and maintained in them (45). The Nt test in tissue culture is influenced to a greater extent by variations in the dose of virus than is the test carried out in the chick embryo. With a 10-fold increase in serum concentration, only 25 times the amount of virus is neutralized in the HeLa cultures, whereas 1000 times the amount of virus is neutralized in the egg test. For performing larger numbers of tests, a microtiter procedure using mumps virus CPE in Vero cells is particularly useful (75).

Interpretation. As stated at the outset, the Nt test is technically complex and thus impractical as a routine diagnostic procedure. On rare occasions, cases have been encountered which failed to develop CF or HAI antibodies, although they were strongly suspected to be due to mumps infection, and only Nt tests employed as a last resort showed significant, but low antibody responses. The presence of Nt antibodies in human serum, even in titers as low as 1:2, generally signifies past experience with mumps and probable immunity (53), although on rare occasions mumps may develop on subsequent exposure.

Other tests

Several new types of tests have been evaluated in recent years for the diagnosis of mumps virus infection. These include a fluorescent-antibody procedure (9), radioimmunoassay (24, 37), hemolysis-in-gel (42, 86), and single radial immunodiffusion (77). Each of these methods requires highly specialized techniques and well-characterized reagents assessed for specificity against one of the standard serologic methods. Methods for detecting cell-mediated immune responses in mumps virus infections have also been described (2, 18, 44); these may be of interest to those working in this specialized area.

References

1. AASE JM, NOREN GR, REDDY DV, and ST GEME JW JR: Mumps virus infection in pregnant women and the immunologic response of their offsprings. N Engl J Med 286:1379–1382, 1972
2. ANDERSSON T, STEJSKAL V, and HARFAST B: An *in vitro* method for study of human-lymphocyte cytotoxicity against mumps-virus-infected target cells. J Immunol 114:237–243, 1975
3. APPLEBAUM IL: Serum amylase in mumps. Ann Intern Med 21:35–43, 1944
4. BANG HO and BANG J: Involvement of the central nervous system in mumps. Acta Med Scand 113:487–505, 1943
5. BERNARD JP and NORTHROP RL: RNA polymerase in mumps virion. J Virol 24:183–186, 1974
6. BEVERIDGE WIB and BURNET FM: The cultivation of viruses and rickettsiae in the chick embryo. Med Res Coun, Spec Rep Ser No. 256, 1946
7. BRANDT CD: Cytopathic action of myxoviruses on cultivated mammalian cells. Virology 14:1–10, 1961
8. BRANDT CD: Inclusion body formation with Newcastle disease and mumps viruses in cultures of chick embryo cells. Virology 5:177–191, 1958
9. BROWN GC, BAUBLIS JV, and O'LEARY TP: Development and duration of mumps fluorescent antibodies in various immunoglobulin fractions of human serum. J Immunol 104:86–94, 1970
10. BRUNELL PA, BRICKMAN A, O'HARE D, and STEINBERG S: Ineffectiveness of isolation of patients as a method of preventing the spread of mumps. N Engl J Med 279:1357–1361, 1968
11. BURNET FM and STONE JD: The receptor-destroying enzyme of *V. cholerae*. Austr J Exp Biol Med Sci 25:227–233, 1947
12. BURR MM and NAGLER FP: Mumps infectivity studies in hamsters. Proc Soc Exp Biol Med 83:714–717, 1953
13. BUYNAK EB and HILLEMAN MR: Live attenuated mumps virus vaccine. Proc Soc Exp Biol Med 123:768–775, 1966
14. BUYNAK EB, WHITMAN JE JR, ROEHM RR, MORTON DH, LAMPSON GP, and HILLEMAN MR: Comparison of neutralization and hemagglutination-inhibition techniques for measuring mumps antibody. Proc Soc Exp Biol Med 125:1068–1071, 1967
15. CANDEL S and WHEELOCK MC: Serum amylase and serum lipase in mumps. Ann Intern Med 25:88–96, 1946
16. CANTELL K: Mumps virus. Adv Virus Res 8:123–164, 1961
17. CHANNOCK RM, JOHNSON KM, COOK MK, WONG DC, and VARGOSKO A: The hemadsorption technique with special reference to the problem of naturally occurring simian parainfluenza virus. Am Rev Resp Dis 83:125–129, 1961
18. CHIBA Y, DZIERBA JL, MORAG A, and OGRA PL: Cell-mediated immune response to mumps virus infection in man. J Immunol 116:12–15, 1976
19. CHIBA Y, OGRA PL, and NAKAO T: Transplacental mumps infection. Am J Obstet Gynecol 122:904–905, 1975
20. CLARKE DH and CASALS J: Techniques for hemagglutination and hemagglutination-inhibition with anthropod-borne viruses. Am J Trop Med Hyg 7:561–573, 1958
21. Commission on Acute Respiratory Diseases: Hemagglutination by amniotic fluid from normal embryonated hen's eggs. Proc Soc Exp Biol Med 62:118–123, 1946
22. COOK MK, ANDREWS BE, FOX HH, TURNER HC, JAMES WD, and CHANOCK RM: Antigenic relationships among the "newer" myxoviruses (parainfluenza). Am J Hyg 69:250–263, 1959
23. COONEY MK, FOX JP, and HALL CE: The Seattle virus watch. Am J Epidemiol 101:532–551, 1975
24. DAUGHARTY H, WARFIELD DT, HEMINGWAY WD, and CASEY HL: Mumps class-specific immunoglobulins in radioimmunoassay and conventional serology. Infect Immun 7:380–385, 1973
25. DEINHARDT F and HENLE G: Determination of neutralizing antibodies against mumps virus in HeLa cell cultures. J Immunol 77:40–46, 1956

26. DEINHARDT F and HENLE G: Studies on the viral spectra of tissue culture lines of human cells. J Immunol 79:60-67, 1957

27. ECKERT HL, PORTNOY B, SALVATORE MA, and KRELL M: The hemagglutination inhibition and complement fixation tests in the serodiagnosis of mumps central nervous system disease. Am J Clin Pathol 47:481-483, 1967

28. ENDERS JF, COHEN S, and KANE LW: Immunity in mumps. II. The development of complement-fixing antibody and dermal hypersensitivity in human beings following mumps. J Exp Med 81:119-135, 1945

29. ENDERS JF and HABEL K: Mumps In Diagnostic Procedures for Virus and Rickettsial Diseases, 2nd edition, Francis T Jr (ed), Am Public Health Assoc, Inc, New York, 1956, pp 281-312

30. ENDERS JF, KANE LW, COHEN S, and LEVENS JH: Immunity in mumps. I. Experiments with monkeys (Macacus mulatta). The development of complement-fixing antibody following infection and experiments on immunization by means of inactivated virus and convalescent human serum. J Exp Med 81:93-117, 1945

31. ENNIS FA: Immunity to mumps in an institutional epidemic. Correlation of insusceptibility to mumps with serum plaque neutralizing and hemagglutination-inhibiting antibodies. J Infect Dis 119:654-657, 1969

32. ENNIS FA, DOUGLAS RD, STEWART GL, HOPPS HE, and MEYER HM JR: A plaque neutralization test for determining mumps antibodies. Proc Soc Exp Biol Med 129:896-899, 1968

33. ENNIS FA and JACKSON D: Isolation of virus during the incubation period of mumps infection. J Pediatr 72:536-537, 1968

34. FELDMAN HA: Mumps In Viral Infections of Humans, Evans AS (ed), Plenum Publishing Corp, New York, 1976, pp 317-336

35. FENNER F: Classification and nomenclature of viruses. Intervirology 7:59, 1976

36. FINNEY DJ: Probit Analysis, 3rd edition, University Press, Cambridge, 1971

37. FORGHANI B, SCHMIDT NJ, and LENNETTE EH: Sensitivity of a radioimmunoassay method for detection of certain viral antibodies in sera and cerebrospinal fluids. J Clin Microbiol 4:470-478, 1976

38. GORDON I, KHORSHED P, and COHEN S: Response of ferrets to mumps virus. J Immunol 76:328-333, 1956

39. GORDON JE and KILHAM L: Ten years in the epidemiology of mumps. Am J Med Sci 218:338-359, 1949

40. GOTLIEB T, BASHE WJ JR, HENLE G, and HENLE W: Studies on the prevention of mumps. V. The development of a neutralization test and its application to convalescent sera. J Immunol 71:66-75, 1953

41. GRESSER I and ENDERS JF: Cytopathogenicity of mumps virus in cultures of chick embryo and human amnion cells. Proc Soc Exp Biol Med 107:804-807, 1961

42. GRILLNER L and BLOMBERG J: Hemolysis-in-gel and neutralization tests for determination of antibodies to mumps virus. J Clin Microbiol 4:11-15, 1976

43. HABEL K: Cultivation of mumps virus in the developing chick embryo and its application to studies of immunity to mumps in man. Public Health Rep 60:201-212, 1945

44. HARFAST B, ANDERSSON T, and PERLMANN P: Human lymphocyte cytotoxicity against mumps virus-infected target cells: requirement for non-T cells. J Immunol 114:1820-1823, 1975

45. HENLE G and DEINHARDT F: Propagation and primary isolation of mumps virus in tissue culture. Proc Soc Exp Biol Med 89:556-560, 1955

46. HENLE G, DEINHARDT F, and GIRARDI A: Cytolytic effects of mumps virus in tissue cultures of epithelial cells. Proc Soc Exp Biol Med 87:386-393, 1954

47. HENLE G, HARRIS S, and HENLE W: The reactivity of various human sera with mumps complement fixation antigens. J Exp Med 88:133-147, 1948

48. HENLE G, HENLE W, BURGOON JS, BASHE WJ JR, and STOKES J JR: Studies on the prevention of mumps. I. The determination of susceptibility. J Immunol 66:535-549, 1951

49. HENLE G, HENLE W, and HARRIS S: The serological differentiation of mumps complement-fixation antigens. Proc Soc Exp Biol Med 64:290-295, 1947

50. HENLE G, HENLE W, WENDELL KK, and ROSENBERG P: Isolation of mumps virus from human beings with induced apparent or inapparent infections. J Exp Med 88:223-232, 1948

51. HENLE G and McDOUGALL CL: Mumps meningo-encephalitis. Isolation in chick embryos of virus from spinal fluid of a patient. Proc Soc Exp Biol Med 66:209–211, 1947

52. HENLE W and ENDERS JF: Mumps virus *In* Viral and Rickettsial Infections of Man, 4th edition, Horsfall FL Jr and Tamm I (eds), Lippincott, Philadelphia, 1965, pp 755–768

53. HILLEMAN MR, WEIBEL RE, BUYNAK EB, STOKES JJ JR, and WHITMAN JE: Live attenuated mumps virus vaccine. 4. Protective efficacy as measured in field evaluation. N Engl J Med 276:252–258, 1967

54. HORNE RW, WATERSON AP, WILDY P, and FARNHAM AE: The structure and composition of the myxoviruses. I. Electron microscope studies of the structure of myxovirus particles by negative staining techniques. Virology 11:79–98, 1960

55. HSIUNG GD, ISACSON P, and TUCKER G: Studies of parainfluenza viruses. II. Serologic interrelationships in humans. Yale J Biol Med 35:534–544, 1963

56. HUMMELER K: Mumps complement fixing antibodies in guinea pigs. J Immunol 79:337–341, 1957

57. JENSIK SC and SILVER S: Polypeptides of mumps virus. J Virol 17:363–373, 1976

58. JOHNSON CD and GOODPASTURE EW: An investigation of the etiology of mumps. J Exp Med 59:1–19, 1934

59. KANE LW and ENDERS JF: Immunity in mumps. III. The complement fixation test as an aid in the diagnosis of mumps meningoencephalitis. J Exp Med 81:137–150, 1945

60. KENNY MT, ALBRIGHT KL, and SANDERSON RP: Microneutralization test for the determination of mumps antibody in vero cells. Appl Microbiol 20:371–373, 1970

61. KENNY MT and SCHELL K: Microassay of measles and mumps virus and antibody in VERO cells. J Biol Stand 3:291–306, 1975

62. KILHAM L: Isolation of mumps virus from the blood of a patient. Proc Soc Exp Biol Med 69:99–100, 1948

63. KILHAM L: Mumps meningoencephalitis with and without parotitis. Am J Dis Child 78:324–333, 1949

64. KILHAM L: Mumps virus in human milk and in milk of infected monkey. J Am Med Assoc 146:1231–1232, 1951

65. KILHAM L and MURPHY HW: Propagation of mumps virus in suckling mice and in mouse embryo tissue cultures. Proc Soc Exp Biol Med 80:495–498, 1952

66. KILHAM L, MURPHY HW, and OVERMAN JR: Performance of mumps neutralization tests in suckling mice. J Immunol 71:183–186, 1953

67. KILHAM L and OVERMAN JR: Natural pathogenicity of mumps virus for suckling hamsters on intracerebral inoculation. J Immunol 70:147–151, 1953

68. KRAVIS LP, SIGEL MM, and HENLE G: Mumps meningoencephalitis with special reference to the use of the complement-fixation test in diagnosis. Pediatrics 8:204–215, 1951

69. LENNETTE DA, EMMONS RW, and LENNETTE EH: Rapid diagnoses of mumps virus infections by immunofluorescence methods. J Clin Microbiol 2:81–84, 1975

70. LENNETTE EH, JENSEN FW, GUENTHER RW, and MAGOFFIN RL: Serologic responses to para-influenza viruses in patients with mumps virus infection. J Lab Clin Med 61:780–788, 1963

71. LEVENS JH and ENDERS JF: The hemagglutinative properties of amniotic fluid from embryonated eggs infected with mumps virus. Science 102:117–120, 1945

72. LEYMASTER GR and WARD TG: Direct isolation of mumps virus in chick embryos. Proc Soc Exp Biol Med 65:346–348, 1947

73. LEYMASTER GR and WARD TG: The effect of complement in the neutralization test of mumps virus. J Immunol 61:95–105, 1949

74. MARIS EP, ENDERS JF, STOKES J JR, and KANE LW: Immunity in mumps. IV. The correlation of the presence of complement-fixing antibody and resistance to mumps in human beings. J Exp Med 84:323–339, 1946

75. MAYNER RE, McDORMAN DJ, MEYER BC, and PARKMAN PD: Automated microtransfer technique for the assay of poliovirus- and mumps-neutralizing antibodies. Appl Microbiol 28:968–971, 1975

76. MONIF GRG: Maternal mumps infection during gestation. Am J Obstet Gynecol 119:549–551, 1974

77. NORRBY E, GRANDIEN M, and ORVELL C: New tests for characterization of mumps virus antibodies: hemolysis inhibition, single radial immunodiffusion with immobilized virions, and mixed hemadsorption. J Clin Microbiol 5:346–352, 1977

78. ROBBINS FC, KILHAM L, LEVENS JH, and ENDERS JF: An evaluation of the test for antihemagglutinin in the diagnosis of infections by the mumps virus. J Immunol 61:235–242, 1949

79. ST GEME JW JR, NOREN GR, and ADAMS P JR: Proposed embryopathic relation between mumps virus and primary endocardial fibroelastosis. N Engl J Med 275:339–347, 1966

80. SATO H, ALBRECHT P, HICKS JT, MEYER BC, and ENNIS FA: Sensitive neutralization test for virus antibody, 1. Mumps antibody. Arch Virol (in press)

81. SHELOKOV A, VOGEL J, and CHI L: Hemadsorption (adsorption-hemagglutination) test for viral agents in tissue culture with special reference to influenza. Proc Soc Exp Biol Med 97:802–809, 1958

82. SULTZ HA, HART BA, ZIELEZNY M, and SCHLESINGER ER: Is mumps virus an etiologic factor in juvenile diabetes mellitus? J Pediatr 86:654–656, 1975

83. US Public Health Service *Ad Hoc* Committee on the Safe Shipment and Handling of Etiologic Agents: Classification of Etiologic Agents on the Basis of Hazard. 2nd edition, Jan. 1970, National Communicable Disease Center, Atlanta, GA 30333

84. UTZ JP, KASEL JA, CRAMBLETT HG, SZWED CF, and PARROT RH: Clinical and laboratory studies of mumps. I. Laboratory diagnosis by tissue culture technics. N Engl J Med 257:497–502, 1957

85. UTZ JP, SZWED CF, and KASEL JA: Clinical and laboratory studies of mumps. II. Detection and duration of excretion of virus in urine. Proc Soc Exp Biol Med 99:259–261, 1958

86. VAANANEN P, HOVI T, HELLE EP, and PENTTINEN K: Determination of mumps and influenza antibodies by haemolysis-in-gel. Arch Virol 52:91–99, 1976

87. VAN DER VEEN J and SONDERKAMP HJA: Secondary antibody response of guinea pigs to parainfluenza and mumps viruses. Arch Gesamte Virusforsch 15:721–734, 1965

88. WARREN WR: Serum amylase and lipase in mumps. Am J Med Sci 230:161–168, 1955

89. WELLER TH and CRAIG JM: The isolation of mumps virus at autopsy. Am J Pathol 25:1105–1115, 1949

90. WOLMAN IJ, EVANS B, LASKER S, and JAEGGE K: Amylase levels during mumps: findings in blood and saliva. Am J Med Sci 213:477–481, 1947

91. ZELMAN S: Blood diastase values in mumps and mumps pancreatitis. Am J Med Sci 207:461–464, 1944

CHAPTER 21

NEWCASTLE DISEASE VIRUS

Paul D. Parkman and Hope E. Hopps

Introduction

Newcastle disease virus (NDV) is a member of the paramyxovirus group of enveloped negative-stranded RNA viruses. It is the etiologic agent of a highly infectious and sometimes lethal disease of domestic and wild fowl. It occasionally causes infection in exposed laboratory and poultry workers. Clinically manifest human infections are commonly associated with a self-limited superficial conjuctivitis. Febrile influenza-like illnesses have also been described in infected persons.

History

The severe form of the disease in chickens was recognized in Indonesia and in Great Britain in 1926 (13, 29). Subsequently, the disease was detected worldwide, and milder forms of the infection were described (5). Human infection was first recognized by Burnet in laboratory workers (7); infections have also been shown to occur in poultry workers.

Clinical aspects

Newcastle disease is a highly infectious disease of fowl (chickens, turkeys, pheasants, guinea fowl, sparrows, crows, parrots and others) caused by a virus affecting the respiratory, gastrointestinal, and central nervous systems. The disease is of commercial importance to poultry producers; mortality in outbreaks in chicken flocks is variable ranging from about 15% to 100% (5). The virus can be recovered from the blood, brain, viscera, feces, and oral and nasal secretions of infected birds. It is occasionally transmitted to persons who handle infected birds such as poultry-house workers and veterinarians (3, 23) or to personnel working with the virus in the laboratory (1, 7, 22, 32, 35). The virus has been used extensively in laboratories as a prototype for studies of paramyxovirus structure and function, for studies of interferon induction, and as a model for studying "defective" viruses. In a review of laboratory associated infections, Pike was able to find evidence of NDV infection in 51 (4.9%) of a total of 1049 instances of viral etiology (34).

It seems likely that the mode of transmission is by droplet spread or by direct introduction of infected material into the eye. Infections have resulted from both virulent strains and attenuated avian vaccine strains (12, 22). The incubation period appears to be 1–4 days. The illness in humans is manifest as an acute, granular conjunctivitis (sometimes hemorrhagic) with scanty exudate and without pseudomembrane formation or corneal involvement. The conjunctivitis is frequently unilateral. The preauricular lymph nodes are commonly enlarged and tender. Fever, when present, is usually low grade. Headache is common, but other systemic symptoms and signs such as malaise, fever and chills are unusual. Infections may be associated with systemic symptoms in the absence of overt conjunctivitis or may be entirely asymptomatic (3, 20). The disease in humans is self-limited, and spontaneous recovery occurs within 2 weeks. Person-to-person transmission has not been described.

Description and Nature of the Agent

NDV has been classified as a member of the paramyxovirus subgroup of the family *Paramyxoviridae* (16). It is a single-strand RNA virus; the molecular weight of the nucleic acid is 7.5×10^6 daltons. Electron microscope observations show typical virions to be spherical and approximately 120–300 nm in diameter (42). The nucleocapsid is contained in a nonrigid outer envelope from which arise spikes containing the hemagglutinin and neuraminidase antigens. The viral envelope is fragile and readily disrupted releasing the flexible coiled nucleoprotein. NDV is of relatively complex chemical composition. The genome RNA is encapsidated by nucleocapsid protein (NP). The virion contains a number of other proteins, including a carbohydrate-free internal membrane protein (M) and 2 glycosylated proteins making up the surface spikes which bear the hemagglutinating and neuraminidase activities (HN) and appear to carry hemolysis and fusion factor (F) activity, respectively (21, 37). In addition, the envelope contains phospholipids derived from the host cell (24). Purified virions also have been shown to contain several enzymes related to transcription of the viral RNA (11).

Virus infectivity is readily inactivated by treatment with ethyl ether, formalin, and ultraviolet light under the same conditions as are other myxoviruses. The virus is less rapidly inactivated at 56 C than other myxoviruses and is stable on storage for years at −60 C, for weeks at −20 C, and for several days at 4 C (31, 33). The virus agglutinates red blood cells (RBC) of many avian and mammalian species; those of chickens, guinea pigs and human type O are most commonly employed. The hemagglutination (HA) reaction is stable at 4 C, but at room temperature or 37 C the virus rapidly elutes from the RBC. At 37 C, the virus may cause hemolysis (19). Both HA and hemolysis are inhibited by specific antibody to the virus; the hemagglutination-inhibition (HAI) technique may be used to quantitate serum antibodies. Specific antibody may also be measured by the complement-fixation (CF) test and the neutralization (Nt) test performed in cell cultures or in embryonated chicken eggs.

NDV multiplies in the allantoic cavity of embryonated chicken eggs (30), in cell cultures of chick embryo origin, and in a variety of primary and heteroploid mammalian cell culture types (6, 9, 38, 44). The virus is pathogenic for its natural avian hosts and can produce encephalitis in intracerebrally inoculated laboratory animals, including mice and rhesus monkeys (40, 45).

Preparation of Immune Serum

Serum for use in identification of virus isolates can be obtained from chickens convalescent from the natural disease or from birds vaccinated with an avirulent virus strain (10). Such reagents cannot be used for CF tests because chicken serum does not fix complement in the presence of antigen. Hyperimmune serum can be prepared by repeated intraperitoneal injection of rabbits (5–10 ml) or guinea pigs (1–5 ml) using allantoic fluid harvests containing high titers of virus. Following initial priming immunization, booster inoculations at 4-week intervals usually elicit a satisfactory antibody response. Blood samples can be collected 10–14 days after the last injection (37). For some purposes, e.g., immunologic analysis of virus components, immunization with purified preparations may be helpful and, in addition, serum may be treated to remove antibodies against heterologous antigens (37).

Collection and Preparation of Specimens for Laboratory Diagnosis

Precautions

NDV has been categorized in Class 1 (the least hazardous category) by the US Public Health Service *Ad Hoc* Committee on the safe shipment and handling of etiologic agents. As with all potentially pathogenic organisms, correct and careful laboratory techniques, including effective decontamination and sterilization procedures, are indicated (39).

Virus isolation specimens

The diagnosis of NDV infections in humans is accomplished most convincingly by isolation of the virus. Exudate from the affected eye is collected with a sterile capillary pipette or a cotton swab and emulsified in a small volume of bacteriologic broth or balanced salt solution. If exudate is not present, saline solution washings of the conjunctiva may be used. Occasional isolates have been reported from pharyngeal washings or saliva and, in patients with the less well-documented generalized systemic form of the infection, from blood and urine. Specimens likely to be contaminated should be treated with penicillin (1000 units/ml) and streptomycin (100 μg/ml). Specimens for isolation should be stored frozen, preferably at -60 C or below.

Specimens for serologic diagnosis

Blood should be collected, and the serum separated aseptically. Serum should be stored frozen at −20 C. Before testing, serum should be subjected to heating at 56 C for 30 min. Both acute- and convalescent-phase sera from the patient should be assayed in the same serologic test run.

Specimens for microscopic examination

Infected cell culture preparations can be examined for typical acidophilic intracytoplasmic inclusions using coverslip cultures fixed in ethanol or Bouin fluid and stained by the Giemsa method. For immunofluorescence microscopy, coverslips are fixed in acetone for 10 min at room temperature, air dried for 30 min, and stained using rabbit antiserum with high HAI antibody titers (25, 43). Electron microscopic observations are most readily made on preparations concentrated and partially purified by differential centrifugation or by adsorption and elution from fowl erythrocytes (RBC). Negative-staining techniques employing collodion and carbon-coated 300-mesh copper grids and 1% sodium phosphotungstate are most commonly used (36, 42).

Laboratory Diagnosis

Direct examination of stained smears of conjunctival exudates or washings shows that mononuclear cells are predominant. There are no pathognomonic changes.

Virus isolation

In embryonated eggs. Inoculation by the allantoic route is the method of choice. Five to 8 embryos at the ninth to eleventh day of development are injected with 0.2 ml of the specimen. Many strains of virus produce infections lethal for the embryo within 48 hr; others kill more slowly and kill a lesser percentage of infected embryos (18). Hemagglutinins usually appear in the allantoic fluid of infected embryos 48–96 hr after inoculation. A second passage using 0.2 ml of allantoic fluid should be performed if the initial isolation attempt is negative.

Care should be taken to exclude embryonated eggs from flocks experiencing natural NDV infection or from flocks receiving NDV vaccine during the preceding month.

In cell cultures. Laboratory strains of virus grow well in many types of cell cultures including chick embryo fibroblast. HeLa, rhesus monkey kidney, bovine kidney, and bovine fibroblasts. Primary chick-embryo cell cultures should be satisfactory for use in primary isolation. Inocula treated with an antibiotic should be allowed to adsorb for approximately 1 hr at 35 C and then removed and maintenance medium added, since streptomycin (10000 μg/ml) may be toxic to the cell cultures. The cytopathic effects (CPE) produced by NDV may include the development of syncytia as well as generalized degenerative changes and resemble those of mumps or certain parainfluenza virus strains. With some NDV strains, prominent cytopathic changes may not develop (14). Infected cultures show the phenomenon of hemadsorption with chicken or guinea pig RBC; 0.2 ml of a 0.4% suspension is added to each culture and allowed to attach at 4 C (41).

Identification of isolates. Isolates may be identified by neutralization of CPE, hemadsorption inhibition (HAdI), hemagglutination inhibition (HAI) with specific hyperimmune animal antiserum, by CF, and by fluorescent-antibody staining with specific reagents. The simplest procedure is HAI (see below); the unknown isolate is passaged in embryonated eggs, and the hemagglutinin produced in the allantoic fluid is inhibited with specific hyperimmune antiserum.

Serologic diagnosis

A serologic diagnosis of NDV infection may be done by testing for Nt, CF, or HAI antibodies. It appears that there are cross-reacting antigens shared between NDV and mumps virus as evidenced by the fact that: (a) serologic responses may develop to both mumps virus and NDV during mumps infection (28, 26); and (b) NDV antibodies have been removed from human serum by adsorption with mumps virus (40, 41). Thus, recent mumps virus infection could give rise to NDV antibody responses. On the other hand, not all persons with clinically apparent NDV conjunctivitis from whom isolates have been recovered have shown diagnostically significant antibody responses. For these reasons NDV serologic results must be interpreted with caution; virus isolation attempts are particularly important in establishing a diagnosis.

Complement-fixation test

Several different CF procedures have been used. Any standardized technique is satisfactory. A CF test adapted to microtiter plates is described below (8).

Preparation of antigen. Nine- to 11-day-old embryonated chicken eggs are injected by the allantoic route with 0.2 ml of appropriately diluted (usually 10^3 to 10^4) allantoic fluid infected with a standard strain of NDV. The eggs are incubated at 35–36 C, chilled at 4 C when the embryos are moribund, and the allantoic fluids are harvested (attenuated vaccine strains may not kill as rapidly or as high a percentage of embryos). Such fluids should exhibit CF-antigen titers from 1:2 to 1:16. CF antigens are stable when stored frozen or at 4 C for many weeks.

Procedure for test. Serial 2-fold dilutions of heat-inactivated serum ranging from 1:4 to 1:512 are prepared in triplicate, using microdiluters. Put NDV antigen (standardized as described for mumps) diluted to contain 2 optimal units into each well in the first row; in the second row normal allantoic fluid (host antigen control), and in the third, saline solution (anticomplementary serum control). Thereafter each mixture receives complement diluted to contain five 50% hemolytic units as determined in the presence of the antigen dilution to be used. After overnight incubation at 4 C, sensitized sheep RBC (an equal mixture of standard dilution of hemolysin and 2% sheep RBC) are added. The test is read after further incubation at 37 C for 30 min. Additional controls must be included in the test: 1) antigen plus saline solution instead of serum to ascertain the absence of anticomplementary effects; 2) known positive and negative sera to determine the specificity and sensitivity of the reactions; and 3) a titration of the complement employed in the absence of serum and antigen to establish the exact unitage of complement in the test. Chicken antiserum cannot be used in the test because serum from this species does not fix complement.

Interpretation of test. The end point is taken as the reciprocal of the highest serum dilution causing 3+ or greater fixation of complement. A 4-fold increase in antibody titer or reproducible evidence of change in serologic status from seronegative to seropositive is presumptive evidence for NDV infection (see general remarks above).

Hemagglutination-inhibition (HAI) test

The same general procedures for the HAI test for influenza or mumps viruses are applicable. Chicken, guinea pig, or human O RBC function satisfactorily in the test. Incubation of the test at 4 C is advisable because some NDV strains elute readily from RBC at higher temperatures.

Preparation of antigen. The same procedures as described above under the CF test may be employed. It should be noted that attenuated vaccine strains may be of low lethality and may fail to cause HA under certain conditions (30), and thus are unsuitable for HA-antigen production (30). Allantoic fluids should exhibit HA titers from 1:320 to 1:2560. The HA antigen is also stable at 4 C and at freezing temperatures.

Procedure for the test. The HAI test may be performed either in tubes, plastic plates, or by the use of microtiter equipment. Serial 2-fold dilutions of heat-inactivated serum are prepared from 1:10 to 1:2560; and allowed to react for 30 min to 1 hr with 4 hemagglutinating units of antigen. The HA-antigen concentration is determined by a titration performed on the same day as the HAI test using the same batch of RBC. An equal volume of an appropriate concentration of RBC is then added. Usually about a 1% suspension will produce satisfactory HA patterns; the exact RBC concentration optimal for the equipment being used should be determined in preliminary experiments. After addition of RBC, the test is incubated at 4 C and is read just after the RBC have settled. The following controls must be included: 1) The lowest serum dilution tested plus saline solution instead of antigen to ascertain the absence of agglutinins in the serum for the RBC employed; 2) the antigen dilution used in the test and 3 further 2-fold dilutions derived from this dilution plus an equal volume of saline (in place of the test serum dilutions) to determine the exact unitage of antigen in the test; 3) known positive and negative control sera to establish the specificity and sensitivity of the test.

Interpretation of test. Serum titers are expressed as the reciprocal of the highest initial serum dilution (before the addition of other reagents) which causes complete inhibition of hemagglutination. A 4-fold increase in antibody titer or reproducible evidence of change in serologic status from sero-negative to seropositive is presumptive evidence for NDV infection (see general remarks above).

Virus neutralization tests

These tests may be carried out either in embryonated eggs using the allantoic route and the same general procedures as employed for influenza or mumps viruses, by the "egg-bit" technique (4), or in cell cultures. Chick embryo fibroblasts or chick kidney cell cultures and other cell cultures including heteroploid cell lines may be used. Plaque reduction in agar overlaid cultures or HAdI or inhibition of CPE in cultures maintained with liquid culture medium have been employed. The last two procedures are the simplest to perform and have been adapted to microculture systems (27, 46).

Neutralization using embryonated eggs and cell cultures. Serial 2-fold dilutions of heat-inactivated serum (1:2 through 1:2048) are tested against a constant amount of virus. In the chick-embryo test, between 1000 to 10,000 lethal doses are employed. Slight variations in dose have little effect on the results because a 1000-fold increase in virus reduces the neutralizing titer of serum only 10-fold (3, 15). For the cell-culture test, approximately 10–100 infectious doses of virus mixed with an equal volume of each serum dilution is incubated for approximately 45 min at 37 C. The serum-virus mixtures are inoculated in 0.2 ml volumes into the allantoic cavity of 5–6 chick embryos at the tenth to eleventh day of incubation, or into 8 microculture wells. An infectivity titration of virus used should be performed in the homologus host system and uninoculated controls should be included. After an appropriate incubation period, the embryonated eggs are examined for evidence of embryo death and HA-antigen production, and the cell culture systems assessed for CPE or hemadsorption with 0.75% chicken RBC suspensions.

Interpretation of test. The serum antibody titers are calculated on the basis of inhibition of virus effect as the serum neutralizing endpoint$_{50}$ using the probit method (17).

Other tests

Since NDV contains a neuraminidase it seems possible that neuraminidase inhibiting antibodies could develop as a result of infection. Such antibodies have not been assessed in human infection to date.

References

1. ANDERSON SG: A note on two laboratory infections with the virus of Newcastle disease of fowls. Med J Aust 1:371, 1946
2. BANG FB and FOARD M: The serology of Newcastle virus infection. II. The antigenic relationships of Newcastle virus. J Immunol 76:348–351, 1956
3. BANG FB and FOARD M: The serology of Newcastle virus infection. J Immunol 76:352–356, 1956
4. BEARD CW: The egg-bit technique for measuring Newcastle disease virus and its neutralizing antibodies. Avian Dis 13:309–320, 1969
5. BRANDLY CA: Recognition of Newcastle disease as a new disease *In* Newcastle Disease Virus, Hanson RP (ed), The Univ of Wisconsin Press, Madison and Milwaukee, 1964, pp 53–69

6. BRANDT CC: Cytopathic action of myxoviruses on cultivated mammalian cells. Virology 14:1-10, 1961
7. BURNET FM: Human infections with the virus of Newcastle disease of fowls. Med J Aust 2:313-314, 1943
8. BUTTERFIELD WK: A microtiter complement-fixation test for detecting and differentiating Newcastle disease virus strains. Avian Dis 19:834-837, 1975
9. CHANOCK RM: Cytopathogenic effect of Newcastle disease virus in monkey kidney cultures and interference with poliomyelitis viruses. Proc Soc Exp Biol Med 89:379-381, 1955
10. CLANCY CF, COX HR, and BOTTORFF CA: Laboratory experiments with living Newcastle disease vaccine. Poult Sci 28:58-62, 1949
11. COLONNO RJ and STONE HO: Isolation of a transcription complex from Newcastle disease virions. J Virol 19:1080-1089, 1976
12. DARDIRI AH, YATES VJ, and FLANAGAN TD: The reaction to infection with the B1 strain of Newcastle disease virus in man. Am J Vet Res 23:918-920, 1962
13. DOYLE TM: A hitherto unrecorded disease of fowls due to a filter-passing virus. J Comp Path Therap 40:144-169, 1927
14. DURAND DP and EISENSTORK A: Influence of host cell type on certain properties of Newcastle disease virus in tissue culture. Am J Vet Res 23:338-342, 1962
15. EVANS AS: Newcastle disease neutralizing antibody in human sera and its relationship to mumps virus. Am J Hyg 60:204-213, 1954
16. FENNER F: Classification and nomenclature of viruses. Intervirology 7:59, 1976
17. FINNEY DJ: Probit Analysis, 3rd edition, University Press, Cambridge, 1971
18. GRANOFF A: Nature of the Newcastle disease virus population In Newcastle Disease Virus, Hanson RP (ed), The Univ of Wisconsin Press, Madison and Milwaukee, 1964, pp 107-118
19. GRANOFF A and HENLE W: Studies on the hemolytic activity of Newcastle disease virus (NDV). J Immunol 72:322-328, 1954
20. HANSON RP and BRANDLY CA: Newcastle disease. Ann NY Acad Sci 70:585-597, 1958
21. HIGHTOWER LE, MORRISON TG, and BRATT MA: Relationships among the polypeptides of Newcastle disease virus. J Virol 16:1599-1607, 1975
22. HUNTER MC, KENNEY AH, and SIGEL MM: Laboratory aspects of an infection with Newcastle disease virus in man. J Infect Dis 88:272-277, 1951
23. INGALLS WL and MAHONEY A: Isolation of the virus of Newcastle disease from human beings. Am J Public Health 39:737-740, 1949
24. ISRAEL A, AUDUBERT F, and SEMMEL M: Phospholipids in Newcastle disease virus infected cells. Biochim Biophys Acta 375:224-235, 1975
25. JOHNSON CF and SCOTT AD: Cytological studies of Newcastle disease virus (NDV) in HEp-2 cells. Proc Soc Exp Biol Med 115:281-286, 1964
26. JORDAN WS JR and FELLER AE: The relationship of complement-fixing and anti-hemagglutinating factors against the viruses of mumps and Newcastle disease. J Lab Clin Med 36:369-377, 1950
27. KATZ D, BEN-MOSHE H, and ALON S: Titration of Newcastle disease virus and its neutralizing antibodies in microplates by a modified hemadsorption and hemadsorption inhibition method. J Clin Microbiol 3:227-232, 1976
28. KILHAM L, JUNGHEER E, and LUGINBUHL RE: Antihemagglutinating and neutralizing factors against Newcastle disease virus (NDV) occurring in sera of patients convalescent from mumps. J Immunol 63:37-49, 1959
29. KRANEVELD FC: Over een in Ned-Indie heerschende Ziekte onder het pluimves. Ned Indisch B1 Diergeneesk 38:448-450, 1926
30. LIU C and BANG FB: An analysis of the difference between a destructive and a vaccine strain of NDV (Newcastle disease virus) in the chick embryo. J Immunol 70:538-548, 1953
31. LOMNICZI B: Thermostability of Newcastle disease virus strains of different virulence. Arch Virol 47:249-255, 1975
32. MUSTAFFA-BABJEE A, IBRAHIM AL, and KHIM TS: A case of human infection with Newcastle disease virus. Southeast Asian J Trop Med Public Health 7:622-624, 1976

33. PICKEN JC JR: Thermostability of Newcastle disease virus *In* Newcastle Disease Virus, Hanson RP (ed), The Univ of Wisconsin Press, Madison and Milwaukee, 1964, pp 167–188

34. PIKE RM: Laboratory-associated infections: summary and analysis of 3921 cases. Health Lab Sci 13:105–114, 1976

35. QUINN RW, HANSON RP, BROWN JW, and BRANDLY CA: Newcastle disease virus in man. Results of studies in five cases. J Lab Clin Med 40:736–743, 1952

36. ROMAN JM and SIMON EH: Morphologic heterogeneity in egg- and monolayer-propagated Newcastle disease virus. Virology 69:287–297, 1976

37. SETO JT, BECHT H, and ROTT R: Effect of specific antibodies on biological functions of the envelope components of Newcastle disease virus. Virology 61:354–360, 1974

38. TYRRELL DAJ: New tissue culture systems for influenza, Newcastle disease and vaccinia viruses. J Immunol 74:293–305, 1955

39. US Public Health *Ad Hoc* Committee on the Safe Shipment and Handling of Etiologic Agents: Classification of Etiologic Agents on the Basis of Hazard. 2nd edition, Jan 1970. National Communicable Disease Center, Atlanta, GA 30333

40. UPTON E, HANSON RP, and BRANDLY CA: Intracerebral inoculation of mice with Newcastle disease virus. III. Serial passage of NDV in suckling mice. J Infect Dis 96:29–33, 1955

41. VOGEL J and SHELOKOV A: Adsorption-hemagglutination test for influenza virus in monkey kidney tissue culture. Science 126:358–359, 1957

42. WATERSON AP and CRUICKSHANK JG: The effect of ether on Newcastle disease virus: a morphological study of eight strains. Z Naturforsch Teil C 186:114–118, 1963

43. WHEELOCK EF and TAMM I: Effect of multiplicity of infection on Newcastle disease virus—HeLa cell interaction. J Exp Med 113:317–337, 1961

44. WHEELOCK EF and TAMM I: Enumeration of cell-infecting particles of Newcastle disease virus by the fluorescent antibody technique. J Exp Med 113:317–337, 1961

45. WENNER HA, MONLEY A, and TODD RN: Studies on Newcastle disease virus encephalitis in rhesus monkeys. J Immunol 64:305–321, 1950

46. WOOLEY RE, BROWN J, GRATZEK JB, KLEVEN SH, and SCOTT TA: Microculture system for detection of Newcastle disease virus antibodies. Appl Microbiol 27:890–895, 1974

CHAPTER 22

MEASLES VIRUS

Anne A. Gershon and Saul Krugman

Introduction

Measles (rubeola) has been a recognized disease for almost 2000 years. However, diagnostic techniques pertaining to this virus infection have been used for only the past 20 years, since these procedures were developed only after it became possible to propagate measles virus *in vitro*. In 1954, Enders and Peebles isolated this virus from patients with measles using tissue cultures of primary human renal cells (30). Since that time a variety of diagnostic techniques for measles has become available, which is fortunate since concomitantly the need for, and dependence on, these techniques has increased.

The licensure of live measles vaccine in 1963 and its subsequent widespread use brought a marked decline in the incidence of clinical measles (56, 67). Consequently, the need for specific diagnostic procedures has increased as clinicians have become less familiar with the disease due to lack of experience with it. In addition, diagnostic virology has become an important tool in evaluation of the immunogenicity and efficacy of live measles vaccine. More recently, as unvaccinated children have reached adolescence and young adulthood, the epidemiology of measles has changed, resulting in an increased incidence of measles in adults (67, 109). Thus, not only pediatricians but internists have need for diagnostic tests for measles. The major importance of diagnostic virology today is to identify measles in vaccinated and unvaccinated persons, especially when the clinician is confronted with an illness atypical for measles.

Recently, diagnostic techniques for measles virus have also become applicable beyond the spectrum of infectious disease, since measles virus has been implicated in certain degenerative diseases of the nervous system and in certain autoimmune diseases. Evidence has linked measles to a progressive malady of the nervous system, subacute sclerosing panencephalitis (SSPE) (7, 16, 17), so that serologic techniques for measles are also used to diagnose this rare disease. Finally, research on systemic lupus erythematosus (124) and multiple sclerosis (2) has suggested a possible etiologic role of measles virus. While serologic tests for measles are not now used for

665

diagnosis, at some time in the future when the pathologic role of measles virus in these diseases is clarified, these tests may well be used.

Clinical aspects

Mode of transmission. Measles virus spreads by the airborne route (59). The virus persists in experimentally produced aerosols for up to 2 hr, particularly under conditions of low relative humidity (18, 19). This pecularity of the virus may account for the observed seasonal increase in the incidence of measles during cold weather when the relative indoor humidity is low (18, 19).

Under experimental conditions, using attenuated live measles vaccine, susceptibles have been infected with measles virus by instillation of a fine aerosol of the agent onto portions of the respiratory epithelium, e.g., the nose and most particularly, the lower respiratory tract (64).

During the prodromal phase of the naturally occurring illness, measles virus has been isolated from leukocytes, throat and conjunctival washings, and urine (30, 42, 43). Transmission of the infection by blood and urine is believed to be minimal; the major source of infectious virus is probably in secretions shed from the respiratory tract during the prodromal phase and the early stages of rash, when cough and coryza are intense (59).

Pathogenesis. Direct observations concerning early multiplication of measles virus in humans are lacking. However, based on experimental infections in animals, it is hypothesized that a biphasic viremia occurs in measles as well as in other exanthematous diseases (32, 59, 118). Following initial multiplication of the virus in the respiratory tract, a primary viremia occurs during which the virus reaches the reticuloendothelial system and the viscera. After further multiplication of the virus, an intense secondary viremic phase follows, possibly due to necrosis of infected cells of the reticuloendothelial system. Shortly afterward the rash develops.

The first sign of measles is a marked leukopenia (6). Since measles virus has been recovered from leukocytes (42) and since the virus may be propagated in human T and B lymphocytes and monocytes (53, 122), it is believed that the leukopenia is a direct result of invasion and destruction of leukocytes by the virus. In addition, infected leukocytes probably serve as a vehicle for transmission of virus to other areas of the body (6).

Incubation period. In children the incubation period of natural measles averages 10 days; in adults it may be slightly longer (68). The next, or prodromal, phase lasts 4–5 days and is believed to represent the period of viral dissemination. The appearance of rash marks the end of the prodrome; the rash lasts an additional 5 days or so.

When measles infection is artificially induced, bypassing the respiratory epithelium, as with injection of live measles vaccine, the incubation period is somewhat shortened, averaging 7 days (55, 105).

Period of infectivity. The infectivity of measles is greatest during the height of the exudative phase of the illness, just before the rash begins to appear (59). This was well illustrated during the 1962 epidemic in Greenland, when susceptibles exposed to an individual with measles rash did not contract the disease. These same individuals developed measles, when several weeks later, they were exposed to another person with prodromal measles (68). In a study of recovery of virus from patients with natural measles, blood and respiratory secretions yielded infectious virus only as long as 42 hr following onset of rash (113).

Recipients of live measles vaccine and children with atypical measles (see following sections) do not transmit the virus to others (8, 36, 56).

Symptoms. The classical symptoms of measles are fever, cough, coryza, conjunctivitis, and rash, appearing in that order over a 5-day period (68). During the early stage of the illness, when only nonspecific respiratory tract symptoms are present, the diagnosis of measles may be made with almost certainty by the observance of Koplik spots. These lesions were originally described as bright red spots with a blue-white central speck (63). They appear on the labial and buccal mucus membranes, often opposite the second molars. Koplik spots have also been likened to "grains of salt sprinkled on a red background" (68). The spots slough off as the rash develops. While Koplik spots are almost exclusively associated with measles, they have been observed, on occasion, in patients with coxsackie A9 virus infections (57).

The rash of measles begins on the head and neck and moves downward to cover the entire body. Initially maculopapular, the rash often becomes confluent on the upper parts of the body (68). The rash is generally the last symptom of measles to develop and, after it has spread to all areas of the skin, the patient begins to improve. The rash begins to clear in the areas where it first appeared, and desquamation may occur in areas where the rash was most intense.

Complications. The most common complications of measles are those which involve the respiratory tract. Some of the so-called complications may actually be part of the illness itself. Invasion of the respiratory epithelium by the virus results in destruction of tissue, with loss of cilia and mucus, often leading to laryngotracheobronchitis, bronchiolitis, pneumonia, and otitis media. X-ray evidence of pneumonia is not uncommon even during apparently "uncomplicated" measles. In addition, tissue damage wrought by measles virus may predispose to bacterial superinfection of any area of the respiratory tract (59).

Leukopenia, possibly induced by infection of leukocytes by measles virus, may also predispose to bacterial superinfection. Depression of cell-mediated immunity after infection with measles virus occurs (120) and may also be secondary to viral invasion of white blood cells (53).

Encephalitis of 2 varieties has been associated with measles virus. The first, an acute encephalitis which occurs during convalescence from measles, has an incidence of 1 in 1000 cases of measles (68). Symptoms include resurgence of fever, headache, seizures, and coma. Although it is unusual to recover measles virus from the cerebrospinal fluid (CSF) of these patients, occasional reports of virus isolation or transmission of measles to laboratory animals by CSF have appeared in the literature (80, 81, 117, 119). Since 50% of children with measles have been reported to have EEG abnormalities (41) and since there is frequently a CSF pleocytosis in children with measles and no symptoms of encephalitis (102), it is believed that the central nervous system is frequently involved by the virus. Therefore, clinical measles encephalitis is believed to result from from hypersensitivity to both measles virus and brain antigen (i. e., altered self) that cause demyelination. This hypothesis seems sensible since host antigens become incorporated into the virus envelope during virus multiplication (23).

A second form of encephalitis apparently caused by measles virus (or a very closely related agent) is SSPE. This disease, which is less common than acute measles encephalitis, presents as a progressive loss of mental and motor function, often beginning with a change in personality or school performance, and eventually leading to seizures, dementia, and usually within a year, decortication and death (108). SSPE occurs years after an attack of measles, and while it has also been reported to occur following live measles vaccine, the incidence of this disease has apparently declined since the introduction of measles vaccine (85). SSPE is associated with extraordinarily high antibody titers to measles virus in both serum and CSF (16, 68). Recently, measles-like virus has been recovered by co-cultivation techniques from the brain and lymph nodes of children who died from SSPE (4, 60, 106, 128). Anergy to measles virus and to other antigens has also been demonstrated in persons with SSPE (40, 108, 129). However, it remains unclear whether SSPE represents an abnormal response to normal virus or an immune response to a defective virus.

Measles in tropical countries has long been recognized to be unusually severe. This is possibly secondary to the high incidence of severe malnutrition which is known to depress cell-mediated immune function (54).

Measles may also be unusually severe in immunocompromised patients, particularly those with defects in cell-mediated immunity. These children may develop giant-cell (Hecht) pneumonia, which may or may not be accompanied by rash (29, 83). In 1959, Enders and his colleagues identified the causative agent of giant-cell pneumonia as measles virus (29). Since the antibody response to measles virus is often minimal in these children (83), cytologic examination of involved tissues and virus isolation assume increased diagnostic importance. Immunocompromised children, who receive live measles vaccine, have also been reported to develop giant-cell pneumonia (84), so that at present, live measles vaccine is contraindicated in these children.

A chronic form of measles encephalitis has also been described in immunocompromised children (3, 9), and children with concomitant giant-cell pneumonia and SSPE have also been described (9).

An atypical form of measles has been observed in children who received killed measles vaccine and who years later were exposed to wild measles virus (36, 111). In atypical measles, the child is acutely ill with a maculopapular, purpuric, and often vesicular rash which begins peripherally. Often there are accompanying pulmonary infiltrates. These children have low or undetectable measles antibody titers when they are exposed to measles, and during convalescence they develop extremely high antibody titers to the virus (36, 68, 69). Atypical measles is believed to result from either humoral or cell-mediated hypersensitivity (or both) to measles virus in a partially immune host (36, 73). Norrby and his colleagues have postulated that killed measles vaccine lacks certain antigens, possibly those which facilitate entry of virus into cells. Vaccination with killed measles virus, therefore, may not result in the formation of antibodies which inhibit this process, possibly explaining the apparent partial immunity to measles these vaccine recipients seem to have (99).

Measles has at times been observed in children who received live measles vaccine in the past. Their signs and symptoms are similar to those of children with regular measles. These children represent vaccine failures—often due to improper storage or administration of the vaccine or administration of live vaccine in the face of low levels of passively acquired antibody (67).

Pathology

Measles, like many viral diseases, is characterized by lymphoid hyperplasia and mononuclear inflammatory exudates in involved organs. This is in keeping with the suggestion that T lymphocytes play an important role in termination of measles (11, 112). It has been postulated that the mechanism underlying eradication of virus is that T cells kill cells which are infected and therefore display measles surface antigen. In addition, it has been suggested that production of interferon from stimulated T cells plays a role in termination of the infection (59). It is unknown whether measles virus is normally maintained in a latent form following an attack of measles. It has been suggested that this may be the case and that latent infection may be responsible for lifelong production of specific antibody, characteristic of an immune individual (114). The site of measles virus latency, if it exists, is unknown. However, Joseph and his colleagues have suggested that leukocytes may be the site (53).

The classic pathologic cell induced by measles virus is the multinucleate giant cell of lymphoid or epithelial origin. Originally described independently in 1931 by Warthin (131) and Finkeldey (33), the giant cell is often referred to as the Warthin-Finkeldey cell. It is pathognomonic of measles virus infection. These cells are found throughout the respiratory tract in measles and, when identified, may be helpful in establishing the diagnosis.

Koplik spots and the measles rash are believed to be the result of similar pathologic processes. However, exactly what this pathologic process is remains uncertain. Suringa and his colleagues (123) have suggested that synthesis of measles virus in epithelial cells accounts for both phenomena; these workers observed multinucleate giant cells containing microtubular aggregates typical of measles virus in these lesions. However, Kimura et al (61, 62) have criticized this concept, pointing out that epithelial giant cells are sparse and not really typical Warthin-Finkeldey cells; these workers could not detect measles antigen on epithelial cell surfaces by immunofluorescence. Therefore they have postulated that both Koplik spots and the rash are due to hypersensitivity to measles antigen in the endothelial cells of dermal capillaries, since they detected measles antigen in the endothelia of dermal blood vessels.

The fact that the rash of measles appears at about the same time as specific antibody is also in keeping with the hypothesis that the rash is due to hypersensitivity to measles virus. However, the observation that patients with agammaglobulinemia and measles develop a rash, while children with severe combined immunodeficiency and measles do not (11), has led to the suggestion that the rash is mediated not by antibody but by T lymphocytes (70).

Giant-cell pneumonia of measles is characterized, in addition to War-thin-Finkeldey cells, by mononuclear lung infiltrates, squamous metaplasia of the bronchial and bronchiolar epithelia, and proliferation of alveolar lung cells (59).

The pathologic lesions seen after measles encephalitis are similar to those seen in encephalitis after other viral infections. The major changes are demyelination of varying degree in the brain and spinal cord, vascular cuffing, gliosis, and the appearance of fat-laden macrophages in or near blood vessel walls (10). Intracytoplasmic and intranuclear inclusion bodies typical of measles virus and multinucleate giant cells have also been reported in the brains of patients who died of measles encephalitis (1).

Description and Nature of the Agent

Common characteristics

Measles virus is classified as a member of the paramyxovirus group which includes the parainfluenza viruses, mumps virus, Newcastle disease virus (NDV), respiratory syncytial virus (RSV), canine distemper virus, and rinderpest virus. Measles virus is most closely related to the last 2 agents. These 3 viruses have morphologic and antigenic similarities, produce similar cytopathic effects (CPE) in tissue culture, and even cause similar diseases in their respective hosts (51, 103).

Size and shape

Electronmicroscopic and ultracentrifugation studies have shown that the measles virion is spherical with a diameter ranging between 120–250 nm (134). The buoyant density in CsCl is 1.23 g/ml (45, 98). The outer surface of the virion consists of an envelope 10–20 nm (134) in thickness. The envelope is composed of glycoproteins and lipids and bears short surface projections (89, 90, 134). The envelope encloses an elongated helical nucleocapsid in which protein units are spirally arranged around ribonucleic acid (RNA). The diameter of the nucleocapsid helix is approximately 17 nm (77, 134).

Chemical composition

It is now well-established that measles virus contains RNA (45, 98, 115, 134), the size of which is compatible with the classification of measles as a paramyxovirus (14, 113). The RNA has been estimated to have a molecular weight of $6.2-6.4 \times 10^6$ daltons (45, 90).

The Edmonston B strain of measles virus subjected to polyacrilamide-gel electrophoresis has been reported to contain 6 polypeptides with molecular weights ranging from $4.57-7.56 \times 10^4$ daltons (45, 46). Two of the polypeptides were glycoproteins associated with the viral envelope. Another single polypeptide with a molecular weight of 6×10^4 was associated with the nucleocapsid (45, 46, 134). The remaining polypeptides were thought to be in some way associated with the viral envelope (45, 46).

Resistance to physical and chemical agents

Measles virus is relatively thermolabile. At 37 C, half of the infectivity is lost within 2 hr, and no detectable infectivity remains after 30 min at 56 C (5).

The virus is stable at pH from $5.0-10.5$, with an optimum around pH 7 (87). Measles virus is inactivated after exposure to ultraviolet and visible light, as well as by other forms of radiation (134). Infectivity is lost at room temperature after 10 min exposure to 20% ethyl ether or 30 min exposure to 50% acetone. Treatment with the detergent Tween 80 followed by ether causes loss of infectivity but preservation of hemagglutinin (92). Treatment with formalin or beta-propiolactone also reduces infectivity but preserves antigenicity (58).

Measles virus is best preserved by storage at -70 C in a suspension medium containing protein. Infectivity may also be maintained at refrigerator temperature (4 C) for several months in protein-containing medium (134). Lyophilization with a protein stabilizer will permit storage at refrigerator temperature for at least 18 months (58).

Classification

Measles virus is so closely related to canine distemper and rinderpest viruses that it has been suggested that the main differences in these agents are their natural hosts (51). Measles infects only primates; distemper infects only dogs, weasels, and related animals; and rinderpest infects only certain ruminants. These 3 agents share envelope antigens; antiserum against each exhibit at least some cross-neutralization against the other 2 agents. In addition to neutralization, shared antigens have been detected with other immunologic tests such as hemagglutination-inhibition (HAI) (103).

Antigenic composition

Number of immunotypes. No strain differences of measles virus have been identified, which is in keeping with the observation that one attack of measles confers lifelong immunity to the virus (114).

Description of the antigens. For purposes of clarity, it is helpful to relate the structural components of measles virus to specific antigens, although some overlap is known to exist. The viral envelope has been associated with the antigens responsible for hemagglutination and hemolysis while complement-fixing (CF) antigens are associated mainly, although not entirely, with the nucleocapsid (134). Nucleocapsid nonhemagglutinating CF activity obtained by Tween-ether splitting of the virion has a buoyant density in CsCl of 1.30–1.32 g/ml and appears to be a soluble antigen (45, 96, 100, 132, 133).

The measles hemagglutinin is present on both the viral envelope and the surface of cells infected with measles virus. The latter situation accounts for the phenomenon of hemadsorption (134). The hemagglutinin is heat stable, it is not inactivated by formalin, and it tolerates a pH range of 4.8–10.1. The antigen agglutinates primate erythrocytes (RBC) (with the exception of those of humans), particularly those of rhesus or African green monkeys (134).

In early studies of measles antigens, both large and small hemagglutinins were found on CsCl density gradients; these probably represented intact virions and either damaged envelopes (96) or possibly defective interfering particles (47). This antigen has now been identified with one glycoprotein having a buoyant density of 1.26 g/ml in CsCl (46).

The antigen responsible for hemolysis has been associated with both glycoproteins and lipids of the viral envelope; it is destroyed by both ether and trypsin (46). This antigen is more sensitive to thermal conditions than is the hemagglutinin, and it is stable at pH 5.6–10, with an optimum of 8. The hemolysin is probably responsible for the syncytial-forming characteristics of measles virus, an activity of the virion quite separate from infectivity (93, 134). Neuraminidase activity has not been associated with measles virus, in contrast to many other paramyxoviruses (49).

Pathogenicity for animals (host range)

Wild measles virus is pathogenic only for humans and certain primates. Humans are probably the natural reservoir of the virus, monkeys acquiring the disease only after capture and removal from the wild to native villages (82). Because monkeys in captivity often develop measles, usually in a mild or even asymptomatic and therefore unrecognized form, early studies on measles which involved monkeys yielded confusing results. Eventually, by using serologic techniques (107) it became possible to identify susceptible monkeys, and valid studies of measles in these animals became possible.

In contrast to wild measles virus which is nonpathogenic for small laboratory animals, tissue-culture-adapted measles virus strains often become pathogenic for them, especially when given by the intracerebral route to an immature animal.

Unadapted virus in monkeys. Laboratory workers have usually used rhesus, cynomolgus, or African green monkeys for infection with measles virus. Monkeys may be infected by a variety of routes, including intranasal instillation or subcutaneous injection of virus (118). The disease is often milder in monkeys than in humans, with fever and rash being somewhat inconstant signs (59). One concrete sign of infection is viremia a few days after inoculation of wild virus (118); vaccine strains do not usually produce viremia (28). However, both wild and vaccine strains stimulate an immune reaction to the virus (27). Therefore, the development of specific antibodies to measles virus is the best indication that infection has taken place. In experiments in which monkeys are to be infected, great care must be taken to isolate them from other laboratory animals which might transmit measles to the experimental animals.

Laboratory-adapted measles virus infections in animals other than primates. Years ago it was reported that the Edmonston strain of measles virus, first passed repeatedly in cell cultures and then intracerebrally in suckling mice, was pathogenic on intracerebral inoculation into young mice, rats, and hamsters (12, 51, 52, 130). More recently, both the original Edmonston strain and the Edmonston strain further attenuated by Schwarz (116) have been reported to cause encephalitis when directly injected intracerebrally into newborn hamsters without further tissue culture passage. This apparently chronic encephalitis in the hamster has been proposed to be a model for SSPE (135). In addition, an SSPE strain of measles virus has been reported to cause giant-cell encephalitis after intracerebral inoculation into newborn hamsters (13). In general, suckling animals are more susceptible to measles encephalitis than weanling animals, and this has been attributed to increasing maturation of cells of the central nervous system rather than to increasing immunologic maturity (44).

Growth in tissue cultures

Propagation of wild measles virus. Isolation of measles virus from blood and throat washings of patients with measles was first accomplished by Enders and Peebles in 1954 with primary human fetal or infant kidney cells (30). Although their report appeared over 20 years ago, these cells, as well as primary adult monkey kidney cells, remain the most sensitive systems in which to propagate wild measles virus.

Unfortunately, problems are encountered with each type of cell culture (77). Primary human fetal or infant kidney cells are difficult to obtain, and primary adult monkey kidney cells, while easily obtainable, may harbor measles virus or simian viruses which cause CPE similar to that of measles virus. While it has been reported that wild measles virus grows very well in fetal rhesus diploid kidney cells (shown to be free of extraneous agents), these cells, too, may not be readily available (34). At one time it seemed that primary cultures of human amnion cells would be acceptable for isolation of wild measles virus. However, it is now clear that these cells are much less sensitive than primary human or rhesus kidney cells for this purpose. Similarly, while wild virus has been isolated on occasion in primary tissue cultures of lower animals such as dog kidney cells, as well as in continuous cell lines, these tissues are not as sensitive for this purpose as primary human or monkey kidney cells (77). Therefore, when available, primary human fetal or infant kidney cells are preferred for isolation of wild measles virus. Alternatively, adult monkey kidney cells may be used provided that there is recognition of the limitations of this tissue culture as described above.

Propagation of laboratory strains. Analogous to the broader susceptibility of laboratory animals to tissue-culture-adapted virus compared to wild virus, vaccine and other laboratory strains of measles virus can be successfully propagated in a wide variety of cell types. Susceptible cells include primary cultures of various organs from primates and other species, as well as stable cell lines of human and nonhuman origin (39, 77, 91, 136).

In tissue culture, measles is a slow growing virus which only begins to appear in intracellular infectious form by 12–18 hr after inoculation. Infectious virus appears in supernatant media later (77). Peak titers of infectivity in primary cells occur in 6–10 days; in cell lines, peak titers are found after 2–4 days. After the peak is reached, there is a relatively constant amount of virus in the supernatant media for several weeks until all the cells have been exhausted. There is always a greater titer of intracellular virus than extracellular virus. Titers from pooled intracellular and extracellular phases above 10^5 $TCID_{50}$/ml rarely occur in primary cultures; in stable cell lines using both the cellular phase and culture media, titers of $10^7 TCID_{50}$/ml may be obtained (57).

Cytopathic effects. Several days after inoculation, CPE begins to appear; 2 types have been described (15, 25, 101). One type, seen after infection with wild virus and with dilute inocula is giant-cell transformation. Multinucleate syncytial giant cells, containing 10–100 nuclei, form as a result of cell fusion induced by the virus. These cultures are usually highly infectious. The second type of CPE, spindle cell transformation, is associated with measles virus which has been passed repeatedly in tissue culture or with repeated passage of undiluted inocula. These cultures appear to have a high degree of hemagglutinin activity, but they are less infectious than cultures exhibiting giant-cell transformation (15, 25, 101). Lessened infectivity may be due to interferon synthesis, which is seen in cells with spindle-cell transformation (25, 79). It may also be due in part to the appearance of defective interfering particles that have been associated with this type of culture (47, 50).

It is important to emphasize that the growth characteristics of a given virus strain are highly dependent on the conditions of passage and that one strain can easily assume a different appearance, depending on how it is passed (48, 57).

In stained preparations of measles infected cells, eosinophilic nuclear and cytoplasmic inclusion bodies are often seen with the light microscope. Examination of these inclusions by electron microscopy suggests that they represent accumulations of nucleocapsid material of the virus (77, 89, 90).

Markers for vaccine and SSPE strains. The Edmonston B vaccine strain originated from one of the first measles virus isolates of Enders and Peebles. The virus was carried through more than 20 passages in both primary human kidney and amnion cells. During the latter passages, spindle-cell transformation was first noted. The virus was then adapted to chick embryo fibroblasts (CEF) after several passages in chick embryos (25). The Schwarz vaccine, which is further attenuated Edmonston B strain, was passed an additional 77 times in CEF (116). At present, vaccine or avirulent strains of measles virus may be distinguished from virulent or wild strains by the ability of the former to grow in CEF and in stable cell lines (25, 26). There is also a significant difference in plaque morphology; vaccine strains that produce feathery elongated plaques on primary monkey kidney cells and CEF, and virulent strains that produce small irregularly round plaques on primary monkey kidney cells only (10). Vaccine strains also induce interferon in tissue-culture cells, while virulent strains do not (26). Indeed, this ability to induce interferon may be related to attenuation of the agent (79). Whether production of defective interfering particles is also involved in attenuation of the virus is unknown.

SSPE strains of measles virus have been found to vary, exhibiting different amounts of infectivity, production of hemagglutinin, and variable CPE. The characteristics of SSPE strains, like other strains of measles virus, are dependent on the conditions of rescue and passage (48). Thus, there are no reliable, consistent markers for SSPE virus strains.

Plaque formation. Infectivity of measles virus may be quantitated by plaque assay using any of the primary cultures or cell lines in which measles virus is known to grow. Usually, primary kidney cells from patas, African green, or rhesus monkeys are used, although plaquing has been successfully accomplished in HeLa, human amnion, HEp-2, and KB cells (77). Plaquing is a rather lengthy process, taking from 1–1.5 weeks. Some workers have utilized 2 successive agar overlays to maintain the tissue culture for so long an interval (21, 77). The process can be shortened by earlier counting of plaques microscopically, utilizing immunofluorescence to identify viral antigens (110). Plaquing can also be accomplished in slanted tubes containing tissue culture cells and liquid medium as in the neutralization (Nt) test (see following section on neutralization).

Electron microscopy. Electron microscopic examination of measles infected HeLa cells has revealed the following sequence of events (89). Approximately 18–20 hr after infection, granular and filamentous cytoplasmic inclusion bodies appear. The granular structures probably represent cross-sections of filaments. At high magnification they appear helical with a width corresponding to that of the measles nucleocapsid, of which they are believed to be a developmental form. Thirty to 40 hr after infection, segments of the cell membrane appear thickened, and aggregates of nucleocapsid material converge below the altered cell membranes. Virus maturation appears to occur at the cell membrane and eventually, mature virions bud off from the infected cell. Ninety-six to 120 hr after infection, intranuclear inclusion bodies similar to the cytoplasic inclusions appear. The role, if any, of these latter structures in formation of new virions is unknown.

Preparation of Immune Serum

A natural source of immune serum is the person who has either recently recovered from a documented case of measles or who has received live measles vaccine in the recent past. Such serum, however, is not suitable for virus identification, since this serum invariably contains antibodies to other viruses. Human serum may be employed as controls in serologic tests but, if they are so used, it is important that pre-measles or preimmunization serum *from the same person* be included as negative controls.

Antiserum may be prepared by inoculation of monkeys with either wild or vaccine measles virus. Antiserum has also been produced in smaller laboratory animals such as rabbits and guinea pigs. For preparation of crude antiserum, guinea pigs have been inoculated either intranasally or intraperitoneally with attenuated measles virus (100). Immune serum has been produced in rabbits injected intramuscularly with measles antigen mixed with Freund complete adjuvant (95).

Antiserum directed against isolated structures of the measles virion, e.g., the envelope or nucleocapsid, has also been prepared. This requires purification of the antigen using nonionic detergent treatment followed by density gradient ultracentrifugation. These partially purified structures have been used to immunize rabbits (96). Hyperimmune serum thus prepared against the measles envelope contained Nt, HAI, and hemolysis-inhibiting antibodies.

Commercially prepared measles antiserum is also available from a number of biological supply houses.

A brief protocol for the preparation of antiserum, free from antibodies to host-cell components, in hamsters follows. Such antiserum may be useful, for example, in immunofluorescence and CF tests for identification of measles virus. Immunizing antigen is prepared by intracerebral inoculation of hamsters with neurotropic measles virus. The brains are homogenized, and the infected brain homogenate is used to immunize additional hamsters. After several "boosters", the immunized hamsters are bled for measles antiserum.

Preparation of measles-virus-infected hamster-brain suspension

Inoculate 3- to 5-day-old hamsters intracerebrally with 0.03 ml of a 2 $\times$ 10^{-2} dilution of neurotropic measles virus in physiologic saline containing penicillin 500 u/ml and streptomycin 500 μg/ml.

Harvest infected hamster brains when animals develop severe neurologic symptoms; this is usually within 3–4 days. Place whole brains in saline to make a 20% suspension and blend in a Sorvall Omnimixer for 2–3 min. Store at 4 C for several hr to allow aerosol to settle.

In a negative-pressure hood, open blender and dispense samples of approximately 12 ml into sterile screw-cap tubes. Store at − 70 C until ready to use. Note: Approximately 60 g of infected hamster brain (30 liters) are required to prepare sufficient antigen to immunize 30 adult hamsters.

Preparation of immunizing antigen

Allowing 1 ml for each animal to be immunized, remove the required amount of frozen hamster brain suspension from the freezer and thaw by immersing the tubes in water at room temperature.

If adjuvant is to be used (see below), prepare adjuvant mixture: 9 parts white mineral oil (Chevron Research Company, No. 3, viscosity 75–85 at 100 C) and 1 part arlacel (specially treated arlacel A, mannide monoleate preparation 5 BCRL No. 67481, Atlas Powder Co. Wilmington, Delaware). Just before immunizing animals, add the measles virus suspension in small increments to an equal volume of adjuvant mixture in a tube, shaking the tube after each addition. Further homogenize the mixture by forcing the material back and forth between 2 syringes connected by a Swinney millipore adapter fitted with a screen.

Animal inoculation schedule

Animals: 30 male hamsters, 6- to 8-weeks-old. One week prior to inoculation, bleed the animals by cardiac puncture; obtain 1 ml blood and save serum at −20 C.

Inoculate animals intraperitoneally for 6 weeks.

Inoculate with 2 ml of measles-infected hamster-brain suspension *with adjuvant* in the first and third week.

Inoculate with 1 ml of brain suspension *without adjuvant* in the second, fourth, fifth, and sixth weeks.

Collection and storage of immune serum

Exanguinate hamsters by cardiac puncture (4–5 ml blood) 14–21 days after the sixth injection. Allow clotted blood to stand overnight at 4 C. Separate serum and store in 10 ml volumes at −20 C until ready for use.

Collection and Preparation of Specimens for Laboratory Diagnosis

Measles is a highly contagious agent so that standard precautions should be taken against creating aerosols with potentially infected fluids, including blood. Individuals with a prior history of measles or live measles vaccine are not at risk to handle infected tissues.

Virus isolation

Measles virus may be isolated from blood, urine, throat, and conjuctivae in the prodromal phase of measles and during the early stages of the rash. However, since measles virus is rather difficult to isolate and since suitable tissue culture may not always be available, attempts to diagnose measles by virus isolation should be reserved for special circumstances. These would include for example, such rare situations as immunocompromised patients dying of interstitial pneumonia without rash (29), encephalitis following measles vaccine (35, 71), and unexplained encephalitis in an immunocompromised individual (3, 9). It is preferable to inoculate 2–3 culture tubes for each specimen. As has been mentioned, it is preferable to inoculate primary human kidney cells but, if these are unavailable, tubes containing primary monkey kidney cells may be used. As a third alternative, tubes containing primary human amnion cells may be inoculated. Control uninoculated tissue culture cells should also be examined to insure that any apparent CPE is not caused by viruses that may be present in the tissue culture itself or by nonspecific degeneration of the cell cultures. Conveniently, most simian viruses such as foamy agent do not hemadsorb, particularly on primary isolation, so that this technique may be used to identify measles virus in simian tissue cultures (114). However, not all measles virus isolates cause hemadsorption, particularly early passage levels. Therefore, immuno-fluorescence is preferable for specific reliable early virus identification. Again, control uninoculated tissue culture cells must be examined, as well as inoculated cultures. Generally, tissue culture cells for virus isolation are grown on slanted tubes although, occasionally, upright tubes are preferable (see below).

Blood. Collect 5-10 ml of blood in a sterile syringe containing approxi-mately 0.5 ml of 1:2000 heparin; 0.1-0.5 ml of blood may be inoculated di-rectly into tubes containing tissue culture cells. However, it is preferable to isolate and inoculate leukocytes, which are known to carry the virus, onto tissue culture. It is best to inoculate tissue cultures with specimens as soon as they are collected. However, if blood or other material must be stored before inoculation, it should be kept at refrigerator temperature, although not for longer than 24 hr.

To isolate white blood cells (WBC), heparinized blood is diluted 1:3 and layered over one-third the volume of ficoll hypaque (Ficoll-Paque, Pharma-cia) in a centrifuge tube. The tube is centrifuged for 45 min at room temper-ature and $1000 \times g$. WBC form an obvious central band in the ficoll hy-paque. The WBC are aspirated, placed in another centrifuge tube, and washed 3 times with Hanks balanced salt solution (BSS) containing antibiot-ics (500 u penicillin/ml and 500 μg streptomycin/ml). The washed WBC are resuspended in approximately 0.01 ml of Hanks BSS and inoculated onto cell cultures. A high percentage of positive isolates using *upright* tube cul-tures of human amnion cells has been reported using this method (42). Cul-tures should be left undisturbed for several days before changing the medi-um. Cultures should be examined daily for syncytia which might be ex-pected to appear 4-12 days after inoculation.

Throat secretions. These may be collected by swabbing the throat with a sterile cotton-tipped swab and placing the swab in 1.0 ml of Hanks BSS containing antibiotics. It is best to inoculate approximately 0.2 ml of the fluid immediately but, if storage is unavoidable, it should be at refrigerator tem-perature. If storage for more than 24 hr is required, secretions should be frozen at -70 C in Hanks BSS containing protein to stabilize the virus (e.g., 1% fetal calf serum or 0.5% gelatin).

In some instances, throat washings may be collected by having the pa-tient gargle a few milliliters of sterilized skim milk, about pH 7. The wash-ings are collected in a sterile bottle to which 500 μg streptomycin and 500 μ penicillin are added. The washings are then centrifuged at 1500 rpm for 35 min and 0.2 ml of supernatant fluid is added to slanted tube cell cultures.

Conjuctival secretions. The conjuctiva is swabbed gently with a sterile cotton applicator, and the specimen is treated as described above for throat swabs.

Urine. As large a volume of urine as possible is collected by "clean catch" into a sterile bottle. The pH is adjusted to about 7 by addition of 5% sodium bicarbonate if necessary. Antibiotics are added to make concentra-tions of penicillin 500 u/ml and streptomycin 500 μg/ml. The urine is then centrifuged for 30 min at 3000 rpm and 4 C. The supernatant fluid is dis-carded, and the sediment is resuspended in 1-2 ml of Hanks BSS; 0.2 ml of the supernatant fluid is inoculated onto slanted cell cultures.

Solid tissues. Fragments of tissues, such as lung or brain, believed to be infected are finely minced under sterile conditions and washed several times with Hanks BSS. The tissue fragments are further broken up by either homogenization or sonication in Hanks BSS. Specimens are then clarified by centrifugation at approximately 1000 rpm, and 0.2 ml of supernatant fluid is inoculated into tubes containing monolayers of cells susceptible to measles virus.

Co-cultivation techniques may be required to isolate measles virus in certain situations such as measles encephalitis (81). In this technique, whole cells from presumably infected tissue (rather than a tissue homogenate) are cultivated together with tissue culture cells (such as primary monkey kidney cells) known to be permissive for the virus.

Serologic diagnosis

For diagnosis of acute measles, approximately 5 ml of whole blood, should be collected as early in the acute phase of illness as possible and 10–14 days later during convalescence. For evaluation of immune status against measles or for diagnosis of SSPE, only one blood sample is necessary. For diagnosis of SSPE, CSF should also be collected for determination of measles virus antibody content.

The RBC should be removed from whole blood promptly by centrifugation. The serum may be stored for short periods at refrigerator temperature and for longer periods at −20 C. It is mandatory to test acute-phase and convalescent-phase sera for antibodies in the same test.

Microscopy

Light microscopy

Samples of presumably infected tissues from patients may be fixed in 10% formalin, embedded in paraffin, sectioned, and stained with hematoxylin and eosin (H & E) (see below).

Direct examination of clinical material. Nasal secretions from patients with suspected measles may be obtained either by aspiration of mucus from the nose with a sterile eye-dropper fitted with a bulb or by swabbing the nasal mucosa with a sterile cotton-tipped applicator (74, 86, 127). Smears are made from the secretions; these are either allowed to air-dry on the slide or preferably are immediately fixed in 50% methanol—50% ether. Air-dried smears are fixed in 95% ethanol for 10 min and stained with either Wright stain or H and E. Smears fixed in alcohol-ether are stained by the standard Papanicolaou technique. Slides prepared by this method are said to give best results (86).

Two possible approaches to the handling of tissue cultures infected with measles virus for microscopy have been described (30, 58).

1. Coverslip preparations—Fix in Bouin solution (see below) and stain with H and E.

2. Tube preparations—Pipette off medium, rinse with Hanks BBS, and add Bouin fixative solution for 5–10 hr. Remove Bouin fixative, dehydrate cells by adding graded alcohols, and finally add a mixture of ether and absolute alcohol. Remove this solution, fill tube with collodion, cap, and leave overnight. Pour off collodion, and drain the tube thoroughly. Rinse tube with water, and gently separate collodion cast from the tube with forceps. Fill the cast with 95% alcohol, twist the top, and place in a 95% alcohol bath. Cut the collodion longitudinally, and place the part of the membrane containing the cells on a stainless-steel wire screen; secure the membrane with a rubber band. Stain with H and E and mount in Permount while still wet with xylene.

H and E staining. Stain in hematoxylin for 10 min; rinse in tap water. Rapidly decolorize in acid alcohol; rinse in water. Dip in dilute ammonia water to blue preparation; rinse in water; dehydrate with 70% and 95% ethanol; stain with eosin for 10 min; rinse rapidly in 95% ethanol; place in oil of origanum, cretic for 5 min; xylene for 5-10 min; mount in Permount while wet with xylene; place on a firm surface with heavy weight on top of cover-glass (38).

Reagents. Bouin fixative, saturated aqueous picric acid (1.2 g in 100 ml of H_2O), 750 ml; formalin (38-40% formaldehyde), 250 ml; glacial acetic acid, 50 ml. Collodion, Merck USP; alcohol 24%-245 g of ether per fluid oz, use as received. Acid alcohol, 1 ml of concentrated HCl in 100 ml of 70% ethanol. Ammonia water, 1-2 drops of NH_4OH in 100 ml of H_2O, or until a faint odor is perceptible. Hematoxylin (Delafield), Eosin, eosin Y (alcoholic solution), saturated solution containing 2% of the dye (Howe and French, Inc.), dilute 1:4 with 95% ethanol. Oil of origanum, cretic (Fritzsche). Permount (Fisher Scientific Co.) (58).

Electron microscopy

Place 1- to 2-mm pieces of tissue to be examined in 2% OsO_4 in Veronal buffer, pH 7.4, at 4 C for 2 hr. Dehydrate tissue in graded ethanols and embed in Epon. Cut ultrathin sections and stain with uranyl acetate and lead citrate.

Immunofluorescence microscopy

Dry infected tissue culture grown on coverslip preparations (or Lab Tek slides, Miles Labs) *in situ* or allow smears from putatively infected specimens to dry on slides. Fix in acetone at −4 C for 10 min. Slides may be stored if necessary at −70 C.

Direct immunofluorescence is preferred for identification of measles virus. For this technique, globulin from measles antiserum is conjugated to fluorescein isothiocyanite by standard methods (88). This conjugated globulin is used to identify measles antigen in cell sheets or smears. Before use for diagnostic purposes, conjugates must be evaluated for sensitivity and specificity. Conjugates should stain tissue culture cells known to be infected with measles virus, but no staining of uninfected cells should occur nor should cells infected with other human paramyxoviruses stain. The highest dilution of conjugate, which yields bright staining of measles infected cells with little or no background staining, should be used.

Antiserum used in immunofluorescence techniques for virus identification is best obtained from small laboratory animals, such as hamsters (see preceding section).

For an indirect test, add appropriately diluted measles antiserum; incubate 30 min at 37 C. Wash thoroughly with phosphate-buffered saline

(PBS), pH 7.2–7.4; re-incubate with fluorescein labeled antihuman globulin (or other homologous antiglobulin, as is necessary) for 30 min at 37 C. Wash with PBS and mount in glycerol—PBS (10:1). Examine slides by fluorescence microscopy. Control slides from similar uninfected tissues should be prepared simultaneously and are of utmost importance. Uninfected tissues should not stain, nor should infected material treated with serum devoid of measles antibody rather than measles antiserum in the first incubation step. Conjugate applied to tissue without an intermediate serum should also cause no staining. Before use, the system must be standardized to determine optimal dilutions of antiserum and fluorescent conjugate. This is done by testing several dilutions of each on tissue culture known to be infected with measles virus. For antiserum, a dilution one tube lower than the last dilution to yield a positive reaction should be selected. For conjugate, the dilution selected for routine use should give no staining of uninfected tissue culture cells, and it should yield bright staining of measles infected tissue culture cells treated with the optimal antiserum dilution.

Laboratory Diagnosis

The most practical method to make a laboratory diagnosis of measles is to obtain acute- and convalescent-phase sera and to demonstrate a $\geq$4-fold rise in specific antibody to measles virus. For more rapid diagnosis, cytologic examination of nasal secretions, with or without demonstration of measles antigen by the fluorescent-antibody technique, may be used. Under the already mentioned special circumstances, virus isolation may be attempted.

Direct examination of clinical material

The demonstration of giant cells of the Warthin-Finkeldey type has been reported by some investigators to be diagnostic for measles (127). Others, however, have contended that giant cells may not necessarily be found in nasal secretions from all patients with measles and that some apparent false-positive results may also occur due to normal shedding of necrotic cells from the respiratory epithelium. These cells often have indistinct borders and, therefore, may be mistaken for giant cells (86).

Another rapid diagnostic approach is to attempt to demonstrate measles antigen(s) on giant cells in nasopharyngeal aspirates by immunofluorescence. In one report utilizing this technique, it was noted that globulin had to be eluted from the cells in approximately half of the cases to demonstrate a positive reaction (38). Elution was performed by incubating fixed smears in Sorenson glycine-hydrochloric acid buffer, 0.1M, pH 2.2, for 2 hr at 37 C and in PBS, pH 7.2, for 30 min before immunofluorescent staining. Positive results occurred in 18 of 24 patients with measles, usually from 2–6 days after onset of rash. Human antiserum, shown to be devoid of antibodies to other paramyxoviruses and myxoviruses, was used for these studies.

Staining of measles-antigen positive cells in urinary sediment by indirect immunofluorescence has also been described (75, 76). In one study (76), urine was obtained and treated as for virus isolation except that sediment was allowed to dry on a slide. Slides were fixed in acetone for 20 min at −20 C and stained by indirect immunofluorescence. Positive results were obtained in 38 of 42 patients with clinical measles from 2 days before to 5 days after appearance of rash. Urinary sediments were also positive for measles antigen in 12 of 14 recipients of live measles vaccine. Sediments from 20 of 20 patients without measles were negative for measles antigen by this method. In these studies, direct immunofluorescence using pooled human globulin containing a high titer of measles antibody and conjugated to fluorescein isothiocyanate was used.

Virus isolation

In tissue cultures. The most sensitive cell cultures which yield accurate results are primary fetal or infant human kidney cells. If these are unavailable, primary monkey kidney cells (somewhat less specific because they may contain extraneous agents) or primary human amnion cells (somewhat less sensitive) may be used. Generally, tissue culture tubes grown in a slanted position are used, except that when attempting to isolate virus from WBC, tubes grown in an upright position are preferable. Human cells may be grown in lactalbumin hydrolysate medium or bovine amniotic fluid medium (58). *Bovine amniotic fluid medium:* Hanks BSS (45%), bovine amniotic fluid (45%), horse serum (5%), bovine embryonic extract (5%). *Lactalbumin hydrolysate* medium: 10% lactalbumin hydrolysate (5%), calf serum (10%), 10X concentrated Hanks BSS (10%), 2.8% $NaHCO_3$ (3%), distilled H_2O (72%). Primary monkey kidney cells may be obtained commercially from Flow Laboratories and, for maintenance of cultures, medium No. 199 containing 2% fetal calf serum is used. These cells may be kept for up to 2 weeks before inoculation.

Cultures should be observed for 30 days for CPE; fresh medium should be added to cultures every third day. Usually CPE develops within 5–10 days after inoculation of wild virus. Apparent negative cultures may be subjected to one blind passage 2 weeks after inoculation; this maneuver may reveal a low-titer positive specimen.

Identification of isolates. Cultures which develop giant-cell or spindle-cell transformation should be regarded as suspicious. As has been mentioned, uninoculated control cultures should always be compared to inoculated cultures. Suspicious cultures may be tested for hemadsorption. A suspension of 0.5% monkey RBC is added to cultures for about 30 min and then the cultures are rinsed with Hanks BSS. If measles virus is present, RBC may adhere to areas of CPE. However, not all measles isolates will cause hemadsorption, and other parainfluenza viruses may also hemadsorb. Therefore, it is preferable to demonstrate measles antigen in cultures exhibiting CPE suggestive of measles virus.

This may be done by several methods. Measles antigen may be looked for in supernatant media by CF, although this is a relatively cumbersome and insensitive technique for this purpose. Measles antigen may be best demonstrated by indirect immunofluorescence. This is probably the most specific and rapid method for identification if reliable antiserum is used. Immunofluorescence assays may be performed in tube cultures using microscopes which have an adequate distance between stage and objective to accommodate a tube. Alternatively, the cells may be removed with trypsin or by the collodion method previously described; in which case, fixation with acetone rather than Bouin solution is recommended. Control uninoculated cultures similarly treated should yield negative results. An attempt may also be made to neutralize an isolate, using known antibody-positive and, antibody-negative (control) measles sera, although this method is unnecessarily time consuming for this purpose.

Serologic diagnosis

Three methods may be used to measure antibody to measles virus. Hemagglutination-inhibition (HAI) is the major method. It is probably the simplest of the tests to perform, and it is the most frequently utilized test for demonstrating measles antibodies. HAI antibodies parallel Nt antibodies to measles virus, except that the HAI test is slightly less sensitive than Nt (55, 114). Measles antibodies may also be demonstrated by the CF technique, an adequate method for demonstrating a significant rise in measles antibody titer between acute-phase and convalescent-phase specimens. However, the CF test is not adequately sensitive for determination of immune status to measles in many instances (114, 126). Virus neutralization is the most sensitive test for determination of measles antibodies, but it is not widely used for diagnostic purposes because it is technically very difficult. In addition, the additional sensitivity of the test is rarely required for diagnostic work. However, on occasion Nt is helpful in determination of immune status. On rare occasions, serum with negative HAI and Nt tests is observed in individuals immune to measles (55, 112). A cellular immune response to measles antigen has been documented in some of these patients (112).

Complement-fixation test

Techniques employed for measles CF tests are similar to CF tests used for other viruses. Usually, the microtiter method is employed because it requires only small amounts of reagents and many serum samples can be handled at one time by this method. The tube method and the drop method of Fulton and Dumbell (37, 58) may also be utilized. Only the microtiter method is described below. Details of the CF test may be found in the US Department of Health, Education and Welfare, Public Health Service Booklet entitled *A Guide to the Performance of the Standard Diagnostic Complement Fixation Method and Adaptation to Micro Test* (22).

Preparation of antigens. Measles antigen may be prepared in any of the previously mentioned cells or cell lines which support growth of the virus. Cell lines may be preferable since they are easier to obtain, free of latent viruses, and higher virus titers may be reached. To prepare a high-titer antigen (58, 114), cultures should be inoculated at as high a multiplicity of infection as is possible. Usually, the Edmonston B measles strain is used; harvest should take place about 7 days after CPE has become extensive. Crude media alone may be harvested as antigen. Inclusion of intracellular virus, as well as extracellular virus in the antigen will include cellular debris, resulting in a more crude but higher titer antigen preparation. Because of the latter consequence, many workers utilize only the fluid phase from infected cultures for preparation of measles antigen. Should it be desired to include intracellular virus, however, this may be accomplished by rapidly freezing and thawing infected cultures before harvest. The antigen is heated to 56 C for 30 min to inactivate the virus, centrifuged at $1000 \times g$ for 15 min, and stored in aliquots at -20 C. Concentration of antigen before use is usually unnecessary.

Serum. Serum obtained from clotted blood is inactivated at 56 C for 30 min; this serum may be stored at -20 C. If serum is anticomplementary (AC), it may be treated as follows (58). Dilute serum 1:2 in Veronal-buffered saline (VBS) and heat to 60 C for 30 min. Chill, then add an equal volume of 10% crystalline bovine serume albumin in VBS. Reheat to 60 C for 20 min. Alternatively, AC activity may be removed by treating serum with complement (125). To 4 volumes of serum, 1 volume of fresh or reconstituted lyophilized guinea pig complement is added. The mixture is kept at 4 C overnight; the next morning it is heated to 37 C in a waterbath for 30 min. Subsequently, diluent is added to give a 1:4 dilution of serum. This is heated to 60 C for 30 min, and the serum is then used in the CF test. Cells: Sheep RBC collected and stored in Alsever solution are used. Before use, RBC are washed 3 times in 0.85% NaCl, Veronal-buffered diluent (VBD). A 2.8% RBC suspension in VBD is used in the test.

Procedure for the test (22). The standard microtiter technique is used. Dilutions of serum (usually doubling, beginning at 1:4) are made in microtiter "U" plate wells with VBD and standard diluting loops which deliver 0.025 ml to each well. Appropriately diluted antigen (0.025 ml) is added to each well. Complement (0.05 ml) is added (usually five 50% hemolytic endpoint units) to each well: the plates are kept at 4 C for 15–18 hr; 0.025 ml of a 2.8% sheep RBC suspension (previously sensitized with a nonhemagglutinating dilution of sheep-cell hemolysin) is added to each well, and plates are incubated 30 min at 37 C. Next the plates are centrifuged at $600 \times g$ for 5 min, and the test is read. Two control wells per serum should be included: serum without antigen and control (uninfected) antigen with serum; there should be complete hemolysis in these wells. The proper dilution of antigen is determined previously by checkerboard titration against a known antiserum.

Interpretation of test. Wells in which no hemolysis is present i.e., CF of complement has taken place, are considered positive; these wells contained measles antibody. The titer of antibody is the reciprocal of the highest positive dilution of serum. The RBC pattern is graded from 0 to 4+, 4+ representing no hemolysis or CF, and 0 representing hemolysis or no fixation. Reactions of 3+ and 4+ are considered positive. Titers >1:4 are consistent with immunity to measles, but titers of <1:4 do not necessarily indicate susceptibility to measles. To make a serologic diagnosis of measles by CF, a ≥4-fold rise in antibody titer in 2 serum samples must be demonstrated.

Hemagglutination-inhibition test

Preparation of antigen. Measles hemagglutinin has been successfully prepared in the following cell systems: KB cells, human embryonic lung fibroblasts, primary monkey kidney, and primary dog kidney cells (114); again cell lines may be expected to result in higher titer antigens. Antigen is prepared by inoculation of tissue culture with as high a multiplicity of infection as is possible using an undiluted inoculum. Usually, the Edmonston B strain is employed. Antigen should be harvested a few days after CPE becomes extensive. Crude supernatant media from cultures may be harvested as antigen. However, for highest titers of antigen, intracellular virus may also be included; this is usually obtained by rapid freezing and thawing of infected cultures and media. Antigen is heated for 30 min at 50 C to inactivate the virus, centrifuged at 15,000 rpm for 20 min, and the supernatant is stored at -20 C in convenient volumes.

Norrby's modification of this procedure for production of hemagglutinin leads to increased yields (4- to 32-fold) of antigen (92), as well as 2-fold higher antibody titers than are found with untreated antigen. In his technique, undiluted virus is propagated on lung fibroblasts or dog kidney cells at 33 C. When there is close to 100% CPE, the cultures are rapidly frozen and thawed 3 times. Tween 80 is added to a concentration of 0.125% with continuous stirring at 4 C. One-half the volume of ether is added, and stirring is continued for 15 min. The mixture is centrifuged at $1000 \times g$ for 20 min or a separatory funnel is used, and the aequeous phase is saved. Residual ether is removed by carefully bubbling N_2 through the liquid.

Commercially available measles HAI antigen can be obtained from a number of biologic supply houses. In some laboratories, commercially prepared measles antigen is apparently used with success.

Serum. Serum should be stored at -20 C or lower. Serum may be inactivated at 56 C for 30 min. Alternatively, serum may be treated with an equal volume of 25% kaolin (wt/vol) in physiologic saline; the mixture is allowed to sit for 20 min at room temperature. The serum-kaolin mixture is then centrifuged at $1000 \times g$ for 10 min, and the supernatant is saved as a 1:2 dilution.

Since some serum contains agglutinins for monkey RBC, it is recommended that each serum (either inactivated or kaolin treated) be adsorbed at 4 C for several hours or overnight with an equal volume of 50% monkey RBC in physiologic saline. The next day the RBC are removed by pipetting off the serum or by centrifugation.

Monkey red blood cells. RBC from the following monkeys may be used: baboon, rhesus, patas, and African green. RBC should be obtained from monkeys which are seronegative against measles virus. In addition, RBC from some animals demonstrate hemagglutination better than others. Therefore, it is necessary to preselect donor animals whose RBC show strongly positive hemagglutination (HA) reactions with measles antigen. RBC are collected and stored for up to 1 week in Alsever solution in the refrigerator. On the day of the test, the RBC are washed 3 times in physiologic saline. A 0.5% suspension of RBC in saline is used in the test.

Procedure for the test. First the titer of hemagglutinin must be obtained. Two-fold serial dilutions of antigen are prepared in physiologic saline with loops in a microtiter "U" plate, resulting in a volume of 0.025 ml of diluted antigen per well. To each well is added 0.025 ml of 0.5% monkey RBC. The plate is shaken and incubated at 37 C for 30 min to 1 hr. The highest dilution of antigen giving complete HA is the endpoint and contains 1 HA unit (HAU).

To perform the test, dilutions of serum usually beginning at 1:8 are made in microtiter plates in physiologic saline. Four HAU of antigen in a volume of 0.025 ml are added to each well. The plates are kept for 1 hr at room temperature after which 0.05 ml of 0.5% monkey RBC is added. Plates are shaken and kept at 37 C for 0.5-2 hr. Titers are recorded as the highest serum dilution resulting in complete HAI. Control wells should include serum without antigen at the lowest dilution and uninfected tissue culture cells; there should be no HA in these wells.

Nonspecific inhibitors of the measles hemagglutinin present in normal human serum have been described. These inhibitors lead to falsely high antibody titers. However, the presence of these inhibitors is usually not as troublesome as when testing for rubella HAI antibody. Such inhibitors, when suspected to be present, may be removed by treatment with 25% kaolin or heparin-$MnCl_2$ (31).

Interpretation of test. To determine immune status to measles, starting dilutions of serum of less than 1:8 may be used in the HAI test. The presence of measles HAI antibody in one serum specimen indicates prior infection with measles virus. Only rarely will immune individuals have no measles antibody (112).

To make a serologic diagnosis of acute measles, a ≥4-fold increase in HAI titer must be demonstrable between acute-phase and convalescent-phase sera. Significant boosts in measles antibody titer in immune persons with low or undetectable antibody who become reinfected with measles without clinical symptoms have been reported (55, 66).

Extremely high measles HAI antibody titers have been reported in blood and CSF of patients with SSPE. In one such patient, for example, a serum titer of 1:16,384 was found (68). The presence of measles HAI antibody in CSF in a patient with clinical symptoms of SSPE is consistent with this diagnosis (16, 68).

Virus neutralization tests in tissue culture

Because of their availability and their sensitivity to tissue culture adapted strains of measles virus, stable cell lines rather than primary cell cultures are recommended for Nt tests. Using these cells, monolayers may be maintained for up to 2 weeks in good condition so that it will be possible to complete the reading of the test.

Virus. The strain used should be standardized as much as possible within the laboratory so that reproducible results may be obtained on successive testing.

Performance of test (58). First, a measles virus titration must be performed to determine the dose of virus to use, as well as when viral cytopathology is maximal and when the test should be read. Too early reading of the Nt test itself will result in apparently false low Nt-antibody titers. Stock virus for Nt in infected tissue culture fluid is aliquoted and stored at −70 C. From the stock, 1 log (or for greater accuracy 0.5 log) dilutions are made in medium No. 199. To each of 3-5 cell cultures, 0.1 ml of each dilution is added, and the cultures are incubated at 37 C. Cultures are observed daily for CPE. The final endpoint is reached when cultures incubated at lower dilutions develop CPE, but CPE does not appear in cultures incubated at higher dilutions. This is usually 2 weeks after incubation. The titer is expressed as log 10 $TCID_{50}/0.1$ ml.

To perform Nt test, stock virus is diluted with medium to a titer of 100 $TCID_{50}/0.1$ ml. An equal amount of serum in serial dilutions beginning at 1:2 or 1:4 is added to tubes containing of virus and allowed to remain at 4 C for 1 hr. Then 0.2 ml of each mixture is added to 3-5 tissue culture tubes at 37 C. Controls should include the following: a) infectivity controls—dilutions of 100 $TCID_{50}$, 10 $TCID_{50}$, 1 $TCID_{50}/0.2$ ml; and b) titration of a known measles antibody-positive serum against measles virus 100 $TCID_{50}/0.1$ ml. Reading of the test is made at the previously determined optimal time.

Two practical modifications of the Nt test seem worth mentioning. Kriel et al (65) have described a microneutralization technique in which secondary rhesus monkey kidney cells, 200,000/ml are seeded into wells of disposable ''U'' microtiter plates (Linbro) and inoculated with serum and 300 $TCID_{50}$ of measles virus. After 5 days of incubation, wells in which the virus had grown were identified by hemadsorption, rather than appearance of CPE, using 0.025 ml of 0.9% African green monkey RBC. Nt titers obtained by this method gave results similar to those obtained by tube Nt tests in similar cells.

A more rapid Nt test, utilizing a continuous line of human amnion cells, has also been described (121). For this test, human amnion cells at a concentration of 200,000 cells/ml are used. Dilutions of serum and the test dose of virus are incubated at room temperature for 1 hr. Then 0.8 ml of the cell suspension plus 0.2 ml of the serum-virus mixtures are inoculated simultaneously into tissue culture tubes. The tubes are evaluated 7 days later for measles virus by the presence of CPE.

Interpretation of the test. The test may be used to confirm a diagnosis of measles, in which case, acute-phase and convalescent-phase sera should be tested simultaneously. As usual, ≥4-fold rises are considered significant.

The Nt test may also be used to determine immune status to measles, in which case, only 1 serum specimen is required. An undiluted sample of serum should also be tested since, occasionally, even Nt titers fall to very low levels years after an attack of measles. Rarely, persons immune to measles may have no detectable Nt antibody (55, 112). This is particularly true in immunocompromised patients, for example, those with leukemia who may also have minimal increases in antibody titer after measles (83).

Other tests

Other serologic tests which have been used for demonstration of measles antibody or antigen include gel precipitation, immunoperoxidase, and immune adherence hemagglutination (IAHA). Experience with these tests has been much less than with the standard tests. However, since these tests may be useful in certain situations a brief description of each follows.

Gel precipitation (20, 94, 104). For this reaction microscope slides are coated with a 0.4 mm high layer of 1% agarose containing 0.01% sodium azide; 0.2-mm holes are made in the gel by aspiration with a Pasteur pipette. Known measles antigen is placed in one well, known positive measles antiserum is placed in antoher, and test serum (or CSF) is placed in a third well. A line (or lines) of identity between the 3 wells indicate the presence of specific measles antibody or antigen; precipitin lines are usually visible within 24-72 hr. Usually, concentration of measles antigen (by ultracentrifugation) and serum or CSF (by vacuum dialysis) are required. Using this method with CSF, increased levels of measles antibody has been demonstrated, and the diagnosis of SSPE has been made (20). Generally, this method is somewhat less sensitive for detection of antigen or antibody than the previously mentioned methods.

Immunoperoxidase (24). This technique may be used to demonstrate the presence of antigen (using a known positive measles serum) or antibody (using tissue culture known to be infected with measles virus). The method is analagous to immunofluorescence, and both direct and indirect techniques are available. The infected tissue culture on a slide or coverslip is fixed in 1% gluteraldehyde and treated with serum, followed by antihuman globulin conjugated with horseradish peroxidase (available commercially from Cappel). The preparation is then treated with diaminobenzidine, a chemical which turns localized peroxidase red-brown. Slides are then dehydrated and mounted in Permount. The advantages of this technique over immunofluorescence are: 1) a fluorescence microscope is unnecessary and 2) this method may also be used to demonstrate immunologic reactions by electron microscopy.

Immune adherence hemagglutination (IAHA). This test, used to detect hepatitis B surface antigen (78), appears to be highly sensitive and simple to perform. For the test, known measles antigen and dilutions of serum are mixed in microtiter plates and incubated together. Later, complement, dithiothreitol, and human type O RBC are added. In the presence of an antigen-antibody reaction, the RBC agglutinate. Using this technique, Lennette and Lennette (72) demonstrated measles antibodies in serum of individuals immune to measles. The IAHA-antibody titers were approximately 2-10 times higher than the measles CF-antibody titers of these sera.

References

1. ADAMS JM, BAIRD C, and FILLOY L: Inclusion bodies in measles encephalitis. J Am Med Assoc 195:290–298, 1966
2. ADAMS JM and IMAGAWA DT: Measles antibodies in multiple sclerosis (27855). Proc Soc Exp Biol Med 111:562–566, 1962
3. AICARDI J, GOUTIERES F, ARSENIO-NUNES ML, and LEBON P: Acute measles encephalitis in children with immunosuppression. Pediatrics 59:232–239, 1977
4. BARBOSA LH, FUCCILLO DA, SEVER JL, and ZEMAN W: Subacute sclerosing panencephalitis: isolation of measles virus from a brain biopsy. Nature 221: 974, 1969
5. BLACK FL: Growth and stability of measles virus. Virology 7:184–192, 1959

6. BLACK FL: Measles: its spread from cell to cell and person to person. Can J Public Health 56:517-520, 1965

7. BOUTEILLE M, FONTAINE C, VEDRENNE C, and DELARUE J: Sur un cas d'encephalite subaiquë a inclusions. Etude Anatomo-Clinique et Ultrastructurale. Rev Neurol 113:454-458, 1965

8. BRANDLING-BENNETT AD, LANDRIGAN PJ, and BAKER EL: Failure of vaccinated children to transmit measles. J Am Med Assoc. 224:616-618, 1973

9. BREITFELD V, HASHIDA Y, SHERMAN FE, ODAGIRI K, and YUNIS EJ: Fatal measles infection in children with leukemia. Lab Invest 28:279-291, 1973

10. BUYNAK EB, PECK HM, CREAMER AA, GOLDNER H, and HILLEMAN MR: Differentiation of virulent from avirulent measles strains. Am J Dis Child 103:460-472, 1962

11. BURNET FM: Measles as an index of immunologic function. Lancet 2:610-613, 1968

12. BURNSTEIN T, FRANKEL, JW, and JENSEN JH: Adaptation of measles virus to suckling hamsters. Fed Proc 17:507, 1958

13. BYINGTON DP, CASTRO AE, and BURNSTEIN T: Adaptation to hamsters of neurotropic measles virus from subacute sclerosing panencephalitis. Nature 225:554-555, 1970

14. CARTER C, SCHLUEDERBERG A, and BLACK FL: Viral RNA synthesis in measles virus-infected cells. Virology 53:379-383, 1973

15. CHIARINI A and NORRBY E: Separation and characterization of products of two measles virus variants. Arch Gesamte Virusforsch 29:205-214, 1970

16. CONNOLLY JH, ALLEN IV, HURWITZ LJ, and MILLAR JHD: Measles-virus antibody and antigen in subacute sclerosing panencephalitis. Lancet 1:542-544, 1967

17. DAYAN AD: Subacute sclerosing panencephalitis. Proc Soc Roy Soc Med 67:1123- 1125, 1974

18. DE JONG JG and WINKLER KC: Survival of measles virus in air. Nature 201:1054-1055, 1964

19. DE JONG JG: The survival of measles virus in air, in relation to the epidemiology of measles. Arch Gesamte Virusforsch 16:97-102, 1965

20. DIETZMAN DE, BARBOSA LH, KREBS HM, MADDEN DL, FUCCILLO DA, and SEVER JL: Diagnosis of subacute sclerosing panencephalitis by a simple spinal fluid gel precipitation test for measles. Pediatrics 49:133-136, 1972

21. DE MAEYER E: Plaque formation by measles virus. Virology 11:634-638, 1960

22. Standardized Diagnostic Complement Fixation Method and Adaptation to Micro Test. US Dept of HEW, 1st edition, 7/1969

23. DRZENIEK R and ROTT R: Host-specific antigens of lipid-containing RNA viruses. Viruses as a carrier of cell-specific antigens. Int arch Allergy 36:146-152 (Suppl), 1969

24. DUBOIS-DALCQ M and BARBOSA LH: Immunoperoxidase stain of measles antigen in tissue culture. J Virol 12:909-918, 1973

25. ENDERS JF: Measles virus, Historical review, Isolation and behavior in various systems. Am J Dis Child 103:282-287, 1962

26. ENDERS JF, KATZ SL, and GROGAN E: Markers for Edmonston measles virus. Am J Dis Child 103:473-474, 1962

27. ENDERS JF, KATZ SL, and Holloway A: Development of attenuated measles virus vaccines. Am J Dis Child 103:335-340, 1962

28. ENDERS JF, KATZ SL, and MEDEARIS DN JR: Perspectives in virology In Recent Advances in Knowledge of the Measles Virus, Pollard M (ed), John Wiley and Sons, New York, 1959, pp 103-120

29. ENDERS JF, McCARTHY K, MITUS A, and CHEATHAM WJ: Isolation of measles virus at autopsy in cases of giant cell pneumonia without rash. N Engl J Med 261:875-881, 1959

30. ENDERS JF and PEEBLES TC: Propagation in tissue cultures of cytopathogenic agents from patients with measles. Proc Soc Exp Biol Med 86:277-286, 1954

31. FELDMAN HA: Heparin-MnCl$_2$ removal of nonspecific serum inhibitor for measles virus hemagglutinin. J Immunol 100:1353-1354, 1968

32. FENNER F: The pathogenesis of the acute exanthems. Lancet 2:915-920, 1948

33. FINKELDEY W: Über riesenzellbefunde in den gaumenmandeln. Zugleich ein beitrag zur histopathologie der mandelverän-derungen im maserninkubationsstadium. Virchows Arch 281:323-329, 1931

34. FORMAN ML, INHORN SL, SHEAFF E, and CHERRY JD: Biological characteristics and viral spectrum of serially cultivated fetal rhesus monkey kidney cells. Proc Soc Exp Biol Med 131:1060-1067, 1969

35. FORMAN ML and CHERRY JD: Isolation of measles virus from the cerebrospinal fluid of a child with encephalitis following measles vaccination. Proceedings of the 77th Meeting of the American Pediatric Society, Atlantic City, 26-29, April 1967. New Haven, American Pediatric Society, Inc, p 32

36. FULGINITI VA, ELLER JJ, DOWNIE AW, and KEMPE CH: Altered reactivity to measles virus. J Am Med Assoc 202: 1075-1080, 1967

37. FULTON F and DUMBELL KR: The serological comparison of strains of influenza virus. J Gen Microbiol 3:97-111, 1949

38. FULTON RE and MIDDLETON PJ: Immunofluorescence in diagnosis of measles infections in children. J Pediatr 86:17-22, 1975

39. GALLAGHER MR and FLANAGAN TD: Replication of measles virus in continuous lymphoid cell lines. J Immunol 116:1084-1088, 1976

40. GERSON KL and HASLAM HA: Subtle immunologic abnormalities in four boys with subacute sclerosing panencephalitis. N Engl J Med 285:78-82, 1971

41. GIBBS FA, GIBBS EL, CARPENTER PR, and SPIES HW: Electroencephalographic changes in "uncomplicated" childhood diseases. J Am Med Assoc 171:1050-1055, 1959

42. GRESSER I and CHANY C: Isolation of measles virus from the washed leucocytic fraction of blood. Proc Soc Exp Bio Med 113:695-698, 1963

43. GRESSER I, and KATZ SL: Isolation of measles virus from urine. N Engl J Med 263:452-454, 1960

44. GRIFFIN DE, MULLINIX J, NARAYAN O, and JOHNSON RT, Age dependence of viral expression: comparative pathogenesis of two rodent-adapted strains of measles virus in mice. Infect Immun 9:690-695, 1974

45. HALL WW and MARTIN SJ: Purification and characterization of measles virus. J Gen Virol 19:175-188, 1973

46. HALL WW and MARTIN SJ: The biochemical and biological characteristics of the surface components of measles virus. J Gen Virol 22:363-374, 1974

47. HALL WW and MARTIN SJ: Defective interfering particles produced during the replication of measles virus. Med Microbiol Immunol 160:155-164, 1974

48. HAMILTON R, BARBOSA LH, and DUBOIS M: Subacute sclerosing panencephalitis measles virus: study of biological markers. J Virol 12:632-642, 1973

49. HOWE C and SCHLUEDERBERG A: Neurminidase associated with measles virus. Biochem Biophys Res Commun 40:606-607, 1970

50. HUANG AS and BALTIMORE D: Defective viral particles and viral disease processes. Nature 226:325-327, 1970

51. IMAGAWA DT: Relationships among measles, canine distemper and rinderpest viruses. Prog Med Virol 10:160-193, 1968

52. IMAGAWA DT and ADAMS JM: Propagation of measles virus in suckling mice. Proc Soc Exp Biol Med 98:567-569, 1958

53. JOSEPH BS, LAMPERT PW, and OLDSTONE MBA: Replication and persistence of measles virus in defined subpopulations of human leukocytes. J Virol 16:1638-1649, 1975

54. KATZ M and STIEHM ER: Host defense in malnutrition. Pediatrics 59:490-495, 1977

55. KATZ SL, ENDERS JF, and HOLLOWAY A: Use of Edmonston attenuated measles strain: a summary of three years experience. Am J Dis Child 103:340-344, 1962

56. KATZ SL: Immunization with live attenuated measles virus vaccines: five years' experience. Arch Gesamte Virusforsch 16:222-230, 1965

57. KATZ SL and ENDERS JF: Measles virus In Viral and Rickettsial Infections of Man. 4th edition, Horsfall FD Jr and Tamm I, (eds), Lippincott, Philadelphia, 1965, pp 784-801

58. KATZ SL and ENDERS JF: Measles virus In Diagnostic Procedures for Viral and Rickettsial Infections, 4th edition, Lennette E and Schmidt N, (eds) Am Public Health Assoc, New York, 1969, pp 504-528

59. KEMPE CH and FULGINITI VA: The pathogenesis of measles virus infection. Arch Gesamte Virusforsch 16:103-128, 1965

60. KETTYLS GD, DUNN HG, DOMBSKY N, and TURNBULL IM: Subacute sclerosing panencephalitis: isolation of a measles-like virus in tissue culture of brain biopsy. Can Med Assoc J 103:1183-1184, 1970

61. KIMURA A, TOSAKA K, and NAKAO T: Measles rash. I. Light and electron microscopic study of skin eruptions. Arch Virol 47:295-307, 1975

62. KIMURA A, TOSAKA K, and NAKAO T: An immunofluorescent and electron microscopic study of measles skin eruptions. Tohoku J Exp Med 117:245-256, 1975

63. KOPLIK H: The diagnosis of the invasion of measles from a study of the exanthemata as it appears on the buccal mucus membrane. Arch Pediatr 13:918-922, 1896

64. KRESS S, SCHLUEDERBERG AE, HORNICK RB, MORSE LJ, COLE JC, SLATER EA, and McCRUMB FR: Studies with live attenuated measles-virus vaccine. Am J Dis Child 101:701-707, 1961

65. KRIEL RL, WULFF H, and CHIN TDY: A microneutralization test for determination of antibodies to rubeola virus. Proc Soc Exp Soc Biol Med 130:107-109, 1969

66. KRUGMAN S, GILES JP, FRIEDMAN H, and STONE S: Studies on immunity to measles. J Pediatr 66:471-488, 1965

67. KRUGMAN S: Present status of measles and rubella immunization in the United States: a medical progress report. J Pediatr 90:1-12, 1977

68. KRUGMAN S, WARD R, and KATZ SL: Infectious diseases of children. 6th edition, The CV Mosby Co, St. Louis, 1977

69. KRUGMAN S: Unpublished data.

70. LACHMANN PJ: Immunopathology of measles. Proc Roy Soc Med 67:12-14, 1974

71. LANDRIGAN PJ, and WITTE JJ: Neurological disorders following live measles-virus vaccination. J Am Med Assoc 223:1459-1462, 1973

72. LENNETTE D and LENNETTE E: Diagnostic Viral Serology by Means of Immune Adherence Hemagglutination. Am Soc Microbiol, Washington, DC, 1977, p 46

73. LENNON RG, ISACSON P, ROSALES T, ELSEA WR, KARZON DT, and WINKELSTEIN W: Skin tests with measles and poliomyelitis vaccines in recipients of inactivated measles virus vaccine: delayed dermal hypersensitivity. J Am Med Assoc 200:275-280, 1967

74. LIGHTWOOD R, NOLAN R, FRANCO M, and WHITE AJS: Epithelial giant cells in measles as an aid in diagnosis. J Pediatr 77:59-64, 1970

75. LIPSEY AI and BOLANDE RP: The exfoliative source of abnormal cells in urine sediment of patients with measles. Am J Dis Child 113:677-682, 1967

76. LLANES-RODAS R and LIU C: Rapid diagnosis of measles from urinary sediments stained with fluorescent antibody. N Engl J Med 275:516-523, 1966

77. MATUMOTO M: Multiplication of measles virus in cell cultures. Bacteriol Rev 30:152-176, 1966

78. MAYUMI M, OKOCHI K, and NISHIOKA K: Detection of Australia antigen by means of immune adherence haemagglutination test. Vox Sang 20:178-181, 1971

79. McCARTHY K: Measles in laboratory hosts and tissue culture systems. Am J Dis Child 103:314-319, 1962

80. McLEAN DM, BEST JM, SMITH PA, LARKE RPB, and McNAUGHTON GA: Viral infections of Toronto children during 1965: II. Measles encephalitis and other complications. Can Med Assoc J 94:905-910, 1966

81. MEULEN VT, MÜLLER D, KÄCKELL Y, KATZ M, and MEYERMANN R: Isolation of infectious measles virus in measles encephalitis. Lancet 2:1172-1175, 1972

82. MEYER HM JR, BROOKS BE, DOUGLAS RD, and ROGERS NG: Ecology of measles in monkeys. Am J Dis Child 103:307-313, 1962

83. MITUS A, ENDERS JF, CRAIG JM, and HOLLOWAY A: Persistence of measles virus and depression of antibody formation in patients with giant cell pneumonia after measles. N Engl J Med 261:882-889, 1959

84. MITUS A, HOLLOWAY A, EVANS AE, and ENDERS JF: Attenuated measles vaccine in children with acute leukemia. Am J Dis Child 103:413-418, 1962

85. MODLIN JF, JABBOUR JT, WITTE JJ, and HALSEY NA: Epidemiologic studies of measles, measles vaccine, and subacute sclerosing panencephalitis. Pediatrics 59:505-512, 1977

86. MOTTET NK and SZANTON V: Exfoliated measles giant cells in nasal secretions. Arch Pathol 72:434-437, 1961

87. MUSSER SJ and UNDERWOOD GE: Studies on Measles virus. II. Physical properties and inactivation studies of measles virus. J Immunol 85:292-297, 1960

88. NAIRN RC: Fluorescent Protein Tracing. 4th edition, Longman Pub Inc, New York, New York, 1976

89. NAKAI M and IMAGAWA DT: Electron microscopy of measles virus replication. J Virol 3:187-197, 1969

90. NAKAI T,, SHAND FL, and HOWATSON AF: Development of measles virus in vitro. Virology 38:50-67, 1969

91. NAKAMURA K, HOMMA M, and ISHIDA N: Growth of measles virus in cultures of rat glioma cells. Infect Immun 12:614-620, 1975

92. NORRBY E: Hemagglutination by measles virus. 4. A simple procedure for production of high potency antigen for hemagglutination-inhibition (HI) tests. Proc Soc Exp Biol Med 111:814-818, 1962

93. NORRBY E: The effect of a carbobenzoxy tripeptide on the biological activities of measles virus. Virology 44:599-608, 1971

94. NORRBY E and GOLLMAR Y: Appearance and persistence of antibodies against different virus components after regular measles infection. Infect Immun 6:240-247, 1972

95. NORRBY E and GOLLMAR Y: Identification of measles virus-specific hemolysis-inhibiting antibodies separate from hemagglutination-inhibiting antibodies. Infect Immun 11:231-239, 1975

96. NORRBY E and HAMMARSKJÖLD B: Structural components of measles virus. Microbios 5:17-29, 1972

97. NORRBY ECJ, MAGNUSSON P, FALKSVEDEN LG, and GRÖNBERG M: Separation of measles virus components by equilibrium sedimentation in CsCl gradients. II. studies on the large and the small haemagglutinin. Arch Gesamte Virusforsch 14:462-473, 1964

98. NORRBY ECJ, MAGNUSSON P, and GRÖNBERG M: The nucleic acid of measles virus. Arch Gesamte Virusforsch 16:81-82, 1965

99. NORRBY E, RUCKLE GE, and MEULEN VT: Differences in the appearance of antibodies to structural components of measles virus after immunization with inactivated and live virus. J Infect Dis 132:262-269, 1975

100. NUMAZAKI Y and KARZON DT: Soluble antigen of measles virus. J Immunol 97:470-476, 1966

101. ODDO FG, et al. On the hemagglutinating and hemolytic activity of measles virus variants. Arch Gesamte Virusforsch 22:35-42, 1967

102. OJALA A: On changes in the cerebrospinal fluid during measles. Ann Med Intern Fenn 36:321-331, 1947

103. ÖRVELL C and NORRBY E: Further studies on the immunologic relationships among measles, distemper, and rinderpest viruses. J Immunol 113:1850-1858, 1974

104. PALOSUO T, SALMI AA, and PETTAY O: Measles antibodies detected by platelet aggregation and gel precipitation in patients with subacute sclerosing panencephalitis. Arch Gesamte Virusforsch 35:45-53, 1971

105. PAPP K: Fixation du virus morbilleux aux leucocytes du sang dans la Période d'incubation de la maladie, Bull Acad Nat Med (Paris) 117:46-51, 1937

106. PAYNE FE, BAUBLIS JV, and ITABASHI HH: Isolation of measles virus from cell cultures of brain from a patient with subacute sclerosing panencephalitis. N Engl J Med 281:585-589, 1969

107. PEEBLES TC, MCCARTHY K, ENDERS JF, and HOLLOWAY A: Behavior of monkeys after inoculation of virus derived from patients with measles and propagation in tissue culture together with observations on spontaneous infections of these animals by an agent exhibiting similar antigenic properties. J Immunol 78:63-74, 1957

108. RABIN ER: Measles and the central nervous system. Mo Med 71:225-229, 1974

109. RAND KH, EMMONS RW, and MERIGAN TC: Measles in adults: an unforseen consequence of immunization? J Am Med Assoc 236:1028-1031, 1976

110. RAPP F, GORDON I, and BAKER RF: Observations of measles virus infection of cultured human cells. I. A study of development and spread of virus antigen by means of immunofluorescence. J Biophys Biochem Cytol 7:43-48, 1960

111. RAUH LW, and SCHMIDT R: Measles immunization with killed virus vaccine. Am J Dis Child 109:232-237, 1965

112. RUCKDESCHEL JC, GRAZIANO KD, and MARDINEY MR: Additional evidence that the cell-associated immune system is the primary host defense against measles (rubeola). Cellular Immunol 17:11-18, 1975

113. RUCKLE G and ROGERS KD: Studies with measles virus. II. Isolation of virus and immunologic studies in persons who have had the natural disease. J Immunol 78:341-355, 1957

114. RUCKLE GE: Methods of determining immunity duration and character of immunity resulting from measles. Arch Gesamte Virusforsch 16:182–207, 1965

115. SCHLUEDERBERG A: Measles virus RNA. Biochem Biophys Res Commun 42:1012–1015, 1971

116. SCHWARZ AJF: Preliminary tests of a highly attenuated measles vaccine. Am J Dis Child 103:386–389, 1962

117. SCOTT TF: Post infectious and vaccinial encephalitis. Med Clin N Am 51:701–717, 1967

118. SERGIEV PG, RYAZANTSEVA NE, and SHROIT IG: The dynamics of pathological processes in experimental measles in monkeys. Acta Virol (Eng) 4:265–273, 1960

119. SHAFFER MF, RAKE G, and HODES HL: Isolation of virus from a patient with fatal encephalitis complicating measles. Am J Dis Child 64:815–819, 1942

120. SMITHWICK EM and BERKOVICH S: *In vitro* suppression of the lymphocyte response to tuberculin by live measles virus. Proc Soc Exp Biol Med 123:276–278, 1966

121. STRAUSS J, ZDRAŽÍLEK J: A more rapid method of measles neutralization test with simultaneous cell inoculation. J Hyg Epidemol Microbiol Immunol 12:47–53, 1968

122. SULLIVAN JL, BARRY DW, LUCAS SJ, and ALBRECHT PL Measles infection of human mononuclear cells I. Acute infection of peripheral blood lymphocytes and monocytes. J Exp Med 142:773–784, 1975

123. SURINGA DWR, BANK LJ, and ACKERMAN AB: Role of measles virus in skin lesions and Koplik's spots. N Engl J Med 283:1139–1142, 1970

124. TANNENBAUM M, HSU K, BUDA J, GRANT JP, LATTES C, and LATTIMER J: Electron microscopic virus-like material in systemic lupus erythematosus with preliminary immunologic observations on presence of measles antigen. J Urol 105:615–619, 1971

125. TARAN A: A simple method for performing a Wasserman test on anticomplementary serum. J Lab Clin Med 31:1037–1039, 1946

126. THIRY L, DACHY A, and LOWENTHAL A: Measles antibodies in patients with various types of measles infection. Arch Gesamte Virusforsch 28:278–284, 1969

127. TOMPKINS VM and MACAULAY JC: A characteristic cell in nasal secretions during prodromal measles. J Am Med Assoc 157:711, 1955

128. UEDA S, OKUNO Y, HAMAMOTO Y, and OHYA H: Subacute sclerosing panencephalitis (SSPE): Isolation of a defective variant of measles virus from brain obtained at autopsy. Biken J 18:113–122, 1975

129. VALDIMARSSON H, AGNARSDOTTIR G, and LACHMANN PJ: Cellular immunity in subacute sclerosing panencephalitis. Proc Roy Soc Med 67:1125–1129, 1974

130. WAKSMAN BH, BURNSTEIN T, and ADAMS RD: Histologic study of the encephalomyelitis produced in hamsters by a neurotropic strain of measles. J Neuropathol Exp Neurol 21:25–49, 1962

131. WARTHIN A: Occurrence of numerous large giant cells in tonsils and paryngeal mucosa in prodromal stage of measles. Report of four cases. Arch Pathol 11:864–874, 1931

132. WATERS DJ, HERSH RT, and BUSSELL RH: Isolation and characterization of measles nucleocapsid from infected cells. Virology 48:278–281, 1972

133. WATERS DJ and BUSSELL RH: Isolation and comparative study of the nucleocapsids of measles and canine distemper viruses from infected cells. Virology 61:64–79, 1974

134. WATERSON AP: Measles virus. Arch Gesamte Virusforsch 16:57–80, 1965

135. WEAR DJ and RAPP F: Encephalitis in newborn hamsters after intracerebral injection of attenuated human measles virus. Nature 227:1347–1348, 1970

136. WEBB HE, ILLAVIA S, and LAWRENCE GW: Measles-vaccine viruses in tissue-culture of non-neuronal cells of human fetal brain. Lancet 2:4–5, 1971

CHAPTER 23

RESPIRATORY SYNCYTIAL VIRUS

Robert H. Parrott, Hyun Wha Kim,
Carl D. Brandt, Marc O. Beem, Linda Richardson,
John L. Gerin, and Robert M. Chanock

Introduction

Strains of respiratory syncytial virus (RSV) were first recognized in 1956 when isolated from chimpanzees with coryzal respiratory illness (50). Although first called the "chimpanzee coryza agent," it was soon evident that the natural habitat of this virus was the human respiratory tract and that extensive syncytial areas developed in cell cultures infected with this virus. Hence the name "respiratory syncytial virus" was selected as being more appropriate (14).

Epidemiology

RSV is now recognized as one of the most important viruses causing acute respiratory illness, especially as the major cause of bronchiolitis and pneumonia in infants and young children. Although worldwide in distribution (35, 44, 49), most of the information about this virus has come from studies conducted among temperate zone urban populations where most persons experience several infections. Initial RSV infections usually occur during infancy and infrequently during the preschool years of life; the chief impact of this virus is in infants both in terms of incidence and severity of illness (4, 5, 11, 28, 36, 40, 52). Seroepidemiologic studies from all parts of the world demonstrate the presence of RSV antibody, and it is likely that similar patterns of infection occur worldwide, possibly modified in degrees by population density. RSV infections occur in annual epidemics during fall, winter, and spring. In several long-term studies there have been alternating short (approximately 7-12 month) and long (approximately 13-16 month) intervals between peaks of successive epidemics (40). Urban epidemics often last approximately 5 months; however, the duration has been shorter in smaller population groups such as nursery schools. The presence of the virus in the community typically is signalled by a sharp increase in the incidence of bronchiolitis and bronchopneumonia among infants and young children (11, 24, 53). In the course of an epidemic, the bronchiolitis and bronchopneumonia caused by RSV may represent 85% and 35%, respectively, of the annual total of these diseases (11, 15, 28, 45). RSV infections are also encountered in older children and adults (32) but less frequently and with a milder "common cold" type of symptomatology. Various reports suggest that RSV infections may be an important cause of acute exacerbations of chronic bronchitis or asthma, an occasional cause of otitis media, a possible cause of heart disease, and that apnea frequently accompanies RSV infection in hospitalized infants (8, 12, 13, 22, 46). Since RSV infection is a virtually universal experience of early childhood, most infections occurring in older children and adults are reinfections. In serologic studies it has been found that approximately half of the infants tested were infected during their first RSV epidemic, and almost all children were infected after living through 2 RSV epidemics (11). These observations suggest that the virus becomes widely disseminated during an epidemic and that the risk of infection for previously uninfected infants and young children is extremely high. A crude estimate for the incidence of bronchiolitis requiring admission to the hospital per 1000 infants 0-12 months of age is 10 and for RSV bronchiolitis the estimate is 4 (11). These estimates lead to a further estimate of 1 hospital admission for RSV bronchiolitis per 100 primary RSV infections during infancy. In England, Sims et al estimated that the risk of hospital admission with RSV infection in the first year of life for city children was about 1 in 50 (59). Of course, the toll of RSV in infancy is considerably higher since for every hospital admission for RSV bronchiolitis there are many other infants who develop respiratory disease which is almost as serious as that seen in the individuals admitted to the hospital. Children may become fully symptomatic on reinfection after as short an interval as 1 year. Reinfection appears to occur because of incomplete host resistance rather than antigenic variation of virus (3).

RSV infection is spread by droplets from the respiratory tract of infected individuals. Following a 3-7 day incubation period (42), virus shedding is demonstrable in 90% of affected hospitalized infants. This shedding may briefly precede onset of clinical symptoms and may continue for as long as 15-27 days in young infants (26, 27). The distribution of the RSV in the body is confined to the respiratory tract; virus has been isolated from exudates of the nose, throat, and middle ear but not from blood or stools.

Clinical aspects

RSV infections that can be identified by virus isolation are almost always symptomatic. Among older children and adults the symptoms may be those of a "cold" and confined to the nose and nasopharynx; in younger children and particularly in infants, lower respiratory tract involvement is the rule, and the extent of this may range from a troublesome cough to severe respiratory distress due to bronchiolitis, bronchopneumonia, or both. The systemic response to the uncomplicated infection is not striking; malaise is mild and the temperature normal or slightly elevated. Neither atypical lymphocytes nor leukopenia characterize this virus infection. The most common complications involve the lower respiratory tract and result from the compromise of the diameter of the lumen of the bronchiole which is slightly larger in diameter during inspiration than it is during expiration. Thus, up to the point of complete obstruction by the inflammatory reaction of the mucosa and secretions in the lumen, air enters alveoli more readily than it exits. This relative expiratory obstruction traps the air in the alveoli, producing respiratory distress characterized by emphysema and expiratory wheezing. Should the obstruction become complete, there is resorption of air distal to that point, and small areas of atelectasis result. As a rule, the involvement of the lower respiratory tract is quite diffuse and, where severe enough to induce respiratory distress, there is usually a spectrum of physical and x-ray findings combining those of atelectasis, emphysema, and pneumonia. Where air trapping is the most prominent feature, the term "bronchiolitis" is applied to the condition; where atelectasis and signs of consolidation are prominent, the condition is termed "bronchopneumonia." In truth, neither term as conventionally used is an accurate description of the condition, and a term such as "RSV disease" might be more appropriate not only to typify the diffuse and diverse pulmonary changes that are truly neither "pneumonia" nor "bronchiolitis" but also to stress the preponderant role that RSV plays in the etiology of such a clinical disease. Fluid accumulation in the middle ear has been described in infants with RSV infection (7, 8), but symptomatic middle-ear infections do not seem to be more common than with other acute respiratory infections. In one study, RSV infection preceded a large proportion of cases of purulent otitis media (Denny F, personal communication).

An immunoprophylactic approach to prevention of RSV infection must recognize that serum antibody does not protect as evident from the study of natural disease and of infections following administration of killed vaccine (53). Local antibody responses occur in natural illness. Possibly, serum antibody in the absence of local antibody plays a part in illness. Thus, current efforts have been directed toward attenuated vaccines. Cold-adapted and temperature-sensitive (ts) mutant RSV vaccines have been studied. Both produced the desired infection as evidenced by virus recovery, serum, and local antibody response. However, both appeared to have had minor residual pathogenicity for young infants. This included mild bronchitis after administration of cold-adapted (26 C) RSV vaccine and mild rhinitis, which might be acceptable, but fever and otitis also occurred in 1 infant who received ts-RSV vaccine. Also, some of the virus recovered from subjects in the ts studies had wild-type growth characteristics. An acceptable RSV vaccine strain will infect without undergoing reversion or other genetic changes, induce resistance to wild-type virus, cause no or very mild inflammatory changes such as the rhinitis associated with the vaccines thus far tried.

Pathology

Cell cultures infected with RSV show the first characteristic morphologic changes with the development of syncytia (6, 41). These contain clusters of nuclei, usually located near the center of the syncytium, and when fixed and stained with Giemsa or hematoxylin-eosin, show cytoplasmic inclusions that are eosinophilic and surrounded by a clear halo. Immunofluorescence studies of infected cells show extensive specific staining confined to the cytoplasm of infected cells and syncytia. Pathology studies on proved human cases are few in number. Holzel and Parker (35) described the findings in a 10-month-old boy with a clinical diagnosis of bronchiolitis from whom RSV was isolated 24 hr prior to death. Grossly there were areas of emphysema, atelectasis, and consolidation of the lungs. On microscopic examination, the lesions of the bronchial mucosa consisted of ballooning of the goblet cells and desquamation of the columnar layers of the epithelium with infiltration of the bronchial wall by lymphocytes and plasma cells. Alveolar exudates consisted primarily of mononuclear cells. Not seen in the tissues of this patient were the multinucleated cells and eosinophilic intracytoplasmic inclusions seen in HEp-2 cells and in the epithelium of ferret turbinates (17) infected with RSV. However, Sheddon and Emery (58) saw such cells in the bronchial epithelium of lung tissues of 4 children who died with "giant cell bronchitis." Immunofluorescence (FA) methods were used to establish the etiology of these illnesses. Interestingly, RSV antigens in those tissues were not destroyed by prolonged formalin fixation and storage at room temperature.

Description and Nature of the Agent

Morphology, stability, and chemical composition

Electron microscope studies of virus propagated in heteroploid cells reveal a highly pleomorphic particle with a helical filamentous inner component surrounded by an envelope with surface projections. Particle shape and size vary greatly. In thin sections of infected HeLa cells, round forms about 65 nm in diameter, and filamentous forms of like diameter and up to 2.5 μ in length have been described (2), while negative stained preparations from infected HEp-2 cells have shown distorted, roughly spherical particles, with overall diameters varying from 90–860 nm and averaging 340 nm (9, 10).

RSV is relatively thermolabile. Stability studies (29) showed that 90% of infectivity is lost in 5 min at 55 C, in 24 hr at 37 C, and in 4 days at 4 C. Infectivity is rapidly lost at pH 3, and the virus appears to have maximal stability at pH 7.5.

RSV appears to be an RNA virus (30, 63, 67) with an outer lipoprotein coat derived from the plasma membrane of the infected cell. The nucleocapsid of RSV is a single-stranded helix with a diameter of 14 nm (33, 66) and a periodicity of 70 Å (10, 38). Single-stranded 50S RNA isolated from the nucleocapsid probably represents the intact viral genome (34). Biochemical analyses of purified virus indicate that RSV consists of 6–7 polypeptides some of which are glycosylated (43). Although the overall morphology of RSV resembles that of the paramyxoviruses, the smaller diameter of the nucleocapsid and the lower molecular weights of the structural polypeptides support the placing of RSV in a separate taxonomic group (48).

Antigenic composition

Antigenic heterogeneity of RSV can be demonstrated by differences in the neutralizing (Nt) but not complement fixing (CF) antibody titer of animal serum for the immunizing virus strain as compared to titers for heterologous strains of virus. The human immune response is usually sufficiently broad to make these differences less apparent (3, 16, 62). Thus, while an animal immune serum may not neutralize all strains of RSV with equal efficiency, this is seldom true of human convalescent-phase serum.

In addition to infectious virus, cell cultures infected with RSV yield smaller antigens that fix complement with human convalescent-phase serum. One of these, termed antigen A by virtue of its early elution in column chromatography of crude material, is stable to ether-Tween treatment and induces both CF and Nt antibodies in the guinea pig; antigen B, eluting later, elicits only CF antibodies. No hemagglutinating activity has yet been demonstrated for RSV.

Pathogenicity for animals

A wide variety of animals including mice, hamsters, guinea pigs, and ferrets can be infected with RSV by intranasal inoculation (17). These infections are virtually asymptomatic, never lethal, and must be identified in tissue culture by isolation of virus from respiratory secretions or tissues, or by serologic responses.

Growth in tissue culture

Continuous cell lines, such as HEp-2 and HeLa, are satisfactory for the isolation and propagation of RSV and also to show the prominent syncytium formation that characterizes this agent (Fig 23.1). Although human diploid fibroblast lines such as WI-38 support the growth of RSV (1), we have found such lines less satisfactory for the primary isolation of RSV. It should be emphasized, however, that cell strains vary significantly in sensitivity to this virus, and that syncytium formation may be influenced by such factors as the medium employed (35) and the density of the cell sheet. Experience shows that a highly sensitive system such as HEp-2 maintained in Eagle minimal essential medium (MEM) plus an equal volume of medium No. 199 with 2% agamma calf serum (RSV antibody free) propagates virus to a titer of 10^6 to 10^7 $TCID_{50}$/ml and shows first cytopathic effect (CPE) from a large dose of high-passage virus within 48 hr. Adsorption of virus from an inoculum of small volume is 90% complete in 2 hr in both HEp-2 (16) and WI-38 (56) cells. Viral antigen demonstrable by FA staining is first evident from 7 to 10 hr after inoculation. Cell-free virus appears in the culture fluids shortly thereafter, but approximately 50% of the virus remains cell-associated at the time peak virus titers are attained (39, 41).

Preparation of Immune Serum

Immune serum that is free of antibodies reacting with tissue culture components can be produced by repeated intranasal infection of susceptible animals, such as guinea pigs or ferrets; 10^4 $TCID_{50}$ of tissue culture-grown virus is instilled into each nostril of an animal lightly anesthetized with ether or pentothal. The ensuing infection can be confirmed by isolation of virus from nasal secretions. CF and Nt antibodies found 3-4 weeks after infection are usually at levels of 1:32-1:256, a range commonly encountered in human convalescent-phase serum. Intranasal inoculation of these animals after an interval of 4-6 months results in reinfection with a boost in antibody levels to the range of 1:256-1:2048. Should such a lengthy immunization schedule not be suitable, serum with high Nt antibody titer can be prepared by repeated parenteral inoculation of RSV antigen. Material that is relatively free of foreign host-cell antigen may be obtained by growing RSV in tissues derived from the species to be immunized or by concentrating and purifying the virus by ultracentrifugation. Several inoculations are required, the number depending upon the potency of the antigen. Two weeks after the last injection, the animals are bled and the serum is tested for Nt antibodies. If the titer is low, injections are resumed.

Collection and Preparation of Specimens

Virus isolation

RSV is found only in the secretions and tissues of the respiratory tract. Material for virus isolation is usually collected from the nose and oropharynx with a cotton swab. However, the quantity and quality of the specimen to be tested can be improved by aspiration from the nose, or from the nasopharynx and oropharynx, using a No. 5-8 plastic disposable premature-infant feeding tube attached to 10-ml syringe, or suction catheter with a mucus trap, or by a "bedside" nasal wash using a 1-oz rubber suction bulb (25). The swabs or aspirates are placed into 2-4 ml of suitable collecting medium such as veal infusion broth (or Eagle MEM) with 0.5% bovine albumin, or Hanks balanced salt solution (BSS) with 0.5% gelatin. Because RSV is relatively unstable, the best isolation results are obtained by avoiding freezing and by minimizing the time between collection of the specimen and inoculation of cell culture. However, good isolation rates may be expected from material held at 4 C for 3-5 hr. Although virus may be recovered from specimens which have been frozen rapidly and stored at −70 C (31), experience shows that inoculation of specimens without prior freezing is best for primary isolation.

Serologic diagnosis

Blood specimens should be obtained as early in the course of illness as possible, followed by a second specimen in 2-4 weeks. Ross et al (55), stressed that the serologic response of the very young may be slow, and significant changes may be missed unless a 4- to 6-week interval is allowed between collection of the first and the second serum specimen.

Laboratory Diagnosis

Direct examination of clinical material

Electron microscopy

The most rapid diagnosis of RSV infection can potentially be accomplished by electron microscopy of nasopharyngeal secretions (18, 37), but this is not commonly attempted, in part because of the general unavailability of electron microscopes.

Immunofluorescence techniques

FA procedures of the indirect (20, 21, 23, 47) and direct (51) types can be used for the rapid diagnosis of RSV infection, provided that the reagents used are both specific and sensitive. Nasopharyngeal secretions are collected by gentle suction, emulsified in 0.5 ml of saline, and centrifuged at low speed for 10 min. The sediment is resuspended in phosphate-buffered saline (PBS) and recentrifuged (20, 21). The resulting pellet is suspended in a few drops of saline and distributed to several areas on each of 2 slides. The slides are allowed to air-dry. Slides are fixed in acetone for 10 min at 4 C. One of the spots containing fixed nasopharyngeal material is overlaid with RSV antiserum, while other spots are overlaid with parainfluenza virus type 1, 2, or 3 antiserum. The slides are incubated at 37 C for 30 min in a moist chamber and then rinsed for 30 min in 3 changes of PBS. Fluorescein-conjugated anti-rabbit globulin is then added and the slides incubated again for 30 min at 37 C. This is followed by a 30 min rinse in 3 changes of PBS and a final wash for 2 min in distilled water. The slides are then viewed by ultraviolet microscopy. Exfoliated cells infected with RSV exhibit cytoplasmic staining. Staining reactions are completely type-specific and the indirect FA technique appears to be as efficient as isolation of virus in tissue culture for diagnosis of RSV infection (20, 21).

Success of this technique is dependent upon the use of rabbit RSV antiserum which is absorbed with human heteroploid cells (i.e., HeLa or HEp-2 cells) in order to remove reactivity against human tissue. Rabbit antiserum is prepared by immunization of animals with virus grown in human heteroploid cells such as HEp-2 (47).

Virus isolation

Although RSV grows in a variety of cell cultures the preferred cell cultures are HEp-2 or Hela maintained on Eagle basal medium plus an equal amount of medium No. 199 with 2% agamma calf serum which is RSV antibody free. Cultures may be incubated at 33–37 C, rolled or stationary. Due to variations in the sensitivity of HEp-2 cells to RSV it may be useful to obtain cells from at least 2 different sources. HEp-2 cultures should have only a light growth of cells when inoculated. For example, 15-mm × 125-mm tubes seeded with 4-6 × 10^4 cells per tube, are usually ideal for inoculation in 24–48 hr when they show scattered areas of confluent cellular growth. In such cell cultures early CPE appears as small syncytia or giant cells, characteristically first seen at the butt of the tube where the glass bends to form the bottom. In tubes containing heavy cellular growth, RSV causes only indistinct rounding which may be overlooked. Virus growth usually becomes apparent between the fifth and seventh day after inoculation, although occasional cultures may show first CPE on the third day and others become positive only on second passage. Development of CPE is accelerated by replacing the medium. When 50–75% of the cell sheet is affected, direct passage (without prior freezing) of 0.2 ml of fluid and cells to a fresh similar cell culture tube is followed in 3–5 days by the appearance of characteristic CPE. In some laboratories, all specimens receive 2 passages which are held for 10 days each before being considered negative.

While strains of other heteroploid cells, such as KB and HeLa may show the morphologic changes described above, the CPE seen in human diploid cells such as WI-38 is less characteristic. Here cell destruction is more evident than syncytium formation. The process, initially focal, soon becomes generalized with destruction of the entire cell sheet and advanced CPE is not unlike nonspecific degeneration.

Identification of isolates

With the possible exception of parainfluenza virus type 2, no other commonly encountered respiratory tract virus produces giant cell and syncytium formation in appropriate heteroploid cells comparable to that produced by RSV. The presumptive identification of an agent as RSV is further strengthened if the virus in question grows poorly and without hemadsorption in monkey kidney cell cultures. Definitive identification may be obtained by infectivity neutralization, FA staining, or by the CF test.

For identification by virus neutralization, infected cell cultures are harvested at the time of maximal CPE. A 1:2 dilution of virus is mixed with an equal volume of antiserum diluted to contain 10–20 units of antibody (1 unit of antibody is equivalent to the Nt titer of that antiserum in a standard test); 1:2 virus dilution is also mixed with diluent as a control. The mixtures are incubated for 1 hr at room temperature, and then 0.2 ml is inoculated into each of 2 cell-culture tubes; these tubes are incubated at 36 C and are examined daily for 3–5 days. If the agent is RSV, the serum prevents development of the typical CPE. A logical endpoint criterion is minimal CPE in the test specimen tubes when controls show 75–100% CPE. It should be noted that strains may be encountered which are not as readily neutralized by immune serum prepared to prototype strains (such as the Long strain) as they are by homotypic antiserum. If this is the case, or if an especially potent virus is used in this test, syncytia may eventually appear in the tubes containing antiserum. However, there is a definite delay in the appearance of CPE compared with that in the control cultures.

Fluorescein-labeled antiserum to RSV can also be used for the definitive identification of virus isolates (20, 21, 23, 47, 57) (See immunofluorescence, above). The method is sensitive, accurate, and is not influenced by strain differences in antigenicity as is the case with the Nt test. For the procedure originally described, FA staining was done on coverslip-grown cells to which virus had been passaged (57); however, preparations made directly from cell-culture tubes can also be used. This is best done with heteroploid cells when about 25% of the cells show CPE. Cells are scraped from the glass, sedimented, and transferred to a slide. After air-drying and 10 min acetone fixation, this preparation (and controls of known positive and negative materials prepared in like fashion) are stained in a manner similar to that for coverslip preparation.

Cultures to be identified by the CF test are harvested at the time of maximal CPE. The fluid, containing cells which can be readily shaken off the glass, can be used as in the next step or can be subjected to several cycles of freezing and thawing, then centrifuged to remove debris. The undiluted supernatant fluid is used as an unknown antigen in the CF test with a pair of human acute- and convalescent-phase sera known to show a rise in antibody titer. Anticomplementary activity which may be present in some preparations can sometimes be eliminated by heating to 56 C for 30 min. The procedure for the CF test is described in detail in Chapter 1; titration of hemolysin and preparation of sensitized cells are carried out as described therein. The antigen titration is omitted, and the complement titration is carried out with the undiluted, unknown antigen. If several viruses are being identified in a single test and if all viruses have been grown for about the same length of time in the same lot of cell cultures, it is not necessary to titrate complement in the presence of each unknown virus. The unit of complement determined for one of the unknowns can be used for all. Should an isolate show fixation, the anticomplementary control included in the test can be retested after titrating complement in its presence. If the unknown virus is RSV, fixation is obtained with the known convalescent-phase serum to approximately the same titer as that seen with a known RSV-positive control antigen. The titer of the convalescent-phase serum with the isolate should be at least 4-fold higher than that of the acute-phase serum.

Serologic diagnosis

For the serologic diagnosis of RSV infections, either the CF or virus Nt test can be employed. Note that it is not unusual to encounter measurable amounts of both CF and Nt antibodies in acute-phase serum specimens. In the very young these represent transplacental antibodies of maternal origin; in older children and adults they are the result of previous RSV infections. Such antibodies do not preclude the development of a significant increase in antibody titer in response to the current infection.

The procedure for the CF test is outlined in Chapter 1. Antigen for the test is prepared by inoculating bottles of HEp-2 cells (maintained in Eagle MEM with 2.5% heat-inactivated fetal bovine serum) with sufficient virus to produce maximal CPE in 4-5 days. Bottles are then shaken vigorously to dislodge the cells into the medium. The fluids are subjected to several cycles of freezing and thawing and then centrifuged to remove cellular debris. The supernatant fluid is titrated for CF activity as described in Chapter 1. If a serum from an adult is employed for standardization of the antigen, it is recommended that 8 rather than 4 units of antigen be employed in testing serum of infants under 1 year of age (15).

The virus Nt test is done in HEp-2 cell cultures with a light growth of cells using the medium and incubation conditions described above; virus used in this test should have an infectivity titer of at least 10^5 TCID$_{50}$/ml when tested in the cell culture system to be employed. This is prepared from seed virus serially passaged in tube cultures until 100% of the cells show CPE within 4 days of inoculation. An 8-oz prescription bottle (seeded the preceding day with 8×10^6 HEp-2 cells in Eagle MEM and 2% fetal calf serum) is drained of growth medium, rinsed twice with 10 ml of maintenance medium (MM), and then inoculated with 2–4 ml of seed virus. Over a 2-hr absorption period at room temperature, the inoculum is periodically redistributed over the cell sheet; then the inoculum is discarded and replaced with 15 ml of MM. The cell cultures are incubated stationary at 36 C. After 72-hr incubation virtually all cells should show morphologic change. At this time the cells are suspended in the medium by shaking; heat-inactivated fetal bovine serum is added to a final concentration of 5%, and the material is distributed into ampules for freezing and storage. For use in the test, the material is rapidly thawed; cellular debris is sedimented by centrifugation, and the supernatant fluid is diluted in MM to contain approximately 10^3 TCID$_{50}$/ml. Serum specimens to be tested are heat-inactivated and then serially diluted in MM. Virus is mixed with an equal volume of serum dilution (for controls with MM) and incubated at room temperature for 2 hr. Then 0.2 ml of each mixture is inoculated into 2 tubes containing HEp-2 cells. After 4 days of incubation, daily checks of the virus control tubes are made; the final reading of the test is done within 24 hr of the time at which these tubes show 75–100% CPE, usually on the fifth or sixth day. Since there may be a definite but incomplete inhibition of virus growth over a 4- to 16-fold range of serum dilutions, an endpoint other than complete virus growth inhibition is chosen.

An endpoint that is readily identified and reproducible is the serum dilution that inhibits the development of more than occasional areas of small syncytium formation or rounding (i.e., 1 + CPE on a scale of 4 where 1+ = 0 to 25% and 4+ = 75 to 100% of cells showing CPE). The final reading of a dilution is the average of the reading of the 2 tubes. Addition of neutral red at a final concentration of 1:80,000, followed by 1-hr incubation at 36 C, causes syncytia to stain red and can aid in the final reading (15).

A more sensitive and precise assay of RSV Nt antibody can be obtained with the plaque reduction test. Using a methyl cellulose overlay with HEp-2 cells, syncytial plaques appear in 4 days; the plaques can be accurately identified and enumerated in the Giemsa-stained monolayer with a dissecting microscope. The test can be designed to quantitate serum activity by a kinetic test which measures the rate of decrease in plaque forming titer (3), or by a serum dilution endpoint test which determines the serum dilution causing a 50% reduction in plaque forming titer (16).

An enzyme-linked immunosorbant assay (ELISA) for detection of serum antibody against RSV has been developed and is reported to be 100 times more sensitive than the CF Test and 2-4 times more sensitive than plaque reduction for detection of antibody (54).

RSV is grown in HEp-2 or primary African green monkey kidney (GMK) cells maintained in Eagle MEM supplemented with 2% agamma calf serum and 0.002 M glutamine. When CPE of the virus is maximal (3-4 days) the cells and fluid are harvested together by quick freezing and are stored at −70 C. Virus suspensions made in this manner contain 10^5-10^6 pfu/ml. A dilution of this virus preparation is used without further manipulation in the ELISA test in order to provide both internal and surface viral antigens for interaction with antibodies.

The globulin fraction of antihuman IgG, gamma-chain specific, goat serum is prepared by sodium sulfate precipitation and coupled to alkaline phosphatase (Sigma type VII) by the method of Engvall and Perlman using 5 mg of enzyme to 2 mg of immunoglobulin (19).

The method used for performing ELISA is that modified from Voller (61). The optimal dilutions of reagents are determined by checkerboard titration. The antigen (RSV grown in HEp-2 or GMK cells) is diluted 1:10 in carbonate buffer (pH 9.8) and 75 μl is added to the wells of round-bottom polyvinyl microtiter plates. Uninfected cells treated in the same manner as virus infected cells serve as control. Plates coated with antigen are then stored for at least 14 hr at 4 C in a moist chamber. Additional storage at 4 C for at least 3 months does not result in measurable loss of activity.

At the time of testing, the plates are washed 3 times in a solution of PBS containing polysorbate (Tween 20) at a concentration of 0.5 ml/liter (PSB-Tween). Four-fold dilutions of serum are made in the antigen-coated plates using PBS-Tween supplemented with 1% fetal calf serum and 10% uninfected cell suspension. The calf serum and control cell suspension are added to the diluent to reduce the nonspecific binding of the test serum. The final volume of diluted serum in each well is 75 μl. After an overnight incubation at 4 C, the plates are washed 3 times with PBS-Tween, and a 75 μl volume of a 1:400 dilution of the enzyme-linked goat antihuman IgG (made in the same diluent as used for dilution of serum) is added. This is allowed to react for 2 hr at 37 C. The plates are again washed 3 times with PBS-Tween, and 75 μl of p-nitrophenyl phosphate substrate (Sigma 104) diluted to contain 1 mg in 1 ml of diethanolamine buffer (pH 9.8) is added (61). After 15-min incubation at 37 C, the amount of yellow produced by the action of the enzyme (bound to the solid phase) on the substrate is measured in a colorimeter which determines the absorbance at 400 nm through the bottom of the microtiter plate (65). The ELISA titer of each serum is determined by comparing the absorbance value of each serum dilution to the value of a known positive human serum standard diluted to its endpoint; this endpoint is usually 1:1000-1:1600 for serum from adults. In each case the absorbance value of the serum in the control well is subtracted from the value obtained in the RSV antigen-coated wells. The diluted standard serum is considered the endpoint in the ELISA test since it usually has an absorbance value of approximately 0.35, while the absorbance value of the next 4-fold dilution of serum is usually only 0.05. Therefore values >0.35 are considered positive. The diluted standard serum is run in each plate to obviate plate-to-plate variation.

References

1. ANDERSON JM and BEEM MO: Use of human diploid cell cultures for primary isolation of respiratory syncytial virus. Proc Soc Exp Biol Med 121:205-209, 1966
2. ARMSTRONG JA, PEREIRA HG, and VALENTINE RC: Morphology and development of respiratory syncytial virus in cell cultures. Nature 196:1179-1181, 1962
3. BEEM MO: Repeated infections with respiratory syncytial virus. J Immunol 98:1115-1122, 1966
4. BEEM MO, EGERER R, and ANDERSON J: Respiratory syncytial virus neutralizing antibodies in persons residing in Chicago, Illinois. Pediatrics 34:761-770, 1964
5. BEEM MO, WRIGHT FH, HAMRE D, EGERER R, and OEHME M: Association of the chimpanzee coryza agent with acute respiratory disease in children. N Engl J Med 263:523-530, 1960
6. BENNETT CR JR and HAMRE D: Growth and serological characteristics of respiratory syncytial virus. J Infect Dis 110:8-16, 1962
7. BERGLUND B, SALMIVALLI A, TOIVANEN P, and WICKSTROM J: Isolation of respiratory syncytial virus from middle ear exudates of infants. Arch Dis Child 41:554-555, 1966
8. BLATTNER RJ: Respiratory syncytial virus: isolation from middle-ear exudates of infants. J Pediatr 70:848-850, 1967
9. BLOTH B, ESPMARK A, NORRBY E, and GARD S: The ultrastructure of respiratory syncytial (RS) virus. Arch Gesamte Virusforsch 13:582-586, 1963
10. BLOTH B and NORRBY E: Electron microscopic analysis of the internal component of respiratory syncytial (RS) virus. Arch Gesamte Virusforsch 21:71-77, 1967
11. BRANDT CD, KIM HW, ARROBIO JO, JEFFRIES BC, WOOD SC, CHANOCK RM, and PARROTT RH: Epidemiology of respiratory syncytial virus infection in Washington, D.C. III. Composite analysis of eleven consecutive yearly epidemics. Am J Epidemiol 98:355-364, 1973
12. BRUHN FW, MOKROHISHY ST, and MCINTOSH K: Apnea associated with respiratory syncytial virus infection in young infants. J Pediatr 90:382-386, 1977
13. CARILLI AD, GOHD RS, and GORDON WA: A virologic study of chronic bronchitis, N Engl J Med 270:123-127, 1964
14. CHANOCK RM and FINBERG L: Recovery from infants with respiratory illness of a virus related to chimpanzee coryza agent (CCA) II. Epidemiologic aspects of infection in infants and young children. Am J Hyg 66:291-300, 1957
15. CHANOCK RM, KIM HW, VARGOSKO AJ, DELEVA A, JOHNSON K, CUMMING C, and PARROTT RH: Respiratory syncytial virus. I. Virus recovery and other observations during 1960 outbreak of bronchiolitis, pneumonia and minor respiratory diseases in children. J Am Med Assoc 176:647-653, 1961
16. COATES HV, ALLING DW, and CHANOCK RM: An antigenic analysis of respiratory syncytial virus isolates by a plaque reduction neutralization test. Am J Epidemiol 83:299-313, 1966
17. COATES HV and CHANOCK RM: Experimental infection with respiratory syncytial virus in several species of animals. Am J Hyg 76:302-312, 1962
18. DOANE FW, ANDERSON N, ZBITNEW A, and RHODES AV: Application of electron microscopy to the diagnosis of virus infections. Can Med Assoc J 100:1043-1049, 1969
19. ENGVALL E and PERLMAN P: Enzyme-linked immunosorbent assay, ELISA III. Quantitation of specific antibodies by enzyme-linked anti-immunoglobulin in antigen-coated tubes. J Immunol 109:129-135, 1972
20. GARDNER PS and MCQUILLIN J: Application of immunofluorescent antibody technique in rapid diagnosis of respiratory syncytial virus infection. Br Med J 3:340-343, 1968
21. GARDNER PS, MCQUILLIN J, and MCGUSKIN R: The late detection of respiratory syncytial virus in cells of respiratory tract by immunofluorescence. J Hyg 68:575-580, 1970
22. GILES TD and GOHD RS: Respiratory syncytial virus and heart disease, a report of two cases. J Am Med Assoc 236:1128-1130, 1976

23. GRAY KG, MACFARLANE DE, and SOMMERVILLE RG: Direct immunofluorescent identification of respiratory syncytial virus in throat swabs from children with respiratory illness. Lancet 1:446-448, 1968

24. GRIST NR, ROSS CAC, and STOTT EJ: Influenza, respiratory syncytial virus and pneumonia in Glasgow, 1962-1965. Br Med J 1:456-457, 1967

25. HALL CB, DOUGLAS RG JR, and GEIMAN JM: Clinically useful method for the isolation of respiratory syncytial virus. J Infec Dis 131:1-5, 1975

26. HALL CB, DOUGLAS RG JR, and GEIMAN JM: Quantitative shedding patterns of respiratory syncytial virus in infants. J Infec Dis 132:151-156, 1975

27. HALL CB, DOUGLAS RG JR, and GEIMAN JM: Respiratory syncytial virus infections in infants: quantitation and duration of shedding. J Pediatr 89:11-15, 1976

28. HAMBLING MH: A survey of antibodies to respiratory syncytial virus in the population. Br Med J 1:1223-1225, 1964

29. HAMBLING MH: Survival of the respiratory syncytial virus during storage under various conditions. Br J Exp Pathol 45:647-655, 1964

30. HAMPARIAN VV, HILLEMAN MR, and KETLER A: Contributions to characterization and classification of animal viruses. Proc Soc Exp Biol Med 112:1040-1050, 1963

31. HAMPARIAN VV, KETLER A, HILLEMAN MR, REILLY CM, MCCLELLAND L, CORNFELD D, and STOKES J JR: Studies of acute respiratory illnesses caused by respiratory syncytial virus. I. Laboratory findings in 109 cases. Proc Soc Exp Biol Med 106:717-722, 1961

32. HAMRE D and PROCKNOW JJ: Viruses isolated from natural common colds in the U.S.A. Br Med J 2:1382-1385, 1961

33. HOFFMAN EJ, FORD EC, and GERIN JL: Isolation and characterization of ribonucleoprotein of respiratory syncytial virus. Abstracts of Annual Meeting, Am Soc Microbiol, Washington, DC, 1975, p 250

34. HOFFMAN EJ, FORD EC, and GERIN JL: Isolation of 50S RNA from respiratory syncytial virus and ribonucleoprotein. Abstracts of Annual Meeting, Am Soc Microbiol, Washington, DC, 1978, p 262

35. HOLZEL A, PARKER L, PATTERSON WH, WHITE LL, THOMPSON KM, and TOBIN JO'H: The isolation of respiratory syncytial virus from children with acute respiratory disease. Lancet 1:295-298, 1963

36. JACKSON GG and MULDOON RL: Viruses causing common respiratory infections in man. III. Respiratory syncytial viruses and coronaviruses. J Infect Dis 128:674-702, 1973

37. JONCAS JH, BERTHIAUME L, WILLIAMS R, BEAUDRY P, and PAVILANIS V: Diagnosis of viral respiratory infections by electron microscopy. Lancet 1:956-959, 1969

38. JONCAS JH, BERTHIAUME L, and PAVILANIS V: The structure of the respiratory syncytial virus. Virology 38:493-496, 1969

39. JORDAN WS JR: Growth characteristics of respiratory syncytial virus. J Immunol 88:581-590, 1962

40. KIM HW, ARROBIO JO, BRANDT CD, JEFFRIES BC, PYLES G, REID JL, CHANOCK RM, and PARROTT RH: Epidemiology of respiratory syncytial virus infection in Washington, D.C. I. Importance of the virus in different respiratory tract disease syndromes and temporal distribution of infection. Am J Epidemiol 98:216-225, 1973

41. KISCH AL, JOHNSON KM, and CHANOCK RM: Immunofluorescence with respiratory syncytial virus. Virology 16:177-189, 1962

42. KRAVETZ HM, KNIGHT V, CHANOCK RM, MORRIS JA, JOHNSON KM, RIFKIND D, and UTZ JP: Respiratory syncytial virus. III. Production of illness and clinical observations in adult volunteers. J Am Med Assoc 176:657-663, 1961

43. LEVINE S: Polypeptides of respiratory syncytial virus. J Virol 21:427-431, 1977

44. LEWIS FA, RAE ML, LEHMANN NI, and FERRIS AA: A syncytial virus associated with epidemic disease of the lower respiratory tract in infants and young children. Med J Aust 2:932-933, 1961

45. MCCLELLAND L, HILLEMAN MR, HAMPARIAN VV, KETLER A, REILLY CM, CORNFELD D, and STOKES J: Studies of acute respiratory illnesses caused by respiratory syncytial virus. II. Epidemiology and assessment of importance. N Engl J Med 264:1169-1175, 1961

46. MCINTOSH K, ELLIS EF, HOFFMAN LS, LYBASS TG, ELLER JJ, and FULGINITI VA: The

association of viral and bacterial infections with exacerbations of wheezing in young asthmatic children. J Pediatr 82:578, 1973

47. McQuillin J and Gardner PS: Rapid diagnosis of respiratory syncytial virus infection by immunofluorescent antibody techniques. Br Med J 1:602–605, 1968

48. Melnick JL: Classification and nomenclature of animal viruses. Prog Med Virol 13:461–484, 1971

49. Monto AS and Johnson KM: A community study of respiratory infections in the tropics. I. Description of the community and observations of the activity of certain respiratory agents. Am J Epidemiol 86:78–92, 1967

50. Morris JA, Blount RE Jr, and Savage RE: Recovery of cytopathogenic agent from chimpanzees with coryza. Proc Soc Exp Biol Med 92:544–549, 1956

51. Nagahama H, Eller JJ, Fulginiti VA, and Marks MI: Direct immunofluorescent studies of infection with respiratory syncytial virus. J Infect Dis 122:260–271, 1970

52. Parrott RH, Kim HW, Arrobio JO, Hodes DS, Murphy BR, Brandt CD, Camargo E, and Chanock RM: Epidemiology of respiratory syncytial virus infection in Washington, D.C. II. Infection and disease with respect to age, immunologic status, race and sex. Am J Epidemiol. 98:289–300, 1973

53. Parrott RH, Kim HW, Brandt CD, and Chanock RM: Respiratory syncytial virus in infants and children. Prev Med 3:473–480, 1974

54. Richardson LS, Yolken RH, Belshe RB, Camargo E, Kim HW, and Chanock RM: Enzyme linked immunosorbent assay (ELISA) for measurement of serologic response to respiratory syncytial virus infection. Infect Immun 20:660–664, 1978

55. Ross CAC, Stott EJ, McMichael S, and Crowther IA: Problems of laboratory diagnosis of respiratory syncytial virus infection in childhood. Arch Gesamte Virusforsch 14:533–562, 1964

56. Schieble JH, Kase A, and Lennette EH: Fluorescent cell counting as an assay method for respiratory syncytial virus. J Virol 1:494–499, 1967

57. Schieble JH, Lennette EH, and Kase A: An immunofluorescent staining method for rapid identification of respiratory syncytial virus. Proc Soc Exp Biol Med 120:203–208, 1965

58. Shedden WIH and Emery JL: Immunofluorescent evidence of respiratory syncytial virus infection in cases of giant-cell bronchiolitis in children. J Pathol Bacteriol 89:343–347, 1965

59. Sims DG, Downham MAPS, McQuillin J, and Gardner PS: Respiratory syncytial virus infection in North-East England. Br Med J 2:1095–1098, 1976

60. Sommerville RG: Respiratory syncytial virus in acute exacerbations of chronic bronchitis. Lancet 2:1247–1248, 1963

61. Voller A, Bidwell D, and Bartlett A: Microplate enzyme immunoassays for the immunodiagnosis of virus infections In Manual of Clinical Immunology, Rose N (ed), Am Soc Microbiol, Washington, DC, 1976, pp 506–512

62. Wulff H, Kidd P, and Wenner HA: Respiratory syncytial virus: observations on antigenic heterogeneity. Proc Soc Exp Biol Med 115:240–243, 1964

63. Wunner WH, Faulkner GP, and Pringle CR: Respiratory syncytial virus: some biological and biochemical properties. In Negative Strand Viruses, Mahy BWJ and Barry RD (eds), Academic Press, London, 1:193–202, 1975

64. Wunner WH and Pringle CR: Respiratory syncytial virus proteins. Virology 73:228–243, 1976

65. Yolken RH, Kim HW, Clem T, Wyatt RG, Kalica AR, Chanock RM, and Kapikian AZ: Enzyme-linked immunosorbent assay (ELISA) for detection of human reovirus-like agent of infantile gastroenteritis. Lancet 2: 263–267, 1977

66. Zakstelskaya LY, Almeida JD, and Bradstreet CMP: The morphological characterization of respiratory syncytial virus by a simple electron microscope technique. Acta Virol (Praha) 11:420–423, 1967

67. Zhadanov VM, Dreizin RS, Yankevici OD, and Astakhova AK: Biophysical characteristics of respiratory syncytial virus. Rev Roum Virol 25:277–280, 1974

CHAPTER 24

CORONAVIRUSES

Jack H. Schieble and Albert Z. Kapikian

Introduction

The coronaviruses were first classified as a distinct virus group in 1968 (13, 42) on the basis of their nucleic acid content, presence of essential lipids, and their characteristic appearance in negative-stained electron micrographs. The various viruses of the group infect man and a variety of animals, including chickens, mice, pigs, rats, calves, turkeys, and dogs. The name was derived from the appearance of widely spaced projections from the outer membranes of the virus, resembling the solar corona (24).

The first human coronavirus was isolated in 1965 (45) from a school boy suffering from a typical common cold. Nasal secretions shown to be infectious by inoculation of human volunteers were inoculated into organ cultures of human nasal epithelium or trachea, serially passaged, and subsequently shown to be infectious for human volunteers. The virus was given a strain designation of B814, and in a later study (1) was found to be morphologically similar to infectious bronchitis virus (IBV), an avian coronavirus.

In 1966, using routine human embryonic kidney cell cultures, another group of investigators working independently isolated 5 viral agents from medical students, 4 of whom had upper respiratory symptoms. The prototype strain, designated 229E, was shown to be ether-labile, contain RNA, and measure approximately 89 nm (16). With the use of human embryonic tracheal organ cultures, 10 virus strains were isolated by several investigators (29, 35, 46), and all except one virus strain, MR, were shown to possess characteristics of coronaviruses. The MR strain is an ether-labile, non-myxovirus that produces colds in volunteers; however, typical coronavirus morphology has not as yet been demonstrated (29, 46), and its identification as a coronavirus is therefore still presumptive. One of these, the LP strain, has been shown to be similar to 229E in subsequent cell culture studies. An additional 17 coronaviruses, all serologically identical to 229E virus, were isolated in routine cell cultures of human embryonic intestine and lung (14, 27, 39).

As a group, the human coronaviruses are extremely fastidious in their host-cell requirements. A summary of the coronaviruses isolated from humans and the host system of primary isolation is shown in Table 24.1. Twenty-two of 32 isolates were recovered with difficulty in cell cultures, and the remaining 10 coronaviruses were initially recovered in organ cultures of human embryonic trachea and could not be isolated initially in monolayer cell cultures (35, 45).

Clinical aspects

It is now well established that coronaviruses are etiologically related to upper respiratory illnesses in humans (4, 16, 27, 29, 35, 45, 46). Information relating to clinical aspects and symptomology of coronavirus infection has developed primarily from volunteer and epidemiologic studies of coronavirus infection in humans (6, 7, 29).

The incubation period, determined from these studies, was found to be 2–5 days with an average duration of approximately 1 week. The clinical picture was manifested principally by malaise, headache, and sore throat in approximately half of the cases, and a cough was present in slightly more than 30% of the volunteers. There appear to be some minor but definite differences in the clinical aspects of common colds resulting from infection with rhinoviruses and with coronaviruses (9, 24). Because of the relationship of animal coronavirus with transmissible gastroenteritis in pigs, there has been renewed interest in the role of coronaviruses in human gastointestinal disease; however, a definitive association of coronaviruses with human enteric disease has not as yet been established.

Further detailed information on the history, epidemiology, and clinical aspects of coronaviruses can be found in several reviews (24, 33, 38).

Description and Nature of the Agent

Common characteristics

The human coronaviruses possess certain common characteristics, including characteristic electron microscopic appearance resembling, but distinct from, myxoviruses; pleomorphism, with a medium size of 80–160 nm; single-stranded RNA; essential lipid components; heat lability; and acid lability (1, 16, 27, 31, 35, 41, 43, 45, 47).

Morphology and morphogenesis

Human coronaviruses examined by the negative staining technique have an overall diameter of 80–160 nm, appear round or elliptical with moderate pleomorphism, and have widely spaced club- or pear-shaped surface projections distributed uniformly on the circumference of the particle (1, 3, 27, 35, 42). These projections are approximately 20-nm long, narrow at the base, and about 10 nm at the outer edge. A representative human

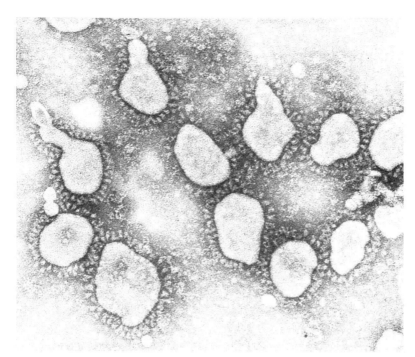

Figure 24.1—Coronavirus found in human embryonic intestine (MA-177) tissue culture negatively stained with phosphotungstic acid. 144,000X.

coronavirus examined by the negative staining technique is shown in Figure 24.1.

Coronaviruses develop within the cytoplasm of infected cells by budding from membranes of the endoplasmic reticulum and cytoplasmic vacuoles (Figure 24.2). This process is also reminiscent of the morphogenesis of myxoviruses, and accounts for the incorporation of host-cell materials into the particles of both virus groups. However, coronaviruses, unlike myxoviruses, have not been observed to bud through the plasma membrane (3, 14, 39). The principal method of egress of coronaviruses appears to be by extrusion of virus-containing vesicles from cells in the lytic state. It is not uncommon in the lytic phase of cellular infection to observe large numbers of coronaviruses adhering to the outer surface of the plasma membrane. It is this feature of the morphogenesis of coronaviruses that provides an explanation of the mechanism of hemadsorption by OC-43 or OC-38 virus and has been called a pseudohemadsorption (11).

Chemical composition and effects of physical and chemical agents

The presence of essential lipids in the outer membrane of coronaviruses is readily demonstrable by the loss of infectivity on exposure to organic solvents. Purified preparations of coronavirus strains 229E and OC-43 have

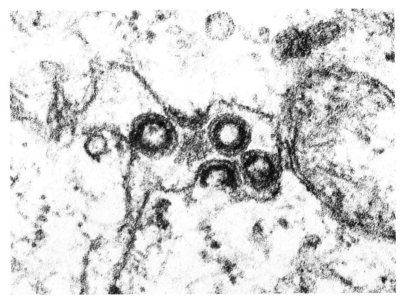

Figure 24.2—Budding and complete coronavirus virions within the cisternae of the endoplasmic reticulum. Human fetal diploid lung cells. 136,000X.

been solubilized with detergents and the polypeptide composition analyzed by polyacrylamide gel electrophoresis; 6–7 polypeptides ranging in size from 15,000 to 196,000 daltons were demonstrated for both viruses (18, 19). Digestion with bromelin removes the projections or "spike" protein, leaving fully enveloped particles. No neuraminidase activity could be demonstrated in purified preparations of the hemagglutinating coronavirus strain OC-43 (19).

DNA inhibitors such as 5-iododeoxyuridine and 5-bromodeoxyuridine have no effect on the replication of human coronaviruses, thus giving indirect evidence of the RNA nature of the virus (16, 27, 34, 42). In addition, the nucleic acid has been reported to exist as a single stranded RNA molecule (41, 43). The infectivity of either crude or purified coronaviruses is destroyed by ether or chloroform, by the detergents sodium lauryl sulfate, deoxycholate, and tween 80, by acid (2 $\log_{10}$ reduction in titer at pH 2–3), heat (56 C 10–15 min), ultraviolet (UV) light, and trypsin (12, 16, 27, 31, 34, 45).

Classification

Recently the Vertebrate Virus Subcommittee of the International Committee on the Taxonomy of Viruses (CTV) proposed a single genus "Coronavirus" within the family *Coronaviridae*, and suggested that the genus be comprised of 7 species, namely avian infectious bronchitis virus (IBV), human coronavirus (HCV), murine hepatitis virus (MHV), porcine transmissible gastroenteritis virus (TGEV), porcine hemagglutinating encephalitis virus (HEV), rat coronavirus (RCV), sialodacryoadenitis virus of rats (SDAV), turkey bluecomb disease virus (TBDV), and neonatal calf diarrhea coronavirus (NCDCV) (43). The family *Coronaviridae* is defined as enveloped particles 80–160 nm in diameter, containing RNA and essential lipids, possessing unique spikes or projections, and developing within the cytoplasm by budding into the cysternae of the endoplasmic reticulum.

Antigenic composition

The antigenic composition of human coronaviruses is not presently well defined, largely because of the great difficulty encountered in their *in vitro* cultivation. Using concentrated preparations of tissue culture-adapted coronaviruses, multiple bands have been observed in immunodiffusion and immunoelectrophoresis tests (5, 19, 36). Although some of these bands result from host-cell antigen-antibody complexes, the data strongly suggest the presence of multiple antigens in human coronaviruses.

Studies on the antigenic relationship among the coronaviruses also suggest that a number of these viruses share common or closely related antigens (5, 28, 29, 30, 36). Of the human coronavirus strains, B814, 229E, OC-38 or OC-43 (serologically identical strains) and probably, strain 692 are distinct coronaviruses. In addition, LP virus isolated in organ culture and later shown to grow in cell culture, also appears to be related to 229E virus (4, 5, 8). OC-44 virus is related to but not identical with OC-38 virus (10, 37). The antigenic relationship among the remaining coronavirus strains listed in Table 24.1 is not currently known.

Description of antigens

Complement-fixing (CF) antigens. CF antigens can be prepared for 2 coronaviruses, 229E and OC-38 (and OC-43), that replicate in monolayer cell cultures. Human fetal diploid cell strains such as WI-38 or similar cell strains can be used. To maintain these cell strains, Eagle minimum essential medium (MEM) or Leibovitz L-15 medium supplemented with 2% fetal bovine serum and appropriate antibiotics can be used. CF antigen is prepared by inoculating the virus into cell cultures, allowing 1 hr for adsorption, and harvesting the infected fluids and cells by freezing and thawing 2–3 times 48–72 hr after inoculation. Early harvest is essential, since it has been shown that the maximal virus is present in infected cell cultures 36–48 hr after inoculation when cytopathology is minimal (3, 15). The infected fluid is clarified by centrifugation at 3000 rpm for 10 min in a refrigerated centrifuge and the supernatant fluid is used as CF antigen.

OC-38 or OC-43 CF antigen can also be prepared in suckling mouse brain. Mouse brain-adapted virus is used for intracranial (ic) inoculation of suckling mice (34, 36). A 10% suspension of infected mouse brain tissue is prepared and clarified by low-speed centrifugation in a refrigerated centrifuge. The clarified supernatant fluid is carefully removed and is used as CF antigen.

Hemagglutinating antigen. Coronavirus OC-38 (or OC-43) is currently the only known hemagglutinating human coronavirus. The hemagglutinin is

TABLE 24.1—HUMAN CORONAVIRUSES

VIRUS DESIGNATION	HOST SYSTEM USED FOR VIRUS ISOLATION	REFERENCE
B814	Human embryonic tracheal organ culture	Tyrrell and Bynoe (45)
229E (5 strains, all serologically similar)	Human embryonic kidney,* WI-38	Hamre and Procknow (16)
OC-16 OC-37 OC-38** OC-43** OC-44 OC-48	Human embryonic tracheal organ culture	McIntosh, et al (36)
LP, EVS	Human embryonic tracheal organ culture	Tyrrell, et al (46)
9 strains, like 229E	Human embryonic intestine cell culture	Kapikian, et al (27)
Linder, like 229E	Human embryonic lung cell culture (L645)	Oshiro, et al (39)
692	Human embryonic tracheal organ culture	Kapikian, et al (29)
7 strains, like 229E	Human embryonic kidney cell culture	Hamre and Beem (14)

*Secondary cell cultures
**Serologically identical strains

directly associated with the virus particle (30), and therefore maximal production of this antigen in either human diploid cell strains or suckling mouse brain closely parallels the period of maximal infectivity production. Thus, the preparation of hemagglutinin in cell cultures is similar to the procedure used for production of CF antigen (30, 34, 36). For the production of hemagglutinin in suckling mouse brain, 3-day-old Swiss mice are inoculated with 100 suckling mouse LD_{50} doses of virus per 0.02 ml, and the brains are harvested when the mice show typical encephalitic symptoms, 48–60 hr after inoculation. A 10% brain suspension is prepared in phosphate-buffered saline (PBS), pH 7.2, and stored at -70 C.

OC-38 (and OC-43) virus hemagglutinates chicken, rat, and mouse erythrocytes (RBC) at 4 C, room temperature, and 37 C; human group O and vervet monkey RBC are also agglutinated, but only at 4 C. The mechanism of hemagglutination by coronaviruses appears to differ from that of myxoviruses, in that coronavirus receptor sites are insensitive to neuraminidase (30).

An indirect hemagglutination test for 229E virus has also been described (32), utilizing tannic acid-treated RBC sensitized with 229E viral antigen.

Pathogenicity for animals

Human embryonic tracheal (HET) OC harvests of coronavirus OC-38 (and OC-43) produce an encephalitic syndrome in suckling mice after either ic or intraperitoneal (ip) inoculation; however, the ic route appears to be more sensitive (34). Weanling mice inoculated similarly do not develop signs of illness; however, asymptomatic infection probably occurs since both CF and neutralizing antibodies are present in serum obtained 3 weeks after inoculation. Coronavirus strains B814, OC-16, OC-37, OC-44, and OC-48 inoculated similarly into suckling mice produced no disease (34, 45).

Growth in cell and organ cultures

Primary isolation of all HCV have been made either in organ cultures or in cell cultures of human embryonic tissues. The HCV strains isolated in cell cultures and the LP strain, which was originally isolated in OC and subsequently isolated in cell cultures, are all similar to the prototype strain 229E and represent a single immunotype. All other HCV strains isolated to date have required organ cultures for initial isolation. The cell cultures used for initial isolation of the 229E-like viruses have been primary, secondary, or semicontinuous diploid cell strains derived from human embryonic kidney, lung, or intestine (14, 16, 27, 39). Coronaviruses B814, LP, and EVS, originally isolated in organ culture, were reported to have been re-isolated from clinical specimens in L-132 cells (4, 8); however, efforts to adapt B814 to this cell line in a subsequent study were unsuccessful (10). It is interesting that 3 HCV strains similar to 229E virus initially isolated in monolayer cultures of human embryonic intestine failed to grow in organ cultures of human embryonic tissues (27). Thus, for the primary isolation of HCV, both organ cultures and sensitive cell cultures must be used.

Efforts to adapt HCV isolated in organ cultures to monolayer cell cultures have been especially successful with OC-38 (and OC-43) virus. This virus has been adapted to grow in suckling mice (34), suckling hamsters (36), cultures of rhesus monkey kidney cells (10), BSC-1 (10), and WI-38 cells (28). Thus, 229E virus and OC-38 (OC-43) virus are the 2 distinct coronavirus immunotypes that grow in monolayer cell cultures and produce a readily recognizable cytopathic effect (CPE). Furthermore, the OC-38 (OC-43) virus also exhibits the phenomenon of hemadsorption, which offers an alternate method for recognition of virus growth (28).

Preparation of Immune Serum

Hyperimmune serum to 229E and OC-43 viruses has been prepared in mice, as serum and ascitic fluid, and in guinea pigs and chickens (3, 16, 19, 34, 36). A simple and successful method is as follows:

Virus preparations containing 10^{-3} to 10^{-5} $TCID_{50}$ per 0.2 ml are clarified by centrifugation at 2000 rpm for 10 min at 4 C; the supernatant fluid containing the virus suspension is removed and emulsified with an equal volume of incomplete Freund adjuvant; 2.0 ml of the antigen-adjuvant mixture is inoculated intramuscularly (im) into a hind leg (or 1.0 ml into each hind leg) of the guinea pig. In 6 weeks the entire procedure is repeated, and the animal is bled 10–14 days after the second injection.

Collection and Preparation of Specimens

Routine laboratory precautions should be observed in the handling of potentially positive or known positive human coronavirus preparations.

Virus isolation

Virus isolation attempts are made from nasal or throat washings or from nasal and throat swabs placed in the same collection medium (16, 27, 35, 45). Comparative data on the sensitivity of nasal washings vs. throat washings are not available. A method for performing nasopharyngeal washings is described in Chapter 17. Data on the influence of the time after onset of symptoms on the isolation rate in naturally occurring coronavirus respiratory illnesses are not available. However, in a study of volunteers inoculated with 229E virus, the peak frequency of virus excretion occurred at about the same time as the onset of clinical symptoms (6). Data are not available on the effect which freezing and thawing clinical specimens before inoculation has on the isolation rates.

Serologic diagnosis

Under aseptic conditions, an acute-phase blood specimen is obtained within the first 2–3 days of onset, and a convalescent-phase serum is collected approximately 2–3 weeks later. The blood is allowed to clot for 1–2 hr; the serum is then separated under aseptic conditions and stored at −20 C until ready for use. If necessary, the serum is centrifuged to remove remaining RBC. Whole blood should not be frozen if it is to be used for antibody studies, since freezing causes hemolysis of RBC. However, whole blood may be refrigerated at 4 C for 24 hr if it is not convenient to separate the serum soon after collection.

Electron microscopy

One to 5 ml of cell culture or OC fluid is clarified by low-speed centrifugation at 2000 rpm for 10–15 min in a refrigerated centrifuge, and the supernatant fluid is centrifuged at $110,000 \times g$ for 60–90 min. The pellet is resuspended in 0.1–0.2 ml of 1% ammonium acetate, negatively stained with 2% phosphotungstic acid (PTA) at pH 5.0 or 7.0, and then spread on formvar-coated copper grids and examined by electron microscopy (27, 35).

An alternate method is to gently grind the OC tissue fragments in a loosely fitting glass homogenizer (Ten Broeck-type) with a few drops of distilled water. In this way, the superficial virus-infected cells are detached while the tissue fragments remain largely intact. A drop of the cell suspension is mixed with an equal volume of 3% PTA adjusted to pH 6.0 with potassium hydroxide. A small volume of this mixture is placed on a carbon formvar-coated grid. After excess fluid is removed with filter paper, the specimen is ready to be examined by electron microscopy (1).

Laboratory Diagnosis

Virus isolation in animals

To date, no HCV has been isolated in an animal system. OC-38 (OC-43) is the only HCV immunotype which has been adapted to grow in an animal model system. An encephalitis syndrome is produced on ic or ip inoculation of 1- to 3-day-old suckling mice. The ic route has proven to be more efficient (34). There is presently no information available relating to the sensitivity of the mouse system for the isolation of OC-38-like viruses from human respiratory specimens. The adaption of OC-38 virus to the mouse required several organ cultures passages and 10-fold concentration followed by 4–5 serial passages in the suckling mouse brain before full adaptation occurred.

Virus isolation in embryonated eggs

No human coronavirus has been reported to multiply in embryonated eggs (16, 33, 45).

Virus isolation in cell cultures

Among the human coronaviruses, only 229E virus was shown to produce CPE on initial passages in cell cultures (16, 27). In one study, noted previously, a semicontinuous human embryonic intestinal cell culture appeared to be more sensitive than cultures of WI-38 cells for the isolation of coronavirus 229E (27). However, this virus was adapted to grow in WI-38 cell cultures, and a semicontinuous human embryonic lung fibroblast culture, similar to WI-38 cells, was used successfully for 229E virus recovery from human respiratory secretions (6, 39).

A suitable growth medium for the above cell cultures consists of Eagle MEM in Earle balanced salt solution (BSS), 10% inactivated (56 C for 10 min) fetal bovine serum, and 100 units of penicillin and 100 μg of streptomycin/ml; for maintenance of cells during isolation attempts, Leibovitz medium (L-15) can be used.

The respiratory specimen is inoculated in 0.2-ml amounts into each of 2 cell-culture tubes and incubated on a roller drum at 35 C, since this temperature also facilitates isolation of rhinoviruses. In virus-positive cultures, a gradual elongation of the cells is evident throughout the monolayer several days after inoculation (27). Gradually, small, granular round cells appear throughout the monolayers, but the cell sheets are rarely destroyed completely on initial isolation.

Virus isolation in organ cultures

Since only a single coronavirus immunotype (229E) has been isolated in monolayer cell culture, organ cultures of human embryonic tissues were essential for all virus isolation attempts and for the subsequent study of these viruses. Several methods used for preparing and maintaining organ cultures are given below (20, 22, 23, 27, 45, 46).

The tracheal or nasal epithelium is cut into square pieces 1- to 3-mm wide; sharp knives are used and the ciliated surface is never touched. Four to 6 tissue fragments, with the mucosal (ciliated) surface up, are placed on the lightly scratched surface of a 60 × 15-mm plastic Petri dish (surface of the dish is scratched to facilitate adherence of the tissue to plastic); 1.25 ml of medium No. 199, containing 0.035 g sodium bicarbonate/100 ml, is added so that the fragment tips are level with or slightly above the fluid level. The medium also contains 100 units of penicillin, 100 μg of streptomycin, and 50 units of mycostatin/ml. The dish is incubated at 33 C in a humidified atmosphere, and the medium is changed daily for 2 days. Before inoculation, the beating cilia on each fragment are observed under the dissecting microscope with reflected light, and only those fragments showing strong ciliary action are used. Cultures are inoculated by distributing about 0.3–0.4 ml of the respiratory specimen on the group of tissue fragments. Each culture is examined for ciliary activity daily, and the medium is harvested daily for approximately 12 days.

Slight modifications of this procedure have been described. In one, maintenance medium consists of Leibovitz Medium (L-15) supplemented with 0.2% bovine albumin, 2.0 mM glutamine, and appropriate antibiotics; pH is adjusted to 7.2 with a few drops of 1N NaOH. In addition, the plates are incubated at 33 C (44). Subpassage of the combined harvests of the second to twelfth days are made by inoculating 0.2–0.5 ml of this pool into fresh organ culture plates.

The presence of virus can be detected by observing whether ciliary action has ceased or diminished in comparison to that in control plates, by electron microscopic examination of concentrated harvests or by virus interference. Ciliary immobilizing effect (CIE) is not a consistent or reliable measure of coronavirus infection. Strain B814 produced a reduction in CIE only in later passages, but this effect was never clear-cut (45). Two of the other coronaviruses isolated in organ cultures had no effect on CIE, even after 3–5 passages, while a third virus lost its CIE after the second passage; the other viruses produced CIE (45). At the present time one of the more practical indicators for the presence of human coronaviruses in organ cultures is examination of harvests under the electron microscope by negative staining (1, 35). More recently, immune electron microscopy has proven to be a very useful technique for detecting the presence of fastidious viruses (2, 25, 26, 29). Briefly, this procedure utilizes convalescent-phase serum by mixing it with fluids from organ cultures inoculated with a respiratory specimen from the same patient and examining the mixture in the electron microscope for aggregated virus. Viral aggregates resulting from specific antigen-antibody complex are more likely to be visualized than are low concentrations of singly dispersed viruses.

In the virus interference test, B814 infected organ cultures were challenged after 5 days of incubation with the Sendai strain of parainfluenza virus type 1, parainfluenza virus type 3, or ECHO virus type 11, and it was found that the titer of the challenge virus was >10-fold lower in the B814-infected organ cultures than in challenged control organ cultures (2). A method for utilizing human embryonic organ cultures in test tubes has been described (17).

Identification of isolates

A presumptive identification of an isolate as a coronavirus can be made by establishing that the isolate has the general characteristics of the family *Coronaviridae;* typical morphology and size by electron microscopy; ether and acid lability; and failure of DNA inhibitors to prevent viral growth.

Coronaviruses isolated in cell cultures (229E)

An isolate suspected of being similar to 229E virus can be identified by a conventional serum neutralization (Nt) test in WI-38 or similar cell strains.

Serum neutralization test. Equal volumes of the unknown virus diluted to contain 100 $TCID_{50}$ and the specific antiserum diluted to contain at least 20 antibody units are mixed and incubated at room temperature for 2 hr. In addition, equal volumes of the unknown virus, diluted as above, and Hanks BSS with 0.5% gelatin are mixed and incubated for 2 hr at room temperature at the same time (simultaneous virus titration). The virus-serum mixture is inoculated in 0.2-ml amounts into each of 2 cell cultures of WI-38 cells maintained with Leibovitz medium (L-15) containing 2% fetal bovine serum and appropriate antibiotics. Ten-fold dilutions of the virus-Hanks BSS are inoculated similarly, but into 4 tubes per dilution. The cultures are rotated on a drum at 12 rph at 33 C and examined at 3-day intervals for approximately 2 weeks. If CPE is present in the virus-serum tubes (and 3-320 $TCID_{50}$ of virus have been used in the test), it can be assumed that the virus is not the same as 229E virus. If CPE is not present, the proper dose of virus is present in the test, and the hyperimmune serum is known to be specific, it can be assumed that the isolate is similar to 229E. At least 20 antibody units of serum prepared against the isolate should also be capable of neutralizing 32-320 $TCID_{50}$ of 229E virus before it can be stated that the isolate is identical to 229E.

Coronavirus isolated in organ cultures

Most of the human coronavirus immunotypes were isolated in organ cultures of human embryonic nasal or tracheal tissues. One of the viruses isolated in organ culture, OC-38 (and the identical OC-43 strain), has been adapted to grow in monolayer cell cultures and the suckling mouse. Thus, efforts to adapt presumptive coronaviruses isolated in organ culture to monolayer cell cultures and the suckling mouse should be made. Successful adaption would suggest that the isolate may be similar to the OC-38 coronavirus immunotype. Final identification can then be accomplished by the serum Nt test in WI-38 cells utilizing hyperimmune anti-OC-38 serum as described for 229E virus.

An alternate procedure is to examine infected cell culture fluids for the presence of hemagglutinins and 'to identify the virus by HAI (30). An indirect fluorescent-antibody test has also been reported for 229E and OC-43 (9, 10, 15, 36).

Serologic diagnosis

Neutralization test. For the serologic diagnosis of 229E or OC-38 (OC-43) virus infections, Nt tests may be performed in WI-38 cell cultures. Serial dilutions of the patient's acute- and convalescent-phase serum (inactivated at 56 C for 30 min) are prepared in Hanks BSS with 0.5% gelatin. An equal volume of virus containing 32-100 $TCID_{50}$ in the same diluent is mixed with each serum dilution and incubated at room temperature for 2 hr. A control virus titration is prepared by mixing an equal volume of virus (diluted to contain 32-100 $TCID_{50}$) with Hanks BSS and incubating for 2 hr at room temperature. After incubation, 0.2 ml from each virus-serum dilution mixture is inoculated into each of 2 cell-culture tubes containing 1.5 ml of maintenance medium (Leibovitz medium L-15, 2% fetal bovine serum, and appropriate antibiotics). The virus control preparation is diluted in serial 10-fold steps in Hanks BSS and similarly inoculated into 4 cell-culture tubes per dilution. If the test is large and many tubes are used, thereby requiring several hours for inoculation, a virus titration should be performed at the beginning of the test and at the conclusion of the test. The cultures are rotated on a drum at 12 rph at 33 C. The test is examined microscopically at 3-day intervals for 2 weeks and the serum Nt-antibody titer is determined according to the Reed and Muench method (40). If 3-100 $TCID_{50}$ of virus is present in the test, as indicated by the control virus titrations, the test is considered satisfactory. A ≥4-fold rise in Nt-antibody titer is considered significant.

Complement-fixation test. For the serologic diagnosis of 229E and OC-38 (or OC-43) infections, CF antigens can be used, and the procedure described in Chapter 1 is followed.

Hemagglutination-inhibition. For the serologic diagnosis of infection with OC-38 or the identical OC-43 virus strain, the following HAI test can be used. Four hemagglutinating units (HAU) of virus are used in the HAI test. To determine the dilution containing 4 HAU, a preliminary hemagglutination (HA) titration is performed. Serial 2-fold dilutions of the virus are made in 0.5-ml volumes of PBS, pH 7.2, and 0.5 ml of 0.5% chicken RBC are added to each virus dilution. An RBC control is prepared by mixing 0.5 ml of 0.5% RBC and 0.5 ml of PBS. The HA titration is shaken and incubated at 4 C until the RBC have settled, i.e., the RBC-control tube has formed a negative pattern. The titration end-point is considered as the last dilution showing complete agglutination; that dilution represents 1 HAU. To calculate the proper dilution of virus to be used in the HAI test, the HA titer is divided by

8. For example, if the HA titer is 1:128 when titrated in 0.5 ml volumes, then a dilution of 1:16 $\left(\dfrac{128}{8}\right)$ would contain 8 HAU/0.5 ml or 4 HAU/0.25 ml. The latter volume of virus is used in the HAI test.

The test is performed by making 0.25-ml volumes of serial 2-fold dilutions of both the acute- and convalescent-phase sera in PBS and adding 0.25 ml volume of virus containing 4 HAU. To test for the presence of RBC agglutinins in the serum, add 0.25-ml volumes of PBS to another series of tubes containing 0.25-ml volumes of the first 4 dilutions of the serum tested. Incubate at room temperature for 30 min and add 0.5 ml of 0.5% chicken RBC. Shake and incubate at 4 C. To check on possible errors in preparing the dilution of virus containing 4 HAU/0.25 ml, the test virus dilution should be back-titrated to insure that 4 HAU are present in the test. To a series of 5 tubes containing 0.5 ml of PBS, add an equal volume of the test dilution of virus to the first tube only. Mix and serially dilute in 2-fold steps, and then add 0.5 ml of 0.5% RBC, shake, and incubate at 4 C. Four HAU are present if the first 3 tubes show complete HA, and the last 2 are negative. The test and controls are read when the RBC have settled and the RBC control tube has formed a negative pattern. The test is considered valid if 4 HAU are present in the test and the serum control tubes do not indicate the presence of agglutinins for the RBC. The antibody titer is considered as the reciprocal of the initial dilution of serum that completely inhibits 4 HAU of virus. A ≥4-fold increase in antibody titer is considered significant and indicates infection with OC-38 virus.

The antigenic relationship among the human coronaviruses is not currently well established because the majority of coronaviruses can only be grown in organ cultures of human embryonic respiratory epithelium, and the problems associated with this technique have precluded a systematic study of these agents. The human coronavirus strains that have been isolated in monolayer cell cultures form a homogenous antigenic group, and all of them appear to be serologically identical to the 229E virus strain and bear little if any relationship to other human coronaviruses. Heterologous reactions have been observed between OC-38 (OC-43) and OC-44 coronavirus by organ culture Nt, CF, and fluorescent-antibody tests. Similarly, heterologous reactivity has been observed between OC-38 (OC-43) and mouse hepatitis virus, a murine coronavirus strain. The remaining human coronaviruses have not been sufficiently studied to determine the cross-reactivity with other human or animal coronaviruses.

References

1. ALMEIDA JD and TYRRELL DAJ: The morphology of three previously uncharacterized human respiratory viruses that grow in organ culture. J Gen Virol 1:175–178, 1967
2. ALMEIDA JD and WATERSON AP: The morphology of virus-antibody reaction. Adv Virus Res 15:307–338, 1969
3. BECKER WB, McINTOSH K, DEES K, and CHANOCK RM: Morphogenesis of avian infectious bronchitis virus and a related human virus (strain 229E). J Virol 1:1019–1027, 1967
4. BRADBURNE AF: Sensitivity of L132 cells to some "new" respiratory viruses. Nature 221:85–86, 1969

5. BRADBURNE AF: Antigenic relationships amongst coronaviruses. Arch Gesamte Virus-forsch 31:352–364, 1970
6. BRADBURNE AF, BYNOE ML, and TYRRELL DAJ: Effects of a "new" human respiratory virus in volunteers. Br Med J 3:767–769, 1967
7. BRADBURNE AF and SOMERSET BA: Coronavirus antibody titer in sera of healthy adults and experimentally infected volunteers. J Hyg 70:235–244, 1972
8. BRADBURNE AF and TYRRELL DAJ: The propagation of coronaviruses in tissue culture. Arch Gesamte Virusforsch 28:133–150, 1969
9. BRADBURNE AF and TYRRELL DAJ: Coronaviruses of man. Prog Med Virol 13:373–403, 1971
10. BRUCKOVA M, McINTOSH K, KAPIKIAN AZ, and CHANOCK RM: The adaptation of two human coronavirus strains (OC-38 and OC-43) to growth in cell monolayers. Proc Soc Exp Biol Med 135:431–435, 1970
11. BUCKNELL RA, KALICA AR, and CHANOCK RM: Intracellular development and mechanism of hemadsorption of a human coronavirus, OC-43. Proc Soc Exp Biol Med 139:811–817, 1972
12. BUCKNELL RA, KING LM, KAPIKIAN AZ, and CHANOCK RM: Studies with human coronaviruses. II. Some properties of strains 229E and OC43. Proc Soc Exp Biol Med 139:722–727, 1972
13. ESTOLA T: Coronaviruses, a new group of animal RNA viruses. Avian Dis 14:330–336, 1970
14. HAMRE D and BEEM M: Virologic studies of acute respiratory disease in young adults. V. Coronavirus 229E infections during six years of surveillance. Am J Epidemiol 96:94–106, 1972
15. HAMRE D, KINDING DA, and MANN J: Growth and intracellular development of a new respiratory virus. J Virol 1:810–816, 1967
16. HAMRE D and PROCKNOW JJ: A new virus isolated from the human respiratory tract. Proc Soc Exp Biol (NY) 121:190–193, 1966
17. HARNET GB and HOOPER WL: Test-tube organ culture of ciliated epithelium for the isolation of respiratory viruses. Lancet 1:339–340, 1968
18. HIERHOLZER JC: Purification and biophysical properties of human coronavirus 229E. Virology 75:155–165, 1976
19. HIERHOLZER JC, PALMER EL, WHITFIELD SG, KAYE HS, and DOWDLE WR: Protein composition of coronavirus OC-43. Virology 48:516–527, 1972
20. HIGGINS PG: The isolation of viruses from acute respiratory infections V. The use of organ cultures of human embryonic nasal and tracheal ciliated epithelium. Mon Bull Minist Public Health Lab Serv 25:283–288, 1966
21. HOORN B: Organ cultures of ciliated epithelium for the study of respiratory viruses. Acta Pathol Microbiol Scand 66 (Suppl. 183):1–37, 1966
22. HOORN B and TYRRELL DAJ: On the growth of certain newer respiratory viruses in organ cultures. Br J Exp Pathol 46:109–118, 1965
23. HOORN B and TYRRELL DAJ: A new virus cultivated only in organ cultures of ciliated epithelium. Arch Gesamte Virusforsch 18:210–225, 1966
24. KAPIKIAN AZ: The coronaviruses. In Chemoprophylaxies and Virus Infections of the Respiratory Tract, JS Oxford (ed), CRC Press, Vol 2, pp 95–117, 1977
25. KAPIKIAN AZ, ALMEIDA JD, and STOTT EJ: Immune electron microscopy of rhinoviruses. J Virol 10:142–146, 1972
26. KAPIKIAN AZ, FEINSTONE SM, PURCELL RH, WYATT RG, THORNHILL TS, KALICA AR, and CHANOCK RM: Detection and identification by immune electron microscopy of fastidious agents associated with respiratory illness, acute nonbacterial gastroenteritis, and hepatitis A. Perspect Virol 9:9–47, the Gustav Stern Symposium, Antiviral mechanisms, M Pollard (ed), Academic Press, New York, 1975
27. KAPIKIAN AZ, JAMES HD, JR, KELLY SJ, DEES JH, TURNER HC, McINTOSH K, KIM HW, PARROTT RH, VINCENT MM, and CHANOCK RM: Isolation from man of "avian infectious bronchitis virus-like" viruses (coronaviruses) similar to 229E virus, with some epidemiological observations. J Infect Dis 119:282–290, 1969
28. KAPIKIAN AZ, JAMES HD, JR, KELLY SJ, KING LM, VAUGHN AL, and CHANOCK RM: Hemadsorption by coronavirus strain OC-43. Proc Soc Exp Biol Med 139:179–186, 1972

29. KAPIKIAN AZ, JAMES HD, JR, KELLY SJ, and VAUGHN AL: Detection of coronavirus strain 692 by immune electron microscopy. Infec Immun 7:111-116, 1973
30. KAYE H and DOWDLE WR: Some characteristics of hemagglutination of certain strains of ''IBV-like'' virus. J Infec Dis 120:576-581, 1969
31. KAYE HS, HIERHOLZER JC, and DOWDLE WR: Purification and further characterization of an IBV-like virus. Proc Soc Exp Biol Med 135:457-463, 1970
32. KAYE HS, ONG SB, and DOWDLE WR: Detection of coronavirus 229E antibody by indirect hemagglutination. Appl Microbiol 24:703-707, 1972
33. MCINTOSH K: Coronaviruses: a comparative review. Curr Top Microbiol Immunol 63:85-129, 1974
34. MCINTOSH K, BECKER WB, and CHANOCK RM: Growth in suckling mouse brain of ''IBV-like'' viruses from patients with upper respiratory tract disease. Proc Nat Acad Sci USA 58:2268-2273, 1967
35. MCINTOSH K, DEES JH, BECKER WB, KAPIKIAN AZ, and CHANOCK RM: Recovery in tracheal organ cultures of novel viruses from patients with respiratory disease. Proc Nat Acad Sci USA 57:933-940, 1967
36. MCINTOSH K, KAPIKIAN AZ, HARDISON KA, HARTLEY JW, and CHANOCK RM: Antigenic relationship among coronaviruses of man and between human and animal coronaviruses. J Immunol 102:1109-1118, 1969
37. MCINTOSH K, KAPIKIAN AZ, TURNER HC, HARTLEY JW, PARROTT RH, and CHANOCK RM: Seroepidemiologic studies of coronavirus infection in adults and children. Am J Epidemiol 95:585-592, 1970
38. MONTO AS: Medical reviews—coronaviruses. Yale J Biol Med 47:234-251, 1974
39. OSHIRO LS, SCHIEBLE JH, and LENNETTE EH: Electron microscopic studies of coronavirus. J Gen Virol 12:161-168, 1971
40. REED LJ and MUENCH H: A simple method for estimating fifty per cent end points. Am J Hyg 27:493-497, 1938
41. TANNOCK GA: The nucleic acid of infectious bronchitis virus. Arch Ges Virusforsch 43:259-271, 1973
42. TYRRELL DAJ, ALMEIDA JD, BERRY DM, CUNNINGHAM CH, HAMRE D, HOFSTAD MS, MALLUCCI L, and MCINTOSH K: Coronaviruses. Nature (London) 220:650, 1968
43. TYRRELL DAJ, ALMEIDA JD, CUNNINGHAM CH, DOWDLE WR, HOFSTAD MS, MCINTOSH K, TAJIMA M, ZAKSTELSKAYA LY, EASTERDAY BC, KAPIKIAN A, and BINGHAM RW: Coronaviridae. Intervirol 5:76-82, 1975
44. TYRRELL DAJ and BLAMIRO CJ: Improvements in a method of growing respiratory viruses in organ cultures. Br J Exp Pathol 48:217-227, 1967
45. TYRRELL DAJ and BYNOE ML: Cultivation of a novel type of common-cold virus in organ cultures. Br Med J 1:1467-1470, 1965
46. TYRRELL DAJ, BYNOE ML, and HOORN B: Cultivation of ''difficult'' viruses from patients with common colds. Br Med J 1:606-610, 1968
47. WATKINS H, REEVE P, and ALEXANDER DJ: The ribonucleic acid of infectious bronchitis virus. Arch Virol 47:279-286, 1975

CHAPTER 25

RUBELLA VIRUS

Kenneth L. Herrmann

Introduction

The clinical disease recognized today as rubella was first described in the German literature over 200 years ago (40). The viral origin of rubella was demonstrated in 1938 by Hiro and Tasaka (77), who transmitted the disease by subcutaneous inoculation of bacteria-free filtrate of throat swabs taken from rubella patients. The description of congenital malformations following rubella infection during pregnancy by Gregg in 1941 (64) established a much more serious significance to this relatively mild exanthematous disease. Since 1962, when the virus was isolated in tissue culture by Weller and Neva (193) and by Parkman et al (122), rubella virus has been studied in many laboratories. The major epidemic of the disease that struck the United States in 1964–1965 (160, 195) was followed by a wave of congenital abnormalities, which greatly increased interest in rubella and provided abundant material for study. Because acquired rubella infection is easily confused with other viral exanthems and because the congenital disease is manifold in its forms, the virologist can give practical and important help to the physician by the laboratory diagnosis of rubella. In addition, since the licensure of rubella vaccine in 1970, the need for practical laboratory methods to identify individuals who are susceptible to rubella and should be vaccinated has become quite evident.

The Disease

Postnatally acquired infection

Clinical features. Rubella virus infection in a child or adult usually is characterized by a mild exanthem with infrequent complications (34, 197). Clinical manifestations may range from inapparent infection to a characteristic clinical picture of rash, lymphadenopathy, and low-grade fever. In adults, however, the disease may be more severe, with polyarthralgia and polyarthritis being present so commonly as to be considered typical of the disease. During the 14- to 21-day incubation period, prodromal symptoms are notably absent in most cases. Lymphadenopathy, however, may precede the onset of rash by several days. The rubella rash is variable and has no feature which is pathognomonic. It is generally maculopapular, erythematous, and mildly pruritic. The rash appears initially on the face and neck and rapidly (usually within 24 hr) spreads to the trunk, arms, and legs. It frequently fades and disappears within 2-4 days.

Although the rash is the most conspicuous feature of this disease, it is of such variable character that it may be confused with that produced by other infections and even by drugs. Except during epidemic periods the clinical diagnosis of rubella is grossly inaccurate. Laboratory study frequently shows "classical" rubella to be another disease or, conversely, identifies atypical cases of true rubella.

Epidemiology and transmission. Before the widespread use of rubella vaccine, rubella was an endemic disease with a seasonal peak in the late winter and early spring and with epidemics occurring at irregular intervals of 5-7 years (195). The last major rubella epidemic in the United States occurred in 1964-1965.

The presence of rubella antibody after clinical or inapparent infection implies protection against subsequent disease. Multiple attacks of clinical rubella have not been documented by prospective virologic study although inapparent reinfection is well recognized (79).

Seroepidemiologic studies (140, 151) show that about 85-90% of adults in the continental United States have detectable rubella antibodies. Much lower seropositivity rates, however, exist in adults in Hawaii (161), Puerto Rico (63), and other island populations (47).

Extensive rubella vaccination of prepubertal children in the United States since 1970 has substantially altered the epidemiologic patterns of the disease. Before 1970, children in elementary-school age groups appeared to be the primary reservoir of rubella disease and the usual source of infection for susceptible pregnant women (195). Since 1974, the greater percentage of cases has occurred in unimmunized older teenagers and in young adults (67).

Rubella is usually transmitted by direct person-to-person contact via respiratory-tract secretions. In most circumstances it is not highly contagious, and casual contacts frequently do not lead to infection. Occasionally, however, specific rubella cases have been highly contagious (72). The factors influencing the spread of rubella infection are still poorly understood.

Pathogenesis. Initial viral invasion begins most commonly in the nasopharyngeal mucosa and is followed by spread of the infection to local lymphatic tissues. Viremia and viral shedding in the throat and nasal secretions may be detected as early as 7 days after initial invasion, reaching a peak near the time of rash onset on about day 14 (Fig 25.1). Viremia is rarely detectable after the onset of rash. Although virus excretion in the throat may continue for up to 2 weeks after the onset of illness, the amount of virus found in respiratory secretions drops very rapidly, making it very difficult to detect the agent when cultures are taken more than 5-6 days after onset of clinical symptoms (39). Urine and stool are unreliable sources of rubella virus.

Viremia has not been detected following reinfection with rubella virus in individuals with natural or vaccine-induced immunity. Local infection of na-

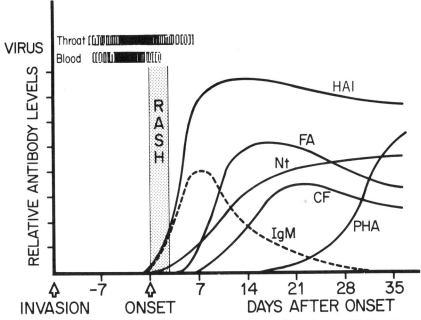

Figure 25.1—Schema of immune response in acute rubella infection. HAI = hemag-
glutination inhibition, FA = immunofluorescence, Nt = neutralization,
CF = complement fixation, PHA = passive hemagglutination, and
IgM = immunoglobulin M.

sopharyngeal tissues with limited shedding of virus has been demonstrated
in these persons (39). Such reinfection in a pregnant woman apparently
poses minimal, if any, risk to the unborn fetus.

   Immunology. In acute rubella infection, antibodies to the virus appear
soon after the onset of illness (Fig 25.1). Initially, both immunoglobulin G
(IgG) and M (IgM) antibodies can be detected. Antibodies of the IgM class
generally do not persist beyond 4–6 weeks after the onset of illness, whereas
IgG antibodies usually persist for the lifetime of the patient. Rubella antibodies can be detected by a number of different methods. Hemagglutination
inhibition (HAI) is the most commonly used assay method for detecting both
IgG and IgM antibodies. HAI antibodies appear early, often while the rash is
still present. Complement-fixing (CF) antibodies become detectable a week
or more after rash onset and do not persist as long as HAI antibodies. The
passive hemagglutination (PHA) test is sensitive only to late IgG antibodies,
which often are not detectable until weeks after a rubella infection. The presence of rubella antibody indicates prior rubella virus infection and implies
immunity against subsequent disease.

   Reinfection with rubella virus can occur but is almost always asymptomatic and can be detected by a rise in antibodies of the IgG class only (141, 183). The attenuated virus vaccines induce the production of IgM
and IgG antibodies similar to those observed with natural infections except

that the titers are not as high, especially the CF-antibody titers (186). Reinfection rates with wild virus are higher among vaccine-immune persons than among those previously infected under natural conditions (79).

Complications. Postinfectious encephalitis is a serious but rare complication of rubella, occurring perhaps once in 6000–10,000 rubella infections (166). Thrombocytopenia purpura is another infrequent complication. Perhaps the most common complications of rubella are arthralgia and arthritis, occurring principally in adults. Rubella arthritis may be acutely disabling, but chronic joint involvement has not been observed (168). Although an association of rubella virus and rheumatoid arthritis has been suggested (117), no conclusive evidence supporting this association has yet been found.

Congenital infection

Incidence. Congenital rubella syndrome is associated with primary maternal rubella infection during the first 3–4 months of gestation. The incidence of fetal infection has been estimated to range from as high as 4–30 cases per 1000 live births during epidemic periods to less than 0.5 cases per 1000 births during nonepidemic periods (3). It is well recognized that the hazard is clearly maximal when maternal infection occurs during the first 8 weeks of gestation. Studies following the 1964–1965 epidemic in the United States showed the risk of defects to be about 50% in infants of mothers infected during the first month of gestation, 22% during the second, 6% during the third, and about 1% during the fourth month (165). In addition to fetal abnormalities, the incidence of spontaneous and therapeutic abortions is higher in pregnancies complicated by rubella and contributes significantly to the fetal wastage (103, 162).

Clinical features. The consequences of rubella *in utero* are varied and unpredictable. Congenital rubella may result in severe involvement with fetal death, live birth with anomalies, or even normal infants without clinical evidence of the infection. The triad of anatomic abnormalities including cataracts, deafness, and congenital heart disease has classically been associated with rubella; but thrombocytopenia, hepatitis, microcephaly, growth retardation, long-bone lesions, retinitis, and encephalitis are also commonly seen as part of the expanded rubella syndrome. Frequently, rubella defects may not be evident until weeks or months after birth. Chronic rubella panencephalitis has been reported as a possible , rare, late-developing manifestation of congenital rubella infection (175, 191).

Pathogenesis. Rubella embryopathy is the result of chronic infection and inhibition of cell multiplication in the developing fetus. Delayed and deranged organogenesis and hypoplastic organ development lead to the characteristic structural organ defects, whereas chronic viral infection in the fetus contributes to the acute illness seen in the newborn period (e.g., bone lesions, hepatitis, encephalitis, and thrombocytopenia purpura) and to the progressive psychomotor retardation often observed as the infant grows older.

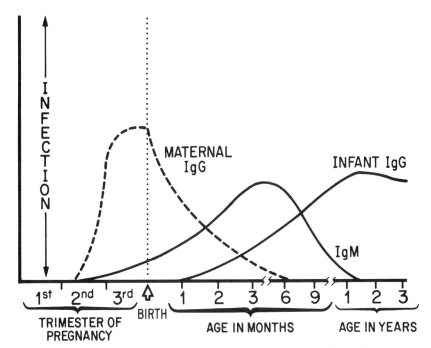

Figure 25.2—Schema of immune response in congenital rubella. IgG = immunoglobulin G, and IgM = immunoglobulin M.

Virology. The infant with congenital rubella may remain chronically infected for months after birth. Virus has been cultured from pharyngeal secretions, urine, cerebrospinal fluid, and virtually every organ. Cooper and
Krugman (33) report that they were able to isolate virus from 31% of children with rubella syndrome at 6 months of age and from 7% at 1 year. By the
end of the second year of life, some children with rubella syndrome are still
excreting virus from the nasopharynx. In addition, virus may be found in
some tissues such as cerebrospinal fluid or cataractous lens months after the
nasopharyngeal excretion has abated (42, 107).

Immunology. The human fetus infected with rubella virus is capable of
producing specific rubella antibodies well before birth (1). This specific rubella antibody is primarily of the IgM class. Since IgM antibody normally
does not pass the placenta, the presence of specific IgM antibody in the
newborn infant is evidence of congenital infection (Fig 25.2). The duration of
presistence of specific IgM antibody appears to be related to the persistence
of the chronic infection. Specific rubella antibody of the IgG class may also
be produced by the infected infant prior to birth, but it is difficult to differentiate from passively transferred maternal IgG rubella antibody, which is
present in considerable quantity at time of birth. Because the half-life of
passively transmitted maternal antibodies is roughly 1 month (5, 75), finding
specific rubella IgG antibodies that persist indefinitely at levels found at birth

is highly suggestive of intrauterine infection (24, 48). Therefore, in addition to the detection of specific rubella antibody in the IgM fraction of globulin, the demonstration of persistence of rubella antibodies can be used to establish a retrospective diagnosis of congenital rubella (187, 192).

The prolonged persistence of congenital infection presumably indicates an impairment of mechanisms concerned with recovery from viral infection. Antibodies apparently have little or no direct role in the termination of infection (2, 109). Depression of delayed-type cellular immune responsiveness may be a much more important factor in these chronic infections.

Pathology. The histopathologic changes are of 2 main types that frequently occur together. First, there are those caused by retardation or inhibition of cell mitosis, and secondly, there is destruction of formed tissues and organs caused by cellular necrosis. Reduced cell division during fetal development appears to be the most probable explanation for the structural malformations (112, 135). Histologically, the characteristic findings include the following: generalized deposits of calcified mucoprotein in the intima of blood vessels, giant-cell hepatitis, splenic fibrosis, necrosis of the organ of Corti, inadequate myelinization, and perivascular cuffing (145, 174). None of the above findings is sufficiently characteristic to be pathognomonic, but in combination they form a recognizable syndrome.

Prevention

The obvious solution to the problem of rubella teratogenesis is widespread use of an effective live-virus vaccine. Live, attenuated rubella virus vaccines have been licensed since 1970. Guidelines for use of these vaccines have been developed by public health and professional advisory groups (6, 29). Mass vaccination of prepubertal children and selective vaccination of susceptible women of childbearing age has been the approach to preventing rubella in the United States. Proper utilization of rubella serologic testing in premarital and prenatal screening programs can be a significant asset to the ultimate elimination of congenital rubella.

The Virus

Size and shape

Electron microscopy studies (16, 111, 118) have shown rubella virus to be a generally spherical particle with a diameter of 60–70 nm (Fig 25.3). Surface projections or spikes 6 nm in length have been reported. The virion contains a dense central nucleoid measuring about 30 nm surrounded by a double-layer envelope acquired during budding of the virus into cytoplasmic vesicles or from the marginal plasma membrane (118).

Chemical composition

Rubella is an ribonucleic acid (RNA) virus. Purified virus preparations reveal no trace of deoxyribonucleic acid (DNA) (11), and inhibitors of DNA

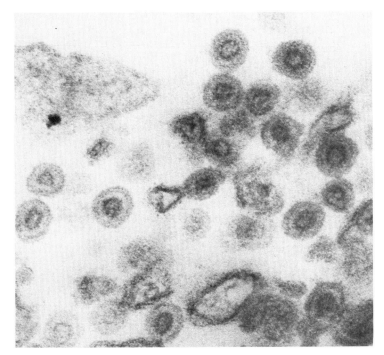

Figure 25.3—Electron micrograph of rubella virus in BHK-21 cells, 192,000X. (Photograph courtesy of FA Murphy and AK Harrison.)

synthesis such as 5-fluorodeoxyuridine and 5-bromodeoxyuridine do not prevent rubella virus synthesis (38, 100, 133). Actinomycin D also fails to prevent rubella virus synthesis (101). The virus envelope contains essential lipid. The genetic information is contained in a single strand of RNA. Eight distinct polypeptides have been identified in purified virus by poly-acrylamide-gel electrophoresis (11).

Resistance to physical and chemical agents

Temperature. Rubella virus is relatively heat labile. At 37 C the half-life of infectivity in 2% serum is 1 hr (123). All infectivity is lost within 30 min at 56 C, within 4 min at 70 C, and within 2 min at 100 C (51).

Rubella virus maintains its infectivity well at refrigerator temperature (4-8 C); titers remain stable for over 1 week in protein-containing solutions (123), and at −60 C the virus will retain its titer for many years (105). At intermediate temperatures (−10 C to −20 C), however, infectivity may be rapidly lost. Rubella virus can be freeze dried without harm.

Hydrogen ion concentration. Rubella virus is sensitive to extremes of pH. Chagnon and Laflamme (30) demonstrated that incubation in solutions of pH <6.8 or >8.1 resulted in rapid loss of infectivity.

Ultraviolet irradiation. Rubella virus infectivity is rapidly destroyed by ultraviolet light (51).

Chemicals. Ether, acetone, chloroform, or deoxycholate (0.1%) destroys the infectivity of rubella virus within 10 min (123). Rubella hemagglutinating (HA) antigen may be protected from ether by pretreatment with Tween 80 (170). Formalin, ethylene oxide, and beta-propiolactone also rapidly inactivate rubella virus with varied effect on the antigenicity of the virus (58, 123).

Rubella is resistant to the action of fluorocarbon (Genetron 113), thiomerosal, and sodium bisulfite. Infectivity is destroyed within minutes by 70% alcohol or 0.5% sodium hypochlorite solution and, to a lesser degree, by benzalkonium chloride.

Rubella virus may be stabilized against heat inactivation by the addition of $MgSO_4$ to virus suspensions (190).

Antiviral agents. Little information is available on the effect of antiviral agents on rubella virus. *In vitro* 1-adamantanamine inhibits the growth of rubella virus as measured by viral synthesis (32) or plaque size (131). The effect appears to be on virus penetration (119). Evidence of clinical effectiveness is, however, lacking.

Classification

Rubella virus has been classified as a togavirus (53). Studies on rubella virus RNA and its structural proteins, however, differentiate rubella from other members of the togavirus family.

Antigenic composition

Number of immunotypes. Only one immunologically distinct type of rubella virus has been described, and no serologic relationship exists between rubella and any other known virus group. Minor biological variations that have been identified in different strains of rubella virus are not reflected in antigenic variations of the virus (15, 55).

Description of the various antigens. Studies of purified rubella virus have provided considerable information regarding the antigenic composition of the virus. A detailed review and discussion of the antigen components of rubella virus have been presented by Vesikari (184). Analysis of the major structural subunits of the rubella virion reveals two main antigenic components, one associated with the viral envelope and the other associated with the ribonucleoprotein core of the virus. The envelope component possesses HA, CF-V, platelet-aggregating (PA-V), and theta precipitinogen activities. The viral RNA core component possesses CF-S, PA-S, and iota precipitinogen activity.

HA antigen. Rubella hemagglutinin was first demonstrated by Stewart et al (170) in fluids from infected tissue cultures maintained with kaolin-treated serum, and by Halonen et al (69) in alkaline extracts of infected cells. To use either method successfully HA inhibitors normally present in serum must be eliminated. A number of other methods for producing the HA antigen have since been developed (see below).

More recent studies associate rubella HA with one of the major proteins for the virus envelope.

Rubella hemagglutinin agglutinates a wide variety of erythrocyte (RBC) species (152). Fowl RBC (newborn chick, adult goose, or pigeon) and human O RBC have been most widely used for rubella HAI testing. The optimal pH for HA is 6.2 (69). HA by rubella virus is unique in that it is dependent on the presence of Ca^{++} ions. If Ca^{++} is removed by addition of versene or ethylenediaminetetraacetate, the HA antigen is unable to attach to the RBC receptors (61, 95). The same Ca^{++} dependent mechanism may also account for the attachment of nonspecific rubella HA inhibitors (20, 149).

Rubella hemagglutinin is stable for months at -20 C, for several weeks at 4 C, and overnight at 37 C, but is destroyed within minutes by heating at 56 C (61, 69).

The nonspecific serum inhibitor of rubella hemagglutination is associated primarily with the beta-lipoproteins; specific removal of this class of protein complexes results in removal of the nonspecific inhibitor.

CF antigens. Cell-associated CF antigen derived from rubella-infected cell cultures was first reported by Sever et al (163). Improved CF antigens were later prepared from alkaline extracts of infected cells (68, 153) or from concentrated fluids from infected cell cultures (154).

The CF activity in rubella virus has been separated into 3 components: a large-particle CF antigen associated with the whole virus particle, a light small-particle antigen that may represent a subunit of the virus envelope, and a third distinct small-particle or "soluble" CF antigen (153, 184). The first two of these antigens appear to be associated with separate viral proteins (156). The major portion of rubella CF activity sediments at about 3S–4S, suggesting association with virus envelope rather than internal components. Some CF activity is associated with a viral component sedimenting at about 150S. This appears to represent the serologic activity of the virus ribonucleoprotein core (179). The latter CF antigen component is quite labile.

Precipitating antigens. Immunodiffusion (ID) studies of rubella virus antigens in concentrates of tissue culture fluids from several different cell systems and in alkaline buffer extracts of infected cells reveal 2 small-size immunoprecipitating antigens, designated "theta" and "iota" by LeBouvier (87). Additional precipitinogens have been suggested by others (147, 158). The theta precipitinogen appears associated with the virus envelope, perhaps with the same proteins that possess CF activity (see above). The iota precipitinogen appears associated with the soluble CF activity and is probably also a component of the ribonucleoprotein core of the rubella virus. ID study results show that natural rubella infections elicit strong precipitating antibody responses to both the theta and the iota antigens, whereas rubella vaccine strains stimulate a strong anti-theta response but a weak anti-iota response. The significance of this difference, as far as rubella immunity is concerned, has not been determined.

PA antigen. Rubella virus antigen and antibody complexes cause aggregation of platelets *in vitro*. The PA test, developed by Penttinen and Myllylä (129), has been used to study rubella antigens and antibodies. The main PA activity in rubella-infected cell cultures is connected with the envelope component of the virus (179). Some PA activity has been detected in the ribonucleoprotein core of the virion, thus representing still another possible activity of the soluble CF antigen mentioned earlier.

Pathogenicity for animals

Rubella virus will grow in primates and in various small laboratory animals. However, in no animal has the acquired or congenital disease been completely reproduced.

Vervet (167) and particularly rhesus monkeys (73, 126) are susceptible to infection by the intranasal, intravenous (iv), or intramuscular (im) routes. Although no rash develops, there is nasopharyngeal virus excretion in all and viremia in 50% of the inoculated monkeys (73, 126). Attempts to produce transplacental infection in pregnant monkeys have been partially successful. Rubella virus has been recovered from the amnion and the placenta, but the embryo itself has not been shown to be consistently infected (127, 164).

The ferret is by far the most useful of the small laboratory animals in rubella studies. Ferret kits are highly sensitive to subcutaneous and particularly to intracerebral inoculations. Virus has been recovered from the heart, liver, spleen, lung, brain, eye, blood, and urine for a month or longer after inoculation, and both neutralizing (Nt) and CF antibodies have developed (50). Ferret kits inoculated at birth develop corneal clouding (50). Virus appears in the fetal ferrets after inoculation of the pregnant animals (10). Rabbits (13, 84), hamsters, guinea pigs (120), and suckling mice (27) have all been infected with rubella virus, but none of these have proven to be a consistent and reliable animal model system for rubella virus studies.

Growth in tissue cultures

Cell systems. A wide variety of cell types support the replication of rubella virus. As a generalization, it may be said that rubella virus grown in primary cells produces interference but no cytopathic effect (CPE), whereas rubella virus grown in continuous cell lines produces CPE that is markedly influenced by environmental variables. Table 25.1 lists cell systems in which rubella virus replicates and the means by which replication is detected.

Interference. Growth of rubella virus in many tissue cultures interferes profoundly with superinfection by other viruses. Parkman et al (123) found that the CPE of enteroviruses, myxoviruses, papovaviruses, herpesviruses, and arboviruses all were blocked in rubella-infected African green monkey kidney (AGMK) tissue cultures. The mechanism of rubella-induced interference is not completely understood. Although interferon production has been described after rubella infection of various cell cultures, evidence suggests that the interference is not based solely on synthesis of interferon (43, 196).

TABLE 25.1—TISSUE CULTURE SYSTEMS IN WHICH RUBELLA VIRUS PROPAGATES

TISSUE CULTURE	MEANS OF DETECTION*		
	INTERFERENCE	CPE	PLAQUES
Primary Cells			
African green monkey kidney	X		
Rhesus monkey kidney			
Patas monkey kidney	X		
Human amnion	X	X	
Human thyroid		X	
Human embryo kidney	X		
Bovine embryo kidney	X		
Bovine skin and muscle			
Rabbit kidney	X	X	
Rabbit embryo kidney		X	
Swine kidney	X		
Canine kidney			
Chick embryo			
Duck embryo			
Cell Strains			
Human diploid fibroblasts			
Rhesus embryo kidney	X		
Cell Lines			
BHK-21 (baby hamster kidney)		X	X
RK$_{13}$ (rabbit kidney)		X	X
RK$_1$ (rabbit kidney)		X	X
SIRC (rabbit cornea)		X	X
BS-C-1 (vervet kidney)	X		
LLC-MK$_2$ (rhesus kidney)	X	X	
Vero (vervet kidney)		X	X
AH-1 (vervet kidney)		X	X
HEp-2 (human carcinoma)			
Chang (liver)			
HeLa (cervical carcinoma)			
FL (human amnion)			

* Growth of rubella in tissue culture systems that do not show interference or cytopathogenic effect (CPE) is detected by subculture into other systems.

Cytopathogenic effect (CPE). The cytopathogenicity of rubella virus is markedly dependent on external conditions. In many cell lines CPE may be subtle and develops slowly. The appearance of CPE is dependent on the composition of the nutrient medium used (91); serum concentration above 2% will depress CPE, as will the addition of vitamins or amino acids either originally or in later changes of medium. Vero and RK-13 cells are most useful for rubella virus propagation when CPE changes are desired (14, 98, 143).

Plaquing. Rubella virus has been plaqued in RK-13 (132, 173), BHK-21 (176), SIRC (144), and Vero (98, 143) cells. Most virus strains are sensitive to agar inhibitors; therefore, adding diethylaminoethyl-dextran or using agarose or carboxymethylcellulose in the overlays promotes accurate titration (55, 177). The differences in plaquing characteristics among strains have been used to develop markers (55, 78, 110).

Preparation of Immune Serum

Antiserum to rubella virus can be produced in a wide variety of animals, including rabbits, monkeys, guinea pigs, ferrets, pigs, and horses. A satisfactory rubella immune antiserum should have an Nt antibody titer of 1:64 and an HAI titer of $\geq 1:512$.

In ferrets and monkeys the antibody response follows multiplication of the virus, and only 1 subcutaneous inoculation of virus is necessary. Serum is collected 4–6 weeks after inoculation.

In other animals multiple injections of virus are required to achieve a satisfactory immune response. The inocula consist of concentrated supernatant fluids from infected tissue cultures or partially purified virus. The virus strain used as antigen is of minor importance as long as it can be grown to high titer in the appropriate cell line. The production of antihost-cell antibody is an important consideration because the rubella virus incorporates host antigens in its structure. Development of antibody against serum components of heterologous species in the inoculum should also be avoided. The use of a totally homologous system is therefore most satisfactory, e.g., inoculation into rabbits of virus grown in RK-13 cells grown and maintained on rabbit serum media. One satisfactory schedule for producing immune serum in rabbits entails inoculating them with 5 ml of concentrated fluid subcutaneously and 1 ml iv, followed by 1-ml booster doses iv weekly for 4–5 weeks. Two weeks after the last inoculation, the serum is collected.

Collection and Preparation of Specimens for Laboratory Diagnosis

Precautions

Laboratory-acquired rubella infections are extremely rare, although considerable concern has been expressed about exposing susceptible women of childbearing age to rubella virus or antigens in the laboratory. It is not known whether pregnancy alters an individual's resistance to rubella infection; therefore, susceptible pregnant women should avoid being exposed to laboratory areas where rubella virus is being studied (28).

Laboratory workers, particularly women, who are found serologically susceptible to rubella and who plan to work in an area where rubella virus may be handled should be vaccinated at an appropriate time when the possibility of pregnancy is essentially nil.

Specimens for virus isolation

Indications. Virus isolation has only limited applicability for routine rubella diagnosis because of the lability of the virus at ambient temperature and the expense and time involved. Most diagnostic situations are better investigated serologically. Clinical situations in which rubella virus isolation is indicated include suspected acute rubella cases with severe complications (e.g., encephalitis) or fatal infections for which serologic confirmation of the etiology would not be possible. In addition, virus isolation with strain characterization of a rubella virus isolate is the most meaningful approach to evaluating rubella-vaccine–related illnesses.

Collection. In general, specimens for rubella virus isolation should be collected as early as possible after the person becomes ill, preferably within 3-4 days after symptoms appear.

1. Respiratory secretions—Both nasal and pharyngeal swabs should be obtained. Nasal swabs should be well soaked with respiratory secretions. Throat swabs are obtained by vigorous rubbing of an ordinary cotton swab over the tonsils and posterior pharynx. The swabs should be placed immediately into tubes containing 1-2 ml of nutrient broth containing antibiotics (penicillin 400 u/ml, streptomycin 400 μg/ml, gentamycin 50 μg/ml, and mycostatin 50 μg/ml). Rubella virus is relatively unstable and requires a protein-protective substance for stabilization. Best results are achieved with a nutrient broth containing 0.5% bovine albumin or 1% gelatin. Throat washings are less satisfactory than nasal-pharyngeal swabs for rubella virus isolation.

2. Blood—Blood for virus isolation is heparinized at time of collection (200 u/ml). After centrifugation, the plasma, leukocyte-rich buffy coat, and RBC pack may be separated for independent inoculation.

3. Cerebrospinal fluid—Cerebrospinal fluid is collected under aseptic conditions. It is one of the best potential sources of virus in congenital rubella cases.

4. Urine—Freshly voided urine is collected in a sterile vessel and neutralized with sodium bicarbonate to give pH 7 as measured with indicator paper.

5. Cataract material and lens fluid—Cataractous lens tissue and fluid should be inoculated directly into tissue culture whenever possible. If direct culture is not possible, the specimen should be kept moist with nutrient broth containing antibodies and transported to the laboratory at 4 C.

6. Tissue specimens—Autopsy tissues, placenta, amniotic fluid, and fetal tissues from spontaneous or surgical abortions should be collected in sterile jars containing sufficient saline or Hanks balanced salt solution (BSS) to prevent drying and transported to the laboratory at 4 C. A separate container should be used for each specimen.

Storage and shipping. In general, all specimens that are to be inoculated within 48 hr of collection should be stored at 4 C and transported to the laboratory on wet ice. At this temperature virus is preserved satisfactorily in protein-containing solutions. However, if inoculation is to be delayed, the specimen should be frozen at −60 C or below immediately after it is collected. Tissue specimens to be used for explant cell cultures must not be frozen.

Specimens that must be mailed to a laboratory for processing must be packed frozen on dry ice in a well-insulated container to insure against thawing en route.

Processing of specimens. Frozen tissue specimens should be thawed slowly before they are processed for inoculation. When completely thawed, the specimen may be dissected and specific parts may be selected for processing. A small portion of the tissue should be removed and ground thoroughly, and a 10% suspension should be made in Hanks BSS containing antibiotics. The suspension can then be centrifuged at slow speed to remove gross debris before inoculation.

Fresh, unfrozen tissue specimens should be processed also for propagation of explant cell cultures (see below). This approach is of particular value in attempts to isolate virus from fetal tissues and organs. No study of tissue specimens for the presence of rubella virus is complete without cultures developed from the specimen tissues themselves since they are more frequently positive for virus than are suspensions of ground tissue (31, 139).

Swab fluids, cerebrospinal fluid, urine, or tissue suspension fluid is inoculated in 0.25-ml amounts into at least 4 tube-cultures of whatever cell system is being used. The cultures are inoculated without maintenance medium, which is added after 1 hr of absorption. To avoid toxicity from urine or tissue specimens, it is often best to remove the original inoculum after adsorption and rinse the cell monolayer before addition of maintenance medium.

Heparinized blood can be tested whole or after separation of plasma. No data are available comparing the isolation rates from plasma and whole blood. The separation and inoculation of buffy coat leukocytes may be of particular value in testing for viremia in cases of congenital rubella or in other situations where circulating antibody may be present. If whole blood or leukocyte-rich buffy coat is inoculated, it should be removed from the tissue culture monolayers after 2 hr of adsorption by rinsing before maintenance medium is added.

Specimens for serologic diagnosis

Collection. Blood is collected in sterile tubes, allowed to clot, and centrifuged to separate the serum. Avoidance of hemolysis is desirable.

Handling, processing, and shipping. Serum should be handled with care to avoid contamination. Bacterial contamination of serum may affect subsequent tests for rubella antibody (19, 25). Specimens for serologic testing can be stored for a limited period at 4 C and can be shipped by mail without refrigeration.

Storage. For extended storage serum should be kept frozen at −10 C to −20 C. Laboratories performing rubella serologic diagnostic tests should store serum specimens after initial testing for at least 6 months to permit retesting of specimens if indicated by subsequent clinical developments.

Laboratory Diagnosis

Virus isolation

Isolation in tissue cultures. Although the list of cell culture systems in which rubella virus replicates is long (Table 25.1), not all lend themselves to recovery of new isolates. For practical purposes primary isolation of rubella virus is done in either primary AGMK, Vero, or RK-13 cell cultures. In the latter two systems, CPE is not always clear on primary isolation, and tissue culture fluids may have to be passaged several times for full detection of virus. Other cell systems are not sufficiently sensitive for primary isolations.

Some lots of calf serum contain inhibitors that interfere with rubella virus growth; therefore, maintenance media for cell cultures used for primary rubella virus isolation should be prepared only with pretested, inhibitor-free fetal calf, chicken, or rabbit serum. Sensitivity of the system used for rubella virus replication should be monitored by titration of virus of known potency.

1. AGMK cells—Isolation of rubella virus in primary cultures of AGMK cells has been considered the standard method since 1962 (122, 123). Virus is detected in these cells by interference with the CPE of a challenge virus. Many still consider this system to be the most sensitive for recovering rubella virus from clinical specimens. A significant disadvantage, however, is that profound differences exist in the sensitivity of different lots of AGMK cells to rubella virus (194). Simian virus contamination may be associated with diminished growth of rubella virus, and individual lots of AGMK cells that appear perfectly normal on microscopic examination may moderately resist rubella virus replication. A standard rubella virus of known titer must be titrated in each lot of AGMK tubes to determine the sensitivity of a particular batch. If the titer of the standard virus is 1 $\log_{10}$ mean tissue culture infectious dose ($TCID_{50}$) or more below the expected titer, the entire test should be considered undersensitive, and samples with negative results should be retested. In addition, since a high percentage of AGMK lots may contain simian viruses such as cytomegalovirus, rubella isolate strains will frequently contain these adventitious agents.

Some simian virus contaminants can be detected early by hemadsorption. Upon receipt, each new lot of AGMK tubes should be tested by randomly selecting 10 tubes, removing growth medium, rinsing with phosphate-buffered saline (PBS), and adding 1 ml of 0.4% guinea pig RBC suspended in PBS to each tube. After 45 min of incubation at 4 C, the tubes are washed several times with PBS and examined for hemadsorption. Cell lots showing the presence of hemadsorbing agents are discarded. Cells obtained from commercial suppliers are generally checked for hemadsorbing agents before distribution.

For rubella virus isolation, each specimen is inoculated into at least 4 tubes. The maintenance medium, added after 1 hr of adsorption, consists of 1.5 ml of Eagle basal medium (BME) with 2% inactivated fetal calf serum and antibiotics. The cultures are incubated at 35 C in stationary racks, and after 5–7 days the medium is changed. At about 10 days after inoculation, the tubes are examined for any cytopathic agent. If none is found, the medium in half of the tubes is changed with maintenance medium containing challenge virus while the other tubes receive maintenance medium only.

Rubella virus interferes with CPE of many different virus types (123); however, those most commonly used as the challenge agent for rubella isolation in AGMK cells include echovirus type 11 or coxsackievirus A9. A challenge dose of 100–1000 $TCID_{50}$ should be able to cause 3+ to 4+ CPE in AGMK cells within 3–4 days.

The tubes are read 3–4 days after challenge. If the challenge virus has produced extensive CPE in control tubes but not in tubes inoculated with specimen material, interference is judged to have occurred. Whether or not interference is present, the cells and fluids of the unchallenged tubes are harvested by freezing for further passage in cell cultures. For general purposes, only 1 blind passage of negative specimens is necessary since an interfering agent not evident earlier is rarely detected after subsequent passage.

2. RK-13 rabbit kidney cell line—RK-13 cells are grown in medium No. 199 with 10% fetal calf serum. The cells should be subcultured weekly with use of a trypsin (0.125%)/versene (0.05%) mixture for cell dispersion. Each tube is seeded with 1–3 × 10^5 cells. Confluent cell monolayers are generally obtained within 2–3 days (14). One disadvantage of RK-13 cells is that most sublines of RK-13 are contaminated with mycoplasmas, which may cause the cells to grow poorly. Fortunately, the presence of mycoplasmas does not usually interfere with the detection of rubella virus.

Maintenance medium consists of medium No. 199 with 2% fetal calf serum and 0.15% sodium bicarbonate. At least 3–4 tubes per specimen should be inoculated. Better adsorption of virus occurs if specimens are inoculated directly onto the cell sheet rather than onto cell cultures on maintenance medium. Cultures are observed up to 10 days for the development of microplaques or general CPE (173). Although CPE has been recognized as early as 3–4 days in some laboratory-adapted rubella strains, not infrequently CPE fails to develop in these cells on first inoculation of a new isolate. At least 3 serial passages of fluids harvested at 7- to 10-day intervals should be made before a specimen can be considered negative.

Some rubella virus strains, notably attenuated vaccine strains derived from the HPV-77 rubella virus (124), produce distinct plaques in RK-13 cells under agar; wild isolate strains do not produce recognizable plaques under similar conditions. Such differential plaquing characteristics can help one distinguish natural wild rubella virus from the vaccine virus (85).

3. Vero continuous vervet monkey kidney cells—Vero cells are highly sensitive to rubella virus although, as with RK-13 cell line, several passages may be required for CPE to develop (98, 143). Vero cells are best grown in Eagle minimal essential medium (MEM) with 5% fetal calf serum and 0.84% sodium bicarbonate. They should be subcultured weekly by dispersing cells with a trypsin/versene mixture and seeding tubes with 1–2 × 10^5 cells per tube. Tubes are fed with fresh medium after 3–4 days and are ready for inoculation after 6–7 days. For maintenance, Eagle MEM with 2% fetal calf serum is used.

Specimens are inoculated into at least 4 tubes. After adsorption of virus, maintenance medium is added, and the tubes are incubated at 35 C. Because of the slow evolution of CPE, especially with new isolates, cultures must be observed for 21 days. Though unadapted rubella virus often fails to produce CPE, it appears to propagate readily in Vero cell cultures. It should be noted that Vero cells are deficient in cell-mediated interference production (44); therefore, challenge of infected cell cultures as described for AGMK cells cannot be used in detecting noncytopathic rubella virus infection in Vero cells.

4. Other cell lines—A number of other cell lines have been used for isolating rubella virus, including human amnion (193), primary rabbit kidney (104), LLC-RK$_1$ continuous rabbit kidney (81), SIRC rabbit cornea (89, 130), BS-C-1 vervet monkey kidney (157), LLC-MK$_2$ rhesus monkey kidney (181), and GMK-AH-1 vervet monkey kidney (65). Because none of these cell lines are as sensitive for primary isolation of rubella virus as the three cell systems described previously in detail, the listed group is not recommended for this purpose.

Isolation from fetal tissues. Rubella virus can best be isolated from fetal tissue specimens by setting up explant cultures, with use of one of the techniques described below.

1. The fetal tissue is cut into small fragments with sterile scissors. After 0.25% trypsin is added, the mixture is incubated in a sealed flask at 37 C. The flask should be checked frequently to see when the fragments dissolve; 30 min may be enough. The suspension is then removed from the flask, and the cells are centrifuged and resuspended at a concentration of 200,000 cells/ml in BME with 10% fetal bovine serum, 0.75% NaHCO$_3$, and antibiotics. The suspension is placed in Petri dishes perfused with 5% CO$_2$ in air or in small tissue culture flasks. When sufficient growth has taken place to produce confluent cell sheets, the medium is harvested and the cells are passaged.

2. The fetal tissue is cut into 1-mm fragments. A metal grid (Frankle Co., Philadelphia) is placed in a Petri dish and covered with a circular piece of teabag paper. Ten milliliters of BME is added with double strength vitamins, amino acids, and 10% fetal bovine serum. The liquid will moisten the paper, which becomes a gas-liquid interphase. Two fragments of fetal tissue are then placed on each paper-covered grid. Fibroblasts will grow out from the fragment and drop through the grid to the surface of the dish, where they will divide. The medium is changed weekly until the monolayer is confluent.

3. A modification of the above, which permits more rapid detection of virus, is to place the grids bearing the fetal fragments on monolayers of rubella-susceptible cells (AGMK, BS-C-1, RK-13, or Vero) in Petri dishes. Virus produced by the fragments then infects the monolayer, where it can be detected by interference or CPE.

With any of these methods supernatant virus released by the fetal tissue is usually detected by subculture in another system, although rubella-carrier cultures of fetal fibroblasts will show interference against vesicular stomatitis virus, poliovirus, or herpesvirus.

Identification of isolates. Methods commonly used for identification of rubella isolates include Nt, HAI, and immunofluorescence (FA).

1. Neutralization—Once rubella virus has been presumptively recognized in a cell system by interference or CPE, the same system can be used for Nt identification. Immune rabbit serum, prepared as described above is diluted to contain a minimum of 4 units of Nt antibody. A normal preimmune (rubella-antibody–free) rabbit serum is diluted similarly for the control titration. The isolate to be tested is diluted in 10-fold steps to 10^{-6}; samples of each dilution are inoculated into 3 cell culture tubes. The 10^{-1}, 10^{-2}, and 10^{-3}

dilutions are also combined with an equal volume of the prediluted rubella antiserum and of the prediluted normal rabbit serum. After 1 hr of incubation at 37 C, 0.2-ml volumes of the mixtures are inoculated into 3-4 tubes. If the cell system is one in which rubella causes CPE, the tubes are read at intervals until the mixtures that *do not* contain rubella antiserum become positive. In an interference-producing cell system, the challenge virus is added routinely at 7-8 days.

The titration of the isolate permits retrospective calculation of the exact amount of virus present in the dilutions that were mixed with serum. The result obtained with the dilution containing between 10 and 100 $TCID_{50}$ is the one by which the Nt is judged. Inhibition of the isolate at this dosage by the immune rabbit serum, but not by the control normal rabbit serum, indicates that the isolate is rubella virus.

2. Hemagglutination-inhibition—To prepare an isolate for identification by HAI, the virus is passaged in BHK-21 cell cultures maintained with Eagle MEM containing 2% kaolin-treated fetal calf serum. After 3-4 days of incubation at 35 C (with change of the medium at day 2), the supernatant fluid is harvested and tested directly for hemagglutinin (see Serologic Diagnosis below for method). One or 2 passages in BHK-21 cultures may be necessary before a hemagglutinin titer sufficient to give a positive test and permit an HAI assay is developed.

When hemagglutinin is detected, it is titrated, and 4 units are then used in an HAI test against known immune and nonimmune sera. Inhibition of agglutination by the immune serum confirms rubella. If 2 passages fail to produce hemagglutinin despite the production of 10^6 $TCID_{50}$/ml or more of virus, the agent is probably not rubella.

3. Immunofluorescence—Schmidt et al (157) have used the FA test to identify rubella isolates. Rubella immune serum made in rabbits and fluorescein-conjugated antirabbit globulin made in goats are used. Their method follows:

Agents to be identified by the FA technique are subpassaged once in the same cell type in which they were isolated, because the original inocula frequently contain bacterial and epithelial cells which stain with the rabbit serum. RK-13 cultures inoculated with the passaged material are harvested on day 5 of incubation; similarly inoculated BS-C-1 or secondary AGMK cell cultures are harvested at 6-7 days. Cells are scraped from the walls of the tubes and centrifuged at 2000 rpm for 5 min. The fluids are then removed, and the sedimented cells are resuspended in 1-2 drops of medium. Thin smears are prepared on microscope slides by spreading approximately 0.01 ml of the heavy cell suspension over an area 5-10 mm in diameter. The smears are allowed to air dry at room temperature; then they are fixed in cold acetone at −20 C for 18-24 hr. Slides are removed from the fixative and dried at room temperature, and the smears are outlined with quick-drying paint.

Immune and preimmune rabbit antisera are inactivated at 56 C for 30 min. The sera are diluted in a 20% suspension of normal mouse or beef brain (to reduce nonspecific staining) to give approximately 4 units of FA antibody as previously determined. A drop of serum is applied to smears of infected cells (and to uninfected cells for controls); the slides are incubated at 36 C in a humidified atmosphere for 20 min. The slides are then washed twice (10 min each washing) in PBS, pH 7.2–7.5. A dilution (prepared in a 20% brain suspension) of the fluorescein-conjugated antirabbit globulin is added to each smear. The appropriate dilution of the conjugate was determined previously by block titrations of the conjugate with immune and normal rabbit sera; a dilution is selected which gives maximal staining with rubella virus-infected cells and minimal background staining. After further incubation at 36 C for 20 min, the slides are washed twice, drained, and mounted with a buffered glycerol-saline solution.

If the cells treated with immune serum fluoresce, but the cells treated with nonimmune serum do not, the isolate is rubella virus. Schmidt et al (157) showed that false-positive test results did not occur.

Flow chart for isolation and identification (Fig 25.4). If clinical material is being examined specifically for rubella virus, one of the sensitive cell culture systems, primary AGMK, Vero, or RK-13 should be used for primary isolation. Since rubella CPE is variable, tissue culture fluids should be subcultured in AGMK cells for interference testing. If feasible, the primary inoculation of both AGMK cells and a continuous line with the clinical material is desirable. Interfering agents detected directly or indirectly can then be identified either in AGMK or in the continuous cell line. If the clinical specimen is obtained for a general virologic examination, rubella virus will usually be detected by its interference in AGMK cultures. Interfering agents are then identified as described above.

Serologic diagnosis

The diagnosis of rubella is best established by serologic methods. The methods available for measuring rubella antibodies include HAI, CF, PHA,

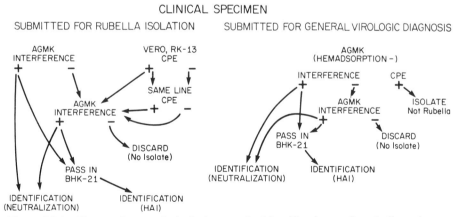

Figure 25.4—Flow chart of isolation and identification of rubella virus. AGMK = African green monkey kidney, CPE = cytopathic effect, and HAI = hemagglutination inhibition.

Nt, indirect FA, gel precipitation, solid-phase radioimmunoassay (RIA), and enzyme-labeled immunosorbent assay (ELISA). The dynamics of the antibody response to rubella infection is illustrated in Figure 25.1.

Hemagglutination inhibition (HAI)

Preparation and storage of antigen. Satisfactory rubella HA antigens are commercially available to most laboratories. In preparing rubella HA antigen, the beta-lipoprotein inhibitors must be removed from the serum used in the maintenance medium of infected tissue cultures (170). A number of techniques have been reported for the production of HA antigen, several of which are summarized below. Which virus strain is used for antigen preparation does not appear to matter as long as it replicates well in the tissue cells, generally either BHK-21 or Vero cultures. A number of techniques for antigen preparation follow.

1. In the method of Stewart et al (170), rubella virus–infected BHK-21 monolayers are maintained with BME containing 2% kaolin-absorbed fetal calf serum. The cultures are washed and fed with fresh medium 24 hr after inoculation. Starting at day 3, supernatant fluid is harvested daily and tested to detect the peak titer of extracellular HA activity. The harvests with highest titers may then be pooled and processed as described below.

2. BHK-21/clone 13 cells (178) grown in suspension may also be used in preparing rubella HA antigen. Cells inoculated with a high concentration of rubella virus particles (0.5–1.0 virus per cell) are maintained on a modified Eagle MEM (178) containing 5% kaolin-treated fetal calf serum or 0.4% bovine albumin (70). Starting at day 3, daily harvests of supernatant fluid are tested to determine the peak of hemagglutinin titer. Harvests with highest titers are further processed as described below.

3. The infected BHK-21/13 cell pack from the suspension culture in 2 above may be extracted with an alkaline 0.1 M glycine-NaOH buffer to produce HA antigen (69). Titers as high as 1:512 can be obtained after 30 hr of extraction, but the volume of antigen is small.

4. The association of HA antigen and beta-lipoprotein inhibitor requires divalent cations; the addition of versene can destroy this bond. If this fact is taken advantage of, maintenance medium for infected cultures can consist of BME with 2% untreated fetal calf serum. One volume of 0.1 M versene is added to 9 volumes of chilled tissue culture fluid harvested 4 or 5 days after inoculation. After incubation for 1 hr at 4 C, the hemagglutinin is sedimented by centrifugation at $32,000 \times g$ for 2 hr. The pellet is resuspended in PBS or 0.4% bovine albumin borate saline (pH 9) to 10% of the original volume, giving titers of 1:160 to 1:640 (60). The final product may be treated as described below with Tween 80 and ether to increase the titer further before storage.

5. Rubella hemagglutinin may also be prepared in Vero cell cultures by the method described by Liebhaber et al (97). Roller bottle cultures of Vero cells are inoculated with a high concentration of rubella virus and maintained with Eagle MEM containing 2% fetal calf serum. Alkaline extraction of the cell monolayers with use of 0.1 M glycine-NaOH buffer followed by low-speed centrifugation to remove gross cellular debris yields satisfactory HA antigen. Treatment with Tween 80 and ether can be used to increase the potency of the antigen further.

By whichever method antigen is made, it can be rendered noninfectious and increased slightly in titer by treatment with Tween 80 and ether, by the method of Norrby (116):

1. Add 0.125 ml Tween 80 solution to 100 ml antigen-containing fluid.
2. Shake or agitate with magnetic stirrer at 4 C for 15 min.
3. Add one-half volume anesthetic-grade ether (i.e., 5 ml ether/10 ml antigen/Tween).
4. Shake at 4 C for 15 min.

5. Centrifuge at 2000 rpm for 10 min; remove and discard the ether phase and the gelatinous interphase.

6. Bubble nitrogen through antigen to remove all residual ether.

7. To improve stability of the HA antigen, adjust the pH to 9 (137) and add versene to a final concentration of 0.001 M.

8. Store at −60 C.

9. Residual ether in the final antigen material will cause instability of the hamagglutinin and gradual loss of HA titer. Freeze drying will remove residual traces of ether and increase the stability of the antigen (129). Rubella HA antigen, free of ether, is stable indefinitely when stored undiluted at −60 C and for several weeks at 4 C.

Test variables. The HAI technique is the primary method for serologic diagnosis of rubella used in laboratories. Much work has been done to define the optimal conditions for the test and to standardize the various steps of the procedure. Each of the variables of the test system has a marked effect on the sensitivity and reliability of the rubella HAI test. These variables include the type of RBC, the type and amount of antigen, the composition of the diluent, the methods used for removing nonspecific inhibitors and natural agglutinins from the serum, and the temperature of incubation (155).

1. Erythrocytes—RBC used as the indicator cells must be highly sensitive to agglutination by rubella virus. A broad variety of RBC species can be agglutinated by rubella; however, baby chick and trypsinized human O cells have been the types most widely used for rubella testing. The sensitivity of the cells to agglutination is greatly influenced by the composition of the diluent (152) and the age of the cells. RBC treated with preservatives to increase their shelf life are available commercially; however, in some instances these are less sensitive than fresh RBC and require an excess of antigen. This in turn may result in low antibody titers and may even give false-negative reactions.

2. Antigen—Satisfactory rubella HA antigens may range in titer from 1:64 to 1:1024. In HAI antibody assays antigens are used at a dilution that contains 4 hemagglutinating units. Excessive antigen in the test system results in low antibody titers, whereas insufficient antigen gives antibody titers that are too high. In every HAI test it is necessary to know whether the proper dose of antigen was used; to confirm dosage the test antigen dilution is "back-titrated." Control sera of known titer are included in each test run to determine the relative sensitivity of each day's test. Qualitative differences in rubella HA antigens also affect the sensitivity of an HAI test; Tween-ether treated HA antigens are more reliable than untreated antigens for demonstrating significant increases in antibody, whereas antigens prepared by alkaline extraction of infected cells tend to give higher antibody titers than concentrated fluid antigens (155).

3. Diluents—The optimal pH for rubella HA is 6.2, and the reaction is enhanced by the presence of 0.001 M Ca^{++} ion. Various diluents have been described for rubella HAI test systems. Some of these (45, 69, 95) have a final pH of 6.2 in the test, whereas others (8, 35, 61, 170) have a final pH of 7.1–7.3. The N-2-hydroxyethyl piperazine-N'-2-ethanesulfonic acid (HEPES) diluent (95) containing 0.025 M HEPES, 0.14 M NaCl, 0.001 M $CaCl_2$, 1.0% bovine albumin, and 0.00025% gelatin (HSAG) has to date most closely approximated the optimal buffer diluent for rubella HAI testing.

4. Removal of nonspecific inhibitors—Nonspecific inhibitors of rubella HA are heat-stable beta-lipoproteins (46, 96, 134). Earlier rubella HAI test procedures used kaolin adsorption for removal of these inhibitors, but this method is not entirely satisfactory because of the tendency of kaolin to adsorb different amounts of specific antibody, particularly IgM immunoglobulins; the lack of reproducibility of HAI titers of kaolin-treated sera; and the variation among batches of kaolin in effectiveness for adsorbing the lipoproteins. Occasional batches do not completely adsorb the nonspecific inhibitors in some sera.

Kaolin adsorption of serum at pH 9 reduces the amount of nonspecific adsorption of immunoglobulin proteins and improves the reliability of beta-lipoprotein removal (155).

A faster and more specific method for removing nonspecific inhibitors is by precipitating them with either heparin-$MnCl_2$ (35, 52, 96, 134) or dextran sulfate-$CaCl_2$ (96, 114). Serum must not be heated before treatment by this latter method because heating alters the serum beta-lipoproteins so that some can no longer be precipitated by these reagents (96). This method is very effective and reliable in removing nonspecific inhibitors from serum for rubella HAI testing; however, one particular problem has been encountered with sufficient frequency to limit its use. In some instances serum treated with heparin-$MnCl_2$ or dextran sulfate-$CaCl_2$ may spontaneously agglutinate the indicator RBC at low serum dilutions (37). The reasons for this reaction are not clear, but an excess of divalent cations (Mn^{++} or Ca^{++}) appears to be central to the problem. If such difficulties are experienced, excess Mn^{++} or Ca^{++} ion can be removed by addition of Na_2CO_3 to the treated serum (18).

Another polyanion/divalent cation combination, sodium polyanetholsulfonate/$CaCl_2$, has also been reported to be effective for removing nonspecific inhibitors of rubella HA (49). In limited studies this method appears to have all the advantages of heparin/$MnCl_2$ treatment and not its disadvantages.

A method in which phospholipase C is used for removing the nonspecific beta-lipoprotein inhibitors by enzymatic hydrolysis has been reported (82). It is simple and rapid and avoids the problems presented by the methods discussed earlier. The method has been insufficiently evaluated to be further commented on at this time.

5. Temperature—Serum-antigen reactions are generally carried out at 4 C in most rubella HAI test systems. For most RBC types, including baby chick, rubella HA proceeds optimally at 4 C. However, temperature dependency for HA of human O RBC has not been demonstrated; no difference in levels of sensitivity is detectable between 4 C and 37 C (136). The presence of cold agglutinins in human sera may cause nonspecific agglutination of human O cells if used at the 4 C incubation temperature, but these agglutinins can easily be removed by prior cell adsorption at 4 C.

Recommended test method. Many variations of rubella HAI test methodology have been described, a number of which are currently in use in clinical laboratories. A standardized reference method was developed in 1970 to incorporate the optimal conditions into a single procedure (121), thus minimizing errors due to the pitfalls inherent in the unstandardized test methods. This method has since been adopted by the National Committee for Clinical Laboratory Standards as their recognized standard reference rubella HAI method (113). This method is described and recommended for routine diagnostic use on the basis of extensive proficiency evaluations (172) that have clearly indicated its greater consistency, sensitivity, specificity, and reproducibility when compared with other rubella HAI methods. The following is an abbreviated outline of this test protocol. The reader is referred to the referenced procedural guides (92, 113, 121) for a detailed description of the method.

1. Reagents—The following reagents for the rubella HAI test may be obtained from commercial sources.

Alsever Solution (Modified)

Dextrose	20.50	g
Sodium citrate, $Na_3C_6H_5O_7.2H_2O$	8.00	g
Citric acid, $C_6H_8O_7$	0.55	g
Sodium chloride	4.20	g
Distilled H_2O q.s.ad	1.00	liter

Sterilize by filtration through Millipore membrane (0.22-μ pore size); pH should be 6.0–6.2. Store at 4 C in convenient aliquots.

Dextrose-Gelatin-Veronal (DGV)

Diethyl barbituric acid (Barbital)	0.58	g
Gelatin	0.60	g
Sodium barbital	0.38	g
$CaCl_2$ (anhydrous)	0.02	g
$MgSO_4.7H_2O$	0.12	g
NaCl	8.50	g
Dextrose	10.00	g
Distilled H_2O q.s.ad	1.00	liter

Dissolve barbital and gelatin in 250 ml of water by heating. Combine this solution with the remaining reagents. Sterilize by filtration through Millipore membrane (0.22-μ pore size); pH should be 7.3. Store at 4 C.

HSAG Diluent

Hepes Saline 5X Stock Solution

HEPES	29.80	g
NaCl	40.95	g
$CaCl_2.2H_2O$	0.74	g
Distilled H_2O q.s.ad	1.00	liter

Dissolve in 900 ml distilled water. Adjust pH of this solution to 6.5 by adding 1 N NaOH (approximately 12 ml). Add distilled water to bring volume of solution to 1 liter. Sterilize by filtration through Millipore membrane. Store at 4 C.

Bovine Serum Albumin 2X Stock Solution

Bovine Albumin Powder (Fraction V)	20.0	g
Distilled H_2O q.s.ad	1.0	liter

Dissolve bovine albumin in 900 ml of water. Adjust volume to 1 liter by adding distilled water. Sterilize by Millipore filtration. Store at 4 C.

Gelatin 10X Stock Solution

Gelatin	25.0	mg
Distilled H_2O q.s.ad	1.0	liter

Dissolve the gelatin, and sterilize the solution by autoclaving for 15 min at 120 C. Store at 4 C.

To Make HSAG Diluent, Combine

HEPES saline 5X stock solution	200	ml
Bovine serum albumin 2X stock solution	500	ml
Gelatin 10X stock solution	100	ml
Sterile distilled H_2O	200	ml

At 25 C the pH of HSAG should be 6.2 ± 0.05. If pH is below 6.2, adjust with 1 N NaOH. If pH is above 6.2, adjust with 1 N HCl. This solution should be stored at 4 C and may be used for 2 months if kept sterile.

Heparin-Manganous Chloride Reagent

Heparin Stock Solution

Sodium heparin (USP)	5000	units/ml

This concentration may be obtained from commercial sources. If heparin is obtained as a more concentrated preparation (10,000 u/ml or more), dilute to 5000 u/ml with distilled water.

1 M Manganous Chloride Solution

$MnCl_2.4H_2O$	39.6	g
Distilled H_2O q.s.ad	200.0	ml

Sterilize by filtration through Millipore membrane (0.22-μ pore size). Store in the dark at 4 C. Discard if brown precipitate appears.

Heparin-$MnCl_2$ 1:1 Working Solution

Combine equal parts heparin (5000 u/ml) and 1 M $MnCl_2$. Store at 4 C no longer than 2 weeks. Keep sterile.

Dextran Sulfate 5% Solution

Dextran sulfate	5	g
Distilled H_2O q.s.ad	100	ml

Sterilize by Millipore filtration. Store at 4 C.

Calcium Chloride—1 M Solution

$CaCl_2.2H_2O$	29.4	g
Distilled H_2O q.s.as	200.0	ml

Sterilize by Millipore filtration. Store at 4 C.

2. Cells—Fresh RBC collected in Alsever solution from 1- to 3-day-old chicks are used in this test. Appropriate RBC can be purchased commercially. Cells can be used in the HAI test for no more than 2 weeks after they are obtained; however, older cells that do not show significant hemolysis can be used for absorbing natural agglutinins. Cell suspensions of 0.25% concentration in HSAG are used to detect HA in the test proper; 50% cell suspensions in HSAG are used for serum adsorption to remove natural agglutinins.

3. HA antigen titration—Antigen is pretitrated in triplicate with use of V-type microtitration plates. All reagents are cooled to 4 C, and the procedures are done at that temperature. A preliminary 1:4 dilution of antigen is prepared by combining 0.1 ml antigen and 0.3 ml cold HSAG diluent. The solution should stand at 4 C for 15 min to permit the hemagglutinin to disaggregate before titration. The HSAG (0.025 ml) is placed in dilution wells from 1:8 to 1:1,024 of the antigen titration and into 3 cell control wells. To the 1:4 dilution well in each row, 0.05 ml antigen is added. Serial 2-fold dilutions of the antigen are prepared with the microtitration diluters. Cold HSAG (0.025 ml) is added to all dilution and control wells, mixed, and placed at 4 C for 5 min. Cold 0.25% RBC suspension (0.05 ml) is added to each well, mixed well, and placed at 4 C for 90 min. The plate is then allowed to stand at room temperature. After 15 min, the agglutination patterns are read. The antigen titer is the highest dilution of antigen causing *complete* agglutination of the cells. This dilution is taken as 1 unit; the 4-fold lower dilution therefore contains 4 units.

  4. Serum treatment—Serum must *not* be heat inactivated before treatment. All test and control serum specimens are treated with heparin-$MnCl_2$ or dextran sulfate-$CaCl_2$ to remove nonspecific inhibitors and are adsorbed with chick RBC to remove natural cell agglutinins before HAI testing. One-tenth milliliter of serum is mixed with 0.15 ml HSAG diluent, 0.1 ml of the 1:1 heparin-$MnCl_2$ working solution, or 0.05 ml each of the 5% dextran sulfate and the 1 M $CaCl_2$, is added and mixed gently. The solution is incubated at 4 C for 15 min. Next, 0.1 ml of 50% chick RBC is added, mixed gently, and incubated at 4 C for 1 hr. Finally, 0.4 ml of HSAG diluent is added and centrifuged at 900 × *g* for 15 min at 4 C. The supernate should be removed carefully so as not to disturb the precipitate and cell pack. This is considered to be a 1:8 dilution of serum and may be stored at 4 C for up to 2 weeks before testing.

  5. Performing the HAI test—A row of 10 wells should be set up for each serum specimen, with 9 wells used for the serum dilutions of 1:8–1:2,048 and the tenth well for the serum control. To all wells except the first in each row, 0.025 ml of cold HSAG should be added. Into the first well containing no diluent, 0.05 ml of each 1:8 treated serum dilution is pipetted, and 0.025 ml is pipetted into the last well (serum control). Serial 2-fold dilutions of the sera are made with 0.025 microtitration diluters from the first well through the ninth well. When serum dilutions are completed, 0.025 ml of antigen dilution containing 4 HA units is added to each well except that containing the serum control. An antigen "back titration" should be set up at this time to check that the antigen dilution used in the test is correct (see below). The plate should be incubated at 4 C for 1 hr. Then 0.05 ml of cold 0.25% chick RBC suspension should be added to each well, mixed thoroughly, and placed at 4 C for 90 min. The plate is then placed at room temperature and read after 15–20 min. The serum antibody titer is the highest dilution of serum which completely inhibits HA.

  6. Controls—*Antigen back titration* is performed in triplicate. Cold HSAG (0.025 ml) is added to wells 2–5 in each of 3 rows. The first well of each row is left empty. To the first and second well of each row, 0.025 ml of the antigen dilution used in the test (4 units) is added. The plate is incubated with the test serum at 4 C for 1 hr. After incubation, with use of a 0.025 -ml diluter, 2-fold dilutions of the antigen are made from wells 2–5. HSAG (0.025 ml) is added to each well. Cold 0.25% chick RBC (0.05 ml) are added, mixed thoroughly, and incubated with the test sera for 90 min at 4 C. The plate is removed to room temperature and read after 15–20 min. Complete agglutination should occur in wells 1, 2, and 3, indicating that 4 units of antigen were used in the test. If <2 or >8 units were actually used, the entire test must be considered invalid.

  Two serum specimens known to contain rubella HAI antibody are to be included in each test as *positive control sera*. They are treated for removal of nonspecific inhibitors and agglutinins and are tested as the test sera were. One serum specimen should have a high antibody titer (≥1:256). The second serum specimen should have a low antibody titer (1:16–1:32). The titers obtained in each test on these positive serum controls must vary no more than ± one 2-fold dilution from the average titer obtained in previous tests with these sera; otherwise the entire test is considered invalid.

Serum containing no rubella HAI antibody but having a nonspecific inhibitor titer ≥1:256 is to be included in each test as the *negative control serum*. It is treated and tested as the test sera were. This serum must show no inhibition of agglutination in any of the dilutions, indicating complete removal of the nonspecific inhibitors; otherwise the entire test is considered invalid.

At least 2 wells containing only HSAG (0.05 ml) and 0.25% chick RBC suspension (0.05 ml) must be included in each test as *cell controls*. No agglutination or hemolysis must occur in these wells for the test to be valid.

The tenth well of each serum titration is the *serum agglutinin control* well. This well contains only the treated serum (1:8 dilution), HSAG, and chick cells. Any HA that occurs in this tenth well indicated incomplete removal of chick cell agglutinins from this serum; such nonspecific agglutination may obscure an HAI endpoint in the antibody titration. Thus, if no inhibition endpoint is observed in titrations of serum with nonspecific agglutination, the serum must be retreated and retested.

Interpretation of test results. The test is valid if the antigen control shows that there were between 2 and 8 units of HA antigen in the test, if the known negative control serum has a titer <1:8, if the known antibody-positive control sera are within ± one 2-fold dilution of their expected titers and show at least a 4-fold difference between the titers, if the test serum controls show no nonspecific agglutination, and if the cell control shows no nonspecific agglutination or hemolysis.

A ≥4-fold rise in serum antibody titer between acute- and convalescent-phase sera is generally accepted as evidence of recent rubella infection. Substantial drops in titer are rarely observed during the convalescent phase in acute rubella infections and, when observed, have no known significance. Because of day-to-day variations in the sensitivity of rubella HAI tests, multiple serum specimens from the same patient must be analyzed in the same test run for differences in titer to be considered significant. Fourfold differences in titers of paired sera tested on different days may reflect only test-to-test variation and not a true change in antibody concentration. Judgments regarding therapy should be withheld until the serum specimens have been reexamined in parallel.

Often acute-phase serum is not collected, and the laboratory is asked to make a diagnosis on a single serum specimen collected during the convalescent phase of the illness. Basing diagnostic interpretations on the HAI titer of a single serum is a dangerous practice (9) and should be strongly discouraged. High rubella HAI titers (≥1:512) cannot be considered to have any diagnostic significance since high titers are found in all population surveys with no known recent rubella infection (184). However, low HAI titers (≤1:16) when found 2 weeks or more after a suspected rubella illness may be given some negative diagnostic value, since acute rubella infections generally produce significantly higher titers.

The presence of HAI antibody at titers $\geq 1{:}8$ in a patient's serum indicates that the patient has been infected with rubella virus at some time and implies immunity to rubella disease. Patients without detectable HAI antibody at a serum dilution of 1:8 are usually susceptible to infection by rubella virus; however, a small percentage of adults may not have detectable HAI antibodies at this dilution and yet be immune. Nt antibodies at low dilutions can usually be detected in the serum of these patients. The lack of a serologic response to rubella virus vaccine in women who do not have detectable HAI antibodies is often caused by low levels of preexisting Nt antibodies (57).

Complement fixation

Preparation and storage of antigens. Although several cell lines, RK-13 (163), GMK-AH-1 (180), LLC-MK$_2$ (169), AGMK (163), and Vero (98), have yielded rubella CF antigens, the most convenient and widely used is the BHK-21 cell system (62, 68, 150, 153). Specific clones have been used, but it is probable that any BHK-21 cell line sensitive to rubella virus will be satisfactory. The sensitivity of the cell line should be checked periodically since changes can occur with multiple passaging.

BHK-21 cells can be grown in suspension (178) or in monolayer cultures (62, 153). The advantage of suspension cultures is that they can be propagated for long periods and yield large amounts of packed cell material for antigen production. The medium used for growth and maintenance of BHK-21 cells is that of Stoker and Macpherson (171).

Satisfactory rubella CF antigens can be produced by lysis or by alkaline extraction of packed infected cells or by concentration of tissue culture fluids. These antigens generally contain both soluble and virus CF components (see above). Control antigens are prepared from uninfected BHK-21 cells cultured and processed in parallel. The antigens should be stored at −70 C for maximal stability.

1. Lysis of packed cells—Cell cultures inoculated with high concentrations of rubella virus particles (1 virus per cell or more) are harvested at 4–5 days after infection. The infected cells are scraped and sedimented by centrifugation at 1000 rpm for 10 min. The sedimented cells are suspended in Veronal-buffered saline to give a 10% suspension. The antigen can then be relaesed by freeze-thawing 3 times in dry ice-alcohol or by sonication. After clarification by centrifugation at 2000 rpm, the resulting supernatant fluid is the antigen.

2. Alkaline extraction of packed cells (68, 153)—Infected BHK-21 cells are harvested 5–7 days after inoculation, centrifuged, and resuspended as a 10% suspension in 0.1 M glycine-NaOH buffer at pH 9. After 8–16 hr of incubation at 35 C, the material is sonicated, and the lysate clarified by centrifugation at 2500 rpm for 30 min. The supernatant lysate may be used directly as the CF antigen, or the antigen may be further purified by ultracentrifuging the supernatant lysate at 30,000 rpm for 3 hr and resuspending the pellet in tris(hydroxymethyl)-aminomethane (Tris) buffer at pH 8.2. The further purification step removes additional cell and medium components that may cause anticomplimentary activity in the crude alkaline-extracted antigen and increases the stability of the final product. Preparation of CF antigen by alkaline extraction of infected cells has the advantages of producing an antigen of high titer, high sensitivity, and high stability.

3. Concentration of culture fluids—Early in the course of infection in tissue culture, CF antigen in supernatant fluid is associated with infectious virus. Later, a noninfectious "soluble" antigen appears (63, 153, 154, 156) (see Antigenic Composition, page 732).

To produce soluble CF antigen, BHK-21 cells are infected as described earlier. The culture fluids are harvested at 7–8 days after inoculation and clarified by centrifugation at 2000 rpm for 20 min. The clarified fluids are then concentrated 100-fold by overnight dialysis at 4 C against polyethylene glycol (Carbowax 20 M), and the final concentrate is used directly as antigen.

Procedures for test. See Chapter 1 for the standard CF procedure by microtitration method.

Interpretation of test results. CF antibodies generally appear later after onset of a rubella infection than do HAI antibodies (74, 93). The test therefore is most useful in combination with the HAI test or as a back-up procedure when the collection of paired sera has been delayed, preventing the demonstration of an HAI titer rise. Testing a single serum sample for rubella CF antibody is of little diagnostic value. After rubella infection, the CF titer remains elevated for a shorter time than does the HAI titer, so that a negative CF report is not always a reliable indicator of the immunity status of an individual. However, rubella CF antibodies may persist for many years; thus, their presence cannot be used as evidence of recent rubella.

Passive hemagglutination

Preparation and storage of test reagents. Stabilized RBC coated with a soluble rubella virus antigen have been used in a 1-stage PHA system for the detection of antibody to rubella virus (H. H. Fricke, personal communication, 71, 146). Methods for sensitization of stabilized RBC with soluble protein and polysaccharide antigens have been reported previously (21, 76). Reagents for the PHA test for rubella antibody detection are available commercially.

Test procedure. Standard microtitration techniques are used for this test. Only serum or recalcified plasma specimens may be used in the PHA test. The specimens must be free of particulate matter but otherwise require no pretreatment before testing. Known positive and negative control sera and a buffer control are included with each test run. The test and control sera are diluted with the test buffer in wells of a V-type microplate. Sensitized RBC are added to each well and thoroughly mixed to insure uniform distribution of the cells. After incubation at room temperature for 2 hr, the test patterns can be read and compared with the patterns of the buffer control and the positive and negative serum controls.

Commercial kits are available for performing the rubella PHA test. Detailed protocols are provided with these test kits and should be followed exactly.

Interpretation of test results. The PHA test is most useful in detecting evidence of serologic immunity from past rubella infection. If a test specimen contains sufficient antibody to the rubella antigen fixed to the carrier RBC, a complex resulting in agglutination of the cells will form. An agglutinated, or dispersed, pattern of the cells after settling indicates the presence of antibody to rubella virus and implies immunity. If there is insufficient or no antibody to react with the coated RBC, they will settle as a sharp, compact button, indicating the absence of antibody and a susceptible status.

The PHA antibody response in acute rubella infections is delayed and may not begin until 15–30 days after appearance of the rash, and maximal titers are now reached for 3–4 months in some cases (M. Goldfield, personal communication). Consequently, the PHA test is not recognized as useful by itself in detecting recent rubella infections.

Neutralization

Test methods. Since the development of the HAI and CF tests, rubella Nt tests are now performed only for special purposes in a few laboratories. Rubella Nt tests are, in general, quite complex and present a number of technical problems that make reproducibility difficult. Variations in tissue cell sensitivity, serum complement concentration, and virus dose used in the test may produce great variation in antibody titer. If insufficient care is taken, false-negative or false-positive antibody titers may result. Assay systems for Nt antibody have been reported in which neutralization of rubella interference (115, 125, 182), of CPE (80, 90, 98, 106, 150), or by plaque reduction (132, 138, 140, 144, 178) was used. Since these procedures are all rarely used in diagnostic laboratories, readers interested in their specific details are referred to the stated references.

Indications for test. Nt tests are rarely used at present because of the complicated nature of the test and the longer period required for assay. They offer no distinctive advantage over other tests for rubella serologic diagnosis or for determining the presence of antibody *per se*. Occasionally, individuals with no detectable HAI antibodies at the lowest dilution tested will not respond to vaccination. Low levels of Nt antibodies can usually be demonstrated in the prevaccination serum, and repeated vaccinations to obtain a "take" are not indicated (57).

Interpretation of test results. The Nt test has generally been considered the reference standard for determining "protective" antibody. The presence or absence of rubella Nt antibody correlates well with immunity or susceptibility to rubella disease. Studies have shown that results from Nt antibody assays also correlate well with those obtained by HAI (54, 93, 99) but offer no advantage over those obtained with the latter assay system.

Indirect FA

An indirect FA technique for rubella antibody assay was first described in which chronically infected LLC-MK$_2$ cells called "RAL" were used (22). Since then FA techniques have been developed for a number of cell systems. Acutely infected BHK-21 (41) or BS-C-1 (94) cells offer the most satisfactory systems for this test now. Because infected tissue culture preparations necessary for the test are not available commercially, the test is limited to those laboratories which are able to prepare their own infected-cell antigen slides and which are proficient in FA techniques. With the necessary equipment and reagents available, the test can be performed rapidly and inexpensively and allows quantitation of specific IgM and IgG antibodies through the use of fluorescein-tagged specific antiheavy chain antibody for the various immunoglobulin classes (36, 56).

Preparation, fixation, and storage of cells. Cells for the FA test are grown either in Leighton tubes containing coverslips or in ordinary bottles and then are trypsinized and deposited on slides to form smears. The cell cultures are infected with a sufficient quantity of stock rubella virus adapted to the particular cell to produce a multiplicity of 1 virus per cell. Normal uninfected cells are grown in parallel as controls. At 4 days, the coverslips or cells are harvested. If smears are to be made, the infected and control cultures are trypsinized. The cells are washed in buffered saline solution, pH 7.3, and centrifuged to produce a pellet of cells. To make the smears, approximately 0.01 ml of cells is spread on 5–10 mm^2 of coverslip. The coverslips are fixed in acetone at -20 C for 30 min, with 1 change of acetone after 10 min. The coverslips are allowed to air dry at room temperature for 30 min. Fixed coverslips can be stored at -60 C for as long as 3 weeks before use (94).

Test procedure. Test and control sera are inactivated at 56 C for 30 min and then diluted from 1:4 through 1:128 in PBS, pH 7.4. One drop of each serial 2-fold dilution of serum is added to separate smears of infected and uninfected cells. After incubation in a moist chamber for 1 hr at 37 C, the smears are washed 3 times in PBS. The smears are covered with 1 drop of the fluorescein-labeled antihuman globulin conjugate (prediluted to its optimal dilution based on prior titration with known positive and negative sera), and reacted for 1 hr at 37 C. After incubation, the smears are again washed 3 times in PBS, rinsed in distilled water, allowed to air dry, and mounted with buffered glycerol (90% glycerol in PBS, pH 8).

Controls. For the FA test each serum specimen must be tested also on uninfected cells. Serum known to be positive for rubella antibodies must be tested on both infected and uninfected cells. Likewise, serum known to be negative for rubella antibody must be tested on both infected and uninfected cells. The PBS diluent must be tested on infected and uninfected cells instead of serum.

Interpretation of test results. Results obtained with the indirect FA method correlate well with those obtained by the Nt test, but technical pitfalls and the availability of the HAI test have limited its use in the general diagnostic laboratory. The main advantage of the test is in identifying the immunoglobulin class of the antibody by use of specific antiheavy chain antibody conjugates for the various immunoglobulin classes. The use of this test in detecting rubella IgM antibodies is discussed on pages 756–757.

Other test methods

Enzyme-linked immunosorbent assay. A micro-ELISA test has been described for detecting and quantitating rubella antibodies (187, 188). The test is carried out in polystyrene microtitration plates sensitized with rubella antigen. It is likely that plates presensitized with rubella antigen and the appropriate enzyme-labeled antiglobulin conjugates will soon be available commercially. IgG and IgM rubella antibody levels can be measured separately with the ELISA test by use of class-specific antiimmunoglobulin conjugates. Alkaline phosphatase-labeled antihuman globulin conjugates have been found most satisfactory in this test system.

Briefly, the test is performed as follows (188): Test and control sera are diluted in PBS, pH 7.2, containing 0.05% Tween 20, added to the wells of the sensitized plate, and incubated for 2 hr at room temperature. After incubation, the plate is washed thoroughly with the Tween-PBS buffer, and 0.2 ml of alkaline phosphatase-labeled antihuman globulin conjugate (prediluted to its optimal dilution based on prior titration with known positive and negative sera) is added to each well. After 3 hr of incubation at room temperature, the plate is emptied and washed again with Tween-PBS, and 0.2 ml of the substrate solution (p-nitrophenyl phosphate 1 mg/ml in 10% diethanolamine buffer, pH 9.8, with 0.5 mmol/l $MgCl_2$) is added to each well. After exactly 30 min, the reaction is stopped by addition of 0.05 ml of 2 N NaOH to each well. The color change may be assessed visually or with a spectrophotometer to measure the absorbance at 400 nm of the contents of each well. The color can then be related to readings from known positive and negative reference sera.

Radioimmunoassay (RIA). A solid-phase RIA method has been developed for measuring rubella antibodies in human serum (83). A distinct advantage of this procedure is that serum can be tested without any pretreatment, since no natural serum inhibitors of the reaction have been demonstrated. Polystyrene has been found to be the most satisfactory material for solid phase for this RIA system. Studies have shown the rubella RIA test to be highly sensitive and specific. When compared with the conventional rubella HAI test, the rubella RIA system has been shown to be 16–256 times more sensitive (83). The RIA technique may be further refined to allow detection of IgM class-specific antibodies. Given the required reagents and equipment, the RIA test is simple to perform and would be feasible for clinical laboratory diagnostic use.

The method described by Kalimo and Meurman (83, 108) follows. Purified rubella virus is adsorbed onto polystyrene balls (6.4 mm in diameter, Precision Plastic Ball Co., Chicago, Ill.) by submerging balls in an antigen solution (protein concentration 50 μg/ml), pH 7.35, at room temperature for 16 hr. The antigen-coated balls are then incubated for 1 hr at 37 C in 2% normal sheep serum, after which they are allowed to air dry and are stored at 4 C until used.

Fourfold serial dilutions of test and control sera are made with PBS, pH 7.35, containing 1% bovine serum albumin, fraction V, and a sensitized polystyrene ball is added to each serum dilution. After incubating at 37 C for 1 hr, the serum dilutions are aspirated off, and the balls washed twice with tap water. Then the balls are incubated for 1 hr at 37 C in a solution of ^{125}I-labelled antihuman gamma-globulin with a specific activity of 10–20 μCi/μg. Thirty thousand counts per minute (cpm) are added to each dilution tube. The radioactive solutions are then aspirated off, and the polystyrene balls washed again in tap water. The balls are then assayed for bond radioactivity in a gamma counter.

Serum titers are calculated by plotting the binding ratios (cpm of test serum dilution ÷ cpm of the negative control serum at the same dilution). The highest serum dilution with a binding ratio of 3 is taken as the endpoint titer.

Immune precipitin assays. Gel immunodiffusion tests for demonstrating rubella-precipitating antibodies have been described by several investigators (87, 148, 158). Despite their diagnostic potential, tests for precipitating antibodies have not been developed for routine diagnostic use because of the difficulties in obtaining suitable reagents. No rubella-precipitating antigens are available commercially, although a method for producing large quantities of rubella theta and iota antigens in Vero cells has been described (26). Tests for rubella-precipitin antibodies have been used in some specialized laboratories to demonstrate qualitative differences in the immune response to natural rubella infection and to rubella vaccines (88).

Given suitable antigen reagents, the immunodiffusion test can be performed easily and rapidly. Tests are conveniently done on glass slides (75- × 25-mm) covered with 2.5 ml of gel consisting of 0.4% agarose in Tris-saline buffer (0.01 M Tris, pH 7.4, and 0.1 M NaCl) and 0.1% sodium azide. Aliquots (20 μl) of reactants are placed in wells 5 mm in diameter and 3 mm apart. The slides are incubated in a moist chamber at room temperature, and the results read after 24 hr.

Precipitin antibodies can be quantitated according to the method described by LeBouvier (86). Serial dilutions of standard antigen and antibody are reacted against each other to determine the equivalence zone for each system (theta or iota). The highest dilution of the standard antibody reactant that gives a distinct band of precipitate in the equivalence zone with any dilution of the homologous standard antigen reactant is assumed to contain 1 unit of the antibody per μl. That dilution of the antigen reactant with which this band of precipitate is obtained is defined as containing 1 unit of antigen per μl. In a given test, unanalyzed sera are compared with 1 or 2 dilutions of the standard antibody reactant to determine the relative position of the precipitate that forms with 2 units of standard antigen reactant per μl. On the basis of this comparison, the titer of a particular serum specimen (units per μl) is assigned.

Serologic diagnosis by identification of IgM antibody

Test methods. Demonstrating specific IgM antibodies to rubella may be a valuable aid in serologic diagnosis of rubella infections. Specific rubella antibodies in the IgM class can be detected by various methods including indirect FA (12), RIA (108), ELISA (188), adsorption of IgG with staphylococcal protein A (7, 102), or physical separation of IgM from IgG by sucrose density gradient ultracentrifugation (17, 185) or column chromatography (23, 66) followed by HAI assay of the fractions. Detection of rubella IgM antibody by degradation with 2-mercaptoethanol is not recommended since specific IgG antibodies are invariably present in greater quantity than are IgM antibodies. The reduction of titer resulting from removing the IgM antibody is generally too slight to be of diagnostic value. With the indirect FA method, IgG antibody present in the serum may compete with the IgM antibody for antigenic sites in the infected cell preparations, thus masking the presence of IgM antibody and decreasing the sensitivity of the technique. In addition, the presence of rheumatoid factor (IgM anti-IgG antibodies) in serum causes false-positive IgM results in indirect FA, RIA, and ELISA test systems (59, 142). The indirect FA, RIA, and ELISA systems for assaying IgM antibody are dependent on absolute purity and specificity of the antiheavy chain (mu) conjugates for reliable results.

Method of choice. Separation of specific rubella IgM antibodies by sucrose gradient fractionation of serum followed by HAI assay of the fractions (185) has generally been considered the procedure of choice because of the proven reliability of this technique in reference laboratories. Given the necessary equipment, the separation procedure is relatively easy to perform.

A linear sucrose gradient is prepared by layering 1.4 ml of 37%, 23%, and 10% (wt/vol) solutions of sucrose in PBS, pH 7.2, on a 0.2 ml cushion of 50% sucrose in a 5-ml cellulose nitrate centrifuge tube. The tube is allowed to mature (diffuse) for 4-6 hr at 4 C. The test serum is diluted 1:1 in PBS, pH 7.2 (0.15 ml of serum mixed with 0.15 ml of PBS). No further serum pretreatment is necessary. A 0.2-ml volume of the diluted serum is carefully layered on top of the gradient, and the gradient is centrifuged at 157,000 × *g* for 16-18 hr in a swinging bucket rotor (SW-39 or SW-50.1). After centrifugation, 10-12 fractions (approximately 0.4 ml each) are collected drop by drop through the bottom of the tube, or by some other acceptable fraction collection method. The fractions are then tested for HAI activity without further treatment, dialysis, or cell adsorption. IgM antibodies will concentrate in the bottom 3-4 fractions. IgG antibodies separate primarily in fractions 6-8, and the nonspecific beta-lipoprotein inhibitors remain in the top layers of the gradient.

Additional modifications of this technique designed to increase its sensitivity and reliability further have been proposed (4, 159). Some of the more recently developed systems for assaying rubella IgM antibody, such as the IgM-RIA method (108) and the IgM-ELISA method (188), may in time prove to have greater sensitivity and reliability than the sucrose gradient fractionation method described in this section. However, insufficient data are available at this time to recommend these last methods until more extensive evaluation studies have been reported.

Interpretation of test results. The detection of rubella IgM antibodies can be of considerable value in diagnosing recent rubella virus infections. Since these antibodies are detectable for only 4-6 weeks after eruption of the rash, their presence implies recent primary rubella infection. Negative results, however, do not exclude a recent infection since detectable rubella IgM antibodies may disappear long before the end of the 4- to 6-week period. Rubella IgM antibodies are not found following reinfection with rubella virus, so this test can be of value in differentiating primary rubella infection from reinfection.

Detection of rubella IgM antibodies can also be of value in diagnosing congenital rubella infection. Since IgM antibody does not pass the placenta,

TABLE 25.2—RECOMMENDED TESTS FOR RUBELLA SEROLOGIC DIAGNOSIS IN SPECIFIC SITUATIONS

CLINICAL SITUATION	PRIMARY METHOD	BACK-UP METHOD
Acute rubella illness (paired sera)	HAI	CF, HAI-IgM*
Acute rubella illness (convalescent-phase serum only)	HAI-IgM*	
Immune status (single serum specimen)	HAI, PHA	
Exposure/no illness (single serum specimen within 7 days) (follow-up serum specimen if negative)	HAI	CF
Exposure/no illness (serum, 7–21 days after exposure plus convalescent-phase > 1 month after exposure)	HAI	CF, HAI-IgM*
Congenital rubella		
Birth–3 months old (single serum specimen)	HAI-IgM*	HAI†
3–6 months old (infant and maternal serum specimen)	HAI	HAI-IgM*
6–12 months old (single serum specimen)	HAI	
Over 12 months old‡ (single serum specimen)	HAI	

NOTE: HAI-hemagglutination inhibition, CF-complement fixation, IgM-immunoglobulin, and PHA-passive hemagglutination

   * Other comparable rubella IgM antibody may be used.

   † Follow-up testing required.

   ‡ Antibody present may be result of acquired natural infection or rubella vaccination.

the presence of such antibody in the blood of a neonate implies congenital infection.

Schema for use of rubella serologic diagnostic tests

A number of different clinical situations may arise with rubella exposure and infection, and knowledge of the comparative values and immune response patterns (Fig 25.1) of the various serologic tests is important to the meaningful diagnostic application of these laboratory tools. A well-equipped diagnostic laboratory should have the following serologic capabilities for rubella diagnosis: HAI testing with standardized methodology, CF testing with soluble or alkaline-extracted rubella antigen, and rubella-specific IgM testing. Table 25.2 shows the serologic tests preferred in different clinical situations. Other test methods described earlier in this section may also be of considerable value in these clinical situations but have not been included in this outline because they have been too recently developed to have been evaluated fully or because they are more applicable to research laboratories than to diagnostic laboratories.

References

1. ALFORD CA: Immunoglobulin determinations in the diagnosis of fetal infection. Pediatr Clin North Am 18:99-113, 1971
2. ALFORD CA JR, NEVA FA, and WELLER RH: Virologic and serologic studies on human products of conception after maternal rubella. N Engl J Med 271:1275-1281, 1964
3. ALFORD CA, STAGNO S, and REYNOLDS DW: Diagnosis of chronic perinatal infections. Am J Dis Child 129:455-463, 1975
4. AL-NAKIB W, BEST JM, and BANATVALA JE: Rubella-specific serum and nasopharyngeal immunologic responses following naturally acquired and vaccine induced infection— prolonged persistence of virus-specific IgM. Lancet 1:182-185, 1975
5. ALTEMEIER WA and SMITH RT: Immunologic aspects of resistance in early life. Pediatr Clin North Am 12:663-686, 1965
6. AMERICAN ACADEMY OF PEDIATRICS: Report of the Committee on Infectious Diseases. Seventeenth edition, Am Acad Pediatr, Evanston, Illinois, 1974, p 153
7. ANKERST J, CHRISTENSEN P, KJELLEN L, and KRONVALL G: A routine diagnostic test for IgA and IgM antibodies to rubella virus: adsorption of IgG with *Staphylococcus aureus*. J Infect Dis 130:268-273, 1974
8. AULETTA AE, GITNICK GL, WHITMIRE CE, and SEVER JL: An improved diluent for rubella hemagglutination and hemagglutination-inhibition tests. Appl Microbiol 16:691-694, 1968
9. BANATVALA JE, BEST JM, BERTRAND J, BOWERN MA, and HUDSON SM: Serological assessment of rubella during pregnancy. Br Med J 3:247-250, 1970
10. BARBOSA L and WARREN J: Studies on the detection of rubella virus and its immunogenicity for animals and man. Semi-annual Contract Progress Report to the National Institute for Neurological Diseases and Blindness. Sept 1, 1966 to Mar 1, 1967
11. BARDELETTI G, KESSLER N, and AYMARD-HENRY M: Morphology, biochemical analysis and neuraminidase activity of rubella virus. Arch Virology 49:175-186, 1975
12. BAUBLIS JV and BROWN GC: Specific responses of the immunoglobulins to rubella infection. Proc Soc Exp Biol Med 128:206-210, 1968
13. BELCOURT RJ, WONG FC, and WALCROFT MJ: Growth of rubella virus in rabbit foetal tissues and cell cultures. Can J Public Health 56:253-254, 1965
14. BEST JM and BANATVALA JE: A comparison of RK_{13}, vervet monkey kidney and patas monkey kidney cell cultures for the isolation of rubella virus. J Hyg 65:263-271, 1967
15. BEST JM and BANATVALA JE: Studies on rubella virus strain variation by kinetic hemagglutination-inhibition tests. J Gen Virol 9:215-223, 1970
16. BEST JM, BANATVALA JE, ALMEIDA JD, and WATERSON AP: Morphological characteristics of rubella virus. Lancet 2:237-239, 1967
17. BEST JM, BANATVALA JE, and WATSON D: Serum IgM and IgG responses in postnatally acquired rubella. Lancet 2:65-69, 1969
18. BIANO SA, CHANG T-W, and DANIELS JB: Rubella hemagglutination inhibition: removal of nonspecific agglutination due to manganous chloride. Appl Microbiol 28:992-994, 1974
19. BIANO S, COCHRAN W, HERRMANN KL, HALL AD, and CHANG T-W: Rubella reinfection during pregnancy. Am J Dis Child 129:1353-1356, 1975
20. BIANO SA, JENKINS CC, and DANIELS JB: Effect of calcium concentration on inhibitors of hemagglutination of rubella virus. J Infect Dis 123:421-425, 1971
21. BOYDEN SV: The adsorption of proteins on erythrocytes treated with tannic acid and subsequent hemagglutination by antiprotein sera. J Exp Med 93:107-120, 1951
22. BROWN GC, MAASSAB HF, VERONELLI JA, and FRANCIS TJ JR: Rubella antibodies in human serum: detection by the indirect fluorescent-antibody technic. Science 145:943-945, 1964
23. BÜRGIN-WOLFF A, HERNANDEZ R, and JUST M: Separation of rubella IgM, IgA, and IgG antibodies by gel filtration on agarose. Lancet 2:1278-1280, 1971
24. BUTLER NR, DUDGEON JA, HAYES K, PECKHAM CS, and WYBAR M: Persistence of rubella antibody with and without embryopathy. A follow-up study of children exposed to maternal rubella. Br Med J 2:1027-1029, 1965
25. CAMPBELL JB, ROMACH M, and ELLINS ML: Rubella hemagglutination-inhibition test: false-positive reactions in sera contaminated with bacteria. J Clin Microbiol 4:389-393, 1976

26. CAPPEL R, SCHLUEDERBERG A, and HORSTMANN D: Large-scale production of rubella precipitinogens and their use in the diagnostic laboratory. J Clin Microbiol 1:201-205, 1975

27. CARVER DH, SETO DSY, MARCUS PI, and RODRIGUES L: Rubella virus replication in the brains of suckling mice. J Virol 1:1089-1090, 1967

28. CENTER FOR DISEASE CONTROL, Laboratory Safety at the Center for Disease Control, U.S. Department of Health, Education, and Welfare, DHEW Publication No. 75-8118, Atlanta, CDC, Revised September 1974

29. CENTER FOR DISEASE CONTROL: Collected Recommendations of the Public Health Service Advisory Committee on Immunization Practices. Morbid Mortal Weekly Rep 21(25):23-25, 1972

30. CHAGNON A and LAFLAMME P: Effect of acidity on rubella virus. Can J Microbiol 10:501-503, 1964

31. CHANG TH, MOOREHEAD PS, BOUE JG, PLOTKIN SA, and HOSKINS JM: Chromosome studies of human cells infected in utero and in vitro with rubella virus. Proc Soc Exp Biol Med 122:236-243, 1966

32. COCHRAN KW and MAASSAB HF: Inhibition of rubella virus by 1-adamantanamine hydrochloride. Fed Proc 23:387, 1964

33. COOPER LZ and KRUGMAN S: Clinical manifestations of postnatal and congenital rubella. Arch Ophth 77:434-439, 1967

34. COOPER LZ and KRUGMAN S: The rubella problem. Disease-a-Month, February 1969, pp 3-38

35. COOPER LZ, MATTERS B, ROSENBLUM JK, and KRUGMAN S: Experience with a modified rubella hemagglutination inhibition antibody test. J Am Med Assoc 207:89-93, 1969

36. CRADOCK-WATSON JE, BOURNE MS, and VANDERVELDE EM: IgG, IgA, and IgM responses in acute rubella determined by the immunofluorescent technique. J Hyg (Camb.) 70:473-485, 1972

37. CREMER NE: Immunodiagnosis of rubella virus infection. Public Health Lab 32:87-97, 1974

38. CUSUMANO CL, SCHIFF GM, SEVER JL, and HUEBNER RJ: Rubella virus: nucleic acid studies using 5-iodo 2'-deoxyuridine. J Pediatr 65:138-140, 1964

39. DAVIS WJ, LARSON HE, SIMSARIAN JP, PARKMAN PD, and MEYER HM: A study of rubella immunity and resistance to infection. J Am Med Assoc 215:600-608, 1971

40. DE BERGEN: cited by Emminghaus, H. Über Rubeolen. Jahrb Kinderheilkd 4:47-59, 1870

41. DEIBEL R, COHEN SM, and DUCHARME CP: Serology of rubella: virus neutralization, immunofluorescence in BHK_{21} cells, and hemagglutination inhibition. NY State J Med 68:1355-1362, 1968

42. DESMOND MM, WILSON GS, MELNICK JL, SINGER DB, ZION TE, RUDOLPH AJ, PINEDA RG, ZIAI MH, and BLATTNER RJ: Congenital rubella encephalitis. Course and early sequelae. J Pediatr 71:311-331, 1967

43. DESMYTER J, DESOMER P, RAWLS WE, and MELNICK JL: The mechanism of rubella virus interference in international symposium on rubella viruses, London 1968, Symposium Series Immunobiol. Standard., Vol 11, Karger, Basel/New York, 1969, pp 139-148

44. DESMYTER J, MELNICK JL, and RAWLS WE: Defectiveness of interferon production and of rubella virus interference in a line of African green monkey kidney cells (Vero). J Virol 2:955-961, 1968

45. DOLD HJ and NORTHROP RL: Analysis of the diluents used for rubella virus hemagglutination and hemagglutination-inhibition tests. Appl Microbiol 18:221-227, 1969

46. DOLD HJ and NORTHROP RL: The nonspecific inhibitors of rubella-virus hemagglutination. Proc Soc Exp Biol Med 128:577-581, 1968

47. DOWDLE WR, FERREIRA W, DESALLES-GOMES LF, KING D, KOURANY M, MADALEN-GOITIA J, PEARSON E, SWANSTON WH, TOSI HC, and VILCHES AM: WHO collaborative study on the sero-epidemiology of rubella in Caribbean and Middle and South American populations in 1968. Bull WHO 42:419-422, 1970

48. DUDGEON JA, BUTLER NR, and PLOTKIN SA: Further serological studies on the rubella syndrome. Br Med J 2:155-160, 1964

49. ELLINS ML and CAMPBELL JB: Use of sodium polyanetholsulfonate/$CaCl_2$ for the removal of serum nonspecific inhibitors of rubella hemagglutination: a comparison with other polyanion/divalent cation combinations. J Clin Microbiol 6:348-358, 1977

50. FABIYI A, GITNICK GL, and SEVER JL: Chronic rubella virus infection in the ferret (*Mustela putorius fero*) puppy. Proc Soc Exp Biol Med 125:766–771, 1967

51. FABIYI A, SEVER JL, RATNER N, and CAPLAN B: Rubella virus: growth characteristics and stability of infectious virus and complement-fixing antigen. Proc Soc Exp Biol Med 122:392–396, 1966

52. FELDMAN HA: Removal by heparin-MnCl₂ of nonspecific rubella hemagglutinin serum inhibitor. Proc Soc Exp Biol Med 127:570–573, 1968

53. FENNER F: The classification and nomenclature of viruses. Intervirology 6:1–12, 1975/76

54. FIELD AM, VANDERVELDE EM, THOMPSON KM, and HUTCHINSON DN: A comparison of the haemagglutination-inhibition test and the neutralization test for the detection of rubella antibody. Lancet 2:182–184, 1967

55. FOGEL A and PLOTKIN SA: Markers of rubella virus strains in RK₁₃ culture. J Virol 3:157–163, 1969

56. FORGHANI B, SCHMIDT NJ, and LENNETTE EH: Demonstration of rubella IgM antibody by indirect fluorescent antibody staining, sucrose density gradient centrifugation and mercaptoethanol reduction. Intervirology 1:48–59, 1973

57. FOX JP, RAINEY HS, HALL CE, RAY CC, and PATTERSON MJ: Rubella vaccine in postpubertal women. J Am Med Assoc 236:837–843, 1976

58. FRANKEL JW: Neutralizing antibody responses of guinea-pigs to inactivated rubella virus vaccine. Nature 204:655–656, 1964

59. FRASER KB, SHIRODARIA PV, and STANFORD CF: Fluorescent staining and human IgM. Br Med J 3:707, 1971

60. FURUKAWA T, PLOTKIN SA, SEDWICK WD, and PROFETA ML: Hemagglutinin of rubella virus. Nature 215:172–173, 1967

61. FURUKAWA T, PLOTKIN SA, SEDWICK WD, and PROFETA ML: Studies on hemagglutination by rubella virus. Proc Soc Exp Biol Med 126:745–750, 1967

62. FURUKAWA T, VAHERI A, and PLOTKIN SA: Growth of rubella virus in BHK-21 cells. III. Production of complement-fixing antigens. Proc Soc Exp Biol Med 125:1098–1102, 1967

63. GREENBERG ER, BLAKE PA, CLINE BL, and HERRMANN KL: Rubella susceptibility among Puerto Rican mothers. Bol Asoc Med PR 65:259–261, 1973

64. GREGG N McA: Congenital cataract following german measles in the mother. Trans Ophthalmol Soc Aust 3:35–46, 1941

65. GÜNALP A: Growth and cytopathic effect of rubella virus in a line of green monkey kidney cells. Proc Soc Exp Biol Med 118:85–90, 1965

66. GUPTA JD, PETERSON VJ, STOUT M, and MURPHY AM: Single-sample diagnosis of recent rubella by fractionation of antibody on sephadex G-200 column. J Clin Pathol 24:547–550, 1971

67. GUYER B, GIANDELIA JW, BISNO AL, SCHAFFNER W, RAY RB, RENDTORFF RC, and HUTCHESON RH: The Memphis State University rubella outbreak: an example of changing rubella epidemiology. J Am Med Assoc 227:1298–1300, 1974

68. HALONEN PE, CASEY HL, STEWART JA, and HALL AD: Rubella complement fixing antigen prepared by alkaline extraction of virus grown in suspension culture of BHK-21 cells. Proc Soc Exp Biol Med 125:167–172, 1967

69. HALONEN PE, RYAN JM, and STEWART JA: Rubella hemagglutinin prepared with alkaline extraction of virus grown in suspension culture of BHK-21 cells. Proc Soc Exp Biol Med 125:162–167, 1967

70. HALONEN PE, STEWART JA, and HALL AD: Rubella hemagglutinin prepared in serum free suspension of BHK-21 cells. Ann Med Exp Fenn 45:182–185, 1967

71. HASSAN SA and COCHRAN KW: Immunohemagglutination test for rapid detection and assay of rubella antibodies. Proc Soc Exp Biol Med 125:430–435, 1967

72. HATTIS RP, HALSTEAD SB, HERRMANN KL, and WITTE JJ: Rubella in an immunized island population. J Am Med Assoc 223:1019–1021, 1973

73. HEGGIE AD and ROBBINS FC: Rubella in naval recruits: a virologic study. N Engl J Med 271:231–234, 1964

74. HERRMANN KL, HALONEN PE, STEWART JA, CASEY HL, RYAN JM, HALL AD, and CASWELL KE: Evaluation of serologic techniques for titration of rubella antibody. Am J Public Health 59:296–304, 1969

75. HERRMANN KL, WENDE RD, and WITTE JJ: Rubella immunization with HPV-77 DE$_5$ vaccine during infancy. Am J Dis Child 121:474-476, 1971

76. HIRATA AA and BRANDRISS MW: Passive hemagglutination procedures for protein and polysaccharide antigens using erythrocytes stabilized by aldehydes. J Immunol 100:641-646, 1968

77. HIRO Y and TASAKA S: Die röteln sind eine viruskrankheit. Monatsschr Kinderheilkd 76:328-332, 1938

78. HOPPS HE, PARKMAN PD, and MEYER HM: Laboratory testing in rubella vaccine control. Am J Dis Child 112:338-346, 1969

79. HORSTMANN DM, LIEBHABER H, LEBOUVIER GL, ROSENBERG DA, and HALSTEAD SB: Rubella: reinfection of vaccinated and naturally immune persons exposed in an epidemic. N Engl J Med 283:771-778, 1970

80. HULL RN and BUTORAC G: The utility of rabbit kidney cell strain, LLC-RK$_1$ to rubella virus studies. Am J Epidemiol 83:509-517, 1966

81. HULL RN, DWYER AC, CHERRY WR, and TRITCH OJ: Development and characteristics of the rabbit kidney cell strain, LLC-RK$_1$. Proc Soc Exp Biol Med 118:1054-1059, 1965

82. IWASA S and HORI M: Improved rubella hemagglutination inhibition test: inactivation of non-immunoglobulin hemagglutination inhibitors by phospholipase C. J Clin Microbiol 4:461-466, 1976

83. KALIMO KOK, MEURMAN OH, HALONEN PE, ZIOLA BR, VILJANEN MK, GRANFORS K, and TOIVANEN P: Solid-phase radioimmunoassay of rubella virus immunoglobulin G and immunoglobulin M antibodies. J Clin Microbiol 4:117-123, 1976

84. KONO R: Antigenic structures of American and Japanese rubella virus strains and experimental vertical transmission of rubella virus in rabbits. International Symposium on Rubella Vaccines, London 1968; Symp Series Immunobiol Standard, Vol 11, Karger, Basel/New York, 1969, pp 195-204

85. LAWRENCE GD and GOULD J: Morphology of rubella plaques in RK$_{13}$ cultures. International Symposium on Rubella Vaccines, London, 1968; Symp Series Immunobiol Standard, Vol 11, Karger, Basel/New York, 1969, pp 177-180

86. LEBOUVIER GL: Poliovirus precipitins. A study by means of diffusion in agar. J Exp Med 102:661-675, 1957

87. LEBOUVIER GL: Precipitinogens of rubella virus infected cells. Proc Soc Exp Biol Med 130:51-54, 1969

88. LEBOUVIER GL and PLOTKIN SA: Precipitin responses to rubella vaccine RA 27/3. J Infect Dis 123:220-223, 1971

89. LEERHØY J: Cytopathic effect of rubella virus in a rabbit-cornea cell line. Science 149:633-634, 1965

90. LEERHØY J: Neutralization of rubella virus in a rabbit cornea cell line (SIRC). Acta Pathol Microbiol Scand 67:158-159, 1966

91. LEERHØY J: The influence of different media on cell morphology and rubella virus titer in a rabbit cornea cell line (SIRC). Arch Gesamte Virusforsch 19:210-220, 1966

92. LENNETTE EH and SCHMIDT NJ: Principles and Performance of the Rubella Hemagglutination Inhibition Test. American Society of Clinical Pathologists, Chicago, 1973

93. LENNETTE EH, SCHMIDT NJ, and MAGOFFIN RL: The hemagglutination inhibition test for rubella: a comparison of its sensitivity to that of neutralization, complement fixation and fluorescent antibody tests for diagnosis of infection and determination of immunity status. J Immunol 99:785-793, 1967

94. LENNETTE EH, WOODIE JD, and SCHMIDT NJ: A modified indirect immunofluorescent staining technique for demonstration of rubella antibodies in human sera. J Lab Clin Med 69:689-695, 1967

95. LIEBHABER H: Measurement of rubella antibody by hemagglutination inhibition. I. Variables affecting rubella hemagglutination. J Immunol 104:818-825, 1970

96. LIEBHABER H: Measurement of rubella antibody by hemagglutination inhibition. II. Characteristics of an improved HAI test employing a new method for removal of non-immunoglobulin HA inhibitors from serum. J Immunol 104:826-834, 1970

97. LIEBHABER H, PAJOT T, and RIORDAN JT: Growth of high titer rubella virus in roller bottle cultures of Vero cells. Proc Soc Exp Biol Med 130:12-14, 1969

98. LIEBHABER H, RIORDAN JT, and HORSTMANN DM: Replication of rubella virus in a continuous line of African green monkey kidney cells (Vero). Proc Soc Exp Biol Med 125:636–643, 1967

99. LOGAN L, CHAGNON A, PODOSKI MO, HATCH LA, McLEOD DH, and deVRIES JD: An evaluation of three serological tests in diagnosing rubella virus infections. Can J Public Health 59:189–192, 1968

100. MAASSAB HF and COCHRAN KW: Influence of 5-fluorodeoxyuridine on growth characteristics of rubella virus. Proc Soc Exp Biol Med 117:410–413, 1964

101. MAES R, VAHERI A, SEDWICK WD, and PLOTKIN SA: Synthesis of virus and macromolecules by rubella-infected cells. Nature 210:384–385, 1966

102. MALLINSON H, ROBERTS C, and BRUCE-WHITE GB: Staphylococcal protein A; its preparation and an application to rubella serology. J Clin Path 29:999–1002, 1976

103. MANSON MM, LOGAN WP, and LOY RM: Rubella and other virus infections during pregnancy. Reports on Public Health and Medical Subjects. No. 101, Ministry of Health, London, 1960, pp 1–101

104. McCARTHY K and TAYLOR-ROBINSON CH: Growth and cytopathic effects of rubella virus in primary rabbit tissue culture. Arch Gesamte Virusforsch 16:415–418, 1965

105. McCARTHY K and TAYLOR-ROBINSON CH: Rubella. Br Med Bull 23:185–191, 1967

106. McCARTHY K, TAYLOR-ROBINSON CH, and PILLINGER SE: Isolation of rubella virus from cases in Britain. Lancet 2:593–598, 1963

107. MENSER M, HARLEY JD, HERTZBERG R, DORMAN DC, and MURPHY AM: Persistence of virus in lens for three years after prenatal rubella. Lancet 2:387–388, 1967

108. MEURMAN OH, VILJANEN MK, and GRANFORS K: Solid-phase radioimmunoassay of rubella virus immunoglobulin M antibodies: comparison with sucrose density gradient centrifugation test. J Clin Microbiol 5:257–262, 1977

109. MONIF GRG, HARDY JH, and SEVER JL: The lack of association between the appearance of complement fixing antibodies and the recovery of virus in a child with congenital rubella. Pediatrics 39:289–291, 1967

110. MORGAN JR: The use of plaque methods for strain comparisons. International Symposium on Rubella Vaccines, London 1968; Symp Series Immunobiol Standard, Vol 11, Karger/Basel, New York, 1969, pp 173–176

111. MURPHY FA, HALONEN PE, and HARRISON AK: Electron microscopy of the development of rubella virus in BHK-21 cells. J Virol 2:1223–1227, 1968

112. NAEYE RL and BLANC W: Pathogenesis of congenital rubella. J Am Med Assoc 194:1277–1283, 1965

113. NATIONAL COMMITTEE FOR CLINICAL LABORATORY STANDARDS (NCCLS). Tentative Standard Rubella HI Test Method TSM-5

114. NELSON DB, QUIRIN EP, and INHORN SL: Improved dextran sulfate-calcium chloride method for the removal of nonspecific inhibitors with modifications for nonspecific agglutinin removal in the rubella hemagglutination-inhibition test. Appl Microbiol 24:264–269, 1972

115. NEVA FA and WELLER TH: Rubella interferon and factors influencing the indirect neutralization test for rubella antibody. J Immunol 93:466–473, 1964

116. NORRBY E: Haemagglutination by measles virus 4. A simple procedure for production of high potency antigen for Hemagglutination-inhibition (HI) tests. Proc Soc Exp Biol Med 111:814–818, 1962

117. OGRA PL, OGRA SS, CHIBA Y, DZIERBA JL, and HERD JK: Rubella-virus infection in juvenile rheumatoid arthritis. Lancet 2:1157–1161, 1975

118. OSHIRO LS, SCHMIDT NJ, and LENNETTE EH: Electron Microscopic studies of rubella virus. J Gen Virol 5:205–210, 1969

119. OXFORD JS, and SCHILD GC: In vitro inhibition of rubella virus by 1-adamantanamine hydrochloride. Arch Gesamte Virusforsch 17:313–329, 1965

120. OXFORD JS: The growth of rubella virus in small laboratory animals. J Immunol 98:697–701, 1967

121. PALMER DF, HERRMANN KL, LINCOLN RE, HEARN MV, and FULLER JM: (EDS): A Procedural Guide to the Performance of the Standardized Rubella Hemagglutination-inhibition Test. Center for Disease Control Immunity Series No. 2, Atlanta, Ga, 1970

122. PARKMAN PD, BUESCHER EL, and ARTENSTEIN MS: Recovery of rubella virus from army recruits. Proc Soc Exp Biol Med 111:225-230, 1962

123. PARKMAN PD, BUESCHER EL, ARTENSTEIN MS, McCOWN JM, MUNDON FK, and DRUZD AD: Studies of rubella. I. Properties of the virus. J Immunol 93:595-607, 1964

124. PARKMAN PD, MEYER HM, KIRSCHSTEIN RL, and HOPPS HE: Attenuated rubella virus. I. Development and laboratory characterization. N Engl J Med 275:569-574, 1966

125. PARKMAN PD, MUNDON FK, McCOWN JM, and BUESCHER EL: Studies of rubella. II. Neutralization of the virus. J Immunol 93:608-617, 1964

126. PARKMAN PD, PHILLIPS PE, KIRSCHSTEIN RL, and MEYER HM JR: Experimental rubella virus infection in the rhesus monkey. J Immunol 95:743-752, 1965

127. PARKMAN PD, PHILLIPS PE, and MEYER HM: Experimental rubella virus infection in pregnant monkeys. Am J Dis Child 110:390-394, 1965

128. PEETERMANS J, HUYGELEN C, and BOUILLET A: Freeze-dried rubella virus hemagglutinating antigen. Appl Microbiol 16:154, 1968

129. PENTTINEN K and MYLLYLÄ G: Interaction of human blood platelets, viruses, and antibodies I. Platelet aggregation test with microequipment. Ann Med Exp Biol Fenn 46:188- 192, 1968

130. PHILLIPS CA, MELNICK JL, and BURKHARDT M: Isolation, propagation and neutralization of rubella virus in cultures of rabbit cornea (SIRC) cells. Proc Soc Exp Biol Med 122:783- 786, 1966

131. PLOTKIN SA: Inhibition of rubella virus by amantadine. Arch Gesamte Virusforsch 16:438-442, 1965

132. PLOTKIN SA: Plaquing of rubella virus in RK$_{13}$ cells. Arch Gesamte Virusforsch 16:423- 425, 1965

133. PLOTKIN SA: Rubella: epidemiology, virology, and immunology. By TH Ingalls, SA Plotkin, HM Meyer, Jr, and PD Parkman. Am J Med Sci 253:356-364, 1967

134. PLOTKIN SA, BECHTEL DJ, and SEDWICK WD: A simple method for removal of rubella hemagglutination inhibitors from serum adaptable to finger-tip blood. Am J Epidemiol 88:301-304, 1968

135. PLOTKIN SA, BOUE A, and BOUE JG: The in vitro growth of rubella virus in human embryo cells. J Epidemiol 81:71-85, 1965

136. QUIRIN EP, NELSON DB, and INHORN SL: Use of trypsin modified human erythrocytes in rubella hemagglutination-inhibition testing. Appl Microbiol 24:353-357, 1972

137. RAFAJKO RR, POLAKAVETZ S, HANDELMAN B, and ZUR-NEDDEN D: Stability of rubella hemagglutinin. Appl Microbiol 16:423, 1968

138. RAWLS WE, DESMYTER J, and MELNICK JL: Rubella virus neutralization by plaque reduction. Proc Soc Exp Biol Med 124:167-172, 1967

139. RAWLS WE, DESMYTER J, and MELNICK JL: Serologic diagnosis and fetal involvement in maternal rubella. Criteria for abortion. J Am Med Assoc 203:627-631, 1968

140. RAWLS WE, MELNICK JL, BRADSTREET CMP, BAILEY M, FERRIS AA, LEHMANN NI, NAGLER FP, FURESZ J, KONO R, OHTAWARA M, HALONEN P, STEWART J, RYAN JM, STRAUSS J, ZDRAZILEK J, LEERHØY J, VON MAGNUS H, SOHIER R, and FERREIRA W: WHO collaborative study on the sero-epidemiology of rubella. Bull WHO 37:79-88, 1967

141. RAWLS WE and PEARSON DA: Rubella virus, In Manual of Clinical Microbiology, 2nd edition, American Society for Microbiology, Washington, DC, 1974, pp 716-722

142. REIMER CB, BLACK CM, PHILLIPS DJ, LOGAN LC, HUNTER EF, PENDER BJ, and McGREW BE: The specificity of fetal IgM: antibody or anti-antibody? Ann NY Acad Sci 254:77-93, 1975

143. RHIM JS and SCHELL K: Cytopathic and plaque assay of rubella virus in a line of African green monkey kidney cells (Vero). Proc Soc Exp Biol Med 125:602-606, 1967

144. RHIM JS, SCHELL K, and HUEBNER RJ: Plaque assays of rubella virus in cultures of rabbit cornea (SIRC) cells. Proc Soc Exp Biol Med 125:1271-1274, 1967

145. RORKE LB and SPIRO AJ: Cerebral lesions in congenital rubella syndrome. J Pediatr 70:243-255, 1967

146. SAFFORD JW JR and WHITTINGTON R: A passive hemagglutination assay for detecting rubella antibody (abstract 3351). Fed Proc 35:813, 1976

147. SALMI AA: Gel precipitation reactions between alkaline extracted rubella antigens and human sera. Acta Pathol Microbiol Scand 76:271-278, 1969
148. SALMI AA: Purification of a soluble gel precipitating antigen of rubella virus and antibody responses to the purified antigen. Acta Pathol Microbiol Scand (Section B) 80:545-558, 1972
149. SATO H: Studies on rubella virus hemagglutination. I. Activation by various treatments. Arch Gesamte Virusforsch 35:256-268, 1971
150. SCHELL K, WONG KT, TURNER HC, and HUEBNER RJ: Production of rubella complement fixing antigen in BHK-21 cells. Proc Soc Exp Biol Med 123:832-836, 1966
151. SCHIFF GM and SEVER JL: Rubella: recent laboratory and clinical advances. Prog Med Virol 8:30-61, 1966
152. SCHMIDT NJ, DENNIS J, and LENNETTE EH: Rubella virus hemagglutination with a wide variety of erythrocyte species. Appl Microbiol 16:469-470, 1968
153. SCHMIDT NJ and LENNETTE EH: Rubella complement-fixing antigens derived from the fluid and cellular phases of infected BHK-21 cells: extraction of cell-associated antigen with alkaline buffers. J Immunol 97:815-821, 1966
154. SCHMIDT NJ and LENNETTE EH: The complement-fixing antigen of rubella virus. Proc Soc Exp Biol Med 121:243-250, 1966
155. SCHMIDT NJ and LENNETTE EH: Variables of the rubella hemagglutination-inhibition test system and their effect on antigen and antibody titers. Appl Microbiol 19:491-504, 1970
156. SCHMIDT NJ, LENNETTE EH, and DENNIS J: Density gradient centrifugation studies on rubella complement-fixing antigens. J Immunol 99:399-405, 1967
157. SCHMIDT NJ, LENNETTE EH, WOODIE JD, and HO HH: Identification of rubella virus isolates by immunofluorescent staining, and a comparison of the sensitivity of three cell culture systems for recovery of virus. J Lab Clin Med 68:502-509, 1966
158. SCHMIDT NJ and STYK B: Immunodiffusion reactions with rubella antigens. J Immunol 101:210-216, 1968
159. SCHMITZ H and KRAINICK-RIECHERT CM: Simple detection of fluorescent stained IgM in sucrose gradients: demonstration of virus-specific IgM. Intervirology 3:353-358, 1974
160. SEVER JL: The epidemiology of rubella. Arch Ophthalmol 77:427-429, 1967
161. SEVER JL: Rubella antibody among pregnant women in Hawaii. Am J Obstet Gynecol 92:1006-1008, 1965
162. SEVER JL: Rubella as a teratogen In Advances in Teratology Vol 2, 1967, pp 127-138
163. SEVER JL, HUEBNER RJ, CASTELLANO GA, SARMA PS, FABIYI A, SCHIFF GM, and CUSUMANO CI: Rubella complement fixation test. Science 148:385-387, 1965
164. SEVER JL, MEIER GW, WINDLE WF, SCHIFF GM, MONIF GR, and FABIYI A: Experimental rubella in pregnant rhesus monkeys. J Infect Dis 116:21-26, 1966
165. SEVER JL and WHITE LR: Intrauterine viral infections. Ann Rev Med 19:471-486, 1968
166. SHERMAN FE, MICHAELS RH, and KENNY FM: Acute encephalopathy (encephalitis) complicating rubella. Report of cases with virologic studies, cortisol-production determinations and observations. J Am Med Assoc 192:675-681, 1965
167. SIGURDARDOTTIR B, GIVAN KF, ROZEE KR, and RHODES AJ: Association of virus with cases of rubella studied in Toronto: propagation of the agent and transmission to monkeys. Can Med Assoc J 88:128-132, 1963
168. SMITH JW and SANFORD JP: Viral arthritis. Ann Int Med 67:651-659, 1967
169. STERN H: Rubella virus complement-fixation test. Nature 208:200-201, 1965
170. STEWART GL, PARKMAN PD, HOPPS HE, DOUGLAS RD, HAMILTON JP, and MEYER HM JR: Rubella-virus hemagglutination-inhibition test. N Engl J Med 276:554-557, 1967
171. STOKER M and MACPHERSON I: Syrian hamster fibroblast cell line BHK-21 and its derivatives. Nature 203:1355-1357, 1964
172. TAYLOR RN, FULFORD KM, PRZYBYSZEWSKI VA, and POPE V: Results of the Center for Disease Control diagnostic immunology proficiency testing program for 1976. J Clin Microbiol (in Press), 1977
173. TAYLOR-ROBINSON CH, MCCARTHY K, GRYLLS SG, and O'RYAN EM: Plaque formation by rubella virus. Lancet 1:1364-1365, 1964
174. TONDURY G and SMITH DW: Fetal rubella pathology. J Pediatr 68:867-879, 1966

175. TOWNSEND JJ, BARINGER JR, WOLINSKY JS, MALAMUD N, MEDNICK JP, PANITCH HS, SCOTT RA, OSHIRO LS, and CREMER NE: Progressive rubella panencephalitis: late onset after congenital rubella. N Engl J Med 292:990-993, 1975

176. VAHERI A, SEDWICK WD, and PLOTKIN SA: Growth of rubella virus in BHK-21 cells. I. Production, assay, and adaptation of virus. Proc Soc Exp Biol Med 125:1086-1092, 1967

177. VAHERI A, SEDWICK WD, and PLOTKIN SA: Growth of rubella virus in BHK-21 cells. II. Enhancing effect of DEAE-dextran, semicarbazide and low doses of metabolic inhibitors. Proc Soc Exp Biol Med 125:1092-1098, 1967

178. VAHERI A, SEDWICK WD, PLOTKIN SA, and MAES R: Cytopathic effect of rubella virus in BHK-21 cells and growth to high titers in suspension culture. Virology 27:239-241, 1965

179. VAHERI A and VESIKARI T: Small size rubella virus antigens and soluble immune complexes, analysis by the platelet aggregation technique. Arch Gesamte Virusforsch 35:10- 24, 1971

180. VERONELLI JA and ECKERT EA: A new technique for preparation of rubella complement fixing antigen. Proc Soc Exp Biol Med 121:1223-1227, 1966

181. VERONELLI JA and MAASSAB HF: Characterization of growth of rubella virus in LLC-MK$_2$ cells. Arch Gesamte Virusforsch 16:426-437, 1965

182. VERONELLI JA, MAASSAB HF, and HENNESSY AV: Isolation in tissue culture of an interfering agent from patients with rubella. Proc Soc Exp Biol Med 111:472-476, 1962

183. VESIKARI T: Antibody response in rubella reinfection. Scand J Infect Dis 4:11-16, 1972

184. VESIKARI T: Immune response in rubella infection. Scand J Infect Dis (Supp 4):1-42, 1972

185. VESIKARI T and VAHERI A: Rubella: a method for rapid diagnosis of a recent infection by demonstration of the IgM antibodies. Br Med J 1:221-223, 1968

186. VESIKARI T, VAHERI A, and LEINIKKI P: Antibody response to rubella virion (V) and soluble (S) antigens in rubella infection and following vaccination with live attenuated rubella virus. Arch Gesamte Virusforsch 35:25-37, 1971

187. VESIKARI T, VAHERI A, PETTAY O, and KUNNAS M: Congenital rubella: immune response of the neonate and diagnosis by demonstration of specific IgM antibodies. J Pediatr 75:658-664, 1969

188. VOLLER A and BIDWELL DE: A simple method for detecting antibodies to rubella. Br J Exp Pathol 56:338-339, 1975

189. VOLLER A and BIDWELL DE: Enzyme immunoassays for antibodies in measles, cytomegalovirus infections, and after rubella vaccination. Br J Exp Pathol 57:243-247, 1976

190. WALLIS C, MELNICK JL, and RAPP F: Different effects of MgCl$_2$ and MgSO$_4$ on the thermostability of viruses. Virology 26:694-699, 1965

191. WEIL ML, ITABASHI HH, CREMER NE, OSHIRO LS, LENNETTE EH, and CARNAY L: Chronic progressive panencephalitis due to rubella virus simulating subacute sclerosing panencephalitis. N Engl J Med 292:994-998, 1975

192. WELLER TH, ALFORD CA JR, and NEVA FA: Retrospective diagnosis by serologic means of congenitally acquired rubella infections. N Engl J Med 270:1039-1041, 1964

193. WELLER TH and NEVA FA: Propagation in tissue culture of cytopathic agents from patients with rubella-like illness. Proc Soc Exp Biol Med 111:215-225, 1962

194. WHITMIRE CE, FUCCILLO DA, GITNICK GL, and SEVER JL: Problems in the detection of rubella virus in African green monkey tissue culture. Proc Soc Exp Biol Med 128:253-257, 1968

195. WITTE JJ, KARCHMER AW, CASE G, HERRMANN KL, ABRUTYN E, KASSANOFF I, NEILL JS: Epidemiology of rubella. Am J Dis Child 118:107-111, 1969

196. WONG KT, BARON S, and WARD TG: Rubella virus: role of interferon during infection of African green monkey kidney tissue cultures. J Immunol 99:1140-1149, 1967

197. ZIRING PR, FLORMAN AF, and COOPER LZ: The diagnosis of rubella. Pediatr Clin North Am 18:87-97, 1971

CHAPTER 26

ARBOVIRUSES

Robert E. Shope and Gladys E. Sather

Introduction

The arboviruses (arthropod-borne animal viruses) are a heterogeneous group of viral agents linked together in classification by certain basic epidemiologic characteristics. In principle, any virus classified as an arbovirus must be maintained in nature principally by a continuous cycle through biological transmission (multiplication and extrinsic incubation period) by an arthropod vector to a vertebrate, producing a viremia which is infectious to another suitable arthropod vector after taking a blood meal. Insofar as it is known, the virus during such a cycle is always acquired by a hemophagous vector from vertebrate blood. Once infective, the vector usually remains so for life. No pathologic histology has been recognized in naturally infected vectors. Evidence supporting these criteria for all the viruses usually included in this group has not been found. Assumptions have been made on the basis of findings for those few viruses adequately studied. Most arboviruses are maintained in a cycle involving arthropod vectors and a lower vertebrate. Infection in humans is not essential to the maintenance and dissemination of most arboviruses, and the diseases which result are therefore considered to be zoonoses.

In addition to those viruses meeting the above criteria many are classified tentatively as arboviruses on incomplete but suggestive evidence, and some are so classified on no epidemiologic evidence whatsoever but on the basis of a serologic relationship to a known arbovirus. Some arboviues maintained in ticks (11), in phlebotomines (61), and mosquito-borne viruses of the California group (68) are transmitted transovarially and, in some instances, venereally (64) in the arthropod. In addition to the principal arthropod-borne methods of transmission, a few well established agents can be transmitted from time to time without the mediation of an arthropod, through throat secretions or other excreta, and arthropod transmission may occasionally be by mechanical rather than by biologic means.

History

Before 1940 only 15 viruses now classified as arboviruses had been isolated or proved to be filterable agents. All of these were obtained directly

767

from sick mammals and most of them after 1930. Only 7 were first isolated from humans, rather than other animals. These 7 included the viruses causing yellow fever, dengue fever, St. Louis encephalitis, Japanese (B) encephalitis, Russian spring-summer encephalitis (RSSE), Bwamba fever, and West Nile fever, in about that order. Since 1950 the numbers isolated have increased rapidly, with a preponderance coming from arthropods and sentinel animals. Today more than 400 viruses are tentatively classified as arthropod-borne (6, 33).

Clinical aspects

As might be expected from such a heterogeneous group of agents the clinical manifestations are diverse in animals and humans. Since this volume is devoted to the diagnosis of disease in humans the manifestations in this host alone are considered (Table 26.1).

Diseases of humans can be divided roughly into 4 large categories: fever, encephalitis, hemorrhagic fever, and polyarthritis.

Fever. The first and largest group of diseases, usually relatively benign, consists of the fevers. Many of these are dengue-like in character with a duration of 3–7 days. The onset is usually abrupt with fever, headache, and general malaise frequently associated with vomiting or only nausea, and pain on moving the eyes. Muscle or joint pains may be conspicuous; a macular or maculopapular rash, or a series of rashes may or may not be present. Lymphadenopathy is also variable. Leukopenia, sometimes very marked, is quite common.

Encephalitis. The second most frequent form of disease is encephalitis or meningoencephalitis, a far more serious syndrome associated with significant case-fatality ratios and residual motor or mental damage. Milder infections with the same viruses frequently greatly outnumber those with central nervous system involvement.

Hemorrhagic fever. This group produces several very serious epidemic diseases with high case-fatality ratios. Yellow fever, with additional heavy liver damage, is included in this group, since it also may have the hemorrhagic manifestations. Again, as in the previous group, many milder infection do not cause obvious bleeding and resemble the milder fevers.

Polyarthritis. Viruses of group A, including Ross River, chikungunya, o'nyong nyong, and Mayaro cause arthritis sometimes without fever and often with rash. The arthritis may be very painful but is generally self-limited.

Pathology

An attempt to describe the many aspects of pathology of these various diseases requires more space than is available. For the fevers, little is known since mortality is rare. Little is known about the lesion responsible for the leukopenia. The encephalitides are produced by destructive and inflammatory type lesions involving neurons. Focal and disseminated involvement tends to vary in pattern with different viruses, but, in general, no specific lesion or pattern observed in a single case permits a specific etiologic diagnosis. Perivascular cuffing is common, and lesions are frequently present in the spinal cord as well as in the cerebrum. Yellow fever has a specific and pathognomonic liver lesion. The hemorrhagic lesions of the various hemorrhagic fevers are not specific. Vascular necrosis is not observed. There is a general and frequently massive diapedesis of erythrocytes (RBC) from capillaries observed in a variety of skin lesions and in many other tissues, including heart and other viscera. Edema and hemorrhage are usually conspicuous. A mild or severe thrombocytopenia is a common finding and appears to be due in part to inactivity of megakaryocytes, apparently present in normal numbers.

Description and Nature of Viruses

Physical and chemical characteristics

The major groups of arboviruses fall into 5 taxons: *alphaviruses, flaviviruses, bunyaviruses, orbiviruses, and rhabdoviruses* (Table 26.1). All contain ssRNA, except the orbiviruses which contain dsRNA. The RNA of bunyaviruses and orbiviruses is segmented. All except the orbiviruses have an essential lipid envelope, making the infectious particle sensitive to ether, chloroform, and sodium deoxycholate. The alphaviruses measure 60 nm in diameter, flaviviruses, 30 nm; bunyaviruses, 95 nm; orbiviruses, 80 nm; and rhabdoviruses 60 × 180 nm. Considerable variation in dimensions is observed, depending on the virus and method of size determination. In general, they are rather unstable viruses, readily inactivated by relatively little heat (37–56 C) and inactivated more readily on the acid side of neutrality than on the alkaline side. They appear to be quite stable at temperatures of about −70 C and, when lyophilized, at 5 C. In neutral or slightly alkaline glycerol (50% at 5 C), tissue containing virus usually remains infective for months and in the case of some arboviruses, for years. Practically all arboviruses produce encephalitis in suckling mice and hamsters, and some produce it in guinea pigs, monkeys, and other animals. Those viruses classed in the immunologic Group A (Table 26.1) are resistant to most proteolytic enzymes, those in group B are not. Similarly, certain sulfhydryl reagents inactivate members of several groups but not of Group A. Arbovirus hemagglutination is inhibited by numerous lipids and lipoproteins. Only a very small proportion of the arboviruses have been subjected to some of these tests and, even within a group, assumptions are frequently made on the basis of the characteristics of a few. Some of these assumptions may prove to be limited in their application.

Classification

The 5 major taxons which contain arboviruses are listed above; in addition, African swine fever is an *iridovirus* and Cotia is a *poxvirus*. These iso-

TABLE 26.1—ARBOVIRUSES PRODUCING DISEASE IN HUMANS, BY IMMUNOLOGIC GROUP, VECTOR, AREA, AND DISEASE SYNDROME

GROUP AND VIRUS	VECTOR	GEOGRAPHIC AREA	DISEASE SYNDROME
TOGAVIRUS			
Group A (alphavirus)			
Chikungunya	Mosquito	Africa, Southeast Asia, Philippines, India	Fever, hemorrhagic fever, arthritis
Eastern equine	Mosquito	Americas	Encephalitis
Everglades	Mosquito	USA	Encephalitis
Mayaro	Mosquito	South America, USA	Fever
Mucambo	Mosquito	South America	Fever
O'nyong nyong	Mosquito	Africa	Fever, arthritis
Ross River	Mosquito	Australia	Polyarthritis
Sindbis	Mosquito	Africa, India, Southeast Asia, Philippines Australia	Fever
Venezuelan equine	Mosquito	South and Central America, Mexico, Florida	Fever, encephalitis
Western equine	Mosquito	Americas	Encephalitis
Group B (flavivirus)			
Banzi	Mosquito	Africa	Fever
Bat Salivary (Rio Bravo)	Unrecognized	North America	Encephalitis
Bussuquara	Mosquito	South America	Fever
Central European encephalitis	Tick	Europe	Encephalitis
Dengue 1	Mosquito	Southeast Asia, India, Pacific Islands, Caribbean, Africa	Fever, hemorrhagic fever
Dengue 2	Mosquito	Southeast Asia, India, Pacific Islands, Caribbean, Africa	Fever, hemorrhagic fever
Dengue 3	Mosquito	Southeast Asia, India, Philippines, Pakistan, Caribbean	Hemorhagic fever, fever
Dengue 4	Mosquito	Southeast Asia, Philippines, India	Hemorrhagic fever, fever
Ilheus	Mosquito	Central and South America	Encephalitis
Japanese B	Mosquito	Eastern and Southeast Asia, Japan, Ryukyus, Taiwan India, Philippines, Guam, Indonesia	Encephalitis
Kunjin	Mosquito	Australia	Fever
Kyasanur Forest	Tick	India	Hemorrhagic fever
Louping ill	Tick	British Isles	Encephalitis
Murray Valley	Mosquito	Australia, New Guinea	Encephalitis
Negishi	Unrecognized	Japan	Encephalitis
Omsk	Tick	Asia	Hemorrhagic fever
Powassan	Tick	North America	Encephalitis
Russian spring summer (TBE)	Tick	Europe, Asia	Encephalitis

TABLE 26.1—ARBOVIRUSES PRODUCING DISEASE IN HUMANS, BY IMMUNOLOGIC GROUP, VECTOR, AREA, AND DISEASE SYNDROME *(Continued)*

GROUP AND VIRUS	VECTOR	GEOGRAPHIC AREA	DISEASE SYNDROME
Sepik	Mosquito	New Guinea	Fever
Spondweni	Mosquito	Africa	Fever
St. Louis	Mosquito	Americas, Jamaica	Encephalitis
Wesselsbron	Mosquito	Africa, Southeast Asia	Fever
West Nile	Mosquito	Africa, Middle East, India, Europe	Fever, encephalitis
Yellow fever	Mosquito	Africa, Central and South America	Hemorrhagic fever
Zika	Mosquito	Africa, Southeast Asia	Fever
BUNYAVIRUS			
Group C			
Apeu	Mosquito	South America	Fever
Caraparu	Mosquito	South America	Fever
Itaqui	Mosquito	South America	Fever
Madrid	Unrecognized	Panama	Fever
Marituba	Mosquito	South America	Fever
Murutucu	Mosquito	South America	Fever
Oriboca	Mosquito	South America	Fever
Ossa	Mosquito	Panama	Fever
Restan	Mosquito	South America	Fever
Bunyamwera group			
Batai (Calovo)	Mosquito	Czechoslovakia, Malaya, India	Fever
Bunyamwera	Mosquito	Africa	Fever
Germiston	Mosquito	Africa	Fever
Guaroa	Mosquito	South America, Panama	Fever
Ilesha	Mosquito	Africa	Fever
Tensaw	Mosquito	USA	Encephalitis
Wyeomyia	Mosquito	South America, Panama	Fever
Bwamba group			
Bwamba	Mosquito	Africa	Fever
California encephalitis group			
California	Mosquito	North America	Encephalitis
Inkoo	Mosquito	Finland	Fever
LaCrosse	Mosquito	North America	Encephalitis
Tahyna	Mosquito	Europe	Fever
Guama group			
Catu	Mosquito	South America	Fever
Guama	Mosquito	South America	Fever
Sandfly fever group			
Candiru	Phlebotomine	Brazil	Fever
Chagres	Phlebotomine	Panama	Fever
Naples sandfly fever	Phlebotomine	Europe, Middle East	Fever
Punta Toro	Unrecognized	Panama	Fever
Sicilian sandfly fever	Phlebotomine	Africa, Middle East, Sicily	Fever

TABLE 26.1—ARBOVIRUSES PRODUCING DISEASE IN HUMANS, BY IMMUNOLOGIC GROUP,
VECTOR, AREA, AND DISEASE SYNDROME *(Continued)*

GROUP AND VIRUS	VECTOR	GEOGRAPHIC AREA	DISEASE SYNDROME
Simbu group			
Oropouche	Mosquito	South America	Fever
Shuni	Mosquito	Africa	Fever
Congo-Crimean hemor-			
rhagic fever group			
Congo-CHF	Tick	Africa, Asia, Europe	Hemorrhagic fever
Nairobi sheep disease			
group:			
Dugbe	Tick	Africa	Fever
Nairobi sheep disease	Tick	India, Africa	Fever
Thogoto group			
Thogoto	Tick	Africa, Europe	Fever
Ungrouped			
Rift Valley fever	Mosquito	Africa	Fever, hemorrhagic fever, encephalitis
Tataguine	Mosquito	Africa	Fever
ORBIVIRUS			
Changuinola group			
Changuinola	Phlebotomine	Panama	Fever
Colorado tick fever group			
Colorado tick fever	Tick	USA	Fever
Kemerovo group			
Kemerovo	Tick	Europe, Africa	Fever
RHABDOVIRUS			
Vesicular stomatitis group			
Vesicular stomatitis-Indiana	Phlebotomine	North and Central America	Fever
Vesicular stomatitis-New Jersey	Phlebotomine	North and Central America	Fever
Chandipura	Mosquito	India, Africa	Fever
POXVIRUS			
Cotia	Mosquito	South America	Fever
UNGROUPED			
Bangui	Unknown	Africa	Fever
Quaranfil	Tick	Africa	Fever
Nyando	Mosquito	Africa	Fever
Zinga	Mosquito	Africa	Fever

SOURCE: References 6 and 33

lated examples of presumed arboviruses outside of the 5 major groups are decidedly unusual.

At the time of this writing, a rough estimate of the probable number of significantly different arboviruses is in excess of 400 (6, 33). By serologic tests—neutralization (Nt), complement fixation (CF) and hemagglutination-inhibition (HAI)—these viruses were classified (principally by Casals and coworkers) into a series of antigenic groups. In general, all viruses showing any significantly detectable immunologic relationship by any of these tests are placed in 1 group. Within a group, several showing the most intimate relationship, one to the other, form a subgroup or complex. The main immunologic groups and their further subdivisions are not yet subject to international nomenclature because regroupings and new groups are continually being established as more types of immunologic tests are performed on a larger number of agents.

A list of those now-classified arboviruses currently believed to produce disease in humans on the basis of one or more naturally acquired clinically apparent infections is presented in Table 26.1 in "groups" based upon their antigenic relationships. This list, even by the time of publication, will be incomplete, and some of the arboviruses listed may be based on erroneous diagnosis or information. Furthermore, classification as shown is not always clear-cut by all tests, and minor overlapping of some member or members in one group with one or more of those in another group has been shown. The listing has several purposes: to indicate antigenic groups believed to be responsible for human disease, to indicate the type of diseases which may be expected from any one virus or members of the group, to indicate the recognized or suspected vector, and to show that viruses are recognized in certain geographic areas. This information may assist in deciding what viruses might be suspected in the patient from whom specimens were submitted.

Hosts Other Than Humans

Vectors

Diagnostic leads can be obtained by epidemiologic considerations other than geographic areas. Vectors known to be present and active at the season of the exposure may furnish useful leads. These also are listed by group (e.g., mosquito, tick, or others) in Table 26.1.

Recognized vectors are in order of frequency as presently known: mosquitoes, ticks, sandflies (*Phlebotomus* and *Lutzomyia*), midges (*Culicoides*), and possibly mites. No viruses producing disease in humans are as yet recognized among those transmitted by midges.

Vertebrate hosts

Two types of vertebrate hosts in nature are of particular importance: those which play an important role as sources of vector infection and those which do not but in which overt disease occurs. Of primary interest from an epidemiologic standpoint are the former which, together with the vector, serve in the role of reservoir-disseminator of arboviruses. The criteria which characterize this role are many but the presence of a high-titer viremia of adequate duration, and attractiveness and availability of the host to the vector are among those of greatest importance. With the exception of arboviruses which cause dengue, urban yellow fever, and chikungunya virus infection—humans do not appear to play an essential or important role in the maintenance and dissemination of arboviruses. When humans are infected, it is usually a biologic accident and a dead-end for the virus. Definite reservoir vertebrates vary for each virus. Many of the zoonotic viruses depend predominantly on avian hosts, some on rodents, and some on larger mammals. Reptiles, amphibians, and bats are suspect as overwintering vertebrate hosts for a few of these viruses.

Preparation of Immune Serum or Ascitic Fluid

The procedures described here basically follow those devised by Casals (12, 14) and Clarke and Casals (21) who found that, because of nonspecific reactions attributable to heterologous host antibodies resulting from use of different species of laboratory animals, it is advisable to use exclusively, if at all possible, the suckling and weanling mouse for the source of virus and antiserum for *in vitro* tests.

A 10^{-2}–10^{-4} dilution of infected suckling mouse brain suspension (stock virus) is inoculated intracerebrally (ic) into a sufficient number of litters of suckling mice, 1- to 3-days of age, to provide infected mouse brains to immunize a group of mice for antiserum or immune ascitic fluid. When definite signs of illness are observed in the inoculated mice and a few of the mice are moribund or dead, the brains are harvested aseptically either by removing the skull cap with scissors and scooping out the brain with a small spatula, scoop, or forceps, or by a closed vacuum system, such as described by Strome (58). The brains are preferably used fresh. Adequate but somewhat lower antibody responses are obtained with brains stored frozen at about −70 C (Revco) in quantities sufficient to prepare at the time of use each immunizing suspension of infected brain. For each immunizing dose, a 10% suspension of infected suckling mouse brain is prepared by homogenizing in a chilled, sealed blender in phosphate-buffered saline (PBS), pH 7.4, or in borate-saline solution, pH 9. This homogenized suspension need not be centrifuged before inoculation.

Whenever possible it is advisable to utilize specific pathogen-free mice for production of immune reagents since the presence of naturally occurring antibodies to other viruses can lead to confusing results.

A variety of protocols are used for mouse immune-serum production. For some viruses, adequate antibody levels are produced after 1–2 injections but for some, additional injections are required. However, for definitive identification and comparative studies a standard procedure should be adopted.

For production of mouse hyperimmune serum, 5- to 6-week-old weanling mice, preferably female, are given a series of 4 intraperitoneal (ip) inoculations (0.2 ml) of a freshly prepared 10% suspension of frozen infected suckling mouse brain at 7-day intervals and bled 7 days after the last inoculation. For those viruses pathogenic for weanling mice by the ip route, inactivated virus is substituted for the live virus for the first two immunizing doses and live virus, prepared as above, is administered for the third and fourth injections. For inactivation with formalin, a total volume of 10% suspension sufficient to inoculate each mouse twice with 0.1 or 0.2 ml is centrifuged at 800 × g for 30 min, and the supernatant fluid is treated with 0.2% formalin for 7 days (held at 4 C and shaken at least once a day). Inactivation by beta-propiolactone (BPL), as devised by Clarke (19), may be substituted. This is performed as follows: a 10% suspension of infected suckling mouse brain is prepared in pH 9, 0.1 M Tris buffer. The buffering to alkalinity is considered important because of the rapid hydrolysis of BPL when diluted, yielding an acid which may be deleterious to the antigenic composition of some arboviruses. Because of this hydrolysis, it is advisable to dilute the BPL in 2 steps. BPL is a colorless fluid in sealed ampules, preserved from decomposition by refrigeration under 0 C, and it should be freshly prepared each time it is used.

BPL is a carcinogen in concentrations of ≥1% and should be handled with gloves in a glove box or exhausted hood. The ampule is opened and 0.5 ml of BPL is withdrawn into a 1.0- or 2.0-ml syringe. This is expressed into 4.5 ml of chilled water in a test tube. Another needle and syringe is used for mixing, and 0.5 ml of this 10% BPL solution is transferred as before to 4.5 ml chilled water to make a 1% BPL solution.

This 1% dilution of the original BPL is then added to the pH 9 infected-brain suspension in appropriate volume to make a final concentration of 0.1% BPL, which is sufficient to inactivate infectivity of most 10% arboviral suspensions held at 4 C for 18 hr. With alphaviruses, a final concentration of 0.3% BPL is recommended. A specially purified grade of BPL should be used (39, 40).

The immunized animals are bled under ether-anesthesia at the appropriate time by cardiac puncture or by jugular or axillary exsanguination. Axillary bleeding is easy to perform and generally results in good serum yields. For this, the body of the anesthetized animal is dipped in a suitable disinfectant, e.g., 70% alcohol, and pinned down ventral side up. The skin at the midline over the chest is slit, pulled to one side with a hemostat and held to form a pocket and to expose the axillary vessels. With sharp scissors the vessels are cut, and as the blood flows into the pocket, it is withdrawn with a 2- to 5-ml syringe attached to a 16–18-gauge needle. By this means up to 2 ml or more of blood can be recovered from a single animal. The blood is pooled in tubes, held at room temperature to clot, and refrigerated overnight for maximal clot retraction. After centrifugation in the cold at 500 × g for 15 min or longer, the supernatant serum is withdrawn, pooled, and stored frozen in multiple portions.

If repeated bleedings are desired, small amounts of blood, no more than 0.5 ml, are obtained by retro-orbital bleeding (42) or by cardiac puncture.

Much larger yields per mouse may be obtained by preparing mouse immune ascitic fluid; the antibody titers in antiserum and immune ascitic fluid are comparable. Immune ascitic fluid is produced by incorporating adjuvants with the immunizing doses (9) or by utilizing a variant ascites cell line, sarcoma 180/TG (TG = thioguanidine resistant) (53, 65). In another satisfactory procedure, Freund complete adjuvant (Difco Laboratories, Detroit, Michigan) and sarcoma 180/TG are combined. Greater yields appear to be obtained from female mice, 5–6 weeks of age at initiation of immunization. A satisfactory protocol is as follows: day 1, 10% infected suckling mouse brain mixed with an equal part of Freund complete adjuvant, 0.2 ml ip; this inoculation is repeated on days 7 and 14; 0.5 ml Freund complete adjuvant is given ip on day 18; day 21, same inoculation as day 1. By day 28 it should be possible to remove ascitic fluid by paracentesis with an 18-gauge needle into a 10-ml syringe. Alternatively, fluid flows freely through a 16-gauge needle into a tube. Generally it is possible to tap the same animals for 3–4 successive weeks. The ascitic fluid is pooled. A fibrin clot will form in the fluid, but this can be removed by centrifugation. The immune ascitic fluid is stored in a manner similar to that used for immune serum. For those viruses pathogenic for weanling mice by the ip route, an injection of inactivated virus is given 7 days before the inoculation of the virus-adjuvant mixture.

In some laboratories, sarcoma 180/TG tumor cells are given on day 28 of the above protocol to obtain an increased volume of ascitic fluid. This technique is satisfactory, although the resulting fluid is somewhat lower in antibody titer, and the mice may develop mouse tissue antibody CF reactions by the tenth day after inoculation of sarcoma 180/TG (7). Mice die 2–3 weeks after implantation of sarcoma 180/TG.

Generally, the sarcoma 180/TG tumor cells are maintained in the peritoneal cavity of mice. Scherer (personal communication) reported successful maintenance of the sarcoma 180/TG cells by freezing them with 10% glycerol on dry ice in a manner similar to that described for the preservation of human HeLa and mouse L cells (54). Cells preserved as long as 227 days have produced ascites and sarcoma within 1–2 weeks in ip-inoculated mice.

It should be emphasized that the procedures outlined for the production of immune serum or ascitic fluids only provide a guide, and for certain viruses modifications are indicated.

Normal control serum or control ascitic fluid is prepared in a similar way, by using normal mouse brain in place of infected mouse brain. The immune serum or ascitic fluid should be characterized by tests in homologous systems utilizing the CF, Nt and, when possible the HAI tests.

Under special circumstances different procedures may have to be used to produce specific sera. For instance, the subtypes of California encephalitis virus are not easily separated by CF testing of hyperimmune mouse serum. Hamster serum taken 10–21 days after single inoculation by the subcutaneous (sc) or ip routes was relatively specific by CF test (57).

Collection and Preparation of Specimens for Laboratory Diagnosis

Precautions

Laboratory infections, with or without clinical disease, have been all too frequent among those working with the arboviruses. A survey of arboviruses and arenaviruses shows 36 viruses to have produced disease in workers in the laboratory, causing 16 deaths (7 viruses) and 428 illnesses (26, 27).

A large number of illnesses have been of serious import, some producing residual clinical manifestations or months of hospitalization, or both. Other patients in still larger numbers have had 3- to 7-day febrile illnesses, generally of a dengue-like nature, but a few have been alarmingly ill. Among the most serious infections have been yellow fever, western equine encephalitis (WEE), eastern equine encephalitis (EEE), St. Louis encephalitis (SLE), and Russian Spring-Summer encephalitis (RSSE), tick-borne encephalitis (TBE), and Rift Valley fever. Venezuelan equine encephalitis (VEE), Kyasanur Forest, louping ill, West Nile, chikungunya, and vesicular stomatitis viruses (VSV) have induced disease with considerable frequency, although not usually resulting in residual changes or death. Clinical cases of dengue and Colorado tick fever virus infection, in addition to a few other diseases, have occurred in more limited numbers. It is important to note that isolation and identification of certain of these viruses, together with antigen preparation and the performance of serologic tests with viable antigens are associated with risks which are sometimes very serious. These risks must be recognized and infection prevented. Such risks differ as to source and route of infection for different arboviruses. Unless the dangers from any virus with which one chooses to work are adequately understood and suitable safeguards are made available and used, the virus should not be introduced into the laboratory and no attempts should be made to isolate it from specimens from suspected cases.

Excreta from mice and certain other animals inoculated with members of the RSSE-TBE complex of agents, including louping ill and Kyasanur Forest viruses, are highly infectious. The same is true for VEE virus. "Wet" chicks (just hatched) inoculated with EEE and WEE viruses have been shown to excrete large amounts of virus.

The Center for Disease Control (CDC) in a bulletin entitled *Classification of Etiologic Agents on the Basis of Hazard* (1976), describes the physical containment recommended for arboviruses. These containment levels are assigned numbers (CDC-2, CDC-3, and CDC-4). The arboviruses listed for CDC-2 containment are Cache Valley, Flanders, Hart Park, Langat, Sindbis, Tensaw, Turlock, and 17 D yellow fever. Those listed for CDC-3 containment include dengue, vesicular stomatitis, yellow fever used *in vitro*, and all strains not CDC-2 or CDC-4. The CDC-4 containment should be used for hemorrhagic fever agents, tick-borne encephalitis virus complex, epidemic strains of Venezuelan encephalitis when used for transmission or animal inoculation experiments, and yellow fever virus when used for transmission or animal inoculation experiments. Precise operational requirements for safe handling of many specific arboviruses are described in DHEW publication CDC 76-8118, *Laboratory Safety at the Center for Disease Control* (1971, reprinted 1975). In general terms, CDC-2 containment involves closed doors, decontamination of work surfaces and experimental materials, mechanical (not mouth) pipetting, prohibition of food or smoking in laboratory, washing of hands, minimizing aerosols, forbidding children in the laboratory, biohazard instruction, rodent and insect control, use of laboratory clothing (not to be worn outside of laboratory), and avoidance of needles and syringes where possible. Biological safety cabinets for procedures producing aerosols and sealed centrifuge heads or cups are used. Contaminated materials are kept in a closed vessel and autoclaved in the same building.

CDC-3 containment is more stringent. In addition to the above measures, CDC-3 containment should have all manipulations done in a safety cabinet, such as a vertical laminar-flow hood, biohazard signs, negative-pressure ventilation in a laboratory restricted to authorized personnel, non-recirculated air with filtered exhaust, an autoclave in the laboratory area, sealed windows, and use of gloves and protective laboratory clothing. Special precautions are recommended for holding infected insects and animals. The insects are secured in screened cages, which, in turn, are in a room secure from escape of insects. Animals are held in filter top cages, in cages enclosed in a laminar-flow hood or room, or in isolators maintained under negative pressure with filtered exhaust air.

Containment classified as CDC-4 is available in only a few laboratories in the world. Completely closed and sealed units serviced by gloves in ports, or sealed units entered by personnel wearing 1-piece positive-pressure isolation suits are required. Elaborate ventilation, chemical disinfection, and safety training make this containment beyond the means of most laboratories.

There is no substitute for intelligent, well-trained laboratory personnel. Commonsense handling of viruses prevents most laboratory infections. Personnel should be immunized against arboviruses for which a vaccine is available. Yellow fever vaccine is licensed in the United States; eastern, western, and Venezuelan encephalitis (41) experimental vaccines are available, as is Rift Valley fever experimental vaccine (49).

Following a known laboratory exposure to a potentially dangerous agent, every attempt should be made to inoculate the person within the next 12–24 hr with an appropriate hyperimmune or convalescent-phase serum or gamma globulin concentrate (69). Supplies of human immune serum for a limited spectrum of arboviruses are available on an emergency basis from CDC. A dose should be administered intramuscularly or intravenously which is calculated to be detectable as free neutralizing antibody in the recipient's blood for about 1 week after injection. Infiltration of serum about the wound, as recommended in rabies prophylaxis, would also appear to be indicated. Tests for sensitivity must be carried out before any heterologous serum or serum product is given. In considering the use of immune human serum or plasma, the risk of hepatitis must always be taken into account.

Virus isolation

The optimal method for determining specific etiology of an arbovirus infection requires isolation of the virus from a specimen obtained from the patient during the acute stage of the disease and the demonstration of a rise in titer of an antibody to the isolate during convalescence. For a number of reasons successful isolation of most arboviruses from specimens from patients is the exception, reasons being that the specimen to be examined is not collected soon enough, is not properly handled, or is not expeditiously transmitted to the virus laboratory for inoculation.

The viremia for many arbovirus infections in humans, if detectable at any stage, ceases by the time of or soon after onset of symptoms—a stage when antibody is often demonstrable. Because some circulating virus may be recoverable and the antibody may be absent, or present in low titer, the acute-phase blood specimen should be collected immediately upon suspicion of a viral etiology. Delay of an hour or so can compromise the chance of virus isolation; the allowable time depends upon the type of complex of viruses involved. For example, mosquito-borne encephalitis viruses such as Japanese B and SLE have very rarely been isolated from the circulating blood of patients, but West Nile, yellow fever, dengue, VEE, and the tick-borne viruses have rather routinely been isolated from serum collected up to several days to a week following onset of symptoms. In a few instances encephalitis viruses may be detected in cerebrospinal fluid (CSF) or even in throat collections if timed properly. Therefore, detection of virus by performance of appropriate laboratory tests and interpretation thereof depend upon the elapsed time after infection in relation to viremia, onset of disease, and development of antibodies. Because of the absence or the transient nature of post-onset viremia with most arboviruses, diagnosis is usually dependent upon a rise in titer of antibodies. During the acute-phase, the most likely sources of virus in order of probability are blood, throat swabs, and CSF, the latter two less frequently.

In general, antibody appears to be the inhibiting factor in the attempt to isolate virus, though interferon may also be involved. To reduce the effect of antibody or interferon, isolation attempts should be made not only with undiluted material but also with dilutions from 1:10 to 1:50. Whole defibrinated blood, serum, plasma or clot may be productive, and one may be more successful than another, depending on the virus, the time of collection, and the means of isolation to be employed. Serum is most frequently used. Portions not immediately used should be held at about −70 C in a series of tubes or ampules for subsequent tests—either for confirmation by reisolation, for tests at varying dilutions, or in another isolation system, as well as for serologic tests for comparison with convalescent-phase specimen.

In fatal illnesses, a variety of tissues should be tested; the most suitable organ and the frequency of success varies with the disease. In the encephalitides, however, the brain and spinal cord frequently contain detectable virus. Principles and methods of preparation of source material are essentially identical with those for isolation of most other viruses. Solid tissues should be thoroughly homogenized in a manner to protect the environment from aerosol and to keep the material near 5 C. A final tissue concentration of 10–20% is generally prepared in a diluent with pH 7.2-8.5 and containing 20–50% animal serum or bovine albumin (Fraction V) ranging from 0.75-2.0% to partially stabilize the virus. The animal serum should be free of antibodies to the virus sought (if known). Rabbit, horse, calf, and monkey sera have all been used. The tissue homogenate is centrifuged at 500-800 $\times g$ for 15-20 min, the supernatant fluid is removed for inoculation at one or more dilutions into a susceptible host or cell culture, and a portion is held frozen at about −70 C for subsequent testing. Tests for bacterial sterility, both aerobic and anaerobic, should be employed routinely. To ensure freedom from other microorganisms capable of producing lesions in the susceptible biologic system employed, the following must be included: asepsis; antibiotics (a final concentration of 200 units penicillin, 40 μg streptomycin, and 10 units polymyxin are satisfactory); centrifugation at 12,000 $\times g$ for 60 min, or filtration, preferably without reduction of the number of virus particles.

Serologic diagnosis

In the diagnostic serology of arbovirus infections, valid test results and their interpretation depend on the cardinal principles of collection, preparation, preservation, and handling of the blood specimens: timely collection with sterile precautions, in adequate quantity, followed by comprehensive and detailed documentation; appropriate refrigeration and proper storage; and expeditious dispatch to the laboratory.

The time to collect an acute-phase blood specimen is as soon as a viral etiology is suspected. Collection of an adequate (substantial) volume of acute-phase blood is essential, for there is only one opportunity to collect this important specimen at the earliest point in time relative to the course of infection. Adequacy of volume may well determine ultimate success in establishing definitive serologic diagnosis in situations where a number of arboviruses are possible etiologic agents or when a variety of serologic tests may be necessary. An adequate quantity of whole blood is considered to be not less than 10 ml, and 15–20 ml are preferred.

The tube is held at room temperature for 20–30 min, the period required for the clot to form. The specimen is then refrigerated at 4 C (on wet ice or in a refrigerator) to accelerate contraction of the clot. Subsequent centrifugation at 270 $\times g$ for 10 min packs the clot for maximal serum yield. With a rubber bulb attached to a sterile Pasteur pipette, the serum is carefully withdrawn from the clot and is transferred to a sterile, well-stoppered tube or to a screw-cap vial.

If the time from collection of a first or acute-phase specimen until dispatch to the laboratory is to be prolonged and the serum is to be examined for virus isolation, the serum is frozen on dry ice or by mechanical refrigeration below −40 C. If frozen on dry ice, the container holding the serum must be tightly sealed to prevent entrance of CO_2 which will inactivate an arbovirus. If submitted only for serologic study, the serum need not be frozen, but the temperature should not exceed 5 C during the temporary holding period. Repeated freezing and thawing, or temperature fluctuation between 0 and −20 C, are particularly deleterious to both viruses and antibodies.

The physician, epidemiologist, virologist, or laboratorian should decide whether circumstances indicate that the single acute-phase specimen should be examined serologically at once or should await collection of a second specimen or of additional serum during convalescence for demonstration of a rise in antibody titer. Serologic examination of paired sera is usually the only requirement. If collected and handled under sterile conditions, tightly sealed containers of serum may be dispatched at ambient temperatures in appropriate packages, by mail or express. Refrigeration is definitely to be preferred, when available. Specific instructions for shipping serum are given in Chapter 1 and are detailed in several available references (22, 35). Labile accessory substance is frequently present and important in antibody tests for a number of arboviruses; therefore, refrigeration during shipment is to be insisted on, when practicable.

Laboratory Diagnosis

Virus isolation

Laboratory rodents. By far the greatest number of successful arbovirus isolations have been made by ic inoculation (0.01 or 0.02 ml) into suckling mice (usually 1–3 days of age) and frequently combined with the subcutaneous or ip route (0.03–0.05 ml) (Fig 26.1). The suckling mouse is considered to be the universal host system. The suckling hamster, when available and compared, has generally given closely comparable results, and in rare instances better results. These 2 species of small suckling rodents are best inoculated without anesthesia, using a 0.25- or 1-ml tuberculin-type syringe with a 25-, 26-, or 27-gauge needle. The inoculation is made slightly lateral to the midline and into the midportion (or slightly anterior to it) of one lateral hemisphere. No antiseptic need be used, and it is probably advantageous not to use any since its presence on the fur might, in contact with the needle, inactivate any extremely small amount of virus present in the fluid being inoculated. The infant mice are also less likely to be rejected by their mother when antiseptics are avoided. All infant mice (up to 6 or 8) of 1 or 2 litters are usually given each type of material to be tested. Litters containing more than 8 infant mice are reduced to 8 in order to equalize litter size and also because the mother will take better care of smaller litters when disturbed. Mice that die in less than 24 hr are usually discarded unless the suspect virus is one of those known to have an extremely short incubation period (several viruses in group A). Generally, nonspecific deaths and cannibalism occur within a few hours of inoculation. After the first 24 hr, careful inspections must be made twice a day, or more frequently, for any signs of abnormal behavior. Great clinical skill is required in this examination to prevent the selection of normal animals for sacrifice or failure to detect illness before death and to prevent possible cannibalism by the mother. In the very young animals a few of the suggestive signs to be watched for are failure to eat (no milk in stomach), unusual color, wasting or runting, unusual activity, tremors, or lying on the side. When animals are somewhat older, paralysis is frequently seen, especially with agents which are poorly mouse adapted. Usually, 15 days is an adequate period of observation, but with certain dengues and a few other viruses another week may be required.

Mice (or other animals) noted to be ill should be euthanized, the skull cap removed aseptically with scissors, and the brain scooped out. The brains are prepared as 20% emulsion in a standard buffered serum or albumin containing diluent between pH 7.2 and 8.0 in the same manner as described above. Portions of this are frozen for subsequent testing. Tests are again

Figure 26.1—Flow chart for virus isolation

	Living Patient	*Autopsy*
Material for inoculation:	1) Blood, serum, plasma (fevers chiefly) 2) Throat secretions (fevers, rare) 3) CSF (encephalitis, rare)	1) Brain, multiple portions of gray areas (encephalitis) 2) Spleen, lung, liver, other organs (hemorrhagic fevers, rare)
Preparation:	Clot homogenized Blood defibrinated or serum or plasma removed from clot. Use undiluted and diluted ≥ 1:10.	Tissue homogenized as 10–20% suspension in buffer with protein stabilizer and antibiotics. Centrifuge at 500–800 × g for 20 min. Use at 10^{-1} and 10^{-2} tissue dilutions.

Inoculation:

1) Suckling mice (1–3 days) ic (0.01–0.02 ml) and sc (0.03 ml)
   and/or
2) Suckling hamsters ic (0.01–0.02 ml)
   and/or
3) Variety of cell cultures—for CPE and/or plaques
4) Chick embryo (for certain group A viruses); yolk sac and/or embryonic stab or chorioallantoic membrane
5) Mosquitoes

Observation:	1) Rodents— Abnormal behavior or death	2) Cell cultures—CPE Plaques FA	3) Chick embryos—Sluggish movement Death	4) Mosquitoes FA CF
Passage material:	1) Brain from suspect rodent (prepare 10% wt/vol as above). 2) Liver—Observe condition (prepare 10% wt/vol as above). Note: Some arboviruses have a higher titer in liver than in brain.	1) Supernatant fluid 2) Supernatant fluid plus cells 3) Agar plug from plaque	Whole chick embryo (with eyes, beak and legs removed) Suspension of chorioallantoic membrane (prepare 10% wt/vol as above).	Subculture in mice or TC Mosquitoes or other TC

Passage for establishment or adaptation of agent:	Inoculate same host, variety of tissue culture systems, and other animals—weanling mice, weanling hamsters, guinea pigs. (Blood survivors may be used for serologic tests.)

Figure 26.2—Flow chart for identification of an isolate

Passage serially in proven susceptible host system until infectivity titer $\geq 10^{-5}$ and incubation period and death or cell injury pattern are regular. Prepare bacteriologically sterile stock as 20% infected-tissue suspension in protein-stabilized diluent.

Identify:

If suspected identity is limited to a few known viruses for which antisera are available:
1) Prepare pH 9 borate saline suspension for CF and HAI tests.
   1. Test for HA and pH range.
   2. Test by CF and/or HAI vs specific antisera.
2) Confirm identity by Nt test or perform Nt test instead of CF or HAI test.
3) If virus belongs in group with cross-reactions:
   a. Prepare purified antigens and immune and hyperimmune sera.
   b. Perform cross-quantitative comparisons with other group members by most discriminating test or tests: CF, HAI, Nt, vaccination-cross challenge.

If identity is not suspected:
1) Demonstrate filterability, or size by filtration or electron-microscopy.
2) Demonstrate ether or sodium deoxycholate sensitivity.
3) Investigate host range.
4) Prepare immune and/or hyperimmune serum.
5) Determine ability to produce HA by sucrose-acetone extraction and sonication.
6) On basis of criteria established test by Nt, CF, and/or HAI against broad group and suspect specific antisera.
   or
   Send with all available data and reagents to regional laboratory for identification.
7) If identified, confirm identity by cross-block CF and Nt, and vaccination cross-challenge tests with known virus.
8) Consider as a new arbovirus, if it fulfills all criteria of an arbovirus but is not antigenically identical or closely related to known viruses or virus groups. Register in *Catalogue of Arthropod-Borne Viruses of the World.*

Reisolate from original material for confirmation.

made for bacterial sterility. A 10^{-1} dilution is prepared and passage is made to 1 or 2 more litters of the same species, and possibly to other animals, including weanling mice, by both the ic and ip routes, or into tissue cultures. If essentially all of the mice have died within a rather short and constant incubation period, procedures usually postponed until adaptation has been established may be carried out (Fig 26.2). At this time it should be determined that the agent is filterable, and the approximate size determined by filtration through membranes of graded sizes.

Chick embryos and newborn chicks. For a few viruses, principally some in Group A, chick embryo inoculation has proved useful and is preferred by some workers, but in most laboratories this system has been abandoned in favor of others. The newborn chick (wet chick) has also been similarly used, but the highly infectious cloacal discharges pose unnecessary dangers.

Cell cultures. Unfortunately, there is still no universal cell culture system for the isolation of arboviruses. However, most arboviruses can be grown with the production of either cytopathic effects (CPE) or plaques, or both, in several or many cell cultures. The number and variety of these are too great to tabulate and do not greatly differ from those described in Chapter 3. However, among those with the widest range for arboviruses are the continuous cell lines, Vero (71), BHK-21 (34), and CER (56), and among the primary cells, hamster kidney, chick embryo and duck embryo. When cell cultures are used, the usual precautions to ensure freedom from living bacteria or mycoplasmas in the test materials must be adhered to with much greater care than necessary with mice. In addition, to prevent excessive toxicity, materials to be tested may require dilution or removal by washing after a period of absorption to the cell sheet.

When CPE or plaques suggest that an agent has been isolated, supernatant fluid from the cell cultures or an agar plug from the latter is collected for culture and passage, and portions are frozen as in the case of mouse tissues.

Mosquito cell culture. Arboviruses may be readily isolated in mosquito tissue culture and in mosquitoes by inoculation. *Aedes albopictus* (Singh) tissue culture is susceptible to a wide variety of agents, however, its sensitivity is slightly less than the baby mouse, and a detection system, such as CF, FA, or infectivity assay in mice or vertebrate tissue culture, must be employed because CPE does not usually occur. Mosquito tissue cultures grow at ambient temperature and can be taken directly into the field when incubators are not available and when specimens cannot be refrigerated. *Aedes pseudoscutellaris* tissue culture has been used for primary isolation of yellow fever virus (66), as well as for dengue virus.

Aedes albopictus tissue culture is maintained on Mitsuhashi-Maramorosch medium (42) with 20% fetal bovine serum, 10,000 units of penicillin, 10,000 μg streptomycin, and 0.05% amphotericin. Infected samples can be tested at 7 days for virus and can be held for as long as 3 or more weeks with virus still detectable by CF, FA, and infectivity in mice.

Mosquitoes. Arboviruses are readily isolated in mosquitoes by intrathoracic inoculation. This is the method of choice when dengue virus is suspected. The mosquito does not sicken, and therefore an indirect method, such as CF, FA, or virus assay, must be used to demonstrate antigen or infectivity, as with mosquito tissue culture.

The method of Rosen and Gubler for dengue viruses is described here (50). Female and male *Aedes albopictus* mosquitoes are equally susceptible; males are preferred for safety reasons. Borosilicate glass tubing of outside diameter 0.7–1.0 mm is drawn to a point after heating, and the tip is broken to form a needle. It may be calibrated if accuracy is needed. The needle is attached to a holder, which is in turn attached by plastic tubing to a syringe with a 3-way stopcock. The needle is filled with the inoculum and the tip introduced into the membranous area anterior to the mesepisternum and below the spiracle in females, or through the neck membrane of male mosquitoes. Mosquitoes are immobilized by cold, CO_2, or smoke. A measured amount is inoculated by gentle pressure on the syringe. Mosquitoes are held for 7–10 days at 32 C with high relative humidity and access to 10% sucrose solution. Infectivity is detected in vertebrate tissue culture. Antigen is demonstrated by testing extracts of pooled mosquitoes by CF (36) or by testing mosquito head squashes by the direct FA technique (37). Since some human sera are toxic for mosquitoes, it is recommended that test sera be inoculated at a 1:5 dilution.

Aedes aegypti and *Toxorhynchites amboinensis* mosquitoes have also been used successfully for isolation of dengue viruses (37). The *Toxorhynchites* is a large mosquito and has the advantage of tolerating a much larger inoculum than does *Aedes*. Both males and females can be used, since safety precautions need not be considered, and a few *Toxorhynchites* produce large quantities of virus, facilitating detection by FA and identification.

Identification of isolates

Occasionally, isolates may be identified at the time of harvest of a suitable tissue from the chosen biologic system but, in general, adaptation must be accomplished by serial passage in a suitable system (Fig 26.2). Adaptation is recognized when deaths, CPE, or plaques occur consistently in an essentially constant incubation period, and a titration in 10-fold dilutions indicates that the lesion is produced by a dilution of the crude harvest tissue at about $\geq 10^{-5}$. Frequently, even higher titers must be obtained, and rarely can satisfactory identification be made with materials of lower titer. Bacteriologic sterility should be demonstrated.

Serologic tests for identification. If the type of arbovirus is suspected from knowledge of the circumstances, a stock antiserum against a prototype strain of that virus may be used at this point, or one may employ several antisera prepared against a few viruses known to be present in the area and in the host from which the specimen was derived. In most areas a few appropriate polyvalent grouping sera like A, B, C, Bunyamwera and California encephalitis (CEV) can prove to be of great value in partially identifying most agents.

It is strongly recommended that personnel of any laboratory planning on isolating or identifying arboviruses acquaint themselves with the known arboviral flora of their area and prepare identifying reagents for such.

Any one of several standard serologic tests described can be employed in this preliminary phase of the identification, i.e., Nt, CF, HA, double diffusion in agar, FA, etc. Some of these are more specific than others, and even the most specific may simply give a group identification. For any virus in a recognized group (Table 26.1) type-specific identification is required, usually a task to be performed in a reference laboratory. However, if other viruses representing the group are known not to be present in the area or not capable of infecting the host involved, comparison is simplified. In any case, complete identification requires serologic comparison between the new isolate and the prototype in both directions with essentially equal results. For this an antiserum must be prepared against the isolate. Nt is usually the preferred and accepted method for such comparisons, but not necessarily so. For viruses in group B, immunization-cross challenge is frequently resorted to for final identification within a subgroup.

The immunization-challenge test is described here for mice although any laboratory animal which succumbs to the effects of the virus may be used. In addition, in animals which do not die but which develop viremia, absence of viremia may be used as an indicator of protection, a system applied specifically to immunization-challenge of monkeys with dengue virus.

Mice 4-6 weeks old are immunized by a single 0.5 ml ip inoculation of a 10% suspension of infected mouse brain in saline or of undiluted infected tissue culture fluid. Usually the immunizing material is the unknown virus to be identified. Approximately 48 mice are immunized and an equal number of litter-mates are held without immunization as a control. Four weeks later the challenge virus is inoculated ic 0.03 ml in 10-fold increasing dilutions each to 6 immunized and 6 control mice. The mice are observed for death for 3 weeks and the log LD_{50} of the titration in immunized mice is subtracted from the log LD_{50} of control mice and expressed as the log protective index, a measure of relatedness of the immunizing to the challenge virus.

The test may be adapted by varying several parameters: the number and route of immunizing inoculations, the use of killed virus vaccine as opposed to live vaccine, and the timing and route of inoculation of the challenge.

If a virus is isolated and proves not to be one of a small number suspected, the task becomes far more complicated, and it is usually wisest to send it to a regional laboratory together with a complete history of the source material and all laboratory results obtained thus far. Nevertheless, a laboratory without a battery of many viruses and identifying antisera may make some helpful progress by using other nonspecific types of characterization, such as the following.

Size determination. This may be roughly determined by the smallest porosity of membrane through which the virus will pass without substantial loss in titer. Most arboviruses will pass a 50-nm size, and still others are larger. Reference sources on sizes would be of assistance here (14).

Ether or sodium deoxycholate sensitivity tests. With the exception of orbiviruses, arboviruses are sensitive to lipid solvents and detergents. If not sensitive and not an orbivirus, the agent is probably not an arbovirus; if it is sensitive, it may possibly be a member of several other groups, such as herpesviruses, myxoviruses, poxviruses, and coronaviruses, which are similarly sensitive, but these viruses are generally larger. Picornaviruses and reoviruses are not sensitive.

The test with ether is the simplest but seemingly is less frequently used (1, 62). Cold diethyl ether is added in a ratio of 1 to 2 or 4 parts of 10% or 20% suspension of a well-centrifuged infected tissue suspension in a buffer system (pH 7.2 to 8.0) with 0.5% bovine albumin. This is shaken, placed in an "explosion proof" refrigerator, or otherwise held at 0-5 C, with occasional shaking, for 12–18 hr. A control sample to which nothing is added is held in the same manner. At the end of the holding period the ether is removed in a separatory funnel followed by vacuum, or by vacuum alone and the remaining aqueous material is tested in 10-fold serial dilutions for infectious virus in a suitable system, simultaneously with the control material.

The more commonly used, but more complicated, sodium deoxycholate (SDC) test was described by Theiler (62). One is cautioned that an excess of protein or particulate matter in the virus suspension may interfere with the action of SDC and lead to erroneous results. A modification of Theiler's method is described here. A 1:500 dilution of commercially available SDC (Fisher, purified) is prepared in 0.75% bovine albumin phosphate-buffered saline solution (BAPS), pH 7.4, and sterilized by filtration. A 20% virus suspension is prepared in 0.75% BAPS and centrifuged at 12,000 $\times$ g for 60 min. The supernatant is used for SDC sensitivity tests. One portion is mixed with an equal volume of 1:500 SDC BAPS (or 1:100 SDC BAPS) and 1 portion (control) is mixed with an equal volume of 0.75% BAPS. These are incubated in a 37 C waterbath for 1 hr; the test and control are titrated in serial 10-fold dilutions in a suitable host system, and the titers are compared.

A loss of ≥ 1.5 log in titer indicates the virus is sensitive to SDC or ether, but does not necessarily mean it is an arbovirus. In some cases, resistant viruses exhibit a higher titer in the presence of SDC or ether than in the control titration. In selecting a test system, one should keep in mind that SDC may be toxic to certain cell culture systems.

Orbiviruses are relatively resistant to ether and sodium deoxycholate. A few strains are readily inactivated, but most lose about 0.5 log ID_{50}. The orbiviruses, in contrast to reoviruses and picornaviruses, are inactivated at pH 3 (8).

Acid sensitivity test. Virus is suspended in modified Eagle medium with 10% newborn calf serum at pH 7.5. To the virus is added pH 2.7 bicarbonate-HCl buffer in Eagle medium until the resulting final pH is 3. Control virus is diluted in the same volume of Eagle medium at pH 7.5. Both control and test specimens are held at 4 C for 3 hr and then diluted and assayed for infectivity (8).

Animal or cell culture host range. Incubation period by various routes of inoculation in mice, susceptibility of weanling mice by the ic or the ip route of inoculation, susceptibility of the guinea pig by ic inoculation, of rabbits by the ic route, of monkeys usually also by the ic route, of the chick embryo by the allantoic membrane or yolk-sac route of inoculation, or the production of CPE or plaques on a variety of primary or continuous cell cultures frequently furnishes an excellent lead in virus identification. These characteristics, however, may vary depending on the number of previous passages and the host used. Also, virus strain variations to host susceptibility may exist in nature.

All animals used in these and subsequent techniques should be cared for in a humane manner, with the principles of laboratory animal care as promulgated by the Animal Health Division, Agricultural Research Service, USDA (32) being observed.

Formation of hemagglutinins. Many arboviruses show only low-titer or no hemagglutinin by the commonly used sucrose-acetone preparation methods when applied to mouse brain. This characteristic may also help in identification, but again, strain variations occur with some viruses and the degree of adaptation to the mouse may play a role.

Electron microscopy. With the greatly increased availability of this laboratory tool, characteristics may be detected which assist in identification. Examinations are made on thin sections of brain, tissue culture, or ultracentrifuge pellets, or by negative staining of purified suspensions or concentrates. Determination of the size and shape of the virus is most useful. All arboviruses studied appear to replicate only in the cytoplasm. Several, like VSV, are elongated or bullet-shaped like rabies virus, and recognition of such characteristics greatly facilitates identification.

Other methods of identification. In special circumstances in which a large number of isolates is being made of a limited number of viruses, many variations and short cuts may be introduced for preliminary or tentative identification. For example, a concentrated emulsion of infected suckling mouse brain is placed in the central well of a micro double gel-diffusion slide of the Ouchterlony type (43, 46), surrounded by antisera (absorbed for removal of antibody to normal tissue components) of several types in the peripheral wells. If a precipitin line occurs between one of the antisera and the mouse brain emulsion, tentative identification is provided and confirming tests can be applied. Another useful procedure, applied when cell culture isolation techniques are utilized, is to inoculate a series of cultures with the inoculum mixed with specific antisera; inhibition by an antiserum indicates the probable identity of the isolate, if the culture without serum or those with other sera show a viral effect.

Confirmation

A virus isolate identified as similar in type to one in use in the laboratory must always be suspect as to origin until confirmation is obtained. If isolated from a living person, an increasing antibody titer to the virus in paired serum samples from the patient may be accepted as partial or adequate confirmation. Lacking this, reisolation from a preserved portion of the original specimen becomes important. Even this, however, may not establish the source, for the original inoculum may have been contaminated while it was being prepared, and the preserved portion would then contain the same contaminant. Prevention of laboratory contamination thus becomes extremely important, and wherever and whenever possible, those engaged in any phase of virus isolation should work only in a room where no known, living viral agents are handled, and at no time should they handle laboratory virus strains or visit areas where they are present.

Confirmation of still another type is occasionally needed to avoid other serious problems. Colonies of laboratory mice or other animals are frequently infected with latent viruses which become clinically apparent in some animals after needle trauma or other stresses. These agents are seldom arboviruses but occasionally have been. Checking of older animals for antibodies can serve as a useful control.

Serologic diagnosis
Techniques available

For diagnostic serologic studies on a patient, for serologic surveys, or for identification of a virus isolate, 1 or more of 3 major serologic techniques can be employed. These, as mentioned before, are Nt, CF, and HAI tests. Other specialized techniques showing promise are Ouchterlony double diffusion in gel (29, 43, 46), immunoelectrophoresis (30), hemadsorption-hemagglutination inhibition (10) and enzyme-linked immunosorbent assay (67). The latter have all been used to advantage in limited studies but have not yet been applied to a large number of the arboviruses and therefore are not discussed here.

The most widely used diagnostic technique in arbovirology is the CF test. Variations in quality and reactivity of antigens, the frequent development of anticomplementary activity in serum collected and stored under widely varying conditions, and difficulties in interpreting results leave much to be desired in the diagnosis of arboviral infection by this technique alone. Since CF antibodies are frequently of relatively brief duration (a few months to a few years), they may have limited application to serologic survey for past infections.

Tests for HAI antibodies were developed more recently and, if properly done, are highly reliable. In general, HAI antibodies tend to be more group-specific and less type-specific; they appear earlier than CF and Nt antibodies, and disappear more rapidly than Nt antibodies. In some arboviral infections they reach a very early peak and then fall rapidly. Most normal sera contain nonspecific HAI substances which must be removed by extraction, and various methods of treatment to eliminate these can have varying effects on the antibody titer, or can remove part or all of the IgM.

The Nt test is the oldest, most tried, most reliable and probably the most readily interpreted of all and usually is the most type-specific. The plaque reduction Nt test is highly quantitative. In general, Nt antibodies last longer than the others and in many instances are life-long, making this test particularly useful for serologic survey of past infections. Although the serum of humans may frequently contain nonspecific virus inactivating substances for certain other groups of viral agents, requiring preliminary heat inactivation, this is not known to be the case for the arboviruses. Unfortunately, a certain labile component or components, as yet undefined, frequently referred to as "accessory substance(s)", are present in some human sera, and their state of preservation or loss, as influenced by storage, may occasionally produce some confusion in interpretation, particularly when undiluted sera are tested.

The FA test offers the possibility of making a rapid diagnosis on biopsy or postmortem tissue of the patient, on arthropod tissue such as a mosquito head-squash, or on infected tissue culture cells or mouse brain or liver after passage of an isolate. The direct FA method is simpler than the indirect (IFA) and is preferable when nonspecific fluorescence is a problem such as with arthropod tissues. The direct technique has been effectively applied to rapid diagnosis of Colorado tick fever by visualization of antigen in RBC (22a) and to West Nile virus in brain (45). The IFA test has the advantage of greater sensitivity and of application when a battery of known reagents such as mouse ascitic fluids is to be tested with a single antigen. The IFA test is also readily applied to detection of antibody using the spot slide test described in Chapter 27.

Complement-fixation test

Preparation of antigens. For many arboviruses, crude antigens for use in both CF and HAI tests may be quickly prepared in pH 9 borate saline solution as 10% infected suckling mouse brain suspensions and centrifuged at 12,000 × g for 1 hr at 4 C. These crude antigens can be used in either type of test for rapid but tentative identification of a virus isolate. They are generally of low titer and more often anticomplementary than more purified antigens and are not recommended for routine diagnostic serology. For some arboviruses, useful HA antigens cannot be prepared by any currently known method, and for others only HA antigens produced by highly refined means can be used. However, satisfactory CF antigens can be prepared for all arboviruses.

Useful CF and HA antigens for certain arboviruses have been made from chick embryo membranes, weanling mouse and hamster brains, and infected tissue culture fluids. However, for the production of high-titer arboviral antigens the suckling mouse is the best and is a universally available source.

To eliminate nonspecific and anticomplementary reactions most effectively, several different lipid solvent extraction techniques have been developed. Clarke and Casals (21) devised the sucrose-acetone method, which preserves the hemagglutinin for many arboviruses as well as the CF antigen. This permits the use of 1 antigen preparation for both CF and HAI tests. Because substantial lipid is not deposited in mouse brain until about 1 week after birth, production of a partially purified, lipid-free antigen is facilitated by the use of suckling mouse brain as a source.

For preparation of a sucrose-acetone antigen, animals from an appropriate number of suckling mouse litters 1–2 days old are inoculated ic and held, and timed for harvest. They are exsanguinated by severing the carotid and jugular vessels; the brains are harvested as described above. The brains are frozen immediately in an open tube or beaker in a dry ice-alcohol bath and then held frozen at about −70 C in a mechanical freezer until the antigen can be prepared. The antigen is prepared with maximal safety precautions. All operations should be carried out in a laminar-flow biological safety cabinet.

The total weight of brain harvest and container is determined and then that of the container after the brains have been transferred to a cold aerosol-tight homogenizer. Four volumes of an 8.5% aqueous solution of sucrose are added, and the brains are homogenized for three 1-min cycles. All manipulations during extraction are carried out in an ice-water bath.

In a proportion of 1 volume of homogenate to 20 volumes of acetone (9 ml to 180 ml), the homogenized mouse brain suspension is expressed rapidly from a syringe with an 18-gauge needle into a container of acetone. The acetone is decanted, leaving the sediment to which 20 volumes of chilled acetone is immediately added. The antigen suspension is shaken vigorously then held 1 hr at 4 C. The supernatant acetone is decanted carefully, and the sediment is dried at room temperature for 1 hr on a vacuum pump, with an intermediate cotton-filled filter flask used as a trap.

The antigen sediment and the supernatant acetone are infectious and dangerous and should be handled under a hood. Because of the volatile nature of the solvents, open flame, sparks, and smoking must be avoided in any room where this antigen extraction is carried out. The discarded acetone is autoclaved or disinfected with hypochlorite solution.

To this dried residue in the container is added sterile 0.1 M Tris buffer, pH 9, in a volume equal to only 0.4 of the original volume of the brain homogenate, or about double the weight of the original brain harvest, which is the key figure in estimating the number of mice required to produce a specified amount of antigen. The container with glass beads is tightly stoppered and vigorously shaken for a few minutes, then placed at 4 C. The sediment should dissolve in 1 or 2 hr, but may be left overnight at 4 C; the latter is preferable for complete hydration. The solution is then centrifuged in the cold at 12,000 $\times$ g for 60 min using the multispeed attachment of the PR2 International Centrifuge, or its equivalent. The supernatant fluid is the antigen. It should be transferred to ampules and frozen at -70 C or lyophilized for storage at 4 C.

Normal mouse brain control reagent is prepared by extracting uninfected suckling mouse brains in the same manner.

The number of antigen controls required can be reduced by using antigens that are prepared from the same type of tissue and in the same manner; therefore mouse brain antigen is most frequently used. However, liver is a more suitable source of antigen for certain viruses.

Antigens may be inactivated with heat (15) or with BPL (55) diluted to a final concentration of 0.3% for alphaviruses and 0.1% for all other arbovirus groups. The BPL-treated antigen is held for 3 days at 4 C before the undiluted antigen and dilutions of 1:10 and 1:100 are tested for safety.

Procedure for test proper. Since a number of antigens must be used to establish a specific etiology in some situations, the volume of the test serum available often prevents complete testing. Therefore, for CF tests one of the microtechniques should be used. One microtechnique is outlined in Chapter 1; another is that of the Center for Disease Control referred to as the Laboratory Branch Complement Fixation (LBCF) technique.

The serum to be tested is inactivated in a 1:4 dilution with the test diluent for 20 min at 60 C for human, monkey, or mouse serum, at 62 C for hamster, and 56 C for guinea pig serum. If the serum is anticomplementary, it is sometimes possible to eliminate this characteristic by inactivaiton at 65 C for 20 min or by inactivating on 2 successive days at 60 C. A modificaiton of the method of Taran (60), with guinea pig complement, is described in Chapter 1. All these methods to remove or reduce the anticomplementary property of the serum may reduce specific titer somewhat, but they should permit interpretation of results more readily, provided any other serum from the same patient is treated in the same manner.

Suitable antigens generally have a titer of 1:32–1:128 or higher. The proper antigen dilution to use in a test is determined by a ''checkerboard'' or "crossblock" titration of varying antigen dilutions tested against varying dilutions of a hyperimmune serum prepared according to a standard protocol. For routine tests use the dilution of antigen which gives the highest serum titer. A 10-fold more concentrated antigen dilution should also be used because some heterologous reactions are detected only with concentrated antigen. Excess antigen tends to inhibit the reaction, and a "zoning" phenomenon may be observed with low dilutions of a high-titer antigen.

In addition to the viral antigens employed, an antigen prepared against normal tissue of the type used for preparing the viral antigens is included for control. Anticomplementary controls are included for each serum and antigen. A preliminary and a test complement control titration are made for each antigen included in the test because tissue antigens vary in their ability to fix complement nonspecifically. During the conduct of the test all reagents are held in an ice-water bath. The test is performed with 2 units of complement and incubated overnight at 4 C before sensitized cells are added (Chapter 1).

Interpretation of CF test. The CF test is usually less specific than the Nt test and tends to show more overlap with other members of the same group. A 4-fold rise or fall in titer is considered diagnostic of infection by a member of the virus group. If a titer of $\geq 1:8$ is obtained in serial sera without a 4-fold difference, it is important to determine the time of specimen collection before stating that the titer derived from some previous infection, because such an antibody level without change in titer, though indicating probable past infection, does not rule out possible etiologic association with the subject's illness; all the sera may have been collected during the phase of maximal antibody titer. A negative result for this test is not an adequate basis for ruling out infection with the test virus in some instances; serum may have been collected too early for CF antibody to be detected. Tests on a later serum or use of another type of test may show diagnostic evidence of infection.

Hemagglutination-inhibition test (HAI)

Preparation and standardization of antigens. Occasionally, particularly with certain group B arboviruses, a crude borate saline antigen contains satisfactory hemagglutinin. Such crude antigens are not recommended for diagnostic or survey serologic testing but only for preliminary identification of isolates. The new virus may be prepared as a 1:10 dilution of the stock (frozen suspension or rehydrated lyophilized stock) in cold (4 C) bovine-albumin-borate solution (BABS), pH 9. All antigen dilutions are made in this diluent. Generally, with new isolates the titer is so low, or the antigenic character is so obscure, that extraction as described below is required.

The same extracted antigens as prepared for CF are routinely used for the diagnostic or survey HAI test, i.e., the sucrose-acetone extracted type. However, the pH range for activity of hemagglutinins from some viruses may be extremely narrow or the HA pattern formed may be unsatisfactory or nonexistent. It has been observed that protamine sulfate treatment (21) of the finished antigen may broaden its pH range, especially toward the acid side and improve the pattern. The effect depends on the virus and type of preparation, and the treatment may produce no effect or an increase or decrease in the HA titer at the optimal pH. The HA properties of an antigen should be determined before this treatment, and it should be applied only to those antigens where it appears desirable to improve the reaction. One is warned that protamine has hemagglutinating activity which is most manifest at low pH (6.0 to 6.4) and low temperature (4 C). This effect appears to be inhibited in the presence of low concentrations of bovine albumin. Therefore, if HA activity is manifest only after protamine treatment and at low pH, it must be viewed with suspicion until demonstrated to be viral.

The sucrose-acetone extracted antigen is chilled in an ice-water bath and treated by adding 0.1 volume of a protamine preparation consisting of 50 mg protamine sulfate per ml of 0.15 M NaCl (protamine sulfate is available from Nutritional Biochemicals Corp., Cleveland, OH). A dense white precipitate forms immediately. The mixture is then held in the ice-water bath for 30 min with occasional shaking and then centrifuged at $800 \times g$ for 15 min at 4 C (PR2 International Centrifuge or equivalent). The clear supernatant fluid is the antigen.

Ardoin and Clarke (3, 4) have reported that sonication produces a marked improvement in the HA titers of group C arboviruses. Their studies, with modifications, have been extended to additional arboviruses and have indicated that not only are marked antigen titer increases obtained in many instances, but that some viruses which did not yield usable HA antigens by other means could now be employed as antigens. Most of the viruses successfully treated are bunyaviruses.

The antigen is prepared by the usual sucrose-acetone extraction method and rehydrated in 0.15 M NaCl overnight at 4 C. This rehydrated antigen is not centrifuged. Low intensity sonication is carried out on the uncentrifuged rehydrated antigen for 1–2 min with 1–2 min cooling periods. The recommended apparatus for sonification is the Branson Sonifer, (Heat Systems Co., Melville, LI, NY). Equipment should include the following: micro-tip for small volumes, rosette cooling cells for good heat exchange, and sealed atmosphere treatment chamber for hazardous viruses. These are repeated 2–3 times. Low-intensity sonication has been used throughout most of the investigative work, with good antigen yields; the effect of higher intensities for sonication has not as yet been adequately determined. The following precautions should be observed. Thin-wall containers should be used, either glass or plastic, to ensure good heat exchange. The temperature should be monitored at the end of each sonication burst to determine that proper control is being maintained. The most effective cooling is achieved by use of NaCl-ice-water bath, with magnetic stirring, but if the salt concentration is too high, the antigen may freeze between sonication bursts. This is probably not harmful to the antigen, but it delays the procedure. The container size must be adjusted to the antigen volume. Too small a volume per container leads to foaming and poor processing. The probe must be centered and deeply immersed to avoid foaming. After sonication the antigen is centrifuged for 10 min at $500 \times g$; a small, well-packed pellet forms. The supernatant fluid is the antigen and it is tested for HA activity over an extended pH range.

If a satisfactory HA antigen has not been obtained at this point, it can be treated with trypsin. For trypsin treatment, 2 preparations have been used: Difco 1:250 crude at a final concentration of 256 μg/ml and Worthington 2X crystallized at a final concentration of 16 μg/ml. Difco trypsin appears to give slightly better results. The trypsin preparation to be used is assayed to ascertain the approximate potency. An assay kit is marketed by Worthington (Determatube TRY, which permits measurement of the rate of splitting of the ester of N-benzoyl-I-arginine). The antigen is treated with approximately 140 units/ml of trypsin for 40 min at room temperature and pH 9. At the end of 40 min the action of trypsin is promptly terminated by adding soybean trypsin inhibitor. Worthington crystalized inhibitor is added at a weight equal to the total weight of Difco trypsin present. If the antigen is turbid, centrifuge it for 10 min at $500 \times g$, and test the supernatant fluid for HA activity over a broad pH range. Resonication (4 times 2 min) at minimal intensity usually improves the post-trypsin titer.

A problem encountered with trypsin-treated antigens is a nonspecific HA, giving a pattern like that of an arbovirus. This pattern has been produced from both normal and infected suckling mouse brains. Presence of a nonspecific HA is suspected when the HA occurs over rather a wide pH range, and it can be proven to be nonspecific by the fact that it is not specifically inhibited by immune ascitic fluid or serum. The production of this HA seems to be favored by incubation at 37 C, as well as by higher trypsin concentration. Because of the phenomenon of nonspecific HA, all antigens must be tested by HAI before diagnostic use, with homologous, heterologous, and normal fluids. Some antigens, on standing at room temperature for a few hours or overnight, or for 1–2 days, show further titer increase. The antigens store well at 4 C and at about −70 C (mechanical freezer). A few treated antigens have been lyophilized after a little bovine albumin has been added without a significant titer loss. Calcium phosphate treatment has been used to increase the sensitivity of group C antigens (2).

An alternative method of antigen preparation which has been quite successful for rhabdoviruses and California encephalitis group viruses (25, 18) employs BHK-21 suspension cell cultures and inhibitor-free medium. BHK-21 cells are suspended in BHK-21 growth medium with 10% heat-inactivated fetal bovine serum and 10% tryptose phosphate broth, and grown for 24 hr in spinner culture flasks at 35 C. The cells are then centrifuged and resuspended to give 1.2×10^9 cells in 100 ml of bovine albumin medium (the fetal bovine serum is replaced with 0.4% Fraction V bovine plasma albumin). The cells are inoculated with virus at a multiplicity of 0.1 or 1.0 and incubated at 35 C for 2 hr, with gentle agitation; then bovine albumin medium is added to bring the volume to 800 ml, and the pH is adjusted with 5% $NaCO_2$ to 7.2. At 24 hr and periodically thereafter, the supernatant culture fluid is tested for HA.

Serum HA antigens, superior in sensitivity to brain or liver-derived antigens, are produced from infected mouse or hamster serum for alpha- and bunyaviruses (20). A technique used successfully in the senior author's laboratory is described here.

Three-day-old mice are inoculated ic with approximately 3 log LD_{50} of virus, and batches of mice are bled by cutting the jugular veins at 24, 36, 48 and 72 hr after inoculation. The optimal time for bleeding varies with the virus. The resulting serum is diluted 1:5 in normal saline and expressed through a 23-gauge needle into 20 volumes of chilled acetone. The mixture is centrifuged by bringing the rotor speed to $500 \times g$ and stopping immediately (excessive packing is deleterious). The supernatant acetone is decanted, and the sediment is resuspended in 20 volumes of chilled acetone, shaken, and held for 1 hr at 4 C. The mixture is then centrifuged at $500 \times g$ for 10 min at 4 C, the acetone decanted, and the sediment dried for 1 hr on a vacuum pump. The sediment is rehydrated at 1:10 the original serum volume in borate saline buffer (BSB), pH 9, and stored lyophilized at 4 C or frozen at -70 C.

Procedure for hemagglutination (HA) titration. The demonstration of HA by arboviruses is pH dependent, and different arboviruses vary in the pH range of optimal activity and the titer produced. Therefore, it is necessary to titrate the antigen in the presence of different pH solutions to determine the HA titer and the dilution to use for demonstrating HA antibodies in diagnostic or survey serum.

A 1:10 antigen dilution is prepared in the antigen diluent (0.4% BABS, pH 9) after it has been thawed or suspended from the lyophilized state. The 1:10 antigen dilution is allowed to stand for at least 1 hr at 4 C before it is used, to permit complete dissociation and exposure of antigenic particles. Serial 2-fold dilutions starting at the 1:10 dilution are prepared in the antigen diluent.

The antigen dilutions are tested at the following pH: 5.75, 6.0, 6.2, 6.4, 6.6, 6.8, 7.0, and 7.4, using goose erythrocytes (RBC) suspended in buffers of the proper pH (see below) as an indicator of HA. The HA titration is performed in plastic plates (Linbro Chemical Co. Inc., New Haven, CT) either by the macrotechnique (0.8 ml total volume) or the microtiter technique (0.1 ml total volume). Eight rows (1 row for each pH) of 9 antigen dilutions (1:10–1:2560) are distributed or prepared on the plates in 0.4 ml or 0.05 ml quantities. The tenth well on the plate should contain an equal amount of diluent to serve as a control for nonspecific agglutination of the RBC at that pH. To each well in each row is added an equal amount of goose RBC suspended at 0.75 OD (optical density) in the proper pH diluent for that row. The goose RBC suspension is prepared just prior to addition to the antigen dilution. The plates are shaken to assure mixing (using a Boerner oscillating platform, A. H. Thomas Co, or a Syntron paper jogger, PJ-4), and incubated at room temperature (approximately 24 C) for 45–60 min. For some viruses, 37 C or 4 C may be a better incubation temperature than 24 C.

A uniformly thin pellicle of RBC following the curvature of the cup bottom is a sign of complete HA and is recorded as $+$. In the higher dilutions, RBC may appear to form a ring associated with a rougher or thinner pellicle. This is partial HA, called a ring, and it is recorded as $\oplus$. At some outer dilutions a button will appear on a thin or scattered pellicle; this indicates minimal HA and is recorded as $\pm$. In those dilutions negative for HA, there is a clearly defined button with no associated film of RBC; this is recorded as $-$.

The endpoint of the HA reaction (1 unit) is the last dilution in which complete $+$ or substantial $\oplus$ HA occurred. In the HA test, only 0.2 or 0.025 ml of antigen is used, instead of 0.4 or 0.05. Thus, to determine the dilution to contain 4 units for use in the HA test, count back 4 dilutions instead of 3 from the endpoint.

The HA of some bunyavirus antigens, in addition to being pH dependent, is salt dependent (32, 6). Addition of 0.4 to 0.8 M NaCl (substituted for the standard 0.15 M NaCl of the phosphate buffer system) to the RBC adjusting diluents enhances the titer of many sucrose-acetone extracted mouse brain antigens, especially in the more acid pH range. This enhancement is additive to that observed after sonication.

HA of some bunyaviruses, especially selected members of the phlebotomus fever group, is also dependent upon RBC type; trypsinized human O cells may be superior to avian cells (23).

RBC and their associated reagents. Porterfield (48) showed that the adult white domestic goose (*Anser cinereus*) is the choice source of RBC for arbovirus HA. Subsequently, cells from other species of goose have been used with no problems. Occasionally, mixing of RBC from several geese may lead to nonspecific agglutination (55). Holden (personal communication) reported that RBC from female geese may, at times, be less sensitive to hemagglutinins than are those of ganders. HA endpoints are generally consistent in the presence of RBC from different ganders. If geese are not available, RBC from 1-day-old chicks (51) or from roosters (52) can be used, though they are somewhat less sensitive than goose RBC. Chick RBC must be used within 1 week.

Withdraw aseptically from the jugular or wing vein of the goose or rooster the amount of blood required to provide RBC for 1–2 weeks. Use a 20-gauge needle attached to a glass syringe containing 1.5 ml acid-citrate-dextrose (ACD) or Alsever solution for each 8.5 ml of blood to be collected. Blood is obtained by decapitating the lightly anesthetized chick and letting the blood drip into a beaker containing Alsever solution (25 ml/12 chicks). All reagents are stored and used at 4 C.

Acid-citrate-dextrose (ACD)

Sodium citrate ($Na_3C_6H_5O_7 \cdot 2H_2O$)	11.26 g
Citric acid ($H_3C_6H_5O_7 \cdot H_2O$)	4.00 g
Dextrose	11.00 g
Distilled water q.s. ad	500.00 ml

Sterilize by autoclaving 10 min at 10 lb pressure.

Alsever solution

Dextrose	20.50 g
NaCl	4.20 g
Citric acid ($H_3C_6H_5O_7 \cdot H_2O$)	0.55 g
Sodium citrate ($Na_3C_6H_5O_7 \cdot 2H_2O$)	8.00 g
Distilled water q.s. ad	1000.00 ml

Sterilize by autoclaving 10 min at 10 lb pressure.

The cells are washed 4 times with dextrose-gelatin-veronal (DGV) solution. All manipulations should be carried out in sterile glassware and with aseptic precautions.

Dextrose-gelatin-veronal (DGV)

Veronal (barbital)	0.58 g
Gelatin	0.60 g
Sodium veronal (sodium barbital)	0.38 g
$CaCl_2$ (anhydrous)	0.02 g
$MgSO_4 \cdot 7H_2O$	0.12 g
NaCl	8.50 g
Dextrose	10.00 g
Distilled water q.s. ad	1000.00 ml

The veronal and gelatin are dissolved in 250 ml of water by heating. This solution is combined with the other reagents. Sterilize by autoclaving 10 min at 10 lb pressure.

For the first wash, 1 volume of whole blood is added to 2.5 volumes of DGV, and subsequent washings are carried out in 3 volumes of DGV. The suspension is centrifuged at $270 \times g$ for 15 min (PR2 International Centrifuge); the supernatant is discarded. After the fourth washing the RBC are suspended in DGV and stored as an 8% suspension; this represents a concentration approximately 24 times higher than the dilution at which they will be used for the HA and HAI tests. In the interest of comparability from test to test and the achievement of optimal conditions for determining HA characteristics of an arbovirus, the dilution of the stock RBC suspension which will give a standardized 0.75 OD should be determined on a Coleman Junior photoelectric or other comparable spectrophotometer at 490 nm. This is measured in a cuvette (tube) of 10 mm internal diameter. To allow for shrinkage of the RBC, the suspension is held for 24 hr at 4 C before this final standardization. Generally, a 1:24 dilution of the 8% suspension gives 0.75 OD. The volume for the final concentration is obtained by this formula:

$$\text{Final volume} = \text{initial volume} \times \frac{\text{observed OD}}{\text{desired OD}}$$

This dilution is not made until just before the RBC are to be added during performance of the test.

To suspend the RBC at the proper pH the following reagents are required:

Stock solutions

1.5 M sodium chloride ($10 \times 0.9\%$ NaCl)
NaCl . . . . 87.68 g
Distilled H_2O q.s. ad . . . . 1000.00 ml
2.0 M dibasic sodium phosphate
Na_2HPO_4 (anhydrous) . . . . 283.96 g
Distilled H_2O q.s. ad . . . . 1000.00 ml
2.0 M monobasic sodium phosphate
$NaH_2PO_4 \cdot H_2O$ . . . . 276.02 g
Distilled H_2O q.s. ad . . . . 1000.00 ml

Adjusting diluents (AD) for addition of cell suspensions: These diluents are 0.15 M NaCl-0.2 M phosphate and are prepared by combining the stock solutions 0.15 M NaCl-0.2 M Na_2HPO_4 and 0.15 M NaCl-0.2 M NaH_2PO_4, as indicated in the table of pH values.

0.15 M NaCl-0.2 M Na_2HPO_4
1.5M NaCl . . . . .100 ml
2.0 M $Na_2 HPO_4$. . . . . .100 ml
Distilled H_2O . . . . .800 ml
0.15 M NaCl-0.2 M NaH_2PO_4
1.5 M NaCl . . . . .100 ml
2.0 M $NaH_2PO_4 \cdot H_2O$ . . . . .100 ml
Distilled H_2O . . . . .800 ml

The following combinations are suggested for preparing adjusting diluents at required pH values for addition of RBC suspension. In practice, minor variations occur, and quantities are adjusted, depending on the measured pH.

Antigen diluents and other reagents used in performing test:

Stock solutions

1.5 M sodium chloride ($10 \times 0.9\%$ NaCl)
NaCl . . . . 87.68 g
Distilled H_2O q.s. ad . . . . 1000.00 ml

Table of pH Values

Final pH*	0.15 M NaCl-0.2 M Na₂HPO₄	0.15 M NaCl-0.2 M NaH₂PO₄
5.75	3.0 ml	97.0 ml
6.0	12.5	87.5
6.2	22.0	78.0
6.4	32.0	68.0
6.6	45.0	55.0
6.8	55.0	45.0
7.0	64.0	36.0
7.2	72.0	28.0
7.4	79.0	21.0

*The pH is that obtained by mixing equal volumes of borate saline, pH 9, and the adjusting diluent. Solutions, pH 5.75-pH 6.6, are stored in the refrigerator at 4 C, but since those pH 6.8 and above may crystallize at refrigerator temperature, they are stored at room temperature.

0.5 M boric acid
    H₃BO₃ . . . .   30.92 g
    Hot distilled H₂O (dissolve then cool) . . . .   700.00 ml
    Distilled H₂O q.s. ad . . . .   1000.00 ml
Borate saline solution, pH 9
    1.5 M NaCl . . . .   80.00 ml
    0.5 M H₃BO₃ . . . .   100.00 ml
    1.0 N NaOH . . . .   24.00 ml
    Distilled H₂O q.s. ad . . . .   1000.00 ml
        (check pH in pH meter)
4% Bovine albumin (Fraction V) (BABS)
    Bovine albumin . . . .   4.00 g
    Borate saline solution, pH 9 (adjust to pH
    9 with 2N NaOH) . . . .   90.00 ml
    Borate saline, pH 9, q.s. . . . .   100.00 ml

This solution may have to be filtered to avoid growth of contaminants on long storage as a stock solution.

Antigen diluent

0.4% bovine-albumin-borate-saline solution (0.4% BABS, pH 9)
    4% bovine albumin, pH 9 . . . . 100 ml
    Borate saline solution, pH 9 . . . . 900 ml

Techniques for treatment of serum. The HAI test measures the ability of a serum to inhibit agglutination of the RBC by 4–8 units of the arbovirus hemagglutinin.

Because normal serum contains nonspecific inhibitors and natural agglutinins, the test serum must be treated either by kaolin adsorption or by acetone extraction, and then by absorption with the RBC type used.

The technique selected depends on the type of serum to be tested and the virus involved. A universally applicable serum treatment system has not been developed. Kaolin treatment has been shown to remove IgM (19S) globulin, but acetone treatment does not affect it. Therefore, acetone treatment would appear to be preferred for acute- or early convalescent-phase serum if the early antibody is to be detected. Neither kaolin nor acetone treatment appears to affect IgG (7S). Many types of nonspecific inhibitors, some thermolabile, have been described which require further special treatment for removal, but most of these are present in serum of birds and mammals other than humans and are not discussed here. Techniques for treatment of test serum are as follows:

Kaolin adsorption—It is important to start with acid-washed kaolin because any other is unlikely to achieve complete adsorption. A slurry is prepared by adding 25 g of the acid-washed kaolin powder to 100 ml of pH 9 borate saline solution, with constant mechanical stirring for maximal suspension. this mixture can be held indefinitely at 4 C. A workable quantity of serum to be tested ranges from 0.2 to 0.7 ml.

To the selected volume of serum are added 4 volumes of pH 9 borate saline solution and 5 volumes of the kaolin mixture. Shake vigorously at 5-min intervals for 20 min at room temperature, and centrifuge at $800 \times g$ for 30 min. The pH 9 supernatant fluid is handled as a 1:10 dilution of the original test serum.

Acetone extraction—The selected volume (0.025–1.0 ml) of serum is diluted 10-fold with isotonic saline solution. The diluted serum cooled in an ice-water bath is expressed into 12 times the diluted serum volume of dry, chilled acetone with an 18-gauge needle. Extraction proceeds for 5 min with intermittent shaking of the solution; then the tube is centrifuged at $500 \times g$ for 5 sec at 4 C. The supernatant fluid is carefully removed and the sediment is resuspended by vigorous shaking with another 12 volumes of chilled acetone. After this mixture has been centrifuged at $800 \times g$ for 5 min at 4 C, the supernatant fluid is carefully removed, and the sediment is dried under vacuum at room temperature; this requires about 60 min. This sediment is resuspended in sufficient pH 9 borate-saline solution to make a 1:10 dilution based on the volume of serum initially introduced. Resuspension occurs at room temperature in a couple of hours, with occasional shaking, or after standing overnight in the refrigerator.

Agglutinin adsorption—Preparation of RBC suspensions has been described. To the kaolin- or acetone-treated 1:10 serum dilutions, cooled in an ice-water bath, is added 0.1 ml of packed RBC of the species to be used in the HAI test per 5.0 ml total volume. The treated serum is held in an ice waterbath to prevent hemolysis. Adsorption occurs during the next 20 min with occasional shaking of the serum, after which time the suspension is centrifuged at $270 \times g$ for 10 min in the cold. The resulting supernatant fluid is the 1:10 serum dilution, ready for testing.

Extracted serum held at 4 C can be used for many weeks in a series of tests against the same antigens without appreciable change in titer. This allows the same serum to be tested with a sequence of arbovirus antigens, the selection of which is determined by the data accumulated as the series proceeds.

Special conditions are required for removal of inhibitors of HA for rhabdoviruses, which are extremely sensitive to inhibitors. Acetone extraction is not satisfactory. Kaolin is preferred; however, several known negative sera should be treated with kaolin along with the test serum to control for complete removal of nonspecific inhibitors.

Procedure for the HAI test. Generally, the microtechnique is employed and is described here. Macrotechniques are described elsewhere (21).

On the morning of the day of the test an ampule (ampules) of the frozen antigen is (are) quickly thawed and held in an ice-water bath. If lyophilized antigen is used, it is rehydrated with cold water and held in an ice-water bath. A dilution of the antigen is prepared in cold C.4% BABS, pH 9, which contains an estimated 4–8 HA units in 0.025 ml at the optimal pH based on the results of the previous HA titration. A sufficient volume is prepared to allow the addition of 0.025 ml to all serum dilutions and to permit performance of a preliminary and final antigen titration. If the desired antigen dilution is high enough, e.g., $\geq$1:80, it is convenient to make an initial dilution of 1:10 and to prepare the desired dilution from the 1:10 dilution. Otherwise, the dilution is made directly from the antigen. The diluted antigen is held in the ice-water bath for about 1 hr before titration to permit complete dissociation of any aggregates. A preliminary titration of each diluted antigen is then made at the predetermined optimal pH and at a pH value above and below that considered optimal. Starting with the diluted antigen, 8 2-fold dilutions are made in 0.05-ml amounts, then 0.05 ml of goose RBC suspension at the proper pH is added to the antigen dilutions, and the test is incubated for 30–60 min at room temperature. The antigen titration is read and recorded as above. If the observed titer indicates that the diluted antigen contains 4–8 units/0.025 ml, no adjustment in the prepared diluted antigen is needed. However, if the observed titer is either too high or too low, it is adjusted by the adding of more diluent or concentrated antigen. There is twice as much antigen in the control titration as in the test proper (0.05 ml vs. 0.025 ml) so 4 units in the test will be shown by reading back 4 dilution wells from the HA endpoint and 8 units by reading back 5 dilutions. The diluted, standardized antigen is held in the cold.

Serum to be tested is extracted and absorbed by one of the methods described above the day before the HAI test is to be performed; otherwise the time and operations involved can result in confusion. Serial 2-fold dilutions of the 1:10 diluted extracted serum are made in 0.4% BABS, pH 9, diluent. Dilutions are made in microwells on plates by using loops or by serologic pipettes in tubes and then the dilutions are transferred to the microplate (0.025 ml). A serum is tested against one or more viral antigens. In addition, a serum control at the 1:10 dilution is included (0.025 ml of the 1:10 dilution is mixed with 0.4% BABS, pH 9, diluent), to assure that the serum is free of nonspecific agglutinins. One serum control is probably adequate if all pH values to be used with the various antigens are quite similar, but if they are widely divergent, more than 1 control should be employed. A positive control serum titrated through its endpoint should be included for each antigen. Generally as a preliminary screen test, serum is tested at dilutions 1:10, 1:20, and 1:40, and if positive at 1:40, it is then titrated for the HAI endpoint through 8–10 dilutions. When all serum dilutions have been made, either on the plates or as master dilutions and then distributed to the plates, the plates are covered to prevent evaporation until the antigen can be added. Then 0.025 ml of each antigen, containing 4–8 units of hemagglutinin, is added to its proper plate of the serum dilutions; the plates are agitated to ensure mixing, and covered to prevent evaporation. The serum-antigen mixtures are incubated overnight (18 hr) in an ordinary refrigerator at 4 C. The diluted antigen is also held in the refrigerator overnight. On the next day, the plates containing the serum-antigen mixtures and the antigens are removed from the refrigerator. A repeat titration to determine hemagglutinin units used in the test is made for each antigen. Goose RBC (0.75 final OD) are suspended at the optimal pH for each antigen, and 0.05 ml is added to the serum-antigen wells (HAI test) and antigen dilutions (HA titration). The tests are incubated for 30–60 min at room temperature (about 24 C) unless otherwise indicated for a specific virus. Inhibition of HA is indicated by a negative HA reaction (button of cells) and is interpreted as positive. The HAI titer is taken as the highest dilution of serum which causes complete or almost complete inhibi-

tion of HA by 4–8 units of antigen. For a test to be considered entirely satisfactory all RBC and serum controls must be negative and each final antigen
titration should show the presence of 4–8 units of hemagglutinin. The number of the tube representing the reciprocal of the extent of the 2-fold dilution
which is inhibited is sometimes used to simplify presentation of serum HAI
titer; thus 1:10 is equivalent to 1; 1:20 to 2; 1:40 to 3; and so forth, with
1:5120 being 10.

Interpretation of HAI test. A 4-fold difference between an acute-phase-
and a convalescent-phase serum is considered a significant rise or fall in titer
and is diagnostic of infection with a virus antigenically related to that used in
the test, provided both sera have been prepared and handled in the same
manner and tested simultaneously.

Neutralization test (Nt)

Types of tests. Nt antibodies may be measured by *in vivo* or *in vitro*
tests, provided a susceptible tissue culture system is available for the latter.
The following two basic procedures are available:

1. Serial virus dilutions with undiluted serum—This is the most commonly applied *in vivo* test, but it is employed less frequently with tissue
culture. The *in vivo* test in which undiluted serum is used has the least technical difficulties and is the easiest to standardize for comparative purposes.
It is recommended principally for use with freshly collected serum or for
those maintained constantly in a frozen state.

If serum has not been kept frozen and the titer is to be compared with
another or other titers, it should all be inactivated (heated at 56 C for 30 min)
or tested after the addition of "accessory substance(s)." This is due to the
loss of heat-labile substance(s), which enhances the neutralization of certain
arboviruses and is present in varying amounts in the serum of many persons.
It is destroyed by heating, and its effect is diminished by diluting the serum
1:5; in tests with serum diluted above 1:5, it usually poses no problem. Re-
storing the accessory substance requires fresh serum, or fresh serum that
has been kept constantly frozen (≤ -60 C), from an individual or suitable
animal demonstrated to possess the specific accessory substance required
for human serum, and yet to be free from any antibody to the virus under
test. The amount of such an additive needed is usually equal to the volume of
the patient's serum used in the test.

Results of the Nt test with undiluted serum and serial dilutions of virus
are expressed as a neutralizaiton index (NI) either as a $\log_{10}$ result or as an
antilog. With fresh serum, or one to which accessory substance has been
added, a log NI of 1.7 is frequently the accepted lower limit for a "positive"
result.

2. Serial serum dilutions with a constant amount of virus. This test
requires minimal amounts of serum. It is applicable to unfrozen sera, provided comparative endpoints for all sera are greater than the 1:5 or 1:10
serum dilution, since at this dilution the accessory substance is diluted out.
However, this test possesses serious disadvantages in an *in vivo* application:

Since only one virus dilution is employed, it is technically difficult to work within the narrow range required in an *in vivo* test. This is less difficult in a tissue culture system. The amount of virus used cannot be either excessive or insufficient.

The endpoints of titrations are likely to be more drawn out and irregular than those with undiluted serum.

The test is not readily subject to standardization for reference to any constant or index, such as the NI.

This test has been less frequently used *in vivo* and less is known about its variables than the test with serial virus dilutions.

Because the accessory factor may be active at dilutions below 1:5 or 1:10, and not above, and because of the frequent toxicity for cells of undiluted serum or serum in low dilutions, a serum dilution method beginning at dilutions of ≥1:5 is preferred for most tissue culture tests. However, because of this dilution of serum, minimal amounts of antibody may not be detected except in certain of the extremely sensitive and quantitative plaque reduction type tests (Chapter 3).

Results are expressed as that dilution of serum which protects 50% of the animals or cultures against a specified amount of virus (LD_{50} or $TCID_{50}$) or reduces the number of plaques by a specified percentage when a specified number of plaque forming units (pfu) have been used. The amount of virus must always be specified as that shown in a control titration in the same test.

Intracerebral (ic) test. In the *in vivo* test the ic route of innoculation is customarily used for both the virus and the serum dilution methods just described. This procedure may fail to demonstrate a rise in antibody between 2 sera of low or moderate titer, when a conspicuous difference is apparent by the ip route. The ic method, however, is the only practical test for most laboratories because weaned mice can be employed for many viruses, and small age differences in the mice are irrelevant.

Intraperitoneal (ip) test. This test has great advantages in differentiating antibody levels in certain sera of relatively low titer, which are not afforded by the ic method. Contrary to general belief, however, the test is usually less specific at such low or equivocal titer levels. With a few viruses in group A, it has been less effective than the ic test in differentiating between antibodies because of the presence of different viruses of the same subgroup. Nevertheless, it is an extremely useful modification which is of critical importance in the solution of some problems. Only suckling mice 1–4 days of age can be used for some arboviruses; older animals do not die from ip inoculation with most of these agents.

Host systems. Animals or tissue cultures used in the Nt test are essentially the same as those described for virus isolation. Suckling mice (usually 1–4 days of age) are suitable with nearly all viruses. Weanlings are employed when adequately susceptible to the specific virus used. In general, unless the virus titers in weanling mice are in excess of 10^{-5} by the route of inoculation selected, sucklings are used. For most viruses almost any strain of mouse is equally suitable, but certain conspicuous exceptions are recognized. For example, a Rockefeller Institute "Princeton" strain is genetically insusceptible to most group B viruses. The SLE virus has a very low titer in almost all mice, except in the genetically selected strain developed by Webster (this mouse strain is known generally as the Webster neurotropic virus strain).

A few arboviruses can readily be used in certain primary cell cultures without special adaptation. In such instances, the various types of tissue culture neutralization systems described in Chapter 3 may be easily and efficiently substituted for the *in vivo* tests. Many of the group A viruses and certain of those in group B can readily be used in 1 or more of 3 primary cell cultures: hamster kidney, chick embryo and duck embryo. Several cell lines, including a special HeLa line (HeLa–TPB) (10), a baby hamster kidney cell line (BHK-21) (34), a porcine kidney cell line (PS) (70), a rhesus monkey kidney cell line (LLC-MK$_2$) (28), an African green monkey kidney cell line (Vero) (71), and CER line (56) have been found useful for the propagation or assay of many arboviruses. Much of this is based on unpublished observations. However, no single cell line is available that meets requirements for routine use with all arboviruses.

Selection of virus strain. The virus strain to be selected for use in any Nt test may be of considerable importance. Some strains are more readily neutralized than others thus providing a more sensitive test for low-titer serum. In other instances slight antigenic differences between strains of the same type render one better suited than another for tests of persons exposed in a given geographic area. In fact, in rare instances in serologic survey work use of an inappropriate strain of virus has led to an erroneous conclusion that a certain virus was not present or active in the area. A locally derived strain or several from elsewhere can be used in preliminary tests to determine which should be used later.

Techniques of tests

Preparation of virus. For most arboviruses the brains of suckling mice 2–4 days of age provide the best source. For a few viruses weanling mice (3–4 weeks of age) can be used for preparation of virus stock, but for antigen preparation the infant mouse is preferred.

Mice are inoculated ic with a dilution of virus-infected material which will regularly produce typical signs of illness and death. The dilution generally ranges from 10^{-2}–10^{-4}, depending on the virus. Weanling mice are given 0.02 ml ic and suckling mice, 0.01 to 0.02 ml ic. The mice are sacrificed when definite signs of infection are observed and after a few have died or are moribund. The brains are removed aseptically and are either stored at about -70 C in a mechanical freezer until the stock suspension can be prepared or are emulsified immediately in a sterile chilled mortar with abrasive or in a mechanical homogenizer with the container held in an ice-water bath. The brains are suspended in a serum or protein diluent such as 50% inactivated rabbit serum-saline solution (pH 7.2–7.5) or whole rabbit serum inactivated at 56 C for 30 min. The serum must be pretested to be certain it contains no neutralizing substance. This diluent is added in sufficient quantity to make a 10% brain suspension, referred to subsequently as the 10^{-1} dilution. The suspension is centrifuged at 500–100 $\times$ g for at least 30 min in the cold (PR2 International Centrifuge), or at 100 $\times$ g for not more than 10 min at room temperature. The supernatant fluid is shell-frozen in a dry ice-alcohol bath in a number of sealed ampules and stored at about -70 C in a dry-ice chest or in a mechanical freezer. In some laboratories lyophilization and storage at higher temperatures are preferred. The virus suspensions can be used for seed virus stock for Nt tests and as a source of virus for antigen and immune serum preparation.

Titration of virus. The following is suggested for a virus expected to have an LD_{50} titer of about $10^{-7.5}$. At the same or at different times, 2 or 3 preliminary titrations are made. The contents of 2 ampules are combined in each test to correct for possible loss of titer in a single portion. Each titration is made under exactly the same conditions as the Nt test. Since each sample is titrated separately and in a manner identical to the other, the description of only one titration is given.

An adequate quantity of cold diluting fluid, such as 10% inactivated rabbit serum-saline solution, is first prepared. Into a set of sterile tubes standing in an ice-water bath, diluent for a series of 9 10-fold dilutions is pipetted accurately. Customarily, 1.8, 4.5 or, 9.0 ml of diluent is used. When this has been done, and not before, the ampules of virus are rapidly thawed by agitating them in water at 37 C or rehydrated with distilled water and combined as above. With a sterile pipette calibrated to deliver 0.2, 0.5, or 1.0 ml, this exact amount of virus (0.2, 0.5, or 1.0 ml of the 10^{-1} dilution) is delivered into the first tube which already contains the diluent. The pipette is discarded.

The virus and diluent are thoroughly mixed with another sterile pipette or on a mechanical mixer; in order not to inactivate the virus, avoid foaming. With the same pipette used for mixing, the proper amount is transferred to the next tube and the pipette discarded. In a similar fashion, all 10-fold dilutions through 10^{-10} are prepared. The actual range of dilutions to be made and tested will be governed by the virus under test.

Next, 6 cork-stoppered, short, wide-mouth tubes (from which 0.25-ml syringes with short needles can be easily filled) are selected for serum-virus mixtures. Into each tube is placed 0.2 ml of chilled normal inactivated rabbit serum or other known negative serum. Agamma rabbit serum in place of whole serum has been found to be quite satisfactory, but a virus diluent less capable of stabilizing a virus at 37 C during incubation should not replace this serum. Then 0.2 ml of the 10^{-5} dilution is added to the first tube, 0.2 ml of the 10^{-6} dilution into the second, and so on through 10^{-10}. A separate pipette is used for each dilution. The final virus dilutions are now $10^{-5.3}$ through $10^{-10.3}$. The 6 stoppered-tubes are then shaken gently for mixing (avoid foaming) and are placed in a 37 C water bath for exactly 2 hr, after which they are transferred to an ice-water bath. Titers of some viruses, such as some dengues, are substantially reduced in 2 hr at 37 C. If this is shown to occur in a titration carried out with a control without incubation, the incubation period must be reduced to 90 or 60 min.

Six weanling mice (the number ranges from 4 to 8, depending on the availability of mice and the desired sensitivity of endpoint) or 1–2 litters of suckling mice are inoculated per serum-virus mixture. Weanling mice are inoculated ic with 0.03 ml while under light ether anesthesia and suckling mice receive 0.01 ml (0.02 ml is used in some laboratories) by the ic route without anesthesia. Antiseptic should not be used on the heads of the mice. The material to be inoculated is drawn into a small syringe attached to a 25-, 26-, or 27-gauge $1/2$-inch or $3/8$-inch needle. Care is taken to fill the syringe without forming air bubbles. Unavoidable bubbles or foam may be expelled through the needle embedded in a sterile cotton pledget. The needle is then introduced into the soft skull of the mouse lateral to the midline to avoid hemorrhage from the superior sagittal sinus; the virus is inoculated, and the needle is withdrawn after a momentary pause. This permits equalization of pressure and minimal loss of material through the needle hole on withdrawal. The suckling mice are returned to their mother for the incubation period. Each suckling mouse in the litter is inoculated with a portion of the same material or dilution.

These mice are examined daily for signs of illness, paralysis and death. The number of days allotted for the titration depends upon the incubation period and the pattern of deaths for the particular virus and mouse strain used. Ten days to 2 weeks is usually a sufficient period of time to observe practically all deaths that will occur from an ic inoculation of a properly adapted virus, provided a suitable, uniformly susceptible strain of mouse is used. There are a few exceptions, notably the dengue group of viruses; for these agents, a 21-day observation period is customary. Deaths are recorded daily. All mice that die within a period of less than the minimal incubation period (determined by experience for each virus) are discounted as having died from extraneous causes. The LD_{50} (50% mortality endpoint) is computed by the method of Reed and Muench as described in Chapter 1. Results of the tests on the 2 or 3 samples are combined before calculating the LD_{50}, or after calculating each separately the results are averaged. Following this preliminary titration with a "normal" serum to determine the LD_{50}, all unknown sera may be tested with a minimal number of dilutions.

Screen test. If series of sera are to be tested from several patients and a report of definitive results is not urgently needed, it is advantageous from the standpoint of economy to test first with one or more selected viruses only the final serum from each patient to determine whether suspected antibodies have developed. If they have not developed, it is not necessary to test the earlier serum. If antibody to one virus is present, this will be confirmed by a titration, including this and an earlier serum. Thus, the results of a comparative titration are obtained.

In the usual screen test, 2 dilutions of each virus are used. Antibodies in some viral infections are slow to form; in some individuals they may not reach a high titer at any time. Therefore, two 10-fold dilutions are usually used, the higher dilution containing about 10–25 LD_{50} and the lower 100–250 LD_{50}. Dilutions are made in the identical manner used previously in the virus titration.

For procedural terminology, the dilution representing between 10 and 25 LD_{50} is called dilution 1. The dilutions containing more virus than dilution 1, by 10-fold sequence are, in order, 2, 3, 4, etc. Those with less virus than dilution 1 are represented in 10-fold sequence as -1, -2, and -3 etc. Dilutions 1 and 2 (10–25 and 100–250 LD_{50}) are used with each unknown serum for the screen test. At the same time, dilutions 2, 1, -1, -2 and -3 are added to an equal amount of normal rabbit serum to determine the LD_{50} endpoint for the control virus titration. Each test should include a control titration in the presence of a negative inactivated rabbit or human serum or other equivalent stabilizer, and another in the presence of a specific positive immune control serum of known titer.

The procedure for the test is essentially that used for the virus titration. First, virus dilution blanks are set up through 2 dilutions beyond the pre-determined LD_{50} of the virus. These are held in an ice-water bath or placed in the refrigerator. Second, a 0.2 ml volume of each serum for each of the virus dilutions included is pipetted into the same type short tubes used for virus titration. These are set up in racks in such a manner that all tubes in 1 row receive 1 virus dilution; those in the second row, the second virus dilu-tion, etc. After the distribution is completed, the tubes are placed in the refrigerator. Then the virus is thawed as described for the virus titration, and transferred to a sterile tube in an ice-water bath. The virus dilution blanks are now held in an ice-water bath. Virus dilutions are made and 0.2-ml amounts of the appropriate dilutions distributed to the serum tubes and gent-ly agitated for mixing. The serum-virus mixtures are placed in a rack in the order they are to be inoculated into mice, with the negative control titration inoculated last. The rack is gently shaken, then placed in a 37 C water bath for 2 hr.

Immediately after incubation the racks of tubes are placed in an ice-water bath and the inoculum is expeditiously administered by using 4, 5, or 6 mice for each unknown serum-virus mixture and 6 for each of the control dilutions. If the control titration indicates that the dilutions are properly made, any serum protecting at least 3 or 4 mice (out of 4) in dilution 1 is tentatively considered as positive. This serum is then scheduled for simulta-neous comparative titration with the earlier serum from the same patient. If too little virus has been used, as confirmed by the control titration endpoint, dilution 2 may possibly be considered significant. If too much virus was used, only occasionally would a significant positive be missed when up to a 5- or 10-fold increase over that expected for dilution 1 was employed. Under these circumstances of significantly more than $10-25$ LD_{50} in dilution 1, the test is repeated, but only with those sera giving suspicious results, e.g., 1 or more mice surviving with dilution 1.

Comparative titrations of serum with serial dilutions of virus. If the titration is to be made by using serial dilutions of virus with undiluted serum, the following technique is used. No change in procedure is necessary if serum is inactivated at 56 C and/or fresh pretested serum containing acces-sory substance is added to test serum, including the controls.

Serial dilutions of the test virus are prepared as for the screen test. In practice, the same set of dilutions is used, and some sera are set up for the screen test at the same time that the previously selected ''positives'' are titrated with their earlier paired sera or series of sera. The number of virus dilutions to be used for each serum is determined by judgment. Each serum is tested against dilutions 1, 2, and 3, at the minimum (10–25, 100–250, 1000–

2500 LD_{50}, respectively), but it may be advisable to test later sera against one or more still lower dilutions (additional log increments of virus in terms of LD_{50}). The LD_{50} virus dilution for each series of serum-virus mixtures, and also that of the control, are computed to one decimal point. The logarithmic LD_{50} is expressed as the exponent of the reciprocal of the endpoint dilution. Thus, if the LD_{50} dilution in the presence of a normal control serum is $10^{-7.8}$, the logarithmic expression of the LD_{50} is 7.8. It is customarily assumed that this is a logarithmic expression and simply stated that the LD_{50} is 7.8.

The log NI of each serum (except those sera failing to protect against dilution 1) is obtained by subtracting its LD_{50} from that of the control. Thus, if the computed LD_{50} dilution in the control is $10^{-7.8}$ (LD_{50} is 7.8) and that in the unknown serum $10^{-4.9}$ (LD_{50} is 4.9), their respective difference (log NI) is 2.9, or the anilog (numerical NI) 800.

Comparative titrations of serum with serial dilutions of serum. If this method is selected there is no change in the manner of handling the test virus, and the same method of preliminary titration of the virus and control serum is employed.

Serum is usually set up in 5-fold dilutions and a constant amount of virus is added to each serum dilution. All serum-virus mixtures are incubated at 37 C for 1 hr before inoculation. When high dilutions of serum are employed, 2 hr of incubation are not recommended. The calculations of the LD_{50} are made on the basis of serum dilutions.

It is usually advisable to employ about 4 serum dilutions (undiluted, 1:5, 1:25, 1:125) with an acute-phase serum, and 6 (undiluted, 1:5, 1:25, 1:125, 1:625 and 1:3125) with a convalescent-phase serum. The number of days after onset that the serum was collected and the usual time required for antibodies to form with the virus in question should be considered as factors influencing the choice of dilutions.

For dilutions of each serum, short wide-mouth tubes are employed. Into each of the first two of a series is placed 0.2 ml of the serum to be tested. To each but the first is added 0.8 ml of a 10% serum-saline solution diluting fluid. After the contents of the second tube (representing a 1:5 dilution) is mixed, 0.2 ml is transferred to the third, etc., in series, and 0.2 is finally discarded from the last. Virus is added to these same tubes; 0.2 ml to the tube of undiluted serum and 0.8 ml to all others. In this manner, a minimum of serum and glassware is required. Virus dilutions are prepared as in the other test. Only one dilution (preferably between 75 and 125 LD_{50}) is employed, except for the control virus titration with normal undiluted rabbit serum. This control series must extend from a dilution which will kill all animals through the one which kills none.

The LD_{50} for each serum is computed again by the method of Reed and Muench, now on the basis of serum dilutions. This measure has no absolute value, as it had in the previously prescribed test, for it depends entirely on the amount of virus present in the test dose. However, 2 sera from the same patient tested simultaneously are readily compared. Comparison is expressed as the arithmetic quotient of the reciprocals of the 2 LD_{50}. For example, if the LD_{50} in the first serum is 1:25 and that in the second is 1:625, there is a 25-fold increase. If that of the first is 1:10 and that of the convalescent-phase specimen 1:32, the apparent change is 3.2-fold.

Intraperitoneal neutralization test. For this test, the technique of Olitsky and Harford (46) or that of Lennette and Koprowski (39) is recommended. Incubation of the serum-virus mixture for 2 hr at 37 C before inoculation increases sensitivity of the test. Serial dilutions of either serum or virus can be used, and calculations are made in the same manner as described for the ic test.

Tissue culture. Serum Nt tests have been effectively carried out with certain arboviruses in tissue culture, and these are performed in a manner similar to those described in Chapter 3. These can be performed with confidence only after the test virus has been adapted to a cell system giving replicable titration results.

Interpretation of test. Difference in NI is the factor by which the serum titer rises or falls. Results of *in vivo* Nt titrations in duplicate tests conducted at the same time may easily vary as much as 1 log. Therefore, changes in titer between 2 sera run in the same test are not considered significant unless the change in titer is in excess of 1 log. Comparative tests on 2 or more serum samples from the same patient should always be run at the same time, but when this is impossible, a difference should not be interpreted as significant unless it is ≥1.7 log. For the same reasons, the NI of any single serum is generally not accepted as definitely positive unless it is at least 1.7 log. Levels of 1.0 to 1.6 log are generally interpreted as equivocal and the tests are repeated if possible. If replicable, they may be highly significant. Because of antigenic differences in strains of the same virus, marked differences in degree of response and time of development of antibodies with different arboviruses, and the lability of antibody under certain storage conditions, absolute lower limits for a significant positive response cannot be set. One fact must be emphasized in interpretation. *No diagnostic significance can be placed on any positive neutralization result with a single convalescent-phase serum.* Mild missed cases are known to occur frequently, and in certain communities a considerable proportion of clinically healthy residents have antibodies to one or several of these viruses. A definite rise in titer between 2 suitably spaced serum samples must be obtained, and the significance of the rise must be evaluated on the basis of several facts, including time of onset, day of serum collection, and temperature of storage of the serum at all times. These data must be available to the laboratorian for intelligent interpretation of test results. Anyone else attempting to interpret the tests must have a thorough understanding of the laboratory procedures involved, the characteristics of the virus strains, and their behavior in the test animals.

A negative Nt result probably has a more clear-cut diagnostic significance than any other test result, at least when as little as 10 or 25 LD_{50} of virus are used with a serum taken 2 months or later after the onset of illness. Individual cases are on record in which Nt antibodies have apparently failed to develop, but in most instances a negative result on a late serum by this test has unchallenged significance: no infection with the virus used in the test.

Of inestimable value in interpretation, in many instances, are the additional results of CF and HAI tests performed on the same sera. If there is any doubt, several types of tests should be performed. Because the Nt test with arboviruses is almost always the most specific, any laboratory should confirm at least a portion of its *in vitro* HAI and CF test results by Nt test.

Indirect immunofluorescence test

Preparation of antigens. For most arboviruses, infected mouse brain impression smears (5) may be prepared on clean laboratory slides and dried for 10 min in air. Alternatively tissue culture antigens may be prepared; the cells are grown in chamber-slides available from Lab-Tek Products, Division of Miles Laboratories, Naperville, IL. The 2-, 4-, or 8-chamber slides are satisfactory for the test. Cell monolayers are infected and used when initial CPE is seen. The maintenance fluid is discarded and the slides are washed in PBS.

Fixation and staining of slides. The indirect staining technique of Gardner and McQuillan (24) is described here. Slides are fixed in acetone at 4 C for 10 min, dried in air at ambient temperature, and stained immediately or stored for months at −60 C before use. A Petri dish humidified with water-soaked cotton pledgets is used to hold the slides. The slides are overlayed with serial dilutions of antibody beginning at 1:4, incubated at 37 C for 30 min in the humidified Petri dish. The antibody is flushed in PBS, then the slides are rinsed in PBS for 10 min each through 3 successive rinses and dried in air. Commercially available fluorescein isothiocyanate-labelled antiglobulin is added using a dilution predetermined in a known positive system. The antiglobulin will be antimouse, antihuman, antiguinea pig, antihamster, or other depending on the species antibody preparation being used. Anti-IgG and anti-IgM may be used to add further specificity to the test. The slides are incubated at 37 C for 30 min in the humidified Petri dish. The conjugate is rinsed off in PBS and the slides are rinsed in PBS for 10 min each through 3 successive rinses, then in distilled water for 2 min. Evans blue counterstain at 1:10,000 may be added to the conjugate to enhance the contrast. Slides to be observed under epi-illumination are dried in air and not covered with a mounting medium; those to be examined under transmitted light are dried and mounted in 9 parts glycerol−1 part PBS, pH 8, under a coverslip.

Controls. Uninfected mouse brain or tissue culture is fixed and stained in parallel with the test antigen. This control should show no fluorescence. In addition a nonimmune serum is used in parallel with the specific antibody and should show no fluorescence when used with infected mouse brain or tissue culture antigens. In cases when specificity is in doubt, a blocking test is done—staining is inhibited by absorption of antibody with homologous virus.

Interpretation of test. The slides are observed under incident or transmitted light using UV or blue excitation light. The specific apple-green fluorescence denoting arboviral antigens is located in the cytoplasm or on the plasma membrane.

Utilization and interpretation of laboratory data

The plethora of possible agents and the variety and complexity of serologic tests that must be considered when an arbovirus etiology of infection and disease is suspected makes expeditious and definitive laboratory diagnosis difficult. This kind of problem is one of the most challenging to the capabilities of a virus diagnostic laboratory.

Isolation and identification of an arbovirus associated with a familiar, previously characterized, clinical illness, followed by a rise in titer of homologous antibody, is the combination of criteria sought but rarely fulfilled. Contributing to the complications are the relatively late suspicion of an arbovirus etiology; the variability in time of appearance and duration of viremia, if it is detectable; the technical difficulties in isolating such agents; and the known variety of viruses of which only one can be the causative agent. Further complicating the laboratory approach is the spectrum of antigenic relationships producing immunologic overlap, which requires selection of appropriate test antigens to be used in an appropriate combination of serologic tests on serum collected during the appropriate phases of an arboviral infection.

The technical information presented in this chapter is intended as a guide to different procedures which must be followed in correct sequence to provide results for proper interpretation. The description herein of the nature of arboviruses covers the wide variety of situations in which they may be encountered. The table of known disease association, geographic distribution, mode of transmission, and immunologic grouping serves to eliminate many possibilities and cause attention to be focused on a few which must be considered.

Information on what happens during the course of infection with regard to viremia and antibody response suggests why and when specimens should be collected and what range of information is obtainable by laboratory tests of these materials. Since Nt and HAI antibodies usually develop early in an arboviral infection, these may be detectable in an early or acute-phase serum specimen. Because HAI antibody is of broad immunologic reactivity, use of a battery of several different or distantly related arbovirus antigens can produce a clue as to what kind of agent is involved. However, the Nt test is usually the most arbovirus-specific and must therefore be used to define as closely as possible the probable identity of the infecting agent.

For the most significant diagnostic results, it is necessary to test simultaneously two or more serial blood specimens collected from the same person during the course of acute illness and convalescence. If the suspected etiologic agent used in the test is the correct one, a significant rise in titer, or at least a substantial antibody level, is usually demonstrated. In general, a 4-fold rise or fall in CF and HAI antibody is considered significant.

When interpreting results, both the time of collection with respect to onset and duration of the acute illness and the interval between collection of specimens must be considered. It is advisable to perform a combination of HAI, CF, and Nt tests because a rise in titer, depending on the time of collection of paired or serial sera, may be demonstrated with one test and not with the others.

Most of the foregoing discussion, despite its apparent complexity, has dealt with a relatively simple phase of the arbovirus diagnostic problem, in that only the antibody responses expected in a primary infection with a virus belonging to any one antigenic group have been considered. Such patients are frequently referred to as having been immunologic virgins for group A, or B, etc. When—as is all too frequently the case particularly in tropical and subtropical areas, or when dealing with an arbovirus-vaccinated population—the patient has had previous experience with one or several antigenically related agents, the antibody responses are quite different from those of the virgin. An excellent discussion of this problem, as applied to yellow fever diagnosis, has been presented by Theiler and Casals (63). An anamnestic rapid rise of titer may make it far more difficult, or impossible, to obtain the first specimen early enough to detect any antibody rise by any one of the classical tests. Furthermore, the group antibody response is frequently so broad that the etiologic agent cannot be specifically identified any closer than its group association, even by using the Nt method. Occasionally, the antigen giving the highest antibody response is the one which was responsible for the first infection in an individual by a virus of the group encountered possibly many years before ("original antigenic sin"). One approach, which may assist in detecting a rise in the group antibody titer when the probable infecting virus shows very elevated but unchanging titer, is to use in its place a related antigen to which the patient has probably never been exposed. For example, an infection with St. Louis encephalitis virus which manifested a constant high titer in a series of sera might show a rising titer if one used a West Nile, Japanese B, or dengue antigen, provided the patient had not been previously infected by that particular virus. The actual agent involved cannot be determined with any reasonable degree of certainty under such circumstances except by isolation of the specific etiologic arbovirus.

References

1. ANDREWES CH and HORSTMANN DM: The susceptibility of viruses to ethyl ether. J Gen Microbiol 3:290–297, 1949
2. ARDOIN P and CLARKE D: The use of sonication and of calcium phosphate chromatography for preparation of group C arbovirus hemagglutinins. Am J Trop Med Hyg 16:357–363, 1967
3. ARDOIN P, CLARKE DH, and HANNOUN C: The preparation of arbovirus hemagglutinin by sonication and trypsin treatment. Am J Trop Med Hyg 18:592–598, 1969
4. ATCHISON RW, ORDONEZ JV, SATHER GE, and HAMMON W McD: Fluorescent antibody and complement fixation method for detection of dengue viruses in mice. J Immunol 96:936–943, 1966
5. BEATY BJ, SHOPE RE, and CLARKE DH: Salt-dependent hemagglutinins with *Bunyaviridae* antigens. J Clin Microbiol 5:548–550, 1977
6. BERGE TO (ed): International Catalogue of Arboviruses. DHEW Publication No. (CDC) 75-8301, second edition, U.S. Government Printing Office, Washington, DC, 1975, 789 pp
7. BERMAN RS and SHOPE RE: Complement-fixing antimouse antibodies found in mice after inoculation of brain, Freund's complete adjuvant, and sarcoma 180/TG cells. Proc Soc Exp Biol Med 138:936–938, 1971
8. BORDEN EC, SHOPE RE, and MURPHY FA: Physicochemical and morphological relationships of some arthropod-borne viruses to bluetongue virus—a new taxonomic group. physicochemical and serological studies. J Gen Virol 13:261–271, 1971
9. BRANDT WE, BUESCHER EL, and HETRICK FM: Production and characterization of arbovirus antibody in mouse ascitic fluid. Am J Trop Med Hyg 16:339–347, 1967
10. BUCKLEY SM: Propagation, cytopathogenicity, and hemagglutination-hemadsorption of some arthropod-borne viruses in tissue culture. Ann NY Acad Sci 81:172–187, 1959

11. BURGDORFER W and VARMA MGR: Trans-stadial and transovarial development of disease agents in arthropods. Annu Rev Entomol 12:347–376, 1967

12. CASALS J: Acetone-ether extracted antigens for complement fixation with certain neurotropic viruses. Proc Soc Exp Biol Med 70:339–343. 1949

13. CASALS J: Filtration of arboviruses through "millipore" membranes. Nature 217:648–649, 1968

14. CASALS J: Complement fixation test with encephalitis viruses. J Immunol 56:337–341, 1947

15. CASALS J: Heated, avirulent antigens for complement-fixation tests with certain encephalitis viruses. Science 102:618–619, 1945

16. CASALS J: Relationships among arthropod-borne animal viruses determined by cross-challenge tests. Am J Trop Med Hyg 12:587–596, 1963

17. CASEY HL: Adaptation of LBCF method of microtechnique In Standard Diagnostic Complement-Fixation Method and Adaptation to Microtest. Public Health Monograph No. 74. Public Health Service Publication No. 1228, US Government Printing Office, Washington, DC, 1965

18. CHAPPELL WA, HALONEN PE, TOOLE RF, CALISHER CH, and CHESTER L: Preparation of LaCrosse virus hemagglutinating antigen in BHK-21 suspension cell cultures. Appl Microbiol 18:433–437, 1969

19. CLARKE DH: Further studies on antigenic relationships among the viruses of the group B tick-borne complex. WHO Bull 31:45–56, 1964

20. CLARKE DH and THEILER M: The hemagglutinins of Semliki Forest and Bunyamwera viruses. Their demonstration and use. J Immunol 75:470–475, 1955

21. CLARKE DH and CASALS J: Techniques for hemagglutination and hemaglutination-inhibition with arthropod-borne viruses. Am J Trop Med Hyg 7:561–573, 1958

22. DAMON SR: Collection, handling and shipment of diagnostic specimens. USPHS, Communicable Disease Center, Atlanta, Ga, 1962, 75 pp

22a. EMMONS RW and LENNETTE EH: Immunofluorescent staining in laboratory diagnosis of Colorado tick fever. J Lab Clin Med 68:923–929, 1966

23. GAIDAMOVICH SY and KURAKHMEDOVA SA: Hemagglutinating properties of viruses of the phlebotomus fever group. Arch Gesamte Virusforsch 45:177–184, 1974

24. GARDNER PS and McQUILLAN J: Rapid Virus Diagnosis: Application of Immunofluorescence. Butterworth and Co, London, 1974

25. HALONEN PE, MURPHY FA, FIELDS BN, and REESE DR: Hemagglutinin of rabies and some other bullet-shaped viruses. Proc Soc Exp Biol Med 127:1037–1042, 1968

26. HAMMON W McD: Human infection acquired in the laboratory. J Am Med Assoc 203:647–648, 1968

27. HANSON RP, SULKIN SE, BUESCHER EL, HAMMON W McD, McKINNEY RW, and WORK TH: Arbovirus infections of laboratory workers. Science 158:1283–1286, 1967

28. HULL RN, CHERRY WR, and JOHNSON IS: The adaptation and maintenance of mammalian cells to continuous growth in tissue culture. Anat Rec 124:490, 1956

29. IBRAHIM AN and HAMMON W McD: Application of Immunodiffusion methods to the antigenic analysis of dengue viruses. I. Precipitin-in-gel diffusion in two dimensions. J Immunol 100:86–92, 1968

30. IBRAHIM AN and HAMMON W McD: Application of immunodiffusion methods to the antigenic analysis of dengue viruses. II. Immunoelectrophoresis. J Immunol 100:93–98, 1968

31. INABA Y: Hemagglutination with Simbu group arboviruses, Akabane, Aino, and Samford. Working Conference on Arboviruses, Dengue Hemorrhagic Fever, and Rabies, Sendai, Japan, August 25–27, 1976

32. IRVING GW JR: Laboratory Animal Welfare. Fed Reg, Part II, 32/37:3270–3282, 1967

33. KARABATSOS N: Supplement to the international catalogue of arboviruses. Am J Trop Med Hyg 27:372–440, 1978

34. KARABATSOS N and BUCKLEY SM: Susceptibility of the baby-hamster kidney-cell line (BHK-21) to infection with arboviruses. Am J Trop Med Hyg 16:99–105, 1967

35. KOKKO UP, STUART J, and TAYLOR G: Mailing of infectious specimens for diagnostic purposes. Public Health Rep 75:979–984, 1960

36. KUBERSKI TT and ROSEN L: Identification of dengue viruses using complement-fixing antigen produced in mosquitoes. Am J Trop Med Hyg 26:538–543, 1977

37. KUBERSKI TT and ROSEN L: A simple technique for the detection of dengue antigen in mosquitoes by immunofluorescence. Am J Trop Med Hyg 26:533-537, 1977

38. LENNETTE EH and KOPROWSKI H: Neutralization tests with certain neurotropic viruses: a comparison of the sensitivity of the extraneural and intracerebral routes of inoculation for the detection of antibodies. J Immunol 49:375-385, 1944

39 LOGRIPPO GA: Investigations of the use of beta-propiolactone in virus inactivation. Ann NY Acad Sci 83:578-594, 1960

40. LOGRIPPO GA: The safety of β-propiolactone as a biologic sterilizing agent. Clinical evaluation with human plasma and homotransplants. Angiology 12:80-83, 1961

41. MCKINNEY RW, BERGE TO, SAWYER WD, TIGERTT WD, and CROZIER D: Use of an attenuated strain of Venezuelan equine encephalomyelitis virus for immunization in man. Am J Trop Med Hyg 12:597-603, 1963

42. MITSUHASHI J and MARAMOROSCH K: Leafhopper tissue culture: embryonic, nymphal and imaginal tissues from aseptic insects. Contributions Boyce Thompson Institute for Plant Research 22:435-460, 1964

43. MURPHY FA and COLEMAN PH: California group arboviruses: immunodiffusion studies. J Immunol 99:276-284, 1967

44. NOYES WF: Visualization of Egypt 101 virus in the mouse's brain and in cultured human carcinoma cells by means of fluorescent antibody. J Exp Med 102:243-248, 1955

45. OLITSKY PK and HARFORD CG: Intraperitoneal and intracerebral routes in serum protection tests with the virus of equine encephalomyelitis. I. Comparison of the two routes in protection tests. J Exp Med 68:173-189, 1938

46. OUCHTERLONY O: Diffusion in gel methods for immunological analysis. Prog Allergy 5:1-78, 1958

47. POKORNY J: Taking blood samples from small animals from the retro-oribital venous plexus. Czech Epidemiol Mikrobiol Immunol 7:212-214, 1958

48. PORTERFIELD JS: Use of goose cells in haemagglutination tests with arthropod-borne viruses. Nature 180:1202, 1957

49. RANDALL R, GIBBS CJ JR, AULISIO CC, BINN LN, and HARRISON VR: The development of a formalin-killed Rift Valley fever virus vaccine for use in man. J Immunol 89:660-671, 1962

50. ROSEN L and GUBLER D: The use of mosquitoes to detect and propagate dengue viruses. Am J Trop Med Hyg 23:1153-1160, 1974

51. SABIN AB: Hemagglutination by viruses affecting the human nervous system. Fed Proc 10:573-578, 1951

52. SALMINEN A: Difference in the agglutinability of rooster and hen erythrocytes by the tick-borne encephalitis virus. Ann Med Exp Biol Fenn 37:400-406, 1959

53. SARTORELLI AC, FISCHER DS, and DOWNS WG: Use of sarcoma 180/TG to prepare hyperimmune ascitic fluid in the mouse. J Immunol 96:676-682, 1966

54. SCHERER WF and HOOGASIAN AC: Preservation at subzero temperatures of mouse fibroblasts (strain L) and human epithelial cells (strain HeLa). Proc Soc Exp Biol Med 87:480-487, 1954

55. SEVER JL, CASTELLANO GA, PELON W, HUEBNER RJ, and WOLMAN F: Inactivation of the infectivity of viral hemagglutinating antigens with the use of betaprone [propiolactone]. J Lab Clin Med 64:983-988, 1964

56. SMITH AL, TIGNOR GH, MIFUNE K, and MOTOHASHI T: Isolation and assay of rabies serogroup viruses in CER Cells. Intervirology 8:92-99, 1977

57. SPRANCE HE and SHOPE RE: Single inoculation immune hamster sera for typing California group arboviruses by the complement-fixation test. Am J Trop Med Hyg 26:544-546, 1977

58. STROME CPA: A closed-vacuum system for harvesting infectious infant mouse-brain material. Proc Soc Exp Biol Med 84:287-288, 1953

59. SUNAGA H, TAYLOR RM, and HENDERSON JR: Comparative sensitivity of viruses to treatment with diethyl ether and sodium desoxycholate. Am J Trop Med Hyg 9:419-424, 1960

60. TARAN A: A simple method for performing a Wassermann test on anticomplementary serum. J Lab Clin Med 31:1037-1039, 1946

61. TESH RB, CHANIOTIS BN, and JOHNSON KM: Vesicular stomatitis virus (Indiana serotype):

transovarial transmission by phlebotomine sandflies. Science 175:1477-1479, 1972
62. THEILER M: Action of sodium desoxycholate on arthropod-borne viruses. Proc Soc Exp Biol Med 96:380-382, 1957
63. THEILER M and CASALS J: The serological reactions in yellow fever. Am J Trop Med Hyg 7:585-594, 1958
64. THOMPSON WH and BEATY BJ: Venereal transmission of LaCrosse (California encephalitis) arbovirus in *Aedes triseriatus* mosquitoes. Science 196:530-531, 1977
65. TIKASINGH ES, SPENCE L, and DOWNS WG: The use of adjuvant and sarcoma 180 cells in the production of mouse hyperimmune ascitic fluids to arboviruses. Am J Trop Med Hyg 15:219-226, 1966
66. VARMA MGR, PUDNEY M, LEAKE CJ, and PERALTA PH: Isolation in a mosquito *(Aedes pseudoscutellaris)* cell line (Mos. 61) of yellow fever virus strains from original field material. Intervirology 6:50-56, 1975/6
67. VOLLER A, BIDWELL DE, and BARTLETT A: Enzyme immunoassays in diagnostic medicine. Bull WHO 53:55-56, 1976
68. WATTS DM, PANTUWATANA S, DEFOLIART GR, YUILL TM, and THOMPSON WH: Transovarial transmission of LaCrosse virus (California encephalitis group) in the mosquito, *Aedes triseriatus*. Science 182:1140-1141, 1973
69. World Health Organization: Arboviruses and human disease, WHO Tech Rep Ser No. 369, 1967
70. WESTAWAY EG: Assessment and application of a cell line from pig kidney for plaque assay and neutralization tests with twelve group B arboviruses. Am J Epidemiol 84:439-456, 1966
71. YASUMURA Y and KAWAKITA Y: Studies on SV40 in relationship with tissue culture. Nippon Rinsho 21:1201-1209, 1963

CHAPTER 27

ARENAVIRUSES

Jordi Casals

Introduction

The arenaviruses or *Arenaviridae* (41) are a group of antigenically related viruses which by electron microscopy (EM) show a unique morphology, including particles of electron-dense material inside the virion that give it the aspect of being sand-sprinkled (Latin, *arenosus*). The oldest recognized member of the group, first isolated in 1933, is lymphocytic choriomeningitis virus (LCMV), and it is therefore considered the type species. The other arenaviruses pathogenic for humans, the disease that they cause, and the year of their first isolation are: Junin virus, Argentinian hemorrhagic fever (AHF), 1958; Machupo virus, Bolivian hemorrhagic fever (BHF), 1963; and Lassa virus, Lassa fever, 1969 (11). Pathogenicity for humans has not been shown for a number of other arenaviruses (Table 27.1).

Clinical aspects

Epidemiology

With the exception of LCMV, all arenaviruses are geographically restricted in their natural distribution. AHF and BHF have been reported only in limited areas of Argentina and Bolivia, respectively; Lassa fever occurs in a larger area but, thus far, the naturally-acquired disease has been observed only in West Africa. LCMV may well have worldwide distribution, although its occurrence in Africa and Australia has not been documented. Similarly restricted distribution is shown by the arenaviruses that are not pathogenic for humans.

Two characteristics of the arenaviruses have important epidemiologic implications. These agents have a limited host range in nature with each virus being associated with 1, some with 2, animal species which constitute the viruses' reservoirs. The reservoirs are rodents, with the exception of Tacaribe virus which is maintained in bats. Secondly, the viruses induce in their natural host or reservoir a persistent tolerant infection with no easily preceptible ill effects, if any, with depressed or no antibody formation and continuing virus excretion.

TABLE 27.1—ARENAVIRUSES

VIRUS	NATURAL HOST RESERVOIR	ENDEMIC AREA
Human Pathogens		
Lassa	*Mastomys natalensis*	Nigeria, Liberia, Sierra Leone
LCM	*Mus musculus*	Worldwide
Junin	*Calomys laucha, C. musculinus*	Argentina
Machupo	*Calomys callosus*	Bolivia
Not Human Pathogens		
Amapari	*Neacomys guianae, Orzyomys goeldii*	Brazil
Be An 293022 (43)	*Oryzomys* spp	Brazil
Latino	*Calomys callosus*	Bolivia
Mozambique	*Mastomys natalensis*	Mozambique
Parana	*Oryzomys buccinatus*	Paraguay
Pichinde	*Oryzomys albigularis*	Colombia
Tacaribe	*Artibeus* l. *palmarum, A.j. trinitatis*	Trinidad
Tamiami	*Sigmodon hispidus*	Florida

The arenaviruses are not arthropod-borne; the few isolations from arthropods which have been reported appear to be of no epidemiologic significance. Maintenance of the viruses in nature and transmission probably occur by transuterine and transovarian routes and postpartum by way of infected milk, urine, and saliva. Horizontal transmission between individual animals is likely; it is also the way by which the infection is propagated to humans. Transmission to humans is by direct or indirect contact with the reservoir or, in some instances, with other infected persons; entry of the virus is by the upper respiratory or digestive route, conjunctiva, or through cuts in the skin.

Pathogenesis

LCMV infection of the adult mouse is the classic example of virus-induced immunopathologic disease; studies with Tamiami virus indicate that the disease caused in mice by this virus can also be immunomediated. Currently there is little to indicate that arenavirus diseases of humans are due to immunopathologic processes; clinical and pathologic observations rather favor the view that direct damage to cells by the virus can best explain the disease (11). The following pathogenesis has been suggested for the infection in humans (31): the virus gains entry by the upper respiratory or upper digestive route, or through cuts or abrasions in the skin, is caught in the local lymphoid tissue or lymph nodes where it first replicates; it then invades the cells of the reticuloendothelial system and the cells involved in the immune response whose functions are, thereby, inhibited. The virus causes extensive capillary damage resulting in capillary fragility, hemorrhagic tendency, and plasma leakage leading to hypovolemic shock. In progressive cases, damage to the organ's cells follows. If the infection regresses, recovery is usually complete, as the organ malfunction may have been induced by capillary damage and edema rather than by cell damage.

The diseases

The incubation period of the several diseases is estimated to be from 6-7 to 14-16 days; shorter incubation periods have been observed.

Lymphocytic choriomeningitis (LCM). There are 3 clinical forms of the disease and there may also be inapparent infections: aseptic meningitis, influenza-like or non-nervous system type, and meningoencephalomyelitic type. The influenza-like and meningeal types occur most frequently. The disease may last for up to 2 weeks and lead to considerable prostration and illness. Most of the specifically diagnosed clinical infections follow a benign course; only a few fatal cases have been reported, either after CNS involvement or hemorrhagic manifestations.

Argentinian hemorrhagic fever (AHF) and Bolivian hemorrhagic fever (BHF). The two diseases are very similar. The onset is insidious with chills, asthenia, malaise, headache, muscular pains which are often pronounced at the costovertebral angle, conjunctival injection, exanthem on face, neck, and upper part of the trunk, and increasing temperature that reaches 38-41 C (102-105 F), with little diurnal variation, remaining at that level at least 5 days. In severe cases, signs and symptoms become more pronounced, with dry tongue, dehydration, oliguria, and hemorrhagic manifestations consisting of petechiae on the trunk and oral mucous membrane and hemorrhages from the gums, nasal cavities, hematemesis, hematuria, and melena; loss of blood, however, is generally not a life-threatening complication. The disease lasts 1-3 weeks and convalescence is long. Mortality varies from 5% to 30% in different outbreaks. Clinically inapparent infections are considered to be uncommon. Transmission from person to person occurs infrequently.

Lassa fever. This is a disease with generalized organ involvement. The infection in humans has a wide spectrum of severity from mild, even clinically inapparent cases, to a prolonged often fatal disease with marked toxemia, capillary leakage, shock, and disfunction of various organs and systems. The onset is insidious with generally nonspecific symptoms which make for a difficult diagnosis; the acute phase of hospitalized patients lasts 2-4 weeks, but is much shorter in milder cases that may go undiagnosed.

A patient in West Africa or one who has recently traveled in that area, presenting with malaise, sore throat, exudative pharyngitis, 4- or 5-day fever unresponsive to antimalarials and antibiotics, myalgias and low or slightly subnormal white cell count must be strongly suspected of having Lassa fever.

On physical examination a patient appears acutely ill, febrile, toxic, dehydrated and somewhat lethargic. There is often conjunctival injection, coated tongue, exudative pharyngitis, lymphadenopathy, pulmonary rales, abdominal and muscular tenderness, and often a maculopapular rash; a temperature of 38-39 C (100-102 F) is usual, although it can go as high as 42 C (106 F). The disease progresses to its severe form in from 35% to 50% of hospitalized patients, with the increased toxicity and dehydration, diffuse capillary fragility as indicated by edema in neck and face, petechiea, rales and suffusions in pleural, peritoneal, and pericardial cavities; these patients usually have a fatal outcome during the second week of illness, the immediate cause of death being shock and cardiovascular collapse. Hemorrhage is not a serious complication of the disease. Mortality is between 35% and 50% of hospitalized patients; overall mortality from all infections, including inapparent, mild, and severe, has been estimated at 3% to 5%.

Pathology

Little is known about localization and type of lesions in humans after LCMV infection. Autopsy of AHF and BHF victims has consistently revealed lymphadenopathy on gross examination and occasional focal hemorrhages in the gastric and intestinal mucosae, lungs, and cerebral cortex. Microscopically, the most consistent abnormality reported in AHF is endothelial swelling in capillaries and arterioles of all organs and depletion of lymphocytes in the spleen. In BHF, hemorrhagic necrosis is observed in the brain and lungs, as well as widespread bronchopneumonia; altered Kupfer cells are seen. In Lassa fever, gross examination reveals congestion and edema of the viscera with effusions in pleural, peritoneal, and pericardial cavities; petechial hemorrhages are seen in the face, neck, and trunk. Microscopically, there is interstitial pneumonitis with edema and congestion. The liver appears to be the main target of the virus; fatty degeneration is observed, but the main and characteristic lesions are eosinophilic necrosis of individual hepatocytes and larger foci of necrosis generally distributed with little inflammation (49).

Description and Properties of the Viruses

Size and shape

The similarities in morphology and morphogenesis of the arenaviruses are marked and distinctive and were the basis for first associating the viruses in the present group (38).

Thin-section EM of infected Vero cells shows all arenaviruses are alike. At the peak of infection a large number of particles are seen in the cultures. The particles are round, oval, or pleomorphic, 60–280 nm in diameter, have a membranous envelope with surface projections or spikes 6-nm long, and contain between 2 and 12 internal electron-dense granules, about 20 nm across, strongly resembling ribosomes; no symmetry has been discerned. The virions mature by budding from plasma membranes; negative-contrast EM shows similar common characteristics of the virus with a slightly larger diameter, between 90 and 350 nm (39).

Chemical composition

All arenaviruses contain RNA. Extensive studies with LCMV and Pichinde virus have shown these 2 viruses have single-strand linear RNA in 4 large segments and 1–3 small segments; 2 of the large pieces with sedimentation coefficients 31S and 22-23S are virus specific, the other two, 28S and 18S are cell-specific, and the small ones, 4-6S are of uncertain origin (41).

Resistance to chemical and physical agents

These viruses are easily inactivated by ethyl ether, chloroform, and sodium deoxycholate. Low concentrations of beta-propiolactone (BPL) (0.1%) completely inactivate infectivity of Lassa fever (8) and other arenaviruses while preserving complement-fixing (CF) activity. The viruses are rapidly inactivated at a pH <5.5 and >8.5, and by heat at 56 C; they are highly sensitive to ultraviolet (UV) and gamma irradiation (41).

Antigenic types

There are currently 12 different arenaviruses recognized (Table 27.1). The viruses are related by immunofluorescence (FA) and CF tests (12, 13, 44, 51) to various degrees, and they are antigenically unrelated to any other agent. Of the human pathogens, Machupo and Junin viruses are closely related by FA and CF tests, while LCMV and Lassa virus are easily separable from each other and from the other two viruses. Neutralization (Nt) test results, either in plaque reduction tests with serum dilutions or by intracerebral inoculation of mice with the virus dilutions are, on the other hand, completely specific (9, 30, 47). There is no evidence to indicate that antigenic variants of the serotypes exist.

Antigens

Early studies with LCMV demonstrated the existence of a CF antigen distinct and separable from the infective particle by centrifugation; it was called soluble antigen. Recent studies have confirmed that virion and CF antigen are different entities. The antigen involved in virus neutralization appears to be located on the virion's surface and is highly type-specific; the CF antigen is not present on the surface (25). No hemagglutinating antigen for erythrocytes (RBC) from any animal species has been reported for arenaviruses.

Pathogenesis for animals

The laboratory animals most commonly used that develop a disease and die following experimental inoculation are for LCMV, adult mouse and guinea pig; for Junin virus, newborn mouse, newborn hamster, and adult guinea pig; for Machupo virus, newborn hamster and, to a lesser extent, newborn mouse; and for Lassa virus, adult mouse, guinea pig, and squirrel monkey. Newborn mice and newborn hamsters are generally susceptible to the nonhuman pathogenic arenaviruses.

Growth in cell cultures

Lassa, Junin, and Machupo viruses replicate well in various cell cultures with visible cytopathic effect (CPE), either in cultures under a fluid medium or under solid overlay for plaque formation; the culture generally used is Vero cells. Other cells such as BHK-21, LLCMK2, and CER can also be used satisfactorily with some of these agents. LCMV replicates to a high titer in nearly all cell cultures tried, but CPE in cultures with a fluid medium or plaque formation are not a dependable feature of its multiplication (32, 42). Lassa virus does not replicate in cultures of *Aedes albopictus* or *A. aegypti* cells (8).

Preparation of Reagents

Immune serum and ascitic fluid

Reference immune reagents can be prepared in inexpensive laboratory animals, and mice, hamsters and guinea pigs are generally used. In order to insure a high titer of antibody, the donor animals are hyperimmunized by giving them 3-5 injections of the vaccinating suspension; to minimize nonspecific reactions, particularly in the CF test, resulting from development of antibodies against the viral substrate, it is advisable to prepare antiserum in the same animal species in which the immunizing virus is propagated. If infected tissues from a heterologous species are used for vaccination, only one inoculation is recommended, for example when using infected mouse brain tissue to immunize guinea pigs.

Virus propagated in cell cultures has not been generally used as a source of vaccinating antigen for preparation of reference immune reagents. However, there is no reason why it should not be satisfactory if the titer is sufficiently high and the virus is banded in a gradient to increase the titer and to eliminate substrate constituents. The simplest procedure, however, is to vaccinate mice or hamsters with mouse or hamster propagated virus, respectively. While serum from mice is difficult to obtain, and the yield is small, these animals can be inoculated with ascites-producing materials (37, 45, and the fluid simply removed by paracentesis; the titer of antibody in ascitic fluid and serum is similar, and the yield of fluid from a mouse is from 5 to 15 ml.

Mice. Different inoculation schedules can be employed, two of which are routinely used in our laboratory.

In one of the schedules, 15-20 60-day-old mice are used; the vaccinating material, freshly prepared each time, consists of a 10% suspension of infected newborn mouse brain tissue in physiologic saline. The first injection of vaccine, given on day 0, is 0.3 ml by the intraperitoneal (ip) route. Some strains of LCMV are lethal for mice at that, or even higher, dilutions; it is advisable in this case to inactivate the virus used in the first injection only, by adding 0.5% formalin to the suspension and holding it at 4 C for 7 days, or by treating with 0.1% BPL for 24 hr at 4 C. On day 20-25, a second similar injection of fully active virus is given; 7 days later the mice are test-bled by cardiac puncture under deep ether anesthesia, using a 26-gauge needle ¼ inch long mounted on a 1-ml tuberculin syringe. Experienced workers obtain an average of 0.6-0.7 ml of blood from each mouse quickly and with a mortality not greater than 10%; workers with no experience should not attempt this technique. On day 45-50 the mice are given a third injection of virus similar to the second injection, followed 2 days later by ip injection of 0.1-0.2 ml of ascites from a mouse bearing sarcoma 180/TG (45); 7-9 days after administration of the sarcoma fluid when the mice begin to develop prominent ascites, the fluid is removed by paracentesis; this can be done several times on succeeding days until the mice die of their tumor. The ascites are pooled, allowed to clot at room temperature, centrifuged at 3200 × g for 30 min in an angle-head centrifuge; the clear supernatant fluid is collected and either lyophilized in 1-ml amounts or stored at −20 C until used. The titers of the serum and fluid by CF test are similar, between 1:64 and 1:512, depending on the virus.

In a second schedule, Freund complete adjuvant is used in order to induce ascites, as well as to enhance antibody titers. Groups of 60-day-old female mice are used; all injections are by the ip route. On day 0 the mice are given 0.2 ml of a mixture of equal parts of virus (a 10% suspension of infected newborn mouse brain tissue) and complete Freund adjuvant (Difco); the 2 components are thoroughly mixed by using a syringe and 18-gauge needle. Similar injections are given on days 7 and 14. On day 21, a fourth injection is given of 0.2 ml of adjuvant alone; on day 26 another injection of antigen and adjuvant, similar to the first injection, is given. Ascites develop and paracenteses are done beginning 6-7 days after the last injection. The amount of ascitic fluid produced is somewhat smaller than that in mice with sarcoma, but since the mice do not die they can be tapped more times. The titers of CF antibodies are similar to those obtained by the first method described.

Hamsters. Repeated inoculations of virus have been used for preparation of high-titer sera to Parana, Latino, and Machupo viruses (47). The schedule calls for 4 weekly ip injections of 0.1 ml of a 10^{-1} suspension in saline of suckling hamster infected brain tissue; the animals are bled 7-10 days after the last injection by cardiac puncture under deep ether anesthesia.

Guinea pigs. Immune sera for Lassa, Junin, and Tacaribe viruses have been prepared in guinea pigs by a single inoculation of virus. With Lassa virus, an ip inoculation of 1 ml of infected Vero cell cultures results in 75% mortality (46); the survivors bled 28-30 days after injection have CF antibody with a titer of 1:128 or 1:256. A second injection of similar material (booster injection) can be given 4 weeks after the first, and the guinea pigs are bled 7 days later. Single inoculations by the ip route of infected newborn mouse brain tissue containing from 10^3 to 10^5 LD_{50} of Junin or Tacaribe viruses, produce serum with a high CF titer (10).

Complement-fixing antigens

The source materials for preparation of CF antigens are newborn mouse and newborn hamster brain tissue and cell cultures infected with the viruses. Brain tissue is harvested 7-8 days after intracerebral inoculation of the virus, whether the animals show signs of disease or not; tissue cultures are harvested when they show moderate to advanced CPE.

Mouse and hamster brain tissue antigens. Antigens can be prepared from newborn mice for Lassa, Junin, Tacaribe, Pichinde, LCM, and Tamiami viruses; and from newborn hamster for Machupo, Parana, and Latino viruses. Various methods for antigen preparation have been described.

Concentrated and partially purified antigens are prepared by the sucrose-acetone method (8, 16). A diluent is prepared consisting of 9 parts of an 8.5% solution of sucrose in distilled water and 1 part of 1 M Tris buffer, pH 9, containing 1% BPL; the final concentration of BPL in the diluent is 0.1%. Brain tissue is homogenized (in a safety cabinet) in 4 ml/mg of chilled diluent using a high-speed blender (Lourdes, Model MM) set at 50% input, for 30 sec; a towel soaked with a diluted 5–6% sodium hypochlorite solution is wrapped around the blender jar before turning on the motor. The towel-wrapped jar is kept at 4 C for 18 hr. After this interval, the sucrose suspension is removed from the jar and added dropwise with mechanical stirring to 20 volumes of chilled acetone, analytic reagent grade. The mixture is centrifuged at 500 × g for 5 min, the supernatant fluid is discarded and to the sediment is added a volume of acetone equal to that first used. The centrifuge bottles containing the suspension are held for 1 hr in an ice-water bath, after which the sediment is easily dispersed by means of a plunger. The suspension is centrifuged as before, the supernatant fluid discarded, and the sediment dried under an oil-pump vacuum. After 3–4 hr the sediment is dry and to it is added a volume of physiologic saline (0.9% NaCl) equal to 40% the volume of the original homogenate. The rehydrated extract, after being held overnight at 4 C, is centrifuged in a preparatory angle-head centrifuge at 12,800 × g for 1 hr. The supernatant fluid is the antigen and is stored lyophilized in 0.5-ml or 1-ml amounts. The yield of final product is about 1.7 ml/g of original brain tissue. Antigens prepared by this method from mouse brain tissue infected with Lassa, LCM, Junin, Tacaribe, Amapari, Pichinde, and Tamiami viruses have CF titers between 1:128 and 1:512, depending on the virus, are avirulent, are not anticomplementary, and give no nonspecific reactions even when used undiluted.

Crude antigens are prepared by making a 10% suspension of infected brain tissue in physiologic saline containing 0.1% BPL. The suspension is homogenized in a high-speed blender as described above, held at 4 C for 18 hr, and centrifuged at 12,800 × g for 1 hr; the supernatant fluid is the antigen. These antigens have a low titer (from 1:4 to 1:16); while satisfactory for identifying isolates, they are not adequate for investigating antigenic relationships among viruses.

An improved crude antigen is prepared as follows. A 20% suspension of brain tissue in physiologic saline containing 0.1% BPL is prepared, homogenized in a high-speed blender, and held at 4 C for 18 hr, as described above. The suspension is next distributed in plastic tubes, 10–12 ml per tube, and immersed alternately for periods of 15 min in dry-ice alcohol at −76 C and water at 37 C; after 3 cycles of freezing and thawing, the suspension is centrifuged in an angle-head centrifuge at 12,800 × g for 1 hr. The clear supernatant fluid is the antigen and it is best preserved lyophilized in 0.5 or 1 ml amounts. The CF titers of these antigens for arenaviruses are between 1:16 and 1:64, depending on the virus; the antigens are not anticomplementary even when used undiluted (13).

Infected cell culture antigens. CF antigens can be prepared for Lassa, LCM, Tacaribe, Pichinde, and probably other arenaviruses using cell cultures, particularly Vero, BHK-21 and L cells. Cultures under fluid medium, either in tubes, 75-cm^2 bottles, or roller tubes, are inoculated at MOIs between 0.1 and 1; the fluids and cellular debris are harvested between the sixth and eighth day, at which time some viruses show marked CPE, others less so. To 9 volumes of the culture material add 1 volume of Tris buffer, pH 9, containing 1% BPL; after 18 hr at 4 C the material is centrifuged at low speed to sediment the cellular debris. The supernatant fluid constitutes the antigen. The CF titers of these antigens vary between 1:4 and 1:16, depending on the virus and time of harvesting of the cultures; they can be concentrated by means of Acquacide (8), or filtration under pressure (Amicon). For Acquacide concentration, the fluid is introduced into dialysis tubing, placed and covered in a bed of Acquacide, and held at room temperature from 4 to 12 hr, depending on the volume and degree of concentration desired. The concentrated fluid is then dialyzed for 24 hr at 4 C against 50–100 volumes of physiologic saline (0.9% NaCl); concentrations between 5- and 10-fold can be easily obtained, giving antigens with titers from 1:20 to 1:160. Excessive concentration may result in anticomplementary preparations.

General reagents

Complement-fixation test

Guinea pig complement, hemolysin, and sheep RBC are commercially supplied; the availability of dependable preparations saves much time, effort, and uncertainty.

Hemolysin is supplied as a 50% antisheep-RBC rabbit serum in glycerol; it is stable for periods of years when kept at 4 C. The titer of each lot of hemolysin must be determined in the system used, after which no further titrations are necessary.

Lyophilized guinea pig complement is available in ampules containing 1 ml, 3 ml, or more; the expiration date is usually 1 year. Complement must be used on the same day that it is rehydrated in the fluid supplied by the manufacturer.

Sheep RBC, washed and stabilized, are supplied as a 10% suspension of packed cells, usually in bottles containing 20 ml. The RBC can reach most laboratories in the United States within 24–48 hr after mailing; their expiration date is 2 weeks. If no such supply is available, they can be procured by bleeding sheep into Alsever solution.

As diluent, Veronal buffer has given consistently good results in our laboratory. Veronal (diethyl barbituric acid) and sodium Veronal (sodium barbiturate) of good quality are commercially available. The formula of the 5X concentrated buffer is 85 g sodium chloride (NaCl); 5.75 g Veronal; 3.75 g sodium Veronal; 1.68 g magnesium chloride (MgCl$_2$ - 6H$_2$0), 0.25 g calcium chloride (CaCl$_2$); and distilled water to 2000 ml. For use in the test, the stock is diluted by adding 4 volumes of distilled water to 1 volume of stock; the pH of the diluted buffer is 7.3–7.4.

Cell culture solutions

The general methodology for cell culture work is described in Chapter 3 of this book. Pertinent details concerning the particular use of cell cultures with arenaviruses are given on pages 828–829; in this section the preparation of reagents that are widely used in this work is described.

Phosphate-buffered saline (PBS). The buffer consists of 8.5 g sodium chloride (NaCl); 1.07 g disodium phosphate (Na_2HPO_4); 0.39 g monosodium phosphate (NaH_2PO_4 - $2H_2O$); distilled water to 1000 ml. Autoclave at 15 lb for 20 min. The buffer has a pH 7.1–7.2.

Growth medium. For Vero and CER cells in bottles the growth medium is 90 ml Eagle minimal essential medium prepared with Hanks or Earle balanced salt solution (EEM-H or EEM-E); 10 ml fetal calf serum; 1-ml mixture of penicillin and streptomycin (10,000 units of penicillin and 10,000 μg of streptomycin/ml). For BHK-21 cells and for stationary tube cultures of all vertebrate cell lines, the growth medium is 80 ml EEM-H; 10 ml fetal calf serum; 10 ml tryptose phosphate broth (Difco); 1-ml mixture of penicillin and streptomycin (10,000 units penicillin and 10,000 μg streptomycin/ml); 0.08 ml kanamycin (500 mg/2 ml).

Maintenance medium (MM). After monolayers have been infected, the MM consists of 97 ml EEM-H; 3 ml fetal calf serum; 1-ml mixture of penicillin (10,000 units) and streptomycin (10,000 μg); 0.08 ml kanamycin (500 mg/2 ml). The pH of the MM is adjusted with 2 M Tris stock solution (24.2 g of Trizma® Base/100 ml) by adding 0.1 ml or 0.2 ml of stock to 200 ml MM.

Overlay medium. A nutrient agar overlay routinely used in this laboratory (7) is as follows. The nutrient part of the overlay contains 18 ml Earle balanced salt solution, with no $NaHCO_3$, concentrated 10X; 3 ml 10% lactalbumin hydrolysate; 1.2 ml 5% yeast extract; 3.6 ml fetal calf serum; 3 ml 0.1% neutral red; 5.4 ml 7.5% $NaHCO_3$; 0.9 ml 2% DEAE-dextran; 1.8 ml penicillin (10,000 units) and streptomycin (10,000 μg/ml); 1.8 ml 100X concentrated fungizone; and sterile distilled, demineralized water to 90 ml volume. The nutrient part is mixed with an equal volume, 90 ml of 2% ion agar, and the overlay applied.

Immunofluorescence supplies

The indirect method of FA is generally used for diagnosis and other studies with arenaviruses. Conjugates of good quality are commercially available, the most commonly used being antihuman, antimouse, antiguinea pig, and antihamster. These reagents are supplied as goat or rabbit anti-gamma globulin for the species required conjugated with fluorescein isothiocyanate (see Chapter 4 for preparation of conjugates).

Tissue culture chamber-slides 75-mm × 25-mm with ≥4 chambers are available (Lab-Tek Products, Division of Miles Laboratories, Naperville, IL). Ordinary size, 75-mm × 25-mm, microscope slides coated with a water-repellent finish (Teflon) except on 10 or 12 circular areas 5 mm in diameter are used in seroepidemiologic surveys (Cel-Line Associates, Inc., Minotola, NJ).

Collection and Shipment of Specimens

Precautions

Junin, Machupo, and Lassa viruses are rated as highly dangerous in the laboratory and have been placed in a high-risk category, Class 4, by current Center for Disease Control (Atlanta, GA) guidelines entitled, *Classification of Etiologic Agents on the Basis of Hazard*; work with Class-4 viruses in the United States is restricted to centers which have a Class-P4 containment facility as defined in *NIH Recombinant DNA Research Guidelines*, July 1976, Fed. Reg. 41: 27911–27943.

Virus isolation

The principal material for isolation of virus from a patient is blood or blood serum collected as soon as possible after onset of illness. The period of viremia can vary with different viruses, but from 3 to 12 days after onset is the best time for successful isolation.

Other clinical specimens that have frequently yielded virus are CSF from LCM patients with meningeal manifestations; throat washings or swabs for Lassa virus, less frequently for Junin and Machupo viruses; and pleural, pericardial, and peritoneal exudates for Lassa virus. In fatal cases, LCMV has been isolated from brain tissue; Junin virus from liver, spleen, kidney, and blood clots; and Machupo virus from spleen and lymph nodes. Lassa virus could probably be recovered from viscera, but no attempts to isolate it from organs taken at autopsy have been recorded.

In order to achieve a rapid diagnosis, direct demonstration of the virus or its antigens in clinical specimens has been urged (2). For Lassa fever diagnosis, the specimens may include conjunctival scrapings, throat secretions and scrapings, blood cells, or various exudates or secretions.

Blood is collected by venipuncture using vacutainers (*Caution:* the stopper is almost always contaminated with blood) in preference to a syringe and needle; about 10 ml is taken, less from a child or infant. If the virology laboratory is nearby, the vacutainer is placed in a water-proof plastic bag, then in a thermos jar or insulated container with wet ice and transported to the laboratory by messenger; if whole blood is frozen, lysis of RBC may result in toxic effects to animals or tissue cultures on inoculation. Other clinical specimens can be handled similarly by placing bits of tissue or throat swabs in tightly stoppered tubes or, preferably, in screw-cap vials; in either case, the closure is covered with adhesive tape, and the containers placed inside water-proof bags.

When long-distance shipping is required, the specimens should be sent frozen on dry ice. Using extreme precautions, the serum is separated from the clot at the local laboratory, placed in a screw-cap plastic tube (Nunc tube) which in turn is placed in a double mailing case, the inside case is made of metal and the outside of cardboard, both screw-cap; the mailing case is placed in a box insulated with polystyrene and containing sufficient dry ice and cotton padding. Shipment of whole blood on dry ice requires that the blood be collected with syringe and needle and placed in a plastic tube; vacutainers made of glass often shatter at very low temperatures or on thawing. Other specimens are shipped similarly to serum, placing them in plastic tubes in preference to glass containers.

Specimens for virus isolation can also be shipped frozen in liquid nitrogen. This method has the advantage that a tankful of nitrogen lasts from 10 to 15 days, thus allowing the tank to be used for storage while collecting field specimens, as well as for shipping; air transportation by common carrier may have to be specially arranged. For liquid nitrogen shipping, the specimens are placed in shatter-proof screw-cap plastic tubes (Nunc tube) which in turn are placed in sturdy plastic bags, sealed, and immersed into the liquid nitrogen.

Special procedures apply to shipping of materials suspected of containing Lassa fever virus (1); this could equally apply to Machupo virus. The added precautions consist of wrapping the metal case that contains the specimen (see above) with absorbent material; the wrapped case is next placed in a plastic bag which is tightly closed or sealed and placed into a cardboard case containing a fair amount of shock absorbing padding material; the case is then closed with a screw cap. The case is placed in a container with dry ice, as described above. Specimens for Lassa fever virus isolation may currently be sent to 2 laboratories: Head of Special Pathogens Unit, Microbiological Research Establishment, Porton Down, Salisbury, Wiltshire SP4 OJG, England; or to, Chief, Special Pathogens Branch, Virology Division, Bureau of Laboratories, CDC, Atlanta, GA 30333, USA. The receiving laboratory must be informed by telegram prior to shipping.

Serologic diagnosis

At least 2 blood samples are collected, one during the early phase of the disease, and the other during convalescent phase. In general, antibodies in arenavirus diseases are late in appearing; the time at which the second sample is positive depends on the virus and on the test used. The Nt or plaque reduction tests have not been generally used for diagnosis of current arenavirus infections; as a matter of routine, the CF test has been employed. However, since about 1973 the FA test is becoming the test of choice for serologic diagnosis of these diseases (18, 23, 40, 50); antibodies are generally detected a few days earlier by FA than by CF and remain positive longer.

The early or acute-phase sample of serum is taken as soon as possible after onset of symptoms; it can be the same sample on which attempts to isolate virus have been carried out, provided that it is not hemolyzed whole blood. The second sample is taken from 25 to 30 days after onset of symptoms and, if negative, a third sample is taken at from 45 to 80 days. Serum for serologic diagnosis is placed in plastic tubes with tight screw caps and placed in plastic bags; in glass vials with screw caps and gaskets; or in sealed glass ampules. They can be sent at ambient temperature if the time needed to reach the diagnostic laboratory is only 2–3 days or in boxes with cold packs.

When serum is sent on dry ice, the use of plastic tubes is advisable to prevent breakage.

Since acute-phase serum may contain virus, they constitute a biohazard and should be handled with due care.

Direct visualization of clinical specimens

No attempts have been described to visualize and identify the virus in clinical specimens in LCM, AHF, or BHF; for Lassa fever, see pages 836–838.

General Considerations for Laboratory Diagnosis

The methods and procedures vary to a certain extent with the different diseases. In this section are described methods of general application; for their use in the specific diseases, see pages 832–838. These methods apply to all arenaviruses, including the nonhuman pathogens; however, procedures that require handling of infectious Class-4 viruses may be performed in the United States only in adequate containment facilities.

Virus isolation methods

Inoculation of animals

Animals routinely used for the diagnosis of arenavirus infections are mice and, to a lesser extent, hamsters and guinea pigs.

Newborn mice, intracerebral inoculation. Litters 1–4 days old are used; except for special studies, Swiss all-purpose mice of outbred stocks are used. The mice are lightly anesthetized in a large jar that contains a wad of cotton soaked with ether. The solution to be inoculated is taken up in a 0.25-ml syringe with 0.01 ml calibrations, fitted with a $^1/_4$-inch, 27-gauge needle with a short bevel. The mouse is gently but securely held flat on to the table in a prone position by holding its head and trunk between thumb and index finger, although the use of forceps is preferable. A fresh pair of forceps (or fresh pair of disposable gloves) should be used for each group of mice; the skin of the head is dabbed with an alcohol-soaked sponge, although this is not an absolute requisite and, holding the syringe at a 45° angle, the needle is gently inserted into the cranium at a point half way between the eye and the ear, lateral to the midline. Applying gentle pressure to the plunger, 0.02 ml of fluid is slowly inoculated, after which the needle is quickly withdrawn; if any oozing occurs at the puncture wound, it is wiped off with a sponge soaked in alcohol.

Newborn hamsters, intracerebral inoculation. Hamsters 1–5 days of age are used and are inoculated exactly as newborn mice.

Adult mice, intracerebral inoculation. The procedure is similar to that used for newborn mice. The age of adult mice is generally 28–60 days when used; with older mice the skull becomes tougher and it requires stronger pressure to penetrate. The mice are put under deep ether anesthesia; a $^1/_4$-ml syringe with 0.01-ml divisions is also used, with a $^1/_4$-inch, 26-gauge needle;

the amount of inoculum is 0.03 ml. For inoculation, mice should be held with large forceps (Russian tissue forceps).

Adult hamsters, intracerebral inoculation. Inoculate in the same manner as for adult mice; the inoculum is 0.03–0.04 ml.

Adult mice, ip inoculation. It is not nessary to anesthetize the mice; 1 person can do the inoculation alone by holding the mouse firmly in 1 gloved hand, by the skin of the neck with thumb and forefinger and by the hind legs and root of the tail with the fourth and fifth finger, while the other hand operates the syringe. The procedure is much faster if a helper holds the mouse. Inoculation is done with a 25- or 26-gauge needle, unless a heavy emulsion in Freund adjuvant is being injected, in which case an 18- or 19-gauge needle is advisable; the needle is $1/3$ or $1/2$ inch. The site of the puncture is in one of the lower quadrants, in a rostral direction; if the puncture is done slowly but steadily there is hardly ever any perforation of the gut. The amount of the inoculum varies depending on the purpose from 0.1 to 1 ml; for routine vaccination, inoculation with 0.3 ml is used.

All animals should be held in isolation cages. Intraperitoneal inoculation of hamsters and guinea pigs is done in a manner similar to that in mice. Foot pad inoculation of guinea pigs or mice is used on certain occasions (LCMV).

Preparation of cell cultures

Several cell types in cultures have been used successfully for propagation of arenaviruses with CPE under fluid medium and plaque formation under an overlay; the main cells are Vero, BHK-21, LLCMK2, and L. CPE and plaque production depend to a great extent on the virus: LCMV, while replicating to a high titer in most cell lines, does not generally give visible CPE or plaques.

The cells generally used in our laboratory are Vero (52) and BHK-21; the following description applies to them but can be used for other cells with adequate modifications.

Cultures of Vero cells are maintained in Roux or 150 cm^2-plastic bottles by weekly transfers. The growth medium consists of Eagle minimum essential medium prepared with Hanks balanced salt solution, 90%; fetal calf serum, 10%; and 1-ml mixture penicillin (10,000 units) and streptomycin (10,000 μg). The bottles, which contain 100 ml of medium, are held at 37 C. Subculture of the cells is described in Chapter 3. For transfer to maintain the cell line, a 1:4 split is used; the cell contents of 1 bottle are resuspended in a total of 400 ml of growth medium and this volume is divided equally into 4 new Roux bottles.

To prepare tubes and smaller bottles, cells are suspended in growth medium to contain between 1×10^5 and 2×10^5 cells/ml. In certain instances, for example to prepare cultures in chamber-slides, cells are used at a concentration of 2.5×10^5 to 4×10^5 /ml.

Tubes are seeded with 1 ml of the suspension and 2- or 3-oz glass or plastic prescription bottles with 8 and 10 ml, respectively. Panels with small wells have been used satisfactorily (48); they are seeded with 0.2 or 0.5 ml of the suspension. Tubes in a stationary position and bottles are incubated at 37 C for 3–4 days at which time they are ready for use; panels are held in a humidified incubator with 4% carbon dioxide and are ready in 2 days.

To inoculate tubes, or bottles under fluid medium, with the virus-containing material, the growth medium is removed, 0.1–0.2 ml of the inoculum is dispensed in the tube or bottle, allowed to adsorb for 1 hr at 37 C, after which the maintenance medium is added, 1 ml to a tube, 8–10 ml to a bottle.

The following procedure is used for inoculation and to overlay monolayers. Two- or 3-oz glass prescription bottles, or equivalent plastic bottles, are seeded as described above; when the monolayers are confluent, in 3–4 days, the fluid medium is removed. The inoculum is diluted, if so required, in 0.75% bovine plasma albumin (BPA) in PBS at pH 7.2, and 0.2 ml is dispensed to a bottle. The inoculum is adsorbed for 1 hr at 37 C after which 8 ml of freshly prepared nutrient agar overlay is added; the cultures are incubated at 37 C in an inverted position for 2 weeks. Plaque counts are made at various times as required.

Serologic tests

Neutralization test

Plaque reduction test. The test has been used routinely with the arenaviruses (31, 47) except LCMV; it has also been used with Lassa virus (3, 8, 26), but there are now conflicting views about its efficacy with this agent (36).

Serum is inactivated at 56 C for 30 min and serial 2- or 4-fold dilutions beginning at 1:4 are made in 0.75% BPA in PBS. A dilution of virus stock estimated to contain 100–200 plaque-forming units/0.1 ml is prepared; 0. 4 ml of virus and 0.4 ml of serum in dilutions are mixed, incubated at 37 C for 1 hr in a water bath and 0.2 ml of the mixture is inoculated into each of two 2-oz glass prescription or equivalent plastic bottles. After 1 hr of adsorption at 37 C, the cell cultures are overlayed with nutrient agar and incubated as described above and on page 824. Serum endpoints are calculated on the basis of 50% reduction of the number of plaques, the titer of a serum being given as the highest dilution that brings about that reduction.

Variations of plaque reduction tests for arenaviruses have been described in which plastic panels with wells of 1-ml or 0.3-ml capacity are used instead of 2-oz prescription bottles; in general, higher and more reproducible counts are demonstrated in bottles than in panels (48).

Mouse Nt test. Inoculation of mixtures of undiluted serum and virus dilutions by the intracerebral route is generally used. Three- to 4-week-old mice are required for LCMV, as newborn mice are not lethally infected by the virus; 1- to 5-day-old mice are used with other arenaviruses, provided that these animals are susceptible. Of the 4 arenaviruses pathogenic for humans, the mouse Nt test has been used only with LCM and Junin viruses.

The virus stock is a 10% suspension of infected newborn mouse brain tissue in 7.5% BPA in PBS kept at −60 C or lower in glass sealed ampules; this type of stock is used even with LCMV which, although not killing newborn mice, replicates to a high titer in their brain tissue. A 1:50 (or 2×10^{-2}) dilution of original infected tissue is prepared from the stock and from it, increasing 10-fold dilutions until a dilution is reached which from previous experience with the virus is known to be about 2 decimal dilutions higher than the anticipated LD_{50}. Dilutions are made with 0.75% BPA in tubes, 100-m × 13-mm, in an ice-water bath.

The test is based upon comparing the titer of the virus in the presence of each unknown serum with its titer when mixed with a known negative serum (control). Sets of tubes for each test serum plus one for the control serum and another one in which diluent will be substituted for serum are placed in wire racks in an ice-water bath; each set consists of as many tubes as there are decimal dilutions in the virus titration, ordinarily 7–8, from 2×10^{-2} to 2×10^{-8} or 2×10^{-9}. Into each tube of a set is measured 0.3 ml of the serum, or 0.3 ml of diluent when required. After the serum is distributed, the virus is added, 0.3 ml to each tube beginning with the highest dilution. The tubes with the mixtures are incubated at 37 C in a water bath for 1–2 hr, after which they are placed in an ice-water bath; the mixtures, beginning with the highest dilution, are inoculated intracerebrally into mice. Generally, 8 mice are inoculated with each serum-virus mixture; the mice are observed for 21 days and deaths recorded. Calculation of endpoint titers or LD_{50} are made by the Reed and Muench formula, or a similar one (see Chapter 26).

Complement-fixation test

Numerous versions of the test exist that differ in detail; one is described in Chapter 1. Another method which has evolved in our laboratory since 1940 (14) for the study of arboviruses and arenaviruses utilizes plastic trays 9″ × 14″ with 96 wells; the total volume of the reagents is 0.15 ml.

Numerous mechanical aids are commercially available for dilution and distribution of reagents, recommended as time-savers, for this and other *in vitro* tests, such as wire-loop diluters, multiple-drop distributors and others; their use is an individual decision.

Immunofluorescence test

The indirect test with incident illumination is being increasingly used; for routine diagnosis, transmitted UV light with fluorescein isothiocyanate as conjugated compound is employed. Techniques for fixation and staining of specimens have been repeatedly described, with minor variations; the procedure followed in our laboratory is given here.

Slide preparation. Antigen-containing preparations for diagnosis of current cases or for seroepidemiologic surveys are prepared on Teflon-coated slides with 12 circular areas or spots. Cell cultures under fluid medium are infected with a virus dilution at a MOI of 0.1–1, with LCM, Junin, or non-human pathogenic arenaviruses in the form of infected newborn mouse brain tissue stock. Five or 6 days later, regardless of presence or absence of CPE, the infected cultures are harvested; the cells are dispersed with 0.25% trypsin (see Chapter 3), washed 3 times with PBS, and resuspended in a volume of this diluent which gives a concentration of $3–4 \times 10^6$ cells/ml. The suspension is taken up in a 0.25 ml syringe with a 27-gauge needle, through which a drop of the suspension is deposited on each spot of the slide; the volume of a drop is approximately 0.01 ml, therefore it contains $3–4 \times 10^4$ cells. The slides are held at 37 C for 15–20 min until the drops dry, then fixed in acetone at 4 C for 10–12 min, dried in air, and stored at −60 C until used. The slides are good for at least 8 months.

Slides for FA test are also prepared in chamber-slides, usually those with 4 chambers. Cell monolayers under fluid medium are grown in the chambers; for 4-chambered slides each chamber is seeded with 2.5×10^5 cells in a volume of 0.8 ml of growth medium. After 2–4 days, depending on the cell—2 days for CER, 4–5 for Vero—the monolayer is ready for infection; the fluid is aspirated and the cells are infected with a virus dilution equivalent to 0.1–1 MOI, or with the material that is being tested for virus. From 4 to 7 days later some arenaviruses produce visible CPE, others none; at that time, the chambers are removed, the slides are thoroughly rinsed with PBS, fixed in acetone at 4 C for 10–12 min, dried in air, and stored at −60 C.

Due to current safety restrictions, no slides for FA have been prepared in our laboratory with Lassa and Machupo viruses; they may be available from the Center for Disease Control, Atlanta, GA.

Staining of slides. The method for indirect staining described by Gardner and McQuillin (22) gives excellent results. The slide is placed in a large Petri dish in which there are a few cotton pledgets soaked with water to maintain high humidity throughout. One or 2 drops of each serum to be tested, usually at dilutions $\geq 1{:}4$, are deposited on a spot; when the spots are filled, the lid is placed on the dish and it is placed in a humidified chamber kept in an incubator or walk-in room at 37 C for 30 min. The drops must not dry at any time during the incubation. The slides are removed, rinsed with PBS, and immersed in succession in 3 changes of PBS, 10 min each time. The slides are next drained and dried in air. The conjugated antiglobulin appropriately diluted is added, 1–2 drops to each spot, and the slide in the Petri dish is returned to the humidified chamber at 37 C where it remains for 30 min. The slides are rinsed with PBS, immersed in 3 changes of PBS each for 10 min, then in distilled water for 2 min, and dried in air. The slides can be observed in the microscope directly; mounting has not been found necessary, which simplifies the operation considerably. The addition of a counterstain, Evans blue at dilution 1:10,000, to the conjugated antiglobulin gives an excellent black-reddish background which increases the ease of viewing.

Microscope. There are commercially available at reasonable prices various makes and models of microscopes that operate with incident or reflected light of the proper wavelength for immunofluorescence; detailed descriptions and operating procedures are supplied by the manufacturers.

Most of the models have a setting for blue fluorescence, with a combination of dichroic mirror and filter that allows the required wavelength light (blue) to strike the preparation on the slide and reflect the light at a somewhat higher wavelength (green). For blue fluorescence the conjugate is made with fluorescein isothiocyanate. A light source that gives good performance is a high-pressure xenon lamp (Osram XBO-150 W) with a lifetime of 1500 hr and the advantage that it can be turned off and on repeatedly without loss of efficiency or need for cooling.

Other serologic tests

Other serologic tests have been used with arenaviruses, but they have not been applied extensively. Among these tests are agar gel diffusion and precipitation (13, 15); immunoelectrophoresis (17); and indirect hemagglutination (21). In the latter, glutaraldehyde-treated sheep RBC are sensitized with immune gamma globulin against a virus, Tacaribe as an example; contact of the sensitized RBC with a Tacaribe antigen causes agglutination of the RBC, which can be specifically inhibited by antibody against the virus.

Application of a solid-phase radioimmunoassay to LCMV has been recently reported (5); its potential requires investigation. There is no hemagglutination-inhibition test reported for these viruses; nor are there at present any reports on the possible application of enzyme-linked immunoassays to these agents.

Laboratory Diagnosis for Particular Diseases

With the arenaviruses as with other pathogens the basis of a specific diagnosis is identification of the virus or detection of antibody development between early-and late-phase serum samples. Virus identification, in general, requires isolation first; however, with some viruses other than arenaviruses, it has been acomplished directly in clinical specimens.

Owing to their restricted geographic distribution and to the characteristic clinical picture presented by severe cases, Lassa fever, AHF, and BHF are often clinically diagnosed with accuracy; clinical specimens for examination are usually available for these diseases. This is not the case with LCM; sporadic or even multiple cases of the influenza-like type may go unrecognized and, as no suspicion is aroused, early clinical specimens are often unavailable. It is only when multiple cases of the disease appear associated with contact with mice or hamsters, and particularly when some of the patients present meningeal manifestations that LCM is suspected and adequate clinical specimens for isolation are available.

Attempts to isolate virus are not generally made when AHF and LCM are suspected; they are made with BHF but are successful in only a small minority of cases; the diagnosis of these diseases is based on serologic tests. With Lassa fever, on the other hand, diagnosis is based on isolation and identification of the virus.

Argentinian hemorrhagic fever

The diagnosis is based on detection of antibody development between early- and late-phase sera. Virus isolation is attempted only in fatal cases, in cases that show antibody conversion to both LCM and Junin viruses, and in cases strongly suspected of being AHF but with serum conversion only to LCMV.

Isolation. Blood or blood serum taken as early as possible is inoculated undiluted and in a dilution of 1:10 by the intracerebral route into newborn mice, 1–2 litters per dilution; viremia in patients is observed between the second and the twelfth day from onset, with the highest frequency between the third and the eighth day (6). If virus is present in the inoculum, the mice appear sick beginning on the eighth or tenth day after inoculation, and they begin to die several days later. The brains from a few mice are removed, and a 10% suspension is prepared; it is advisable to make a second intracerebral passage in similar mice in order to improve the uniformity of infection. The stock suspension, first or second mouse passage, is kept wet, frozen at -60 C or lower temperature in sealed glass ampules.

In fatal cases, a pool is made with fragments of several viscera, kidney, liver, spleen, abdominal lymph nodes, and blood clots; the tissues are suspended in diluent to a 10% dilution, centrifuged lightly and the supernatant fluid is inoculated intracerebrally into mice as with the serum. As deaths of mice due to trauma may follow inoculation of a 10^{-1} dilution, it is advisable to inoculate other mice with dilution 10^{-2}. If mice appear sick, proceed as after serum inoculation.

Hamsters and guinea pigs have also been used for virus isolation; adult guinea pigs are as susceptible as newborn mice, even when inoculated ip. However, the use of these animals has no advantage over the newborn mice.

Isolation attempts directly in cultures of BHK-21 and Vero cells have been made; the available information about their success is scant and conflicting.

Serologic diagnosis. The routine procedure followed to confirm suspected cases is the CF test; since 1975, the FA test has also been used. In the CF test, serum is as a rule tested against Junin virus and LCMV antigens prepared by the sucrose-acetone method. The Nt test in newborn mice is not generally used to confirm cases during AHF outbreaks, as it is considered too costly and not entirely without technical difficulties. The plaque reduction test, although possible and sensitive (47), is not generally used as a diagnostic procedure.

Two samples of serum are requested: the first taken as soon as possible after onset, and this serum may be used for isolation attempts. Since extremely few sera are positive 15 days after onset, the second sample is taken 30 days after onset and, if it is negative, a third sample is taken at 60 days. The first dilution of serum used in both CF and FA is 1:4.

For some patients, conversion takes even longer than 60 days, particularly by CF test. Although of only recent application, it appears that the FA technique has definite advantages over the CF test for diagnosis in that the number of conversions are higher and detected earlier (4, 23, 53).

Identification of strains. Strains isolated from humans or from wild-caught rodents, suspected of being Junin virus are identified by CF. Crude saline extracts and sucrose-acetone antigens prepared with the strains are tested with reference immune serum or ascitic fluids for Junin virus; since LCMV is present in the endemic area for AHF, a test should include also an anti-LCMV serum. For complete and final identification a plaque Nt test easily separates Junin from Machupo and other arenaviruses (31).

Serologic surveys. No extensive surveys of the general population have been reported for this virus; they should be done by intracerebral Nt test in mice or by plaque reduction test in Vero cells. Possibly the FA test can give good information, but not the CF test since antibodies detected by this method are not long lasting.

Bolivian hemorrhagic fever

Specific diagnosis of the disease in nonfatal cases is difficult due to the fact that viremia is at a low titer, making virus isolation difficult, and antibodies take a long time to appear. Therefore, the patient is either dead or out of the hospital before serology is of any use. In fatal cases, virus isolation from the spleen is a reliable means of diagnosis.

Isolation. Newborn hamsters are more susceptible to the virus than are newborn mice. Blood or blood serum, also oral and throat swabs, taken from the acutely ill patient are inoculated simultaneously intracerebrally and ip to litters of hamsters. The isolation rate is positive in only about 20% of samples in serologically confirmed or subsequently fatal cases; the highest frequency of virus recovery is 7–12 days after onset (30).

Vero cell cultures are susceptible to the virus but less so than newborn hamsters. It may be profitable to inoculate hamsters and Vero cell cultures in chamber-slides, and to test brain sections or impressions and cell monolayers for the presence of Machupo antigen by FA; this approach may reduce the time needed for a diagnosis as in the case of Lassa fever (Johnson KM, personal communication).

For isolation from fatal cases, spleen tissue is suspended, with mortar and pestle or tissue grinder, in PBS with 0.75% bovine plasma albumin to a concentration of 10%; the suspension clarified by light centrifugation is inoculated simultaneously by intracerebral and ip routes into 2- to 5-day-old hamsters. With positive specimens, animals become sick 6–7 days after inoculation and even as late as 14 days.

Serologic diagnosis. The measurement of antibodies by CF and now, preferably by FA, is the most efficient and convenient means of establishing a specific diagnosis. Two samples of serum are required, one taken early and the second, 40–80 days after onset. Serum can be positive by CF as early as 14 days after onset, but the optimum diagnostic efficiency is shown at the 40- to 80-day period (34). FA and plaque reduction tests shorten somewhat the time needed to detect seroconversion but not to the point of giving an early diagnosis (40).

Identification of strains. The simplest methods for identification of Machupo virus strains are CF and FA tests; however, owing to the marked overlap among South American arenaviruses in these tests, final identification is made by plaque reduction test in Vero cell monolayers, using hyperimmune serum or ascitic fluid (30).

Serologic surveys. No large serologic surveys have been reported for Machupo virus; the opinion is that inapparent infections with the virus are rare. Seroepidemiologic surveys should be done by plaque reduction test or, more simply although less specifically, by the FA test; the CF test is not recommended as antibody becomes undetectable within a relatively short time.

Lymphocytic choriomeningitis

From a practical point of view the diagnosis of LCM in humans is based on determination of antibody development; virus isolation is rarely attempted.

Isolation. The most sensitive medium for detection of LCMV is a living animal, usually a mouse. Attempts to isolate the virus are carried out by intracerebral inoculation of the test materials into mice 4- to 6-weeks old; tissue culture systems are not satisfactory for routine diagnosis. The material of choice for virus isolation is the cerebrospinal fluid (CSF) from patients with meningeal signs, taken during the first week after onset; early-phase serum, while positive on occasion, appears to be less productive. Brain, spleen, liver, kidney, lung, and blood clots are the source for virus recovery from rodents; a 10% suspension of single or pooled organs is made in PBS containing 0.75% bovine plasma albumin and clarified by centrifugation at $1000 \times g$ for 10 min. The inoculated mice are observed for at least 14 days; in positive specimens a characteristic disease appears 6–8 days after inoculation, with tremors, convulsions, respiratory paralysis, and death, but the agent must be characterized serologically. Stocks of virus are prepared from the brain tissue resuspended to a 10% concentration in the above diluent.

There is some variability in the response of mice to different strains of virus; with some strains, they show convulsions and die in 6–7 days; with others, the mice may develop a somewhat lingering disease and die 10–20 days later, or even survive. The time needed for virus isolation can be shortened by giving the mice an ip injection of 100 μg of *Escherichia coli* endotoxin (Difco) in a 0.2 ml volume of PBS, 4–7 days after the intracerebral inoculation of the test material. In the presence of incipient LCMV infection the mice will sicken and die 24 hr after inoculation of the endotoxin (29).

Inoculation of 0.1 ml of a virus-containing specimen into the footpad of mice 4- to 6-weeks old results in foot swelling 10–14 days later; these mice, when challenged 2 weeks later with an intracerebral inoculation of an LCMV reference strain at dilution 10^{-2} or 10^{-3} will survive. For footpad inoculation, a ¼ inch, 26- or 27-gauge needle is used; the injection is made in the subcutaneous tissue of the plantar aspect of the foot.

Serologic diagnosis. The more readily available test in the immediate past has been the CF test; antigens and positive reference sera are commercially available. This test, however, is less sensitive than the indirect FA test, particularly in the early phase of the disease (18, 28). The Nt test, either by intracerebral inoculation in young adult mice, or in cell cultures (27) is more sensitive than either CF and FA for late-phase serum samples, but it is much too costly and elaborate for routine use. It appears that indirect FA is the test of choice for early serologic diagnosis of the disease in humans (33); if FA is not available the CF test is used.

Two serum samples are taken, one during the first week of illness and the second 20–30 days later. As an antigen source for the FA test, BHK-21 cells infected with a reference strain of LCMV in chamber-slides or spot-slides are used.

A plaque reduction test for assay of Nt antibodies to LCMV is the microplaque reduction, which differs substantially from other such tests. The test as described (27) is as follows.

The test is carried out in panels with microtiter cups 5 mm in diameter; serial increasing 2-fold dilutions of the test serum in 0.025-ml amounts are made in a diluent consisting of 1% bovine serum albumin (BSA) in distilled water beginning at 1:4 ending at 1:512, using microdiluters. LCMV consisting of infected BHK-21 fluid diluted in BSA so as to contain 3×10^5 pfu/ml, is added to the cups in 0.025-ml amounts. The mixture of serum and virus is incubated at 37 C for 1 hr. Then 0.05 ml of 1% agarose in water, previously boiled and cooled to 45 C is dropped into each cup and allowed to harden for 10 min. In the meantime a BHK-21 cell suspension is prepared and adjusted to contain 1.2×10^7 cells/ml; a mixture of equal parts of the cell suspension in Earle double-strength medium and 1% melted agarose in water is made and used immediately; 0.025 ml of the mixture is added to the cup and allowed to harden. The panels are incubated at 37 C in a humidified atmosphere of 5% CO_2 in air for 4 days. On the fourth day, 0.05 ml of 1% agarose containing 0.2% neutral red is added to each cup, incubated an additional 4 hr and read. Cups with control non-neutralized virus show 6-10 small plaques.

Identification of strains. Once a strain presumed to be LCMV is isolated, the method of choice for its identification is the CF test; cross-reactivity with other arenaviruses is minimal in this test. Antigens for the new isolate are prepared from infected BHK-21 cell cultures, or from infected newborn mouse brain tissue (24).

Serologic surveys. These are conducted by intracerebral inoculation into 4- to 6-week-old mice of mixutres of undiluted serum and virus dilutions. A plaque reduction test (27) may be the choice method for surveys of the general population, as antibodies can be demonstrated longer by Nt than by FA and CF tests, but there is little reported about its application.

Lassa fever

The diagnosis of Lassa fever is based primarily on virus isolation and identification; secondarily, on demonstration of seroconversion.

Isolation. Clinical specimens for virus isolation are blood serum, throat washings or swabs, and urine. Collection of blood and, particularly, throat specimens must be done with great precaution in order to minimize the risk of contact or droplet infection. The virus is also isolated from pleural and peritoneal exudates. Collection of visceral tissues at autopsy for virus isolation should be held at a minimum because of the risk involved.

Serum and urine, the latter treated with antibiotics, are inoculated undiluted, and in 1 or 2 decimal dilutions; throat washings are collected by gargling 1-2 ml of saline, which is then added to 4-5 ml of PBS with antibiotics, and inoculated. The method of choice for isolation, in fact almost the only method used, is by inoculation of Vero cell cultures; stationary tubes are generally used, but monolayers on 2-oz prescription bottles with an overlay, or monolayers in chamber-slides under fluid medium are also used. CPE is visible in tubes as early as 4 days after inoculation. Soon after CPE is definite, a virus stock is made with the fluid of the first set of tubes inoculated or after a subpassage (8).

The virus in the culture tubes is identified by CF; the whole culture is frozen and thawed, centrifuged lightly, and the supernatant fluid is used as an antigen against known immune serum.

A rapid diagnostic method combines isolation of the virus in Vero cells and identification in the cultures by IF. Chamber-slides with confluent, 2- or 3-day-old monolayers, are inoculated with 0.1 ml of the suspect material, usually serum; at daily intervals a slide is processed for indirect FA. Under most favorable circumstances a specific diagnosis can be made 24 hr after the specimen reaches the laboratory, in many instances by the third day; CPE does not become visible in these cultures until 2–3 days after identification is made by FA staining (50).

Virus is best isolated from serum collected within 14 days after onset, with 94% positives in that period in an observed series; virus has been isolated up to 19 days after onset. Throat washings are positive in about 50% of the cases during the same period; virus is found in the urine in a relatively small proportion of specimens, but it persists for as long as 32 days (35).

Serologic diagnosis. Owing to the delay in development of antibodies for this disease, serologic diagnosis does not provide an early answer. Currently, FA is the test that detects antibodies earliest; they can be observed 7–10 days after onset, even in viremic serum (50). CF is reasonably accurate and efficient but gives results late; antibodies are seldom seen before the fourteenth day after onset and remain positive for a much shorter time than by FA (12, 50). The Nt test has not been used for either early or delayed diagnosis (36).

Identification of strains. This is done by CF, using fluids from infected cell cultures or by FA with isolates propagated in chamber-slides or Leighton tubes. Strains of Lassa fever are easily separable from other known arenaviruses; all strains of the virus are indistinguishable from each other by these two tests. Plaque reduction tests have not been used successfully in attempts to detect possible antigenic differences between isolates form diverse areas (36).

Serologic surveys. In spite of reports of successful surveys by plaque reduction (3, 8, 26), the test has not been applied much to the problem, because there appear to exist unresolved difficulties with the test, as shown by the fact that serum with high CF titers may have no neutralizing capacity (36). Current surveys are done by CF test (19, 20) which probably reveals only recent infections, and by FA (Frame and Casals, 1977, unpublished observations) which is more efficient.

Rapid or early diagnosis. Owing to the relative frequency with which severe secondary cases of Lassa fever occur, it is advisable to have a specific diagnosis as soon as possible. At the moment, the earliest diagnosis is accomplished by isolation of the virus in cell cultures in chamber-slides and daily FA tests; in general, 3 days are required as a minimum.

Direct detection of the virus in clinical specimens, cells, tissues, blood, and secretions and excretions from the patient with no previous isolation, would be the fastest method. EM of a liver biopsy taken shortly after death of a patient (49) revealed Lassa virions associated with hepatocytes; the method is not recommended in the living patient as it may result in serious hemorrhage, nor is it type-specific. Observation of blood cells and urine sediments have given equivocal results. FA staining of conjunctival cells

obtained by scraping the everted upper eyelid in cases with prominent conjunctivitis has given a successful specific diagnosis in a number of patients,
within 2-3 hr after collecting the specimens (Johnson KM and Cannon RO,
personal communication).

Summary

Isolation of arenaviruses from humans, with the exception of Lassa fever virus, is dependent on inoculation of live animals (mouse, hamster, and
guinea pig) with clinical specimens; the use of cell cultures for direct isolation should be investigated and promoted.

Serologic diagnosis of current clinical cases has been based to a large
extent on the CF test; technical improvements and commercial availability
of good conjugates has now made indirect FA the test of choice. In comparative tests with serum from patients, the FA test has shown a higher proportion of positives, earlier seroconversion, and increased persistence of
antibodies than did the CF test. A similar comparison with the Nt test is
generally lacking. In fact, even if the Nt test proved to be better than FA, its
use may be limited for reasons of economy and safety. The possible application of other serologic tests, radioimmunoassay and enzyme-linked immunoassay, awaits trial.

In view of the frequency with which person-to-person transmission occurs in Lassa fever and of the problems created by evacuation of suspect
cases, early diagnosis is essential in this disease. Detection of viral antigen in
clinical specimens and its identification by FA—possibly also by immunoenzyme tests or immuno-electronmicroscopy—appears to be the answer.

AHF and LCM viruses co-exist in the same area; this results in serologic diagnostic problems deriving from the cross-relationship between the
viruses and the possible anamnestic booster responses easily detected by CF
and FA. This problem may become greater as additional arenaviruses, pathogenic or nonpathogenic for humans, are discovered.

Acknowledgement

In writing the section dealing with the actual procedures followed in
practice by the persons in charge of arenavirus laboratory diagnosis, the
author has had the benefit of the invaluable advice of: Dr. J. G. Barrera Oro,
Instituto Nacional de Microbiologia, Buenos Aires, Argentina; Dr. M. S.
Sabattini, Instituto de Virologia de Cordoba, Argentina; Dr. K. M. Johnson,
CDC, Atlanta, GA, USA; Dr. J. Hotchin, NY State Department of
Health, Albany, NY; and Dr. J. P. Woodall, San Juan Laboratories, CDC,
Puerto Rico. The writer expresses his deep appreciation to these individuals.

References

1. ANONYMOUS: Despatch of clinical specimens for laboratory examination for the diagnosis
   of Lassa fever. Wkly Epidem Rec 51:129, 1976

2. ANONYMOUS: Rapid laboratory diagnosis of virus diseases. Wkly Epidem Rec 52:77-78, 1977
3. ARNOLD RB and GARY GW: A neutralization test survey for Lassa fever activity in Lassa, Nigeria. Trans Roy Soc Trop Med Hyg 71:152-154, 1977
4. BARRERA ORO JG, GRELA ME, ZANNOLI VH, and GARCIA CA: Investigacion de anticuerpos contra virus Junin y LCM en casos presuntivos de FHA. Medicina (Buenos Aires), 37, Suppl No. 3:69-77, 1977
5. BLECHSCHMIDT M, GERLICH W, and THOMSSEN R: Radioimmunoassay for LCM virus antigens and anti-LCM virus antibodies and its application in an epidemiologic survey of people exposed to Syrian hamsters. Med Microbiol Immunol 163:67-76, 1977
6. BOXACA MC, GUERRERO LB, PARODI AS, RUGIERO HR, and GONZALEZ S: Viremia en enfermos de fiebre hemorragica Argentina. Rev Assoc Med Argentina 79:230-238, 1965
7. BUCKLEY SM: Cross plaque neutralization tests with cloned Crimean hemorrhagic fever-Congo (CHF-C) and Hazara viruses. Proc Soc Exp Biol Med 146:594-600, 1974
8. BUCKLEY SM and CASALS J: Lassa fever, a new virus disease of man from West Africa. III. Isolation and characterization of the virus. Am J Trop Med Hyg 19:680-691, 1970
9. CALISHER CH, TZIANABOS T, LORD RD, and COLEMAN PH: Tamiami virus, a new member of the Tacaribe group. Am J Trop Med Hyg 19:520-526, 1970
10. CASALS J: Serological studies on Junin and Tacaribe viruses. Am J Trop Med Hyg 14:794-796, 1965
11. CASALS J: Arenaviruses. Yale J Biol Med 48:115-140, 1975
12. CASALS J: Serological reactions with arenaviruses. Medicina (Buenos Aires), 37, Suppl No. 3:59-68, 1977
13. CASALS J, BUCKLEY SM, and CEDENO R: Antigenic properties of the arenaviruses. Bull WHO 52:421-427, 1975
14. CASALS J: Immunological techniques for animal viruses In Methods in Virology, Maramorosch K and Koprowski H (eds), Vol 3, Academic Press, New York-London, 1967, pp 113-198
15. CHASTEL C: Interet des techniques d'immunoprecipitation en gel (Immunodiffusion double, immunoelectrophorese) pour l'etude des arbovirus et des arenavirus. Rev Epid Med Soc 22:231-254, 1974
16. CLARKE DH and CASALS J: Techniques for hemagglutination and hemagglutination-inhibition with arthropod-borne viruses. Am J Trop Med Hyg 7:561-573, 1958
17. CUADRADO RR and CASALS J: Differentiation of arboviruses by immunoelectrophoresis. J Immunol 98:314-320, 1967
18. DEIBEL R, WOODALL JP, DECHER WJ, and SCHRYVER GD: Lymphocytic choriomeningitis virus in man. J Am Med Assoc 232:501-504, 1975
19. FABIYI A and TOMORI O: Use of the complement-fixation (CF) test in Lassa fever surveillance. Bull WHO 52:605-608, 1975
20. FRAME JD: Surveillance of Lassa fever in missionaries stationed in West Africa. Bull WHO 52:593-598, 1975
21. GAJDAMOVIC SJA, KLISENKO GA, KOCEROVSKAJA MJU, and SANOJAN NK: Antigenic relationships of lymphocytic choriomeningitis virus and Tacaribe virus in the indirect haemagglutination test. Bull WHO 52:437-439, 1975
22. GARDNER PS and McQUILLIN J: Rapid Virus Diagnosis, Application of Immunofluorescence, Butterworth and Co, London, 1974
23. GRELA ME, GARCIA CA, ZANNOLI VH, and BARRERA ORO JG: Serologia de la fiebre hemorragica Argentina. II. Comparacion de la prueba indirecta de anticuerpos fluorescentes con la de fijacion de complemento. Acta Bioquim Clin Latinoamericana 9:141-146, 1975
24. GRESIKOVA M and CASALS J: A simple method of preparing a complement-fixing antigen for lymphocytic choriomeningitis virus. Acta Virol 7:380, 1963
25. GSHWENDER HH and LEHMANN-GRUBE F: Antigenic properties of the LCM virus: virion and complement-fixing antigen In Lymphocytic Choriomeningitis Virus and Other Arenaviruses, Lehmann-Grube F (ed), Springer-Verlag, Berlin, 1973, pp 26-35
26. HENDERSON BE, GARY GW JR, KISSLING RE, FRAME JD, and CAREY DE: Lassa fever. Virological and serological studies. Trans Roy Soc Trop Med Hyg 66:409-416, 1972

27. HOTCHIN J and KINCH W: Microplaque reduction: new assay for neutralizing antibody to lymphocytic choriomeningitis virus. J Infect Dis 131:186–188, 1975
28. HOTCHIN J and SIKORA E: Laboratory diagnosis of lymphocytic choriomeningitis. Bull WHO 52:555–559, 1975
29. HOTCHIN J, SIKORA E, KINCH W, HINMAN A, and WOODALL J: Lymphocytic choriomeningitis in a hamster colony causes infection of hospital personnel. Science 185:1173–1174, 1974
30. JOHNSON KM, HALSTEAD SB, and COHEN SN: Hemorrhagic fevers of Southeast Asia and South America: a comparative appraisal. Prog Med Virol 9:105–158, 1967
31. JOHNSON KM, WEBB PA, and JUSTINES G: Biology of Tacaribe-complex viruses In Lymphocytic Choriomeningitis Virus and Other Arenaviruses, Lehmann-Grube F (ed), Springer-Verlag, Berlin, 1973, pp 241–258
32. LEHMANN-GRUBE F: Lymphocytic choriomeningitis virus. Virol Monogr 10:1–173, Springer-Verlag, New York, 1971
33. LEWIS VJ, WALTER PD, THACKER WL, and WINKLER WG: Comparison of three tests for the serological diagnosis of lymphocytic choriomeningitis virus infection. J Clin Microbiol 2:193–197, 1975
34. MACKENZIE RB, WEBB PA, and JOHNSON KM: Detection of complement-fixing antibody after Bolivian hemorrhagic fever, employing Machupo, Junin and Tacaribe virus antigens. Am J Trop Med Hyg 14:1079–1084, 1965
35. MONATH TP and CASALS J: Diagnosis of Lassa fever and the isolation and management of patients. Bull WHO 52:707–715, 1975
36. MONATH TP, MERTENS PE, PATTON R, MOSER CR, BAUM JJ, PINNEO L, GARY GW, and KISSLING RE: A hospital epidemic of Lassa fever in Zorzor, Liberia, March-April 1972. Am J Trop Med Hyg 22:773–779, 1973
37. MUNOZ J: Production in mice of large volumes of ascites fluid containing antibodies. Proc Soc Exp Biol Med 95:757–759, 1957
38. MURPHY FA, WEBB PA, JOHNSON KM, and WHITFIELD SG: Morphological comparison of Machupo with lymphocytic choriomeningitis virus: basis for a new taxonomic group. J Virol 4:535–541, 1969
39. MURPHY FA, WHITFIELD SG, WEBB PA, and JOHNSON JM: Ultrastructural studies of arenaviruses In Lymphocytic Choriomeningitis Virus and Other Arenaviruses, Lehmann-Grube F (ed), Springer-Verlag, Berlin, 1973, pp 273–285
40. PETERS CJ, WEBB PA, and JOHNSON KM: Measurement of antibodies to Machupo virus by the indirect fluorescent technique. Proc Soc Exp Biol Med 142:526–531, 1973
41. PFAU CJ, BERGOLD GH, CASALS J, JOHNSON KM, MURPHY FA, PEDERSEN IR, RAWLS WE, ROWE WP, WEBB PA, and WEISSENBACHER MC: Arenaviruses. Intervirology 4:207–213, 1974
42. PFAU CJ, WELSH RW, and TROWBRIDGE RS: Plaque assays and current concepts of regulation in arenavirus infections In Lymphocytic Choriomeningitis Virus and Other Arenaviruses, Lehmann-Grube F (ed), Springer-Verlag, Berlin, 1973, pp 101–111
43. PINHEIRO FP, WOODALL JP, TRAVASSOS DA ROSA APA, and TRAVASSOS DA ROSA JF: Studies on arenaviruses in Brazil. Medicina (Buenos Aires), 37, Suppl No. 3:175–181, 1977
44. ROWE WP, PUGH WE, WEBB PA, and PETERS CJ: Serological relationship of the Tacaribe complex of viruses to lymphocytic choriomeningitis virus. J Virol 5:289–292, 1970
45. SARTORELLI AC, FISCHER DS, and DOWNS WG: Use of sarcoma 180/TG to prepare hyperimmune ascitic fluid in the mouse. J Immunol 96:676–682, 1966
46. WALKER DH, WULFF H, LANGE JV, and MURPHY FA: Comparative pathology of Lassa virus infection in monkeys, guinea pigs, and Mastomys natalensis. Bull WHO 52:523–534, 1975
47. WEBB PA, JOHNSON KM, HIBBS JB, and KUNS ML: Parana, a new Tacaribe complex virus from Paraguay. Arch Gesamte Virusforsch 32:379–388, 1970
48. WEBB PA, JOHNSON KM, and MACKENZIE RB: The measurement of specific antibodies in Bolivian hemorrhagic fever by neutralization of virus plaques. Proc Soc Exp Biol Med 130:1013–1019, 1969
49. WINN WC JR, MONATH TP, MURPHY FA, and WHITFIELD SG: Lassa virus hepatitis: observation on a fatal case from the 1972 Sierra Leone epidemic. Arch Pathol 99:599–604, 1975

50. WULFF H and LANGE JV: Indirect immunofluorescence for the diagnosis of Lassa fever infection. Bull WHO 52:429–436, 1975

51. WULFF H, LANGE JV, and WEBB PA: Interrelationships among arenaviruses measured by indirect immunofluorescence. Intervirology, 9:344–350, 1978

52. YASUMURA Y and YAWAKITA Y: Research into SV40 virus by tissue culture. Nippon Rin-sho 21:1201, 1963

53. ZANNOLI VH, GRELA ME, GARCIA CA, and BARRERA ORO JG: Serologia de la fiebre hemorragica Argentina I. Prueba indirecta de anticuerpos fluorescentes. Acta Bioquim Clin Latinoam 9:133–140, 1975

CHAPTER 28

RABIES VIRUS

Harald Norlin Johnson

Introduction

Rabies is one of the zoonotic diseases, related to man's association with dogs. When infected with rabies virus, animals ordinarily docile or timid of man can become extremely vicious and aggressive; hence the name rabies, meaning furious, raging, mad, or frantic. The disease has been known since ancient times, and there is a history of periodic outbreaks of rabies in wolves, foxes, coyotes, and jackals. During such outbreaks people working in the fields or walking on the roads are attacked by rabid animals, and dogs as well as other domesticated animals become infected with the disease. Rabies in humans, also called hydrophobia, was relatively rare until the increase in the number of dogs in urban centers. Since the beginning of the eighteenth century the canine population in most large cities has been large enough to maintain the disease by dog-to-dog transmission for an indefinite period unless quarantine or vaccination of dogs against rabies is practiced. Infected dogs and cats are the common source of human infection.

The current widespread epidemic of rabies in wildlife, which extends from the Arctic Circle to the Tropics in both the Old and New Worlds, is an example of the cyclical character of diseases derived from wildlife. About 100 years ago there was a similar outbreak of rabies. The animal reservoir of rabies is not known, but the natural history of the disease indicates that the permanent hosts of the virus are the weasel, civet, mongoose, and skunk families. In the United States the spotted skunk and the weasel are occasionally found infected with rabies in regions where the disease is otherwise unknown. Such sporadic cases of rabies are of particular interest as regards the natural history of the virus because they indicate the probable source of the virus (35).

In the United States, dog rabies is relatively rare due to the enforcement of control regulations, especially the requirement that dogs be immunized with an approved rabies virus vaccine if allowed at large in a region where the disease is active in wildlife. There have been recurrent outbreaks of dog rabies in the United States-Mexico border region, one in the Nogales, Arizona area in 1972; another in the El Paso, Texas area in 1973-1975; and a recent outbreak in the Laredo, Texas area in 1976-1977. In 1976, of 3146 laboratory-confirmed rabies cases in the United States, only 116 were in dogs. There were cases in 1468 skunks, 737 bats, 187 foxes, 277 raccoons, 40 mongooses (Puerto Rico), 106 domestic cats, 164 cattle, 30 horses and mules, 3 swine, and 1 goat. Two people died from rabies in 1976, one in Maryland, exposed by the bite of a big brown bat, *Eptesicus fuscus*, the other in Texas, exposed by the bite of a stray dog while visiting in Mexico (78). There have been 9 cases of human rabies from skunk bite in the United States and 2 in Canada since 1951. Four of these occurred in South Dakota, 2 in California, 1 in Ohio, 1 in Minnesota, 1 in Arizona, and 2 in Ontario. There have been 10 cases of human rabies from bat-bite exposure in the United States and one in Canada since 1950. One of the victims, a 6-year-old boy who developed rabies in 1970, recovered completely from the disease (28). The rabies epidemic in wildlife in Canada is similar to that in the United States. There were 1696 laboratory-confirmed rabies cases in Canada during 1976; these were in 775 foxes, 269 cattle, 334 skunks, 89 dogs, 83 cats, 56 bats, 41 horses, 22 sheep, 10 swine, 4 wolves, 5 raccoons, 4 coyotes, 2 goats, 1 deer, and 1 rabbit. In Mexico and much of Central and South America, rabies is present as an endemic infection of dogs. In 1976 there were 4525 laboratory-confirmed cases of rabies in Mexico, and 3940 of these were in dogs (78). The epidemic of fox rabies in Europe continues to spread southward and westward. There does not seem to be any bat-to-bat transmission of rabies in Europe, Africa, or Asia.

Clinical aspects

Mode of transmission. Rabies ordinarily is transmitted by bite from animal to animal and from animal to humans. Dog rabies is an example of aberrant parasitism where the natural capacity of the virus to produce encephalitis becomes the means by which it can adapt to the host, that is, by increasing the tendency of this host to bite. In turn, this mode of transmission selects a virus population which can reach and multiply in the submaxillary salivary glands and be excreted in the saliva of the rabid animal. The lungs may be infected by rabies virus, and the natural history of the disease indicates that the infection is maintained in some natural host as an asymptomatic infection of the respiratory tract. Two cases of rabies in humans were related to non-bite exposure to rabies virus in a cave in Texas (15). The mode of transmission of rabies virus in this cave bat population seems to have selected a variant of the virus which is transmitted more readily by aerosol exposure than the rabies virus found in dogs. This hypothesis was confirmed by the occurrence of an outbreak of non-bite transmission of rabies in laboratory-held foxes and coyotes, some of which had been held for a time in a bat cave (74). In 1972, a veterinary microbiologist died of rabies (14). There was no history of animal bite, but 12 days prior to the onset of the disease this person had prepared an experimental lot of rabies vaccine from goat brain tissue infected with the Pasteur rabbit-brain-fixed rabies virus. There was no indication of a laboratory accident; however, the type of blender used to homogenize the brain tissue could have produced an aerosol containing the rabies virus. The virus isolated from the patient was similar to the rabies virus used for the production of the vaccine (14, 29). In 1977, a laboratory technician contracted rabies and survived the infection. There was no history of animal bite or accidental exposure to rabies, but 13 and 14 days prior to the onset of the disease this person had worked with an aerosol-producing machine in the course of preparing a live-virus vaccine for immunization of animals. The vaccine virus used was the Street-Alabama-Dufferin (SAD) commercial veterinary rabies virus strain (66, 67). These laboratory-associated cases of rabies illustrate the danger of inhaling aerosols containing rabies virus. Special precautions must be used in processing tissue suspensions in blenders and in the course of transfer of infected tissue suspensions from one container to another.

Pathogenesis. Rabies is an acute, often fatal, infectious disease of the central nervous system (CNS) which is apt to be characterized by abnormal behavior or madness, a type of infectious insanity. The relationship of the early sensory and motor symptoms to the site of bite exposure is evidence for the invasion of the CNS by way of the nerve pathways. Studies of the pathogenesis of rabies in experimental animals have shown that the infection may begin in striated muscle cells. Neuromuscular and neurotendonal spindles near the site of inoculation are involved secondarily, the infection progressing along peripheral nerves to the brain (49). Following intramuscular inoculation with rabies virus, administration of an adrenocorticotropic hormone can reactivate a latent infection (61). This indicates that the virus can infect and remain localized at the inoculation site for several months. The virus may invade and multiply in the submaxillary salivary glands, the parotid salivary glands, the lachrymal glands, the mammary glands, the lungs, kidneys, and pancreas. The virus has been isolated from the epithelial lining of the intestine (35). The rabies virus antigen can be demonstrated by the fluorescent rabies antibody (FRA) test in the cornea, nasal mucosa, and in nerve-end organs of the mouth (16, 50, 55).

The ability of rabies virus to multiply in the lungs and various mucus-secreting tissues of the respiratory tract makes it possible for the virus to be dispersed as an aerosol from the nose and mouth. The demonstration of rabies virus in the kidneys in some infected animals shows that the virus may be excreted in the urine. The virus has been isolated from the urine of a child that had rabies (9). Virus from the pancreas and intestine can be eliminated in the feces, and virus from the mammary glands in the milk. There are, thus, a variety of means for the virus to set up cycles of infection not associated with encephalitis.

The use of infant mice in testing for rabies virus furnishes an example of infection by ingestion of the virus. A high percentage of mother mice develop rabies if they eat the infant mice that die of rabies. This shows that carnivorous animals can be infected by eating carcasses infected with rabies virus. This route of exposure must be considered in the investigation of isolated cases of rabies in animals. For example, carnivores such as skunks, foxes, dogs, and cats presumably could become infected from eating bats that have rabies. This could explain some of the isolated cases of rabies observed in cats. There is no evidence to indicate that rabies virus will be present in the blood or blood-forming organs of rabid animals. In experimentally infected animals the blood is negative for rabies virus during the incubation period, as well as after the onset of the disease. The presence of rabies virus in epithelial tissues of various organs is always associated with infection of the CNS, and studies of field specimens of bats do not confirm the alleged carrier state of rabies in bats reported in the literature (35).

Rabies virus has been isolated from the spinal fluid of humans with rabies, but this is an unusual finding. If street rabies virus produces a local infection of muscle tissue as the result of experimental inoculation, the secretory organs appear to be invaded only as the result of centrifugal spread from the CNS (50). This suggests that local infection of muscle tissue alone would not result in transmission of the disease.

Incubation period. The incubation period is usually from 1 to 3 months but may vary from 10 days to >1 year. An incubation period of <30 days can be expected in about 20% of the cases of untreated rabies in humans. Passive immunization by administration of rabies hyperimmune serum usually prevents the development of the disease until immunity is obtained from the vaccine treatment. The usual incubation period for natually exposed dogs is 21–60 days.

Period of infectivity. Rabies virus may be present in the saliva of dogs as early as 3 days before obvious symptoms of rabies appear. A dog or other animal, although apparently healthy, that has bitten a person must be confined in a veterinary hospital or animal pound for 7–10 days, depending on local regulations, to permit observation for signs of rabies and to insure that the animal does not escape. If the biting animal is apprehended and can be kept under observation for 5 days and remains healthy, one can conclude that exposure to rabies did not occur (69). Wild animals and obviously ill domestic animals that have bitten someone should be killed and tested for rabies virus.

Symptoms and signs. If a patient is known to have been bitten by a rabid animal and the symptomatology is characteristic, there is little or no difficulty in making a correct clinical diagnosis. However, in some cases it is impossible to obtain a history of exposure, due largely to the failure of a patient or his relatives to recollect a minor wound produced by an apparently healthy dog. At times the clinical course of rabies may be very similar to that of poliomyelitis or encephalitis produced by other viral agents. The disease in humans is called hydrophobia because it commonly results in episodes of painful spasmodic contractions of the throat muscles following attempts to swallow water. The symptomatology is dependent on the relative excitation or depression of the CNS. In most instances death occurs during a convulsive seizure or following the onset of coma. Sometimes the disease is characterized by progressive ascending paralysis without a prodromal excitation phase. Abnormal sensations at the site of infection occur in about 80% of the cases.

For practical purposes, rabies in dogs is classified as furious or dumb, depending on the signs shown. In the former type, the excitation phase is prolonged, while in the latter the paralytic phase develops early. Most infected dogs show some manifestation of both types, that is, a short excitation phase characterized by restlessness, nervousness, and viciousness, followed rapidly by depression and paralysis. Sudden death of dogs from rabies, without appreciable signs of illness, is not uncommon. Dogs with the furious type of the disease usually die within 5 days after the onset of symptoms. In an exceptional case the rabid dog may live for 2–3 weeks after the onset of illness, and experimentally infected dogs are known to recover after a classic paralytic illness (4). Dogs that develop a paralytic disease following inoculation with rabies virus and recover show a high titer of rabies antibodies in the cerebrospinal fluid (CSF) as well as in the blood serum (7). Prolonged survival as well as recovery from rabies in humans has been proved by serologic tests (20, 28, 53). An immediate laboratory diagnosis of rabies by FRA tests of corneal impressions can be made in some cases (13, 55). Saliva and mouth swab specimens and CSF should be taken for virus isolation studies. Blood should be taken for serologic studies, and fecal specimens for examination for enteroviruses.

Complications. The major complication in cases of rabies is hypoxia which is accentuated during convulsive seizures and coma. Tracheostomy and the use of a respirator are necessary to treat this complication. Cardiac arrest or arrythmia may occur. These complications require special treatment in an intensive care unit.

Pathology

A diagnosis of rabies cannot be made with certainty on the basis of the pathologic picture because the lesions produced by the virus are similar to those found in other viral encephalitides. The cell count in the CSF usually is within normal limits. Examination of the urine may show a slight albuminuria, and hyaline and cellular casts may be found in the sediment. A reaction to glucose and acetone is noted in most cases. The white blood cell count is apt to be elevated.

Description and Nature of Rabies Virus

Common characteristics

Rabies virus is a neurotropic virus, having the ability to propagate along nerve pathways to the CNS and to produce encephalitis. It has also an affinity for mucus-secreting tissues, especially those associated with the respiratory system. The general biological characteristics of rabies virus are similar to those of subgroup II of the myxoviruses. On the basis of electron microscopy, rabies virus has been classified as a rhabdovirus (8). The members of this group, found in the United States, include Hart Park, Kern Canyon, Klamath, and vesicular stomatitis viruses. There is no serologic evidence of relationship between these viruses and rabies virus.

The recently described rabies-like viruses, Mokola and Lagos Bat viruses, are characterized by unexplained serologic relationships to rabiesvirus and to other viruses that belong to the rhabdovirus group. Mokola virus shows antigenic relationship to Obodhiang virus, isolated from mosquitos, and Kotonkan virus, isolated from culicoides flies (6, 59). It seems possible that Mokola virus consists of a rabies ribonucleoprotein core with an envelope of glycoprotein that contains antigenic determinants derived from another virus.

Hybridization is known to occur between viruses of morphologically different types, as well as different members of the same group (77). Mice infected by intracerebral inoculation of Mokola virus are positive for rabies by the FRA test. However, standard rabies immune serum obtained from hamsters immunized with the standard strain (CVS) of Pasteur rabies virus, which has a log neutralization index (LNI) of >5 with CVS rabies virus, shows a LNI of <2 with Mokola virus. Furthermore, mice immunized by intracerebral inoculation with HEP-Flury strain rabies virus, that are solidly immune to intracerebral challenge with CVS rabies virus, are uniformly susceptible when challenged by intracerebral inoculation with Mokola virus (36). It is important to have confirmation of the existence in nature of rabies virus strains such as Mokola and Lagos Bat viruses. It is obvious that rabies immunization as practiced does not produce immunity to these viruses, and there is a potential danger of working with such viruses in the laboratory despite prior immunization against rabies.

The presence of rabies-like viruses in rodents in Czechoslovakia has been reported (62). Here again, we are confronted by an unexplained serologic relationship to rabies virus. There were 121 strains of virus isolated from 928 wild small animals. Ten of these strains were identified as rabies virus. These viruses were obtained from 4 different species, *Microtus arvalis*, *Mus musculus*, *Apodemus flavicollis*, and *Clethrionomys glareolus*. The problems of identification included low-titer, weak, or atypical fluorescent-antibody staining and low immunogenicity. Here again, it is important to have confirmation of the existence of rabies-like viruses from such a variety of species. We know that lymphocytic choriomeningitis virus (LCMV) is present in house mice, *Mus musculus*, in Germany, and that LCMV had become established in commercial hamster colonies and children have been infected with LCMV by exposure to pet hamsters (1, 2). It is therefore possible that LCMV could have been involved in the studies reported in Czechoslovakia. The ectromelia-vaccine virus complex is readily introduced into mouse colonies and animals associated with them, and this can lead to similar complications in virus isolation and identification studies.

The occurrence of LCMV in association with several different strains of rabies virus maintained in different cell culture systems has been reported (70, 71). The association of rabies virus and LCMV resulted in a rapid and uniform infection of the human diploid WI-38 cell cultures as determined by the FRA test. It is otherwise difficult to establish and maintain rabies virus in the WI-38 cell line. The LCMV was described as having an enhancing effect for infection of the WI-38 cells. On the basis of what is known about hybridization of viruses, it seems possible that an antigenic determinant derived from LCMV had been added to the rabies virus and so increased its ability to enter and infect the WI-38 cells (72).

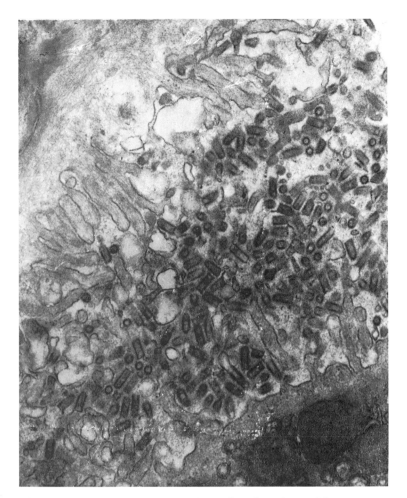

Figure 28.1—Longitudinal section of rabies virus virion.

Size and shape

In electron microscopy studies, the rabies virus virion is found in matrices replacing normal cytoplasmic structures, in cytoplasmic vacuoles, or budding from the cell surface. In cross section, the virion is cylindrical, with a diameter of 75–80 nm. In longitudinal section it is 180–200 nm and has a bacillary form (Fig 28.1). The virions occur singly or are arranged in closely packed arrays which tend to a geometric pattern. There are filamentous forms to >1000 nm which exhibit breaks at about 200 nm. The surface or envelope of the virion contains spikes or protrusions 6–8 nm long and which appear knoblike in some preparations. These are arranged in a honeycomb-like structure. It has been calculated that a virion 200-nm long would contain

580 hexagons (41). The inner helical component of the virion is similar to the nucleoprotein helix of the paramyxovirus group. It is a single-strand, right-handed helix, with a diameter of 16 nm and a periodicity of 7.5 nm. The intracytoplasmic ground substance, or matrix, associated with the development of rabies virus, which is specific for viral nucleoprotein by the FRA test, can be identified as virus-specific by means of ferritin-labeled antibodies. This filamentous matrix consists of strands about 15 nm in diameter, and the assembly of the virions in and around such masses of matrix is similar to that of some paramyxoviruses, such as parainfluenza type 2 or SV5 (30, 31).

Chemical composition

Rabies virus is a ribonucleic acid (RNA) virus. The envelope of the virion with its surface projections contains a glycoprotein (GP) which elicits virus neutralizing (Nt) antibodies in immunized animals. This GP has an isoelectric point of 3.7 (51). Immunization with this substance produces little or no resistance to infection in immunized animals. The ribonucleoprotein (RNP) contains about 5% ribonucleic acid. The disrupted virions contain polypeptides of a molecular weight of about 62,000. Immune serum from animals immunized with the RNP of rabies virus contains virus-specific complement-fixing (CF), precipitating, and immunofluorescent (IF) antibodies, but no virus neutralizing capacity (56). The virus envelope contains lipid, and lipid solvents destroy the infectivity of the virus. The chemical nature of the lipid fraction has not been determined (68). The growth of rabies virus is not inhibited by actinomycin D, mitomycin C, or 5-fluorodeoxyuridine. Arabinosylcytosine, fluorophenylalanine, and cyclohexamide inhibit the replication of rabies virus, and the inhibitory effect of fluorophenylalanine can be reversed by the addition of phenylalanine to the phenylalanine-free medium. The inhibitory effect of arabinosylcytosine can be reversed by the addition of deoxyribosylcytosine and cytidine. This action of cytidine may be related to the phospholipid metabolism, that is, preventing the inhibitory action of arabinosylcytosine on the formation of phospholipids necessary for the formation of the lipid coat of the virion (11, 46). Rabies virus is inactivated by phospholipase C (68). It has been suggested that the receptor of rabies virus may be a lipid or lipoprotein (40).

Resistance to physical and chemical agents

When infected tissues are stored in undiluted neutral glycerol or 50% glycerol in physiologic phosphate-buffered saline (PBS) solution, rabies virus retains its infectivity for several weeks at 25 C, or for months at 4 C. In dilutions containing less than 0.1% tissue extract, the virus deteriorates rapidly unless a stabilizing protein material is added to the diluent. Physiologic PBS at pH 7–9, containing at least 2% inactivated normal guinea pig, hamster, or horse serum, or 0.75% bovalbumin fraction V, is a satisfactory diluent for rabies virus; there is no significant loss of infectivity in the higher dilutions over a period of a few hours at room temperature or 24 hr at 4 C.

When exposed to a temperature of 37 C, only a trace of active virus can be demonstrated at 24 hr. Aqueous suspensions of the virus are inactivated in 5 min at 60 C (68). The best method for preserving the virus is by dessication while in the frozen state, followed by storage at 4 C; under such conditions virus will remain infective for many years.

The virus is destroyed rapidly by sunlight or by ultraviolet irradiation, and virus suspensions should be protected from exposure to sunlight and unnecessary exposure to electric light. The virus is inactivated rapidly by bichloride of mercury and strong acids and bases. Benzalkonium chloride is an effective chemosterilant. It is used in a concentration of 1% for local treatment of wounds, but has a virucidal effect to a dilution of 1:5000 (18). Lipid solvents such as ether, chloroform, and sodium deoxycholate inactivate the virus. The virus is resistant to phenol and can remain infective in tissue suspensions containing 0.5% phenol for several months at 4 C. The common antibiotics do not harm the virus. Na^+ and Mg^+ ions at 0.5-2.0 M concentration are detrimental to the stability of the virus. A virus suspension having a titer of $10^{-4.5}$ LD_{50} is inactivated in 2 hr by a concentration of 1:6000 beta-propiolactone and within 7 hr by a concentration of 0.05% formalin at 33 C (38). The virus is stable at pH 5-10 but is inactivated at pH 3 (68).

Antigenic composition

Number of immunotypes. All strains of rabies virus isolated from natural sources are closely related, that is, immunization with any one of these produces immunity to the other (see Description and Nature of Rabies Virus, page 847). Furthermore, rabies vaccine prepared from the Pasteur rabbit-fixed rabies virus appears to be effective against all of the various natural strains of rabies virus. However, it has been shown that there are differences in the antigenicity and invasiveness of different strains of the Pasteur rabbit-fixed rabies virus (26). Therefore, the most antigenic strain of this rabies virus has been chosen for vaccine production, and a standard strain (CVS) of the Pasteur rabies virus is used for testing the potency of rabies vaccine. There are differences also when we compare a street rabies virus with the Pasteur rabies virus by the serum-virus neutralization (Nt), complement fixation (CF) and cross-protection (CP) tests (33). The RNP antigen of the various strains of rabies virus isolated from wildlife is group specific by the CF and FRA tests, but the envelope antigens differ. Therefore, the Nt is the best for studying strain variation (56). There are soluble (S) and RNP virion-related (V) CF antigens. The hemagglutinating (HA) antigen is associated with the virion. Rabies virus forms strong complexes with host-cell debris, and with some serum components. This formation is indicated by the masking of the HA activity of the infectious extracellular virus in the presence of serum and the marked inhibition of the HA in homogenates of infected cells. The formation of complexes with cell fragments can be suppressed by ethylenediaminetetraacetate (EDTA). When the cell debris is removed in the presence of EDTA, the HA activity of the intracellular virus is unmasked. This binding of the virions to cell debris and serum components leads to aggregation of the virions in crude virus preparations. This phenomenon should be considered in studies of heterogeneity of virus strains (63). It has been known for a long time that the supernatant fluid of suspensions of virions that have been subjected to centrifugation at >10,000 rpm for 1 hr give more accurate results in the serum-virus Nt.

Soluble antigen. The S-antigen can be separated from the V-antigen by high-speed centrifugation (22, 51, 52, 54, 56, 64). The S-antigen obtained by different methods of disrupting the virion does not seem to be a pure antigen but is composed of both envelope GP and virion RNP material. The CF antigen associated with the S-antigen is heat stable at pH 6-10. The HA reaction is not observed with the S-antigen (40).

Viral antigen. The V-antigen associated with the nucleocapsids obtained from disrupted virions sedimented by high-speed centrifugation elicits CF, precipitating, and IF antibodies which are group specific for all strains of rabies virus. The RNP antiserum did not neutralize the homologous rabies virus (56). The complete virion antigen does produce virus-Nt antibodies indicating that the virus envelope S-antigen contains the component that elicits Nt antibodies (51). The lytic antibody against rabies-infected cells parallels the presence of virus-Nt antibody, indicating its relationship to the S-antigen of the virus envelope (73). Rabies-specific HA is bound exclusively to the virions (63).

Pathogenicity for animals (host range)

The street rabies virus, as obtained from dogs during epidemics of rabies, is pathogenic for all mammals that have been tested, when given by intracerebral inoculation. Injection of the virus into the peritoneal cavity, skin, subcutaneous tissue, muscle, or nervous tissue, in that order, is increasingly efficacious in producing encephalitis. Intranasal inoculation is almost as effective as intramuscular inoculation in producing the disease. Young chickens ordinarily develop a fatal paralytic disease following intracerebral inoculation with the virus, but recovery from the disease produced in this way is relatively frequent in mature chickens. Certain strains of rabies virus obtained from skunks have little pathogenicity for mature mice (35). Rabies virus obtained from vampire bats is not very pathogenic for dogs (33). The avianized Flury-HEP strain of rabies virus which has been used as a live virus vaccine in humans, dogs, cattle, and cats is not pathogenic for mature mice. This strain must be titrated in 1- to 2-day-old mice. The animals commonly used for experimental studies of rabies are the mouse, rat, guinea pig, hamster, rabbit, and dog. The infant mouse is the most sensitive experimental host for virus isolation studies. Intracerebral passage of rabies virus selects a highly neurotropic variant of the virus, and the high-passage brain-fixed strains of the virus do not invade and multiply in the submaxillary salivary glands or other organs usually found infected with street rabies virus.

Growth in chicken and duck embryos

Chicken embryos can be infected by the chorioallantoic membrane, allantoic sac, or yolk-sac inoculation routes. For the preparation of the Flury strain live-virus canine vaccine, the virus is inoculated by the yolk-sac route in 7-day-old embryos, and the entire embryo is harvested 9–10 days later. The temperature of incubation is 35 C. The virus is not pathogenic for embryos inoculated at this age (39). Infection of 1-day-old chicken embryos by yolk-sac inoculation results in death of the embryos in 4–5 days (76). The Flury strain of rabies virus used for immunization of dogs was derived from a human with rabies. It has been passaged 138 times in 1-day-old chickens, using the intracerebral route of inoculation, and 40–50 times in chicken embryos inoculated into the yolk sac. This is the low-egg-passage (LEP) variant. It is pathogenic for mature mice. The high-egg-passage (HEP) variant has been passed more than 180 times in chicken embryos by yolk-sac inoculation, and it is not pathogenic for mature mice and must be titrated in infant mice. The technique for cultivation of rabies virus in duck embryos is the same as for chicken embryos.

Growth in tissue cultures

Primary hamster kidney cell cultures have been used extensively in the study of rabies virus (38). Rabies vaccine has been prepared from the virus cultivated in hamster kidney cell culture (23). Knowing that hemadsorbing viruses, such as the parainfluenza viruses, may be encountered in hamster kidney cell cultures, care should be taken to monitor all strains of rabies virus which have been adapted to hamster kidney cell culture for extraneous viruses. Rabies virus has been cultivated in a continuous diploid cell line derived from human fetal lung (24). The part played by LCMV in the adaption of rabies virus to this cell line has been reviewed in subsequent papers (see Description and Nature of Rabies Virus, page 847). The BHK-21/13S line of hamster kidney cells is an excellent cell line for the cultivation of rabies virus, and it is possible to do a plaque reduction Nt test in this system (57). The virus can be cultivated in chicken embryo cell culture and a canine vaccine prepared from the Flury-LEP strain of rabies virus cultivated in this type of cell has been tested in dogs and found to be antigenic (19). A plaque assay of rabies virus has been described using the Flury-HEP strain cultivated in chicken embryo cells (75). The Flury-HEP strain of rabies virus is cultivated in canine kidney cells for vaccine production (10). There are live-virus vaccines for veterinary use prepared from canine kidney, bovine kidney, and porcine kidney cells infected with the SAD strain of rabies virus (12). Primary skunk kidney and ferret kidney cell cultures are suitable for cultivation of rabies virus (36).

Preparation of Immune Serum

Specific high-titer antiserum to the CVS or Flury-LEP strains of rabies-virus, appropriate for virus Nt tests or conjugation with fluorescein, has been prepared using homologous host immunizing antigens in hamsters, guinea pigs, and rabbits. Rabies immune serum prepared by immunization of large animals (horse, sheep, goat) raised in a "barnyard" environment contain antibodies to numerous viruses and bacteria; these may cause nonspecific fluorescent staining reaction in animal brains submitted for rabies diagnosis by the FRA examination. The hamster is an excellent host for the preparation of antiserum for use in the FRA test.

Inoculate 3-week-old hamsters intracerebrally with 0.03 ml of a 1:50 dilution of stock CVS rabies virus, and harvest the brains 3–5 days later when the animals show moderate symptoms of rabies virus infection. For primary immunization, prepare a 20% suspension of the rabies-infected hamster brain in physiologic saline solution. Inactivate the virus by adding an equal volume of 0.4% beta-propiolactone (BPL) freshly prepared in cold physiologic saline solution containing 1.68 g/dl of $NaHCO_3$ and phenol red indicator. Adjust the pH to 7.2–7.4 with 1 M disodium acid phosphate. Incubate this mixture for 2 hr at 37 C. Test for active virus in mice and then store at −20 C until used. At weekly intervals give male hamsters, 6–8 weeks old, 4 intraperitoneal (ip) injections of 2 ml each of a mixture of equal parts of adjuvant (1.5 parts Arlacel A and 8.5 parts Standard Oil Co. No. 3 white mineral oil, viscosity 75–85 at 100 F) and the BPL-treated brain-virus suspension. After a rest period of 10–14 days, give an ip injection of 1 ml of a 5% suspension of the virus. After another interval of 10–14 days, give an ip injection of 1 ml of a 10% suspension of the live-virus suspension. Bleed the hamsters at 10–14 days after the last injection, pool the serum, and store at −20 C. The surviving animals may be held for a month and given another booster injection of live virus and then bled again as noted above (21, 43, 44, 45).

Collection and Preparation of Specimens

Precautions

All persons who are expected to work in a laboratory processing street rabies virus specimens must be immunized with rabies vaccine. The method of immunization is to give 2 injections of killed-virus rabies vaccine, a month apart, followed by a booster dose 6 months later, then demonstration of specific antibodies by the serum-virus Nt. Additional booster doses of vaccine should be given until an antibody response is achieved, and then periodic boosters (annually or biannually) sufficient to maintain an antibody level at ≥1:8 (≥1:16 according to methods used at the Center for Disease Control).

There are certain safety precautions which should be observed in working with pathogenic viruses. Pipetting is done with a Propipette to avoid aerosol exposure. Plastic face shields are worn when opening the calvaria of large animals, when cutting or breaking open sealed glass ampules, or when grinding specimens in a mortar, if the procedure is not done in a hood. Mice to be used for test virus inoculation are handled with forceps. Screw-cap closures are used for test tubes so that the hand will not be contaminated with virus. The basic rule is to avoid any possibility of getting virus on the skin, or in the mouth, nose, or eyes. Carry out each procedure on a clean working surface such as can be obtained with absorbent paper having a polyethylene backing, or by using a sheet of aluminum foil covered with a sheet of absorbent paper. This is especially important when inoculating animals so that virus from one specimen does not contaminate the working surface for another specimen. Large animals must be handled with heavy-duty rubber gloves. The use of surgical-type rubber gloves is not recommended for laboratory workers removing brain specimens. Those engaged in opening containers and removing brains and other tissues from large animals should wear heavy-duty, industrial-type rubber gloves.

Specimens for isolation of virus

Knowledge of when exposure to rabies occurred makes it possible to immunize and protect a high percentage of exposed individuals during the relatively long incubation period of the disease. Administration of rabies hyperimmune serum offers an added safeguard by giving temporary protection. The serum alone may not prevent the disease, but it at least lengthens the incubation period sufficiently to allow for development of active immunity induced by the vaccine.

The frequency with which people are bitten by dogs makes it impossible to give the rabies vaccine treatment to all cases of dog-bite exposure, even in regions where the disease is known to be prevalent. It therefore becomes important to have a method of assessing the probability of exposure.

The question whether or not exposure has occurred must be determined by what happens to the biting animal. For example, if a dog that has bitten someone can be restrained and kept under observation for at least 5 days and remains healthy, one may conclude that exposure to rabies has not occurred. If the biting animal has symptoms of rabies, it should be killed and examined for rabies. It is no longer necessary to hold animals until they die because the FRA test will be positive at any stage of the disease. Wild animals which have bitten someone should be killed immediately and examined for rabies.

In addition to infecting the CNS, rabies virus can invade and multiply in the submaxillary salivary glands, parotid salivary glands, lungs, kidneys, pancreas, mammary glands, and muscle tissue. The laboratory diagnosis of rabies from clinical specimens depends on isolation of the virus from sputum, saliva, nasal swab, eye swab, throat swab, urine, or spinal fluid. In addition, impressions of the cornea may be examined by the FRA test for rabies virus antigen. A negative saliva test does not rule out rabies infection because the virus may fail to become established in the salivary glands or in other tissues of the upper respiratory tract.

Rabies is a disease of the CNS; therefore, the postmortem diagnosis of rabies depends on the demonstration of Negri bodies, or rabies virus antigen, or infectious virus in the brain. The Ammon horn of the hippocampus is best for the demonstration of Negri bodies and of rabies virus antigen, but in cases of suspected rabies in humans, portions of frontal and parietal cortex, cerebellar cortex, thalamus, pons, and medulla should be taken also for examination.

In cases of exposure by animal bite, it is helpful to know whether the submaxillary salivary glands contained rabies virus. These glands can be examined for rabies virus antigen by the FRA test and by animal inoculation. If the submaxillary salivary glands are to be examined, they should be removed before opening the calvaria; if the animal had rabies, the head after decapitation will be superficially contaminated with virus released by severing of the spinal cord, resulting in contamination of the submaxillary salivary glands if they are exposed in the process of removing the head.

Clinical and postmortem specimens

It is important that clinical specimens be collected early in the course of the disease. The acute-phase blood specimen is taken as soon as convenient after the patient is admitted. Should the patient survive for several days, a second specimen is taken. If the patient recovers, another blood specimen is taken before the patient is discharged from the hospital. A portion of the spinal fluid obtained by diagnostic lumbar puncture is saved for virus studies. Sputum is collected because the virus may be excreted by mucus glands of the eyes, nose, and throat as well as from the lung parenchyma. Saliva is obtained from under the tongue where the ducts of the submaxillary salivary glands enter the mouth. The best way for doing this is to use 5-ml screw-cap serum vials containing 2-3 ml tissue culture medium. Wet a sterile cotton swab with the medium, and roll it against the side of the tube to express the excess fluid; then swab under the tongue. Rinse the swab in the medium. Similar specimens are taken from the nose and throat. Discard the contaminated swabs into a metal pan for sterilization. Urine is saved for virus studies. A fresh specimen is required. The sediment is collected immediately by centrifugation and taken up in 2 ml of tissue culture medium. The virus is preserved best by mixing the urine with an equal amount of tissue culture medium as soon as it is obtained so as to protect the cellular sediment during centrifugation and processing. Stool specimens are collected as for enterovirus studies.

Postmortem specimens are placed into sterile, plastic, screw-cap wide-mouth bottles. Blocks of tissue about 1 cm^2 are taken from the hippocampus, thalamus, pons, medulla, cerebellum, and frontal and parietal cortex. In testing for rabies virus in organs other than the brain, it is essential to use separate sets of sterile instruments for each organ. The submaxillary salivary glands usually are the best source of rabies virus from tissues other than that of the CNS, and these glands may contain more virus per gram of tissue than the brain. Parotid gland, lachrymal gland, lung, kidney, pancreas, and muscle also are taken for virus studies. The mammary gland, if active, and intestinal mucosa may contain the virus.

Typewritten labels such as the self-sticking vinyl-coated labels are preferable so that the information does not become illegible on handling and from moisture.

If the specimens are to be tested within 24 hr, it is preferable to keep them at 4 C. If the specimens are to be shipped, they should be refrigerated on dry ice. For prolonged storage prepare a 20% suspension of the tissues as noted elsewhere and save 1-ml portions of this material in flame-sealed glass ampules at ≤ -60 C.

Wild animals submitted for rabies examination should be correctly identified. For example, it is very important to know whether an animal is a striped skunk, *Mephitis mephitis,* or a spotted skunk, *Spilogale putorius.* Small mammals such as rodents and bats are saved until the diagnosis is completed. It is a good idea to preserve bat specimens in formalin or 50% ethyl alcohol, for identification, after the proper specimens are taken, because it is important to know the species of the rabies-negative specimens as well as that of the positive specimens.

Specimens for microscopy

Specimens are kept under refrigeration at 4 C prior to processing for pathology; freezing alters the structure and staining reaction. When it is necessary to ship the entire carcass of a small animal or an animal head specimen for diagnosis, the specimen is placed in a watertight metal container. This, in turn, is placed in a larger container of sufficient size to allow space for 1 or 2 containers of plastic or metal, filled with refrigerant solution that has been cooled in the freezer compartment of an ordinary refrigerator.

If there are ectoparasites, such as fleas and ticks, on the animal specimen, place the specimen in a container and immobilize the parasites with chloroform. Subsequently, the skin surface may be moistened with a 0.001% solution of benzalkonium chloride or 70% ethyl alcohol. Most of the specimens received will be dog heads. The salivary glands must be removed first if they are to be tested for virus. When the skin is reflected from a ventral midline neck incision, the submaxillary salivary glands will be exposed at the angle of the jaw. These are firm, well-demarcated, pale reddish-brown, lobulated glands about $1.5 \times 2.5 \times 3.5$ cm. Place these glands in a Petri dish or screw-cap wide-mouth bottle. Plastic containers are preferred to avoid the danger of breakage.

When removing the brain of the dog, have an assistant hold the head firmly by grasping the lower jaw with a lion-jawed bone-holding forceps. The operator exposes the calvaria with a midline longitudinal incision, reflects the skin laterally, and cuts away the muscle tissue to the base of the ears. The skull is opened with a sharp butcher's cleaver, hammer and chisel, or a bone saw, by a cut first across the occipital area, then laterally on each side, and finally transversely just behind the eyes. The calvaria is then pried up from the front and broken backward, thereby exposing the brain. For small animals, scissors are used for opening the calvaria. Do not use power-operated circular saws because they will contaminate the work area and are difficult to decontaminate. In removing large brains, reflect the meninges laterally, have the assistant hold the muzzle of the head upright, and then the brain can be removed without handling, by cutting under the frontal lobes and finally severing the cranial nerves and brain stem, letting the brain fall onto a disposable plastic or aluminum plate. Another plate inverted over the first one and sealed with masking tape provides a convenient means of handling and storing such specimens prior to processing. It is necessary to use separate sets of sterile instruments for each animal specimen and to work on a large tray covered with absorbent paper with a polyethylene liner or another sheet of aluminum foil so that the work surface can be decontaminated between each specimen. Separate sets of instruments must be used for different organs.

Although specimens subjected to freezing are not as good for the Negri body examination and general pathologic studies, such material is satisfactory for the FRA test and for virus isolation. Material preserved in 50% glycerol in phosphate buffer solution, pH 7.4, is not suitable for the Negri body examination but is satisfactory for the FRA test and for virus isolation studies.

Laboratory Diagnosis

Direct examination of clinical material

The examination of corneal epithelial cells for rabies antigen is a new test for the clinical diagnosis of rabies (13, 55). This is done by gently pressing a glass slide against the cornea of both eyes, after application of a local anesthetic. The slides are then air-dried, fixed in acetone, and processed for the FRA test in the usual manner. The cornea test can be used for the clinical diagnosis of rabies in dogs and laboratory animals. A negative test does not rule out rabies.

The direct microscopic examination of brain tissue for Negri bodies and rabies virus antigen is one of the common laboratory procedures in public health laboratories. Although the FRA test has largely supplanted other methods of diagnosis, the examination for Negri bodies in the brain is still a useful method for rapid diagnosis.

Examination for Negri bodies

The Ammon horn of the hippocampus is the best part of the brain for the demonstration of Negri bodies and also for rabies virus antigen by the FRA test. It is advisable to also examine the cerebral and cerebellar cortex for Negri bodies. With a pair of straight scissors, cut through the Ammon horn transversely removing a cross section about 2-mm thick. Use this for preparation of impressions. This can be done by placing the section on one end of a tongue depressor, holding a clean glass slide between the thumb and forefinger, applying the slide gently against the cut surface of the tissue that is exposed, and removing quickly. This leaves a thin film of tissue on the slide—a mirror image of the cross section. This type of specimen is suitable for staining with Seller stain for Negri bodies, for routine histologic stains, for staining with Giemsa stain as for malaria parasites, and for the FRA test.

For smear preparations, cut out portions of tissue about 1 mm^2 from the Ammon horn, cerebral and cerebellar cortex, and other brain areas; place each near one end of a glass slide. Superimpose a second slide on the first; flatten the tissue by gentle pressure; then draw the top slide lengthwise over the bottom slide, leaving a thin elongated smear on both slides. The thicker smear should be stained immediately with Seller stain, while the other is saved for the FRA test. When testing human brains and those of large animals, such smears should be prepared from each of several different parts of the brain since the distribution of viral antigen may be scanty or irregular: cerebral cortex bilaterally, cerebellar cortex, both Ammon horns, medulla, etc.

The paraffin section method is not recommended for routine diagnosis. For demonstration of Negri bodies in paraffin sections, fix the brain tissue in Zenker fixative. Add glacial acetic acid to a concentration of 5% just before use. Stain with eosin and methylene blue or Giemsa stain. Tissue fixed in formalin and stained with hematoxylin and eosin is not satisfactory for the demonstration of Negri bodies or for the FRA test.

The wet impressions or smears of brain tissue are fixed and stained at the same time by covering the tissue with Seller stain. This stain is a mixture of basic fuchsin and methylene blue. Each stock stain is prepared as a 1 g/dl solution in absolute acetone-free methyl alcohol. The basic fuchsin should be color index No. 677 and the methylene blue, color index No. 922, or equivalent. Store the stock stains in brown bottles in a cabinet where they are protected from light. To prepare the working stain solution, take 1 part of the basic fuchsin and 2 parts of the methylene blue stock stain solutions; for example, 25 ml of basic fuchsin and 50 ml of methylene blue solution. Mix but do not filter. The stain may be kept in a dropper bottle so that the staining process can be done over a metal container which can be sterilized by boiling. While the tissue on the glass slide is still moist, cover it with Seller stain and leave this on for 10–30 sec. Then rinse the stain from the slide with M/150 phosphate buffer at pH 7-7.5. Air dry, and the preparation is ready for examination. *Handle the slide as contaminated material* because it is possible that there may be some active virus left in the tissue.

The properly stained tissue should appear reddish-violet or purplish-blue, depending on the density of the tissue. The cytoplasm of the neurons will be blue or purplish-blue, the nuclei and nucleoli a deeper blue, the stroma rose-pink, and nerve fibers a deeper pink; bacteria, if present, stain an intense blue and erythrocytes stain copper color. Negri bodies, the specific cytoplasmic inclusion bodies of rabies, are found in the cytoplasm of large neurons. The Negri body is a sharply defined spherical, oval, or elongated body, ordinarily 2-10 μ in diameter. Several inclusion bodies, usually of variable size, may be present in one neuron. The larger Negri bodies contain blue-staining granules or inner bodies, often arranged in concentric layers; the ground substance of the inclusion body is finely granular, takes the fuchsin stain, and appears cherry-red. In smear preparations, the Negri bodies often appear to be outside the neurons because the cytoplasm of the neuron has been ruptured. The intracellular location of Negri bodies need not be demonstrated because the staining reaction with Seller stain is characteristic, and they may be identified outside as well as inside the neurons.

Cytoplasmic inclusion bodies caused by viruses other than rabies and which stain red with Seller stain may be found in dog, cat, skunk, and mouse brains. An example that may be cited is the inclusion body found in dogs infected with distemper virus. Many of the wildlife viruses produce cytoplasmic inclusion bodies in the brains of animals inoculated intracerebrally;

for example, the Tacaribe virus and LCMV of the arenavirus group, the Rio Bravo virus of bats, and the Modoc virus of *Peromyscus* mice.

Electron microscopy

Studies have been made of rabies virus as it is found in infected mouse brain, in BHK21/13S cells and chicken embryo cell culture (17, 30, 31, 47). The variation in the appearance and recorded size of the virion can be the result of the method of fixation, dehydration, and staining of the material. Cell cultures or small slices of tissue are fixed in 1–4% glutaraldehyde, depending on the thickness of the tissue. The glutaraldehyde is made up in 0.1 M buffer at pH 7.2, and fixation is done for 1–2 hr at 4 C. The tissue is then washed and dehydrated and embedded in epoxy resin. Some workers use an additional postfixation treatment with 1% osmium tetroxide in 0.1 M buffer for 1 hr. Primary fixation with osmic acid or osmium tetroxide is sometimes used for cell culture material. After sectioning, the tissue may be stained with uranyl acetate or lead citrate. Cell suspensions or small fragments of tissue may be stained with 2% phosphotungstic acid or 2% sodium silicotungstate (3, 5, 30, 31, 48).

Immunofluorescent examination

The FRA test, when used with proper controls, makes possible a prompt diagnosis in cases of animal rabies, and the accuracy of the test is equal to that of isolation of the virus by animal inoculation. There will be certain instances where the mouse inoculation test fails because there is little or no infectious virus in the brain as the result of inactivation of the virus by antibodies or from exposure to heat. Furthermore, some strains of rabies virus are of low pathogenicity, and there is little invasion of the brain by the virus. The FRA test demonstrates rabies virus antigen where the infectivity has been lost, and this test is of particular value in identifying natural strains of rabies virus of low pathogenicity. The mouse inoculation test should be used for confirmation of the FRA test when this test shows only a ± or 1 + positive result, or when the circumstances warrant confirmation of the FRA test.

Rabies immune serum conjugate. The best results are obtained with the use of rabies immune serum from hamsters hyperimmunized with the CVS strain of fixed rabies virus using homologous tissue antigen. The globulin fraction of the rabies immune serum is precipitated by adding an equal volume of saturated ammonium sulfate (final concentration equals 50% saturated) in distilled water at 4 C; permit the precipitation reaction to continue for at least 12 hr at 4 C. Centrifuge the treated serum in a refrigerated centrifuge at 3000–5000 rpm for 30 min and discard the supernatant fluid. Add distilled water to the sediment to equal the original volume of serum; then add an equal volume of the cold saturated ammonium sulfate solution. After thorough mixing, centrifuge as before and discard the supernatant fluid. Take up the sediment in distilled water, and for a third time treat with ammonium sulfate. Take up the sedimented globulin fraction in distilled water to about 40–50% of the original volume of serum. Dialyze the globulin solution at 4 C in 3 changes of physiologic NaCl solution over a period of 18 hr. Determine protein content of the globulin solution by the biuret method. Adjust pH of the globulin solution to 8.7–8.8 with carbonate buffer (stock solution A is a 5.3 g/dl solution of Na_2CO_3; solution B, a 4.2 g/dl solution of $NaHCO_3$. To 100 ml of solution B add solution A until the pH is about 8.8. This usually takes about 7–12 ml of solution A). Take an amount of the buffer solution equal to 15% of volume of the globulin solution and mix the globulin and buffer solutions. Next, add 1 mg of chromatographically pure fluorescein isothiocyanate (Baltimore Biological Laboratories) to each 50 mg of protein in the globulin solution. Agitate the dye-treated globulin solution at 4 C overnight with a magnetic stirrer run at slow speed. The residual uncoupled fluorescein dye is removed by dialysis against 0.01 M phosphate-buffered saline (PBS) solution pH 7.2–7.5 or, preferably, pass the conjugate through a Sephadex G-50 column (Pharmacia Fine Chemicals). Prepare Sephadex gel by suspending 0.075 g dry Sephadex G-50 per ml of PBS; usually 80–160 ml are required. A glass column about 15 × 400 mm suffices for filtration of 5–20 ml of conjugate, using 80 ml of gel; a column about 20 × 450 mm is suitable for conjugate volumes of 20–40 ml, using about 160 ml of gel. Insert a wad of glass wool into the column opening. Put a short piece of sterile tubing on the end of the column, and close it with a plastic pinchcock clamp or screw-compression clamp. Add PBS to a height of 2–3 inches in the column. Add Sephadex slurry and allow to stand until the Sephadex begins to settle. Gradually release the clamp until the pressure diminishes; clear PBS should drip steadily from the column. Allow dripping to continue until the top of the column of saline begins to disappear into the top of the gel column. Pipette the conjugate onto the top of the column. The tagged globulin can be observed moving down the column. As the conjugated globulin reaches the end of the column, discard the first 1 ml; then collect the eluate to the volume of conjugate solution added to the column. Place the tagged globulin in 1- to 2-ml ampules, and store at −20 C or lower.

For titration of conjugate potency prepare 2-fold dilutions of the globulin-dye conjugate in a 20% normal mouse brain suspension in PBS; beginning with 1:10, test each dilution for its staining quality for a control positive smear. The highest 2-fold dilution of the globulin conjugate which gives 3+ to 4+ staining is used for the FRA test. An average conjugate stains satisfactorily at a dilution of 1:40. A glaring yellow/green fluorescence is a 4+ reaction; a bright yellow-green fluorescence without glare is 3+; a dull yellow-green fluorescence is 2+; a very dim but still noticeable yellow-green fluorescence is 1+.

Staining smears with fluorescent antibody. Regular glass slides 25 × 75 mm and 0.9–1.1 mm in thickness are used for the FRA test. The impression or smear preparations are fixed in acetone at 4 C for 4 hr, or overnight at −20 C. In emergency situations fixation for 10 min in acetone at room temperature gives satisfactory results, but the overnight test should be done also. Prepare a stock of whole individual mouse brains infected with street rabies virus, and hold these at −50 C in small screw-cap vials. Prepare a set of 20 slides, which should be enough for a month; air dry and store at −20 C in acetone. Be sure to keep the acetone level over the tissue preparation. As needed, take one of these slides for use as a positive control. It is also necessary to have a negative control prepared the same day from normal mouse brain. Specimens of brain tissue submitted in 50% glycerol-saline solution are washed 3 times in saline solution for 20-min periods and drained on sterile filter paper before preparing smears of the tissue.

After taking the slides out of the acetone, air dry them for 10–15 min; place the slides on a tray covered with a sheet of moistened absorbent paper with polyethylene backing. Handle all slides as contaminated material, and decontaminate the paper by burning or autoclaving when finished. Use forceps for handling slides. Make a circle about 12–15 mm in diameter in the mid-portion of the tissue smear or around the impression with a marking pen (Tri-Chem liquid embroidery pen). With a pipette, drop about 0.1 ml of the appropriate dilution of the tagged antibody onto the tissue preparation so as to cover the entire marked circle. Cover each tray with an inverted tray and place in an incubator at 37 C for 20 min. Place slides in a carrier and rinse for 10 min in each of 2 changes of PBS. Rinse again with distilled water and air dry in a blower unit or with a fan. Mount a 22- × 40-mm No. 1 coverslip on the tissue preparation, using 25% glycerol in PBS. Examine the slides with a microscope equipped with a Osram HB0200 ultraviolet light source in conjunction with a Schott UG-1 excitor filter giving a peak transmission at 360 nm and a Zeiss 41 or comparable (W2A) barrier filter in the eyepiece. Nonfluorescent immersion oil (type A) is placed between the condenser and the slide.

The presence of FRA antigen in the specimen is diagnostic for rabies. The fluorescent material can vary from small particles <1 μ to masses 2–10 μ in diameter. Nerve cells may be outlined by the fluorescent material (43). It is advisable to prepare 3 or more smears or impressions from each specimen, for example, hippocampus, cerebellum, and cortex.

Appropriate positive and negative controls are used each time the test is performed, and specificity tests for the presence of the virus are needed when the fluorescence is only 1+ or uncertain (43, 45). A portion of every specimen tested must be saved for repeat tests if needed, or for forwarding to a reference laboratory.

Interpretation of observations

The demonstration of Negri bodies in a brain specimen makes it possible to make a diagnosis of rabies. The demonstration of Negri bodies in the brains of mice inoculated with brain specimens of dogs or other animals was the standard specificity test prior to the development of the FRA test. The microscopic examination for Negri bodies identifies about 90% of the cases of rabies in dogs (32). However, rabies in wildlife, especially in skunks and free-living bats, is apt to be caused by strains of rabies virus which do not produce Negri bodies. Nevertheless, the examination for Negri bodies with Sellers stain is a useful adjunct to the FRA test. It does show bacteria if present and gives some information about the general pathology in the brain. In a study at the California Department of Health, the FRA test, examination for Negri bodies, and the mouse inoculation test using mature mice were compared for the diagnosis of rabies. A total of 363 of 4200 specimens were positive for rabies by one or another test, of which 361 (99.4%) were detected by the FRA test, 357 (98.3%) by inoculation of mice, and 239 (65.8%) by the presence of Negri bodies (43). The relatively low rate of positives by the Negri body examination is due to the large number of cases of skunk rabies which are included in this series, and <50% of the skunks that have rabies are positive by the Negri body examination. Rabies virus strains isolated from Mexican freetail bats are very similar to those encountered in dogs; that is, they produce the disease in mice following a short incubation period, and Negri bodies are found in large numbers in the infected mice. The strains of rabies virus found in noncolonial bats are similar to those isolated from skunks; that is, the incubation period is long, the virus is apt to be more pathogenic for infant than for adult mice, and mice infected with the virus are not apt to have Negri bodies in the brain.

Do not report a specimen as questionably positive or suspiciously positive for rabies by the Negri body or FRA tests. If not definitely positive report as negative pending additional FRA tests, and infant mice should be inoculated with the specimen. Some of these may be killed in 4–5 days and examined for rabies virus antigen by the FRA test. It is customary to report rabies-positive specimens by telephone whether or not this has been requested. In addition, the results of the examination must be reported by mail.

Virus isolation

Host systems

The white laboratory mouse is the best experimental host for the isolation and identification of rabies virus. There are a number of types of rabies-virus strains, such as the Flury-HEP vaccine virus, which are nonpathogenic for mature mice. There are some strains of rabies virus found in nature which are much more pathogenic for infant mice than for adult mice (35). Therefore, to demonstrate minimal amounts of virus, 1- to 2-day-old mice should be used as test animals in addition to adult mice. There are other advantages in using infant mice; that is, they are cheaper per test animal and they are easier to handle and inoculate. In testing brain and other organs from human autopsies, as well as spinal fluid, saliva, and throat swab specimens from patients, it is essential to use an experimental animal with a broad range of susceptibility to viruses, and the infant mouse is the best animal for such specimens.

Preparation of specimens

Spinal fluid and blood serum specimens are suitable for testing without processing; it is preferable to test such specimens without the addition of antibiotics because the test system will then pick up bacteria and other parasitic organisms which would be missed if antibiotics are used. Saliva, nose swab, throat swab, and urine specimens should be made up to 2 ml with PBS solution containing 0.75% bovine albumin fraction V or 2% inactivated horse, guinea pig, or hamster serum. After centrifugation at 2500 rpm for about 10 min, the supernatant fluid is taken off for test inoculation. As mentioned previously, the sediment of the urine is the most likely to yield rabies virus. The same is true for the spinal fluid. Therefore, in processing such specimens, freeze and thaw the suspension once in order to break up the cells. A portion of each specimen is saved for reference and stored in a sealed glass ampule at −60 C. Antibiotics are added to the material to be tested—usually 1 mg streptomycin and 500 or 1000 units penicillin/ml. Stool specimens are ground in a mortar to make a 10% suspension by weight. After preliminary centrifugation at 2500 rpm for 10 min, antibiotics as given above are added at double strength to the supernatant fluid. If high-speed centrifugation equipment is available, the supernatant fluid is spun at 10,000 rpm for 1 hr in a refrigerated centrifuge; the supernatant fluid is saved for testing. Autopsy specimens are ground in a mortar using an abrasive such as sterile alundum and diluted to a 10% suspension in PBS solution containing a stabilizer as noted above. A portion is saved for reference, and antibiotics are added to the material to be tested as noted above. The Neutraglass 2-ml ampules are suitable for storage of specimens; 0.5 or 1.0 ml is placed in each ampule. Antibiotics are usually made up at 10X strength and stored at − 60 C; it is then a simple procedure to add 0.1 ml of this to each 0.9 ml of the supernatant fluid to be tested. Incubate for 1 hr at 4 C before testing. Tissue specimens are usually made up as 10% suspensions by weight; that is, the weight of the tissue in grams multiplied by 9 gives the amount of diluent to be used.

The mouse inoculation test

For the inoculations, the mice are placed on a sheet of absorbent paper with polyethylene backing or an additional layer of aluminum foil. Any droplets of virus left on the paper will then be decontaminated by burning or autoclaving the paper. A clean work surface is essential so that virus is not carried over from one specimen to another. The miniature aluminum pie plates are excellent for restricting the movement of infant mice during the inoculation procedure; plastic Petri dishes are also satisfactory for this purpose. It is advisable to work on metal trays lined with plastic-backed paper as noted above and to sterilize the trays by autoclaving.

A 0.25-ml tuberculin syringe and a $1/4$–$1/2$ inch 27-gauge needle are used for inoculating mice. Working over the tray, fill the syringe by placing the needle point just inside the lip of the tube, and tip the tube until the fluid can be withdrawn without contaminating the barrel of the syringe. Use screw-cap tubes to avoid contaminating the hands. Have a jar of sterile dental rolls, cut in half, for use in clearing the bubble from the syringe barrel after taking up the fluid into the syringe. If this is not done, there will be loss of some of the suspension from the needle as it is withdrawn because of expansion of the gas left in the syringe.

With sterile $4^{1}/_{2}$ inch grasping forceps pick up the section of dental roll, put this on the needle of the syringe, and with gentle pressure express the bubble into the cotton roll. Place the cotton roll on the paper work surface, and with the forceps hold the infant mice for inoculation. Hold the syringe with the index finger on the plunger, and support the barrel between the thumb and third and fourth finger; the forearm should rest on the table to stabilize the arm. Introduce the needle to a depth of 1–2 mm into the central part of the upper parietal area of the calvaria. The dose for infant and adult mice is 0.015 ml. No antiseptic is necessary or desirable over the inoculation site. It is preferable to use only 6 infant mice so that the mother mouse will be able to feed them well. Place the inoculated mice into a properly labeled box to the side of the operator opposite the hand holding the syringe, to avoid the necessity of crossing hands, a motion which might result in catching the fingers of one hand on the needle attached to the syringe held by the opposite hand. The arm must be bare because a sleeve may pick up virus from the work area and contaminate the person, as well as spread the virus in the laboratory. The record card should be visible to the operator as the mice are inoculated, to check the information with that on the box. Type all labels; vinyl-backed labels are excellent for this purpose.

It is recommended that for urine and stool specimens one group of 1- to 2-day-old mice be used for the intracerebral test and another group for an intraperitoneal test, giving 0.03 ml by the latter route. It is possible to give the test material by both routes to the same group of mice. The testing of the stool specimen is to rule out coxsackieviruses and other viruses pathogenic for infant mice as well as for testing for rabiesvirus.

In testing specimens from humans it is advisable to also inoculate a group of 4-6 young adult mice, because certain viruses, such as LCMV and type 2 poliovirus, can be pathogenic for adult mice and not for infant mice. For inoculation of adult mice, use female mice if the animals are to be held for more than 14 days. Mature male mice are apt to kill each other. For handling adult mice, use 6-inch Russian tissue forceps. Adult mice must be etherized; once a mouse is placed on the working area it is considered to be contaminated and must not be put back into the ether jar unless the ether jar is changed for each specimen and sterilized.

When the test inoculation is completed, the syringe and needle may be rinsed with water, provided the needle is kept below the surface of the water to avoid producing an aerosol. After rinsing the syringe, put the cotton dental roll on the needle and place the syringe in a dry pan. If syringes and other instruments are put into a pan of water, there will be splashing of virus onto the work table. Separate sterile forceps must be used for each group of mice. Two metal pans are placed on the work table, one containing a small amount of water for rinsing the syringes and the other left dry, for the syringes and forceps. After completion of the inoculations, the pans are removed to the sterilizing room; water is poured gently over the instruments, and sterilization is accomplished by boiling the water for a minimal period of 5 min. Ten-inch forceps are used for checking mice; separate sterile forceps must be used for each box. Forceps are sterilized easily by autoclaving or by boiling for 5 min in a stainless steel jar containing a 500-watt electric heating unit.

Observation of inoculated mice

If the specimen contains rabies virus, some of the inoculated mice usually show tremulous muscular activity, incoordination, excitation, or paralysis between 5 and 15 days after inoculation. It is customary to observe the inoculated mice for 28 days. The incubation period in adult mice is longer and more variable. The affected mice usually die within 5 days after the onset of symptoms. Certain strains of rabies virus isolated from skunks produce a spastic paralysis in adult mice followed by recovery in a high percentage of the infected mice. The specificity of these infections can be determined by killing some of the affected mice at the onset of symptoms and others at different intervals after they recover. Rabies virus antigen can be demonstrated by the FRA test in the brain of mice that recover, sometimes as long as several months later. However, infectious virus can be isolated only during the symptomatic phase of the infection. Recovery from rabies in infant mice is observed also with some strains of street rabies virus (35).

Harvesting mouse brain specimens

To remove the brain from a dead mouse or one that has been killed with carbon dioxide or chloroform, place the dead mouse on a metal tray covered with absorbent paper backed with polyethylene or on a sheet of aluminum foil covered with a sheet of absorbent paper. Moisten the head with 70% ethyl alcohol, and expose the skull by reflecting the skin from the midline using 110- or 120-mm forceps and 115-mm scissors with curved points. With another set of instruments cut around the calvaria to expose the brain; remove the brain and place it in a small plastic Petri dish, which is suitable for this type of specimen. Seal the dish with tape to prevent accidental opening. Have a typed label on the lid of the dish to avoid errors resulting in mix-ups of specimens. The use of peg boards is dangerous. If used, the pegs and board must be sterilized between each specimen. There is also the danger of someone pricking themselves with a peg pin.

The microscopic specificity test

The microscopic examination of mouse brains for Negri bodies, and for rabies virus antigen by the FRA test, is necessary to establish a diagnosis of rabies. In studying wildlife specimens, it is useful to stain one of the mouse brain impressions with Giemsa stain to reveal parasites which will not be recognized with the Seller stain or by the FRA test, for example, toxoplasma, certain bacteria, *Borrellia*, ornithosis agents, and rickettsia. In addition, this type of preparation shows polymorphonuclear and mononuclear cells and the pathology of degenerating cells. The method recommended is: fix the impressions of mouse brain with absolute methyl alcohol; stain in a solution of 5 ml Giemsa stain to which is added 20 ml absolute methyl alcohol and 80 ml M/150 PBS, pH 7.2–7.4; filter through coarse filter paper, such as Whatman No. 12; after mixing, pour onto the slides and stain for 2 hr; rinse with PBS and air dry. The slide can be examined directly with immersion oil or prepared for permanent reference with neutral mounting medium. The impression preparations are made from a cross section of the brain taken in the region of the hippocampus, and smears are prepared from the same region.

Passage and titration of the virus

A positive FRA test with proper controls is sufficient to identify a strain of rabies virus under ordinary circumstances. If further studies are indicated, or if the virus is not identified as rabies virus, it is necessary to prepare a stock virus. To do this, prepare a 20% suspension of infected infant mouse brain tissue, using a diluent of PBS solution containing 0.075% bovine albumin fraction V, or 2% inactivated guinea pig or hamster serum. For unidentified viruses, it is best not to use horse serum because it may contain antibodies to the virus. Place 0.5 ml or 1.0 ml in ampules, flame seal, and store at − 60 C. Use typewritten labels for permanent mounts, giving the specimen number, name of individual or animal, type of tissue, percentage suspension, amount, and date.

For titration prepare a series of 13- × 100-mm screw-cap test tubes, labeling them 10^{-1}, 10^{-2} in 10-fold steps through 10^{-8}. If the stock virus is a 20% suspension, add 0.5 ml of the diluent to the tube labeled 10^{-1} and 2.7 ml to the other tubes. Add 0.5 ml of the 20% stock virus to the tube labeled 10^{-1} to make a 10% suspension; with a 1.0-ml pipette calibrated to 0.01 ml, mix by filling and emptying the pipette 10 times; transfer 0.3 ml to the tube labeled 10^{-2} and discard the pipette. Mix with a clean pipette as for the previous tube, transfer 0.3 ml to the tube labeled 10^{-3}, and discard the pipette; mix and transfer in this manner until the series is completed, using a different sterile pipette for each dilution. The pipettes are filled and the transfer done with Propipette bulbs. The pipettes are placed in a dry stainless steel catheter tray and sterilized by boiling after completion of the test. It is best to work over a stainless steel tray covered with absorbent paper backed with polyethylene or a sheet of aluminum foil covered with absorbent paper. It is also preferable to work in a hood with open ports, and equipped with an ultraviolet light sterilizing system. Mouth pipetting should not be allowed.

For inoculation of mice, begin with the highest dilution, that is, 10^{-8}. Use a separate syringe and needle for each dilution. Inoculate 6 infant mice with each dilution, injecting 0.015 ml intracerebrally as described previously. The LD_{50} of the virus is determined by the Reed-Muench method described in Chapter I.

Pathogens to be ruled out

Mice inoculated intracerebrally with brain and other organ specimens from humans and animals can become infected with a variety of specific viruses and other pathogens which produce encephalitis or meningitis. Viruses can be isolated which are derived from the test mice. Among the viruses that may be encountered are herpesvirus hominis, simiae, and suis; LCM, ectromelia-vaccinia group viruses, Western and Eastern encephalomyelitis, California and St. Louis encephalitis; Rio Bravo, Modoc, Klamath, Kern Canyon, Colorado Tick Fever, Powassan, Cache Valley, Tacaribe, poliovirus type 2, coxsackievirus, reovirus, encephalomyocarditis virus, mouse encephalomyelitis (GD-7 type), and many other viruses less well known. Among bacterial parasites, *Leptospira*, *Borrelia*, *Listerella*, *Yersinia*, tularemia, and meningococcus organisms may be encountered. Toxoplasma parasites may be isolated from brain specimens.

Isolation in embryonated eggs and tissue culture

These host systems are not used for diagnostic studies. The passage of rabies virus in chicken embryos has been used for phenotypic selection of variants of the virus in a search for a live-virus vaccine. For example, the avianized Flury-LEP human strain of rabies virus, used as a live virus vaccine for dogs, was passaged 138 times in 1- to 2-day-old chickens by the intracerebral route; and the fortieth to fiftieth chicken embryo yolk-sac passage of this strain is used for the production of vaccine. The Flury-HEP variant, used for vaccination of dogs, cats, and cattle, has been passaged >180 times in chicken embryos and is characterized by lack of pathogenicity for adult mice. This is not a stable character because intracerebral passage in infant mice restores the pathogenicity for adult mice. The duck embryo rabies vaccine used for postexposure immunization is prepared from duck embryos inoculated by the yolk-sac route with the Pasteur rabbit-fixed rabies virus. The seed virus for this vaccine is prepared from infected mouse brain. The virus is inactivated with beta-propiolactone. It is a Semple-type vaccine.

Primary hamster kidney cell cultures and the BHK-21/13S cell line have been used extensively for the study of rabies virus. The primary hamster cell culture system is well suited for isolation and maintenance of non-neuro-adapted strains of street rabies virus (34). When used for challenge inoculation, such strains are less virulent than the brain-passaged strains of the virus. There is no need for special media: Hanks balanced salt solution with 0.5% lactalbumin hydrolysate and Eagle minimal essential medium (MEM) can be used for both outgrowth and maintenance medium. Horse serum seems to be better than bovine serum for use in cell culture medium.

Diethylaminoethyl (DEAE) dextran is used to increase virus adsorption and penetration of the cells (63). All primary hamster kidney cell cultures should be screened for hemadsorbing viruses which are apt to be present in hamster colonies.

Serologic diagnosis

The serologic diagnosis of rabies is possible by the serum-virus neutralization (Nt) test in mice, by plaque reduction in cell culture, by indirect FRA (IFA), by fluorescent focus inhibition test (FFIT), or by CF tests. In addition to identification of rabies in humans, these various tests are used for assaying the immunity state of an individual or animal following pre-exposure or post-exposure vaccination and characterization of strains of rabies virus.

The serum-virus neutralization test in mice

This test is useful for the characterization of strains of rabies virus, for checking stock strains of rabiesvirus for viral contaminants, and for demonstrating antibodies to rabies in human or animal serum. The development of antibodies to rabies virus in the blood serum and spinal fluid of individuals infected with rabies makes it possible to obtain a clinical diagnosis of rabies. The test should be run in parallel with other serologic tests in all cases of suspected rabies in humans.

In order to identify an unknown virus by the serum-virus Nt test, titrate the virus in normal and in rabies hyperimmune serum. If the unknown virus is neutralized by the rabies immune serum and not by the normal control serum, it is assumed to be rabies. The difference in titer must be $>$ a log neutralization index (LNI) of 2 to be significant, and the expected difference is 4 or more. Neutralizing-activity against rabies virus may be found in the blood of humans, dogs, and cattle, and where there is no record of immunization against rabies. This may reflect the presence of antibody resulting from infection with viruses having a serologic relationship, or can be due to nonspecific inhibitors. The IFA test can be used to show that antibody activity resides in the gamma globulin fraction of the serum. Interferon produced by other infections or biologics can also result in neutralization of rabies virus in the Nt test. This could explain the early appearance and subsequent rapid drop in Nt antibodies in persons given vaccines containing a high concentration of nonviral protein.

It is necessary to have a standard virus for the serum-virus Nt test. The CVS strain is the standard reference rabiesvirus. Prepare a 20% suspension of brain tissue from infant mice infected with a moderate dosage of this virus, for example, 3-4 $\log_{10}$ LD$_{50}$. Use a diluent of 0.01 M PBS solution containing 0.75% bovine albumin fraction V, or 2% inactivated guinea pig, hamster or horse serum. Place 1 ml in ampules, flame seal, and store at $-$ 60 C, or lower. The use of a 20% suspension by weight of brain tissue simplifies titration of the virus in normal and rabies immune serum; that is, when 0.2 ml of serum has been added to each tube of a titration series, the addition of 0.2 ml of the 10-fold virus dilution gives a final tissue dilution of 10^{-1}, 10^{-2}, etc. When using high-titer virus prepared from infant mouse brain, the titration series should include 10-fold dilutions through 10^{-8}.

It is essential to have a rabies immune serum of known potency, previously tested to show that it possesses Nt antibody. Prepare rows of 13-mm $\times$100-mm screw-cap test tubes, to include 10-fold dilutions of 10^{-2} through the expected endpoint of the virus. Prepare typed labels reading N-2, N-3, etc., for the normal serum series, ordinarily guinea pig or hamster serum; RI-2, RI-3, etc., for the rabies immune serum; and the initials and dilution of the other sera to be tested. Place 0.2 ml of the serum in the tubes, measured from a 1-ml pipette, graduated in divisions of 0.01 ml. Use a separate pipette for each serum.

Stock virus. The stock virus is diluted in 0.75% bovine albumin fraction V in PBS solution as noted previously. Prepare a set of tubes labeled S-1, S-2, etc., through 10^{-8}. In order to obtain final dilutions of 10^{-2}, 10^{-3}, etc., in the serum-virus mixture, make 10-fold dilutions (2×10^{-2}, 2×10^{-3}, etc.,) of the stock 20% suspension. Transfer 2.7 ml of the diluent to each of the tubes except S-1 which contains the 20% stock suspension. Take a sterile 1-ml pipette, mix this suspension, transfer 0.3 ml to the tube labeled S-2, and discard the pipette; take another sterile pipette and mix this suspension by filling and emptying the pipette 10 times; transfer 0.3 ml to the tube labeled S-3; mix and transfer in this manner until the series is completed, using a different pipette for each dilution. A routine should be established whereby the tube to which the virus has been added is moved 2 spaces along the rack before mixing to make it evident that this mixture is to be pipetted before transfer to the next tube. Use a Propipette for transferring the virus mixtures to avoid aerosol exposure. Work over a tray covered with polyethylene-backed absorbent paper. If a large amount of stock virus is needed, use the proper 10-fold multiple, that is, 3.6 ml plus 0.4 ml etc.

Serum-virus mixture. Beginning with the highest 10-fold dilution of the stock virus, transfer 0.2 ml to the N tube, the serum to be tested bearing the same dilution number, and the RI tube, in that order. Taking a sterile pipette, transfer 0.2 ml of the next 10-fold dilution to the serum tubes bearing the same dilution number, in the same order as before, and so on until the series is completed. Shake the serum-virus mixtures gently and place in an incubator at 35–37 C for 1 hr. Thereafter, transfer the rack to a refrigerator at 4 C to chill the serum-virus mixtures quickly; hold at this temperature until required for inoculation into mice.

Inoculation of mice. Inoculate each of 4–6 young adult mice or a litter of 6 infant mice intracerebrally with each serum-virus mixture, using the technique described previously. Complete the inoculation of the rabies immune serum and the serum to be tested before doing the normal control series. A different syringe and needle must be used for each serum-virus mixture. It is preferable to use an inoculum of 0.015 ml for both infant and adult mice. The usual observation period for inoculated mice is 21 days.

Interpretation of results. The titer of the virus in normal serum and rabies immune serum is calculated as described elsewhere. The LNI is obtained by subtracting the log number of the LD_{50} titer of the virus in rabies immune serum from that in normal serum, and the LNI of the other sera tested is determined in the same way. The dilution of the serum is not calculated on the final dilution after mixing with the virus suspension because the amount of antibody in the serum remains the same. For more accurate results, undiluted serum may be tested against 0.5 log dilutions of the stock virus.

Maximal neutralization is obtained in tests of fresh serum specimens. In testing serum specimens which have been stored for some time, it is advisable to add the so-called "fresh serum factor." When testing undiluted serum against 10-fold dilutions of the virus, the serum to be tested is mixed with an equal amount of fresh hamster or guinea pig serum to make a 2-fold dilution of the serum. When testing serum dilutions against a standard virus suspension, the first dilution of the serum is made in the fresh normal serum and subsequent dilutions in 0.75% bovine albumin fraction V in PBS solution.

Another Nt method is to test various dilutions of serum, usually 2-fold, against a constant amount of virus. This method is recommended for testing the potency of rabies immune serum and for testing the serum of persons or animals to determine the immunity obtained after vaccination or for diagnosis in cases of rabies in humans. Knowing the titer of the stock virus, dilute this so that 0.015 ml contains about 200 LD_{50}. When this is mixed with an equal volume of serum or serum dilution, 0.015 ml contains about 100 LD_{50} of virus.

Infant mice are susceptible to certain strains of rabies virus given by ip inoculation, and the titer by this route is about 2 log_{10} less than by intracerebral inoculation. Non-neuroadapted strains of rabies virus are suitable for use in the ip serum-virus Nt in infant mice. The use of this route of inoculation increases the effectiveness of the neutralization of viruses by immune serum.

Indirect fluorescent-antibody test

The IFA test has proved to be very useful in studies of human serum after treatment with hyperimmune rabies antiserum (equine) and rabies vaccine. The test reveals the individual's active antibody response to vaccination rather than passive immunity, since there is no cross-reaction between equine and human gamma globulin. The test was done originally with smears or impressions of mouse brain infected with the standard CVS strain of rabies virus (42). There was considerable variation in the amount of rabies virus antigen in such preparations, and more consistent results have been obtained by using cell cultures infected with rabies virus (37, 45, 65). The technique described here is that used currently at the California Department of Health Viral and Rickettsial Disease Laboratory (45). This is a modification of the test developed for demonstration of rubella antibodies (44). Cultures of baby hamster kidney cells (line 0853) derived at this laboratory are grown in 8-oz (240 ml) prescription bottles with Eagle MEM containing 10% fetal bovine serum (FBS) as the outgrowth medium (OGM). When a complete sheet of cells is obtained, the cell sheet is infected with Flury-LEP strain rabiesvirus, derived from a commercial dog vaccine by a single passage in infant mice. Each bottle receives an inoculum of 0.1 ml containing about 10^6 LD_{50} of the virus. This virus suspension is added to the 10 ml of Eagle MEM containing 2% FBS, which is the maintenance medium (MM). Additional uninoculated cell cultures are maintained on MM for use as normal cells. On the third day after inoculation, the infected cell cultures are trypsinized and, as the cell sheet begins to slip, the trypsin solution is removed. Normal cells are mixed with infected cells in a ratio of 3:1, to adjust the proportion of antigen-containing cells. The cells from 3 bottles of uninfected cells are mixed with the cells from 1 bottle of infected cells. This is done by adding 10 ml of PBS containing 2% FBS to 1 bottle of uninfected cells. After mixing, this same medium is used to take up the cells from the other uninfected bottles and the infected bottle. The mixture of normal and infected cells is then centrifuged. The cell sediment is carefully mixed with PBS containing 2% FBS, using increments of 1 ml, until a uniform suspension is obtained, which takes about 0.5 ml per bottle. The final suspension of 2 ml of infected and normal cells is used to make a series of slides with three 5-mm spots, marked as for routine FRA tests. The inoculum is about 0.005 ml/spot. Twelve to 14 slides can be made with 0.1 ml. A series of slides of normal cells are prepared with 3 spots of cells on each slide. The cell preparations are then air-dried and fixed with acetone. If kept below − 50 C, they will be satisfactory for 1 year. One normal and 2 or more infected cell slides are used for each serum dilution to be tested; 2-fold dilutions prepared in 20% beef brain suspension in PBS, of 1:4–1:16 for the normal cells, and of from 1:4 to ≥1:128 for the infected cells; and an inoculum of about 0.05 ml of the serum dilution per spot. The slides are incubated for 20 min, washed twice in PBS solution, rinsed with distilled water, and air dried. An appropriate working dilution (determined previously by box titration, as the lowest dilution of antihuman IgG conjugate giving the maximal reaction on virus-infected cell smears and a minimal reaction on normal uninfected cell smears) of anti-human IgG conjugate is added to each spot in a volume of about 0.05 ml. The slides are incubated again for 20 min, washed twice in PBS for 5 min, rinsed with distilled water, and air dried. After mounting with 25% glycerol in PBS, the slides are examined with a fluorescence-equipped microscope, as described previously, and the degree of fluorescence demonstrated by each serum dilution is recorded. The rabies IFA titer of the serum is recorded as the highest serum dilution demonstrating a 1+ degree fluorescence reaction. This test is used routinely in testing serum from people who have received prophylactic immunization against rabies and also for testing the level of immunity in persons because of exposure to rabies (45).

Fluorescent focus inhibition test (FFIT)

The FFIT is given as done at the California Department of Health Viral and Rickettsial Disease Laboratory (45). Microcultures of baby hamster kidney cells (line 0853) are prepared on the standard glass slides used for routine FRA tests. About 100 slides are placed on a paper surface, with 2 culture sites on each marked by 15-mm coverslips. The slides are sprayed with Fluoroglide (Chemplast Inc., Wayne, NJ), after which the coverslips are removed. Disks of filter paper are used to cover the bottom of 150-mm Petri dishes, and 5 of the prepared slides are placed in each dish. The covers are replaced and the dishes are sterilized by autoclaving. In preparation for the addition of the cells, the filter paper in the Petri dishes is wet with sterile distilled water. The baby hamster kidney cells are dispersed in Eagle OGM, and 0.1 ml is pipetted onto each of the clear spots on the slides. The seeded microcultures are incubated in a CO_2 incubator at 35 C for 48 hr. The serum to be tested is inactivated at 56 C for 30 min, and 2-fold dilutions, from 1:4–1:128, are prepared in Eagle MM. On the basis of preliminary titration, the Flury-LEP strain of rabies virus, obtained from a suspension of infected mouse brain representing the second mouse brain passage of a commercial chick-embryo-derived dog vaccine, is diluted in Eagle MEM to give 100–300 rabies fluorescent foci/50 (RFF/50) units per 0.1 ml, when mixed with an equal amount of serum dilution. Titration endpoints (RFF/50) are calculated according to the method of Reed and Muench, as described in Chapter I. A volume of 0.2 ml of the virus suspension is added to 0.2 ml of the serum dilution. After mixing by shaking, the tubes are incubated at 37 C for 90 min. The OGM is then aspirated from the microcultures with a vacuum suction system. Each serum-virus mixture is inoculated, in a volume of 0.1 ml, onto 2 microcultures. The cultures are incubated for 4 days at 35 C in the CO_2 incubator. The medium is then aspirated, and the slides fixed in acetone, air dried, and stained with conjugated rabies immune serum according to the routine FRA system. Test controls consist of normal uninoculated cell cultures, normal human serum diluted 1:4 and 1:8, and several appropriate dilutions covering the neutralization endpoint of a known and standardized rabies immune serum. The antibody titer endpoint is given as the highest dilution of a serum which is able to inhibit the development of fluorescent foci to only 1 or 2 in 20–40 high-power fields. There will be a few single infected cells representing secondary seeding in dilutions of serum which contain very little Nt antibody. As noted previously under serologic diagnosis, the serum dilution is the dilution prior to addition of equal volumes of virus, not the "final dilution" of serum in the serum-virus mixture. Unfortunately, the "final dilution" has been used in some reports (60). The reader should be aware that rabies antibody titers can differ by a 2-fold dilution in reports from various laboratories, and that the way in which the calculation is made is not always specified in publications and reports. The FFIT has shown good agreement with the standard Nt test in mice. There are other procedures for the FFIT using different strains of virus and different methods for cultivating the cells (37, 60).

Plaque-reduction test

Certain strains of rabies virus produce plaques in a test system of BHK-21/13S cells suspended in agarose. Titrations of rabies virus in normal and test sera are done in the usual 2-fold dilutions and inoculated in 0.1-ml amounts onto Petri dishes containing the BHK-21/13S cells suspended in agarose. A final overlay of agarose containing 1:10,000 neutral red is done on the sixth or seventh day, and the plaques are counted after 4 hr (57). A similar system has been described using chick embryo cells (75).

The complement-fixation test

The CF test, in which antigen derived from infant mouse brain or BHK cell cultures is used, is applicable to the study of rabies virus strains. When used to determine antigenic response to vaccination, uninfected antigen prepared from the same host tissue as the vaccine antigen must be tested against the serum to establish that any reactivity with the specific test antigen is not due to the presence of host material. It is preferable to use a test antigen that is derived from a host source different from the one employed for the immunizing antigen. The technique of the CF test for rabies is the same as that given for routine use with viral and rickettsial agents (see Chapter I). The group-specific CF antigen of rabies virus is found associated with the nucleoprotein fraction after disruption of the virus particles (56).

Other serologic tests

The hemagglutination (HA) test (27, 40), the passive hemagglutination test (25), and the hemadsorption test (58) have not proved satisfactory for routine laboratory diagnosis.

The cross-protection test

The cross-protection test is the most certain method of determining the relationship of 2 viruses. If immunization with one virus produces resistance to infection with another virus, they are classified as the same organism. Further classification as to strain depends on serologic tests and tests of pathogenicity for various experimental host systems.

Mice inoculated intracerebrally at 4–6 weeks of age with the Flury-HEP rabies virus strain do not sicken or die, but are resistant to infection with the more pathogenic varieties of rabiesvirus when infected by the same route. Using about 3 log 10 LD_{50}, determined by titration in infant mice, vaccinate a group of 6 female mice by intracerebral inoculation and set aside a control group of the same age and sex. At 1 month after vaccination, challenge the vaccinated and control mice by giving them an intracerebral inoculation of 0.015 ml of the 10^{-2} dilution of the unknown virus prepared from infected mouse brain and having a titer of more than 10^{-5} LD_{50}. Use a separate syringe and needle for each group. If the vaccinated mice survive and the control mice die, you can be certain that the unknown virus is rabies virus.

The Flury-HEP strain vaccine virus is available commercially as prepared for immunization of dogs, cats, and cattle. The antigenic titer of such vaccines can be determined by intracerebral inoculation of adult mice with 10-fold dilutions of the vaccine virus in parallel with a titration of the vaccine virus in infant mice. At 1 month after vaccination challenge all the vaccinated mice with a standard dose of 3 log_{10} LD_{50} of the CVS rabies virus. Only a single control group is needed for the standard challenge dose, but it is advisable to obtain an endpoint by testing the next two 10-fold dilutions of the challenge virus.

A recently isolated virus called Mokola virus shows a serologic relationship to rabies virus. However, there is no cross-protection between the 2 viruses (36). Therefore, Mokola virus cannot be classified as rabies virus (see Description and Nature of Rabies Virus, page 847).

The Flury-LEP rabies virus, derived in the United States, has proved to be effective as a vaccine virus for the control of dog rabies in Europe, Africa, Asia, Central and South America, as well as in North America. The Pasteur rabbit-fixed rabies virus, derived in France, has been used on a worldwide basis for the postexposure immunization of humans against rabies. The 2 viruses appear identical by the usual serologic tests and cross-protection tests (36, 56). This shows that the rabies virus strains which cause disease in humans and dogs on the various continents are closely related.

References

1. ACKERMANN R, BLOEDHORN H, KUPPER B, WINKENS I, and SCHEID W: Über die verbreitung des virus der lymphocytären choriomeningitis unter den mäusen in Westdeutschland I. Untersuchungen uberwiegend an hausmausen (*Mus musculus*). Zentralbl Bakteriol Parasitenkd Infektionskr Hyg 194:407–430, 1964
2. ACKERMANN R, STILLE W, BLUMENTHAL W, HELM EB, KELLER K, and BALDUS O: Syrische Goldhamster als Übertrager von Lymphozytärer Choriomeningitis. Dtsch Med Wochenschr 45:1725–1731, 1972
3. ALMEIDA JD, HOWATSON AF, PINTERIC L, and FENJE P: Electron microscope observations on rabies virus by negative staining. Virology 18:147–151, 1962
4. ARKO RJ, SCHNEIDER LG, and BAER GM. Nonfatal canine rabies. Am J Vet Res 34:937–938, 1973
5. ATANASIU P and SISMAN J: Rage. l'aspect morphologique du virion rabique. Bull Off Int Epizoot 67:521–533, 1967
6. BAUER SP and MURPHY FA: Relationship of two arthropod-borne rhabdoviruses (Kotonkan and Obodhiang) to the rabies serogroup. Infect Immun 12:1157–1172, 1975
7. BELL JF, SANCHO MI, DIAZ AM, and MOORE GJ: Nonfatal rabies in an enzootic area: results of a survey and evaluation of techniques. Am J Epidemiol 95:190–198, 1972

8. BENNETT JA, RABIN ER, WENDE RD, and MELNICK JL: A comparative light and electron microscope study of rabies and Hart Park virus encephalitis. Exp Molec Pathol 7:1–10, 1967

9. BHATT DR, HATTWICK MAW, GERDSEN R, EMMONS RW, and JOHNSON HN: Human rabies: diagnosis, complications, and management. Am J Dis Child 127:862–869, 1974

10. BROWN AL, MERRY DL, and BECKENHAUER WH: Modified live-virus rabies vaccine produced from flury high-egg-passage virus grown in an established canine-kidney line: three-year duration-of-immunity study in dogs. Am J Vet Res 34:1427–1432, 1973

11. CAMPBELL JB, MAES RF, WIKTOR TJ, and KOPROWSKI H: The inhibition of rabies virus by arabinosylcytosine. Studies on the mechanism and specificity of action. Virology 34:701–708, 1968

12. CENTER FOR DISEASE CONTROL: Compendium of Animal Rabies Vaccines, 1977, Veterinary Public Health Notes. Center for Disease Control, Atlanta, GA, February, 1977

13. CIFUENTES E, CALDERON E, and BIJLENGA G: Rabies in a child diagnosed by a new intravitam method: the cornea test. J Trop Med Hyg 74:23–25, 1971

14. CONOMY JP, LEIBOVITZ A, MCCOMBS W, and STINSON J: Airborne rabies encephalitis: demonstration of rabies virus in the human central nervous system. Neurology 27:67–69, 1977

15. CONSTANTINE DG: Rabies transmission by non-bite route. Public Health Rep 77:287–289, 1962

16. CONSTANTINE DG, EMMONS RW, and WOODIE JD: Rabies virus in nasal mucosa of naturally infected bats. Science 175:1255–1256, 1972

17. DAVIES MC, ENGLERT ME, SHARPLESS GR, and CABASSO VJ: The electron microscopy of rabies virus in cultures of chicken embryo tissues. Virology 21:642–651, 1963

18. DEAN DJ, BAER GM, and THOMPSON WR: Studies on the local treatment of rabies-infected wounds. Bull WHO 28:477–486, 1963

19. DEAN DJ, EVANS WM, and THOMPSON WR: Studies on the low-egg-passage Flury strain of modified live rabies virus produced in embryonated chicken eggs and tissue culture. Am J Vet Res 25:756–763, 1964

20. EMMONS RW, LEONARD LL, DEGENARO F JR, PROTAS ES, BAZELEY PL, GIAMMONA ST, and STURCKOW K: A case of human rabies with prolonged survival. Intervirology 1:60–72, 1973

21. EMMONS RW and RIGGS JL: Application of immunofluorescence to diagnosis of viral infections, *In* Methods in Virology, Vol 6, Maramorosch K and Koprowski H (eds), Academic Press, New York, 1977, p 1–28

22. ENDE M, POLSON A, and TURNER GS: Experiments with the soluble antigen of rabies in suckling mouse brain. J Hyg 55:361–373, 1957

23. FENJE P: A rabies vaccine from hamster kidney tissue cultures: preparation and evaluation in animals. Can J Microbiol 6:605–609, 1960

24. FERNANDES MV, WIKTOR TJ, and KOPROWSKI H: Mechanism of the cytopathic effect of rabies virus in tissue culture. Virology 21:128–131, 1963

25. GOUGH PM, and DIERKS RE: Passive haemagglutination test for antibodies against rabies virus. Bull WHO 45:741–745, 1971

26. HABEL K and WRIGHT JT: Some factors influencing the mouse potency test for rabies vaccine. Public Health Rep 63:44–55, 1948

27. HALONEN PE, MURPHY FA, FIELDS BN, and REESE DR: Hemagglutinin of rabies and some other bullet-shaped viruses. Proc Soc Exp Biol Med 127:1037–1042, 1968

28. HATTWICK MA, WEIS TT, STECHSCHULTE CJ, BAER GM, and GREGG MB: Recovery from rabies. A case report. Ann Intern Med 76:931–942, 1972

29. HOWARD P, LIEBOVITZ A, BEYSON J, and DICKERSON MS: Epidemiologic notes and reports. Human rabies-Texas, Morbid Mortal Weekly Rep 21:113–114, 1972

30. HUMMELER K, KOPROWSKI H, and WIKTOR TJ: Structure and development of rabies virus in tissue culture. J Virol 1:152–170, 1967

31. HUMMELER K, TOMASSINI N, SOKOL F, KUWERT E, and KOPROWSKI H: Morphology of the nucleoprotein component of rabies virus. J Virol 2:1191–1199, 1968

32. JOHNSON HN: The significance of the Negri Body in the diagnosis and epidemiology of rabies. Ill Med J 81:382–388, 1942

33. JOHNSON HN: Derriengue; vampire bat rabies in Mexico. Am J Hyg. 47:189–204, 1948
34. JOHNSON HN: The role of the spotted skunk in rabies. Proc 63rd Ann Meeting US Livestock San Assoc, 1959, pp 267–274
35. JOHNSON HN: Sporadic cases of rabies in wildlife: relation to rabies in domestic animals and character of virus. Proc Nat Rabies Symposium, Center for Disease Control, Atlanta, GA, 1966, pp 25–30
36. JOHNSON HN: Unpublished information
37. KING DA, CROGHAN DL, and SHAW EL: A rapid quantitive in vitro serum neutralization test for rabies antibody. Can Vet J 6:187–193, 1965
38. KISSLING RE, and REESE DR: Anti-rabies vaccine of tissue culture origin. J Immunol 91:362–368, 1963
39. KOPROWSKI H and COX HR: Studies on chick embryo adapted rabies virus I. Culture characteristics and pathogenicity. J Immunol 60:533–554, 1948
40. KUWERT E, WIKTOR TJ, SOKOL F, and KOPROWSKI H: Hemagglutination by rabies virus. J Virol 2:1381–1392, 1968
41. KUWERT E, BÖHME U, LICKFELD KG, and BÖHME W: Zur oberflächenstruktur des tollwutvirion (TWV). On the surface structure of rabies virus. Zentralbl Bakteriol Parasitenkund Infektionkr Hyg I Abt Orig A 219:39–45, 1972
42. LEFFINGWELL L and IRONS JV: Rabies antibodies in human serums titrated by the indirect FA method. Public Health Rep 80:999–1004, 1965
43. LENNETTE EH, WOODIE JD, NAKAMURA K, and MAGOFFIN RL: The diagnosis of rabies by fluorescent antibody method (FRA) employing immune hamster serum. Health Lab Sci 2:24–34, 1965
44. LENNETTE EH, WOODIE JD, and SCHMIDT NJ: A modified indirect immunofluorescent staining technique for the demonstration of rubella antibodies in human sera. J Lab Clin Med 69:689–695, 1967
45. LENNETTE EH and EMMONS RW: The laboratory diagnosis of rabies: review and prospective In Rabies, Nagano Y and Davenport FM (eds), University Park Press, Baltimore, 1971, pp 77–90
46. MAES RF, KAPLAN MM, WIKTOR TJ, CAMPBELL JB, and KOPROWSKI H: Inhibitory effect of a cytidine analog on the growth of rabies virus: comparative studies with other metabolic inhibitors In The Molecular Biology of Viruses, Academic Press, Inc, New York, 1967, pp 449–462
47. MATSUMOTO S: Electron microscope studies of rabies virus in mouse brain. J Cell Biol 19:565–591, 1963
48. MURPHY FA and FIELDS BN: Kern Canyon virus: electron microscopic and immunological studies. Virology 33:625–637, 1967
49. MURPHY FA, BAUER SP, HARRISON AK, and WINN WC JR: Comparative pathogenesis of rabies and rabies-like viruses. Viral infection and transit from inoculation site to the central nervous system. Lab Invest 28:361–376, 1973
50. MURPHY FA, HARRISON AK, WINN WC, and BAUER SP: Comparative pathogenesis of rabies and rabies-like viruses. Infection of the central nervous system and centrifugal spread of virus to peripheral tissues. Lab Invest 29:1–16, 1973
51. NEURATH AR, VERNON SK, WIENER FP, HARTZELL RW, and RUBIN BA: The rabies virus glycoprotein: partial purification and some properties. Microbios 7:7–15, 1973
52. POLSON A and WESSELS P: Particle size of soluble antigen of rabies virus. Proc Soc Exp Biol Med 84:317–320, 1953
53. PORRAS C, BARBOZA JJ, FUENZALIDA E, LOPEZ-ADAROS H, OVIEDO DE DIAZ AM, and FURST J: Recovery from rabies in man. Ann Int Med 85:44–48, 1976
54. SCHLUMBERGER HD, WIKTOR TJ, and KOPROWSKI H: Antigenic and immunogenic properties of components contained in rabies virus-infected tissue culture fluids. J Immunol 105:201–298, 1970
55. SCHNEIDER LG: The cornea test; a new method for the intra-vitam diagnosis of rabies. Zentralbl Veterinaermed 16:24–31, 1969
56. SCHNEIDER LG, DIETZSCHOLD B, DIERKS RE, MATTHAEUS W, ENZMANN PJ, and STROHMAIER K: Rabies group-specific ribonucleoprotein antigen and a test system for grouping and typing rhabdoviruses. J Virol 11:748–755, 1973
57. SEDWICK WD, and WIKTOR TJ: Reproducible plaquing system for rabies, lymphocytic choriomeningitis and other ribonucleic acid viruses in BHK-21/13S agarose suspensions. J Virol 1:1224–1226, 1967

58. SELIMOV MA and ILJASOVA RS: Phenomenon of hemadsorption provoked by street rabies virus adapted to tissue culture. Prob Virol 13:76-80, 1968

59. SHOPE RE, MURPHY FA, HARRISON AK, CAUSEY OR, KEMP GE, SIMPSON DIH, and MOORE DL: Two African viruses serologically and morphologically related to rabies virus. J Virol 6:690-692, 1970

60. SMITH JS, YAGER PA, and BAER GM: A rapid reproducible test for determining rabies neutralizing antibody. Bull WHO 48:535-541, 1973

61. SOAVE OA, JOHNSON HN, and NAKAMURA K: Reactivation of rabies virus infection with adrenocorticotropic hormones. Science 133:1360-1631, 1961

62. SODIA I, LIM D, and MATOUCH O: Isolation of rabies virus from small wild rodents. J Hyg Epidemiol Microbiol Immunol 15:271-277, 1971

63. SOKOL F, KUWERT E, WIKTOR TJ, HUMMELER K, and KOPROWSKI H: Purification of rabies virus grown in tissue culture. J Virol 2:836-849, 1968

64. SOKOL F, SCHLUMBERGER HD, WIKTOR TJ, KOPROWSKI H, and HUMMELER K: Biochemical and biophysical studies on the nucleocapsid and on the RNA of rabies virus. Virology 38:651-665, 1969

65. THOMAS JB, SIKES RK, and RICKER AS: Evaluation of indirect fluorescent antibody technique for detection of rabies antibody in human sera. J Immunol 91:721-723, 1963

66. TILLOTSON JR, AXELROD D, and LYMAN DO: Rabies in a laboratory worker—New York, Morbid Mortal Weekly Rep 26:183-184, 1977

67. TILLOTSON JR, AXELROD D, and LYMAN DO: Follow-up on rabies—New York, Morbid Mortal Weekly Rep 26:249-250, 1977

68. TURNER GS and KAPLAN C: Some properties of fixed rabies virus. J Gen Virol 1:537-551, 1967

69. VAUGHN JB, GERHARDT P, and NEWELL KW: Excretion of street rabies virus in the saliva of dogs. J Am Med Assoc 193:363-368, 1965

70. WIKTOR TJ, FERNANDES MV, and KOPROWSKI H: Cultivation of rabies virus in human diploid cell strain WI-38. J Immunol 93:353-366, 1964

71. WIKTOR TJ, FERNANDES MV, and KOPROWSKI H: Detection of a lymphocytic choriomeningitis component in rabies virus preparation. J Bact 90:1494-1495, 1965

72. WIKTOR TJ, KAPLAN MM, and KOPROWSKI H: Rabies and lymphocytic choriomeningitis virus (LCMV). Infection of tissue culture; enhancing effect of LCMV. Ann Med Intern Fenn 44:290-296, 1966

73. WIKTOR TJ, KUWERT E, and KOPROWSKI H: Immune lysis of rabies-infected cells. J Immunol 101:1271-1282, 1968

74. WINKLER WG, BAKER EF, and HOPKINS CC: An outbreak of non-bite transmitted rabies in a laboratory animal colony. Am J Epidemiol 95:267-277, 1972

75. YOSHINO K, TANIGUCHI S, and ARAI K: Plaque assay of rabies virus in chick embryo cells. Arch Gesamte Virusforsch 18:370-373, 1966

76. YOSHINO K: One-day egg culture of animal viruses with special reference to the production of anti-rabies vaccine. Jpn J Med Sci Biol 20:111-125, 1967

77. ZAVADA J: Assay methods for viral pseudotypes In Methods in Virology, Vol 6 Maramorosch K and Koprowski H (eds) Academic Press, New York, 1977, pp 109-140

78. ZOONOSES SURVEILLANCE, Annual Summary Rabies 1976, Center for Disease Control, Atlanta, GA, October, 1977

CHAPTER 29

HEPATITIS A AND B

Stephen M. Feinstone, Lewellys F. Barker and Robert H. Purcell

Introduction

Although the existence of hepatitis has been recognized since antiquity, many illnesses which included jaundice as a symptom were probably grouped together. There were several well-documented reports of epidemics of jaundice, most likely type A hepatitis (HAV), dating from the seventeenth and eighteenth centuries. The first evidence for transmissible, blood-borne, long-incubation hepatitis (almost surely type B disease) came from an outbreak of hepatitis in shipyard workers in Bremen, Germany, in 1885. The disease occurred in individuals who had been vaccinated against smallpox several months previously with lymph obtained from the vesicles of other vaccinated humans. Other outbreaks of parenterally transmitted hepatitis were reported in the first half of the twentieth century. These included epidemics among patients attending diabetes clinics or venereal disease clinics, where inadequately sterilized needles and syringes were the apparent vehicles of transmission, and outbreaks of hepatitis among recipients of yellow-fever vaccine, which contained human immune serum, and recipients of human immune plasma for measles and mumps prophylaxis (146).

Proof that serum hepatitis (type B hepatitis) was distinct from infectious hepatitis (type A hepatitis) came from a series of epidemiologic studies and experiments conducted in human volunteers during the 1940s (83, 97). Concepts derived from these studies were refined and expanded in additional extensive human volunteer studies in adults and children during the 1950s and the 1960s (70, 71, 95, 133). Much of our understanding of the nature of viral hepatitis stems from these studies and subsequent re-analysis of specimens obtained from them.

Prior to the late 1960s, intensive efforts to isolate the hepatitis B virus (HBV) *in vitro* or to demonstrate an antigen-antibody reaction specific for this disease were unsuccessful. Furthermore, attempts to transmit HBV to many species of animals and birds were also unsuccessful, and inoculation of human volunteers remained the only method of demonstrating the presence of the HBV agent. However, the discovery of "Australia antigen", now termed hepatitis B surface antigen (HBsAg), by Blumberg in 1965 and its subsequent association with type B hepatitis provided the first specific antigenic marker of HBV infection and stimulated a resurgence of viral hepatitis research (3, 19, 20, 52, 80, 105). The antigen was found in the blood of 30–60% of adults with acute viral hepatitis and also in approximately 0.1% of normal individuals in the United States and Western Europe and in 5–20% of apparently healthy individuals in parts of Asia, Africa, and South America. In 1968, Bayer et al (17) demonstrated that HBsAg was physically associated with particles 20 nm in diameter and filaments of similar diameter and variable length, and it was postulated that HBsAg, previously thought to be a serum protein polymorphism (18), was the HBV. However, Dane et al (27) described 42-nm virus-like particles that were associated with HBsAg particles and shared the antigenic specificity of these particles (Figs 29.1–3). He proposed that the larger, more complex, virus-like particles were, in fact, the HB virions. In 1971, Almeida et al (1) described a second antigen-antibody system associated with HBV infection. This antigen was on the surface of the core-like structure inside the particle noted by Dane and could be released by treatment with detergent or lipid solvent; it is called hepatitis B core antigen (HBcAg). The immune responses to HBsAg and HBcAg by HBV-infected patients were quite distinct in magnitude and temporal relationship and provided additional evidence that the Dane particle was the HBV (61). The intrahepatic localization of HBV antigens was demonstrated by immunofluorescence (FA) techniques by Edgington and his colleagues

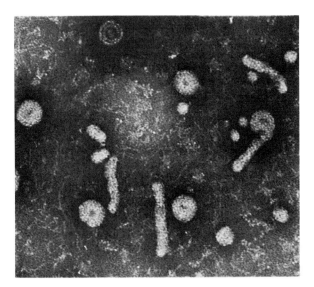

Figure 29.1—An electron micrograph illustrating the 3 morphologic forms associated with the HBV. This preparation is highly enriched for the 42-nm Dane particles thought to represent the actual HBV. The 22-nm diameter spherical and filamentous forms contain the determinants of HBsAg as does the surface of the 42-nm structure. 1% phosphotungstic acid, 150,000X (Courtesy E Ford and J Gerin)

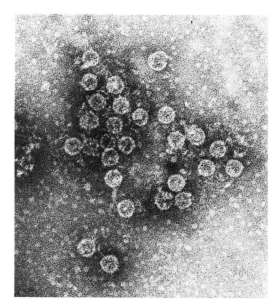

Figure 29.2—An electron micrograph of 27-nm core particles purified from HBV particles seen in Figure 29.1. 1% phosphotungstic acid, 150,000X (Courtesy E Ford and J Gerin)

(12, 39). HBsAg was found in the cytoplasm of hepatocytes, and HBcAg was localized to the nucleus, thus confirming electron microscopic observations of virus-like particles by others (64, 99).

Advances have also been made recently in HAV research. These have greatly expanded our knowledge of this disease and its causative agent. In 1969, Holmes et al conclusively showed that marmoset monkeys were susceptible to infection with HAV (60). Lorenz et al (81) and Mascoli et al (86) extended these observations and, using the marmoset model, it was possible to perform a neutralization (Nt) test as a measure of serum antibody (59, 108). In 1973, Feinstone, Kapikian, and Purcell reported the detection by immune electron microscopy (IEM) of 27-nm virus-like particles in filtrates of acute-phase stools from patients with HAV (Fig 29.4). The particles could be serologically associated with the illness, and by using these particles as an antigen, antibody could be detected in a quantitative way. Though IEM is a difficult technique to perform, it is sensitive, specific, and has been useful for serologic studies. By purifying the HAV particles from human stool or marmoset livers for use as an antigen, new tests which are easy to perform, as well as sensitive, have recently been devised to measure antibody to hepatitis A virus. These tests have been applied to diagnostic uses as well as to seroepidemiologic surveys.

The ability to accurately make a diagnosis of HAV or HBV infection in individual patients has changed many concepts about viral hepatitis. One of the most important recent developments has been the conclusive demon-

HEPATITIS B VIRAL COMPONENTS

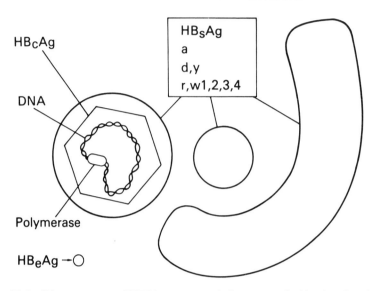

Figure 29.3—The structure of HBV represented diagrammatically showing the position of the various antigens, the double-strand circular DNA and the DNA dependent DNA polymerase after completion of the polymerase reaction. Before the reaction approximately 30% of the DNA is single strand.

stration that many patients with a viral hepatitis syndrome have neither HAV or HBV infection. Since little is presently known about the etiology of this hepatitis, we prefer to call it non-A, non-B hepatitis.

Hepatitis B

Clinical aspects

Mode of transmission

Early epidemiologic and volunteer studies of HBV transmission suggested that this virus was exclusively transmitted by percutaneous means, including the infusion of contaminated blood and blood products and the inoculation of minute quantities of contaminated blood via the use of improperly sterilized needles and syringes. However, the development of sensitive tests for HBsAg and antibody to it (anti-HBs) led to the recognition that HBV infection was relatively widespread in many populations, including individuals with no history of hepatitis or percutaneous exposure to HBV. It is now recognized that HBV can be transmitted by non-percutaneous means. HBsAg has been detected in virtually every type of excretion and secretion, and infectious virus has been demonstrated in saliva, and probably semen, by transmission experiments in chimpanzees or gibbons (10, 12). Epidemiologic evidence also is consistent with spread of the virus through intimate oral and/or genital contact: HBV attack rates are higher among spouses of index cases than among other family members and are particularly high among male homosexuals (134, 137). So called "verti-

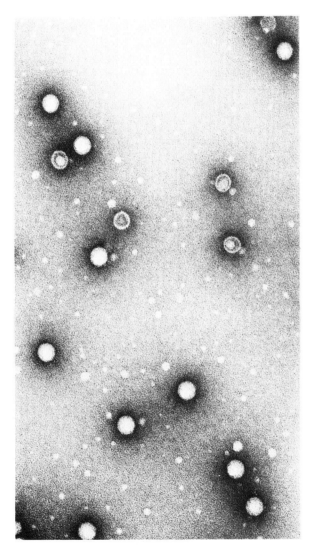

Figure 29.4—An electron micrograph of 27-nm HAV particles highly purified from human stool. 1% phosphotungstic acid 150,000X (Courtesy E Ford, Y Moritsugu, and J Gerin)

cal transmission'' from HBV infected mothers to their offspring is also well recognized (16, 100, 126, 134, 136, 137). This type of transmission is not a true vertical transmission but, more likely, transmission to the offspring at time of birth via exposure to the mother's contaminated blood. The likelihood of transmission to offspring from mothers acutely infected with HBV in the United States is greater than transmission from the chronically infected mothers. In contrast, transmission to offspring from both the acutely and chronically infected mother is common in Asia.

Pathogenesis

The pathogenesis of HBV infection is poorly understood. The temporal relationship of the humoral immune responses to HBV antigens and the results of various studies of *in vitro* correlates of cellular immunity in patients with hepatitis has led to the theory that the nature of the host's immune response dictates the course and severity of HBV infection (38). Thus, the development of the immune response would lead to damage of infected liver cells that might have hepatitis viral antigens expressed on their surface. It is believed that the cellular component of the response is more important in this regard than the humoral component. However, recent studies suggest-

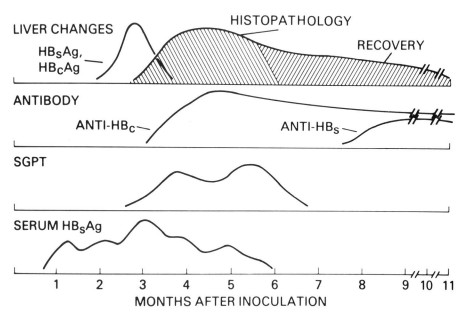

TYPE B HEPATITIS (CHIMP 1640)

Figure 29.5—Diagrammatic illustration of the clinical and serologic events in a typical case of acute type B hepatitis in a chimpanzee. These events are similar to the course of human hepatitis type B.

ing that HBV is heterogeneous, consisting of populations of particles resembling defective interfering particles, as well as fully infectious particles suggests that clinical response may be complex and modulated by both the virus and the host (48, 66, 123).

Incubation period

The incubation period of HBV infection is quite variable, ranging from approximately 2 weeks to 6 months from time of exposure to appearance of HBsAg in the blood and from 3–4 weeks to 6 months from exposure to illness. The incubation period is inversely related to the dose of infecting virus (13, 14). At present the average incubation period for HBV posttransfusion hepatitis is approximately 12–14 weeks.

Period of infectivity

The period of infectivity of the acutely infected patient probably extends at least from the time that HBsAg can first be detected until it disappears. All chronically infected individuals may be infectious, regardless of whether they have clinical disease or are inapparent carriers of HBsAg. However, patients whose serum contains the hepatitis B e antigen (HBeAg), demonstrable viral DNA polymerase actively, and detectable HB virions have been shown to be more infectious in situations of small volume blood transmission (inadvertent needlesticks, etc.) and in perinatal transmission (6, 100).

Symptoms

The signs and symptoms of acute viral hepatitis include fever, anorexia, nausea, vomiting, abdominal distress, diffuse tenderness of the liver and, frequently, jaundice (121). However, severity may range from completely inapparent infection to massive necrosis of the liver leading to death (fulminant hepatitis). In addition, approximately 5–10% of cases of clinical HBV infection progress to a chronic state. Chronic HBV infection may be inapparent, with normal liver function tests, or may be characterized by chronic hepatitis that is well tolerated by the patient or progresses to cirrhosis and death. Late sequelae of chronic HBV infection are thought to include hepatic cell carcinoma, especially in parts of Africa, Asia, and Southern Europe (139, 142). Whether the association is etiologic or the result of chronic inflammation of the liver has not been established. The laboratory diagnosis of hepatitis is most frequently made by demonstrating abnormalities of liver function tests, especially serum alanine amino transferase (ALT) and serum aspartate amino transferase (AST) activity. Serum bilirubin levels may also be elevated, particularly in more severe cases.

Certain extrahepatic manifestations of HBV infection have been reported (50). These include a serum sickness-like syndrome occurring during the late-incubation period and early-acute phase of HBV infection. Signs and symptoms include fever, arthralgia, and skin rashes. Occasionally patients in the early-acute stage of HBV infection are first seen in rheumatology clinics for evaluation of acute arthritis. Periarteritis nodosa and glomerulone-

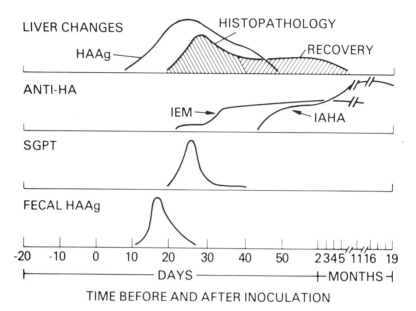

Figure 29.6—Diagrammatic illustration of the clinical and serologic events in a typical case of type A hepatitis in a chimpanzee. These events are similar to the course of human hepatitis type A.

phritis have both been associated infrequently with HBV infection and are thought to result from the deposition of immune complexes of HBsAg and antibody in arterial walls and glomeruli, respectively. Acrodermatitis (Gianotti-Crosti syndrome) may be a rare complication of HBV infection, particularly following infection with the *ayw* subtype of HBV. Aplastic anemia is also a rare complication of hepatitis but is not limited to HBV infection.

Pathology

Histopathologic changes in the liver during acute HBV infection have not been distinguished from those of acute HAV infection, except by special stains that reveal the presence of HBsAg or HBcAg. The histologic picture varies with the severity of the disease, ranging from loss of scattered individual hepatocytes and replacement by inflammatory cells to massive necrosis of whole lobules of the liver (103). Characteristic lesions include acidophilic bodies (the dehydrated remains of individual liver cells, sometimes with pycnotic nuclei), hepatocytolysis, "ballooned" hepatocytes that appear swollen and pale, excess lipofuscin pigment (resulting from breakdown of liver cells), and scattered or portal inflammation consisting of accumulations of Kupffer cells, lymphocytes, plasma cells, eosinophils, and fibroblasts. Chronic hepatitis may contain some of these elements and, in addition, varying degrees of fibrosis. Virus inclusion bodies are not seen in acute or chronic viral hepatitis.

Description and nature of hepatitis B virus

General characteristics

HBV is a deoxyribonucleic acid (DNA)-containing virus. The intact virion is approximately 42 nm in diameter and consists of a 27-nm nucleocapsid core particle which possesses the HBcAg surrounded by an outer coat which possesses the HBsAg (Figs 29.1–3). Early studies revealed that HBsAg was predominantly protein, but the presence of lipid was shown by staining (3). The major phospholipids identified in HBsAg preparations are phosphatidyl choline and sphingomyelin (69, 131). Carbohydrate, apparently as glycoprotein and perhaps also glycolipid, has been found in purified HBsAg preparations (24, 25, 49).

Circular, double-strand DNA with a molecular weight of approximately 2.0×10^6 has been isolated from the core of HBV, and the cores have also been found to possess DNA-dependent DNA polymerase activity (54, 68, 82, 123, 124). This enzyme synthesizes new DNA, presumably using as template the double-strand circular DNA. Approximately 30% of the circular DNA molecule is single-strand, and it is apparently the complementary strand of this single-strand DNA portion that is synthesized by the polymerase *in vitro*. The nature of this single-strand region is not well understood, but restriction endonuclease analysis of HBV DNA indicates that the sum of the recognizable DNA fragments is greater than the total molecular weight of the undigested circular DNA. These findings, coupled with the finding of subpopulations of HB virions with densities in CsCl of 1.22 and 1.20 g/cm^3, in which the heavier particles are associated with polymerase activity and a larger DNA, strongly suggests that defective interfering particles exist that may play a role in the modulation of infection. Nucleocapsid cores are synthesized in the nuclei of infected cells (Fig 29.2), and the outer lipoprotein coat material is synthesized in the cytoplasm and attached to the cores before release of the fully synthesized virions. At present it cannot be classified on morphologic, immunologic, or biochemical bases with any other group of animal viruses. Recently, however, a virus with characteristics very similar to HBV has been found in woodchucks. (Summers, unpublished).

Resistance

Early attempts to inactivate HBV were made on human plasma known to be contaminated with infectious virus and were evaluated by injection of the treated material into human volunteers (46, 95). Under these conditions, infectivity was not eliminated by up to 4 hr of heating at 60 C, or by ultraviolet irradiation, or betapropiolactone treatment; lengthening of the incubation times in recipients of the treated material compared with recipients of the untreated plasma suggested that all of these measures partially inactivated HBV, which was present at a high titer in the untreated plasma. Although there is no cell culture system available for evaluation of the inactivation kinetics of HBV, it is now possible to use the chimpanzee animal model as an indicator for infectivity. In this system it has been shown that the virus can be inactivated by formalin treatment of purified suspensions of HBsAg prepared for experimental vaccine development (56, 114). As HBsAg is rapidly destroyed by sodium hypochlorite (Chlorox), this probably is a reliable solution for inactivating HBV in laboratory and clinical settings, as is heat sterilization in an autoclave for 30–60 min. The ability of other solutions, including alcohol, quaternary ammonium compounds, and iodophors, to inactivate HBV has not been demonstrated.

Antigens

The antigenic complexity of HBsAg, first suspected from the study of Raunio et al (120), was proven by the discovery of the *d* and *y* determinants by LeBouvier (74) and the *w* and *r* determinants by Bancroft et al (9) in the early 1970s. The *d-y* and *w-r* determinants were shown to be allelic in nature and to be associated with a group-reactive determinant, *a*, that defined all HBsAg particles. All of these antigenic determinants were found on the surface of the 22-nm spherical and filamentous particles, as well as the 42-nm virus-like particles. A number of other antigenic determinants have been associated with particulate HBsAg. The best characterized of these are the "*a* subdeterminants" of Soulier and Courouce-Pauty (130) that are now interpreted as being subdeterminants of *w* and are referred to as *w*-1, *w*-2, *w*-3, and *w*-4 (144). These, like the *d-y* and *w-r* determinants, have distinct geographic distributions and epidemiologic significance: contact cases of hepatitis are associated with HBsAg of the same subtype as the index case. Thus, the genetic information necessary for the synthesis of these antigens is carried by the virus and not the host.

A third HBV antigen (or antigens) was described in 1972 (85). This antigen complex, HBeAg, was associated with a soluble protein found in the serum of some patients acutely or chronically infected with HBV. At least two and possibly three, HBeAg components exist; Williams and LeBouvier (143) have defined two of these as *e*-1 and *e*-2.

A possible fourth HBV-associated antigen has recently been described (122). This antigen, called delta antigen, has been demonstrated by immunofluorescence in the nuclei of hepatocytes from certain patients with HBV infection. The new antigen may be allelic with HBcAg: liver tissue that contains HBcAg does not contain delta antigen and *vice versa*.

Pathogenicity for animals (host range)

Chimpanzees and gibbons are highly susceptible to experimental infection with HBV (10, 12, 13, 90). In both species the serologic and biochemical events closely resemble those that occur in mild hepatitis in humans. Chimpanzees have been infected with each of the 4 major HBsAg subtypes (*adw*, *ayw*, *adr*, and *ayr*) and have been used for infectivity titrations, as well as studies of virus inactivation, passive and active immunization, and reagent preparation. Rhesus monkeys and woolly monkeys are also susceptible to HBV infection, but virus adaptation appears to be necessary for studies in these animals; in any case, they are clearly much less sensitive than chimpanzees and gibbons.

Preparation of immune serum

Numerous sources of antiserum for hepatitis B antigen (anti-HBs) are available. Anti-HBs of sufficient titer for use in serologic tests described below can be obtained from multiply transfused patients (hemophiliacs, thalassemics, etc.) or from patients previously infected with HBV who developed an anamnestic response following infusion of blood or blood products. Anti-HBs is also available from a number of commercial sources. Hyperimmune anti-HBs can be prepared in a variety of laboratory animals, including guinea pigs, rabbits, mice, monkeys, and chimpanzees, and in larger animals such as horses, sheep, and goats. Purification of HBsAg for antibody production is laborious and requires expertise in ultracentrifugation if removal of most or all of the contaminating serum proteins is to be achieved. Even after meticulous purification of HBsAg, resultant antiserum often requires absorption to remove low levels of antihuman serum antibodies.

One successful method of purification involves collection of human or chimpanzee plasma containing a high titer of HBsAg from a chronic HBsAg carrier. HBsAg-positive plasma is layered onto a cesium chloride (CsCl) (density gradient ranging from 1.1 to 1.6 g/cm^3) and centrifuged in an SW 40 rotor at 5 C for 18 hr at 152,000 $\times$ g. After fractionation, the gradient is monitored for HBsAg by one of the serologic tests listed below and the fractions containing peak HBsAg activity (at a density of approximately 1.20 g/cm^3) are pooled and rebanded in a second CsCl density gradient. The HBsAg peak is identified, pooled and purified by rate zonal separation in a 5–20% (wt/wt) sucrose gradient at 5 C and 200,000 $\times$ g). After fractionation, the HBsAg is identified serologically, and peak fractions are pooled. At this stage of purification most of the serum proteins have been removed (49, 116). However, greater purity can be achieved by a third isopycnic banding in a CsCl density gradient. Purified HBsAg is stable when stored at -70 C in CsCl. However, some aggregation or loss of antigen activity through nonspecific adsorption to surfaces may occur when stored in sucrose or in dilute form in certain buffers.

A number of immunization procedures have been successfully employed. One such is the immunization of seronegative guinea pigs by the footpad inoculation method (116). Prescreened guinea pigs are inoculated in each hind footpad with 1 ml of a 50% emulsion of Freund complete adjuvant and 10–50 μg of purified HBsAg; 4–6 weeks after inoculation the animals are test-bled and inoculated ip with 1 ml of aqueous purified HBsAg. The guinea pigs are bled weekly and given booster inoculations of aqueous HBsAg ipevery other week until satisfactory titers are obtained.

Serum with a high titer of anti-HBc is readily obtained from chronic carriers of HBsAg. Patients with accompanying chronic hepatitis are more likely to have higher titers of anti-HBc because of more active virus replication in these patients. Hyperimmune anti-HBc can be prepared in laboratory animals, but acquisition and purification of HBcAg for immunization is difficult. Human or chimpanzee liver obtained at necropsy from a case of acute or chronic HBV infection is the usual source of HBcAg for this purpose. Best results have been obtained when the patient or chimpanzee lacked anti-HBc; chimpanzees have been experimentally infected with HBV for the purpose of obtaining HBcAg-rich livers (61).

Purification of HBcAg

The following procedure has proven suitable for purifying HBcAg for immunization of animals (61). A 20% (wt/vol) homogenate of HBcAg-rich liver in hypotonic (0.45%) saline is prepared in a Waring Blendor and clarified by centrifugation for 30 minutes at $1100 \times g$. The supernatant fluid is centrifuged for 2 hr at 4 C and $75,000 \times g$ and the resultant pellet resuspended in approximately 10% of the original volume of distilled water. The high-speed centrifugation and resuspension of the pellet in distilled water is repeated, and the final suspension is again clarified by centrifugation for 30 min at 4 C and $1100 \times g$. The clarified supernatant fluid is then layered onto a continuous CsCl gradient (density 1.2–1.5 g/cm^3) and centrifuged for 16 hr at 4 C and $75,000 \times g$. After fractionation, peak HBcAg activity is located by one of the serologic tests described below, and appropriate fractions are pooled and dialyzed for 2 days at 4 C against phosphate-buffered saline (PBS), pH 7.4. HBcAg from liver bands at a density of approximately 1.30–1.33 g/cm^3. Excellent anti-HBc has been prepared from HBcAg purified in this manner, but additional purity can be achieved by repeating the isopyonic banding in CsCl and rate-zonal separation in sucrose as described above for the purification of HBsAg. An alternative method for purifying HBcAg from plasma containing Dane particles is described on page 898.

To produce anti-HBc, guinea pigs are inoculated subcutaneously with 0.2 ml of purified HBcAg emulsified in an equal volume of complete Freund adjuvant and given booster inoculations in a similar manner with HBcAg emulsified in incomplete Freund adjuvant at 14 days (47, 61). The animals are test-bled at 21 days and weekly thereafter until suitable anti-HBc titers are obtained.

Anti-HBe is obtained from chronic carriers of HBsAg who demonstrate such antibody. These patients often have antibody to both e-1 and e-2 components of the HBeAg complex. Methods for the purification of HBeAg and the preparation of hyperimmune anti-HBe are still being developed and are beyond the scope of this chapter.

Collection and preparation of specimens for laboratory diagnosis

Precautions

HBV is highly infectious when exposure is by percutaneous means: titers of virus as high as 10^8 infectious particles/ml have been documented in transmission studies to humans and chimpanzees (13, 15). Although transmissible by nonpercutaneous means, the virus appears to be less infectious by these routes ("nonpercutaneous" transmission may represent covert percutaneous transmission through minute cuts, abrasions, etc.), and there is scanty evidence for infection via aerosol. Therefore, precautions consist primarily of preventing exposure of bare skin and mucous membranes to potentially infectious material, but additional precautions should be considered when procedures that might generate aerosols of highly infectious material (purification and concentration of antigens, homogenization of infected liver tissue, etc.) are employed. Gowns and gloves (preferably disposable) should be worn, and smoking and eating in the laboratory should be prohibited. The use of hypodermic needles and other sharp objects should be minimized and, where their use is necessary, they should be disposed of in such a way as to prevent inadvertent needlesticks. Serum samples should be collected from all personnel at intervals (monthly in the authors' laboratories) and tested for biochemical and serologic evidence of HBV infection. Samples of serum should also be stored frozen.

Virus isolation

HBV has not been successfully cultivated *in vitro*, and the only biologic means of demonstrating its presence is by inoculation of seronegative chimpanzees or gibbons. Serum or plasma specimens collected for future virus isolation are best stored undiluted at -70 C or lower. The intravenous route of inoculation of suitable primates is preferred; biochemical, histologic, and serologic indicators of HBV infection in the chimpanzee and the gibbon are similar to those in humans.

Serologic diagnosis

Serologic diagnosis can be made by testing the serum from acute or chronic cases for the presence of HBsAg or for development of anti-HBs or anti-HBc. Serum is stored undiluted at -20 C or lower. Enzymes of certain bacteria can destroy HBsAg, and bacterial contamination can make serum anticomplementary and introduce new antigens that make serologic diagnosis difficult. Therefore serum should be collected and stored aseptically or protected from contamination by the addition of 0.1% sodium azide.

Microscopy

The diagnosis of HBV infection cannot usually be accomplished by ordinary light microscopy, but both FA and, to a lesser extent, EM are useful for diagnosis.

Immunofluorescence microscopy. Liver tissue is placed on a disk of cork and covered with several drops of Tissue-Tek (Lab-Tek Products, Napavilla, Illinois) or other suitable cryo-embedding medium and gently lowered into liquid nitrogen. The frozen sample is stored at -70 C or lower. Four-micron sections are cut on a cryostat, transferred to a clean microscope slide, and used immediately or stored at -70 C.

Electron microscopy. For thin-section electron microscopy, approximately 1-mm cubes of liver tissue are fixed in 2.5% gluteraldehyde with 0.1 M sodium cacodylate, pH 7.3, for 1 hr, transferred to buffered 4% sucrose in cacodylate buffer, and stored until embedding, preferably within hours. Alternatively, tissue is fixed in buffered 10% formalin, pH 7.0, in which it can be stored until embedding.

Laboratory diagnosis

Although virus isolation techniques by propagation in one or another small animal host or cell culture system are not currently available for the diagnosis of HBV infection, a wide variety of serologic techniques have been applied to the detection of HBsAg, anti-HBs and anti-HBc. The presence of HBsAg in a patient's blood is diagnostic of active HBV infection, either acute or chronic; anti-HBs is an indicator of recovery from active infection, whereas anti-HBc may be detected during active infection or during convalescence. Conversion from seronegative to seropositive or a significant rise in titer for either anti-HBs or anti-HBc may be used to diagnose recent HBV infection.

Serologic techniques for detection of HBsAg and anti-HBs

Frequently used serologic techniques for HBsAg and anti-HBs detection are listed in Table 29.1. They have been classified, in the case of HBsAg, as first, second, and third generation techniques, according to relative sensitivity. As the third generation methods, radioimmunoassay (RIA), hemagglutination (HA), and enzyme-linked immunosorbent assay (ELISA) are the most sensitive, they are the preferred methods for most diagnostic applications. All commercially available reagents for HBsAg and anti-HBs detection are subject to federal licensure and are accompanied by detailed directions for use. A list of licensed manufacturers of the reagents for various test methods can be obtained by writing to the Director, Bureau of Biologics, Food and Drug Administration, 8800 Rockville Pike, Bethesda, MD 20014. Reference reagents for research use can be obtained from the Reference Resources Branch, National Institute of Allergy, and Infectious

TABLE 29.1—METHODS FOR DETECTION OF HBsAG AND ANTI-HBS

First generation (1X)	Agar gel diffusion
Second generation (5–10X)	Counterelectrophoresis
	Rheophoresis
	Complement fixation
	Reverse passive latex agglutination
Third generation (50–100X)	Radioimmunoassay
	Reverse passive hemagglutination (HBsAg) and passive hemagglutination (anti-HBs)
	Immune adherence hemagglutination
	Enzyme-linked immunosorbent assay
Research laboratory	Immune electron microscopy
	Immunofluorescence microscopy

SUBTYPING OF HEPATITIS B ANTIGENS

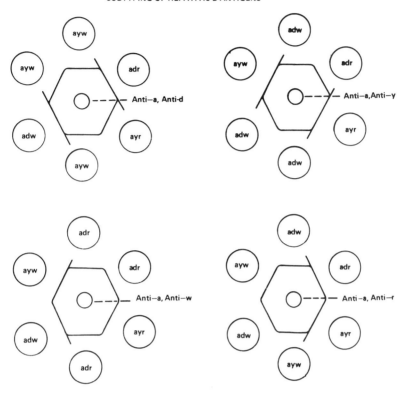

Figure 29.7—Diagrammatic illustration of the use of the agar gel diffusion technique to subtype HBsAg. The center well in each case contains antibody to the group antigen, *a*, as well as antibody to one of the subtype antigens *d*, *y*, *w*, or *r*. All the outer wells contain HBsAg. A common precipitin line completely surrounds the central well and represents the *a*/anti-*a* reaction. A spur is formed where wells contain the subtype antigen of the same specificity as the subtype antibody in the central well and where the adjoining well does not contain this antigenic specificity.

Disease, National Institutes of Health, 9000 Rockville Pike, Bethesda, MD 20014.

Agar gel diffusion (AGD). The AGD technique is relatively insensitive, but continues to be valuable for detecting and characterizing certain HBsAg subtype determinants (Fig 29.7) and also for seeking strong, precipitating antibodies which are valuable for reagent purposes and for preparation of hyperimmune globulin (19, 74, 105). See appendix for method.

Counterelectrophoresis (CEP). CEP is a practical method with the advantages of greater speed and sensitivity than AGD (4, 51, 102, 106). For several years it was the most commonly used method to test samples from blood donors for HBsAg, but it was eventually replaced by more sensitive techniques. See appendix for method.

Rheophoresis. Rheophoresis uses the same principle as AGD but achieves greater sensitivity, so that it is similar in this regard to CEP (65). This method has been particularly valuable for achieving increased sensitivity in the study of HBsAg subtypes. See appendix for method.

Complement fixation (CF). The microtiter CF technique may be used to detect and quantitate HBsAg with slightly greater sensitivity than CEP or rheophoresis (116, 117, 127). A potent and specific CF antiserum of human or animal origin is a prerequisite; many precipitating antisera are not satisfactory for use in CF, which appears to be less sensitive than the precipitation methods for anti-HBs detection.

Reverse passive latex agglutination. Agglutination of latex particles coated with anti-HBs provides a rapid and simple method for HBsAg detec-

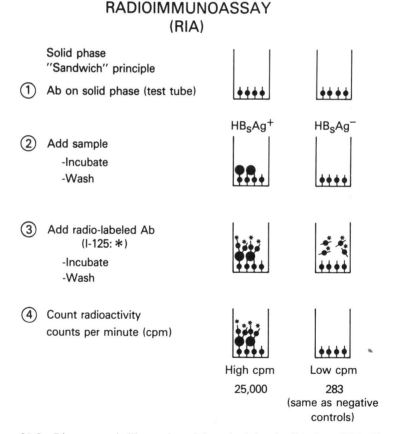

Figure 29.8—Diagrammatic illustration of the principle of solid-phase RIA. The technique has been useful for detecting all the HAAg and HBsAg. ELISA techniques are similar except that an enzyme-conjugated antibody replaces the radiolabeled antibody, and the binding is measured by adding the substrate and measuring the reaction product colorimetrically.

tion (73). The sensitivity of this method is approximately that of CEP; false-positive reactions are quite common because of the prevalence of substances other than HBsAg which agglutinate globulin-coated latex particles. Therefore the test is rarely used.

Radioimmunoassay (RIA). A number of different RIA techniques have been developed for detection of both HBsAg and anti-HBs; these techniques provide the highest sensitivity of the various available serologic methods. The main disadvantages of RIA methods are the short shelf-life (30–60 days) of the radiolabeled reagents and the hazards and inconvenience associated with radioactive materials.

Because of its simplicity, solid-phase RIA (SPRIA) has come into widespread use for a variety of applications. There are several commercially available SPRIA kits for HBsAg detection, and at least one for anti-HBs detection. In all instances the sandwich principle is used (Fig 29.8) (58, 76, 118). For HBsAg detection, the solid phase, usually plastic beads or tubes, is coated with anti-HBs; test samples are added to this solid phase. After an appropriate incubation period, usually 1–2 hr, the sample is removed, the solid phase is washed, and ^{125}I-radiolabeled anti-HBs is added for a second incubation phase. Following removal of the radiolabeled reagent and another washing step, the solid phase is counted in a gamma counter and the amount of ^{125}I-labeled anti-HBs bound to the bead or tube is compared with counts produced in the same system by a negative control serum which contains no detectable HBsAg. When a test sample gives counts significantly higher than the negative control it is desirable to repeat the test, as technical errors occasionally give false-positive results that are not reproducible. A sample which gives reproducible positive results should be evaluated to see whether the reaction is inhibited by unlabeled anti-HBs as a means of determining the specificity of the reaction. The same principle is applied to serum for detection of anti-HBs, but in this case the solid phase is coated with HBsAg and the radioactive reagent is ^{125}I-labeled HBsAg. By using specific antibody and antigen reagents for inhibition of the SPRIA reaction it is possible to apply these methods to subtyping HBsAg and anti-HBs in test samples with a high degree of sensitivity (62).

The double-antibody or radio-immunoprecipitation method has also been widely used for detection of both HBsAg and anti-HBs (58, 72). For HBsAg detection, test samples are mixed with a known quantity of ^{125}I-labeled HBsAg and anti-HBs, and then antigen-antibody complexes are precipitated by a second antibody directed against the anti-HBs reagent. If HBsAg is present in the test sample, then it competitively inhibits the reaction between the ^{125}I-HBsAg and anti-HBs in the reaction mixture resulting in a higher ratio of free ^{125}I-HBsAg in the test sample to bound and precipitated ^{125}I-HBsAg than would be found when negative control samples containing no detectable HBsAg are tested. Testing for anti-HBs is accomplished by mixing the test samples with ^{125}I-HBsAg alone followed by the precipitation step to determine how much of the ^{125}I-HBsAg is bound by anti-HBs. Both of these RIA methods (solid-phase and double-antibody) are in the order of 100- to 1000-fold more sensitive than the second generation methods such as CEP. See appendix for SPRIA methods.

Passive hemagglutination. Agglutination of human group O erythro-cytes (RBC) coated with purified HBsAg provides a rapid and sensitive pas-sive HA method for detecting anti-HBs (104, 141). The RBC coating step is done in the presence of chromic chloride; checker-board titration of the puri-fied antigen preparation and $CrCl_3$ at several concentrations is necessary to establish the optimal coating conditions. This system may be used to detect HBsAg as well, by looking for inhibition by test samples of the reaction between coated RBC and a small amount of anti-HBs; the sensitivity of this method for HBsAg detection is approximately the same as the sensitivity of CEP. Subtype-specific inhibition of anti-HBs reactions in this system pro-vides a simple method for determining the subtype specificity of antibodies in test samples (53, 107).

Reverse passive hemagglutination, in which RBC coated with anti-HBs are reacted with test samples for HBsAg detection, provides sensitivity al-most equivalent to RIA (104). Anti-HBs-coated RBC have been prepared commercially and distributed in the freeze-dried state for this reverse pas-sive hemagglutination method. The propensity for false-positive reactions to occur makes it necessary to evaluate positive results for specificity in a man-ner similar to that applied to RIA tests.

Immune adherence hemagglutination (IAHA). The same IAHA method useful for detection of anti-HAV and anti-HBc can be adapted to HBsAg, anti-HBs, HBeAg, and anti-HBe detection (91, 140). Purified HBsAg is re-quired for this test which is probably somewhat more sensitive than CF for HBsAg detection and similar in sensitivity to passive hemagglutination for anti-HBs detection. As the test sensitivity and specificity require delicate adjustments of a number of variables, however, it has not achieved as wide-spread acceptance and use as other equally sensitive but less complex tests for HBsAg and anti-HBs. See appendix for method.

Enzyme-linked immunosorbent assay (ELISA). Adaptation of the ELISA to HBsAg detection has been accomplished by preparing conjugates of anti-HBs and an enzyme such as peroxidase or alkaline phospha-tase (40, 145). The principle of the test is the same as for the SPRIA except that a substrate for the enzyme in the conjugate, which gives a color change when the enzyme is present, is used as the indicator system instead of a radioisotope. For this test, therefore, a final incubation of the substrate with the solid phase is necessary to determine whether an (anti-HBs)—HBsAg-(enzyme-labeled anti-HBs) sandwich reaction has taken place. The color change can be detected by visual inspection or, more objectively, by reading in a spectrophotometer. The ELISA method appears to have sensitivity equivalent to SPRIA systems; the stability and consequent long shelf-life of the enzyme-conjugated anti-HBs reagent and the simplicity of the equipment needed for reading the reactions provide some practical advantages over RIA methods. See appendix for method.

Immune electron microscopy (IEM) and immunofluorescence (FA) mi-croscopy. Aggregation of HBsAg particles by anti-HBs to facilitate their identification by EM was a critical early research step in the characterization of HBsAg (1, 17). Localization of HBsAg in the cytoplasm of infected he-patocytes was accomplished by the application of standard FA microscopy techniques with potent conjugated antiserum (39). Because a variety of simple and sensitive serologic techniques for diagnostic applications are available, use of these methods has been confined to research applications.

Serologic techniques for detection of HBcAg and anti-HBc

A number of procedures for detecting HBcAg and anti-HBc have been developed. The most useful of these, from the standpoint of diagnosis and epidemiology, are tests for anti-HBc. Methods appropriate to the routine diagnostic laboratory have been developed and commercial tests for anti-HBc are becoming available. An advantage of tests for anti-HBc over tests for anti-HBs in the diagnosis of HBV infection is that anti-HBc develops early during the infection, often in the acute phase of disease, and a rising titer of anti-HBc at this time is diagnostic, even in the absence of detectable serum HBsAg. In contrast, anti-HBs often does not develop until weeks or

TABLE 29.2—SEROLOGICAL TECHNIQUES FOR DETECTING HEPATITIS ANTIGENS AND ANTIBODIES

TECHNIQUE	RELATIVE SENSITIVITY* FOR DETECTING						
	HBsAg	Anti-HBs	HBcAg	Anti-HBc	HBeAg AND Anti-HBe	HAV	Anti-HA
Agar gel diffusion	+	+			+		
Counterelectrophoresis	++	++	+	+	+		
Complement fixation	++	++	+	+		++	++
Rheophoresis	++	++	+	+	+		
Reverse passive latex agglutination	++						
Passive hemagglutination	++**	+++			++		
Immune adherence hemagglutination	+++	++	++	+++		++	+++
Immune electron microscopy	+++	+++	+++	++		++	++
Immunofluorescence microscopy	++	++	+++	++		+++	++
Reverse passive hemagglutination	+++						
Solid-phase radioimmunoassay	++++	++++	++++	++++	+++	++++	++++
Radioimmunoprecipitation	++++	++++		++++			
Enzyme-linked immunoassay	++++		++++	++++	+++	++++	++++

*Estimated gradation from least sensitive (+) to most sensitive (++++). These gradations do not give any indication of the relative specificity of the techniques.

**HBsAg detected by inhibition of passive hemagglutination.

months after loss of HBsAg, making early serologic diagnosis difficult in some cases.

Suitable tests for HBcAg and anti-HBc are listed in Table 29.2. Although there are considerable differences in sensitivity among the various tests for anti-HBc, the immune response to HBcAg is usually brisk and detectable with most of the tests described.

Purification of HBcAg. Several of the tests for anti-HBc require partially purified HBcAg. This can be derived from 2 sources: liver tissue and plasma of a human or a chimpanzee acutely or chronically infected with HBV. HBcAg from liver is purified as described above for preparation of immunizing antigen; HBcAg derived from HBV particles (Dane particles) in plasma is purified as follows.

Purification of HBcAg from Dane particles (96). A HBsAg-positive plasma or serum sample rich in HB virions is selected for purification. Selection can be made on the basis of direct visualization of virions by EM or by detection of HBeAg or HBV-specific DNA polymerase activity, both of which correlate with presence of HB virions. HB virions are concentrated by pelleting through a cushion of 10% (wt/wt) sucrose in 0.01 M Tris, pH 8, with 0.15 M NaCl, 1% bovine serum albumin, and 0.1% sodium azide (BSA-Tris-saline). The supernatant, usually containing a high titer of anti-HBc, is carefully removed and the pellet is resuspended in BSA-Tris-saline to 2% of the original volume. Centrifugation through sucrose is repeated and the resuspended pellet is then mixed with NP-40 (final concentration 3%) and incubated at 37 C for 4 hr. The detergent-treated HBV concentrate is subjected to isopycnic banding in a preformed CsCl density gradient (1.0–1.5 g/cm³) and centrifuged for 18 hr at 5 C and 160,000 × *g*. After fractionation, the fractions are tested for HBcAg and HBsAg. Peaks of HBcAg activity may be found at densities of 1.30–1.33 g/cm³ and 1.35–1.37 g/cm³. In some cases a peak of HBcAg is detected at an intermediate density. The low density HBcAg peak is generally devoid of DNA polymerase activity and is thought to represent empty nucleocapsids. The high-density peak is strongly DNA polymerase positive and is thought to contain the nucleocapsids of fully infectious virions. The intermediate peak, when present, is weakly DNA-polymerase positive and is thought to contain the nucleocapsids of defective interfering-like virions that lack a portion of the HBV genome (48, 66, Kaplan unpublished). HBcAg from all 3 peaks is suitable for serologic tests. It is important that the HB virions be completely separated from anti-HBc-containing plasma before release of the nucleocapsids by treatment with detergent to prevent attachment of anti-HBc to the nucleocapsids. It is also important to completely remove HBsAg from the nucleocapsids with detergent; otherwise the HBcAg preparation will react with anti-HBs. The HBcAg preparation must be carefully tested for specificity by demonstrating that it reacts with anti-HBc but not anti-HBs or antihuman immunoglobulin. Purified HBcAg is stable at −70 C in BSA-Tris-saline.

Complement fixation (CF). CF has been the most widely used and perhaps best characterized serologic technique for detecting anti-HBc (61). This technique detects anti-HBc following most clinical acute HBV infections, but is not sufficiently sensitive to diagnosis many subclinical and inapparent infections. Almost all patients with chronic infection, whether clinical or subclinical, have anti-HBc when tested by CF. A disadvantage of the CF test is the relatively large quantity of antigen required when compared with other serologic tests for anti-HBc. The CF test for HBcAg and anti-HBc is performed by a standard CF technique as described in Chapter 1.

Counterelectrophoresis (CEP). CEP is approximately as sensitive as CF for detecting HBcAg and anti-HBc but provides results within 2 hr. As with CF, the test requires relatively large quantities of HBcAg. See appendix for method.

Immune Adherence hemagglutination (IAHA). IAHA is approximately 10 times as sensitive as CF and CEP for detecting HBcAg and anti-HBc (140). It uses relatively small quantities of antigen and, therefore, can be performed with HBcAg purified from plasma, as well as with antigen derived from liver. The test is performed as described for HAV (see below). The IAHA test is very sensitive to slight variations in the quality of the reagent, and therefore it is necessary to preselect human RBC for their sensitivity as indicators of hemagglutination in the test. See appendix for method.

Radioiummunoassay (RIA). The most sensitive methods for detecting HBcAg and anti-HBc are RIAs (115). The SPRIA for detection of HBcAg is similar to one of the methods used for detecting HBsAg. The test is performed as described for HAV. This test has been modified for the detection of anti-HBc, and RIAs utilizing the wells of microtiter plates or plastic beads have been developed. The latter RIA has been developed as a commercial test. SPRIA has the advantage of permitting use of relatively impure nucleocapsids (HBV concentrates that have been treated with detergent but not further purified) if the antibody used for coating of the solid phase and for radiolabeling is specific for anti-HBc; other antigen-antibody reactions that might be present such as HBsAg-anti-HBs are not detected. The test also uses very small quantities of reagents. A disadvantage is that quantitation of anti-HBc is somewhat more difficult than with CF or IAHA. See appendix for method.

Radioimmunoprecipitation test (RIP). Perhaps the most sensitive test for anti-HBc is a double-antibody RIP test utilizing tritium-labeled HBcAg (55, 94).

Although extremely sensitive and, from a theoretical standpoint, extremely specific, the RIP for anti-HBc detects an antibody that binds to the labeled HBcAg in many human and other primate sera. This does not appear to be a nonspecific reaction, but rather, one that measures a cross-reacting antibody that is widely distributed. Titers of this antibody as high as 1:1000 have been detected in normal serum, thereby seriously limiting the usefulness of this test for seroepidemiologic studies. Although the test is useful for detecting weak immune responses to HBcAg, changing titers of the cross-reacting antibody have also been detected, making interpretation of results difficult in some cases. Nevertheless the RIP test is approximately 300 times more sensitive than CF for detecting anti-HBc.

Immunofluorescence (FA). FA is a sensitive test for HBcAg and can be modified for detection of anti-HBc (12, 84). Liver is the only tissue demonstrated to contain HBcAg, which is localized to the nuclei of hepatocytes. Liver tissue from a human or chimpanzee infected with HBV serves as the substrate. Chronic infections that lack evidence of chronic hepatitis are less likely to yield HBcAg-positive liver tissue than are infections with associated hepatitis. Liver tissue obtained during the acute phase of HBV infection from chimpanzees is usually positive for HBcAg. See appendix for method.

HBeAg. Serologic tests for HBeAg and anti-HBe are still somewhat limited in scope and sensitivity. Although RIA and passive hemagglutination assays are being developed, virtually all testing is currently performed by AGD or rheophoresis (41, 85).

Two distinct bands, HBeAg/1 and HBeAg/2 can be visualized in approximately one-third of sera positive for HBeAg by AGD. Occasionally a third precipitin line can also be visualized. The advantage of AGD for detecting HBeAg and anti-HBe is its ability to demonstrate lines of identity with reference reagents and to distinguish between HBeAg/1 and HBeAg/2, as well as being inexpensive and relatively simple to perform. Its disadvantages are those of relative insensitivity and long incubation before results can be obtained. See appendix for method.

Rheophoresis is approximately as sensitive as AGD and is suitable for demonstrating both HBeAg/1 and HBeAg/2. However, it is less suitable for studying antigenic relationships than is AGD. It shares with AGD the disadvantages of insensitivity and prolonged incubation times. See appendix for method.

DNA polymerase. HBV-specific DNA-dependent DNA-polymerase activity has become an important marker, with HBeAg, of active HBV synthesis and relative infectivity (7, 8, 67). See appendix for method.

Hepatitis A

Clinical aspects

Mode of transmission

HAV infection is commonly transmitted by the fecal-oral route. Food and water contaminated by human waste are most frequently implicated as the vehicle of transmission of the virus in epidemics, however, close personal contact such as within families, or institutions and contact with infected primates have all been related to outbreaks of HAV infection (112). In addition, a significant proportion of sporadic cases of hepatitis with no known exposure have been shown to be due to HAV (28). It is possible to transmit HAV parenterally in experimental situations (31, 60, 70, 81), but, parenteral transmission such as by blood transfusion, illicit intravenous drug use, or biting insects has never been documented (44, 132, 135). Respiratory transmission has been suggested, but volunteer studies failed to confirm the presence of virus in the nasopharyngeal secretions (83, 97).

Pathogenesis

The pathogenesis of HAV infection is not fully elucidated. The virus probably enters the portal blood from the intestine and is thereby transmitted to the liver. Whether HAV infects intestinal cells or is transported by some other means to the liver is not known. In experimentally infected chimpanzees and marmosets, hepatitis A antigen (HA Ag) has not been detected in intestinal cells by FA during the acute illness (87, 88), but this does not rule out an earlier intestinal phase of replication. Viral antigen is detectable by FA in the cytoplasm of chimpanzee and marmoset hepatocytes beginning about 2 weeks after experimental inoculation and continuing for 3-6 weeks. This viral antigen is usually detectable about 1 week prior to either liver enzyme elevations in the serum or histopathologic evidence of hepatitis. Although no chronic carrier state has ever been documented in humans, viral antigen has been shown to persist in hepatocytes of a few marmosets for 3-4 months after inoculation (87). Virus is not detectable serologically in the stools of these animals, but it is not presently known whether they continue to excrete infectious virus at a low level during the extended period of hepatic antigen. Shedding of antigen in the stools usually ceases at about the time of the appearance of serum antibody.

Incubation period

The incubation period of HAV infection determined from naturally occurring epidemics and human volunteer studies is 2-6 weeks (71). Similar incubation periods have been reported for experimentally infected chimpanzees and marmosets, and there is one report of a 7-day incubation period in marmosets using a strain of HAV which was adapted to that animal (31, 60, 110).

Period of infectivity

The period of infectivity has not been precisely worked out and is probably variable. Krugman and Ward reported the period of infectivity to be from 2-3 weeks before jaundice to 1 week after the cessation of jaundice (71). The period of viremia probably begins at about the time of or before shedding of virus in the stools but does not last as long (71).

Symptoms

The symptoms of HAV infection are much like those of HBV infections. The disease may be asymptomatic (diagnosable only by liver function tests), symptomatic without jaundice, or symptomatic with jaundice. It is not known what factors determine how the infection will be manifested in any individual. Children generally have a mild form of the disease—often inapparent. The rate of icteric hepatitis varies from one outbreak to another, and what factors other than age determine the severity of the disease are not known. However, the size of the inoculum as well as virus-determined virulence factors may also be important.

The onset of symptoms in HAV infection can occur within a 24-hr period, but HBV symptoms usually develop more insidiously. Flu-like symptoms of fever or feverishness, chilliness, and headache frequently occur early. Gastrointestinal symptoms often begin slightly later with anorexia and nausea predominating. Vomiting frequently occurs but is not usually severe or protracted. Right upper-quadrant abdominal pain or discomfort is often experienced and is exacerbated by jarring the liver. Most patients with jaundice report a "dark" change in their urine color. Curiously, many of the symptoms disappear at the onset of jaundice. Whether symptoms such as arthralgia and rash which occasionally are reported in patients with HBV infection and are attributed to immune-complex disease also occur in HAV infection may be confused in the old literature because of the inability to accurately separate the two diseases.

Complications

The case-fatality ratio for HAV infection is very low, probably less than 0.1% of icteric cases. Fulminant hepatitis with coma has now been documented in HAV infection, (28) but this is also apparently very rare.

Infections by HAV do not appear to lead to chronic hepatitis nor to a chronic carrier state. Prolonged hepatitis was reported to have occurred in 2 children, one 11 months and one 28 months old at the time their illness began. Their illness was felt to be HAV infection because their stools, taken 5 months and 16 months after the onset of illness, induced a typical short incubation hepatitis in volunteers (133). In the recent epidemic among Naval recruits in San Diego in which 133 people were clinically affected, 11 had abnormal enzymes lasting longer than 3 months. However, all abnormal enzymes had returned to normal by 6 months (37). Other epidemiologic studies also indicate that a carrier state of HAV must be very rare.

Pathology

The use of needle aspiration biopsy has greatly advanced knowledge of the pathologic changes found in viral hepatitis. However, the only justification for this procedure to be performed on patients with HAV infection is to help distinguish viral hepatitis from some other clinical entity for which a specific therapy especially surgery might be indicated. In HBV infection there are other reasons to biopsy, but these indications usually occur after the acute stage of the disease. Acute HAV and HBV infections cannot ordinarily be distinguished by histopathologic criteria. However, as far as is known, HAV infection has no chronic stage, and the lesions described in chronic viral hepatitis do not apply to HAV infection.

In experimental studies in chimpanzees, some differences between the hepatic lesions of HAV and HBV infections have been noted (34). In HAV infections, the alteration in the hepatocytes was primarily in the periportal areas and the parenchymal changes were less severe than the portal inflammation. HBV infection, on the other hand, tended to involve the entire lobular parenchyma but was predominantly centrolobular. The portal areas were less affected in HBV than in HAV infection. These differences may also exist in human hepatitis (H Popper, personal communication), but a large number of biopsies from humans with HAV infection have not been examined.

Other histopathologic methods are useful to distinguish types of viral hepatitis. The ground-glass cells and the orcein-staining cells, both of which are seen in chronic hepatitis and have been shown to contain HBsAg, should not be present in HAV-infected livers. Furthermore, immunologic techniques, notably FA and immunoperoxidase staining, can be used to distinguish HAV from HBV in liver tissue (see Appendix, page 911).

Description of the nature of the agent

Common characteristics

All HAV studied thus far seem identical by morphologic and serologic criteria. Perhaps multiple serotypes or subtypes may be found when large scale purification permits a finer serologic analysis.

Size and shape

The HAV has a mean diameter of approximately 27 nm as determined in both negatively stained EM preparations and thin-section EM of infected chimpanzee or marmoset livers (Fig 29.4). The particles have no envelopes and have cubic symmetry. Both full and empty particles are seen, and full particles are often noted to have an electron-dense central area. In CsCl density gradients, 2 peaks are often found with the major peak at about 1.34 g/cm^3 and a lesser peak at about 1.4 g/cm^3. The significance of these 2 densities is not known, but the particles with a density of 1.4 g/cm^3 seem to be less stable than the lighter density particles. Both densities contain particles which are immunologically reactive (27, 36, 42, 93, 111). Siegl and Frösner determined the sedimentation coefficient of HAV to be 160 (128).

Chemical composition

The nature of the nucleic acid of HAV is not known, but there is mounting evidence that suggests HAV contains RNA. Provost et al showed orange-red staining of partially purified virus by acridine orange and partial destruction of infectivity by treatment with pancreatic RNase for 1 hr at 60 C (111). In addition, both FA and EM techniques have demonstrated HAV only in the cytoplasm of infected chimp or marmoset liver cells (88, 111, 125). In recent studies, Siegl and Frösner have shown that the nucleic acid from highly purified HAV appeared by EM to be linear and single strand with a molecular weight of approximately 1.96 daltons (129). In addition it was hydrolyzed as readily as poliovirus RNA by alkali treatment of pH 12.9, while single-strand DNA resisted hydrolysis by this treatment and double-strand DNA was denatured to single strands but not further hydrolysed (129).

In a recent report, Coulepis et al have shown that SDS polyacrylamide gel electrophoretic analysis of the proteins of purified HAV revealed 3 polypeptides which have molecular weights similar to VP_1, VP_2, and VP_3 of poliovirus. Poliovirus VP_4 was not detected by the methods they used (26). Studies in our laboratory have generally confirmed these findings.

Resistance to physical and chemical agents

HAV is acid and ether stable. It is inactivated by heating to 100 C for 5 min but only partially inactivated by heating to 60 C for 1 hr. HAV is inactivated by ultraviolet radiation and by treatment with 1:4000 formalin at 37 C for 3 days (111).

Classification

HAV is certainly picornavirus-like. The small differences reported between HAV and poliovirus in the size of the RNA and the structural polypeptides may or may not prove to be significant.

Antigenic composition

Number of immunotypes. There is only 1 known immunotype of HAV. All isolates tested thus far have cross-reacted with all other isolates. It is not known if subtypes exist.

Description of the antigen. IEM detects surface viral antigens, and the other immunologic tests probably do also. Whether more than one antigen exists on the surface is not known. The virus has not been shown to agglutinate RBC.

Pathogenicity for animals

HAV has been shown conclusively to infect humans, chimpanzees, and several species of marmosets (tamarins), most notably *Saguinus mystax*. The disease produced in these primates resembles that in humans but is usually milder. Other primate species may indeed by susceptable to infection as evidenced by antibody detected in jungle caught animals (92, 112).

Growth in tissue culture

HAV has never been shown to replicate in any *in vitro* system, including embryonated eggs, organ culture, and primary and continuous cell lines of any species. However, sensitive techniques for detecting HAV have only recently been developed, and many *in vitro* culture systems are now being re-examined for their ability to support the growth of HAV.

Preparation of immune serum

The most common source of immune serum has been from convalescent humans who have a high titer of anti-HA. Chimpanzee serum has also been used in a similar way, and it has been possible to boost the antibody titer in a convalescent chimpanzee by inoculating partially purified HA Ag (35). Anti-HA has been produced in rabbits and guinea pigs using HA Ag partially purified from stool and emulsified in complete Freund adjuvant (36). This serum is of low titer and not specific for HA Ag as it contains large amounts of antibody to stool contaminants. Highly purified antigen in sufficient quantities to raise a specific hyperimmune antibody in laboratory animals is presently being produced.

Collection and preparation of specimens for laboratory diagnosis

Precautions

Because there are no easy and rapid tests for infectivity, all specimens obtained from acutely ill, recently ill, or potentially ill humans or primates must be considered infectious. As HAV is infectious by the oral route, gloves, gowns, and possibly masks should be worn when working with any potentially infectious material. When specimens are transported at least double containment is warranted. Laboratory workers who have frequent, close exposure to HAV should consider taking immune serum globulin if they have no serum anti-HA.

Virus isolation, collection, storage, and processing

Stools and serum (or plasma) are the main clinical specimens collected for the isolation of HAV. Liver and bile are very useful to collect from experimental animals.

Serial stool specimens should be collected beginning as early as possible in the course of the illness. If there are close contacts of an index case, stool collections from them should begin as soon as they are identified. The virus shedding in stools peaks early in the illness, usually before jaundice and occasionally even before any identifiable symptoms. Stool containers should be well-sealed and stored at −70 C until use. Frequent freeze-thawings should be avoided as some loss of antigen has been noted after repeated freeze-thaw cycles. The effect of freeze-thawing on infectivity is unknown. Stool suspensions in an appropriate buffer in concentrations ranging from 2% to 40% (wt/vol) are generally used for various procedures for HAV identification and isolation. In addition micropore filtrates of stool suspensions produce the best material for IEM.

Serologic diagnosis

Blood specimens for serologic diagnosis should be collected as early as possible in the illness and even prior to illness from known exposed individuals. The first serum should ideally be followed by an early convalescent-phase specimen taken 3–4 weeks after the peak of illness and a late convalescent-phase serum obtained about 2–3 months after illness. Some tests for anti-HA, notably IEM, SPRIA, and ELISA, detect antibody (probably IgM and early IgG) usually as early as the peak of illness. The IAHA does not detect this early antibody and often does not become positive for 4–6 weeks after illness. Therefore the method of testing determines to some degree when serum specimens are ideally obtained. Heavy hemolysis and repeated freeze-thaw cycles often cause serum to give nonspecific false-positive results in IAHA testing. The nonspecific activity can often be eliminated by further dilutions of the serum or by centrifugation at 35,000 rpm in a 40.2 rotor for 2 hr.

Microscopy

Light microscopy. Liver biopsy or necropsy material is handled in the standard fashion for histopathology.

Electron microscopy (EM). HA Ag was first described by the technique of IEM using stool filtrates from infected volunteers as the source of antigen (43, 78). A 2% (wt/vol) stool suspension is prepared by vigorously shaking the stool in veal infusion broth with 0.5% bovine serum albumin and glass beads to facilitate breaking up the stool particles. Many other methods such as tissue homogenizers may be used, but adequate containment must always be considered. The stool suspension is then centrifuged at 3000 rpm for 1 hr, and the supernatant fluid is filtered first through a 1.2 μm and then a 0.45 μm micropore filter. This filtrate is placed in a vial in 1- to 2-ml amounts and stored at -70 C until used for IEM.

Twenty-seven-nm virus-like particles have been visualized in the cytoplasm of chimpanzee hepatocytes during the acute phase of illness. Liver biopsy specimens for thin-section EM are fixed in 1% gluteraldehyde by standard procedure or alternatively in phosphate-buffered, neutral 10% formalin.

Immunofluorescence (FA) microscopy. HA Ag has been detected in chimpanzee and marmoset hepatocyte cytoplasm by direct FA (87, 88). Small pieces of liver biopsy or necropsy material are placed on corks in an embedding medium of 10% gelatin in PBS or some commercial embedding medium and then snap frozen in liquid nitrogen or an alcohol dry-ice mixture for cryostat sectioning as described in the chapter on FA techniques. Fluorescein-labeled conjugates are best prepared from high-titer convalescent-phase human or chimpanzee serum. Indirect FA has not yet been adequately evaluated.

Laboratory diagnosis

Direct examination of clinical material

Since HAV cannot be grown in any *in vitro* system, direct examination of clinical specimens by a variety of methods is the only practical way of detecting the virus. Although chimpanzee and marmoset inoculations are quite sensitive for detecting HAV, it is an obviously impractical method except for answering certain research questions which require infectivity data.

Immune electron microscopy (IEM). By using IEM, specific particulate antigen can be distinguished from other morphologically similar particles in a suspension by the presence of antibody on the surface of the particle and by the formation of immune aggregates (43). Although this type of test is very laborious to perform, time consuming, somewhat subjective, and requires expensive equipment, it is also an extremely powerful tool because it adds specificity to the morphologic identification of virus-like particles, and it increases the sensitivity of EM for detecting these particles. IEM is useful for detecting antigen by using a known antibody and for detecting antibody (see section on serologic diagnosis) by using a known antigen suspension and reacting it with a serum of unknown antibody content. See appendix for method.

Radioimmunoassay (RIA). RIA is a sensitive technique that is relatively easy to perform (57, 119). It does however require a gamma radiation counter and the ability to purify and radiolabel IgG. An RIA test for anti-HA may soon be commercially available in a kit form. RIA is most useful for detecting HA Ag during purification steps. However, it can also be useful for detecting antigen in crude stool preparations, but only if nonspecific false positives are carefully excluded.

The test as performed in this laboratory is a modification of the microtiter SPRIA (micro-SPRIA) developed for the detection of HBsAg and HBcAg. See appendix for method.

Enzyme linked immunosorbent assay (ELISA). An ELISA test based precisely on the same principles as the micro-SPRIA test has recently been developed (89). In an ELISA test, the antibody is conjugated to an enzyme, in this case horseradish peroxidase, instead of a radioisotope. The conjugated antibody can be followed by adding substrate and measuring the reaction product most commonly by colorimetric means. The advantages over RIA are that there is no radiation hazard, visual determination of the results is usually adequate unless quantitative data or high sensitivity is required, and the conjugates are usually stable for long periods of time. ELISA tests have been shown in several systems to have sensitivity equivalent to RIA.

The ELISA test has proved useful not only for detecting HA Ag in purified specimens but also in crude stool suspensions. However, stools from humans frequently contain substances, presumably antigens, that give a positive reaction when tested against many sera. Therefore it is necessary to show that any positive reaction is specific for HA Ag. In the ELISA test this is done by blocking with buffer (unblocked), a preinfection serum which will block only the nonspecific reaction, and an HAV convalescent-phase serum from the same individual, which blocks both the nonspecific reaction and the specific HAV reaction. Thus, if a stool were positive when unblocked but negative when blocked by pre-serum (and convalescent-phase serum), all the positive reaction would be considered nonspecific for HA Ag. If a stool were positive when unblocked, not blocked, or only partially blocked by pre-serum and completely blocked by the convalescent-phase serum, the reaction would be considered specific for HA Ag. See appendix for method.

Virus isolation

HAV has never been shown to replicate in any *in vitro* system.

Serologic diagnosis

Infection by HAV is most frequently proved serologically. There are presently several techniques available for this purpose, all of which have been used primarily for experimental and epidemiologic purposes due to the lack of easily accessible antigen. Although there are differences in sensitivity among the techniques for detecting anti-HA, these differences are generally not important because the antibody response in both humans and experimentally infected animals is generally sufficient to be detected by all the techniques discussed below. However, there are some qualitative differences between these methods in their ability to detect early (presumably IgM) antibody. The IAHA, which is very sensitive and well adapted to most laboratories, often does not detect antibody until 4- to 6-weeks after illness. RIA and ELISA blocking tests, as well as IEM, can all detect antibody very early in the infection, usually by the time the clinical disease is fully expressed.

It would be desirable to be able to diagnose HAV infection with a single serum sample from an acutely ill patient. A test to measure anti-HA of the IgM class (which should be present only in an acutely or recently ill patient) would permit this. Such tests have been described (22, 77), but at present there is no practical, laboratory test specific for IgM. Mosely has proposed using a test which measures both IgG and IgM anti-HA, such as RIA plus the IAHA test which measures only late-developing antibody. This approach is generally useful, but some patients do have anti-HA detectable by IAHA at the time of their acute illness. Even when acute- and convalescent-phase sera are available, making a serologic diagnosis can be difficult since an increase in titer may not be detected due to the large, early IgM response which decreases as the IgG anti-HA is increasing. This shift from IgM to IgG may give the appearance of a stable titer between acute- and convalescent-phase sera.

The techniques of practical importance for detection of anti-HA are IEM, IAHA, CF, RIA blocking, and ELISA blocking. FA blocking can also be used to detect anti-HA, but this test requires a plentiful supply of infected primate liver. In addition, it is possible to do a Nt test in marmosets, but such a test presently has little practical value.

Immune electron microscopy (IEM). The technique of IEM is discussed above and in the appendix. For detection of antibody it is necessary to have an antigen preparation—either a stool filtrate or an antigen partially purified from stool or marmoset liver—which has sufficient particles in it so the microscopist will have confidence that any negative samples are so only because no antibody is present to identify HAV particles. If there are so few particles in the antigen preparation that they are difficult to find even with a high-titer antibody, false negatives can occur due just to sampling error. If there are approximately 50 HAV particles observable per 400-mesh EM grid square, the test becomes highly reliable. IEM can be used qualitatively to determine simply the presence or absence of antibody, or it can be used semi-quantitatively to determine the amount of antibody. For this purpose an antibody rating system of 0 to 4+ has been used. Although this type of rating system does not give an actual titer, it is useful for comparing acute-phase and convalescent-phase serum. A rating of 4+ has been found to correlate roughly with an IAHA titer >1:5000. If an actual endpoint titer is required, dilution of the serum can be made, but such an IEM experiment is laborious, time consuming, and wasteful of antigen. See appendix for method.

Immune adherence hemagglutination (IAHA). IAHA is sensitive, quantitative, and easy to perform using routine laboratory equipment. The disadvantages are that it requires partially purified antigen and that it is quite insensitive for detecting early (presumably IgM) antibody.

Preparation of antigen. IAHA antigen has been prepared from acutely infected marmoset liver (92) and human stool (93). As human stool is the most available source, the procedure for extraction and purification of HA Ag from human stool is described here. Fifty grams of stool containing HA Ag is placed in a 250-ml polycarbonate bottle to which is added 200 ml of 0.01 M Tris buffer, pH 8, and 20 g of glass beads, 4 mm in diameter. The bottle is shaken for 5 min, centrifuged at 2700 rpm for 45 min, and the supernatant fluid is carefully removed. The supernatant fluid is replaced with an equal volume of fresh buffer, and the procedure is repeated several times. The supernatant fluids of the several extractions are pooled and clarified by centrifugation in a Beckman 21 rotor at 10,000 rpm for 1 hr. HA Ag is pelleted from the clarified supernatant fluid by centrifuging in a 21 rotor at 20,000 rpm for 16 hr, and the resulting pellet is resuspended in 0.01 M Tris buffer at one-tenth of the starting volume. This suspension is clarified again by centrifuging in a 30 rotor at 15,000 rpm for 45 min. A portion of the supernatant fluid is layered on a preformed discontinuous CsCl density gradient (1.1–1.5 g/cm³) prepared in an SW40 rotor centrifuge tube, centrifuged at 35,000 rpm for 18 hr, fractionated, and the density of each fraction determined by a refractometer or by direct weighing of a measured volume. The HA Ag content of each fraction is determined by IEM, SPRIA, or IAHA, and the fractions (usually at approximately 1.34 g/cm³) with high HA Ag activity are pooled. The CsCl may be removed and the HA Ag concentrated by ultrafiltration (Amicon Diafilter with an XM300 membrane). This material is layered on top of a linear 10–30% sucrose gradient with a 60% sucrose cushion on the bottom in an SW27 rotor centrifuge tube and centrifuged at 25,000 rpm for 150 min. Fractions from this centrifuge run are tested for HA Ag by SPRIA or IAHA, and the fractions with sufficient activity are pooled and assayed in IAHA for use as antigen.

To improve the yield the nonionic detergent, NP-40, can be incorporated into both gradients at a concentration of 0.1%. See appendix for method.

Complement fixation (CF). A CF test for anti-HA has been described using antigen from acutely infected marmoset livers (109). It is advantageous in that it uses a routine laboratory procedure. However, it is less sensitive than IAHA and requires more antigen and it therefore is not often used.

Solid-phase radioimmunoassay blocking test (SPRIA-blocking). A SPRIA-blocking test is quite useful and sensitive for detecting anti-HA. It is best performed with a purified antigen prepared in the same manner as the antigen for IAHA or by other purification procedures (35, 119). The principle of the test is to block the binding of the radiolabeled antibody by incubating the serum to be tested for anti-HA in the wells of the microtiter plate before adding the radioactive anti-HA. If 40% or more of the control counts are blocked by the serum, it is considered positive for anti-HA. A commercial RIA for anti-HA may soon be available. See appendix for method.

Enzyme-linked immunosorbent assay blocking test (ELISA-blocking). An ELISA-blocking test for antibody is performed as described in the section on the ELISA test for antigen detection. A crude stool suspension containing HA Ag which has no nonspecific activity is suitable as antigen.

Other tests. It is possible to detect antibody by an IF blocking test, but this is not generally practical due to the difficulty in obtaining tissue containing a suitable amount of antigen.

A virus Nt test in marmosets is described (59, 108) but has little practical importance at this time. Since a tissue culture system has not been developed an *in vitro* Nt test is not possible.

Non-A, Non-B Hepatitis

As a result of the development of sensitive serologic tests to diagnose HAV and HBV infections, it became clear that certain patients with hepatitis had no evidence of infection by either of these agents (44, 45). When other viruses such as cytomegalovirus and Epstein-Barr viruses, which have the potential of causing a hepatitis syndrome, are excluded as the cause of illness in these non-A, non-B hepatitis cases, there remain many cases presumably caused by heretofore unrecognized hepatitis viruses.

Seroepidemiologic studies performed by excluding HAV and HBV have shown that non-A, non-B hepatitis resembles HBV infection in many ways. First, non-A, non-B hepatitis occurs frequently after transfusion. In fact, in transfusion centers which use only volunteer blood donors and screen all blood for HBsAg by third generation tests, 80–100% of the transfusion-associated hepatitis appears to be due to non-A, non-B agents. HAV has never been associated with post-transfusion hepatitis except under extremely rare circumstances. The implication of this non-B post-transfusion hepatitis is that it is probably transmitted by a relatively healthy chronic carrier of the infectious agent. Indeed, a high proportion of patients who develop non-B hepatitis develop some form of chronic hepatitis, including chronic active hepatitis and cirrhosis. Non-A, non-B hepatitis has also been found to account for a significant proportion of sporadic hepatitis cases where there is no known parenteral exposure or contact with persons known to have hepatitis. However, it does not appear that non-A, non-B hepatitis is easily transmitted by personal contact as judged by the infrequency of secondary cases.

Although there is presently intensive research underway on this important type of hepatitis, there is very little known about it to date. Recent studies have shown that chimpanzees may be infected with the agent(s) of non-A, non-B hepatitis (5, 138). In other studies, an antigen has been found in the blood of a limited number of patients with this disease. The appearance of this antigen is temporally related to the illness, but whether or not it is related to the infecting agent is not presently known (113). Since there are as yet no direct methods of detecting non-A, non-B hepatitis, its diagnosis is presently one of exclusion. If HAV and HBV infection have been ruled out by the methods described in this chapter, there is no evidence for infection by some other known hepatitis-inducing agent, and the epidemiologic circumstances are compatible, then a diagnosis of non-A, non-B hepatitis can be made.

Appendix of Methods

Agar gel diffusion (AGD) and rheophoresis
(Useful for HBsAg, anti-HBs, HBsAg subtyping, HBeAg, and anti-HBe)

Reagents for HBsAg, anti-HBs and HBsAg subtyping

Agarose (L'Industrie Biologique Francoise, Gennevilliers, France) 1% in 0.1 M Tris, 0.1 M NaCl, and 0.001 M EDTA, pH 9.6

Reagents for HBeAg and anti-HBe

1. Agarose 0.4% in 0.05 M tris, 0.15 M NaCl, 1% Dextran pH 7.6
2. Coomassie Brilliant Blue R-250 (Bio-Rad, Richmond, Cal) 0.5% in 25% methanol, 7% acetic acid, and 68% distilled water

AGD for HBsAg, anti-HBs and HBsAg subtyping. Glass microscope slides, 2.5-cm × 7.5-cm, are layered with with 1.3 ml of molten agarose on a level surface. The agarose is allowed to harden overnight in a humidified box. A 2-mm diameter central well is cut with a punch, and 6 peripheral 2-mm wells are cut 5 mm apart (center to center). The central well is filled with a known antiserum. Two opposite peripheral wells are filled with known positive antigen controls and the remaining 4 wells are filled with serum to be tested for antigen. The method for subtyping antigens is illustrated in Figure 29.7.

When testing for anti-HBs, the central well contains the known HBsAg, and the peripheral wells the serum to be tested for anti-HBs. This method is very insensitive compared to second and third generation tests described in this chapter.

AGD for HBeAg and anti-HBe. Agarose is prepared as described above; 1.3 ml of molten agarose solution is carefully pipetted onto a 2.5-cm × 7.5-cm microscope slide and allowed to harden overnight in the cold. Antigen wells of 3-mm diameter and antibody wells of 3-mm diameter are cut in the agarose, and excess agarose surrounding the wells is cut away and removed from the slide leaving a thin rim of gel at the periphery of the wells to minimize outward diffusion of reactants. All wells are filled with reactants at least 2–3 times during the first few hours. The gels are read after 48–72 hr and may be kept for up to 1 week for a periodic rereading.

Rheophoresis is a modification of AGD which is run either in Petri dishes or in special plates (Abbott Laboratories, North Chicago, IL) that have an outer moat around the agar and a central hole in the lid for evaporation. The moat is filled with Tris buffer, the central well is filled twice with the antibody, and the outer wells with reference antigen or serum to be tested for antigen. Migration of reagents toward the center well is accelerated by evaporation through the central hole.

The plates are incubated in a humid chamber at room temperature for at least 48 hr. Improved visualization of precipitin lines can be achieved by staining. Rheophoresis plates that have been incubated for 72 hr are washed extensively in saline with 0.02% sodium azide followed by washing in distilled water. The washed gel is transferred to a glass slide and air dried.

Dried gels are stained for 10 min at room temperature in Coomassie brilliant blue. The gel is destained in methanol-acetic acid-distilled water without Coomassie brilliant blue until the background has cleared. AGD plates made with low concentrations of agarose are very difficult to stain because they are fragile.

References: 19, 41, 65, 75, 105

Counterelectrophoresis (CEP)
(Useful for HBsAg, anti-HBs, HBcAg, and anti-HBc)

Reagents

1% Agarose (L'Industrie Biologique Francaise, Gennevilliers, France) in 0.01 M Tris, 0.1 M NaCl, and 0.001 M EDTA, pH 9.6 (Tris-Saline-EDTA) or 0.05 M barbital-buffer, pH 8.6

Glass lantern slides (8.5-cm × 10-cm) are coated with 10-16 ml of molten agarose. Double rows of parallel wells are cut in the agar with well diameters of 3-5 mm, 3 mm between adjacent wells, and 3-6 mm between the antigen and antibody containing rows of wells. Reagent antiserum or serum samples to be tested for antibody are added to wells on the anode (positive) side of the plate and serum samples to be tested for antigen or reagent antigens are added to wells on the cathode (negative) side of the plate. The wells are filled to the brim using capillary pipettes. The plates are connected to troughs containing 0.05 M barbital buffer, pH 8.6, in an electrophoresis cell by chromatographic paper wicks (Schleicher and Schuell, No. 470C). Electrophoresis is carried out at 30 mA constant current across each slide for 1 hr. The plates are examined with indirect, transmitted light against a dark background 2 hr and 24 hr after electrophoresis. Positive controls for antigen and antibody are included on each plate. Many successful variations on the technique have been described in the literature.

References: 4, 51, 102, 108

Immune adherence hemagglutination (IAHA)
(Useful for HA Ag, anti-HA, HBsAg, anti-HBs, HBcAg, and anti-HBc)

Reagents

1. Veronal-buffered saline, pH 7.5, with 0.1% bovine serum albumin (BVB)
2. Dithiothreitol (DTT), 3 mg/ml in 2 parts 0.1 M EDTA plus 3 parts BVB
3. Human type O RBC
4. Guinea pig complement

The concentration of complement to be employed is determined by checkerboard titration of complement and antigen and/or antibody (see chapter on complement fixation). The appropriate complement concentration is the highest dilution that gives 4+ hemagglutination with antigen-antibody complexes but no nonspecific hemagglutination.

IAHA is performed in a microtiter system using "v" bottom plates. Both the 25-μl and 10-μl microtiter systems have been used successfully, the latter to conserve antigen and serum. However, the 10-μl system requires considerable practice before the small volumes can be accurately dispensed into the bottom of the microtiter plate wells. The sensitivity of the 2 systems is equal. The 25-μl system is described below.

Serum should be heat-inactivated at 56 C for 30 min prior to testing. Since titers of serum cover a wide range and prozones are a frequent occurrence, serum is prescreened at 1:10, 1:100 and 1:1000 dilutions and then, if an endpoint is required, titered in serial 2-fold dilutions from the last positive screening dilution. Dilutions are made in BVB. All sera are tested with a buffer control, as well as with antigen to detect nonspecific hemagglutination. Twenty-five μl of the appropriate serum dilution are added to duplicate wells followed by 4–8 units of antigen (determined in a previous test) diluted to 25 μl in BVB. The plate is shaken a few seconds on a vibrator and then incubated in a humidified box overnight at 4 C. The next day 25 μl of an appropriate dilution of guinea pig complement is added, the plate is shaken and incubated at 37 C for 40 min. After incubation 25 μl of freshly prepared DTT is added to each well. Twenty-five μl of human type O RBC washed once in EDTA-BVB and made up to 1% by volume is added to each well while the plate is on the vibrator. The plate is then incubated at room temperature and may be read anytime after 1 hr. It is important to note that human O RBC differ greatly in their ability to agglutinate in this system. Therefore it is necessary to screen many donors to find one whose cells are sensitive indicators. The results are read on a 0 to 4+ scale of hemagglutination and only 3+ and 4+ are considered positive. All positives must be compared to the buffer control as some sera cause nonspecific hemagglutination.
References: 91, 92, 93, 140

Solid-phase radioimmunoassay (SPRIA)
(*Useful for HA Ag, anti-HA, HBsAg, anti-HBs, HBcAg, anti-HBc, HBeAg, and anti-HBe*)

Reagents

1. 0.15 M NaCl with 0.1% sodium azide (saline)
2. Saline with 1% bovine serum albumin (BSA)
3. High-titer convalescent-phase or hyperimmune anti-serum
4. ^{125}I labeled IgG purified from 3

IgG is purified from as little as 0.5 ml of serum by precipitation of globulins with an equal volume of saturated ammonium sulfate and dialysis against 0.005 M phosphate buffer, pH 8, with 0.1% sodium azide, followed by chromatography on a diethyl amino ethyl-cellulose column equilibrated with the same buffer. The first (void volume) protein peak consists of IgG and is concentrated by membrane filtration to approximately 2 mg/ml and stored at 4 C or −70 C. IgG is labeled by the chloramine T method. Add, in order, to a small conical vessel, the following: 20 µl 0.25 M phosphate buffer, pH 7.4 (PB); 200 µCi of carrier-free ^{125}I (in 1–2 µl as sodium iodide); 10 µg of the IgG (in approximately 5 µl); 15 µl of freshly prepared chloramine T (3.5 µg/µl) in PB; 20 µl of freshly prepared sodium metabisulfite (4.8 µg/µl) in PB; and 20 µl of a solution of sucrose (22.5%) and potassium iodide (2 mg/ml) in PB. After addition of the chloramine T, the reaction is allowed to proceed for 15 sec before addition of the sodium metabisulfite. The mixture is chromatographed through a small Sephadex G-25 column equilibrated with PBS, pH 7.4, with 0.1% sodium azide. The first (void volume) peak of radioactivity is diluted with an equal volume of fetal calf serum pretested to be free to antibodies to the test antigen and stored at 4 C for up to 2 weeks.

The SPRIA can be adapted to a variety of antigen-antibody systems. Several commercial kits are available or soon will be available for detecting various hepatitis antigens and antibodies. The assay described here is a modification that utilizes the microtiter system (Micro-SPRIA).

Wells of polyvinyl microtiter plates (Cooke Engineering Inc., Alexandria, Virginia) are coated with 75 µl of a dilution in saline of a convalescent-phase or hyperimmune serum to the test antigen, the appropriate dilution (usually between 10^{-2} and 10^{-4}) having been determined in a previous titration of this precoat serum. After 4 hr of incubation at 4 C, the wells are washed twice and secondarily coated overnight with 250 µl of 1% BSA in saline, washed twice, and inoculated with 25 µl of the sample to be tested for antigen. A series of wells is inoculated with saline to serve as a negative control. The plates are incubated for 1–2 days at 4 C, washed 5 times with saline and inoculated in duplicate with 50 µl of ^{125}I-labeled IgG. The plates are then incubated at 37 C for 4–6 hr on a rocker platform. The radioactive IgG is aspirated, the wells are washed 5 times, the plates are cut apart, and the individual wells are transferred to gamma counting tubes to measure the bound radioactivity in a gamma spectrometer. The residual radioactivity (cpm) in wells that received test samples is divided by the mean residual cpm in wells that received negative control samples to calculate the positive/negative (P/N) value. P/N values of ≥2.1 are considered positive for the presence of antigen. All tests should be performed in duplicate and the results averaged. Nonspecificity can be detected by blocking tests as described under the section on ELISA.

For measuring antibody, standard antigen is used in the test and incubated and washed as in the test for antigen; 50 µl of decimal dilutions in PBS of serum to be tested for antibody is mixed with 50 µl of ^{125}I-IgG, added to duplicate wells, and incubated overnight at 4 C. The wells are washed 5 times and counted as described above for detecting antigen. Forty percent or greater reduction in residual radioactivity by a serum when compared to an antibody-negative serum is considered as evidence for the presence of antibody.

References: 57, 58, 62, 118, 119

Enzyme-linked immunosorbent assay (ELISA)

(Useful for HA Ag, anti-HA, HBsAg, anti-HBs, HBcAg, anti-HBc, HBeAg, and anti-HBe)

Reagents

1. Phosphate-buffered saline plus 0.5% Tween −20 (PBS-T)
2. Citrate buffer, pH 5, (0.1 M citric acid, 98.6 parts plus 0.2 M Na_2HPO_4, 101.4 parts)
3. Orthophenylenediamine, hydrogen peroxide substrate (OPD/H_2O_2), 0.4 mg/ml with 0.006% H_2O_2 in citrate buffer
4. 2 M Sulfuric acid
5. Peroxidase conjugated anti-HA IgG

The method developed for HA Ag and anti-HA is detailed below. Modifications of this method can be used for the other hepatitis antigens and antibodies.

Wells of polyvinyl microtiter plates (Cooke Engineering, Inc., Alexandria, VA) are precoated with 75 μl of anti-HA serum diluted in PBS at a predetermined level to give the maximum binding of antigen. After 4 hr of incubation in a humidified box at 4 C the wells are washed for 5 min 3 times with PBS-T. Each well is then completely filled with PBS containing 1% BSA and the plates are left overnight at 4 C in a humidified box. After 1 additional washing, 25 μl of the samples to be tested for HA Ag are added and the plates are incubated for 20–24 hr at 4 C. After another washing, 25 μl of either PBS-T, pre- or convalescent-phase serum used for specificity testing is added, and the plates are left for 15 min at room temperature. Without emptying the wells, 25 μl of the anti-HA peroxidase conjugate diluted in 50% bovine serum in PBS is added, and the plates incubated at room temperature for 2 hr. After washing (3 times for 5 min with PBS-T), 100 μl of freshly prepared OPD/H_2O_2 is added, and the plates incubated in the dark at room temperature. After 30 min, 50 μl of 2 M sulfuric acid is added to each well to stop the reaction and the optical density (OD) at 493 nm is measured. For specificity testing (see above) 6 wells (duplicate wells blocked by PBS-T, preinfection- and convalescent-phase serum) are prepared.

Because the OD in control wells (diluent without test sample) is often elevated by adding the preinfection- or convalescent-phase blocking serum compared to adding only PBS-T, the following ratio may be used to calculate the results:

$$\text{ratio} = \frac{^{OD}\text{test well} - ^{OD}\text{control well}}{^{OD}\text{blank well}}$$

where the "control well" is the well with diluent instead of the test sample but blocked in the same way as the "test well", and the "blank well" has diluent instead of the test sample but is blocked only with PBS-T. A value of a ratio >1.1 is considered positive, but the sample can only be considered to contain the specific antigen if the reaction is completely blocked by the convalescent-phase serum but incompletely blocked by the preinfection serum. Antibody can be measured in this system by using an antigen preparation known not to contain any nonspecificity. The serum to be tested for antibody is used in place of the convalescent-phase blocking serum. If the ratio with the test serum in reduced by more than 50% compared to the negative control serum, the test serum is considered positive for antibody.

The peroxidase conjugate is best prepared by the method of Nakane et al. (96). The IgG fraction of a convalescent-phase serum or hyperimmune animal serum is first isolated by ammonium sulfate precipitation and diethylaminoethyl cellulose column chromatography (see appendix on RIA). Five mg of horseradish peroxidase (HRPO) (Sigma HRPO type VI) is dissolved in 1 ml of 0.3 M sodium bicarbonate; 25 μl of 0.32% p-formaldehyde is added and stirred for 30 min at room temperature. One ml of 0.04 M NaIO$_4$ is added and stirred for another 30 min. Then 1 ml of 0.16 M ethylene glycol is added and stirred for 1 hr. This solution is then dialyzed against 1 liter of 0.01 M sodium bicarbonate buffer, pH 9.5, overnight at 4 C. The next day, 10 mg of IgG in 1 ml of 0.01 M bicarbonate buffer is added to the solution, and the mixture is stirred for 2 hr at room temperature. After cooling the solution to 4 C in an icebath, 5 mg NaBH$_4$ is added, and the solution is left at 4 C for 2 hr. This IgG peroxidase solution is then dialyzed against PBS, pH 7.4, and chromatographed through a Sephadex G-100 column, 85 cm $\times$ 1.5 cm, to separate the conjugate from free HRPO. The OD^{280} and OD^{430} are measured on the fractions recovered from the column. The RZ value

$$\frac{OD^{403}}{OD^{280}}$$

is calculated on the fractions from the first OD^{280} peak, and those fractions which have an RZ of approximately 0.6 (HRPO: IgG molar ratio approximately equal to 2) are pooled.
References: 40, 89, 96, 145

Immunofluorescence (FA)
(Useful for HBsAg, HBcAg, and HA Ag)

Materials and reagents

1. Fluorescein-isothyocyanate (FITC) conjugated specific antibodies
2. Phosphate-buffered saline, pH 7.4 (PBS)
3. Cryostat
4. Fluorescence microscope

Four-μm thick cryostat sections of frozen liver tissue are dried for 5 min at 37 C and fixed for 3 min (HBcAg) or 30 sec (HBsAg) in acetone at room temperature or left unfixed (HA Ag); 20 μl of an appropriate dilution of FITC-labeled antibody is added to the slide which is incubated in a humidified chamber at room temperature for 40 min. The slide is rinsed in PBS for 15 sec and washed for 5 min each in 3 rinses of PBS. After washing, excess PBS is drained from the slide and a coverslip applied over a mounting medium consisting of 90% glycerin-10% Tris buffer, pH 9.5. Normal liver tissue from a human, chimpanzee, or marmoset serves as a negative control. The tissue sections are evaluated with a fluorescence microscope and either transmitted light (HBcAg, HBsAg) or incident light (all 3 antigens) optics. Unlike HA Ag, HBcAg and HBsAg are readily detected with most lighting systems appropriate for FA. HA Ag, however, requires incident illumination. The following combination has proven useful: a 200 W mercury bulb, KP490 (interference) and 2-mm LP455 (glass) exciter filters and 2-mm LP530 and LP510 (glass) barrier filters.

Sections positive for HBcAg demonstrate granular intranuclear fluorescence in scattered hepatocytes. Sometimes the majority of hepatocytes have fluorescent nuclei; often only a few cells are positive. Sections positive for HBsAg demonstrate diffuse cytoplasmic fluorescence either uniformly distributed or marginated along the cell membrane. The former pattern is usually limited to scattered hepatocytes and Kupffer cells; the latter may be seen in every hepatocyte. There is no strict correspondence between HBcAg- and HBsAg-positive cells: many hepatocytes contain HBsAg but not HBcAg. Hepatocytes and Kupffer cells positive for HA Ag contain a very fine, granular cytoplasmic fluorescence that coalesces somewhat late in the infection. From very few to every cell may be positive, at least in non-human primates, in which this has been studied in detail.

Specificity of the FA can be confirmed by mixing the conjugated anti-serum with unconjugated preinfection-phase or convalescent-phase serum before incubation with the liver section and determining if only the con-valescent-phase serum blocks the fluorescence.

References: 39, 88, 99

Immune electron microscopy (IEM)
(Useful for HA Ag, anti-HA, HBsAg, anti-HBs, HBcAg, and anti-HBc)

Reagents

1. PBS
2. Phosphotungstic acid, 3%, pH 7, (neutralized with NaOH) (PTA)

IEM has been most useful for detecting HA Ag in stools. Briefly, 0.9 ml of a 2% stool filtrate to be tested for HA Ag is incubated for 1 hr with 0.1 ml of an appropriate dilution of serum known to contain anti-HA. The serum should be diluted at least 1:5 but, when looking for HAV particles, enough antibody should be used to produce a relative antibody excess. This will insure small aggregates of particles or single particles which will be ran-domly distributed rather than a few large aggregates of particles which may be missed by EM observation due to sampling error. After incubation, the suspension is centrifuged at $23,000 \times g$ for 90 min, the supernatant fluid drawn off, and all excess fluid removed from the inverted tube with a piece of filter paper. The pellet is resuspended in 1 drop (or more if the pellet is large) of distilled water and mixed with an equal volume of PTA. A drop of this mixture is placed on a Formvar-carbon-coated EM grid, allowed to sit for 30 sec to 1 min, and the excess fluid is drawn off by touching the edge of the grid with a piece of filter paper. If all conditions are held constant, IEM can be roughly quantitative. All particles in a set number of grid squares can be counted and different samples can thereby be compared for the amount of virus present. Such particle counts have been shown to have at least a rough correlation with other immunologic methods of detecting HAV.

For measuring antibody, a stool filtrate or other antigen preparation which contains at least 50 HAV particles per grid square should be used. The test serum should be used at a dilution of 1:10. If antibody coated particles are seen, the serum is considered positive for anti-HA. For more detail on this method see Chapter 30.

IEM may be used in a similar fashion for HBsAg, anti-HBs, HBcAg and anti-HBc.

References: 1, 17, 43

DNA polymerase test

Reagents

1. NP-40 and mercaptoethanol (NP 40-ME) mixture: 0.47 ml distilled H_2O, 1 ml 10% NP-40 in H_2O, 0.03 ml 2-mercaptoethanol. Prepare fresh and under a chemical hood.

2. Reaction mixture (quantity necessary for 1 sample) 65 μl distilled water, 20 μl Tris-MgCl$_2$ (16.5 ml 1 M Tris, pH 7.5, 3.5 ml 1 M MgCl$_2$), 6 μl 2.0 M NH$_4$Cl, 2.5 μl *each* of the following: 0.02 μ (in distilled H_2O) solutions of deoxyadenosine-5'-triphosphate, deoxyctidine-5'-triphosphate and deoxyguanosine-5'-triphosphate, and 5^{3}H-thymidine-5'triphosphate (approximately 50 Ci/m mol).

Label two small Whatman No. 3 filter disks per sample to be tested: one for 0 reaction time and one for 3 hr reaction time. Pipette 25 μl of sample to be tested into a 10-mm × 75-mm plastic tube or well of a microtiter plate. Add 5 μl of NP 40-ME mixture and shake tube gently. Add 100 μl of reaction mixture and shake tube gently. For 0 reaction times, spot 50 μl of the mixture on the 0-time filter disk and incubate the remaining 80 μl at 37 C for 3 hr. Pipette 50 μl of incubated mixture onto the 3-hr reaction time filter disk. As soon as the mixture is absorbed into the filter disk, the disk is dropped into a beaker containing 5% trichloroacetic acid and 0.1 M sodium pyrophosphate, tetra, in distilled water. Wash for 1 hr by agitating disk at room temperature. Briefly drain filter disks on a paper towel and transfer to a second 5% TCA-0.1 M sodium pryophosphate wash for 1 hr. Drain and transfer to 25% TCA wash for 30 min. Drain and transfer to 95% ethyl alcohol for 15 min. Drain, transfer filter disks to an aluminum foil tray and dry in an oven at 100 C for 5 min. Place into scintillation vials, add counting fluid (Econofluor, New England Nuclear, Boston, MA) and count in a beta scintillation spectrometer. Handle filter disks with forceps and dispose of all wash solutions as appropriate for radioactive waste.

Every polymerase test should include 2 HBV-specific DNA polymerase positive control sera, 2 polymerase negative control sera, and 1 reagent blank in which PBS, pH 7.4, is substituted for a serum sample.

Subtract time-0 cpm from the cpm obtained after 3-hr incubation. Calculate ratio of mean cpm obtained with test serum to mean cpm obtained with normal serum (P/N). A P/N >2 is considered positive for DNA polymerase activity.

Bacterial contamination can cause false-positive reactions in the polymerase test. This false positivity can sometimes be removed by filtration or low-speed centrifugation of the serum. Specificity of the reaction should be confirmed by preincubating separate aliquots of the serum sample with normal serum and anti-HBs respectively, adding anti-IgG to augment the precipitation, centrifuging at low speed, and performing the polymerase test on the supernatant fluids. Polymerase specific for HBV is precipitated by anti-HBs but not normal serum.

References: 54, 67, 68

References

1. ALMEIDA JD, RUBENSTEIN D, and STOTT EJ: New antigen-antibody system in Australia antigen positive hepatitis. Lancet 2:1224–1227, 1971
2. ALMEIDA JD and WATERSON AP: Immune complexes in hepatitis. Lancet 2:304–306, 1969
3. ALTER HJ and BLUMBERG BS: Further studies on a new human isoprecipitin system (Australia antigen). Blood 27:297–309, 1966
4. ALTER HJ, HOLLAND PV, and PURCELL RH: Counterelectrophoresis for detection of hepatitis-associated antigen: methodology and comparison with gel diffusion and complement fixation. J Lab Clin Med 77:1000–1010, 1971
5. ALTER HJ, HOLLAND PV, PURCELL RH, and POPPER H: Transmissible agent in non-A, non-B hepatitis. Lancet 1:459–463, 1978
6. ALTER HJ, PURCELL, RH, GERIN JL, LONDON WT, KAPLAN PM, MCAULIFFE VJ, WAGNER J, and HOLLAND PV: Transmission of hepatitis B to chimpanzees by hepatitis B surface antigen-positive saliva and semen. Infect Immun 16:928–933, 1977
7. ALTER HJ, SEEFF LB, KAPLAN PM, MCAULIFFE VJ, WRIGHT EC, GERIN JL, PURCELL RH, HOLLAND PV, and ZIMMERMAN HJ: Type B hepatitis: the infectivity of blood positive for e antigen and DNA polymerase after accidental needlestick exposure. N Engl J Med 295:909–913, 1976
8. ARNOLD W, HESS G, PURCELL RH, KAPLAN PM, GERIN JL, and MEYER ZUM BÜSCHENFELDE KH: Anti-HBc, HBeAg and DNA polymerase activity in healthy HBsAg carriers and patients with inflammatory liver diseases. Klin Wochenschr 56:297–303, 1978
9. BANCROFT WH, MUNDON FK, and RUSSELL PK: Detection of additional antigenic determinants of hepatitis B antigen. J Immunol 109:842–848, 1972
10. BANCROFT WH, SNITBHAN R, SCOTT RM, TINGPALAPONG M, WATSON WT, TANTICHAROENYOS P, KARWACKI JJ, and SRIMARUT S: Transmission of hepatitis B virus to gibbons by exposure to human saliva containing hepatitis B surface antigen. J Infect Dis 135:79–85, 1977
11. BARKER LF, ALMEIDA JD, HOOFNAGLE JH, GERETY RJ, JACKSON DR, and MCGRATH PP: Hepatitis B core antigen: Immunology and electron microscopy. J Virol 14:1552–1558, 1974
12. BARKER LF, CHISARI FV, MCGRATH PP, DALGARD DW, KIRCHSTEIN RL, ALMEIDA JD, EDGINGTON TS, SHARP DG, and PETERSON MR: Transmission of type B viral hepatitis to chimpanzees. J Infect Dis 127:648–662, 1973
13. BARKER LF, MAYNARD JE, PURCELL RH, HOOFNAGLE JH, BERQUIST KR, LONDON WT, GERETY RJ, and KRUSHAK DH: Hepatitis B virus infection in chimpanzees: titration of subtypes. J Infect Dis 132:451–458, 1975

14. BARKER LF, MAYNARD JE, PURCELL RH, HOOFNAGLE JH, BERQUIST KR, and LONDON WT: Viral hepatitis, type B, in experimental animals. Am J Med Sci 270:189-195, 1975

15. BARKER LF and MURRAY R: Relationship of virus dose to incubation time of clinical hepatitis and time of appearance of hepatitis-associated antigen. Am J Med Sci 263:27-33, 1971

16. BEASLEY RP, TREPO C, STEVENS CE, and SZMUNESS W: The e antigen and vertical transmission of hepatitis B surface antigen. Am J Epidemiol 105:94-98, 1977

17. BAYER ME, BLUMBERG BS, and WERNER B: Particles associated with Australia antigen in the sera of patients with leukemia, Down's syndrome and hepatitis. Nature 218:1057-1059, 1968

18. BLUMBERG BS: Polymorphisms of the serum proteins and the development of isoprecipitins in transfused patients. Bull NY Acad Med 40:377-386, 1964

19. BLUMBERG BS, ALTER HJ, and VISNICH S: A "new" antigen in leukemia sera. J Am Med Assoc 191:541-546, 1965

20. BLUMBERG BS, SUTNICK AI, and LONDON WT: Hepatitis and leukemia. Their relation to Australia antigen. Bull NY Acad Med 44:1566-1586, 1968

21. BOGGS JD, MELNICK JL, CONRAD ME, and FELSHER BF: Viral hepatitis. Clinical and tissue culture studies. J Am Med Assoc 214:1041-1046, 1970

22. BRADLEY DW, HORNBECK CL, GRAVELLE CR, COOK EH, and MAYNARD JE: CsCl banding of hepatitis A-associated virus-like particles. J Infect Dis 131:304-306, 1975

23. BRADLEY DW, MAYNARD JE, HINDMAN SH, HORNBECK CL, FIELDS HA, McCAUSTLAND KA, and COOK EH JR: Serodiagnosis of viral hepatitis A: detection of acute-phase immunoglobulin M anti-hepatitis A virus by radioimmunoassay. J Clin Microbiol 5:521-530, 1977

24. BURRELL CJ, PROUDFOOT E, KEEN GA, and MARMION BP: Carbohydrates in hepatitis B antigen. Nature (London) New Biol 243:260-262, 1973

25. CHAIREZ R, STEINER S, MELNICK JL, and DREESMAN GR: Glycoproteins associated with hepatitis B antigen. Intervirology 1:224-228, 1973

26. COULEPIS AG, LOCARNINI SA, FERRIS AA, LEHMANN NI, and GUST ID: The polypeptides of hepatitis A virus. Intervirology 10:24-31, 1978

27. DANE DS, CAMERON CH, and BRIGGS M: Virus-like particles in serum of patients with Australia-antigen-associated hepatitis. Lancet 1:695-698, 1970

28. DIENSTAG JL, ALAAMA A, MOSLEY JW, REDEKER AG, and PURCELL RH: Etiology of sporadic hepatitis B surface antigen-negative hepatitis. Ann Int Med 87:1-6, 1977

29. DIENSTAG JL, DAVENPORT FM, McCOLLUM RW, HENNESSY AV, KLATSKIN G, and PURCELL RH: Nonhuman primate-associated viral hepatitis type A. Serologic evidence of hepatitis A virus infection. J Am Med Assoc 236:462-464, 1976

30. DIENSTAG JL, FEINSTONE SM, KAPIKIAN AZ, PURCELL RH, BOGGS JD, and CONRAD ME: Faecal shedding of hepatitis A antigen. Lancet 1:765-767, 1975

31. DIENSTAG JL, FEINSTONE SM, PURCELL RH, HOOFNAGLE JH, BARKER LF, LONDON WT, POPPER H, PETERSON JM, and KAPIKIAN AZ: Experimental infection of chimpanzees with hepatitis A virus. J Infect Dis 132:532-545, 1975

32. DIENSTAG JL, KRUGMAN S, WONG DC, and PURCELL RH: Comparison of serological tests for antibody to hepatitis A antigen, using coded specimens from individuals infected with the MS-1 strain of hepatitis A virus. Infect Immun 14:1000-1003, 1976

33. DIENSTAG JL, LUCAS CR, GUST ID, WONG DC, and PURCELL RH: Mussel-associated viral hepatitis type A: serological confirmation. Lancet 1:561-564, 1976

34. DIENSTAG JL, POPPER H, PURCELL RH: The pathology of viral hepatitis types A and B in chimpanzees: a comparison. Am J Pathol 85:131-148, 1976

35. DIENSTAG JL, PURCELL RH: Viral hepatitis, type A: etiology and epidemiology. Rush-Presbyter-St. Luke's Med Bull 15:104-114, 1976

36. DIENSTAG JL, SCHULMAN AN, GERETY RJ, HOOFNAGLE JH, LORENZ DE, PURCELL RH, and BARKER LF: Hepatitis A antigen isolated from liver and stool: immunologic comparison of antisera prepared in guinea pigs. J Immunol 11:876-881, 1976

37. DIENSTAG JL, SZMUNESS W, STEVENS CE, and PURCELL RH: Hepatitis A virus infection: new insights from seroepidemiologic studies. J Infect Dis 137:328-340, 1978

38. EDGINGTON TS and CHISARI FV: Immunological aspects of hepatitis B virus infection. Am J Med Sci 270:213-227, 1975

39. EDGINGTON TS and RITT DJ: Intrahepatic expression of serum hepatitis virus-associated antigens. J Exp Med 134:871-885, 1971

40. ENGVALL E and PERLMANN P: Enzyme-linked immunosorbent assay, ELISA, III. Quantitation of specific antibodies by enzyme-labeled anti-immunoglobulin in antigen-coated tubes. J Immunol 109:129-135, 1972

41. FEINMAN SV, BERRIS B, SINCLAIR JC, WROBEL DM, MURPHY BL, and MAYNARD JE: *e* antigen and anti-*e* in HBsAg carriers. Lancet 2:1173-1174, 1975

42. FEINSTONE SM, KAPIKIAN AZ, GERIN JL, and PURCELL RH: Buoyant density of the hepatitis A virus-like particle in cesium chloride. J Virol 13:1412-1414, 1974

43. FEINSTONE SM, KAPIKIAN AZ, and PURCELL RH: Hepatitis A: detection by immune electron microscopy of a virus-like antigen associated with acute illness. Science 182:1026-1028, 1973

44. FEINSTONE SM, KAPIKIAN AZ, PURCELL RH, ALTER HJ, and HOLLAND PV: Transfusion-associated hepatitis not due to viral hepatitis type A or B. N Engl J Med 292:767-770, 1975

45. FEINSTONE SM and PURCELL RH: Non-A, non-B hepatitis. Annu Rev Med 29:359-366, 1978

46. GELLIS SS, NEEFE JR, STOKES J JR, STRONG LE, JANEWAY CA, and SCATCHARD G: Chemical, clinical and immunological studies on products of human plasma fractionation. Inactivation of virus of homologous serum albumin by means of heat. J Clin Invest 27:239-244, 1948

47. GERETY RJ, HOOFNAGLE JH, and BARKER LF: Humoral and cell-mediated immune responses to two hepatitis B virus antigens in guinea pigs. J Immunol 113:1223-1229, 1974

48. GERIN JL, FORD EC, and PURCELL RH: Biochemical characterization of Australia antigen. Evidence for defective particles of hepatitis B virus. Am J Pathol 81:651-667, 1975

49. GERIN JL, HOLLAND PV, and PURCELL RH: Australia antigen: large-scale purification from human serum and biochemical studies of its proteins. J Virol 7:569-576, 1971

50. GOCKE DJ: Extrahepatic manifestations of viral hepatitis. Am J Med Sci 270:49-52, 1975

51. GOCKE DJ and HOWE C: Rapid detection of Australia antigen by counterelectrophoresis. J Immunol 104:1031-1034, 1970

52. GOCKE DJ and KAVEY NB: Hepatitis antigen: correlation with disease and infectivity of blood donors. Lancet 1:1055-1059, 1969

53. GOLD JW, ALTER HJ, HOLLAND PV, GERIN JL, and PURCELL RH: Passive hemagglutination assay for antibody to subtypes of hepatitis B antigen. J Immunol 112:1100-1106, 1974

54. GREENMAN RL and ROBINSON WS: DNA polymerase in the core of the human hepatitis B virus candidate. J Virol 13:1231-1236, 1974

55. GREENMAN RL, ROBINSON WS, and VYAS GN: A sensitive test for antibody against the hepatitis B core antigen (anti-HBc). Vox Sang 29:77-80, 1975

56. HILLEMAN MR, BUYNAK EB, ROEHM RR, TYTELL AA, BERTLAND AU, and LAMPSON GP: Purified and inactivated human hepatitis B vaccine: progress report. Am J Med Sci 270:401-404, 1975

57. HOLLINGER FB, BRADLEY DW, MAYNARD JE, DREESMAN GR, and MELNICK JL: Detection of hepatitis A viral antigen by radioimmunoassay. J Immunol 115:1464-1466, 1975

58. HOLLINGER FB, VORNDAM V, and DREESMAN GR: Assay of Australia antigen and antibody employing double-antibody and solid-phase radioimmunoassay techniques and comparison with the passive hemagglutination methods. J Immunol 107:1099-1111, 1971

59. HOLMES AW, DEINHARDT F, WOLFE L, FROESNER G, PETERSON D, CASTO B, and CONRAD M: Specific neutralization of human hepatitis type A in marmoset monkeys. Nature (Lond) 243:419-420, 1973

60. HOLMES AW, WOLFE L, ROSENBLATE H, and DEINHARDT F: Hepatitis in marmosets: inducation of disease with coded specimens from a human volunteer study. Science 165:816–817, 1969

61. HOOFNAGLE JH, GERETY RJ, and BARKER LF: Antibody to hepatitis B virus core in man. Lancet 2:869–873, 1973

62. HOOFNAGLE JH, GERETY RJ, SMALLWOOD LA, and BARKER LF: Subtyping hepatitis B antigen and antibody by radioimmunoassay. Gastroenterology 72:290–296, 1977

63. HOOPER RR, JUELS CW, ROUTENBERG JA, HARRISON WO, KILPATRICK ME, KENDRA SJ, and DIENSTAG JL: An outbreak of type A viral hepatitis at the Naval Training Center, San Diego: epidemiologic evaluation. Am J Epidemiol 105:148–155, 1977

64. HUANG S: Hepatitis-associated antigen hepatitis. An electron microscopic study of virus-like particles in liver cells. Am J Pathol 64:483–492, 1971

65. JAMBAZIAN A and HOLPER JC: Rheophoresis: a sensitive immunodiffusion method for detection of hepatitis associated antigen. Proc Soc Exp Biol Med 140:560–564, 1972

66. KAPLAN PM, FORD EC, PURCELL RH, and GERIN JL: Demonstration of subpopulations of Dane particles. J Virol 17:885–893, 1976

67. KAPLAN PM, GERIN JL, and ALTER HJ: Hepatitis B-specific DNA polymerase activity during post-transfusion hepatitis. Nature 249:762–764, 1974

68. KAPLAN PM, GREENMAN RL, GERIN JL, PURCELL RH, and ROBINSON WS: DNA polymerase associated with human hepatitis B antigen. J Virol 12:995–1005, 1973

69. KIM CY, BISSELL DM: Stability of the lipid and protein of hepatitis-associated (Australia) antigen. J Infect Dis 123:470–476, 1971

70. KRUGMAN S, GILES JP, and HAMMOND J: Infectious hepatitis. Evidence for two distinctive clinical, epidemiological and immunological types of infection. J Am Med Assoc 200:365–373, 1967

71. KRUGMAN S, WARD R, and GILES JP: The natural history of infectious hepatitis. Am J Med 32:717–728, 1962

72. LANDER JJ, ALTER HJ, and PURCELL RH: Frequency of antibody to hepatitis-associated antigen as measured by a new radioimmunoassay technique. J Immunol 106:1166–1171, 1971

73. LEACH JM and RUCK BJ: Detection of hepatitis associated antigen by the latex agglutination test. Br Med J 4:597–598, 1971

74. LEBOUVIER GL: The heterogeneity of Australia antigen. J Infect Dis 123:671–675, 1971

75. LEBOUVIER G and WILLIAMS A: Serotypes of hepatitis B antigen (HBsAg): The problem of "new" determinants, as exemplified by "t". Am J Med Sci 270:165–171, 1975

76. LING CM and OVERBY LR: Prevalence of hepatitis B virus antigen as revealed by direct radioimmunoassay with ^{125}I-antibody. J Immunol 109:834–841, 1972

77. LOCARNINI SA, FERRIS AA, LEHMANN NI, and GUST ID: The antibody response following hepatitis A infection. Intervirology 8:309–318, 1977

78. LOCARNINI SA, FERRIS AA, STOTT AC, and GUST ID: The relationship between a 27-nm virus-like particle and hepatitis A as demonstrated by immune electron microscopy. Intervirology 4:110–118, 1974

79. LOCARNINI SA, GUST ID, FERRIS AA, STOTT AC, and WONG ML: A prospective study of acute viral hepatitis with particular reference to hepatitis A. Bull WHO 54:199–206, 1976

80. LONDON WS, SUTNICK AI, and BLUMBERG BS: Australia antigen and acute viral hepatitis. Ann Intern Med 70:55–59, 1969

81. LORENZ D, BARKER L, STEVENS D, PETERSON M, and KIRSCHSTEIN RL: Hepatitis in the marmoset, *Saguinus mystax*. Proc Soc Exp Biol Med 135:348–354, 1970

82. LUTWICK LI and ROBINSON WS: DNA synthesized in the hepatitis B Dane particle DNA polymerase reaction. J Virol 21:96–104, 1977

83. MACCALLUM FO: Hepatitis. Am J Dis Child 123:332–335, 1971

84. MADALINSKI K, BUDKOWSKA A, MICHALAK T, and TREPO C: Immunofluorescent test for the detection of anti-HBc. Bibl Haematol 42:65–70, 1976

85. MAGNIUS LO and ESPMARK JA: New specificities in Australia antigen positive sera distinct from the LeBouvier determinants. J Immunol 109:1017–1021, 1972

86. MASCOLI CC, ITTENSOHN OL, VILLAREJOS VM, ARGUEDAS GJA, PROVOST PJ, and HILLEMAN MR: Recovery of hepatitis agents in the marmoset from human cases occurring in Costa Rica. Proc Soc Exp Biol Med 142:276–282, 1973

87. MATHIESEN LR, DRUCKER J, LORENZ D, WAGNER JA, GERETY RJ, and PURCELL RH: Localization of hepatitis A antigen in marmoset organs during acute infection with hepatitis A virus. J Infect Dis 138:369–377, 1978

88. MATHIESEN LR, FEINSTONE SM, PURCELL RH, and WAGNER JA: Detection of hepatitis A antigen by immunofluorescence. Infect Immun 18:524–530, 1977

89. MATHIESEN LR, FEINSTONE SM, WONG DC, SKINHOEJ P, and PURCELL RH: Enzyme-linked immunosorbent assay for detection of hepatitis A antigen in stool and antibody to hepatitis A antigen in sera: comparison with solid-phase radioimmunoassay, immune electron microscopy, and immune adherence hemagglutination assay. J Clin Microbiol 7:184–193, 1978

90. MAYNARD JE, BERQUIST KR, KRUSHAK DH, and PURCELL RH: Experimental infection of chimpanzees with the virus of hepatitis B. Nature 237:514–515, 1972

91. MAYUMI M, OKOCHI K, and NISHIOKA K: Detection of Australia antigen by means of immune adherence haemagglutination test. Vox Sang 20:178–181, 1971

92. MILLER WJ, PROVOST PJ, MCALEER WJ, ITTENSOHN OL, VILLAREJOS VM, and HILLEMAN MR: Specific immune adherence assay for human hepatitis A. Application to diagnostic and epidemiologic investigations. Proc Soc Exp Biol Med 149:254–261, 1975

93. MORITSUGU Y, DIENSTAG JL, VALDESUSO J, WONG DC, WAGNER J, ROUTENBERG JA, and PURCELL RH: Purification of hepatitis A antigen from feces and detection of antigen and antibody by immune adherence hemagglutination. Infect Immun 13:898–908, 1976

94. MORITSUGU Y, GOLD JWM, WAGNER J, DODD RY, and PURCELL RH: Hepatitis B core antigen: detection of antibody by radioimmunoprecipitation. J Immunol 114:1792–1798, 1975

95. MURRAY R: Viral hepatitis. Bull NY Acad Med 31:341–358, 1955

96. NAKANE PK and KAWAOI A: Peroxidase-labeled antibody, A new method of conjugation. J Histochem Cytochem 22:1084–1091, 1974

97. NEEFE JR, GELLIS SS, and STOKES J: Homologous serum hepatitis and infectious (epidemic) hepatitis. Studies in volunteers bearing on immunologic and other characteristics of the etiologic agents. Am J Med 1:3–22, 1946

98. NEEFE JR, NORRIS RF, REINHOLD JG, MITCHELL CB, and HOWELL DS: Carriers of hepatitis virus in the blood and viral hepatitis in whole blood recipients. J Am Med Assoc 154:1066–1074, 1954

99. NOWOSLAWSKI A, BRZOSKO WJ, MADALINSKI K, and KRAWCZYNSKI K: Cellular localization or Australia antigen in the liver of patients with lymphoproliferative disorders. Lancet 1:494–497, 1970

100. OKADA K, KAMIYAMA I, INOMATA M, IMAI M, MIYAKAWA Y, and MAYUMI M: e antigen and anti-e in the serum of asymptomatic carrier mothers as indicators of positive and negative transmission of hepatitis B virus to their infants. N Engl J Med 294:746–749, 1976

101. OKOCHI K and MURAKAMI S: Observations on Australia antigen in Japan. Vox Sang 15:374–385, 1968

102. PESENDORFER F, KRASSNITZKY O, and WEWALKA F: Immunoelectrophoretischer nachweis von "Hepatitis-associated-antigen" (Au/SH-antigen). Klin Wochenschr 48:58–59, 1970

103. PETERS RL: Viral hepatitis: a pathologic spectrum. Am J Med Sci 270:17–31, 1975

104. PETERSON DA, FROESNER GG, and DEINHARDT FW: Evaluation of passive hemagglutination, solid-phase radioimmunoassay, and immunoelectroosmorphoresis for the detection of hepatitis B antigen. Appl Microbiol 26:376–380, 1973

105. PRINCE AM: An antigen detected in the blood during the incubation period of serum hepatitis. Proc Nat Acad Sci USA 60:814–821, 1968

106. PRINCE AM and BURKE K: Serum hepatitis antigen (SH): rapid detection by high voltage immunoelectroosmophoresis. Science 169:593–595, 1970

107. PRINCE AM, SZMUNESS W, BROTMAN B, IKRAM H, LIPPIN A, STRYKER M, EHRICH C, and FINLAYSON NCDC: Hepatitis and Blood Transfusion In Hepatitis B Immune Globulin, Vyas GN, Perkins HA, and Schmid RS (eds), Grune and Stratton, New York, 1972, pp 335–347

108. PROVOST PJ, ITTENSOHN OL, VILLAREJOS VM, ARGUEDAS GJA, and HILLEMAN MR: Etiologic relationship of marmoset-propagated CR326 hepatitis A virus to hepatitis in man. Proc Soc Exp Biol Med 142:1257-1267, 1973

109. PROVOST PJ, ITTENSOHN QL, VILLAREJOS VM, and HILLEMAN MR: A specific complement-fixation test for human hepatitis A employing CR326 virus antigen. Diagnosis and epidemiology. Proc Soc Exp Biol Med 148:962-969, 1975

110. PROVOST PJ, VILLAREJOS VM, and HILLEMAN MR: Suitability of the rufiventer marmoset as a host animal for human hepatitis A virus. Proc Soc Exp Biol Med 155:283-286, 1977

111. PROVOST PJ, WOLANSKI BS, MILLER WJ, ITTENSOHN OL, MCALEER WJ, and HILLEMAN MR: Physical, chemical and morphologic dimensions of human hepatitis A virus strain CR326. Proc Soc Exp Biol Med 148:532-539, 1975

112. PURCELL RH, DIENSTAG JL, FEINSTONE SM, and KAPIKIAN AZ: Relationship of hepatitis A antigen to viral hepatitis. Am J Med Sci 270:61-71, 1975

113. PURCELL RH, FEINSTONE SM, ALTER HJ, and WONG DC: Detection of a novel antigen in two cases of non-A non-B hepatitis, a recently recognized persistent infection of probable viral origin In Proceedings of the 1978 ICN-UCLA Symposium on Persistent Viruses, Vol XI, Stevens JG, Todaro GJ and Fox CF (eds), Academic Press, New York, 1978, pp 535-549

114. PURCELL RH and GERIN JL: Hepatitis B subunit vaccine: a preliminary report of safety and efficacy tests in chimpanzees. Am J Med Sci 270:395-399, 1975

115. PURCELL RH, GERIN JL, ALMEIDA JD, and HOLLAND PV: Radioimmunoassay for the detection of the internal component of the DNA particle and antibody to it. Intervirology 2:231-243, 1974

116. PURCELL RH, GERIN JL, HOLLAND PV, CLINE WL, and CHANOCK RM: Preparation and characterization of complement-fixing hepatitis-associated antigen and antiserum. J Infect Dis 121:222-226, 1970

117. PURCELL RH, HOLLAND PV, WALSH JH, WONG DC, MORROW AG, and CHANOCK RM: A complement-fixation test for measuring Australia antigen and antibody. J Infect Dis 120:383-386, 1969

118. PURCELL RH, WONG DC, ALTER HJ, and HOLLAND PV: Microtiter solid-phase radioimmunoassay for hepatitis B antigen. Appl Microbiol 26:478-484, 1973

119. PURCELL RH, WONG DC, MORITSUGU Y, DIENSTAG JL, ROUTENBERG JA, and BOGGS JD: A microtiter solid-phase radioimmunoassay for hepatitis A antigen and antibody. J Immunol 116:349-356, 1976

120. RAUNIO VK, LONDON WT, SUTNICK AI, MILLMAN IS, and BLUMBERG BS: Specificities of human antibodies to Australia antigen. Proc Soc Exp Biol Med 134:548-557, 1970

121. REDEKER AG: Viral hepatitis: clinical aspects. Am J Med Sci 270:9-16, 1975

122. RIZZETTO M, CANESE MG, ARICO S, CRIVELLI O, TREPO C, BONINO F, and VERME G: Immunofluorescence detection of new antigen-antibody system (δ/anti-δ) associated to hepatitis B virus in liver and in serum of HBsAg carriers. Gut 18:997-1003, 1977

123. ROBINSON WS: The genome of hepatitis B virus. Annu Rev Microbiol 31:357-377, 1977

124. ROBINSON WS, CLAYTON DA, and GREENMAN RL: DNA of a human hepatitis B virus candidate. J Virol 14:384-391, 1974

125. SCHULMAN AN, DIENSTAG JL, JACKSON DR, HOOFNAGLE JH, GERETY RJ, PURCELL RH, and BARKER LF: Hepatitis A antigen particles in liver, bile, and stool of chimpanzees. J Infect Dis 134:80-84, 1976

126. SCHWEITZER IL: Vertical transmission of the hepatitis B surface antigen. Am J Med Sci 270:287-291, 1975

127. SHULMAN NR, BARKER LR: Virus-like antigen, antibody, and antigen-antibody complexes in hepatitis measured by complement fixation. Science 165:304-306, 1969

128. SIEGL G and FRÖSNER GG: Characterization and classification of virus particles associated with hepatitis A I. Size, density, and sedimentation. J Virol 26:40-47, 1978

129. SIEGL G and FRÖSNER GG: Characterization and classification of virus particles associated with hepatitis A. II. Type and Configuration of nucleic acid. J Virol 26:48-53, 1978

130. SOULIER JP and COUROUCE-PAUTY AM: New determinants of hepatitis B antigen (Au or HB antigen). Vox Sang 25:212-234, 1973

131. STEINER S, HUEBNER MT, and DREESMAN GR: Major polar lipids of hepatitis B antigen preparations: evidence of the presence of a glycosphingo lipid. J Virol 14:572–577, 1974

132. STEVENS CE, SILBERT JA, MILLER DR, DIENSTAG JL, PURCELL RH, SZMUNESS W: Serologic evidence of hepatitis A and B virus infections in thalassemia patients: a retrospective study. Transfusion 18:94–98, 1978

133. STOKES J JR, BERK JE, MALAMUT LL, DRAKE ME, BARONDESS JA, BASHE WJ, WOLMAN IJ, FARQUHER JD, BEVAN B, DRUMMOND RJ, MAYCOCK WD'A, CAPPS RB: The carrier state in viral hepatitis. J Am Med Assoc 154:1059–1065, 1954

134. SZMUNESS W: Recent advances in the study of the epidemiology of hepatitis B. Am J Pathol 81:629–649, 1975

135. SZMUNESS W, DIENSTAG JL, PURCELL RH, PRINCE AM, STEVENS CE, LEVINE RW: Hepatitis type A and hemodialysis: a seroepidemiologic study in 15 U.S. centers. Ann Intern Med 87:8–12, 1977

136. SZMUNESS W, HARLEY EJ, and PRINCE AM: Intrafamilial spread of asymptomatic hepatitis B. Am J Med Sci 270:293–304, 1975

137. SZMUNESS W, MUCH MI, PRINCE AM, HOOFNAGLE JH, CHERUBIN CE, HARLEY EJ, BLOCK GH: On the role of sexual behavior in the spread of hepatitis B infection. Ann Intern Med 83:489–495, 1975

138. TABOR E, DRUCKER JA, HOOFNAGLE JH, APRIL M, GERETY RJ, SEEFF LB, JACKSON DR, BARKER LF, and PINEDA-TAMONDONG G: Transmission of non-A non-B hepatitis from man to chimpanzee. Lancet 1:463–466, 1978

139. TABOR E, GERETY RJ, VOGEL CL, BAYLEY A, and BARKER LF: Type B hepatitis and primary hepatocellular carcinoma. J Natl Cancer Inst 58:1197–2900, 1977

140. TSUDA F, TAKAHASHI T, TAKAHASHI Y, MIYAKAWA Y, and MAYUMI M: Determination of antibody to hepatitis B core antigen by means of immune adherence hemagglutination. J Immunol 115:834–838, 1975

141. VYAS GN and SHULMAN NR: Hemagglutination assay for antigen and antibody associated with viral hepatitis. Science 170:332–333, 1970

142. WILLIAMS AO: Hepatitis B surface antigen and liver cell carcinoma. Am J Med Sci 270:53–56, 1975

143. WILLIAMS A and LEBOUVIER G: Heterogeneity and thermostability of 'e'. Bibl Haematol 42:71–75, 1976

144. WHO Expert Committee on Viral Hepatitis: Terminology of hepatitis viruses and antigens. Intervirology 8:65–67, 1977

145. WOLTERS G, KUIJPERS L, KACAKI J, and SCHUURS A: Solid-phase enzyme-immunoassay for detection of hepatitis B surface antigen. J Clin Pathol 29:873–879, 1976

146. ZUCKERMAN AJ: Twenty-five centuries of viral hepatitis. Rush-Presbyter St Luke's Med Bull 15:57–82, 1976

CHAPTER 30

GASTROENTERITIS VIRUSES

Albert Z. Kapikian, Robert H. Yolken, Harry B. Greenberg, Richard G. Wyatt, Anthony R. Kalica, Robert M. Chanock, and Hyun Wha Kim

Introduction

Up until the 1970s, etiologic agents of acute infectious nonbacterial gastroenteritis were indeed elusive. Before 1972, not a single virus had been implicated as a potentially important cause of acute gastroenteritis. This was especially frustrating since studies of infants and young children hospitalized with nonepidemic sporadic gastroenteritis, or studies of outbreaks of "winter vomiting disease," or epidemic diarrhea and vomiting etc. consistently failed to reveal a causative agent in the majority of instances, and it was frequently assumed by exclusion that viruses were responsible for these gastroenteritides of unknown etiology. This frustration was compounded by the knowledge that during this golden age of virology, when the use of tissue cultures had led to the discovery of literally hundreds of new viruses, many of which were associated with important diseases, not one could be implicated as a major etiologic agent of gastroenteritis. Even viruses which were capable of multiplying quite efficiently in the enteric tract, such as the many echoviruses which were discovered as a direct consequence of this tissue culture era and which held great promise as important etiologic agents of gastroenteritis, disappointingly, have turned out not to be the long sought after agents of gastroenteritis (47, 48, 99, 110, 170, 279).

However, discoveries made since 1972 of 2 new groups of agents associated with nonbacterial gastroenteritis have led to an abundance of new information about the etiology of this disease. The first group, of which the 27-nm Norwalk particle is the prototype, has been associated with outbreaks of viral gastroenteritis which occurred in school, community, or family settings, infecting school-age children, adults, family contacts, and some young children as well (10, 12, 23, 125, 232). The other group, the 70-nm rotaviruses, has been shown to be associated with up to 50% of the acute diarrheal diseases in hospitalized infants and young children and is the major known etiologic agent of infantile gastroenteritis in many parts of the world (5, 19, 20, 21, 28, 29, 33, 34, 51, 58, 59, 62, 63, 69, 75, 121, 124, 133, 168, 179, 200, 207, 209, 241, 268).

It is remarkable that in this era of tissue culture virology that both of these groups of agents were identified initially without the use of any *in vitro* tissue culture system. The Norwalk group of agents has still not been propagated definitively in any *in vitro* system, including tissue and organ cultures (23, 54, 55). The human rotaviruses have been cultivated in only a limited fashion in tissue or organ cultures, and attempts to serially propagate human rotaviruses from clinical specimens in cell culture systems have been almost uniformly unsuccessful (6, 261, 263, 266). The methods used to study these agents have highlighted a concept which was used successfully for studies of hepatitis B antigens and for the discovery of the 27 nm Norwalk and hepatitis A virus particles (73, 125, 259); such methods might be termed "direct virology", i.e., studying the natural history of infection with viral agents by considering the virus as an entity which can be visualized, concentrated, coated with antibody, or used in numerous assay systems as an antigen, all without the necessity of its *in vitro* or *in vivo* cultivation (8, 115, 116). The initial studies which described the detection of the Norwalk group of agents, the human rotavirus (and the hepatitis A virus, as well) relied exclusively on the use of electron microscopy (EM) for virus detection and for demonstration of serologic responses to these agents (10, 12, 19, 20, 21, 23, 73, 75, 125, 232). Although EM is still of importance in studying these agents, second and third generation tests have been developed to study infection with them. The Norwalk agent was visualized in an infectious stool filtrate derived from an outbreak of gastroenteritis which affected students and teachers in an elementary school, along with family contacts (3, 23, 53, 54, 125). The technique of immune electron microscopy (IEM) was essential for the recognition of this agent (116, 125). Other morphologically similar particles (Hawaii, MC, Ditchling, W, and cockle) have been detected from individuals with gastroenteritis by IEM or conventional EM (10, 12, 232). The human rotavirus was first visualized in duodenal biopsies obtained from acutely ill infants and young children with diarrhea (19, 20). Rotavirus was later observed in stool preparations by EM (21, 28, 75, 121, 168). The reader is referred to several recent review articles for a comprehensive review of viral gastroenteritis agents (82, 122, 123, 126, 127, 212, 246, 263–265).

Clinical aspects

Viral gastroenteritis appears to consist of 2 clinical entities with quite different epidemiologic characteristics. One, which is designated epidemic viral gastroenteritis and is associated with the Norwalk group, is usually self-limited, lasting approximately 24–48 hr, affecting school-age children, adults, and some young children as well; it occurs in family, school, or communitywide outbreaks (23, 53, 280). In antibody prevalence studies of the metropolitan Washington D.C. area with the newly developed immune adherence hemagglutination assay (IAHA) for the Norwalk agent, it was found that Norwalk antibody was acquired gradually, beginning slowly in childhood and accelerating in the adult period so that by the fifth decade 50% of the population has the antibody (118). This pattern contrasted markedly with that of the human rotavirus, thus adding further support to the view that the Norwalk agent is not an important cause of gastroenteritis in infants and young children but rather is associated with such illness in older children and adults. In the original Norwalk outbreak acute gastroenteritis occurred in 50% of the students and teachers in an elementary school, and a secondary attack rate of about 32% was observed among family contacts (3). A filtrate made from a rectal swab obtained from a person with a secondary case was administered orally to adult volunteers, and it produced disease; it also was successfully passaged serially (54, 55, 260). The Norwalk agent was visualized by IEM in the infectious stool filtrate of an inoculated volunteer. Of the 604 persons with primary or secondary cases in Norwalk, Ohio, 85% had nausea, 84% vomiting, 62% abdominal cramps, 57% lethargy, 44% diarrhea, 32% fever, and 5% chills (3). Symptoms lasted 12–24 hr; none of the patients was hospitalized. The average incubation period was 48 hr (3). Signs and symptoms of illness observed in published reports of 32 of 55 volunteers who developed illness following administration of 2% filtrates of stools containing the Norwalk agent were similar to those observed under natural conditions: incubation period, 10–51 hr, fever ($\geq$99.4 F) in 16 (50%), diarrhea in 27 (84%), vomiting in 20 (63%), abdominal discomfort in 23 (72%), anorexia in 30 (94%), headache in 27 (84%), and myalgias or malaise in 20 (63%); clinical manifestations usually lasted 24–48 hr (260). The illness was generally mild and self-limited although a volunteer who vomited approximately 20 times within a 24-hr period required parenteral administration of fluid (55). Shedding patterns of the Norwalk particle in volunteers as determined by IEM, revealed that shedding was maximal during the first 72 hr after onset of clinical illness and occurred only infrequently afterwards (231). Signs and symptoms of illness observed in volunteers following administration of the Hawaii, MC, and W agents were similar to those observed with the Norwalk agent (42, 232, 260).

The other clinical form of viral gastroenteritis has been associated with rotavirus infection and is characterized by a severe diarrhea which occurs predominantly in infants and young children and may require hospitalization and parenteral fluid therapy (34, 41, 51, 121, 164, 196, 215, 228, 233). The illness rate among family contacts of patients with this form of gastroenteritis is low, although subclinical infections in contacts occur frequently (60, 121, 130, 164, 180, 199, 228, 243). In contrast to the Norwalk agent, rotavirus antibody is acquired early in life, in a pattern similar to that for respiratory syncytial and parainfluenza type 3 viruses (22, 65, 93, 118, 131, 193). Rotavirus is the major etiologic agent of infantile gastroenteritis and is associated with up to 50% of the hospitalized cases of diarrheal illness in infants and young children in many countries with temperate climates (5, 34, 51, 92, 121, 164, 168). Rotavirus infection has an unusual epidemiologic feature as it is prevalent predominantly or is at its peak in the cooler months of the year in the temperate climates (18, 34, 51, 92, 121, 164, 168). This pattern is not applicable in all situations as a significant number of rotavirus infections has been reported throughout the year in South Africa, during the summer in Taiwan, during the "small rains" period in Ethiopia, during the summer in a newborn nursery in England, and all seasons in a newborn nursery in Australia (57, 85, 175, 207, 209, 226). In both of the newborn nurseries most virus-positive infants were symptom free. Rotaviruses also appear to be of major clinical importance in tropical countries as well (97a, 145, 200). The incubation period is about 1-3 days (51, 215, Kapikian et al, unpublished studies).

A study of hospitalized gastroenteritis patients in Children's Hospital National Medical Center (Washington, DC) revealed that 83% of study patients with rotavirus infection had dehydration as compared to 40% of the gastroenteritis patients without such infection (196). Dehydration was mild to moderate in both groups, being isotonic in 95% of the rotavirus group and in 77% of the rotavirus-negative group. As determined from admission history and hospitalization record, 96% of the rotavirus-infected patients had vomiting (duration 2.6 days) whereas only 58% of the rotavirus-negative group had this symptom (duration, 0.9 days) (196). Diarrhea started later and lasted longer than vomiting (duration of 5 days vs. 2.6 days) in the rotavirus-infected patients. Once the patient was hospitalized, diarrhea was observed for an average of 2.6 days (range 1-9 days) in the rotavirus group and 3.8 days (range 1-16 days) in the rotavirus-negative group. Patients were managed essentially by restriction of oral fluids and administration of parenteral fluid. Oral fluid was restricted an average of 24 hr for the rotavirus group and 16.5 hr for the others, whereas the mean duration of intravenous fluid therapy was essentially the same in both groups (about 2 days). Duration of hospitalization ranged from 2-14 days for the rotavirus group (mean 4 days) (196). Recovery usually is complete and uneventful, although brief readmissions to the hospital for recurring diarrhea after initial rotavirus infection have been described (228). A recent study indicates that oral rehydration can also be effective in rotavirus diarrhea (175a, 200a).

Deaths have been reported among infants and young children with rotavirus infection (51, 164, 168). In one study in Canada, 21 such fatal cases were identified between May 1972 and March 1977 (37a). Ten patients were dead on arrival at a hospital and 10 were moribund and received resuscitative measures on reaching a hospital but such measures were unsuccessful; one patient had underlying congestive cardiomyopathy and acquired rotavirus disease while hospitalized and died as an inpatient. The mean age of the 21 patients was 11 months with a range of 4-30 months. Death occurred within 3 days of onset of symptoms. The major factor causing death was believed to be dehydration and electrolyte imbalance in 16 cases; aspiration of vomitus was found in 3 individuals and in the remaining 2, seizures were a contributory factor (37a). Rotavirus infections have also been observed in infants and young children with intussusception and with self-limited gastrointestinal bleeding (51a, 134). In another study, a child with rotavirus-associated gastroenteritis developed a fatal Reye syndrome, and a second child with rotavirus associated gastroenteritis developed encephalitis and was having a slow recovery (202). Studies of rotavirus infection in gastroenteritis patients not requiring hospitalization have been few; however, rotaviruses appear also to play an important role in such episodes of gastroenteritis (29). Since subclinical rotavirus infections occur quite commonly in adult contacts of patients with rotavirus infection, it has been suggested that infected adults may be the source of infection for very young infants who are not normally in contact with other infants or young children (121, 130). Rotavirus infection with associated gastroenteritis has been reported in older children and adults (25-27, 95, 96, 121, 130, 163, 180, 228, 243, 284). Finally, rotavirus has been administered to volunteers and found to induce gastroenteritis in certain susceptible individuals (168, Kapikian et al. unpublished studies).

Pathology

In volunteers challenged with the Norwalk or Hawaii agents, characteristically, there is broadening and blunting of the villi of the jejunal mucosa; the mucosa itself is histologically intact (4, 56, 210, 211). Moderate mononuclear cell infiltration and cytoplasmic vacuolization of epithelial cells have also been observed. Examination of thin sections of the jejunal mucosa by transmission EM has characteristically revealed intact epithelial cells with shortening of microvilli; convalescent-phase biopsies have been normal (4, 56, 210, 211). During illness caused by the Norwalk agent, the gastric mucosa appears normal histologically (252). Brush border small intestinal enzyme studies (including alkaline phosphatase, sucrase, and trehalase) revealed a decrease in comparison to baseline and convalescent-phase values, whereas adenylate cyclase activity in jejunal mucosa during illness with Norwalk or Hawaii agents was not found to be elevated as occurs in diarrhea associated with cholera or enterotoxigenic *Escherichia coli* heat-labile toxins (4, 140, 201).

Rotaviruses have been detected in stool material of numerous animals, including calves, infant mice, piglets, foals, lambs, rabbits, deer, antelopes, apes, turkeys, chickens, young goats, kittens, a normal monkey, in intestinal washings of sheep and cattle and by immunofluorescence of bison calf intestine (13a, 16a, 31, 36, 46, 76, 103a, 146, 153a, 159, 174, 191, 193, 212a, 217a, 219, 220, 245, 254). In addition, the human rotavirus has been administered to various newborn colostrum-deprived animals and has induced a diarrheal illness in gnotobiotic calves, gnotobiotic and conventional piglets, rhesus monkeys, and gnotobiotic lambs (99, 136, 138, 162, 167, 169, 218, 238, 239, 267). Also, it infected but did not induce illness in newborn puppies (244). In the newborn calf the morphologic changes observed in the small intestine following human rotavirus infection appear to proceed in a cephalocaudad direction (161). The progression of events includes infection of the absorptive villous epithelial cells, replacement of the tall columnar villous epithelial cells with cuboidal and squamous cells, villous shortening, reticular cell enlargement, infiltration of the villous lamina propria with lymphocytes and, finally, repair (161). Histopathologic studies of humans with rotavirus infection are few and include limited biopsy studies of hospitalized infants and young children. Small intestinal mucosal changes included shortening of the villi, mononuclear cell infiltration of the lamina propria, distended cisternae of the endoplasmic reticulum, mitochondrial swelling, and sparse and irregular microvilli (101, 227). Patients with gastroenteritis whose intestinal fluid was positive for rotavirus appeared to have impaired d-xylose absorption (152). Studies in piglets with experimental human rotavirus infection revealed that in the villous epithelial cells of the small intestine glucose-coupled Na^+ transport was impaired, sucrase activity diminished, and thymidine kinase activity increased, whereas adenylate cyclase activity was not stimulated and cyclic AMP levels were not increased (49, 86).

Description and Nature of the Norwalk and Norwalk-like Agents

General characteristics

The Norwalk group of agents has been detected in the stool of patients with gastroenteritis (10, 12, 125, 232). They have not yet been propagated definitively *in vitro*, and therefore must be detected by EM or in addition, for the Norwalk agent, by the recently developed radioimmunoassay (RIA) and IAHA (10, 12, 23, 90, 91, 118, 125, 232). Some common characteristics of this group are shown in Table 30.1.

Agents in this group have a diameter of 25–27 nm (shortest diameter) (10, 12, 125, 232). They are not perfectly round as, for example, the Norwalk agent averages 27 nm in its shortest diameter and 32 nm in its longest (125); they are similar morphologically to the picorna- or parvoviruses and the hepatitis A virus (73, 116, 125, 232). A clear-cut substructure is not visible by EM. The characteristic appearance of Norwalk agent is shown in Figure 30.1A.

This group of agents has a buoyant density in cesium chloride of 1.37–1.41 g/cm^3 as determined by ultracentrifugation and EM or IEM (10, 12, 117, 232). The nucleic acid content and number of proteins is unknown.

The Norwalk agent is stable when exposed to pH 2.7 for 3 hr at room temperature as determined from infectivity studies in volunteers (54). The Norwalk and W agents are stable when exposed to 20% ether at 4 C for 24 or 18 hr, respectively, as determined from infectivity studies in volunteers (42, 54). The Norwalk agent is relatively heat stable; after heating at 60 C for 30 min it retained infectivity for volunteers (54).

These agents have not yet been classified. However, because the Norwalk agent shares certain characteristics with the parvoviruses, such as morphology and density, and ether, acid, and relative heat stability, it was suggested to be parvovirus-like (54, 125). It should be emphasized, however, that the nucleic acid content of none of these agents has been determined; thus, they cannot be classified in any group.

The Norwalk agent represents the prototype strain (Table 30.1) of this group of agents (125). Particles resembling the Norwalk agent in morphology and density were discovered by IEM in individuals in 2 family outbreaks of gastroenteritis, one in Hawaii (Hawaii agent) and the other in Montgomery County (MC agent), Maryland (232). By IEM and cross-challenge studies, the Hawaii and Norwalk agents were found to be distinct, the Norwalk and MC agents to be related, and the relationship between the Hawaii and MC agents was inconclusive (125, 232, 260). Viruses resembling the Norwalk agent in morphology and density have been observed in fecal specimens from a gastroenteritis outbreak in a primary school in Ditchling, England (10); from a volunteer who became ill after administration of the W agent which was obtained from a boy who developed gastroenteritis during a

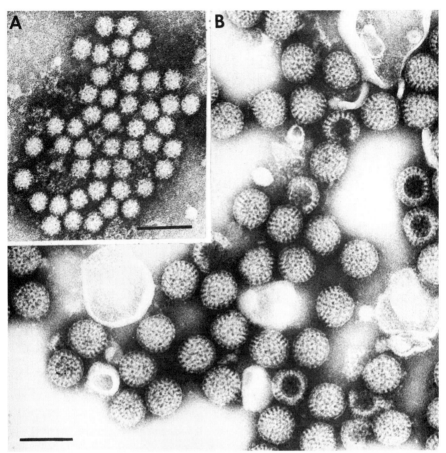

Figure 30.1—A. The Norwalk particle. An aggregate observed after incubation of 0.8
ml of Norwalk stool filtrate (prepared from a stool of a volunteer administered the Norwalk agent), with 0.2 ml of a 1:5 dilution of a volunteer's
prechallenge serum and further preparation for EM. The quantity of
antibody on these particles was rated as 1+. The bar = 100 nm. (After
ref 125) B. The human rotavirus. Rotavirus particles observed in a stool
filtrate (prepared from a stool of an infant with gastroenteritis), after
incubation with PBS and further preparation for EM. The particles appear to have a double-shelled capsid. Occasional "empty" particles are
seen. The bar = 100 nm. (From ref 124)

boy's boarding school outbreak (10, 42); and from individuals developing
gastroenteritis after eating cockles (12). By IEM the Ditchling and W agents
are related to each other but distinct from Hawaii and Norwalk agents,
whereas the cockle agent appears to be distinct from the Norwalk
agent (10, 12, 116). The relationship of the cockle agent with the other
agents is inconclusive. Thus, as shown in Table 30.1 there appear to be 3
and, possibly 4, serotypes of this group of agents.

TABLE 30.1—Characteristics of Parvovirus-like Agents Associated with Acute Epidemic Nonbacterial Gastroenteritis in Humans

Agent	Size (nm)	Buoyant density in cesium chloride (g/cm³)	Growth in cell culture	Agent induces illness in		Particle identified by	Serologic studies by	Antigenic relationships
				Humans	Animals			
Norwalk (54, 55, 117, 125, 262)	27 × 32*	1.38-1.41	No	Yes	No	IEM**	IEM	Distinct
Hawaii (56, 125, 232, 260)	26 × 29*	1.37-1.39	No	Yes	No	IEM	IEM	Distinct
Montgomery County (125, 232, 260)	27 × 32*	1.37-1.41	No	Yes	No	IEM	IEM	Related to Norwalk agent by IEM and cross-challenge studies
Ditchling (10)	25-26	1.38-1.40	No	NT†	No	EM	IEM	Ditchling and W agents related to each other but appear to be distinct from Norwalk and Hawaii agents by IEM
W (10, 42, 116)	25-26	1.38-1.40	No	Yes	NT	EM	IEM	
Cockle (12)	25-26	1.40	No	NT	NT	EM	IEM	Appears to be distinct from Norwalk agent by IEM

*Shortest × longest diameter.
**Immune electron microscopy.
†NT = not tested.

The surface antigens of the Norwalk, Hawaii, and MC particles which react with specific antibody have been important in enabling the recognition of these agents by IEM (125, 232). In the case of Norwalk agent, they have also permitted the successful development of an IAHA and RIA (91, 118). In addition, during attempts to purify the Norwalk particle from stool, a large amount of virus-specific antigen was found in soluble form (90). A hemagglutinin has not been found.

Norwalk agent has been administered to mice, guinea pigs, rabbits, kittens, calves, baboons, chimpanzees, and rhesus, marmoset, owl, patas, and cebus monkeys (23, 54, 55, 262, 264, Wyatt et al, unpublished studies). None of the animals developed illness. Paired sera from monkeys, baboons, and chimpanzees were examined for a seroresponse to the Norwalk agent, and only the chimpanzee developed such a response (91, 116, 262). Chimpanzees were also found by RIA to be shedding Norwalk antigen after challenge (91, 262).

None of these agents has been propagated in tissue cultures or conclusively in organ cultures (10, 12, 23, 54, 55).

Description and Nature of the Rotaviruses

Common characteristics

Human rotaviruses can be found in the feces of infants and young children with acute gastroenteritis (58, 59, 62). They have also been observed in duodenal or small intestinal aspirates (152, 168). Much less often, they can be found in feces of older children and adults with acute gastroenteritis (25–27, 95, 96, 121, 130, 163, 228, 284). Rotaviruses have also been found in numerous animals, including calves, mice, piglets, foals, lambs, rabbits, deer, antelopes, a monkey, apes, bison, turkeys, chickens, young goats and kittens (Table 30.2) (13a, 16a, 31, 36, 46, 76, 103a, 146, 153a, 159, 174, 191, 193, 212a, 217a, 219, 245, 254). Each, except the monkey rotavirus (SA-11), causes severe diarrhea in newborns of each respective group. SA-11 has not been administered by the alimentary route to monkeys; however, it has been shown to induce diarrheal illness in young calves and gnotobiotic piglets (195). Rotavirus strains recovered from clinical specimens are generally quite fastidious and, thus at least initially, grow poorly, if at all (168, 261, 263, 266). Virus replication, when observed, occurs in the cytoplasm where viral antigen may be detected by immunofluorescence (FA) or EM (6, 261, 263, 266).

Size and shape

Complete rotavirus particles possess a double capsid and measure about 70 nm in diameter; particles without the outer layer of the double capsid measure approximately 55 nm, whereas the core, which may be hexagonal in outline, has a diameter of approximately 37 nm (64, 81, 101, 147, 181, 186, 194, 255). The particles have 32 capsomeres and have a rather distinctive appearance by negative-stain EM (Fig 30.1B) (147). The term

TABLE 30.2—SOME GENERAL CHARACTERISTICS OF ROTAVIRUSES VISUALIZED IN STOOLS* OF HUMANS AND ANIMALS

ROTAVIRUS SOURCE	DESCRIPTIVE NAMES OR DESIGNATION	CLINICAL SYNDROME	SERIAL PASSAGE (>2×) IN CELL CULTURE
Human infant (6, 21, 51, 58, 75, 94, 190, 261)	Reovirus-like (RVL) agent, rotavirus duovirus, infantile gastroenteritis virus	Diarrheal illness	Yes (limited)
Calf (bovine) (157, 159, 255)	Nebraska calf diarrhea virus (NCDV), neonatal calf diarrhea reovirus-like agent, rotavirus	Diarrheal illness	Yes
Infant mouse (174)	Epizootic diarrhea of infant mice (EDIM), rotavirus	Diarrheal illness	No
Piglet (138, 154, 193, 230, 256)	Rotavirus	Diarrheal illness	Yes
Foal (76)	Rotavirus	Diarrheal illness	No
Lamb (219)	Rotavirus	Diarrheal illness	No
Young rabbit (36, 46)	Rotavirus	Diarrheal illness	Not known
Monkey (146)	Simian agent (SA)-11, rotavirus	None	Yes
Sheep and calves (146)	Offal (O) agent, rotavirus	(Derived from mixed intestinal washings from abattoir waste)	Yes
Newborn deer (245)	Rotavirus	Diarrheal illness	Yes (6 passages)
Newborn antelope (191)	Rotavirus	Diarrheal illness	Not known
Young chimpanzee (13a)	Rotavirus	Diarrheal illness	Not known
Young gorilla (13a)	Rotavirus	Diarrheal illness	Not known
Young turkey (16a, 153a)	Rotavirus	Diarrheal illness	Not known
Chicken (103a)	Rotavirus	Diarrheal illness	Not known
Young goat (212a)	Rotavirus	Diarrheal illness	Not known
Young kitten (217a)	Rotavirus	Diarrheal illness	Not known

*O agent derived from mixed intestinal washings of sheep and calves from abattoir waste (146). Rotavirus antigen has also been detected by IF in bison calf intestine (245). In addition, serologic evidence of rotavirus infection has been detected in guinea pigs.

"rotavirus" is derived from the Latin word *rota* meaning wheel, which was suggested since the sharply defined circular outline of the outer capsid gives the appearance of the rim of a wheel placed on short spokes radiating from a wide hub (74, 79). Rotaviruses resemble the reoviruses and orbiviruses but differ in their fine structure (178, 263). The distinctive outer capsid of the rotavirus differs from the amorphous outer capsid of orbiviruses; the sharply defined outer capsid margin surrounding the spoke-like capsomeres is said to differentiate rotaviruses from orthoreoviruses (178). The latter distinction is not always clearcut. A small proportion of human rotavirus preparations has been described as containing flattened tubular structures 54–100 nm (mean 70 nm) in width and of varying length; such structures have been shown to be antigenically related to the virion by IEM (69, 81, 101, 132). It has been suggested that they may be formed by the aberrant assembly of viral capsid material (132). The complete tubular forms have a cap-like structure on either end and are about 1000 nm in length (132).

Chemical composition

The genome of rotavirus is comprised of 11 segments of double-stranded RNA ranging in molecular weights from 0.2 to 2.2×10^6 daltons, with a total molecular weight of 11 to 14×10^6 daltons (104, 107, 108, 178, 194, 204, 237). The 11-segmented RNA genome distinguishes rotaviruses from orthoreoviruses and orbiviruses, both of which have only 10 segments of RNA in their genome (82, 263). The migration patterns of the RNA segments in polyacrylamide gel electrophoresis have served as one means of differentiating human and animal rotaviruses and various human rotavirus strains as well (104, 107). Eight to 10 polypeptides with molecular weights of 14,000 to 133,000 have been described with 5 as components of the inner shell and 3, or possibly 4, being associated with the outer shell of the double-shelled capsid (177, 178, 194, 195, 237). The major components of the outer shell have been identified as glycoproteins (100, 195, 206). The double-stranded RNA has a buoyant density in Cs_2SO_4 of 1.57 g/ml (187). RNA polymerase activity has been detected with Nebraska calf diarrhea virus (NCDV) and human rotavirus (45, 102).

Density

Complete rotavirus particles with the double capsid have a density of approximately 1.36 g/cm³ and a sedimentation coefficient of 520–530S (89, 114, 120, 186, 187, 194, 195, 229). Incomplete particles which lack the double capsid (core particles) have a density of approximately 1.38 g/cm³, whereas "empty" particles (penetrated by negative stain) have a density of approximately 1.29–1.30 g/cm³ (64, 194, 229). Infectivity, as measured by fluorescent foci in cell culture, of the higher density (1.38 g/cm³) incomplete particles was compared with that of the lower density (1.36 g/cm³) complete particles (64). The greatest infectivity coincided with the complete particles at the 1.36 g/cm³ density, even though greater numbers of particles were observed at the 1.38 g/cm³ fraction. However, since the fraction with pre-

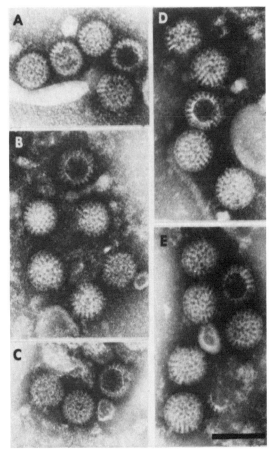

Figure 30.2—Rotavirus particles observed in preparations of 5 rotavirus CF antigens.
One milliliter of each rotavirus CF antigen shown in Table 30.3 was
centrifuged for 1.5 hr at 17,000 rpm. A. Human rotavirus. B. Calf rotavirus (NCDV). C. Mouse rotavirus (EDIM). D. Monkey rotavirus (SA-
11). E. O agent. The bar = 100 nm. (From ref 113)

dominantly incomplete particles also contained a small number of complete
particles, it could not be ascertained whether the incomplete particles had
little or no infectivity (64).

Resistance to physical and chemical agents

Calf rotavirus (NCDV strain) is acid- and ether-stable and relatively
heat-stable (250). SA-11 was clumped or degraded to amorphous form at pH
3 and 4 as observed by EM (195). Calf rotavirus [United Kingdom/Comp-
ton strain (UK)] was studied under a variety of conditions for inactivation by
ultraviolet (UV) light, and resistance to complete inactivation was ob-

served (255, 259a). The structure of rotaviruses is very stable, as human rotavirus stored 9 years at −20 C and another rotavirus strain of uncertain source lyophilized over 30 years previously were recognized morphologically by EM after long storage (5, 98). In addition, purified rotavirus could be detected by counter-immunoelectro-osmophoresis after storage at 4 C for 1 month, whereas after boiling or autoclaving, it could not be detected by this technique (166). It should be noted, however, that extensive purification may lead to instability of rotavirus structure (Kalica et al, unpublished studies). The morphologic appearance of purified human rotavirus was unchanged after being subjected to heat (56 C for 1 hr), centrifugal force (100,000 × g), high salt concentration (50% potassium tartrate), pH 3 and 10, or after treatment with chymotrypsin, papain, pepsin, a halogenated hydrocarbon (Genesolv-D), and nonionic detergents (181). In contrast, however, at pH <3, human rotavirus was unstable and the outer layer of the capsid collapsed, but particles did not disintegrate (181). In addition, human rotavirus was extremely labile after treatment with versene-trypsin (0.125%) for 2 hr at 37 C, as particles were completely degraded to unrecognizable form (181). In another study, the double-shelled human rotavirus retained its morphologic appearance after reaction with papain, pronase, and trypsin but was degraded to a single-shelled form by α-chymotrypsin in the presence of cesium (195). Neither the human nor simian rotavirus was altered morphologically by β-galactosidase, whereas double-shelled calf rotavirus was degraded at least partially to the single-shell form on some occasions (195).

Classification

The human rotaviruses have been designated by a variety of names, including, orbivirus, orbivirus-like, reovirus-like, duovirus, and infantile gastroenteritis virus (20, 51, 57, 81, 94, 121, 187). The name rotavirus was recently accepted by the International Committee on Nomenclature of Viruses as a new genus to be included in the family *Reoviridae* (79, 82, 148a). Rotaviruses have been shown to be distinct serologically from the 3 human reoviruses and also from the orbiviruses with which they have been tested (50, 81, 106, 113, 114, 124, 277).

Antigenic composition

Until very recently, it was assumed on epidemiologic grounds that there was only one human serotype. Such evidence included the rapid acquisition of antibody early in life, the highest frequency of rotavirus illness in the 6- to 24-month age group, and the frequency of subclinical infection in adults (51, 114, 121, 130). However, it now appears that there are at least two serotypes of human rotavirus as detected by CF, IEM, neutralization of immunofluorescent foci (NIFF), and enzyme-linked immunosorbent assay (ELISA) (83, 197, 234, 273, 281). The two serotypes have been designated type 1 and type 2. The various animal and human rotaviruses are similar, if not identical, by CF and immunofluorescence (FA) (common antigen) (Table 30.3) (5, 79, 113, 114, 257); however, by NIFF and ELISA, the human rota-

TABLE 30.3—ANTIGENIC RELATIONSHIPS AMONG THE HUMAN ROTAVIRUS (HRV), NCDV, EDIM VIRUS, SA-11, AND O AGENT WITH HYPERIMMUNE ANIMAL AND CONVALESCENT-PHASE HUMAN SERA BY COMPLEMENT FIXATION*

VIRUS	SOURCE OF CF ANTIGEN**,†	RECIPROCAL OF SERUM ANTIBODY TITER TO INDICATED VIRUS†† (SOURCE OF SERUM)					RECIPROCAL OF CHILD'S ACUTE/ CONVALESCENT-PHASE SERUM			
		HRV (GUINEA PIG)	NCDV (GUINEA PIG)	EDIM (MICE)	SA-11 (GUINEA PIG)	O (GUINEA PIG)	CHILD 1	CHILD 2	CHILD 3	CHILD 4
HRV	Stool filtrate (Da1A)	640	1024	1280	512	2048	<4/128	<4/64	<4/128	<4/128
NCDV	BEK cell cultures	1280	2048	1280	2048	8192	<4/32	<4/16	<4/32	<4/32
EDIM	Intestines of suckling mice	640	512	320	1024	4096	<4/32	<4/<4	<4/32	4/32
SA-11	African green monkey kidney cell cultures	1280	2048	2560	2048	8192	<4/32	<4/8	<4/16	<4/16
O	African green monkey kidney cell cultures	1280	2048	640	2048	4096	<4/32	<4/8	<4/32	<4/16

*All results in table obtained in same test.

**Titer of each antigen (0.025 ml) as calculated in simultaneous (straight line) titration in this test: HRV, 2 units (tested with 2 of the convalescent-phase human sera shown); NCDV, 1–2 units (tested with 2 convalescent-phase NCDV calf sera); EDIM virus, 64 units; SA-11, 16 units; O agent, 32 units. EDIM, SA-11, and O viruses tested with the homologous hyperimmune animal serum shown. In a subsequent titration which included the same sera plus the hyperimmune animal sera for the HRV and NCDV shown, the titers of the 5 viruses were as follows: HRV, 2 units with convalescent-phase human sera, 4 units with homologous hyperimmune animal serum; NCDV, 8 units with convalescent-phase calf sera and 64 units with hyperimmune animal serum; EDIM virus, 64 units; SA-11, 16 units; and O agent, 32 units.

†Control antigens were employed for each viral antigen and tested against each serum. Antibody was not detected in tests with pre- and postimmunization animal sera; in tests with human paired sera, antibody was not detected with control calf, control murine, and control simian antigens, while with control human stool filtrate antigen, antibody (1:8–1:32) was detected but without significant seroresponses.

††Antibody was not detected in any of the preimmunization sera in tests with all 5 reovirus-like antigens.

(From ref 113)

virus can be distinguished from various animal rotaviruses (235, 271). In addition, by 1-way neutralization (Nt) and hemagglutination-inhibition (HAI) tests, the human rotavirus can be distinguished from calf rotavirus (72, 150); by IAHA the two are similar (150). The existence of different serotypes among animal rotaviruses from individual species has not yet been described.

Rotaviruses possess common CF (Table 30.3) and FA antigens (5, 79, 113, 114, 235, 257). CF activity is closely associated with the virion (114). IEM studies suggest that the inner-capsid antigens are the common group antigens and the outer-capsid antigens are type specific (32, 79, 148, 257). With calf rotavirus, the CF activity was more strongly associated with virus particles lacking the outer capsid layer than with the complete virion (72). However, type-specific antigens can also be detected by CF if the appropriate sera are available (281). Two human rotavirus serotypes were distinguished by CF and at least 2 and possibly 4 serotypes were identified by the NIFF assay (81a, 234, 281). The existence of at least two serotypes has been confirmed by ELISA (273). The human, calf (NCDV strain), and monkey (SA-11) rotaviruses each possess a hemagglutinin (72, 105, 216, 223). The calf and SA-11 hemagglutinins appear to reside in the outer capsid, as peak hemagglutination (HA) activity is associated with the double-capsid particle (72, 105, 223). It appears from studies with the human and calf rotaviruses, that the hemagglutinins of these agents detect a specific rather than a group antibody response (72, 216, 223).

Pathogenicity for animals

The human rotavirus induces a diarrheal illness in newborn colostrum-deprived animals, including gnotobiotic calves, gnotobiotic and conventional piglets, rhesus monkeys and gnotobiotic lambs (99, 136, 138, 162, 167, 169, 218, 238, 239, 267). The human rotavirus is also able to infect but not induce illness in newborn puppies (244). Thus far, only newborn or young animals develop diarrhea after challenge with the human rotavirus; older animals appear to be resistant.

Growth in tissue culture

The human rotaviruses have proven to be fastidious agents as they have been very difficult to propagate in any culture system. Three of 15 strains tested of human rotaviruses have been propagated *in vitro* in human embryonic intestinal organ cultures using FA techniques to detect viral antigens (266). Virus replication was not very efficient. Attempts to propagate human rotaviruses in cell cultures have met with only very limited success (6, 261, 263). A few strains of human rotavirus have been passaged successfully in cultures of bovine or human embryonic kidney cells. Once again, however, growth of the virus was not efficient. The cytopathic effect (CPE) develops irregularly and cannot be used consistently for virus detection. Thus, virus propagation is detected by FA or EM and, more recently, by RIA or ELISA (106, 261, 266, 272, 277). With one human strain, in HEK cells, only about 1% of the cells were infected, and the virus population consisted uniformly of subviral particles which lacked the outer capsid (261). Human rotaviruses have been detected efficiently from clinical specimens by centrifugation of rotavirus-containing material onto cell monolayers and examining the cells by FA after appropriate incubation (16, 35, 240). This method has also been used to study antigenic relationships among rotaviruses noted above (235, 257). The calf, piglet, monkey (SA-11) rotaviruses and the O agent have been adapted to grow, or grow readily in, cell cultures, whereas the mouse rotavirus (EDIM) has been cultivated only in organ cultures of mouse embryonic intestine (Table 30.2) (15, 153, 157, 198, 230, 245). The ability to propagate calf rotavirus has led to the development of a commercially available calf rotavirus vaccine (1, 160). Approaches to the development of a human rotavirus vaccine have been described (41, 113, 114). It is noteworthy that calf rotavirus (strain NCDV) was the first of the reovirus-like agents to be recognized as reovirus-like by EM and associated with diarrheal illness, whereas the EDIM was the first to be detected by ultrathin-section EM (2, 159).

Miscellaneous Enteric Agents

Coronaviruses are well known as etiologic agents of diarrheal disease in newborn piglets (transmissible gastroenteritis virus [TGE]), calves, turkeys, and dogs (17, 24, 68, 111, 129, 158, 192, 225), but they have not been implicated conclusively as etiologic agents of human infantile gastroenteritis. However, one report describes the detection by EM of coronaviruses in stools obtained from 3 outbreaks of nonbacterial gastroenteritis in adults; the particles in a stool from one of the outbreaks have been propagated in organ and cell cultures (38–40). Nt antibody to the calf coronavirus has been reported in human serum; however, since the calf coronavirus shares some antigenic relationship with the human respiratory coronavirus, OC43, it is not known whether this antibody is related to OC43 or a related virus, or to an enteric human coronavirus (128, 214).

Astroviruses are approximately 28 nm in diameter and have been shown by negative staining to have 5- or 6-pointed star-shaped surface configuration by negative staining in approximately 10% of the particles (141, 142, 144, 164, 205). They have been seen in stools of infants, young children, and adults with diarrhea but can also be found in symptom-free babies. Serologic evidence of infection has been demonstrated by IEM (135). Astrovirus antigens have been detected in infected monolayers of human embryonic kidney by FA (137). Astroviruses have not only been detected in stools of lambs with diarrhea but have also been successfully passaged in this animal (221).

Other viruses observed in stools of patients with diarrhea include: adenoviruses [the second most commonly found virus in stools or rectal swabs in 6 cross-sectional gastroenteritis studies (18, 34, 51, 57, 121, 241) and with which an outbreak of gastroenteritis in a long-stay children's ward has been associated (77)]; and caliciviruses, minireoviruses, and other small (30 nm) round viruses (11, 33, 34, 37, 42a, 51, 57, 69, 78, 80, 85, 92, 121, 143, 144, 152, 156, 164, 172, 184a, b, 269). Many of the adenoviruses seen by EM in stools are rather fastidious and do not grow or grow with difficulty by conventional cell culture methods. Adenovirus has also been found in small intestinal fluid of pediatric patients with acute gastroenteritis (152). In patients with adenovirus in small intestinal fluids, d-xylose absorption appears to have been impaired (152). Adenovirus infection has also been associated with intussusception (43, 87). Further investigation of these miscellaneous enteric agents is needed to evaluate their role in the etiology of human gastroenteritis.

Preparation of Immune Serum to the Norwalk Agent and to Rotavirus

The preparation of high-titered hyperimmune serum has not been reported for the Norwalk group, since sufficient antigen has not been available for this purpose. However, chimpanzees inoculated with Norwalk agent via the alimentary route develop serologic responses by IEM, IAHA, and RIA (91, 116, 118, 262). Such infection serum is not generally available.

Preparation of immune sera to the human rotaviruses has been accomplished by various methods and in various animals. The critical element in making antiserum to human rotavirus is the availability of sufficient quantities of immunizing antigen since, as indicated earlier, the virus does not grow efficiently in cell culture. Thus, the source of human rotavirus antigen has continued to be a problem in laboratories. The usual source of this fastidious agent has been human stools rich in rotavirus particles. Although rotavirus particles from such stools have been used satisfactorily as immunizing antigen in many studies, they may present a problem in certain tests if immunoglobulins are attached to their surface, as the immunized animal will then develop not only rotavirus antibody but antibodies to immunoglobulins as well (248, 249). Stools from gnotobiotic animals infected with the human rotavirus are an excellent source of antigen; however, this source is not available to most laboratories.

Hyperimmune sera to human rotaviruses have been prepared in guinea pigs, rabbits, and goats by various methods. Large animals have the obvious advantage of providing large amounts of serum; high homologous serum antibody titers are readily achieved in both small and large animals. Preimmunization serum must be screened for rotavirus antibody by one or more of the available serologic tests to assure that the animal does not have rotavirus antibody.

In our laboratory, to prepare goat antiserum the particle-rich stool preparation is made into an approximate 10% suspension, clarified at low speed and purified by rate zonal centrifugation in a sucrose gradient (Kalica et al, unpublished studies). Fractions containing the most antigen, as demonstrated by one or more of the detection methods, such as CF, are pooled. Equal volumes of purified virus and incomplete Freund's adjuvant are mixed; 1 ml of the antigen-adjuvant mixture is inoculated intramuscularly (im). Goats receive the 1-ml inoculation at one site. Blood may be obtained and checked for rotavirus antibody at weekly intervals. Four weeks after initial inoculation, 0.5 ml of the antigen-adjuvant mixture is administered im as a booster. The animal may be bled at weekly intervals.

In other immunization attempts in our laboratory in goats and guinea pigs, sucrose gradient purified rotavirus has been further purified by isopycnic banding in cesium chloride followed by dialysis before emulsifying with incomplete Freund's adjuvant and administering to the appropriate animal (Kalica et al, unpublished studies). The route and dose for immunization was the same as above except that for the guinea pig 0.5 ml of the antigen-adjuvant mixture is administered in each hind leg rather than the total amount at a single site. Guinea pig antirotavirus serum prepared in this way has been used successfully in RIA and ELISA procedures described later. However, it has been observed that such more highly purified virus may be less effective for raising Nt antibody (to calf rotavirus) than the singly purified antigen, suggesting that the more vigorous purification procedure may in certain instances remove viral antigens essential for induction of Nt antibody; it was noteworthy however, that similar CF antibody titers were achieved by virus prepared by single or double purification methods. Since live virus is used for immunization, it may be desirable to keep animals in isolation, depending on the facilities available. Fecal samples collected for 10 days following im inoculation of goats with singly purified human rotavirus as described above did not reveal the presence of rotavirus by ELISA.

Recent studies indicate that conventional methods of rotavirus antigen preparation will yield serum containing antibody to the common, as well as the type-specific antigenic determinants. Recently, two distinct human rotavirus serotypes were detected by CF (281). Each of the two type-specific antisera was prepared with an approximate 30% suspension of human feces rich in rotavirus particles. The suspensions were clarified by centrifugation twice for 10 min; the rotavirus containing supernatant fluid was sedimented through a 60%/45%/30% sucrose gradient at $100,000 \times g$ for 2.5 hr (281). Rotavirus particles with complete double capsids banding at a density of 1.22 were used as immunizing antigen for each of the 2 suspensions (281). Guinea pigs were inoculated according to a previously described method employing complete Freund's adjuvant in one of the inoculations (155). If necessary, the specificity of typing sera may be further enhanced by adsorption with high titered animal rotavirus or heterotypic human rotavirus suspensions in order to remove or decrease antibody to common antigenic determinants (197, 273).

Postinfection sera to human rotavirus may be produced in calves, lambs, monkeys and piglets after inoculation of such animals via the alimentary route (99, 136, 138, 162, 167, 169, 218, 238, 239, 267). Piglet serum does not react satisfactorily in the CF test. Antisera to certain animal rotaviruses such as NCDV or UK from calves, SA-11 from a monkey, piglet rotavirus, and the O agent may be produced relatively easily since these strains may be propagated efficiently in cell culture (146, 157, 255). However, the morphology of the particles should be monitored by EM if antibody to certain viral components is desired.

Collection and Preparation of Specimens for Laboratory Diagnosis

Precautions

Stool and serum specimens obtained from areas where exotic viruses such as Lassa Fever may be prevalent should be handled with extreme caution, as in a recent study it was found that signs and symptoms of certain cases of Lassa Fever may be indistinguishable clinically from viral or non-specific acute gastroenteritis (McCormick JB, Bryan JA, Webb PA, Johnson KM, presentation at Am Epidemiol Soc Meeting, 1978). Thus, specimens coming from those parts of the world where exotic viruses occur should not be handled in the routine laboratory setting but should be studied under appropriate containment conditions. Specimens from areas where such exotic agents do not occur should also be handled with care since the possibility that they may contain other hazardous agents such as hepatitis viruses should be considered.

In addition, well-ventilated areas should be employed when fluoroalkanes (such as trichlorotrifluoroethane or commercially known preparations such as Genetron, Arcton, Freon, Isotron, Ucon, etc.) are used for various preparative procedures of stool material, since serious cardiotoxicity has been reported to be associated with fluoroalkanes (97).

Detection of virus—collection, storage and processing

After collection, stool samples may be stored at −20 C or ideally at −70 C. The physical structure of the rotavirus is extremely stable since, as noted above, they are recognizable by EM after long periods of storage. The effect of lengthy storage at various temperatures on infectivity is not known. However, even if specimens have been kept at ambient temperature they would most likely be suitable for antigen detection studies. Rectal swabs immersed in a fluid medium are acceptable for rotavirus detection but are not nearly as suitable as stool suspensions for direct examination by EM without centrifugation (Brandt CD, et al, unpublished studies). For initial screening tests by EM, as well as by other methods, a stool specimen may be prepared as a 2% suspension by mixing approximately 200 mg of stool with 10 ml of veal infusion broth containing 0.5% bovine serum albumin. (The bovine serum albumin should, of course, be free of a contaminant such as rotavirus antibody.) The suspension is then homogenized by shaking with glass beads for about 10 min; it is then clarified in a refrigerated centrifuge at 3000 rpm for a variable period to remove debris. The suspension is then ready for examination. Appropriate containment facilities should be available for the various steps involved in the preparation of the stool suspension especially if the presence of hazardous agents is suspected.

Two percent stool suspensions have been used for the detection of Norwalk agent by RIA (91); 2%, 10% and 20% stool suspensions have been used successfully for detection of rotaviruses by RIA or ELISA (106, 272, 277).

Alternatively, for rotavirus detection the stool may be kept at 4 C or frozen until ready for direct examination by negative stain EM (see below).

Serologic diagnosis

Two blood samples are needed for demonstrating an antibody response. An acute-phase blood specimen should be obtained within the first few days of onset of illness and a convalescent-phase blood specimen about 3 weeks after onset. The blood is allowed to clot and the serum is separated by centrifugation. Serum is stored at -20 C or lower until ready for use. For antibody studies, whole blood should not be frozen after collection since the blood cells will hemolyze. However, whole blood may be kept at 4 C for about 12–24 hours, and the serum then separated with or without centrifugation if it is not practical to separate the serum from whole blood by centrifugation as described above.

Microscopy

There is no test for examination of stools for viral gastroenteritis agents by direct light microscopy. Stools may be examined directly or after appropriate centrifugation or other procedures for gastrointestinal viral agents by negative stain EM as suspensions or filtrates (10, 12, 21, 34, 51, 57, 78, 88, 124, 164, 168, 181, 188). Rectal swab suspensions may also be examined (121). Stools may also be examined for gastrointestinal viral agents by IEM as suspensions or filtrates (125, 232). Examination of stool smears for rotaviruses directly by FA techniques has resulted in frequent nonspecific reactions, thus preventing the successful implementation of this method (253). Stool suspensions or filtrates have been examined successfully for rotavirus by a fluorescence virus precipitin test (84, 185, 276).

Laboratory Diagnosis of Norwalk and Norwalk-like Agents

Direct examination of the fecal material

Electron microscopy

This group of agents does not have a distinct enough morphology to permit their identification from stool directly by EM (116). However, the Ditchling, W, and cockle agents were visualized after concentration by ultracentrifugation, followed by density gradient centrifugation in cesium chloride (CsCl); for EM, a drop of fluid from a fraction was placed on a slide covered with 0.9% agarose and a grid was placed on the drop for 30 min to permit the CsCl to diffuse into the agarose, followed by staining of the grid with PTA (10, 12).

Immune electron microscopy

This technique was first described in 1941 when electron microscopy was in its infancy (9, 13). In spite of the development of electron microscopes with greater resolving power and of techniques such as negative staining that increased contrast markedly, this technique was relatively underutilized (8, 30, 73a-c, 115, 116). IEM which may be defined as the direct observation of antigen-antibody interaction by EM had been used predominantly with purified antigens (8). However, it has been employed more recently for detecting fastidious viral agents since it has facilitated or enabled their recognition (115, 116). In this technique, antibody directed against an antigen can be observed on the surface of the antigen and, under appropriate conditions, such an antibody causes aggregation of the particles (8, 116). Antibody coated particles and/or specifically aggregated particles may be differentiated from nonspecific matter. IEM has been used recently for the detection of a respiratory coronavirus, Norwalk and Norwalk-like agents, hepatitis A virus, and rotaviruses (73, 116, 119, 124, 125). However, IEM is not essential for the detection of rotavirus in stools since this agent has such a distinctive morphologic appearance it does not need the additional recognition furnished by an antibody coat and/or aggregation (124).

For detection of Norwalk virus particles in stool material, the following technique may be employed (115, 125). Add 0.2 ml of a 1:5 dilution of convalescent Norwalk serum (or if such serum is not available, use a 1:5 dilution of commercially available immune human serum globulin) to an appropriate tube. As a control, add 0.2 ml of 0.01M phosphate-buffered saline (PBS) to another tube. Add 0.8 ml of a 2% stool suspension to each tube, seal tightly, and mix by inverting 15 to 20 times. The mixture is incubated at room temperature for 1 hr. The mixture is then centrifuged at 17,000 rpm for 90 min in a Sorvall RC-2B centrifuge with an SS-34 fixed-angle rotor or in another comparable centrifuge. The supernatant fluid is removed carefully and discarded, and the tubes are inverted in a beaker layered with tissue paper to allow the remaining fluid to drain. The pellet or sediment is resuspended with a few drops of distilled water, stained with 2% phosphotungstic acid, pH 7.2, and placed on a 400-mesh Formvar carbon-coated grid. The excess fluid is removed with the edge of a filter paper disk. The grid is examined at a magnification of about 40,000 with EM. In the preparation of specimens for EM examination, appropriate containment facilities should be available, especially if the presence of a hazardous agent is suspected.

The detection of particles coated with antibody or antibody-like material or the presence of aggregates of particles does not necessarily mean that the particles are of any significance. The specificity of the reaction must be ascertained in further IEM experiments since stools contain much particulate matter which can lead to considerable confusion. Thus, if considering the possibility that a particle is the Norwalk agent, a serologic test must be carried out with the particle as antigen and a specific paired acute- or pre- and post-Norwalk infection sera from a volunteer or from a chimpanzee known by IEM to have developed a seroresponse. Since this method of identification is essentially the same as that used for serologic diagnosis of infection by IEM, it is described in that section later in the chapter.

Radioimmunoassay

RIA for detection of Norwalk agent in fecal specimens has recently been developed (90, 91). This method appears to be even more efficient than IEM for detection of this agent (90, 91). The success of this technique is dependent on the availability of specific reagents. Currently, the only available satisfactory antisera to the Norwalk agent are human or chimpanzee postinfection sera. High-titered convalescent-phase serum and antibody-negative preinfection serum from the same person or chimpanzee must be identified (by IEM or IAHA). At present, these sera are not generally available. As the need dictates, hopefully such reagents will become available commercially or through the National Institutes of Health (NIH). The materials and preparatory methods needed for RIA are as follows (91):

1. High-titered convalescent-phase serum and antibody-negative preinfection Norwalk sera from the same source. These will be replaced by monospecific hyperimmune animal sera when available.

2. IgG fraction of convalescent-phase Norwalk serum. This is prepared by ammonium sulfate precipitation and DEAE-cellulose ion exchange chromatography. This IgG is iodinated with ^{125}I by a modification of the Hunter and Greenwood method (103, 189). Unreacted ^{125}I is removed by chromatography on G50 Sephadex.

3. Norwalk particles to use as a test antigen. 2% stool filtrate or suspension positive for Norwalk agent particles can be used as a positive control test antigen.

4. Polyvinyl microtiter plates.

5. PBS (0.01M with respect to phosphates, 0.15M with respect to NaCl) with 0.1% sodium azide (pH 7.4).

6. PBS with 0.1% sodium azide and 1% bovine serum albumin (PBS-BSA).

7. Test stool suspensions. These suspensions are made as described earlier in PBS, BSA, or in veal infusion broth with 0.5% BSA at a concentration of approximately 2% wt/vol.

The RIA for Norwalk agent is based on the differential binding of stool suspensions containing Norwalk particles to microtiter wells coated with either convalescent-phase or preinfection-phase serum. By this method, nonspecific interaction between infection serum and stools can be differentiated from specific Norwalk particle binding. A diagram of the principle of the Norwalk radioimmunoassay is shown in Figure 30.3.

Test procedure (91). The wells of a microtiter plate are coated with 100 μl of either preinfection-phase or convalescent-phase anti-Norwalk serum. The optimal dilution (in PBS) for precoating is determined by checkerboard titration using the known positive control test antigen. Usually dilutions used for precoating are in the range of 1:1000 to 1:100,000. After 12 hr, the wells are washed 5 times and filled with PBS-BSA for an additional 12 hr or until used; 50-μl volumes of the test samples, as well as positive control test antigen and negative buffer controls, are inoculated in duplicate wells, which had been precoated with either preinfection-phase or convalescent-phase serum. The test is incubated for 18 hr at room temperature. The plate is then washed 5 times, and the wells are inoculated with 50 μl of I^{125} antiNorwalk IgG, approximately 200,000 counts per minute (cpm) per well. Tests are incubated at 37 C for 4 hr. The plate is again washed, and then individual wells are cut apart with scissors, transferred to appropriate tubes for measurement of radioactivity in a gamma counter. The ratio of counts bound to wells coated with convalescent-phase serum, to counts bound to wells coated with preinfection sera is used to determine Norwalk antigen activity. A ratio of positive/negative (P/N) of ≥ 2 is considered indicative of Norwalk antigen activity. This type of assay is at least as sensitive as IEM for detecting Norwalk antigen in stools of volunteers (91). The assay may detect soluble viral antigen as well as particulate material (90). Some stool specimens have high nonspecific activity which masks specific

RADIOIMMUNOASSAY FOR NORWALK ANTIGEN DETECTION

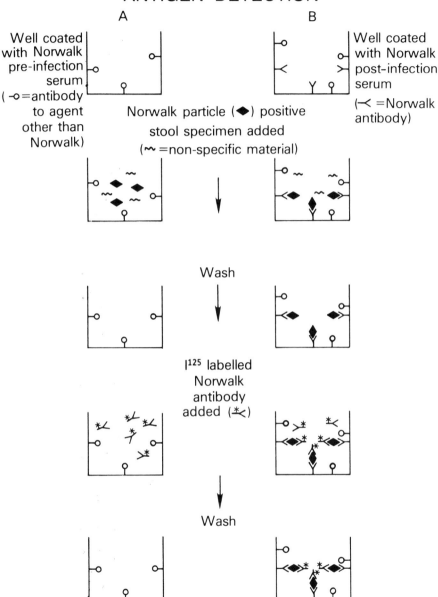

If counts per minute of B/A ⩾ 2 then specimen considered positive for Norwalk agent.

Figure 30.3—Schematic diagram for radioimmunoassay for Norwalk antigen detection.

Norwalk antigen binding. This occurs in fewer than 5% of stool preparations (91).

Virus isolation

The Norwalk agent has not been found to induce illness in any animal model (23, 54, 55, 264). However, chimpanzees inoculated via the alimentary route develop Norwalk infection as demonstrated by virus shedding and serologic response (90, 116, 262). Studies in eggs with the Norwalk agent have not been reported. The Norwalk group of agents has not grown in cell cultures or conclusively in organ cultures (23, 54). The Norwalk group of agents is identified by IEM with appropriate sera bracketing an infection as described below for serologic diagnosis (115, 116, 125). The Norwalk agent is also identified by the RIA as outlined above (91).

Serologic diagnosis
Immune electron microscopy

Up until recently the only method for detecting a serologic response to the Norwalk agent was by IEM (115, 116, 125, 182). In this method, the stool filtrate (or suspension) containing particles is incubated with a standard dilution of antiserum and the amount of antibody coating the particles is rated on a scale of 0 to 4+. The use of IEM for detecting a serologic response has had application in the study of various fastidious viruses such as the Norwalk agent, hepatitis A virus, and rotaviruses (73, 115, 116, 124, 125). In addition, since IEM is employed to facilitate or permit the detection and recognition of fastidious agents as outlined previously, an IEM serologic assay with appropriate paired sera is essential to help determine the significance of a particle observed following reaction with convalescent-phase serum or immune serum globulin (ISG).

The particle-containing suspension is reacted with an acute-phase or preillness-phase serum, and with the convalescent-phase serum (the latter may have been used in the initial IEM study in which the particle was detected) in an attempt to demonstrate a serologic response. In addition, especially if only 2 specimens are being examined, the particle-containing suspension should ideally be reacted with PBS as a control. Each of the paired sera is routinely used at a dilution of 1:5 [or 1:10 in the case of hepatitis A (73)], and the procedure outlined above for the detection of Norwalk agent is utilized (115, 116, 125). The essential factor in such a serologic assay is in the interpretation of the amount of antibody coating the particles. Thus, it is important that critical studies be performed under code to eliminate the possibility of bias in interpretation. Five squares of each grid are routinely examined, and the relative amount of antibody coating the particles is determined on a scale of 0 to 4+. A 0 rating indicates that antibody was not observed coating the particles, whereas a 4+ rating indicates that the particles were so heavily coated with antibody that they were somewhat obscured (Fig 30.4 B & C); a rating of 3+ indicates the presence of a heavy antibody coat but less than 4+, whereas 2+ and 1+ ratings indicate still

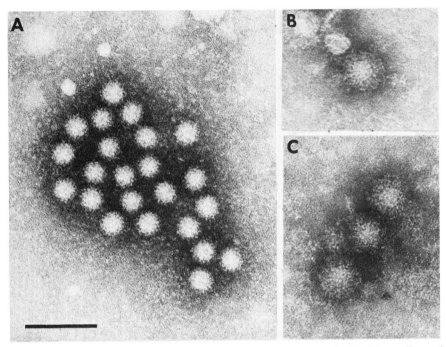

Figure 30.4—A. An aggregate observed after incubation of 0.8 ml of the Norwalk stool
    filtrate with 0.2 ml of a 1:5 dilution of a volunteer's prechallenge serum
    and further preparation for EM. This volunteer developed gastroente-
    ritis following challenge with a second-passage Norwalk filtrate which
    had been heated for 30 min at 60C (54). The quantity of antibody on the
    particles in this aggregate was rated $1-2$ to $2+$ and this prechallenge
    serum was given an overall rating of $1+$ to $2+$.
    B. and C. Single particle (B) and 3 single particles (C) observed after
    incubting 0.8 ml of the Norwalk stool filtrate with 0.2 ml of a dilution
    of the same volunteer's convalescent-phase serum and further prepara-
    tion for EM. These particles are very heavily coated with antibody.
    The quantity of antibody on these particles was rated $4+$ and the serum
    was given an overall rating of $4+$, also. The difference in the quantity
    of antibody coating the particles in the prechallenge and postchallenge
    sera is clearly evident. The bar = 100 nm for each figure. (From ref 116)

lesser amounts (Fig 30.4 A). A $1+$ change in antibody rating between paired
sera is considered significant. As a general rule when $4+$ ratings are observed, the particles are assembled in small aggregates, doublets, or individual particles heavily coated with antibody, whereas with $1+$ to $2+$ ratings
the particles are usually present in larger aggregates.

    When determining by IEM whether a serologic response has occurred
to a known antigen such as Norwalk, the procedures and interpretations are
identical to those outlined above. An example of a significant seroresponse
with a 2% Norwalk stool filtrate as antigen, and pre- and post-challenge sera

from a volunteer who developed illness after administration of the Norwalk agent is shown in Figure 30.4. There is no question that the particles reacted with the convalescent-phase serum have acquired significantly more antibody than those reacted with the prechallenge serum (116).

Pitfalls in IEM studies. Caution must be exercised when interpreting the significance of virus aggregation since certain particles (such as Norwalk) will aggregate spontaneously. Thus, it is critical to determine the amount of antibody coating the particles. If there is question about the specificity of aggregation, the dilutions of antigen or antibody may be varied; this should affect both the size of the aggregates and the amount of antibody coating the particles as the reaction goes from antigen-excess to antibody-excess (52). As noted earlier, particles usually occur predominantly as single units or as doublets in antibody excess, whereas at approximate antigen-antibody equivalence large aggregates of particles lightly coated with antibody are observed, and at antigen-excess single particles, without antibody, may be seen (but not recognized with certainty since numerous other similar structures may be present). In examining paired sera, nonspecific aggregation is not usually a problem since the same conditions exist for each specimen. However, when examining a single serum in IEM tests with the Norwalk agent, antibody ratings of less than 3+ cannot be considered significant, since incubation with PBS may yield a similar rating depending upon the preparation.

A further complication of IEM studies is the presence of other particles which may be confused with a significant agent. For example, groups of 22-nm particles may occasionally be observed in stool specimens. These particles appear to have little or no antibody on them, do not generally change in group size in tests with pre- or acute- and convalescent-phase sera, and do not acquire a significant increase in antibody coating in tests with paired acute- and convalescent-phase sera. Such particles are quite homogeneous in appearance and may be confused with a significant particle if only examining a single specimen. Thus, the mere observation by IEM of virus-like particles in stools does not necessarily mean that they are significant (7, 74, 78, 115, 116, 184).

Many bacteriophage particles are also found in stools (78). Tailed particles are easily identified, whereas those without tails may be more difficult to identify. However, the principles outlined above should be applied to such agents if there is any question about their significance.

Filamentous objects are present in almost all stool preparations. They probably are bacterial flagellae or pili (78). They are easily recognized and should present no problems in interpretation. It is of interest that in isopycnic density gradient centrifugation studies these filamentous objects usually appear in greatest concentration at a density of approximately 1.33–1.35 g/cm^3 in CsCl (Kapikian et al, unpublished studies).

General considerations. The IEM test is reproducible, sensitive, and specific. In a recent study it was shown that for a serially diluted serum sample, 1+ differences in IEM rating represented approximately 10-fold differences in antibody titer (52). In a study with hepatitis A antigen it was found that a 1:64 dilution of a convalescent-phase serum from a patient naturally infected with hepatitis A virus had an IEM rating of 3+ to 4+, the 1:640 dilution a rating of 2+ to 3+, the 1:6400 dilution a rating of 1+, and a 1:64,000 dilution only a trace of antibody (52). In addition, for hepatitis A the IEM ratings of a single dilution of serum were compared with IAHA titers on serial 2-fold dilutions of 92 serum samples from individuals with hepatitis or other illnesses; excellent agreement in antibody quantitation was achieved by the two methods (52). In even more recent studies, for the Norwalk agent, IEM ratings of a single dilution of serum were compared with IAHA and RIA titers on serial dilutions of sera from individuals with Norwalk or other illness; there was a high degree of concordance with serologic responses previously observed by IEM (91, 118). As noted below for human rotavirus, excellent agreement was observed between IEM ratings on single dilutions of serum and CF-antibody titers on serial dilutions of sera from individuals with rotavirus gastroenteritis (112).

Immune adherence hemagglutination assay

Preparation of antigen. The preparation of the IAHA Norwalk antigen from a human stool was similar, but not identical to, that employed for hepatitis A (173). Briefly, stools known to contain Norwalk agent by IEM were made into 20–25% stool suspensions in TN buffer, pH 8 (0.01 M trishydroxymethylaminomethane, 0.15 M NaCl (118). Equal volumes of the stool suspension and trichlorotrifluoroethane (Genetron 113, Allied Chemical Corp. Morristown, NJ) were mixed in a blender at high speed for 1 min and centrifuged for 10 min at 4000 rpm. The aqueous layer was removed and stored. Several additional aqueous extractions with buffer, of the Genetron and stool suspension mixture were also performed. The supernatant fluids were pooled and centrifuged at 5000 rpm for 0.5 hr and the pellet discarded. The Genetron extracted supernatant fluid was centrifuged for 12 hr at 96,000 × *g* using an SW 27 rotor. The supernatant fluid was discarded and approximately 0.5 ml of buffer was added to the pellet. The mixture was stored at 4 C overnight to soften the pellet. The pellet was resuspended in approximately 20–25% of the starting volume of TN buffer and further purified by isopycnic banding in a discontinuous CsCl gradient (1.10 g/cm^3 – 1.60 g/cm^3) at 96,000 × *g* for 18 to 24 hr, in an SW 27 rotor. Routinely, fractions containing the particle (at densities 1.34–1.41 g/cm^3 as detected generally by IEM) were combined and dialyzed in an Amicon ultrafiltration cell and a portion was layered onto a 10–30% sucrose gradient and centrifuged at 152,000 × *g* for 90 min in a SW-40 rotor. The sucrose gradient fractions were tested for IAHA activity using pre- and post-Norwalk-challenge sera from a chimpanzee which was known to have developed a serologic response by IEM.

Test procedure. The test was performed as described for hepatitis A virus extracted from stools (173). Briefly, human sera were heated at 56 C for 30 min and chimpanzee sera at 60 for 30 min. Guinea pig complement was used at a 1:60 dilution. Veronal-buffered saline (VBS), pH 7.5, with 0.1% bovine serum albumin (BSA) was used as diluent for the antigen, serum, and complement. Ethylenediaminetetraacetic acid (EDTA) diluent solution (40 mM) was prepared by mixing 2 parts of 100 mM EDTA (pH 7.5) with 3 parts BSA-VBS. Dithiothreitol solution (3 mg/ml) was made in EDTA-BSA-VBS.

Human group O erythrocytes (RBC) were used as a 1% suspension prepared in the EDTA-BSA-VBS. The Norwalk antigen was standardized, initially by checkerboard titration with pre- and post-Norwalk-infection sera of a chimpanzee or later by testing serial antigen dilutions with 1 or 2 antibody units of the post-infection chimpanzee sera and the same dilution of the preinfection serum (118).

Twenty-five microliters of serum and 25 μl of Norwalk antigen were added to wells of a U-bottom microtiter plate and incubated overnight at 4 C. Twenty-five microliters of a freshly prepared 1:60 dilution (in BSA-VBS) of guinea pig complement was added to the antigen-serum mixture and incubated at 37 C for 40 min; 25 μl of dithiothreitol solution was added to each well, followed by the addition of 25 μl of the 1% human group O RBC suspension. The plate was shaken with a microtiter mixer and then incubated at room temperature. Routinely, hemagglutination patterns were scored on a 0, +/−, and + scale (with 0 and +/− being considered negative and + as positive) when control wells routinely containing each serum dilution with diluent in lieu of antigen, as well as antigen and RBC controls, had developed negative patterns. Patterns usually developed within 1–3 hr and remained essentially the same for several days. Routinely 1–4 units of antigen were used; however, higher-titered preparations had to be used on occasion to increase the sensitivity of the test. The IAHA test was quite efficient for detecting serologic responses as it showed a high degree of concordance with IEM and RIA (see below), but the IEM and RIA were slightly more efficient (91, 118). In addition, the IAHA could not be used successfully to detect Norwalk antigen in stools although purified relatively high titered virus would be detected by this technique (118). A major drawback with the use of IAHA for serologic studies is the lack of an adequate supply of Norwalk antigen to carry out tests routinely. Although IAHA requires considerably less antigen than CF (139), it still utilizes considerably more than the RIA test described below. It should also be noted that not all human group O RBC react comparably in the IAHA; it may be necessary to screen numerous donors' RBC before finding one that reacts sensitively enough with a known antigen.

Radioimmunoassay blocking test (RIA-BL)

The RIA test for Norwalk antigen as described above has been modified to identify Norwalk antibody (91). The assay is based on the ability of a test serum to block the binding of [125]I IgG antiNorwalk to Norwalk antigen. The RIA blocking test (RIA-BL) is highly sensitive and specific. IEM and RIA-BL are equally efficient (both slightly greater than IAHA) at detecting serologic responses in volunteers inoculated with Norwalk agent. The RIA-BL is amenable to large scale studies and can theoretically be used to detect antibody in body fluids other than serum (i.e., intestinal secretions or milk). The reagents and materials needed for RIA-BL are similar to those needed for the RIA for detecting Norwalk antigen: high-titer antiNorwalk serum identified by IEM or IAHA; IgG fraction of antiNorwalk serum, iodinated as described above; partially purified Norwalk particles prepared as described previously or, alternately, suitable crude Norwalk stool suspension which reacts specifically (90); polyvinyl microtiter plates; PBS, and PBS-BSA; and test specimens to be examined for antibody.

A schematic diagram of the RIA-BL test is shown in Figure 30.5, and it is performed as follows (91). The wells of a polyvinyl microtiter plate are precoated with 100 μl of diluted (in PBS) antiNorwalk serum. The optimal dilution is determined by checkerboard titration. This dilution should give the highest binding of a partially purified antigen preparation. The plates are

BLOCKING RADIOIMMUNOASSAY
FOR NORWALK ANTIBODY MEASUREMENT

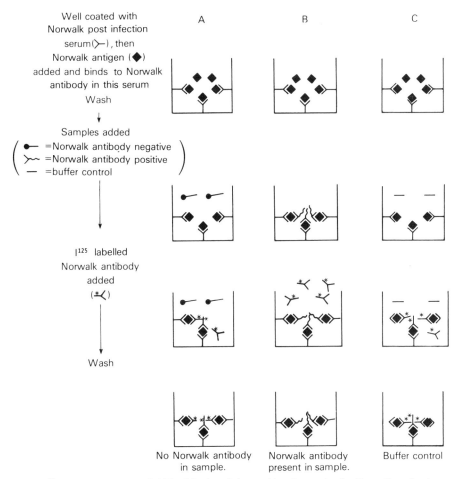

If counts per minute of A/C >0.5, then A is considered negative for Norwalk antibody.

If counts per minute of B/C ≤ 0.5, then B is considered positive for Norwalk antibody.

Figure 30.5—Schematic diagram for blocking radioimmunoassay for Norwalk antibody detection.

incubated for 12 hr at room temperature, washed, and filled with PBS-BSA until used. The plates are washed, and 25 μl of a standard Norwalk antigen preparation is added to all wells. This antigen preparation should have at least 4 binding units and have a P/N ratio in an antigen test of ≥4. The antigen is allowed to absorb to the plates overnight, and the unbound antigen is removed by washing. Then 50 μl of serial 2- or 4-fold dilutions of serum (in PBS-BSA) or buffer controls are added to the wells and incubated at 37 C for 2 hr or overnight. Next 25 μl of ¹²⁵I anti-Norwalk IgG (approximately 200,000 cpm per well) is added to each well. The plates are shaken and the incubation is continued for 4 hr. The plates are then washed and the counts determined as described above. A 50% reduction in residual bound radio-activity produced by a serum compared to a buffer control is taken as evidence of Norwalk antibody. This test requires a less pure and less concentrated antigen preparation than does the IAHA, an important consideration since the source of antigen is so limited (90).

Laboratory Diagnosis of Rotaviruses

Direct examination of fecal material

Electron microscopy

Although the technique was available for decades, it was only recently that stools were examined directly for the presence of viral agents (73a-c, 159). This simple procedure represents an important practical advance in virology. A stool suspension may be examined directly by EM, by taking a small amount of stool and transferring it to a microscope slide and mixing with distilled water (168). A small drop of this suspension is placed on an EM grid stained with PTA, and examined by EM. With these simple techniques the diagnosis of rotavirus infection may be made in just a few minutes after the specimen has been obtained (168). In another method 10–20% stool suspensions are made in distilled water, stained with an equal volume of PTA and examined directly by EM (29). Stool suspensions prepared as outlined previously may also be centrifuged at 17,000 rpm for 1.5 hr, and the pellet reconstituted with distilled water and examined by negative stain EM by methods outlined above (124). The above methods are satisfactory for the detection of rotavirus in pediatric populations studied. However, direct examination, without centrifugation, by negative stain EM of a rectal swab suspension is significantly less efficient for rotavirus detection than is incubation of such a suspension with ISG for 1 hr at room temperature, centrifugation at about 20,000 rpm for 1.5 hr, and examination by negative stain EM (Brandt CD, et al, unpublished studies). Centrifugation of the rectal swab suspension without the addition of ISG would most likely result in a comparable high degree of efficiency for rotavirus detection. Stools should be obtained during the acute phase of illness although shedding for at least 14 days or as long as 23 days after onset of symptoms has been reported (33, 77). However, in one study, rotavirus was not observed in stools obtained after 8 days from onset of symptoms (51).

There are numerous variations to the methods already outlined on the preparation of stools for EM study. Some of these include:

1. Clarifying a 10–20% stool suspension by centrifuging at 3000 rpm for 10 min, followed by 7000 rpm for 30 min, and then centrifuging the supernatant fluid at 30,000 or 50,000 rpm for 0.5 hr or 1 hr, respectively, and examining the resuspended pellet (in distilled water) by negative stain EM (34, 78).

2. Mixing a stool in a homogenizer initially with distilled water, followed by the addition of trifluorotrichlorethane, and further homogenization; the homogenate is centrifuged at 10,000 rpm at 4 C for 30 min to remove fecal debris. Eight percent polyethylene glycol 6000 is added to the supernatant fluid to precipitate virus particles, and the mixture is held overnight at 4 C. The mixture is then centrifuged at $4000 \times g$ for 30 min, and the supernatant fluid is discarded. The deposit is resuspended in distilled water and layered onto 45% sucrose and centrifuged at $100,000 \times g$ for 75–150 min. The pellet is resuspended in distilled water, stained with PTA, and examined by EM. This method was chosen to pellet rotavirus and leave enteroviruses and other small agents in the supernatant fluid (21, 51). With this method patients' stools had 10^7 or 10^9 rotavirus particles/ml (51); $<10^5$ particles/ml would probably not be detected by EM (51, 74). For diagnostic purposes, PTA was preferred because it gave greater contrast, but for studies of fine virus structure, ammonium molybdate staining was preferred (101).

3. Extraction with fluorocarbon and processing for EM by the pseudo-replica technique (57, 88, 181, 188).

Immune electron microscopy

Although it has been utilized successfully for detection of rotaviruses from stool specimens, IEM is not necessary for rotavirus detection in such specimens (124); these agents have such a distinctive morphologic appearance they can be readily identified by conventional EM. However, in research studies in which the role of all agents is being considered, IEM should be utilized since certain agents, like the Norwalk group (and hepatitis A) cannot be identified by conventional EM; in addition, the recognition of as yet undetected agents might be facilitated or enabled by IEM. The IEM procedure and its interpretation have been described in detail above for the Norwalk agent. A description of the use of IEM for rotavirus detection from rectal swab specimens is outlined above under EM.

Counter immunoelectroosmophoresis (CIEOP) (18, 89, 166, 224, 242)

A CIEOP test for detection of rotavirus was developed during early studies with rotaviruses as a possible practical alternative to EM in a clinical virology service; it was later also evaluated in epidemiologic studies (166). Basically, a stool suspension is placed in a well on an agarose slide and human or calf rotavirus antiserum is placed in an adjacent well. A precipitin line develops between the wells of the rotavirus positive sample and rotavirus antiserum after incubation and application of an electrical current.

Staining with tannic acid or Coomassie brilliant blue further increased sensitivity in two of the studies (166, 242).

Radioimmunoassay

RIA, direct or indirect method, was applied to the study of rotaviruses in stool suspensions or filtrates as a detection technique which could be used in large scale studies (106, 165). The test is dependent on the availability of specific and sensitive hyperimmune sera, radioactively labeled IgG, and a gamma radiation counter.

To perform the direct test (106), wells of a microtiter plate are coated with 75 μl of hyperimmune serum. The optimal dilution is determined by checkerboard titration with a known positive antigen. The usual range is a 1:1000 to 1:10,000 serum dilution. After 4 hr, the precoated wells are washed and saturated at 4 C with a PBS-BSA solution for 12 hr or until used. A 25-μl volume of test sample is added to duplicate wells and incubated for 40-48 hr at 4 C. The incubation of antigen can be carried out for shorter periods (1–4 hr) at 37 C. The test sample is removed and the well washed 5 times with PBS; 50 μl of ^{125}I labeled antirotavirus IgG (approx. 2 × 10^5 cpm/well) is added and allowed to incubate for 1-4 hr at 37 C. The wells are washed 5 times with PBS to remove the unbound conjugate. Each well is cut out and placed in a tube to be counted in a gamma counter. A P/N value is calculated by using cpm from known negative specimens as a denominator for the test samples. A P/N of ≥2 is considered positive. A blocking test can be used to demonstrate specificity, especially for borderline positive samples. In the indirect RIA, polystyrene "tissue culture" tubes were precoated with rabbit antihuman rotavirus globulin (capture antibody) which bound the rotavirus to the solid phase; the second antibody (detector antibody) was guinea pig antihuman rotavirus globulin, and the third antibody (indicator antibody) was an ^{125}I labeled goat antiguinea pig IgG (165). The test was standardized so that results could be obtained on the same day the test was started. In the indirect RIA, a single indicator antibody can be used for a variety of agents as long as the detector antibody is derived from the same host, whereas in the direct RIA, detector-indicator antibody must be labeled for each virus being studied. A filter paper solid-phase RIA for rotavirus has also been described using human rotavirus antiserum or SA-11 antiserum (249). Rotaviruses covered with antibody were found in clinical specimens, and it was suggested that this would interfere with the RIA system employed (248). A direct microtiter RIA employing guinea pig SA-11 antiserum as the precoat and ^{125}I labeled anti-SA-11 guinea pig IgG as the second antibody has been developed; it appears to be sensitive and specific for human rotavirus detection (21a, 48a). It has the practical advantage of utilizing antiserum prepared with a readily available cell culture grown rotavirus.

Enzyme-linked immunosorbent assay

The ELISA is similar in principle to the RIA except that it uses a color change induced by an enzyme acting on a substrate as the indicator system rather than the measurement of radioactivity (61, 247). Its success depends on the knowledge that antigen or antibody can be attached to a solid-phase and still retain immunologic activity and the assumption that antibody can be linked to an enzyme, and that the antibody-enzyme complex still retains immunologic and enzymatic activity (247). Thus, an enzyme, such as alkaline phosphatase or peroxidase, is used as an immunoglobulin marker, and the enzyme-labeled immunoglobulin is quantitated by measuring the amount of reaction with a specific substrate (247). Since a single molecule of enzyme can react with many molecules of substrate, very small amounts of immunoglobulin can be detected.

For rotavirus antigen detection, a direct and an indirect ELISA have been developed (66, 67, 203, 272, 277). In the direct test, wells of polyvinyl microtiter plates are precoated with antirotavirus antibody (capture antibody). The second antibody is conjugated with the enzyme; it may be derived from the same host as the precoat antibody (272). The direct test is shown schematically in Figure 30.6.

In the indirect ELISA, the wells are precoated with the capture antibody as above, but the second antibody (detector antibody) must be derived from a different host than the precoat antibody (277); otherwise the antiglobulin-enzyme conjugate (indicator antibody) directed against the second antibody would combine nonspecifically with the precoat antibody. The indirect test is shown schematically in Figure 30.7. The indirect test has the advantage of additional amplification because a single molecule of the second antibody can react with several molecules of the antiglobulin-enzyme conjugate. In addition, a single antiglobulin-enzyme conjugate can be used in ELISA for a variety of agents as long as the second antibody is derived from the same host. The direct ELISA has the disadvantage of requiring the preparation of an enzyme-conjugated antiserum for each virus being studied.

Performance of the indirect ELISA (272, 277).

1. Use only the inner 60 wells of a polyvinyl microtiter plate; fill the outer wells with PBS Tween at each step to insure even heat distribution.

2. By checkerboard titration, the optimal dilution of the antirotavirus serum used for precoating (capture antibody) is determined. In our laboratory, rotavirus antiserum produced in a goat is used at a dilution of 1:10,000 to 1:100,000 depending upon the sensitivity of the test at different times. Add 100 μl of this antiserum to the inner wells of a soft round-bottom polyvinyl microtiter plate. Place at 4 C for at least 24 hr before using; plates may be stored at 4 C for at least 6 months.

3. Just prior to use, wash 3 times in PBS-Tween.

4. Add 50 μl of PBS-Tween containing 1% fetal calf serum and 0.5% goat serum followed by 50 μl of the stool suspension (2–10%). (The sera should be rotavirus antibody negative, or at least negative at the dilutions used.) Incubate at 37 C for 1 hr followed by overnight at 4 C for maximum sensitivity; shorter periods of incubation (e.g., 1 hr at 37 C) may also be employed for rapid diagnosis.

5. Wash 3 times with PBS.

6. Add 100 μl of guinea pig antirotavirus serum (detector antibody) at an optimal dilution which has been determined by checkerboard titration. In our laboratory a 1:3000–1:6000 dilution is employed. This serum is diluted in PBS-Tween containing 1% fetal calf serum and 0.5% goat serum. Incubate 1 hr at 37 C.

7. Wash three times with PBS-Tween.

8. Add 100 μl of alkaline phosphatase labeled antiguinea pig serum (indicator antibody) at an optimal dilution which has been determined by testing at various dilutions for sensitivity. The conjugate is diluted in PBS-Tween containing 1% fetal calf serum and 0.5% normal goat serum (dilution of conjugate used in our laboratory 1:600). Incubate at 37 C for 1 hr.

9. Wash 3 times with PBS-Tween.

10. Add 100 μl of p-nitrophenyl phosphate substrate solution (1 tablet of Sigma 104 substrate for each 5 ml of 10% diethanolamine buffer). Incubate at 37 C until yellow color appears in the positive control.

DIRECT ELISA FOR ANTIGEN MEASUREMENT

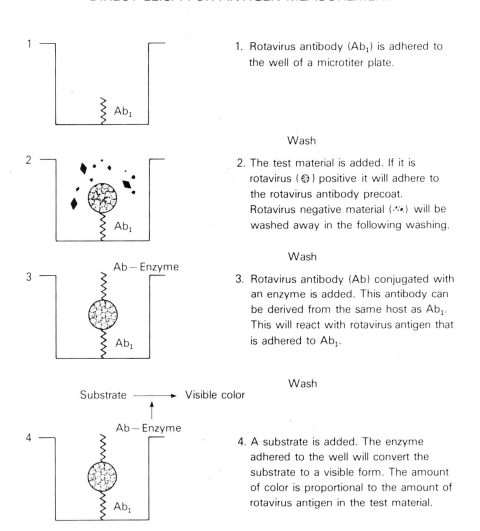

1. Rotavirus antibody (Ab$_1$) is adhered to the well of a microtiter plate.

Wash

2. The test material is added. If it is rotavirus (⊕) positive it will adhere to the rotavirus antibody precoat. Rotavirus negative material (·⁙·) will be washed away in the following washing.

Wash

3. Rotavirus antibody (Ab) conjugated with an enzyme is added. This antibody can be derived from the same host as Ab$_1$. This will react with rotavirus antigen that is adhered to Ab$_1$.

Wash

4. A substrate is added. The enzyme adhered to the well will convert the substrate to a visible form. The amount of color is proportional to the amount of rotavirus antigen in the test material.

Figure 30.6—Schematic diagram for direct ELISA for rotavirus detection.

INDIRECT ELISA FOR ROTAVIRUS ANTIGEN MEASUREMENT

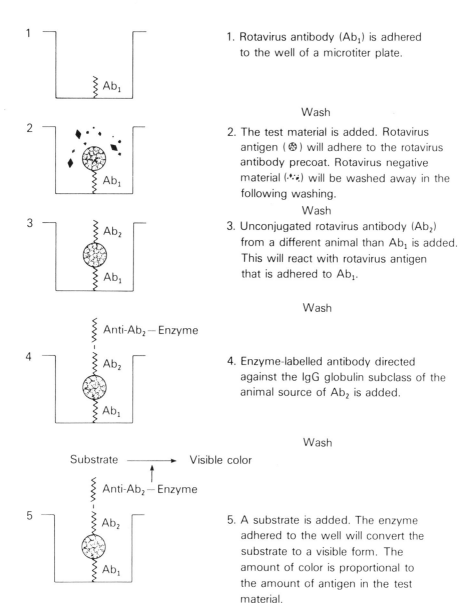

1. Rotavirus antibody (Ab_1) is adhered to the well of a microtiter plate.

Wash

2. The test material is added. Rotavirus antigen (✿) will adhere to the rotavirus antibody precoat. Rotavirus negative material (˙·˙:) will be washed away in the following washing.

Wash

3. Unconjugated rotavirus antibody (Ab_2) from a different animal than Ab_1 is added. This will react with rotavirus antigen that is adhered to Ab_1.

Wash

4. Enzyme-labelled antibody directed against the IgG globulin subclass of the animal source of Ab_2 is added.

Wash

5. A substrate is added. The enzyme adhered to the well will convert the substrate to a visible form. The amount of color is proportional to the amount of antigen in the test material.

Figure 30.7—Schematic diagram for indirect ELISA for rotavirus detection.

Reading the ELISA test. One advantage of ELISA is that the endpoint of the reaction is a visible color (yellow with alkaline phosphatase, and red-brown with peroxidase). Thus, the test can be read with the unaided eye by comparing the color observed in the test well with that of a positive standard of known strength and, if available, with negative controls. In addition, a permanent record of the test can be kept by means of a color photograph. Spectrophotometric techniques may be employed if a numerical reading is desired. Conventional spectrophotometers are not practical for reading large numbers of test specimens because it is cumbersome and time consuming to transfer the reactant solution to the cuvette of the machine. In addition, the transfer of large numbers of specimens raises the potential problem of error in handling. To overcome these problems, an ELISA reader, which is capable of reading the color intensity [optical density (OD)] of a test well through the bottom of the microtiter plate has recently been developed (44, 272). Such a reader can be built from plans available from BEID, NIH, Bethesda, MD or can be purchased from a commercial source. Initially, the standard deviation of the assay system in tests with 15 negative specimens was found to be 0.45 (P/N theoretically = 1 for negative specimens). Therefore a P/N value at least 2 standard deviations above 0.45 (i.e., 1.9) may be used as a cutoff value for possible positivity. The P/N value is determined by testing approximately 4 negative controls in each test and dividing the OD of the test specimen by that of the mean of the negatives. Specimens with a P/N ≥2 may be positive and thus should be blocked as outlined below to determine if the reaction is specific (272). (However, the "N" value should ideally be at least 2 standard deviations greater than the intrinsic variation of the test system). Alternatively, a weakly positive standard can be included and the OD of the test specimen can be compared with the OD of the standard. Such a system has the advantage of requiring fewer control specimens but has the disadvantage of limiting the sensitivity of the test to that of the positive standard; such a system is preferred when visual readings are employed. However, all presumed positive reactions should be blocked as outlined below.

Confirmation of positive results. The specificity of the positive reaction should be confirmed by means of a blocking test as outlined schematically in Figure 30.8 (247). The test specimen is incubated with a serum with, and a serum without, rotavirus antibody. The antibody containing serum should block the ELISA activity more than the serum without specific antibody. The test is performed as follows (247):

1. Add 75 µl of the specimen to be blocked to 75 µl of prerotavirus-infection serum (or if this is not available use a serum negative for rotavirus antibody) diluted 1:5 in PBS-Tween. (This dilution should be adjusted depending on the titer of the standard positive serum). Add 75 µl of the specimen to be blocked to 75 µl of the standard postinfection serum diluted 1:5 in PBS-Tween. The specimen-serum mixtures should be mixed well. (A low serum dilution is usually preferred so that high-titer antigen can be adequately blocked). The serum used for precoating or as the second antibody should not be used as the blocking serum.

2. Incubate for 2 hr at 37 C.

ELISA BLOCKING ASSAY

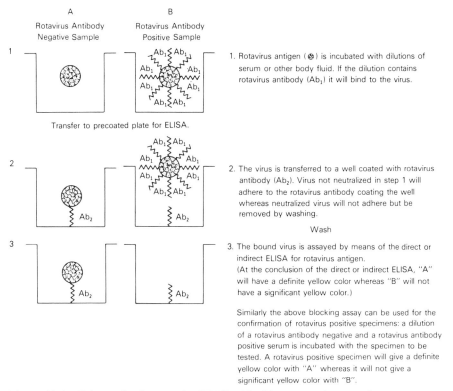

A
Rotavirus Antibody
Negative Sample

B
Rotavirus Antibody
Positive Sample

Transfer to precoated plate for ELISA.

Wash

1. Rotavirus antigen (⊛) is incubated with dilutions of serum or other body fluid. If the dilution contains rotavirus antibody (Ab_1) it will bind to the virus.

2. The virus is transferred to a well coated with rotavirus antibody (Ab_2). Virus not neutralized in step 1 will adhere to the rotavirus antibody coating the well whereas neutralized virus will not adhere but be removed by washing.

3. The bound virus is assayed by means of the direct or indirect ELISA for rotavirus antigen.
   (At the conclusion of the direct or indirect ELISA, "A" will have a definite yellow color whereas "B" will not have a significant yellow color.)

   Similarly the above blocking assay can be used for the confirmation of rotavirus positive specimens: a dilution of a rotavirus antibody negative and a rotavirus antibody positive serum is incubated with the specimen to be tested. A rotavirus positive specimen will give a definite yellow color with "A" whereas it will not give a significant yellow color with "B".

Figure 30.8—Schematic diagram for ELISA blocking assay for rotavirus.

3. Transfer 50 μl to duplicate wells of a microtiter plate coated with goat antirotavirus serum and process as outlined by indirect (or direct) ELISA for rotavirus detection.

4. Rotavirus-containing specimens should demonstrate at least a 50% reduction in the amount of yellow color after incubation with postinfection serum as compared to that with preinfection serum (271, 272). The reduction in color should be observed readily with the unaided eye. Inclusion of a weakly positive control specimen in the blocking test is helpful in evaluating the color change by the unaided eye. If reading by machine the % blocking is calculated as follows (271):

$$\% \text{ blocking} = \frac{\text{OD with preinfection serum} - \text{OD with postinfection serum}}{\text{OD with preinfection serum}} \times 100$$

where the OD pre- and postinfection serum are the OD at 400 nm. Fifty percent blocking by the postinfection serum is considered confirmation that the test sample contained rotavirus antigen. If 50% blocking is not achieved with a specimen which appears to be more than questionably positive (by virtue of a high P/N value and/or a bright yellow color in the test), the specimen should be diluted and retested to determine if the failure to block is due to antigen excess.

An alternate method for detection of rotavirus and confirmation of positive result in a single test by indirect ELISA

The technique is basically the same as above for performance of the indirect ELISA with a few modifications as follows:

1. One row of wells is precoated with a rotavirus antibody negative serum (or at least negative at the dilution employed); an adjacent row is precoated with an optimal dilution of rotavirus antibody positive serum. (The same dilution for precoating is used with the negative serum as for the positive serum). In our laboratory 1:10,000 dilutions of pre- and post-human rotavirus immunization goat sera (from the same goat) have been employed.

2. The stool suspension is placed in 2 wells coated with rotavirus antibody negative serum and in 2 wells coated with rotavirus antibody positive serum.

3. If the OD with rotavirus antibody positive serum is at least 2 standard deviations greater than the OD with the rotavirus antibody negative serum the specimen is considered to be rotavirus positive.

4. If specimens react with intense yellow color with both sera, the yellow colored mixtures should be diluted to determine if there is a dilution at which a significant difference in OD occurs between the 2 sera.

5. If the OD with the rotavirus positive serum is not twice that with the rotavirus negative serum, the specimen is considered to be negative.

6. When this method is used the normal goat serum may be omitted from the diluent, since false positive reactions due to goat antibody in stool should not occur because such antibody should bind equally to rotavirus antibody negative and positive sera (see below).

ELISA for detection of rotavirus serotypes

Serotypes of human rotavirus can also be differentiated by ELISA if type-specific antiserum is available (273). In the ELISAs outlined above, both the goat and the guinea pig antirotavirus sera were prepared with a rotavirus strain which is now known to be type 2. However, no attempt was made to produce a type-specific serum since the existence of serotypes was unknown. Therefore, these sera are broadly reactive, containing antibody to the common as well as the type specific antigenic determinants and are thus quite effective for rotavirus screening purposes; but they cannot differentiate between type 1 and type 2 rotavirus. However, if a rotavirus-specific antiserum is employed as the second antibody (e.g., guinea pig serum prepared for typing purposes as outlined previously) in the indirect ELISA, the same test as described above can be utilized to identify a serotype. The relative type-specificity of this serum will determine whether or not a heterologous serotype will also react with it. However, even if the specificity of the serum is not absolute, a specimen may be tested with a type 1 and type 2 serum, and the P/N value will be significantly greater with the homologous antiserum (273). Adsorption of the guinea pig serum with heterotypic human rotavirus or an animal rotavirus (containing common antigenic determinants) might increase the effectiveness of the typing procedure.

Blocking ELISA for identification of rotavirus from different species

ELISA may also be employed to distinguish rotaviruses from different host species by means of a blocking test outlined above (271). The blocking sera are the key reagents for differentiating the human rotavirus from various animal rotaviruses and various animal rotaviruses from each other. The availability of sera containing antibody induced initially or solely by infection with each rotavirus strain being tested is essential for differentiating the various rotaviruses since hyperimmune antisera prepared with antigen containing the species-specific and common determinants will react about equally with both human and animal rotaviruses (271).

In this test, the post-infection serum and preinfection or normal newborn serum are diluted in 4-fold serial dilutions (starting at 1:10) and incubated at 37 C for 2 hr with an equal volume of the rotavirus suspension (271). The unbound (unblocked) virus is assayed by the basic indirect ELISA using the hyperimmune goat serum for precoating and the hyperimmune guinea pig serum as the second antibody. To insure comparability of the various antigens and sera in the blocking procedure the antigen is first assayed by indirect ELISA as outlined above and the endpoint titer determined and 10 times this dilution is employed (10 units) in the blocking step; each serum is assayed with 10 units of the homologous virus to determine the dilution at which it achieves about 50% blocking. In the initial study for uniformity the sera were diluted if necessary, so that a working dilution of 1:1000 resulted in approximately 50% blocking of the homologous virus (271). The dilution where 50% blocking is achieved is calculated in a manner similar to that above (271).

Infection (or at least initial infection) serum blocked (50%) the homologous virus at a dilution which was 50- to 100-fold greater than that at which it blocked the heterologous virus. By this method the human and bovine strains could be distinguished from each other and from the porcine, equine, simian, and murine rotaviruses, and the O agent (271). The porcine, equine, simian, and murine rotavirus antisera demonstrated a similar specific pattern (271). Infection sera were not available for the SA-11 and O agents.

Thus, ELISA can be used to determine the source of a rotavirus strain. This is of more than academic interest since the host of origin must be ascertained for many reasons. Thus any rotavirus preparation can be tested with a battery of postinfection antisera to ascertain if one blocks it at a dilution at least 10-fold greater than that at which it blocks the others (271). Similarly, antiserum to a rotavirus can be checked with a battery of rotavirus antigens to ascertain which one induced the antibody.

Potential false-positive reactions. Although the ELISA for rotavirus is efficient, sensitive, and specific, false-positive reactions occur if the antigen, antiserum, or conjugate bind nonspecifically to the solid-phase. One way to avoid this is to employ a careful washing technique so that the nonspecifically adhering substances will be washed away and also spillover between wells does not occur. False-positive reactions also occur if the stool preparation contains antibody against the serum used for precoating. For example, it was found that certain stools from Bangladesh gave a positive reaction in the absence of rotavirus (277). Further investigation revealed that these false-positive reactions were most likely due to the presence of antibodies to goat protein, presumably a result of the ingestion of goat meat, and goat milk (277). Such antibodies were binding to the goat antirotavirus precoat and then to the enzyme-labeled goat antiguinea pig serum, thus giving rise to the characteristic yellow color; however, the reaction was not blocked by the addition of antirotavirus serum. Such false-positive reactions could however be blocked by the addition of excess normal goat serum as diluent as outlined previously, since normal goat serum acted to absorb the antibody to goat protein in the stool (277). Thus, all stools tested for rotavirus are diluted in the well in a solution containing 0.5% normal goat serum since this concentration of goat serum is about 50 times the concentration of the goat antirotavirus serum used for precoating. The antigoat antibody in the stool should bind to the normal goat serum in the liquid phase and be removed in the washing step. It is important that the normal goat serum used as a diluent not have detectable rotavirus antibody at the dilution used, as such antibody would bind rotavirus present in the stool and might block its reaction with the goat antirotavirus precoat (resulting in an inadvertent positive blocking test). Fetal calf serum is added to the diluent in the various steps outlined to block unbound sites on the solid-phase. This serum should be tested to establish that it does not have contaminating rotavirus antibody at the dilution used. Preincubation of the stool suspension with an equal volume of 20% N-acetyl cysteine may be helpful in decreasing the number of false positive reactions (41a, Yolken, unpublished studies).

If the alternate method of rotavirus detection is not employed, all positive reactions achieved by the conventional indirect ELISA should be blocked to assure the specificity of the reaction.

Reagents. ELISA systems outlined above are relatively easy to perform; however, the availability of reagents for such tests is a major obstacle for most laboratories. Appropriate hyperimmune sera may be prepared as outlined earlier if suitable antigens are available. It is anticipated that suitable sera for the basic ELISA will be prepared under NIH and commercial auspices.

For preparation of conjugate the following materials are needed: glutaraldehyde, 25%; alkaline phosphatase (Sigma type VII, 1000 units per cc); sodium sulfate 36%, 24%, 18%, and 12%; phosphate-buffered saline (PBS), pH 7.4; and the antiserum to be conjugated.

To perform the conjugation procedure (247): 1 ml of antiserum is diluted with 1 ml of PBS; 2 ml of 36% sodium sulfate is added to the diluted serum. The resulting precipitate is centrifuged at 2000 rpm and washed with 18% sodium sulfate. The precipitate is then redissolved in 1 ml of PBS and reprecipitated with an equal volume of 24% sodium sulfate. The precipitate is again centrifuged at 2000 rpm and washed with 12% sodium sulfate. The remaining precipitate is redissolved in 1 ml of PBS and dialyzed against PBS with 4 changes of buffer. The remaining solution is centrifuged at 6000 rpm for 15 min, the supernatant fluid is saved, and the pelleted euglobulin is discarded. The globulin concentration of the supernatant fluid is determined by measuring the OD at 260 nm and 280 nm with the result read from a standard nomograph (249a). An amount of this solution containing 2 mg of globulin determined as above is transferred to a test tube, and PBS is added to make up a final volume of 1 ml. One milliliter of the enzyme solution is centrifuged at 2000 rpm ror 10 min, and the supernatant fluid is discarded. One milliliter of the solution prepared above containing 2 mg of globulin is added. After the precipitate is dissolved, the solution is transferred to a dialysis bag and dialyzed against PBS with 4 changes of buffer. The solution is then removed from the dialysis bag, and glutaraldehyde is added to a final concentration of 0.2%. The mixture is left at room temperature until a slight yellow appears in the solution. The usual time for this reaction is 1 to 1.5 hr. The mixture is then transferred to a dialysis bag and dialyzed again against PBS at 4 C with 4 changes of buffer. This solution is then dialyzed in the same bag against 0.05 M Tris buffer, pH 8, with 4 changes of buffer. The resulting solution is diluted to a final concentration of 4 ml with 0.05 M Tris containing 1% fetal calf serum and 0.2% sodium azide. This conjugate is dispensed into 1-ml amounts and stored at 4 C in brown vials or vials covered with tin foil to prevent exposure to light.

The potency of the conjugate may be tested by checkerboard titration. However, a practical way of establishing the correct dilution to use is to carry out an ELISA using known positive and negative specimens and to determine the most dilute strength of conjugate which identifies all of the positive specimens. In general, we have found that antiguinea pig IgG and antihuman IgG conjugates are active in the range of 1:400 to 1:800, and antihuman IgA, antihuman IgM, antirabbit IgG, and antigoat IgG are active at dilutions ranging from 1:200 to 1:400. An antihuman IgG conjugated with alkaline phosphatase is currently available commercially. Alternatively, a conjugate may be used which utilizes horseradish peroxidase as the enzyme instead of alkaline phosphatase. In reported rotavirus ELISA studies with horseradish peroxidase as the enzyme, hydrogen peroxide has been used as the substrate along with a coloragen (66, 67, 87a). It should be noted that various coloragens have been described as having carcinogenic and teratogenic properties (16b, 70a, 175b, 205a). With a peroxidase conjugate bacteriostatic agents such as sodium azide should be omitted from the buffers as they will substantially inhibit peroxidase activity.

Summary of methods available for rotavirus detection and evaluation of their efficiency and practicality

Table 30.4 shows numerous methods that have been described for detection of rotaviruses and rates them on a 1+ to 4+ scale with 1+ indicating a low degree of efficiency or practicality and 4+ a high degree. The description presented above has highlighted the ELISA for detection of rotavirus. Although EM and IEM are very efficient and have been the standard by which all other tests are judged, they are not practical for large scale epidemiologic studies. ELISA, on the other hand, is practical, efficient, and does not require sophisticated equipment. Thus, it is the method of choice in

TABLE 30.4—EFFICIENCY AND PRACTICALITY OF METHODS AVAILABLE FOR DETECTING
HUMAN ROTAVIRUSES IN STOOL SPECIMENS

METHOD	EFFICIENCY*	PRACTICALITY*†
Electron microscopy (21, 75, 124, 168, 188)	4+	1+
Immune electron microscopy (121, 124)	4+	<1+
Complement-fixation (conventional) (88, 133, 168, 209, 222, 241)	1+	4+
Human fetal intestinal organ culture (with FA) (266)	1+	0
Counterimmunoelectro-osmophoresis (18, 89, 166, 222, 224, 242)	3+ to 4+	4+
Fluorescent virus precipitin test (84, 185, 276)	4+	1+
Cell culture (cytopathic effect) (171, 261)	<1+	2+ to 3+
Cell culture (with FA) (6, 171, 190, 261)	1+	<1+
Cell culture (with EM) (6, 190, 261)	<1+	<1+
Centrifugation onto cell culture (with FA) (16, 35, 235, 240)	3+ to 4+	1+
Gel diffusion (257)	1+	4+
Smears (with FA) (253)	1+	4+
Radioimmunoassay (21a, 48a, 106, 165)	4+	3-4+
Enzyme-linked immunosorbent assay (ELISA) (272, 277)	4+	4+
Immune adherence hemagglutination assay (151)	3+	2-3+
RNA electrophoresis patterns in gels (70)	3+	1+
Modified complement-fixation (283)	3+ to 4+	2-3+

*On a scale of 1+ to 4+ where 1+ indicates low degree of efficiency or practicality, and 4+ indicates a high degree of efficiency or practicality.

†For large-scale epidemiologic studies, assuming 4+ efficiency.

our laboratory for testing large numbers of specimens. CIEOP has in general been very efficient and quite practical for large scale studies. However, its efficiency has varied from 37% to 100% for detecting rotavirus in specimens known to be positive by EM (18, 166, 222, 224, 242). In one report, it was more sensitive and efficient than EM (89). It may be the method of choice in laboratories, where its efficiency is about that of EM. Screening of stool material by conventional CF has occasionally provided a simple way to detect rotavirus (166, 209, 222, 242, Kapikian et al, unpublished studies). However, this technique has been limited, in general, by low sensitivity, the high percentage of stools which are anticomplementary, and the necessity for some type of purification or clarification procedure.

Recently, however, a modified CF technique which appears to be considerably more sensitive than the conventional CF test has been shown to distinguish rotavirus serotypes, to be as efficient as EM and IEM for detection of rotaviruses in stool suspensions and to provide a quantitative measurement of virus excretion (281–283). The stool specimens were prepared as 30% suspensions and clarified by centrifuging at 5000 rpm for 10 min; the supernatant fluid was centrifuged again the same way, and the clarified supernatant was used as antigen (283). Moreover, anticomplementary (AC) activity of clarified stool suspensions was usually removed by absorption with fetal calf serum. This modified CF technique employed 0.25% sheep RBC, 2 HD_{100} (hemolytic dose) of complement and 1 optimal sensitizing dose of he-molytic serum. After incubation overnight at 4 C the sensitized RBC were added, and the mixtures incubated at 37 C for 1 hr. They were then centri-fuged for 30 seconds at 3000 rpm; the latter resulted in definite buttons of RBC in appropriate wells (283). Although this technique appears promising it is not as practical as ELISA, since clarification of stool suspensions ap-pears to be necessary. In addition, anticomplementary activity may persist in an occasional specimen. This CF system was used to differentiate the two rotavirus serotypes employing appropriate type-specific antisera (83, 281). With rotavirus antisera which have both the common and type-specific determinants, both serotypes are detected by CF (281).

An IAHA for detection of rotavirus antigen in stools has been de-scribed (151). The test was less sensitive and slightly less efficient than EM for detecting rotavirus. The IAHA was usually positive when the number of rotavirus particles by EM exceeded 1×10^9/ml (151). A limitation on the use of IAHA for antigen detection is that the stool specimens must frequently be clarified and/or fluorocarbon extracted to eliminate nonspecific agglutination and/or AC activity. The fluorescent virus precipitin test, which invloves the detection of virus-antibody complexes by epifluorescence microscopy, has been shown to be efficient for detection of rotaviruses but is not practical for large scale studies (84, 185, 276). As described previously and again later, cell culture methods with one exception have not been efficient for rotavirus detection (6, 190, 261, 263, 266). The exception consists of the inoculation of 20% fecal filtrates onto confluent pig kidney (IB-RS-2) or monkey kidney (LLC-MK2) monolayers, centrifugation of the inoculated cultures at low speed for 2 hr at 4 C followed by examination by indirect FA tech-niques (16, 35, 235, 240). This method has proved to be relatively efficient but is impractical for large scale epidemiologic studies. Centrifugation at somewhat higher speeds further increased efficiency (240). Gel diffusion has been low in efficiency for rotavirus detection (257). Examination of fecal smears by FA has yielded variable results mainly on account of nonspecific reactions (253). The RIA which was the precursor of the ELISA for rota-virus detection is both efficient and practical (106, 165). It can be carried out with similar reagents as the ELISA, except that radioactive-labeled con-jugate is used instead of an enzyme label. It has the disadvantage of requir-ing special equipment and involves the use of radioactive-labeled reagents both of which may not be available in field situations. Rotavirus has also been identified from clinical specimens by determining RNA electrophoresis patterns in gels (70). However, the technique was not as efficient as EM, as 20% of the clinical specimens positive by EM did not demonstrate viral RNA after electrophoresis (70).

It is astounding that in this era of tissue culture virology almost all of the techniques outlined above for virus detection do not require *in vitro* cultiva-tion but rather use the concept of ''direct virology'' outlined earlier. Each has been described in detail elsewhere and the interested reader is referred to the appropriate references shown for further details.

Virus isolation

Isolation in animals and eggs

Disease has not been observed in small laboratory animals such as rats, hamsters, guinea pigs, and normal or "nude" thymus deficient suckling mice inoculated with human rotavirus (32, 168, Wyatt et al, unpublished studies). As noted earlier, human rotavirus induces a diarrheal illness in newborn animals such as calves, piglets, lambs, and monkeys. However, for diagnostic purposes, the use of animals would not be necessary or practical. Animal studies are helpful in studies of virulence and pathogenesis in addition to providing useful reagents (antigen and antibody). Animals maintained under gnotobiotic conditions are inoculated either orally or by the intraduodenal route (in calves) (161, 162, 218, 238). Monkeys are inoculated by stomach tube (267) or by direct instillation into the duodenum and stomach. (136, 169). Diarrhea occurred within 24 hr of inoculation in calves, from 2 to 5 days in the monkeys, 2–7 days in piglets, and 2 days in lambs. Virus infection could be documented by presence of rotavirus in feces and by a serum antibody response. Viral antigens stainable by FA were found in intestinal epithelial cells of infected animals. Rotavirus has not been successfully propagated in embryonated eggs (168).

Isolation in tissue or organ cultures

Isolation of rotavirus from clinical specimens is not currently practical as a means of diagnosing infection. The following techniques have, however, proved useful for limited study of strains of human and animal rotaviruses.

Human embryonic intestinal organ culture. Villous epithelial cells of explants of human embryonic intestine supported the growth of 3 of 15 human rotavirus strains (266). Viral antigens were located in the cytoplasm of single infected cells or in small foci of cells and were detected using indirect FA as described below. Frozen sections 12 μm in thickness were fixed in cold acetone for 10 min and were stored at −70 C until used.

LLC-MK2 and IB-RS-2. The detection of human rotaviruses in established cell lines (LLC-MK2 and IB-RS-2) inoculated in the following manner has been described (16, 35, 235, 240). Stool filtrates are inoculated onto coverslip preparations or into microtiter plates containing confluent cell monolayers. Inoculated cells are spun at 1200–3000 $\times$ g for 1–2 hr (centrifugation at 10,000 $\times$ g further increases sensitivity and efficiency) (240). After 18–24 hr incubation at 37 C, cultures are fixed in methanol or acetone, and preparations are stained for detection of rotaviral antigens using indirect FA techniques. While serial passage of rotavirus has not been reported using these techniques, they may be of limited usefulness as a diagnostic alternative.

Monolayer cultures of embryonic gut. Both trypsinized human and bovine embryonic gut monolayer cultures have been used in attempts to propagate human rotavirus (6, 190). Cytoplasmic fluorescent viral antigens were detected in human gut cultures grown in medium No. 199; in this system additional gut cells were added at 6- to 7-day intervals and antigens were detected at 18 days after inoculation (190). Bovine gut monolayers maintained in minimal essential medium (MEM) with 1% fetal calf serum supported limited virus growth which usually diminished on passage (6).

Human embryonic kidney cell culture. Limited growth of a single strain of human rotavirus has been accomplished in HEK cultures for up to 24 serial passages (171, 261, 263). Commercially-obtained primary HEK roller-tube cultures were washed (3X) to remove serum and were refed with a medium of either Earle's balanced salt solution (BSS) with 0.5% lactalbumin hydrolysate plus 0.1% "Yeastolate" and antibiotics, or "Serumless Medium" (as described by Neuman and Tytell) in higher passages (176, 261). Then 0.2 ml of inoculum was added to each tube and incubated at 35 C for 7–32 days until the cells deteriorated (261). A questionable and inconsistent CPE was observed periodically. Virus was detected using negative stain EM of fluid and/or cell harvests and/or by indirect FA. For FA testing, cells were removed from the glass wall of the cell culture tube with trypsin EDTA, centrifuged, and the concentrated cells placed on microscope slides. Air-dried slides were fixed in cold acetone for 10 min. Rotavirus antibody containing serum from humans or animals was incubated on the tissues for 30 min in a moist chamber. After washing in PBS for 15 min, an appropriate antispecies globulin conjugated with fluorescein isothiocyanate was added for 30 min. After another washing in PBS, the preparations were mounted using buffered glycerol and examined for fluorescence. Generally, by this method fewer than 1% of the cells were shown to be infected and the virus particles observed by EM were "incomplete" as they lacked the morphologically distinct outer capsid (261).

Plaque assay. Calf rotavirus (NCDV and UK) and simian rotavirus (SA-11) have been plaqued successfully in various cell cultures (149, 259a). The first reported plaque test for bovine rotavirus (NCDV) required the addition of trypsin and DEAE-dextran to the medium before inoculation into MA 104 cells (149). Subsequently, bovine rotavirus (UK) has been plaqued without the use of trypsin in AGMK, CV-1, and MA-104 cells (259a). L-15 medium with 0.9% methylcellulose comprises the overlay with 5% agamma calf serum, glutamine, and antibiotics added. Simian rotavirus (SA-11) plaques in primary AGMK or CV-1 cells using L-15 or Eagle's medium with 0.9% agarose, glutamine, 5% agamma or fetal calf serum, and antibiotics added (259a).

The test procedures used in our laboratory are as follows: 6-well culture dishes with confluent monolayers are washed 3 times to remove serum. Virus for inoculation is diluted 10-fold in L-15 medium with 0.5% gelatin and antibiotics added. One milliliter volumes are inoculated into the wells and adsorbed for 90 min at 38 C. After one wash with L-15 medium, the overlay is added. Plates are incubated in humidified plastic bags at 38 C in an air incubator without CO_2. After 7 days the cells are fixed with 10% formalin for a minimum of 1 hr and stained with hematoxylin and eosin. Plaques are read with an inverted microscope or with the unaided eye. The titer of virus is enhanced by the use of trypsin, either by the addition of approximately 2 μg of trypsin to each virus dilution prior to inoculation, or preincubation of undiluted virus plus trypsin (10 μg/ml) for 90 min at 38 C prior to dilution and subsequent inoculation. This results in a 10- to 32-fold increase in virus titer (259a, Wyatt et al, unpublished studies).

Identification of isolates

Polyacrylamide gel electrophoresis (PAGE). Since the RNA genome of rotaviruses is segmented it can be readily and reproducibly fractionated by PAGE (104, 107, 108, 178, 194, 204, 237). This technique is a sensitive method for distinguishing animal and human rotavirus strains in stools or in *in vitro* systems (104, 107, 108). Infected cell culture fluid or fecal material is treated with fluorocarbons to release cell-associated virus. The virus is purified by density-gradient centrifugation in sucrose and/or CsCl, and the RNA is obtained by treatment of purified virus with phenol-chloroform. Rotavirus strains are distinguished by comparison of their RNA migration patterns following coelectrophoresis in slab gels of low concentration polyacrylamide (2.5%). By this method 3 distinct human rotavirus patterns have been recognized from among 8 strains which had been passaged in gnotobiotic calves (107, 108). The human strains were also distinct from 6 animal rotavirus strains derived from calves, monkey, and piglets (107, 108). An example of a comparison of electrophoretic RNA migration from a human and calf rotavirus is shown in Figure 30.9 (107). The differences in migration patterns are clearly illustrated as migration differences were observed in 7 of the 11 RNA segments. This method may be employed in helping to identify rotaviruses following *in vivo* or *in vitro* passage. It can be of value in determining whether or not cross-contamination with other rotaviruses has occurred.

Additional methods described in other sections of this chapter have also been employed to identify isolates: inhibition of fluorescent foci, IEM, CF, and ELISA have been used to serotype human strains (81a, 83, 197, 234, 273, 281); the ELISA, IEM, inhibition of fluorescent foci, neutralization and HI tests have been employed to distinguish between certain animal and human rotaviruses (32, 72, 79, 150, 208, 216, 223, 235, 257, 271, 281).

Serologic diagnosis

Immune electron microscopy

This was the first method by which serologic responses to the human rotavirus were detected (124). In this test, which is essentially the same as that for the Norwalk agent outlined above, 0.8 ml of a stool filtrate rich in rotavirus particles is used as antigen and 1:5 dilutions of acute- and convalescent-phase sera as the source of antibody (124). One modification in the rotavirus IEM test is a longer incubation of the virus-serum mixture; incubation is at room temperature for 1 hr and then overnight at 4 C since the longer incubation period appears to increase the amount of antibody on the particles (124). An example of a serologic response by IEM for rotavirus is shown in Figure 30.10 (124). Visualization of antibody on rotavirus particles

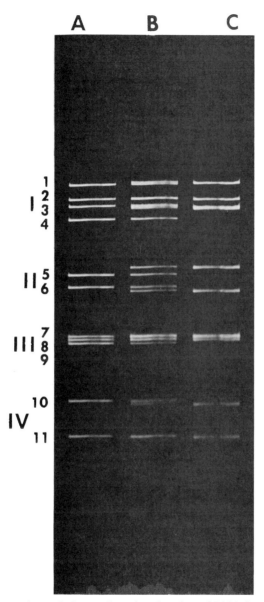

Figure 30.9—Comparison of electrophoretic migration of RNA from a human and a calf rotavirus. A. RNA pattern of human strain "M". B. Pattern from a mixture of human rotavirus strain "M" RNA and calf rotavirus strain "UK" RNA. C. RNA pattern of calf rotavirus strain "UK". (From ref 107)

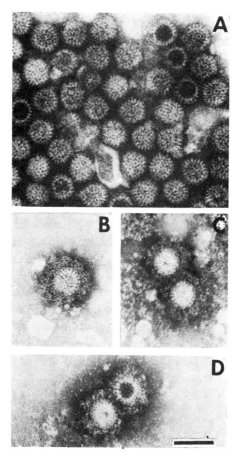

Figure 30.10—A. Rotavirus particles observed after the stool filtrate of a patient (who was hospitalized with gastroenteritis) was incubated with a 1:5 dilution of this same patient's acute-phase serum, and further preparation for EM. No definite antibody was seen on these particles. This serum was given an overall rating of 1+ for antibody to the human rotavirus. B., C., and D. Rotavirus particles observed after the stool filtrate of same patient in A was incubated with 1:5 dilution of this patient's convalescent-phase serum and further preparation for EM. The particles appear to be heavily coated with antibody. The quantity of antibody on these particles was scored as 4+. This convalescent-phase serum was given an overall rating of 4+ for antibody to the human rotavirus. Bar = 100 nm and applies to A–D. (From ref 124)

is more difficult than on the Norwalk-agent particles as the antibody coat does not stand out as clearly on rotaviruses, possibly because of the shorter antibody-length-to-particle-diameter ratio of rotaviruses when compared to the Norwalk agent (e.g., approximately 10 nm/70 nm vs 10 nm/27 nm). In addition to using IEM for detection of rotavirus serologic responses with paired sera (27, 77, 124, 133), this technique has been employed to examine antigenic relationships among human and various animal rotaviruses (32, 79, 208, 251, 281). Such studies have demonstrated antigenic differences among animal rotaviruses, between animal and human rotaviruses, and between human rotaviruses. It has been suggested that type-specific antigens reside on the outer capsid, and the group antigens reside on the inner capsid surrounding the core (32, 79, 208, 257, 281).

Since IEM is so time-consuming it was soon superseded by the CF test for detection of serologic responses in humans. Additional serologic assays, such as ELISA, have also proven to be of great value in studying rotavirus infection especially in select groups as described below.

Complement fixation

CF antigens consist essentially of rotavirus-rich stool preparations derived from gastroenteritis patients (57, 65, 88, 96, 113, 114, 121, 124, 133). The stools may be prepared as 2% filtrates or as clarified suspensions for use directly in CF. The drawback to these simple methods is that stools are frequently anticomplementary or may contain <2 units of antigen. CF antigen may also be prepared from particle-rich stools by purification procedures. One method of purification which yielded satisfactory CF antigen involves clarification by centrifugation at $10,000 \times g$ for 15 min at 4 C; layering approximately 12 ml of supernatant fluid onto a 2-ml cushion of 45% (wt/vol) sucrose in tris-(hydroxymethyl) aminomethane buffer and centrifuging at $100,000 \times g$ for 1.5 hr; resuspending the pellet to one-eighth the original volume and then adjusting the pH to 7.2 (93).

A limitation of the routine use of CF antigen from human stools is that this source of antigen is limited, as the amount of particle-rich stool obtained from patients is generally not sufficient to carry out more than a limited number of tests. However, animal rotaviruses which grow in cell culture may be used as substitute antigens to detect serologic responses to the human agent (27, 113, 114, 121, 241). NCDV was the first such substitute antigen employed; it is not as efficient as some other animal rotaviruses and in addition, in our laboratory at least, does not grow to a high enough titer to be used unconcentrated from cell culture harvests (113, 114). In our laboratory, the antigen is routinely grown in BEK cells and must be concentrated approximately 25-fold (by Amicon ultrafiltration cell) to achieve a minimum of 4 units (114). The O agent is the substitute antigen of choice since it grows readily in AGMK cells (146), achieving a minimum of 4 units of antigen without concentration and is about as efficient as the human rotavirus for detecting serologic responses (113). However, distribution of the O agent which was isolated from intestinal washings of sheep and cattle in South Africa (146) is not permitted in the United States at this time, since it has not yet been cleared for general distribution by the Department of Agriculture. In the meantime, other propagatable animal rotaviruses without distribution problems may be used as substitute CF antigen.

Another source of human rotavirus antigen is the stools of animals infected with human rotavirus as described earlier. Such stools may be made into 2% clarified suspensions and used as antigen if they are not anticomplementary. They may also be purified by rate-zonal and/or density-gradient centrifugation procedures.

A routine CF procedure is employed (213, Chapter 1). Human sera are inactivated at 56 C for 30 min, and routinely tested at 2-fold dilutions (1:4–1:64); a ≥4-fold rise in antibody titer is considered to be significant. If the quantity of serum is sufficient, the initial dilution can be decreased to 1:2. In one study, CF antibody was detected as early as 3 days after onset of illness, with peak levels occurring 10–20 days after onset (133). Antibody in acute and early-convalescent phases was sensitive to mercaptoethanol (133).

A modified CF test described above has recently been developed which can discriminate between the two rotavirus serotypes when using type-specific antisera (281–283).

Immune adherence hemagglutination assay

Serologic responses can also be detected by IAHA (118, 150, 151). Antigens for this test are identical to those used for CF. A major advantage of IAHA over CF is its greater sensitivity (139). Antigen and antibody titers are about 10-fold greater by IAHA when compared to CF. However, comparisons of the efficiency of IAHA with other tests for detecting rotavirus serologic responses have not been reported. The methods for IAHA were described earlier for Norwalk agent.

Hemagglutination-inhibition test

The human rotavirus has very recently been shown to hemagglutinate chicken RBC (216). The antigen was purified from particle positive stools of infants and young children. Examination of paired sera for hemagglutination-inhibition (HAI) and CF responses revealed that the CF test was more efficient than HAI for detecting serologic responses (216). The HAI test may have been measuring serologic responses to the type-specific antigen, whereas the CF test was detecting the broader response (216). A calf rotavirus recovered in Canada and the NCDV both agglutinate human group O and guinea pig RBC (72, 223). With calf rotavirus antigens also, the HAI test appears to be less efficient than CF for detecting serologic responses in human paired sera (72, 223). In addition, simian rotavirus (SA-11) hemagglutinates human group O and guinea pig RBC (105).

Inhibition (neutralization) of fluorescent foci

This technique involves the inoculation of fecal filtrates onto confluent monolayer cell cultures followed by centrifugation, incubation, fixation, and detection of viral antigens by fluorescence microscopy (35, 235, 236). This method has been used to detect antigenic differences among animal rotaviruses, between animal and human rotaviruses, and between human strains (235). It has also been shown to be a sensitive method for determining the prevalence of human rotavirus antibody (65).

Neutralization tests in cell culture

Since the human rotavirus grows so inefficiently in cell culture, a neutralization test is not practical. Attempts have been made to employ NCDV as a substitute antigen in cell culture for neutralization tests with human sera with variable results (65, 79, 96, 114, 257, Kapikian et al, unpublished studies). Plaque neutralization with calf rotavirus has not been as sensitive as CF for demonstrating serologic responses (149).

Immunofluorescence (FA)

Indirect FA techniques can be used as a sensitive and efficient indicator of rotavirus antibody (50, 65, 79, 114, 130, 162, 168, 171, 179, 235, 257, 261, 264, 266). FA antibody directed against rotavirus is broadly cross-reactive, thereby permitting the use of animal rotavirus antigens to test for antibody to the human rotavirus.

Preparation of antigens. Rotavirus antigen can be prepared in the form of cell monolayers infected with rotavirus adapted to cell culture, e.g., BEK cells infected 24 hr earlier with NCDV *or* frozen sections of small intestinal tissues from experimentally infected animals, e.g., human rotavirus infected calves, piglets, or monkeys harvested at the onset of illness (130, 263, 264). In earlier studies, human rotavirus-infected human embryonic intestinal organ cultures were utilized (266). Tissues containing antigens are fixed in cold acetone for 10 min before storage at −70 C and subsequent testing.

Test procedure. Human or animal serum is diluted 2- to 4-fold beginning at 1:10 in PBS, and each dilution is incubated with the antigen on a slide or coverslip for 30 min at 35 C (130, 263, 264). After washing in PBS, an appropriate antispecies IgG conjugated with fluoroscein isothiocyanate is added and incubated for 30 min. Difficulty has been encountered in finding conjugates free of rotavirus antibody due to the frequent occurrence of rotavirus infection in animals used for preparation of hyperimmune sera. A small amount of rotavirus antibody in the conjugate may not interfere with the test if it cannot be detected at the working dilution. After washing the preparations again in PBS, they are mounted with buffered glycerol and examined for fluorescence. Appropriate controls include test serum plus uninfected tissue to test for nonvirus-specific antibody directed against tissue; known positive serum with infected and uninfected tissue to control for the presence of specific antigen; and conjugate alone at the working dilution on infected and uninfected tissue to test for rotavirus antibody or nonspecific reactivity in the conjugate. This step should actually be done as a preliminary step to the use of any conjugate (130, 263, 264).

Interpretation of test. Fluorescence indicates the presence of antibody if all controls are reacting satisfactorily. Titers range from 1:10 to 1:1280 following primary infection. Interpretation is subjective, and therefore evaluation of tests under code is preferable. The use of 4-fold dilutions not only decreases the number of preparations required but also makes the evaluation of endpoints easier. FA antigens characteristically appear as finely to coarsely granular fluorescent areas in the cytoplasm of infected cells. Localization of antigens in villous epithelial cells of infected intestinal sections prepared sequentially offers an advantage since the observer knows the location of antigens and can discount nonspecific fluorescence, for example in smooth muscle cells.

Enzyme-linked immunosorbent assay (203, 270, 274, 278)

Binding test. The indirect ELISA for antigen detection was adapted for use in antibody detection (278). A schematic diagram for measuring rotavirus antibody in serum or body fluids is shown in Figure 30.11. In this assay, titers of specific IgA, IgM, or IgG antibodies can be determined by using the appropriate antiglobulin (274). This is especially useful in antibody studies of colostrum, milk, intestinal fluids, and saliva, since IgA, the princi-

ELISA FOR ROTAVIRUS ANTIBODY MEASUREMENT
(Binding Assay)

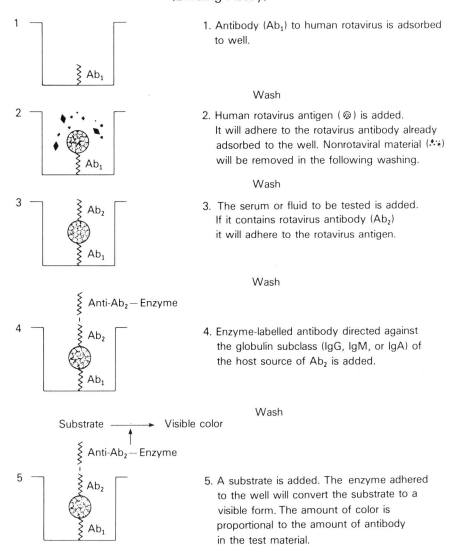

1. Antibody (Ab$_1$) to human rotavirus is adsorbed to well.

Wash

2. Human rotavirus antigen (⊕) is added.
   It will adhere to the rotavirus antibody already adsorbed to the well. Nonrotaviral material (⋰) will be removed in the following washing.

Wash

3. The serum or fluid to be tested is added.
   If it contains rotavirus antibody (Ab$_2$) it will adhere to the rotavirus antigen.

Wash

4. Enzyme-labelled antibody directed against the globulin subclass (IgG, IgM, or IgA) of the host source of Ab$_2$ is added.

Wash

5. A substrate is added. The enzyme adhered to the well will convert the substrate to a visible form. The amount of color is proportional to the amount of antibody in the test material.

Figure 30.11—Schematic diagram for ELISA for rotavirus antibody detection.

pal immunoglobulin of these fluids, does not fix complement. In addition, studies of Nt antibody in such fluids cannot be carried out with human rotavirus since it grows so inefficiently in cell cultures and, as noted above, substitute antigens have yielded variable results in Nt tests.

Preparation of antigen. As outlined above, human rotavirus antigen is needed for this antibody test, in addition to the reagents employed for rotavirus detection (278). Since this agent does not grow efficiently in cell culture an alternate source must be found. Although it can be purified from particle-rich human stools, such virus might be bound with antibody as noted earlier, thus complicating interpretation of the ELISA. An ideal human rotavirus antigen for this assay can be prepared from a stool from a gnotobiotic animal (such as the calf) experimentally infected with human rotavirus. Antigen is prepared either as 2% or 10% bacteria-free filtrates or 2-10% suspensions with 0.1% sodium azide. An alternate source of rotavirus antigen might be one of the animal rotaviruses which grow readily in cell cultures. However, for ELISA antibody studies it appears that NCDV is not as efficient as the human rotavirus for detecting seroresponses (Yolken et al, unpublished studies). In a recent study, however, SA-11 was shown to be an efficient substitute antigen for detecting human rotavirus antibody by ELISA (87a).

Test procedure (274, 278). Coat polyvinyl microtiter plate (Cooke-220-24 or equivalent) with antirotavirus serum diluted in carbonate buffer. Incubate at least overnight at 4 C. The dilution of antiserum for precoating has usually been established previously by checkerboard titration for virus detection studies. In our laboratory, the guinea pig antirotavirus serum is diluted 1:10,000. Wash the plate; add rotavirus antigen diluted in PBS-Tween, and to the companion row add a control antigen, if available, treated similarly. If not available, add diluent only and employ as the "control antigen." Incubate for 2 hr at 37 C and/or overnight at 4 C. The optimum antigen dilution should be determined by checkerboard titration; approximately 10 units of antigen are employed. Wash the plate; add the test serum or fluid diluted in PBS-Tween and 1% fetal calf serum plus 0.5% normal goat serum. (The goat and calf serum should be free of rotavirus antibody.) Sera can be diluted in 2- to 4-fold dilutions beginning at 1:20 to 1:100 and ending at about 1:10,240; dilutions can be made in the precoated plates by means of a Titer Tek® multichannel pipette. [Although the ELISA binding titers were proportional to those measured by CF and FA, the ELISA binding test was found to be about 4 times as sensitive as FA and 10 times as sensitive as CF (278).] Incubate for 2 hr at 37 C and/or overnight at 4 C. Wash the plate; add appropriate enzyme-labeled conjugate diluted in PBS-Tween plus 1% fetal calf serum plus 0.5% goat serum. Incubate 1-2 hr (depending on conjugate) at 37 C. Wash the plate; add substrate. Compare color with that of a positive control containing 10 units of antigen to determine when to read the test.

Interpretation of results. When determining color change with the unaided eye, the endpoint is that dilution at which the test antigen-antibody mixture turned yellow, whereas the control antigen-antibody mixture did not, or had a definitely lower intensity of yellow color. By machine reading, a P/N value of 2 is considered significant, where P = OD at the dilution with test antigen and N = OD at the dilution with control antigen. (However, the N value should be at least 2 standard deviations greater than the intrinsic variation of the test system.) Measurement of OD with a colorimeter is preferable to reading with the unaided eye in this assay.

Blocking test for antibody measurement

A simple method for measuring antibody to rotaviruses is achieved by adaptation of the blocking technique outlined previously (271, 275). A schematic representation of this method is shown in Figure 30.8. The reagents used are identical to those employed in the basic ELISA antigen detection assay. Thus, only one set of reagents is required for antigen and antibody detection. In addition, virus obtained from human stool can be employed, an obvious advantage over the binding assay which optimally requires antigen from infected gnotobiotic animals (278). The blocking antibody test can also be read quite effectively by the unaided eye whereas, ideally for the binding assay, a colorimeter is employed. Titers achieved by binding assay are higher than by the blocking test, but the efficiency for detecting a serologic response is comparable (275). However, the binding assay is required for measuring immunoglobulin subclasses since the blocking assay as outlined will not differentiate such subclasses.

Test procedure (275). Incubate 75 μl of 4-fold dilutions of serum (starting at about 1:5 and ending at about 1:2560) with an equal volume of approximately 4 units of rotavirus antigen for 2 hr at 37 C. Any form of human rotavirus antigen including crude stool suspensions can be used. Dilute the serum and virus in PBS-Tween containing 1% fetal calf serum and 0.5% normal goat serum (both should be rotavirus antibody-negative). Transfer 100 μl of the above mixture to a plate precoated with goat antirotavirus hyperimmune serum and process as for detection of rotavirus antigen by the basic ELISA shown schematically in Figure 30.7. A rotavirus antibody positive serum is incubated with rotavirus antigen as above as a positive control for the blocking procedure. In addition, diluent is incubated with or without rotavirus as above as controls for the antigen and diluent.

When reading with the unaided eye, a dilution is considered antibody positive if it has a markedly reduced color when compared to the control rotavirus-diluent wells. With machine readings, a dilution which has an OD which is at least 50% less than the OD of the rotavirus-diluent control well is considered to be antibody positive.

General considerations. With this method, most infants with rotavirus infection have an acute-phase serum titer of <1:10 and a convalescent phase serum titer of 1:40–1:160 (275). Most adults with rotavirus infection have acute-phase serum titers of <1:10–1:160 and convalescent-phase serum titers of 1:640–1:10,240. The serum titers in the binding assay are about 10-fold higher than in the blocking assay (275).

ELISA for antirotavirus serotype specific antibody

Blocking assay. This assay is similar to the previously outlined blocking assay except that the type-specific rotavirus antigen (type 1 or 2) is used as the blocking antigen with the appropriate serum dilutions (197). In addition, how-ever, cross-reactive antigenic sites on the type 1 antigen (used at 10 units) are blocked by the addition of convalescent-phase serum (4 units) from a type 2 infected calf. The type 2 antigen is treated similarly with the heterologous type 1 calf serum (197). (Alternatively, the type 1 and type 2 antigens may be reacted with calf rotavirus antiserum to block common antigenic determi-nants.) This method has the advantage of permitting the use of identical reagents as outlined previously for the basic ELISA outlined in Figure 30.7.

Binding assay. This assay is similar to the previously described binding assay for antibody detection with a few modifications (273): a type-specific hyperimmune-guinea pig serum is used for precoating; rotavirus of the same serotype as the precoating is added as the antigen; the common determinants on the type-specific antigen are blocked by the addition of a bovine rotavirus postinfection serum or a serum with antibody to the other serotype as well as antibody to the common determinants; the human serum or fluid is added and if it contains antibody to the unblocked type-specific antigenic deter-minants, it adheres; the type-specific human rotavirus antibody is quantitated by the color change induced by the reaction of the enzyme linked antihuman immunoglobulin with substrate. Appropriate washings are carried out as outlined previously.

Comparison of efficiency and practicality of methods available for detecting serologic evidence of rotavirus infection

A comparison of the efficiency and practicality of the various rotavirus antibody test systems is shown in Table 30.5. The ELISA blocking and bind-ing assays are more efficient than CF for detecting antibody responses in infants under the age of 6 months and also in adults. However, for those 6–24 months of age, the CF, ELISA binding, and ELISA blocking assays are comparable in efficiency (275). FA assay is almost as efficient as ELISA for detecting serologic responses (275). However, the ELISA appears to be the most efficient of the available methods for serologic diagnosis (275). The CF test may be more practical in laboratories where this method is already used routinely if the limits in the efficiency of this test are recognized and appropri-ate alternate tests are available when necessary. An indirect solid-phase RIA for detecting bovine rotavirus antibody has been described (14). Bovine rota-virus is cultured in a microtiter plate, fixed with ethanol, thus serving as the solid-phase antigen for the indirect RIA (14). This technique appeared sensi-tive for rotavirus antibody detection in bovine sera; however, the efficiency of the bovine antigen for detecting antibody to human rotavirus by RIA has not been evaluated.

Again, most of the serologic assays outlined above in which human rota-virus is employed as antigen demonstrate the approach of direct virology, an approach which bypasses the necessity of cultivating a viral agent *in vitro* or *in vivo* before it can be identified and characterized, and its epidemiology eluci-dated.

TABLE 30.5—EFFICIENCY AND PRACTICALITY OF METHODS AVAILABLE FOR DETECTING
EVIDENCE OF HUMAN ROTAVIRUS INFECTION IN SERUM

METHOD	EFFICIENCY*	PRACTICALITY*†
Immune electron microscopy (27, 77, 121, 124, 133)	4+	<1+
Complement-fixation (27, 57, 65, 93, 96, 113, 114, 121, 124)	3+ to 4+	4+
Immunofluorescence (50, 65, 79, 114, 130, 171, 179, 266)	4+	1+
Gel diffusion (257)	?	2+
Counterimmunoelectro-osmophoresis (47a, 166)	Variable	2+
Neutralization of calf rotavirus in cell culture (79, 96, 114, 149, 257)	2+	1+
Radioimmunoassay (21a)	Not known	3+
Enzyme-linked immunosorbent assay (217, 273-275, 278)	4+	3+ to 4+
Inhibition (neutralization) of fluorescent foci (35, 65, 235-237)	Not known	1+
Immune adherence hemagglutination assay (118, 150, 151)	3+ to 4+	4+
Hemagglutination-inhibition (72, 216, 223)	2+ to 3+	4+

*On a scale of 1+ to 4+ where 1+ indicates a low degree of efficiency or practicality, and 4+ indicates a high degree of efficiency or practicality.

†For large-scale epidemiologic studies, assuming 4+ efficiency.

References

1. ACRES SD and RADOSTITS OM: The efficacy of a modified live reo-like virus vaccine and an *E. coli* bacterin for prevention of acute undifferentiated neonatal diarrhea of beef calves. Can Vet J 17:197-212, 1976
2. ADAMS WR and KRAFT LM: Epizootic diarrhea of infant mice: identification of the etiologic agent. Science 141:359-360, 1963
3. ADLER I and ZICKL R: Winter vomiting disease. J Infect Dis 119:668-673, 1969
4. AGUS SG, DOLIN R, WYATT RG, TOUSIMIS AJ, and NORTHRUP RS: Acute infectious nonbacterial gastroenteritis: intestinal histopathology. Histologic and enzymatic alterations during illness produced by the Norwalk agent in man. Ann Intern Med 79:18-25, 1973
5. ALBREY MB and MURPHY AM: Rotavirus and acute gastroenteritis of infants and children. Med J Aust 1:82-85, 1976
6. ALBREY MB and MURPHY AM: Rotavirus growth in bovine monolayers. Lancet 1:753, 1976
7. ALMEIDA JD, DEINHARDT F, and ZUCKERMAN AJ: Virus-like particles in hepatitis A - positive fecal extracts. Lancet 2:1083-1084, 1974
8. ALMEIDA JD and WATERSON AP: The morphology of virus antibody interaction. Adv Virus Res 15:207-228, 1969
9. ANDERSON TF and STANLEY WM: A study by means of the electron microscope of the reaction between tobacco mosaic virus and its antiserum. J Biol Chem 139:339-344, 1941
10. APPLETON H, BUCKLEY M, THOM BT, COTTON JL, and HENDERSON S: Virus-like particles in winter vomiting disease. Lancet 1:409-411, 1977

11. APPLETON H and HIGGINS PG: Viruses and gastroenteritis in infants. Lancet 1:1297, 1975
12. APPLETON H and PEREIRA MS: A possible virus etiology in outbreaks of food-poisoning from cockles. Lancet 1:780–781, 1977
13. ARDENNE M VON, FRIEDRICH-FRESKA H, and SCHRAMM G: Electronenmikroskopischen untersuchung der Pracipitin Reaktion von Tabakmosaik Virus mit Kaninchem Anti-serum. Arch Gesamte Virusforsch 2:80–86, 1941
13a. ASHLEY CR, CAUL EO, CLARK SKR, CORNER BD and DUNN S: Rotavirus infections of apes. Lancet 2:477, 1979
14. BABIUK LA, ACRES D, and ROUSE BT: Solid-phase radioimmunoassay for detecting bovine (neonatal calf and diarrhea) rotavirus antibody. J Clin Microbiol 6:10–15, 1977
15. BABIUK LA, MOHAMMED K, SPENCE L, FAUVEL M, and PETRO R: Rotavirus isolation and cultivation in the presence of trypsin. J Clin Microbiol 6:610–617, 1977
16. BANATVALA JE, TOTTERDELL B, CHRYSTIE IL, and WOODE GN: In vitro detection of human rotaviruses. Lancet 2:821, 1975
16a. BERGELAND ME, MCADARAGH JP, and STOTZ I: Proceedings of the 26th Western Poultry Disease Conference at University of California, Davis, 1977, pp 129–130
16b. BIDWELL DE, BUCK AA, DIESFELD HJ, ENDERS B, HAWARTH J, HULDT G, KENT NH, KIRSTEN C, MATTERN P, RUITENBERG EJ, and VOLLER A: The enzyme-linked immunosorbent assay (ELISA). Bull WHO 54:129–139, 1976
17. BINN LN, LAZAR EC, KEENAN KP, HUXSOLL DL, MARCHWICKI RH, and STRANO AJ: Discovery and characterization of a coronavirus from military dogs with diarrhea. Proc 78th Annu Meeting US Animal Health Association, 1974, p 359
18. BIRCH CJ, LEWIS FA, KENNETT ML, HOMOLA M, and PRITCHARD H: A study of prevalence of rotavirus infection in children with gastroenteritis admitted to an infectious diseases hospital. J Med Virol 1:69–77, 1977
19. BISHOP RF, DAVIDSON GP, HOLMES IH, and RUCK BJ: Evidence for viral gastroenteritis. N Engl J Med 289:1096–1097, 1973
20. BISHOP RF, DAVIDSON GP, HOLMES IH, and RUCK BJ: Virus particles in epithelial cells of duodenal mucosa from children with acute gastroenteritis. Lancet 2:1281–1283, 1973
21. BISHOP RF, DAVIDSON GP, HOLMES IH, and RUCK BJ: Detection of a new virus by electron microscopy of fecal extracts from children with acute gastroenteritis. Lancet 1:149–151, 1974
21a. BLACKLOW NR, CUKOR G, PANJAVANI Z, CAPOZZA F, and BEDNARCK F: Simplified radioimmunoassay for detection of rotavirus in pediatric and adult stools, for assessment of duration of antibody to rotavirus in human breast milk. (Abstract) Fourth International Congress for Virology, The Hague, 1978
22. BLACKLOW NR, ECHEVERRIA P, and SMITH DA: Serological studies with reovirus-like agents. Infect Immun 13:1563–1566, 1976
23. BLACKLOW NR, DOLIN R, FEDSON DS, DuPONT H, NORTHRUP RS, HORNICK RB, and CHANOCK RM: Acute infectious nonbacterial gastroenteritis: etiology and pathogenesis. A combined clinical staff conference at the Clinical Center of the National Institutes of health. Ann Intern Med 76:993–1008, 1972
24. BOHL EH: In Transmissible Gastroenteritis in Diseases of Swine, 3rd edition, DUNNE HW (ed), Iowa State University Press, Ames, 1970, pp 158
25. BOLIVAR R, COUKLIN RH, VOLLET JJ, PICKERING LK, DUPONT HL, WALTERS DL, and KOHL S: Rotavirus in travelers' diarrhea: study of an adult student population in Mexico. J Infect Dis 137:324–327, 1978
26. BONSDORFF CH VON, HOVI T, MAKELA P, HOVI L, and TEVALUSTO-AARNIO M: Rotavirus associated with acute gastroenteritis in adults. Lancet 2:423, 1976
27. BONSDORFF CH VON, HOVI T, MAKELA P, and MORTTINEN A: Rotavirus infections in adults in association with acute gastroenteritis. J Med Virol 2:21–28, 1978
28. BORTOLUSSI R, SZYMANSKI M, HAMILTON R, and MIDDLETON P: Studies on the etiology of acute infantile diarrhea. Pediatr Res 8:379, 1974
29. BRANDT CD, KIM HW, RODRIGUEZ WJ, ARROBIO JO, KAPIKIAN AZ, WYATT RG, CHANOCK RM, and PARROTT RH: Gastroenteritis and human reovirus-like agent infection during the 1975–76 outbreak: an electron microscopic study. Clin Proc, Child Hosp Natl Med Center 33:21–26, 1977
30. BRENNER S and HORNE RW: A negative staining method for high resolution electron microscopy of viruses. Biochem Biophys Acta 34:103–110, 1959
31. BRIDGER JC and WOODE GN: Neonatal calf diarrhea: identification of a reovirus-like (rotavirus) agent in feces by immunofluorescence and immune electron microscopy. Br Vet J 131:528–535, 1975

32. BRIDGER JC, WOODE GN, JONES JM, FLEWETT TH, BRYDEN AS, and DAVIES H: Transmission of human rotaviruses to gnotobiotic piglets. J Med Microbiol 8:565-569, 1975

33. BRUCE-WHITE GB, ASHTON CI, ROBERTS C, and PARRY HE: Rotavirus in gastroenteritis. Lancet 2:726, 1974

34. BRYDEN AS, DAVIES HA, HADLEY RE, FLEWETT TH, MORRIS CA, and OLIVER P: Rotavirus enteritis in the West Midlands during 1974. Lancet 2:241-243, 1974

35. BRYDEN AS, DAVIES HA, THOULESS ME, and FLEWETT TH: Diagnosis of rotavirus infection by cell culture. J Med Microbiol 10:121-125, 1977

36. BRYDEN AS, THOULESS ME, and FLEWETT TH: Rotavirus in rabbits. Vet Rec 99:323, 1976

37. CAMERON DJS, BISHOP RF, VEENSTRA AA, BARNES GL, HOLMES IH, and RUCK BJ: Pattern of shedding of two noncultivable viruses in stools of newborn babies. J Med Virol 2:7-13, 1978

37a.CARLSON JAK, MIDDLETON PJ, SZYMANSKI M, HUBER J, and PETRIC M: Fatal rotavirus gastroenteritis. An analysis of 21 cases. Am J Dis Child 132: 477-479, 1978

38. CAUL FO and CLARK SKR: Coronavirus propogated from patient with nonbacterial gastroenteritis. Lancet 2:753, 1975

39. CAUL EO and EGGLESTONE SI: Further studies on human enteric coronaviruses. Arch Virol 54:107-117, 1977

40. CAUL EO, PAVER WK, and CLARKE SKR: Coronavirus particles in faeces from patients with gastroenteritis. Lancet 1:1192, 1975

41. CHANOCK RM, WYATT RG and KAPIKIAN AZ: Immunization of infants and young children against rotavirus gastroenteritis: prospects and problems. J Am Vet Med Assoc 173:570-572, 1978

41a.CHAO RK, FISHAUT M, SCHWARTZMAN JD, McINTOSH K: Detection of respiratory syncytial virus in nasal secretions from infants by enzyme-linked immunosorbent assay. J Inf Dis 139:483-486, 1979

42. CLARKE SKR, COOK GT, EGGLESTONE SI, HALL TS, MILLER DL, REED SE, RUBENSTEIN D, SMITH AJ, and TYRRELL DAJ: A virus from epidemic vomiting disease. Br Med J 3:86-89, 1972

42a.CLARKE SKR, FAVER WK and CAUL EO: The 22nm human faecal virus. International Virology 3 Abstracts, Third Int'l Congress for Virology, Madrid, 1975, p 70

43. CLARKE EJ JR, PHILLIPS IA, and ALEXANDER ER: Adenovirus infection in intussusception in children in Taiwan. J Am Med Assoc 208:1671-1674, 1969

44. CLEM TR and YOLKEN RH: Practical colorimeter for direct measurement of microplates in enzyme immunoassay systems. J Clin Microbiol 7:55-58, 1978

45. COHEN J: Ribonucleic-acid polymerase activity associated with purified calf rotavirus. J Gen Virol 36:395-402, 1977

46. COMMUNICABLE DISEASE REPORT No. 32, Aug 13, 1976 (England)

47. CONNOR JD and BARRETT-CONNOR E: Infectious diarrheas. Pediatr Clin North Am 14:197-221, 1967

47a.COOK DA, ZBITNEW A, DEMPSTER G, and GERRARD JW: Detection of antibody to rotavirus by counterimmunoelectrophoresis in human serum, colostrum and milk. J Ped 93:967-970, 1978

48. CRAMBLETT HJ and SIEWERS CMF: The etiology of gastroenteritis in infants and children with emphasis on the occurrence of simultaneous mixed viral-bacterial infection. Pediatrics 35:885-889, 1965

48a.CUKOR G, BERRY MK, and BLACKLOW NR: Simplified radioimmunoassay for detection of human rotavirus in stools. J Infect Dis 138:906-910, 1978

49. DAVIDSON GP, BUTLER DG, GALL DG, PETRIC M, and HAMILTON JR: Ion transport in enteritis caused by human rotavirus. Am Soc Microbiol Ann Meeting, Abstract A-20/1043, May, 1977, Am Soc Microbiol, Washington, DC, 1977

50. DAVIDSON GP, GOLLER, I, BISHOP RF, TOWNLEY, RRW, HOLMES IH, and RUCK BJ: Immunofluorescence in duodenal mucosa of children with acute enteritis due to a new virus. J Clin Path 28:263-266, 1975

51. DAVIDSON GP, BISHOP RF, TOWNLEY RR, HOLMES IH, and RUCK BJ: Importance of a new virus in acute sporadic enteritis in children. Lancet 1:242-245, 1975

51a.DELAGE G, McLAUGHLIN B, and BESTHAUME L: A clinical study of rotavirus gastroenteritis. J Ped 93:455-457, 1978

52. DIENSTAG JL, ALLING DW, and PURCELL RH: Quantitation of antibody to hepatitis A antigen by immune electron microscopy. Infect Immun 13:1209-1213, 1976

53. DINGLE JH, BADGER GF, and JORDAN WS: Illness in the home. A study of 25,000 illnesses in a group of Cleveland families. The Press of Western Reserve Univ, Cleveland, 1964, p 19

54. DOLIN R, BLACKLOW NR, DuPONT H, BUSCHO RF, WYATT RG, KASEL JA, HORNICK R, and CHANOCK RM: Biological properties of Norwalk agent of acute infectious nonbacterial gastroenteritis. Proc Soc Exp Biol Med 140:578-583, 1972

55. DOLIN R, BLACKLOW NR, DuPONT H, FORMAL S, BUSCHO RF, KASEL JA, CHAMES RP, HORNICK R, and CHANOCK RM: Transmission of acute infectious nonbacterial gastroenteritis to volunteers by oral administration of stool filtrates. J Infect Dis 123:307-312, 1971

56. DOLIN R, LEVY AG, WYATT RG, THORNHILL TS, and GARDNER JD: Viral gastroenteritis induced by the Hawaii agent. Jejunal histopathology and seroresponse. Am J Med 59:761, 1975

57. ECHEVERRIA P, HO MT, BLACKLOW NR, QUINNAN G, PORTNOY B, OLSON JG, CONKLIN R, DuPONT HL, and CROSS JH: Relative importance of viruses and bacteria in the etiology of pediatric diarrhea in Taiwan. J Infect Dis 136:383-390, 1977

58. Editorial: Rotaviruses of man and animals. Lancet 1:257-259, 1975

59. Editorial: Viruses of infantile gastroenteritis. Br Med J 3:555, 1975

60. Editorial: Viral cross-infections in wards. Lancet 1:1391-1393, 1976

61. Editorial. ELISA: A replacement for radioimmunoassay? Lancet 2:406-407, 1976

62. Editorial: Rotavirus gastroenteritis. Br Med J 2:784-785, 1977

63. Editorial: Reovirus-like agent as a cause of human diarrheal disease. South Med J 70:390-392, 1977

64. ELIAS MM: Separation and infectivity of two particle types of human rotavirus. J Gen Virol 37:191-194, 1977

65. ELIAS MM: Distribution and titers of rotavirus antibodies in different age groups. J Hyg Camb 79:365-372, 1977

66. ELLENS DJ and DE LEEUW PW: Detection of infantile gastroenteritis virus (rotavirus) by ELISA. Lancet 1:1363, 1977

67. ELLENS DJ and DE LEEUW PW: Enzyme-linked immunosorbent assay for diagnosis of rotavirus infections in calves. J Clin Microbiol 6:530-532, 1977

68. ELLENS DJ: ELISA for detection of bovine coronavirus in faeces. Abstract of the Fourth International Congress for Virology, No. 627, The Hague, 1978

69. ESPARZA J, VIERA DE TORRES B, PINERO A, CARMONA FO, and MAZZALI DE ILJA R: Rotavirus in Venezuelan children with gastroenteritis. Am J Trop Med Hyg 26:148-151, 1977

70. ESPEJO RT, CALDERON E, and GONZALEZ N: Distinct reovirus-like agents associated with acute infantile gastroenteritis. J Clin Microbiol 6:502-506, 1977

70a.FAIRCHILD, EJ (ed.): Registry of toxic effects of chemical substances. USDHEW, National Institute of Occupational Safety and Health (NIOSH), Cincinnati, OH. Vols. I and II, 1977

71. FARRAH SR, GTOYAL SM, GERBA CP, CONKLIN RH, WALLIS C, MELNICK JL, and DuPONT HL: A simple method for concentration of enteroviruses and rotaviruses from cell culture harvests using membrane filters. Intervirology 9:56-59, 1978

72. FAUVEL M, SPENCE L, BABIUK LA, PETRO R, and BLOCH S: Hemagglutination and hemagglutination inhibition studies with a strain of Nebraska calf diarrhea virus (bovine rotavirus). Intervirology 9:95-105, 1978

73. FEINSTONE SM, KAPIKIAN AZ, and PURCELL RH: Hepatitis A: detection by immune electron microscopy of a virus-like antigen associated with acute illness. Science 182:1026-1028, 1973

73a.FERRIS AA: Antigen in infectious hepatitis. Brit M Bull 28:131-133, 1972

73b.FERRIS AA, KALDOR J, GUST ID, and CROSS G: Fecal antigen in viral hepatitis. Lancet 2:243-244, 1970

73c.FERNELIUS AL, RITCHIE AE, CLASSICK LG, NORMAN JO and MEBUS CA: Cell culture adaption and propagation of a reovirus-like agent of calf diarrhea from a field outbreak in Nebraska. Arch Ges Virusforsch 37:114-130, 1972

74. FLEWETT TH: Diagnosis of enteritis virus. Proc Roy Soc Med 69:693-696, 1976

75. FLEWETT TH, BRYDEN AS, and DAVIES H: Virus particles in gastroenteritis. Lancet 2:1497, 1973
76. FLEWETT TH, BRYDEN AS, and DAVIES H: Virus diarrhea in foals and other animals. Vet Rec 97:477, 1975
77. FLEWETT TH, BRYDEN AS, and DAVIES H: Epidemic viral enteritis in a long-stay children's ward. Lancet 1:4-5, 1975
78. FLEWETT TH, BRYDEN AS, and DAVIES H: Diagnostic electron microscopy of faeces. I. The viral flora of the faeces as seen by electron microscopy. J Clin Pathol 27:603-608, 1974
79. FLEWETT TH, BRYDEN AS, DAVIES H, WOODE GN, BRIDGER JC, and DERRICK JM: Relation between viruses from acute gastroenteritis of children and newborn calves. Lancet 2:61-63, 1974
80. FLEWETT TH and DAVIES H: Caliciviruses in man. Lancet 1:311, 1976
81. FLEWETT TH, DAVIES H, BRYDEN AS, and ROBERTSON MJ: Diagnostic electron microscopy of faeces. II. Acute gastroenteritis associated with reovirus-like particles. J Clin Path 27:608-614, 1974
81a. FLEWETT TH, THOULESS ME, PILFORD JN, BRYDEN AS, CANDEIAS JAS: More serotypes of human rotavirus. Lancet 2:632, 1978
82. FLEWETT TH and WOODE GN: The rotaviruses. Brief review. Arch Virol 57:1-23, 1978
83. FONTEYNE J, ZISSIS G, and LAMBERT JP: Recurrent rotavirus gastroenteritis. Lancet 1:983, 1978
84. FOSTER LG, PETERSON H, and SPENDLOVE RS: Fluorescent virus precipitin test. Proc Soc Exp Biol Med 150:155-160, 1975
85. FREIMAN I, HARTMAN E, KASSEL H, ROBINS-BROWNE RM, SCHOUB BD, KOORNHOF HJ, LECATSAS G, and PROZESKY OW: A microbiological study of gastroenteritis in black infants. S Afr Med J 52:261-265, 1977
86. GALL DG: Pathophysiology of viral diarrhea. In Proc 73rd Ross Conference on Pediatric Research: Etiology, pathology, and treatment of acute gastroenteritis, Ponte Vedra Beach, Florida, March 20-22, 1977
87. GARDNER PS, KNOX EG, COURT SDM, and GREEN CA: Virus infection and intussusception in childhood. Br Med J 2:697-700, 1962
87a. GHOSE LH, SCHNAGL RD, and HOLMES IH: Comparison of an enzyme-linked immunosorbent assay for quantitation of rotavirus antibodies with complement fixation in an epidemiological survey. J Clin Micro 8:268-276, 1978
88. GOMEZ-BARRETO J, PALMER E, NAHMIAS AJ, HATCH MH: Acute enteritis associated with reovirus-like agents. J Am Med Assoc 235:1857-1860, 1976
89. GRAUBALLE PC, GENNER J, MEYLING A, and HORNSLETH A: Rapid diagnosis of rotavirus infections: comparison of electron microscopy and immunoelectro-osmophoresis for the detection of rotavirus in human infantile gastroenteritis. J Gen Virol 35:203-218, 1977
90. GREENBERG HB and KAPIKIAN AZ: Detection of Norwalk agent antibody and antigen by solid-phase radioimmunoassay and immune adherence hemagglutination assay. J Am Vet Med Assoc 173:620, 1978
91. GREENBERG HB, WYATT RG, VALDESUSO J, KALICA AR, LONDON WT, CHANOCK RM, and KAPIKIAN AZ: Solid-phase microtiter radioimmunoassay for detection of the Norwalk strain of acute nonbacterial epidemic gastroenteritis virus and its antibodies. J Med Virol 2:97-108, 1978
92. GURWITH MJ and WILLIAMS TW: Gastroenteritis in children: A two year review in Manitoba. I. Etiology. J Infect Dis 136:239-247, 1977
93. GUST ID, PRINGLE RC, BARNES GL, DAVIDSON GP, and BISHOP RF: Complement-fixing antibody response to rotavirus infection. J Clin Microbiol 5:125-130, 1977
94. HAMILTON JR, GALL DG, KERZNER B, BUTLER DG, and MIDDLETON PJ: Recent developments in viral gastroenteritis. Pediatr Clin N Am 22:747-755, 1975
95. HARA M, MUKOYAMA J, TSURUHARA T, SAITO Y, and TAGAYA I: Duovirus in school children with gastroenteritis. Lancet 1:311, 1976
96. HARA M, MUKOYAMA J, TSURUHARA T, ASHIWARA Y, SAITO Y, and TAGAYA I: Acute gastroenteritis among school children associated with reovirus-like agent. Am J Epidemiol 107:161-169, 1978
97. HARRIS WS: Toxic effects of aerosol propellants on the heart. Arch Int Med 131:162-166, 1973

97a. HIEBER JP, SHELTON S, NELSON JD, LEON J, MOHS E: Comparison of human rotavirus disease in tropical and temperate settings. Am J Dis Child 132:853-858, 1978

98. HODES HL: American Pediatric Society Presidential Address. Pediatr Res 10:201-204, 1976

99. HOLMES IH, MATHAN M, BHAT P, ALBERT MJ, SWAMINATHAN SP, MAIYA PP, PEREIRA SM, and BAKER SJ: Orbiviruses and gastroenteritis. Lancet 2:658-659, 1974

100. HOLMES IH, RODGER SM, SCHNAGL RD, RUCK BJ, GUST ID, BISHOP RF, and BARNES GL: Is lactase the receptor and uncoating enzyme for infantile enteritis (Rota) viruses. Lancet 1:1387-1388, 1976

101. HOLMES IH, RUCK BJ, BISHOP RF, and DAVIDSON GP: Infantile enteritis viruses: morphogenesis and morphology. J Virol 16:937-943, 1975

102. HRUSKA JF, NOTTER MFD, MENEGUS MA, and STEINHOFF MC: RNA polymerase associated with human rotavirus in diarrhea stools. J Virol 26:544-546, 1978

103. HUNTER WM and GREENWOOD FC: Preparation of iodine-131 labeled human growth hormone of high specific activity. Nature 194:495-501, 1962

103a. JONES RC, HUGHES CS, and HENRY RR: Rotavirus infection in commercial laying hens. Vet Rec 104:22, 1979

104. KALICA AR, GARON CF, WYATT RG, MEBUS CA, VAN KIRK DH, CHANOCK RM, and KAPIKIAN AZ: Differentiation of human and calf reovirus-like agents associated with diarrhea using polyacrylamide gel electrophoresis of RNA. Virology 74:86-92, 1976

105. KALICA AR, JAMES HD JR, and KAPIKIAN AZ: Hemagglutination by simian rotavirus. J Clin Microbiol 7:314-315, 1978

106. KALICA AR, PURCELL RH, SERENO MM, WYATT RG, KIM HW, CHANOCK RM, and KAPIKIAN AZ: A microtiter solid phase radioimmunoassay for detection of the human reovirus-like agent in stools. J Immunol 118:1275-1279, 1977

107. KALICA AR, SERENO MM, WYATT RG, MEBUS CA, CHANOCK RM, and KAPIKIAN AZ: Comparison of human and animal rotavirus strains by gel electrophoresis of RNA. Virology 87:247-255, 1978

108. KALICA AR, WYATT RG, and KAPIKIAN AZ: Detection of differences among human and animal rotaviruses using analysis of viral RNA. J Am Vet Med Assoc 173:531-537, 1978

109. KAPIKIAN AZ: Viral gastroenteritis. Prev Med 3:535-542, 1974

110. KAPIKIAN AZ: Enteroviral diseases In Beeson-McDermott Textbook of Medicine, 14th edition. WB Saunders Co, Philadelphia, 1975, pp 216-222

111. KAPIKIAN AZ: The Coronaviruses In CRC Chemoprophylaxis and Virus Infections of the Respiratory Tract. Vol II. OXFORD JS (ed) CRC Press Inc, Cleveland, Ohio, 1977, pp 95-117

112. KAPIKIAN AZ: Identification and serology [of rotaviruses, Norwalk and Norwalk-like viruses.] Proceedings of the Seventy-Fourth Ross Conference on Pediatric Research, Ross Laboratories, Columbus, Ohio, 1978, pp 50-71

113. KAPIKIAN AZ, CLINE WL, KIM HW, KALICA AR, WYATT RG, VANKIRK DH, CHANOCK RM, JAMES HD JR, and VAUGHN AL: Antigenic relationships among five reovirus-like (RVL) agents by complement-fixation (CF) and development of a new substitute CF antigen for the human RVL agent of infantile gastroenteritis. Proc Soc Exp Biol Med 152:535-539, 1976

114. KAPIKIAN AZ, CLINE WL, MEBUS CA, WYATT RG, KALICA AR, JAMES HD JR, VANKIRK D, CHANOCK RM, and KIM HW: New complement-fixation test for the human reovirus-like agent of infantile gastroenteritis. Nebraska calf diarrhea virus used as antigen. Lancet 1:1056-1069, 1975

115. KAPIKIAN AZ, DIENSTAG JL, and PURCELL RH: Immune electron microscopy as a method for the detection, identification, and characterization of agents not cultivable in an In Vitro system In Manual of Clinical Immunology, ROSE NR and FRIEDMAN H (eds), Am Soc Microbiol, Washington, DC, 1976, pp 467-480

116. KAPIKIAN AZ, FEINSTONE SM, PURCELL RH, WYATT RG, THORNHILL TS, KALICA AR, and CHANOCK RM: Detection and identification by immune electron microscopy of fastidious agents associated with respiratory illness, acute nonbacterial gastroenteritis, and hepatitis A. Perspect Virol 9:9-47, 1975

117. KAPIKIAN AZ, GERIN JL, WYATT RG, THORNHILL TS, and CHANOCK RM: Density in cesium chloride of the 27-nm "8FIIa" particle associated with acute infectious nonbacterial gastroenteritis: determination by ultracentrifugation and immune electron microscopy. J Infect Dis 129:709-714, 1974

118. KAPIKIAN AZ, GREENBERG HB, CLINE WL, KALICA AR, WYATT RG, JAMES HD JR, LLOYD NL, CHANOCK RM, RYDER RW, and KIM HW: Prevalence of antibody to the Norwalk agent by a newly developed immune adherence hemagglutination assay. J Med Virol 2:281–294, 1978

119. KAPIKIAN AZ, JAMES HD JR, KELLY SJ, and VAUGHN AL: Detection of coronavirus strain 692 by immune electron microscopy. Infect Immun 7:111–116, 1973

120. KAPIKIAN AZ, KALICA AR, SHIH JW, CLINE WL, THORNHILL TS, WYATT RG, CHAN- OCK RM, KIM HW, and GERIN JL: Buoyant density in cesium chloride of the human reovirus-like agent of infantile gastroenteritis by ultracentrifugation, electron micros- copy, and complement-fixation. Virology 70:564–569, 1976

121. KAPIKIAN AZ, KIM HW, WYATT RG, CLINE WL, ARROBIO JO, BRANDT CD, RODRIGUEZ WJ, SACK DA, CHANOCK RM, and PARROTT RH: Human reovirus-like agent as the major pathogen associated with "winter" gastroenteritis in hospitalized infants and young children. N Engl J Med 294:965–972, 1976

122. KAPIKIAN AZ, KIM HW, WYATT RG, CLINE WL, CHANOCK RM, PARROTT RH, ARROBIO JA, BRANDT CD, RODRIGUEZ WJ, KALICA AR, and VANKIRK DH: Studies with the human reovirus-like agent of infantile gastroenteritis. Report No. 1 of the WHO Col- laborating Centre for Collection and Evaluation of Data on Comparative Virology, Munich, W Germany, 1976, pp 191–206

123. KAPIKIAN AZ, KIM HW, WYATT RG, CLINE WL, PARROTT RH, CHANOCK RM, ARROBIO JO, BRANDT CD, RODRIGUEZ WJ, KALICA AR, and VANKIRK DH: Recent advances in the aetiology of viral gastroenteritis. In Acute Diarrhea in Childhood. Ciba Founda- tion Symposium 42 (new series), 1976, pp 273–309

124. KAPIKIAN AZ, KIM HW, WYATT RG, RODRIGUEZ WJ, ROSS S, CLINE WL, PARROTT RH, and CHANOCK RM: Reovirus-like agent in stools: association with infantile diarrhea and development of serologic tests. Science 185:1049–1053, 1974

125. KAPIKIAN AZ, WYATT RG, DOLIN R, THORNHILL TS, KALICA AR, and CHANOCK RM: Visualization by immune electron microscopy of a 27nm particle associated with acute infectious non-bacterial gastroenteritis. J Virology 10:1075–1081, 1972

126. KAPIKIAN AZ, WYATT RG, KALICA AR, CHANOCK RM, and MEBUS CA: Rotavirus, Nor- walk and Norwalk-like viruses: Experimental animals and in vitro systems. In Pro- ceedings of the International Symposium on Experimental Animals and "In Vitro" systems in Medical Microbiology. Edited by WHO Collaborating Centre for Collec- tion and Evaluation of Data on Comparative Virology, Munich, 1977, pp 53–85

127. KAPIKIAN AZ, YOLKEN RH, WYATT RG, KALICA AZ, CHANOCK RM, and KIM HW: Viral diarrhea: etiology and control. Am J Clin Nutr 31:2219–2236, 1978

128. KAYE HS, HARBROUGH WB, and REED CJ: Calf diarrhea coronavirus. Lancet 2:509, 1975

129. KEENAN KP, JERVIS HR, MARCHWICKI RH, and BINN LN: Intestinal infection of neo- natal dogs and canine coronavirus 1-71: studies by virologic, histologic, histochemi- cal and immunofluorescent techniques. Am J Vet Res 37:247, 1976

130. KIM HW, BRANDT CD, KAPIKIAN AZ, WYATT RG, ARROBIO JO, RODRIGUEZ WJ, CHAN- OCK RM, and PARROTT RH: Human reovirus-like agent (HRVLA) infection. Occur- rence in adult contacts of pediatric patients with gastroenteritis. J Am Med Assoc 237:404–407, 1977

131. KIM HW, ARROBIO JO, BRANDT CD, JEFFRIES BC, PYLES G, REID JL, CHANOCK RM, and PARROTT RH: Epidemiology of respiratory syncytial virus infection in Washing- ton, D.C. Am J Epidemiol 98:216–225, 1973

132. KIMURA T and MURAKAMI T: Tubular structures associated with acute nonbacterial gas- troenteritis in young children. Infect Immun 17:157–160, 1977

133. KONNO T, SUZUKI H, IMAI A, and ISHIDA N: Reovirus-like agent in acute epidemic gas- troenteritis in Japanese infants: fecal shedding and serologic response. J Infect Dis 135:259–266, 1977

134. KONNO T, SUZUKI H, KUTSUZAWA T, IMAI A, KATUSUSHIMA M, SAKAMOTO M, and KITAOKA S: Human rotavirus and intussusception. N Engl J Med 297:945, 1977

135. KURTZ JB, LEE TW, and PICKERING D: Astrovirus associated gastroenteritis in a chil- dren's ward. J Clin Pathol 30:948–952, 1977

136. LAMBETH L and MITCHELL JD: Transmission of human gastroenteritis virus to a monkey. (Abstract), Aust Paediatr J 11:127–128, 1975

137. LEE TW and KURTZ JB: Astroviruses detected by immunofluorescence. Lancet 2:406, 1977

138. LECCE JG, KING MW, and MOCK R: Reovirus-like agent associated with fatal diarrhea in neonatal pigs. Infect Immun 14:816-825, 1976

139. LENNETTE ET and LENNETTE DA: Immune adherence hemagglutination: alternative to complement-fixation serology. J Clin Microbiol 7:282-285, 1978

140. LEVY AG, WIDERLITE L, SCHWARTZ CJ, DOLIN R, BLACKLOW NR, GARDNER J, KIMBERG DV, and TRIER JS: Jejunal adenylate cyclase activity in human subjects during viral gastroenteritis. Gastroenterology 70:321-325, 1976

141. MADELEY CR and COSGROVE BP: Viruses in infantile gastroenteritis. Lancet 2:124, 1975

142. MADELEY CR and COSGROVE BP: 28nm particles in faeces in infantile gastroenteritis. Lancet 2:451-452, 1975

143. MADELEY CR and COSGROVE BP: Caliciviruses in man. Lancet 1:199-200, 1976

144. MADELEY CR, CROSGROVE BP, BELL EJ, and FALLON RJ: Stool viruses in babies in Glasgow. I. Hospital admissions with diarrhea. J Hyg Camb 78:261-273, 1977

145. MAIYA PP, PEREIRA SM, MATHAN M, BHAT P, ALBERT MJ, and BAKER JJ: Aetiology of acute gastroenteritis in infancy and early childhood in Southern India. Arch Dis Child 52:482-485, 1977

146. MALHERBE HH and STRICKLAND-CHOLMLEY M: Simian virus SA-11 and the related "O" agent. Arch Gesamte Virusforsch 22:235-245, 1967

147. MARTIN ML, PALMER EL, and MIDDLETON PJ: Ultrastructure of infantile gastroenteritis virus. Virology 68:146-153, 1975

148. MATHAN M, ALMEIDA ID, and COLE J: An antigenic subunit present in rotavirus infected faeces. J Gen Virol 34:325-329, 1977

148a.MATTHEWS REF: The classification and nomenclature of viruses. Summary of results of meetings of The International Committee on Taxonomy of Viruses in The Hague, September 1978. Intervirology 11:133-135, 1979

149. MATSUNO S, INOUYE S, and KONO R: Plaque assay of neonatal calf diarrhea virus and the neutralizing antibody in human sera. J Clin Microbiol 5:1-4, 1977

150. MATSUNO S, INOUYE S, and KONO R: Antigenic relationship between human and bovine rotaviruses as determined by neutralization, immune adherence hemagglutination and complement-fixation tests. Infect Immun 17:661-662, 1977

151. MATSUNO S and NAGAYOSHI S: Quantitative estimation of infantile gastroenteritis virus antigens in stools by immune adherence hemagglutination test. J Clin Microbiol 7:310-311, 1978

152. MAVROMICHALIS J, EVANS N, MCNEISH AS, BRYDEN AS, DAVIES HA, and FLEWETT TH: Intestinal damage in rotavirus and adenovirus gastroenteritis assessed by D-xylose malabsorption. Arch Pediatr 52:589-591, 1977

153. MCNULTY MS, ALLAN GM, CURRAN WL, and MCFERRAN JB: Comparison of methods for diagnosis of rotavirus infection of calves. Vet Rec 98:463-464, 1976

153a.MCNULTY MS, ALLAN GM, and STUART JC: Rotavirus infection in avian species. Vet Rec, 103:319-320, 1978

154. MCNULTY MS, PEARSON GR, MCFERRAN JB, COLLINS DS, and ALLAN GM: A reovirus-like agent (rotavirus) associated with diarrhea in neonatal pigs. Vet Microbiol 1:55-63, 1976

155. MCLURE AR, MACFARLANE DE, and SOMMERVILLE RG: An intersecting anti-serum pool system for the immunofluorescent identification of respiratory viruses. Arch Gesamte Virusforsch 37:6-11, 1972

156. MCSWIGGAN DA, CUBITT D, and MOORE W: Calicivirus associated with winter vomiting disease. Lancet 2:1215, 1978

157. MEBUS CA, KONO M, UNDERDAHL NR, and TWIEHAUS MJ: Cell culture propagation of neonatal calf diarrhea (Scours) virus. Can Vet J 12:69-72, 1971

158. MEBUS CA, STAIR EL, RHODES MB, and TWIEHAUS MJ: Pathology of neonatal calf diarrhea induced by a coronavirus-like agent. Vet Pathol 10:45, 1973

159. MEBUS CA, UNDERDAHL NR, RHODES MB, and TWIEHAUS MJ: Calf diarrhea (scours): reproduced with a virus from a field outbreak. Univ Neb Res Bull 233:1-16, 1969

160. MEBUS CA, WHITE RG, BASS EP, and TWIEHAUS MJ: Immunity to neonatal calf diarrhea virus. J Am Vet Med Assoc 163:880-883, 1973

161. MEBUS CA, WYATT RG, and KAPIKIAN AZ: Pathology of diarrhea in gnotobiotic calves induced by the human reovirus-like agent of infantile gastroenteritis. Vet Pathol 14:273–282, 1977

162. MEBUS CA, WYATT RG, SHARPEE RL, SERENO MM, KALICA AR, KAPIKIAN AZ, and TWIEHAUS MJ: Diarrhea in gnotobiotic calves caused by the reovirus-like agent of human infantile gastroenteritis. Infect Immun 14:471–474, 1976

163. MEURMAN OH and LAINE MJ: Rotavirus epidemic in adults. N Eng J Med 296:1298–1299, 1977

164. MIDDLETON PJ: Analysis of the pattern of viral infection. *In* Report of the 74th Ross Conference on Pediatric Research: Etiology, Pathology, and Treatment of Acute Gastroenteritis. Ponte Vedra Beach, Florida, March 20–22, 1977

165. MIDDLETON PJ, HOLDAWAY MD, PETORE M, SZYMANSKI MT, and TAM JS: Solid-phase radioimmunoassay for the detection of rotavirus. Infect Immun 16:439–444, 1977

166. MIDDLETON PJ, PETRIC M, HEWITT CM, SZYMANSKI MT, and TAM JS: Counter-immuno-electro-osmophoresis for the detection of infantile gastroenteritis virus (orbi-group) antigen and antibody. J Clin Pathol 29:191–197, 1976

167. MIDDLETON PJ, PETRIC M, and SZYMANSKI MT: Propagation of infantile gastroenteritis virus (orbi-group) in conventional and germfree piglets. Infect Immun 12:1276–1280, 1975

168. MIDDLETON PJ, SZYMANSKI MT, ABBOTT GD, BORTOLUSSI R, and HAMILTON JR: Orbi-virus acute gastroenteritis of infancy. Lancet 1:1241–1244, 1974

169. MITCHELL JD, LAMBETH LA, SOSULA L, MURPHY A, and ALBREY M: Transmission of rotavirus gastroenteritis from children to a monkey. Gut 18:156–160, 1977

170. MOFFET HL, SHULENBERGER HK, and BURKHOLDER ER: Epidemiology and etiology of severe infantile diarrhea. J Pediatr 72:1–14, 1968

171. MORISHIMA T, NAGAYOSHI S, OZAKI T, ISOMURA S, and SUZUKI S: Immunofluorescence of human reovirus-like agent of infantile diarrhea. Lancet 2:695–696, 1976

172. MORITA S, SATO Y, HARADA S, SHOJI K, KIN T, AMANO Y, SUDO T, and ISHIDA N: Sero-epidemiological study of the causative agent of emesis-diarrhea syndrome occurred at a kindergarten and RVLA Aichi-Ken Eisei Kenkyushoho 21:57–64, 1977

173. MORITSUGU Y, DIENSTAG JL, VALDESUSO J, WONG DC, WAGNER J, ROUTENBERG JA, and PURCELL RH: Purification of hepatitis A antigen from feces and detection of antigen and antibody by immune adherence hemagglutination. Infect Immun 13:898–908, 1976

174. MUCH D and ZAJAC I: Purification and characterization of epizootic diarrhea of infant mice virus. Infect Immun 6:1019–1024, 1972

175. MURPHY AM, ALBREY MB, and CREWE EB: Rotavirus infections of neonates. Lancet 2:1149–1150, 1977

175a.NALIN DR, LEVINE MM, MATA L, DE CESPEDES C, LIZANO C, SIMHON A, and MOHS E: Comparison of sucrose with glucose in oral therapy of infant diarrhea. Lancet 2:277–279, 1978

175b.National Institute of Environmental Health Science: Environmental teratology information center file. Research Triangle Park, NC

176. NEUMAN RE and TYTELL AA: Serumless medium for cultivation of cells of normal and malignant origin. Proc Soc Exp Biol Med 104:252–256, 1960

177. NEWMAN JFE, BROWN F, BRIDGER JC, and WOODE GN: Characterization of a rotavirus. Nature (London) 258:631–633, 1975

178. OBIJESKI JF, PALMER EL, and MARTIN ML: Biochemical characterization of infantile gastroenteritis virus (IGV). J Gen Virol 34:485–497, 1977

179. OSTRAVIK I, FIGENSCHAU KJ, HAUG KW, and ULSTRUP JC: A reovirus-like agent (rotavirus) in gastroenteritis of children. Scand J Infect Dis 8:1–5, 1976

180. OSTRAUIK I, HAUG KW, and SOUDE A: Rotavirus-associated gastroenteritis in two adults probably caused by virus reinfection. Scand J Infect Dis 8:277–278, 1976

181. PALMER EL, MARTIN ML, and MURPHY FA: Morphology and stability of infantile gastroenteritis virus: comparison with reovirus and blue tongue virus. J Gen Virol 35:403–414, 1977

182. PARRINO TA, SCHREIBER DS, TRIER JS, KAPIKIAN AZ, and BLACKLOW NR: Clinical immunity in acute gastroenteritis caused by the Norwalk agent. N Engl J Med 297:86–89, 1977

183. PARROTT RH, VARGOSKO AJ, KIM HW, BELLANTI JA, and CHANOCK RM: Myxovirus: parainfluenza. Am J Public Health 52:907–917, 1962

184. PATTERSON S, PARRY J, MATTHEWS THJ, DOURMASHKIN RR, TYRRELL DAJ, WHITE-
HEAD RG, and ROWLAND MGM: Viruses and gastroenteritis. Lancet 2:451, 1975

184a.PAUER WK, CAUL EO, ASHLEY CR, CLARKE SKR: A small virus in human faeces.
Lancet 1:237–240, 1973

184b.PAUER WK, CLARKE SKR: Comparison of human fecal and serum parvo-like viruses.
J Clin Micro 4:67–70, 1976

185. PETERSON MW, SPENDLOVE RS, and SMART RA: Detection of neonatal calf diarrhea virus, infant reovirus-like diarrhea virus and a coronavirus using the fluorescent virus
precipitin test. J Clin Microbiol 3:376, 1976

186. PETRIC M, SZYMANSKI MT, and MIDDLETON PJ: Purification and preliminary characterization of infantile gastroenteritis virus (orbivirus group). Intervirology 5:233–238,
1975

187. PETRIC M, TAM JS, and MIDDLETON PJ: Preliminary characterization of the nucleic acid
of infantile gastroenteritis virus (orbivirus group) Intervirology 7:176–180, 1976

188. PORTNOY BL, CONKLIN RH, MENN M, OLARTE J, and DUPONT HL: Reliable identification of reovirus-like agent in diarrheal stools. J Lab Clin Med 89:560–563, 1977

189. PURCELL RH, WONG DC, ALTER HJ, and HOLLAND PV: Microtiter solid-phase radioimmunoassay for hepatitis B antigen. Appl Microbiol 26:478–484, 1973

190. PURDHAM DR, PURDHAM PA, EVANS N, and McNEISH AS: Isolation of human rotavirus
using human embryonic gut monolayers. Lancet 2:977, 1975

191. REED DE, DALEY CA, and SHAVE HJ: Reovirus-like agent associated with neonatal diarrhea in pronghorn antelope. J Wildl Dis 12:488–491, 1976

192. RITCHIE AE, DESHMUKH DR, LARSEN CT, and POMEROY BS: Electron microscopy of
coronavirus-like particles characteristic of turkey bluecomb disease. Avian Dis
17:546, 1973

193. RODGER SM, CRAVEN JA, and WILLIAM I: Demonstration of reovirus-like particles in
intestinal contents of piglets. Am Vet J 51:536, 1975

194. RODGER SM, SCHNAGL RD, and HOLMES IH: Biochemical and biophysical characterization of diarrhea viruses of human and calf origin. J Virol 16:1229–1235, 1975

195. RODGER SM, SCHNAGL R, and HOLMES IH: Further biochemical characterization, including the detection of surface glycoproteins, of human, calf, and simian rotaviruses. J
Virol 24:91–98, 1977

196. RODRIGUEZ WJ, KIM HW, ARROBIO JO, BRANDT CD, CHANOCK RM, KAPIKIAN AZ,
WYATT RG, and PARROTT RH: Clinical features of acute gastroenteritis associated
with human reovirus-like agent in infants and young children. J Pediatr 91:188–193,
1977

197. RODRIGUEZ WJ, KIM HW, BRANDT CD, YOLKEN RH, ARROBIO JO, KAPIKIAN AZ, and
CHANOCK RM: Sequential enteric illnesses associated with different rotavirus serotypes. Lancet 2:37, 1978

198. RUBENSTEIN D, MILNE RG, BUCKLAND R, and TYRRELL DAJ: The growth of the virus of
epidemic diarrhea of infant mice (EDIM) in organ cultures of intestinal epithelium. Br
J Exp Pathol 52:447–445, 1971

199. RYDER RW, McGOWAN JE, HATCH MH, and PALMER EL: Reovirus-like agent as a cause
of nosocomial diarrhea in infants. J Pediatr 90:698–702, 1977

200. RYDER RW, SACK DA, KAPIKIAN AZ, McLAUGHLIN JC, CHAKRABORTY J, WELLS JG,
MIZANUR RAHMAN ASM, and MERSON MH: Enterotoxigenic Esch. coli and reovirus-
like agent in rural Bangladesh. Lancet 1:659–663, 1976

200a.SACK DA, CHOWDHURY AMAK, EUSOF A, ALI MD. A, MERSON MH, ISLAM S, BLACK
RE, and BROWN KH: Oral hydration in rotavirus diarrhea: a double blind comparison
of sucrose with glucose electrolyte solution. Lancet 2:280–283, 1978

201. SACK RB: Human diarrheal disease caused by enterotoxigenic Escherichia coli. Ann Rev
Microbiol 29:333–353, 1975

202. SALMI TT, ARSTILA P, and KOIVIKKO A: Central nervous system involvement in patients
with rotavirus gastroenteritis. Scand J Infect Dis 10:29–31, 1978

203. SCHERRER R and BERNARD: Application d'une technique immunoenzymologique (ELISA)
a la detection du rotavirus bovin et des anticorps diriges contre lui. Ann Microbiol
(Paris) 128A:499–510, 1977

204. SCHNAGL RD and HOLMES IH: Characteristics of the genome of human infantile enteritis
(rota) virus. J Virol 19:267–270, 1976

205. SCHNAGL R, HOLMES IH, MOORE B, LEE P, DICKINSON-JONES F, and GUST ID: An extensive rotavirus outbreak in aboriginal infants in Central Australia. Med J Aust 1:259-260, 1977

205a. SCHOTTENFELD D and HAAS JF: Carcinogens in the workplace. Ca—A cancer journal for clinicians, Am Cancer Soc 29:144-168, 1979

206. SCHOUB BD, JENKINS T, and ROBINS-BROWNE RM: Rotavirus infection in high-incidence lactase-deficiency population. Lancet 1:328, 1978

207. SCHOUB BD, KOORNOF HJ, LECATSAS G, PROZESKY OW, FREIMAN I, HARTMAN E, and KUSSEL H: Viruses in acute summer gastroenteritis in black infants. Lancet 1:1093-1094, 1975

208. SCHOUB BD, LECATSAS G, and PROZESKY OW: Antigenic relationship between human and simian rotavirus. J Med Microbiol 10:1-6, 1977

209. SCHOUB BD, NEL JD, LECATSAS G, GREEF AS, PROZESKY OW, HAY IT, and PRINSLOO JG: Rotavirus as a cause of gastroenteritis in black South African infants. S Afr Med J 50:1124, 1976

210. SCHREIBER DS, BLACKLOW NR, and TRIER JS: The mucosal lesion of the proximal small intestine in acute infectious nonbacterial gastroenteritis. N Engl J Med 288:1318-1323, 1973

211. SCHREIBER DS, BLACKLOW NR, and TRIER JS: The small intestinal lesion induced by Hawaii agent acute infectious nonbacterial gastroenteritis. J Infect Dis 129:705-708, 1974

212. SCHRIBER DS, TRIER JS, and BLACKLOW NR: Recent advances in viral gastroenteritis. Gastroenterology 73:174-183, 1977

212a. SCOTT AC, LUDDINGTON J, and LUCAS M: Rotavirus in goats. Vet Rec, 103:145, 1978

213. SEVER JL: Application of a microtechnique to viral serological investigations. J Immunol 88:320-329, 1969

214. SHARPEE R and MEBUS CA: Rotaviruses (sic) of man and animals. Lancet 1:639, 1975

215. SHEPHERD RW, TRUSLOW S, WALKER-SMITH JA, BIRD K, CUTTING W, DARNELL R, and BARKER CM: Infantile gastroenteritis: a clinical study of reovirus-like agent infection. Lancet 2:1082-1084, 1975

216. SHINOZAKI T, FUJII R, SATO K, TAKAHASHI E, ITO Y, and INABA Y: Hemagglutinin from human reovirus-like agent. Lancet 1:878, 1978

217. SIMHON A and MATA L: Anti-rotavirus antibody in human colostrum. Lancet 1:39-40, 1978

217a. SNODGRASS DR, ANGUS KW, and GRAY EW: A rotavirus from kittens. Vet Rec, 104:223, 1979

218. SNODGRASS DR, MADELEY CR, WELLS PW, and ANGUS KW: Human rotavirus in lambs: infection and passive protection. Infect Immun 16:268-270, 1977

219. SNODGRASS DR, SMITH W, GRAY EW, and HERRING JA: A rotavirus in lambs with diarrhea. Res Vet Sci 20:113-114, 1976

220. SNODGRASS DR and WELLS PW: Rotavirus infection in lambs: studies on passive protection. Arch Virol 52:201-205, 1976

221. SNODGRASS DR and GRAY EW: Detection and transmission of 30 nm virus particles (astroviruses) in faeces of lambs with diarrhea. Arch Virol 55:286-291, 1977

222. SPENCE L, FAUVEL M, BOUCHARD S, BABIUK L, and SAUNDERS JR: Test for reovirus-like agent. Lancet 2:322, 1975

223. SPENCE L, FAUVEL M, PETRO R, and BLOCH S: Hemagglutinin from rotavirus. Lancet 2:1023, 1976

224. SPENCE L, FAUVEL M, PETRO R, and BLOCH S: Comparison of counter-immuno-electrophoresis and electron microscopy for laboratory diagnosis of human reovirus-like agent-associated infantile gastroenteritis. J Clin Microbiol 5:248-249, 1977

225. STAIR EL, RHODES MB, WHITE RG, and MEBUS CA: Neonatal calf diarrhea: purification and electron microscopy of a coronavirus-like agent. Am J Vet Res 33:1147-1156, 1972

226. STINTZING G, TUFUESSON B, HABTE D, BACK E, JOHNSSON T, and WADSTROM T: Aetiology of acute diarrhoeal disease in infancy and childhood during the peak season Addis Ababa 1977: a preliminary report. Ethiop Med J 15:141-146, 1977

227. SUZUKI H and KONNO T: Reovirus-like particles in jejunal mucosa of a Japanese infant with acute infectious non-bacterial gastroenteritis. Tohoku J Exp Med 115:119-211, 1975

228. TALLETT S, MACKENZIE C, MIDDLETON P, KERZNER B, and HAMILTON R: Clinical, laboratory, and epidemiological features of a viral gastroenteritis in infants and children. Pediatrics 60:217–222, 1977

229. TAM JS, SZYMANSKI MT, MIDDLETON PJ, and PETRIC M: Studies on the particles of infantile gastroenteritis virus (orbivirus group). Intervirology 7:181–191, 1976

230. THEIL KW, BOHL EH, and AGNES AG: Cell culture propagation of porcine rotavirus (reovirus-like agent). Am J Vet Res 38:1765–1768, 1977

231. THORNHILL TS, KALICA AR, WYATT RG, KAPIKIAN AZ, and CHANOCK RM: Pattern of shedding of the Norwalk particle in stools during experimentally induced gastroenteritis in volunteers as determined by immune electron microscopy. J Infect Dis 132:28–34, 1975

232. THORNHILL TS, WYATT RG, KALICA AR, DOLIN R, CHANOCK RM, and KAPIKIAN AZ: Detection by immune electron microscopy of 26–27nm virus-like particles associated with two family outbreaks of gastroenteritis. J Infect Dis 135:20–27, 1977

233. THORNTON A and ZUCKERMAN AJ: The virus of acute diarrhea. Nature 254:557–558, 1975

234. THOULESS ME, BRYDEN AS, and FLEWETT TH: Serotypes of human rotavirus. Lancet 1:39, 1978

235. THOULESS ME, BRYDEN AS, FLEWETT TH, WOODE GN, BRIDGER JC, SNODGRASS GR, and HERRING JA: Serological relationships between rotaviruses from different species as studied by complement-fixation and neutralization. Arch Virol 53:287–294, 1977

236. THOULESS ME, BRYDEN AS, and FLEWETT TH: Rotavirus neutralization by human milk. Br Med J 2:1390, 1977

237. TODD D and MCNULTY MS: Biochemical studies on a reovirus-like agent (rotavirus) from lambs. J Virol 21:1215–1218, 1977

238. TORRES-MEDINA A, WYATT RG, MEBUS CA, UNDERDAHL NR, and KAPIKIAN AZ: Diarrhea in gnotobiotic piglets caused by the human reovirus-like agent of infantile gastroenteritis. J Infect Dis 133:22–27, 1976

239. TORRES-MEDINA A, WYATT RG, TWIEHAUS CA, UNDERDAHL NR, and KAPIKIAN AZ: Patterns of shedding of human reovirus-like agent in gnotobiotic newborn piglets with experimentally-induced diarrhea. Intervirology 7:250–255, 1976

240. TOTTERDELL BM, CHRYSTIE IL, and BANATVALA JE: Rotavirus infections in a maternity unit. Arch Dis Child 51:924–928, 1976

241. TUFVESSON B and JOHNSSON T: Occurrence of reo-like viruses in young children with acute gastroenteritis. Acta Pathol Microbiol Scand [B] 84:22–28, 1976

242. TUFVESSON B and JOHNSSON T: Immunoelectro-osmophoresis for detection of reo-like virus: methodology and comparison with electron microscopy. Acta Pathol Microbiol Scand. [B] 84:225–228, 1976

243. TUFESSON B, JOHNSON T, and PETERSON B: Family infections by reo-like virus. Scand J Inf Dis 9:257–261, 1977

244. TZIPORI S: Human rotavirus in young dogs. Med J Aust 2:922, 1977

245. TZIPORI S, CAPLE IW, and BUTLER R: Isolation of a rotavirus from deer. Vet Rec 99:398, 1976

245a. TZIPORI S and WALKER M: Isolation of rotavirus from foals with diarrhea. Austr J Exp Biol Med Sci 56:453, 1978

246. VANKIRK DH, KAPIKIAN AZ, WYATT RG, and KALICA AR: Viral digestive tract infections In CRC Handbook Series in Clinical Laboratory Science (D. SELIGSON Editor-in-Chief) Section H: Virology and Rickettsiology, Volume 1, Part 2 (Section editors GD HSIUNG and RH GREEN). CRC Press Inc., West Palm Beach, FL, pp 211–233, 1978

247. VOLLER A, BIDWELL DE, and BARTLETT A: Microplate enzyme immunoassays for the immunodiagnosis of virus infections. In Manual of Clinical Immunoassay, ROSE NR and FRIEDMAN H (eds), Am Soc Microbiol, Washington, DC, 1976, pp 506–512

248. WANATABE H, GUST ID, and HOLMES IH: Human rotavirus and its antibody: their co-existence in faeces of infants. J Clin Microbiol 7:405–409, 1978

249. WANATABE H and HOLMES IH: Filter paper solid-phase radioimmunoassay for human rotavirus surface immunoglobulins. J Clin Microbiol 6:319–324, 1977

249a. WARBURG O and CHRISTIAN W: Isolierung und kristallisation des gärungsferments enolase. Biochemische Zeitschrift 310: 384–421, 1942

250. WELCH AB and THOMPSON TL: Physicochemical characterization of a neonatal calf diarrhea virus. Can J Comp Med 37:295–301, 1973

251. WELCH AB and TWIEHAUS MJ: Cell culture studies of a neonatal calf diarrhea virus. Can J Comp Med 37:287–294, 1973

252. WIDERLITE L, TRIER JS, BLACKLOW NR, and SCHREIBER DS: Structure of the gastric mucosa in acute infectious nonbacterial gastroenteritis. Gastroenterology 68:425–430, 1975

253. WILLIAMS T, BOURKE P, and GURWITH M: Program Abstracts, 15th Intersci Conf Antimicrob Agents Chemother, Washington, DC Abst 234:232, 1975

254. WOODE GN and BRIDGER JC: Viral enteritis of calves. Vet Rec 96:85–88, 1975

255. WOODE GN, BRIDGER JC, HALL G, and DENNIS MJ: The isolation of a reovirus-like agent associated with diarrhea in colostrum-deprived calves in Great Britain. Res Vet Sci 16:102–105, 1974

256. WOODE GN, BRIDGER J, HALL GA, JONES JM, and JACKSON G: The isolation of reovirus-like agents (rotavirus) from acute gastroenteritis of piglets. J Med Microbiol 9:203–209, 1976

257. WOODE GN, BRIDGER JC, JONES JM, FLEWETT TH, BRYDEN AS, DAVIES HA, and WHITE GBB: Morphological and antigenic relationships between viruses (rotaviruses) from acute gastroenteritis of children, calves, piglets, mice, and foals. Infect Immun 14:804–810, 1976

258. WOODE GN, JONES J, and BRIDGER J: Levels of colostral antibodies against neonatal calf diarrhea virus. Vet Rec 97:148–149, 1975

259. WHO STUDY GROUP: Viral hepatitis and tests for the Australia (hepatitis-associated) antigen and antibody. Bull WHO 42:951–952, 1970

259a. WYATT RG, CHANOCK RM, and JAMES WD: Characterization of rotavirus using plaque assay. (Abstract) Fourth International Congress for Virology, The Hague, 1978

260. WYATT RG, DOLIN R, BLACKLOW NR, DuPONT HL BUSCHO RF, THORNHILL TS, KAPIKIAN AZ, and CHANOCK RM: Comparison of three agents of acute infectious nonbacterial gastroenteritis by cross-challenge in volunteers. J Infect Dis 129:709–724, 1974

261. WYATT RG, GILL VW, SERENO MM, KALICA AR, VANKIRK DH, CHANOCK RM, and KAPIKIAN AZ: Probable *in vitro* cultivation of human reovirus-like agent of infantile diarrhea. Lancet 1:98, 1976

262. WYATT RG, GREENBERG HB, DALGARD DW, ALLEN WP, SLY DL, THORNHILL TS, CHANOCK RM, and KAPIKIAN AZ: Experimental infection of chimpanzees with the Norwalk agent of epidemic viral gastroenteritis. J Med Virology 2:89–96, 1978

263. WYATT RG, KALICA AR, MEBUS CA, KIM HW, LONDON WT, CHANOCK RM, and KAPIKIAN AZ: Reovirus-like agents (rotaviruses) associated with diarrheal illness in animals and man. *In* Perspectives in Virology X, POLLARD M (ed), Raven Press, 10:121–145, 1978

264. WYATT RG and KAPIKIAN AZ: Viral agents associated with acute gastroenteritis in humans. Am J Clin Nutr 30:1857–1870, 1977

265. WYATT RG and KAPIKIAN AZ: Viral gastrointestinal infections *In* Textbook of Pediatric Infectious Diseases. FEIGIN and CHERRY (eds), WB Saunders Co, Philadelphia (in press) 1980

266. WYATT RG, KAPIKIAN AZ, THORNHILL TS, SERENO MM, KIM HW, and CHANOCK RM: *In vitro* cultivation in human fetal intestinal organ culture of a reovirus-like agent associated with nonbacterial gastroenteritis in infants and children. J Infect Dis 130:523–528, 1974

267. WYATT RG, SLY DL, LONDON WT, PALMER AE, KALICA AR, VANKIRK DH, CHANOCK RM, and KAPIKIAN AZ: Induction of diarrhea in colostrum-deprived newborn rhesus monkeys with the human reovirus-like agent of infantile gastroenteritis. Arch Virol 50:17–27, 1976

268. WYATT RG, YOLKEN RH, URRUTIA JJ, MATA L, GREENBERG HB, CHANOCK RM, and KAPIKIAN AZ: Diarrhea associated with rotavirus in rural Guatemala: a longitudinal study of 24 infants and young children. Am J Trop Med Hyg 28(2):325–328, 1979

269. WYN-JONES AP: Virus-associated gastroenteritis in children. Lancet 2:559, 1975

270. YOLKEN RH, BARBOUR BA, WYATT RG, and KAPIKIAN AZ: Immune responses to human rotaviral infections. J Am Vet Med Assoc 173:552–554, 1978

271. YOLKEN RH, BARBOUR B, WYATT RG, KALICA AR, KAPIKIAN AZ, and CHANOCK RM: Enzyme-linked immunosorbent assay (ELISA) for identification of rotaviruses from different animal species. Science 201:259–262, 1978

272. YOLKEN RH, KIM HW, CLEM T, WYATT RG, KALICA AR, CHANOCK RM, and KAPIKIAN AZ: Enzyme linked immunosorbent assay (ELISA) for detection of human reovirus-like agent of infantile gastroenteritis. Lancet 2:263–267, 1977

273. YOLKEN RH, WYATT RG, ZISSIS GP, BRANDT CD, RODRIGUEZ WJ, KIM HW, PARROTT RH, KAPIKIAN AZ, and CHANOCK RM: Epidemiology of human rotavirus types 1 and 2 as studied by enzyme-linked immunosorbent assay. N Engl J Med 299:1156–1161, 1978

274. YOLKEN RH, MATA L, GARCIA B, URRUTIA JJ, WYATT RG, CHANOCK RM, and KAPIKIAN AZ: Secretory antibody directed against rotavirus in human milk: measurement by means of enzyme linked immunosorbent assay. J Pediatr 93:916–921, 1978

275. YOLKEN RH, WYATT RG, BARBOUR BA, KIM HW, KAPIKIAN AZ, and CHANOCK RM: Measurement of anti-rotavirus antibody by an enzyme-linked immunosorbent (ELISA) blocking assay. J Clin Micro 8:283–287, 1978

276. YOLKEN RH, WYATT RG, KALICA AR, KIM HW, BRANDT CD, PARROTT RH, KAPIKIAN AZ, and CHANOCK RM: Use of a free viral immunofluorescence assay to detect human reovirus-like agent in human stools. Infect Immun 16:467–470, 1977

277. YOLKEN RH, WYATT RG, and KAPIKIAN AZ: ELISA for rotavirus. Lancet 2:818, 1977

278. YOLKEN RH, WYATT RG, KIM HW, KAPIKIAN AZ, and CHANOCK RM: Immunological response to infection with human reovirus-like agent: measurement of anti-human reovirus-like agent immunoglobulin G and M levels by the method of enzyme-linked immunosorbent assay. Infect Immun 19:540–546, 1978

279. YOW MD, MELNICK JL, BLATTNER RJ, STEPHENSON WB, ROBINSON NM, and BURKHARDT MA: The association of viruses and bacteria with infantile diarrhea. Am J Epidemiol 92:33–39, 1970

280. ZAHORSKY J: Hyperemesis hiemis or the winter vomiting disease. Arch Pediatr 46:391–395, 1929

281. ZISSIS G and LAMBERT JP: Different serotypes of human rotaviruses. Lancet 1:38–39, 1978

282. ZISSIS G and CLINET G: Viral-antibody detection by a more sensitive complement-fixation reaction. Lancet 1:754–755, 1978

283. ZISSIS G, LAMBERT JP, and DEKEGEL D: Routine diagnosis of human rotavirus in stools. J Clin Path 31:175–178, 1978

284. ZISSIS G, LAMBERT JP, FONTEYNE J, and DE KEGEL D: Child-mother transmission of rotavirus. Lancet 1:96, 1976

CHAPTER 31

MISCELLANEOUS VIRUSES

Joel Warren

Marburg and Ebola Virus Disease

(African Hemorrhagic Fever)

All laboratory procedures with suspected Marburg or Ebola virus material should be conducted only by virologists experienced in biohazard methodology and in appropriate containment facilities.

In the summer of 1967, a severe illness of hitherto unreported nature occurred almost simultaneously in the personnel of laboratories in Marburg, Frankfurt, and Belgrade (3, 8, 10). After an incubation period of 4–9 days, major clinical symptoms of marked malaise, high fever, headache, diarrhea, and loss of consciousness developed. This was accompanied by a characteristic rickettsial-like rash with severe hemorrhagic diathesis. Signs of central nervous system (CNS) involvement were common. There were 5 fatalities among the 23 cases in Germany (10).

Direct contact with organs and tissues of freshly imported *Cercopithecus aethiops* monkeys from Uganda had occurred in most of the cases, although secondary human-contact infections apparently from blood were also established. At autopsy, practically all of the organs of the body were found to have areas of severe necrosis surrounded by a band of unusual cytoplasmic inclusions.

After an interval of 8 years, 3 additional cases of Marburg disease occurred, this time in South Africa. The primary case, in a young man, was fatal, whereas two contacts, his female traveling companion and an attending nurse, recovered after a severe illness (2). One year later, over 500 cases of an acute hemorrhagic fever simultaneously appeared in Sudan and Zaire in equatorial Africa. This outbreak had a mortality of 70%. The clinical picture in the 1976 outbreak closely resembled the original Marburg disease, and secondary cases in attending medical and nursing personnel were frequent (1, 7). Although the virus was morphologically identical with the Marburg agent, it was antigenically different. The agent is tentatively designated as "Ebola virus" after a river valley in Zaire where the disease first appeared (5). There was no history of contact with monkeys in this epidemic, and the term "Green Monkey Disease" now seems inappropriate (5).

Clinical aspects

In addition to transmission by exposure to infected green monkeys, direct contact with sick patients, their blood, tissues, or excreta is a source of infection. *Strict barrier nursing should be instituted whenever Marburg or Ebola virus disease is suspected.* After a short incubation period the presenting clinical signs include:

1. Malaise, headache, and myalgia.
2. Nausea and vomiting, abdominal pain, and profuse watery diarrhea.
3. A characteristic maculopapular rash and erythema which appear on the trunk, face, and arms on about the fifth day of illness.
4. Severe gastrointestinal or pulmonary bleeding, jaundice, and a marked thrombocytopenia may accompany the above. Detailed clinical records can be found in the report of Grear et al (2).

Because virus has been isolated from patients as long as 2–9 months after the onset of illness, the advisability of prolonged quarantine is obvious.

Pathology

The necropsy findings are those common to the acute, fulminating, viral hemorrhagic fevers and are comprised of extensive necrosis of the spleen, liver, kidney, and gastrointestinal tract, accompanied by massive bleeding into these organs. A unique and frequent finding is the presence of eosinophilic cytoplasmic inclusion bodies surrounding areas of necrosis in the major viscera. (For photographs, see Refs 1 and 5). Laboratory findings of an elevated serum glutamic-oxaloacetic transaminase (SGOT), a leukopenia, and a marked drop in plasma protein are all indicative of a loss of vascular integrity.

Description of agent

The virus has a bizarre, filamentous, tube-like appearance with regular surface projections and, when stained, has internal cross-bands suggestive of a helical core structure (5). The virions average 100μ in diameter and a length between $300–3000\mu$ (1). They are sensitive to ether and are not inhibited by 5-bromodeoxyuridine suggesting that the virus contains RNA. Marburg and Ebola viruses are related but have no antigenic relationship to any other known viruses. Their extreme length distinguishes them from other animal viruses. Although Marburg virus has been tentatively assigned to the rhabdovirus group by Howatson (4), subsequent ultrastructural studies by Murphy et al suggest that it remain unclassified (6).

Virions from the European and African cases have a similar appearance. However, there is some question as to the degree of cross-immunity between the disease in these two areas. When reciprocal cross-titrations by indirect immunofluorescence (IFA) were performed by Johnson et al, the Marburg and Ebola convalescent-phase sera gave higher homologous and weaker cross-reactions (5). Similarly, previous infection with Marburg virus does not confer resistance to a subsequent infection with Ebola virus and *vice versa* (9). Both strains are pathogenic for guinea pigs, causing a nonfatal, febrile disease after an incubation period of 4–7 days (7). Inoculation of suckling mice with acute-phase serum caused a fatal illness, but its identity was unconfirmed (1). Vero (African green monkey) and human amnion cell cultures develop focal rounding and changed refractility in 3–5 days after inoculation with infectious blood or tissues. The agent can be serially passaged in these systems.

Preparation of immune serum

Convalescent-phase human or guinea pig sera can be used for FA tests (5). Both direct and indirect procedures have been used.

Collection and preparation of specimens

Little is known regarding the stability or optimum storage conditions of these agents. Because of their high infectivity and capacity to cause mortal illness, they are best transported in double-sealed, soldered metal containers, refrigerated with dry ice. Blood or tissues have yielded positive isolates in cell culture with a high frequency and are the specimens of choice for diagnosis. Throat swabs, urine, and feces from two of the Johannesburg patients also yielded virus (2).

Laboratory diagnosis

The presence of large eosinophilic, smooth, refractile, and sharply defined inclusion bodies in hepatocytes or parenchymal cells of the spleen or lung is suggestive of this disease (5). Virus has been directly observed by electron microscopy (EM) in liver, lung, and spleen tissues and in Vero cell cultures (2, 5). Its filamentous shape, occasional branching, and extreme length are unique and characteristic. The intraperitoneal inoculation of young guinea pigs (200–250 g) yields highly infectious material in which characteristic virions have been detected by EM or by FA with human or animal immune (convalescent) serum (5). Specimens of blood, throat swabs, urine, and tissues removed at autopsy can rapidly infect Vero or human amnion cells. FA reactions, employing convalescent-phase guinea pig or human antimonkey virus serum, can be positive as early as the second day after infection of a monolayer culture (11). It was also possible to visualize Marburg-type virions in culture fluids inoculated with serum or blood from the Zaire epidemic (1).

References

1. BOWEN ET, PLATT GS, LLOYD G, BASKERVILLE A, HARRIS W, and VELLA EE: Viral hemorrhagic fever in southern Sudan and northern Zaire. Lancet 1:571–572, 1977
2. GEAR JSS, CASSEL GA, GEAR AJ, TRAPPLER B, CLAUSEN L, MEYERS AM, KEW MC, BOTHWELL TH, SHER R, MILLER GB, SCHNEIDER J, KOORNHOF HJ, GOMPERTZ GD, ISAACSON M, and GEAR JHS: Outbreak of Marburg Disease in Johannesburg. Br Med J 4:489–493, 1975
3. HENNESSEN W, BONIN O, and MAULER R: Epidemiologie der Erkrankung von Menschen durch Affen. Deut Med Wochenschr 12a:582–589, 1968
4. HOWATSON AF: Vesicular stomatitis and related viruses. Adv Virus Res 16:195–256, 1970

5. JOHNSON KM, WEBB PA, LANGE JV, and MURPHY FA: Isolation and partial characterization of new virus causing acute hemorrhagic fever in Zaire. Lancet 1:569–571, 1977
6. MURPHY FA, SIMPSON DIH, WHITFIELD SG, ZLOTNIM I, and CARTER GB: Marburg virus
   infection in monkeys. Ultrastructural studies. Lab Invest 24:279–291, 1971
7. PATTYN S, JACOB W, VAN DER GROEN G, PIOT P, and COURTEILLE G: Isolation of a Mar-
   burg-like virus from a case of hemorrhagic fever in Zaire. Lancet 1:573–574, 1977
8. SIEGERT R: Marburg Virus. Virology Monograph, No 11, 1972. Springer-Verlag, Berlin
9. SIMPSON DIH and ZUCKERMAN AJ: Marburg and Ebola: viruses in search of a relation.
   Nature, 266:217–218, 1977
10. STILLE W, BOHLE E, HELM E, VAN REY W, and SIEDE W: Uber eine durch *Cercopithecus
    aethiops* ubertragene Infektionskrankheit. Deut Med Wochenschr 12a:572–582, 1968
11. VELLA EE: Marburg Disease. Nurs Times 14:120–122, 1977

Papovavirus Infections

(Wart Virus Verruca, Myrmecia, BK and JC Viruses)

Warts were among the first diseases to be recognized as being of viral etiology by Ciuffo in 1907 (4). Melnick, in 1962, suggested the family *Papovaviridae* for a group of viruses comprised of the human papilloma virus (wart virus), rabbit papillomavirus (Shope virus), mouse polyoma virus, and simian virus 40 (vacuolating virus) (11). In 1971 there were several simultaneous isolations from human subjects of papovaviruses which were unrelated to each other and to the human papillomaviruses (13). Certain of these, together with SV-40 virus, form a subgroup of primate papovaviruses. These agents, of relatively small size, have a supercoiled, covalently closed, double-strand DNA, and produce transformation of cells in culture.

The human papillomaviruses induce several different histologic and chronic types of benign epithelial papillomata. The most frequently recognized forms are common, juvenile, filiform, digitate, or genital warts, and laryngeal papillomata. The lesions of molluscum contagiosum (see Chapter 8) caused by a virus of the pox family, can resemble common warts but are easily distinguished by their histology (2).

Intranuclear inclusions are easily visualized and can be eosinophilic or basophilic depending upon location in the skin. Virions are demonstrable in most, but not all, warts by optical and EM and by staining with fluorescein-conjugated antibody. The concentration of virus in human warts seems to parallel the incidence of basophilic inclusions (1).

The occasional transmissibility of warts from one individual to another after a long incubation period has been recognized for at least 150 years (5). Entrance of the virus occurs directly or through the skin via abrasions, but there is no information as to the presence or persistence of virus outside of the wart tissue. A tabulation of experiments on the transmission of warts to humans is found in the article by Rowson and Mahy (17).

BK virus (BKV), a human papovavirus, was discovered by Gardner et al in the urine of a patient receiving immunosuppressive therapy (7). Based on serologic surveys, subclinical infection occurs early in life and probably is spread by the oral route from viruses in the urine or feces. Viruria, however, has not been reported in healthy children or adults. Although there are studies which ascribe an oncogenic potential to BKV, the matter remains unsettled (14).

JC virus (JCV) was first isolated by Padgett et al from the brain of a patient with progressive multifocal leukoencephalopathy (PML) (13). Since then it has been identified in brain tissues of over 25 patients with PML (15). JCV has a minor antigenic relationship with SV-40 and BKV, although it multiplies only in cultures of human fetal glial cells. Like BKV, there is serologic evidence of widespread (75%) occult infection in the general population, and it is generally acquired in childhood (14). Padgett et al found antibody to JCV in human serum obtained prior to 1950, thus eliminating the possibility that antibody was produced by SV-40 virus present in the poliovirus vaccine introduced in 1954 (15). There is no evidence that these human strains have an animal reservoir in nature, although the JCV agent produces tumors in newborn Syrian hamsters.

Description of the agents

Human and animal papovaviruses are characterized by a well-defined capsid of 42 or 72 capsomeres arranged in cubic symmetry (8). All strains are predominantly spherical, 40–45 μ in diameter, and ether-resistant. The genomes of these agents have molecular weights between 5.0×10^6 and 5.25×10^6 daltons, depending upon the strain. The papillomaviruses are quite stable, and infectivity is retained after proteinase digestion in water, 50% glycerol-saline, or at -60 C for long periods. Human wart virus was prepared as a killed phenolized vaccine by heating at 56–60 C for 2 hr (17). Its survival in the dried state is unknown.

By means of restriction enzyme analysis and RNA-DNA hybridization, at least two antigenically different types of papillomaviruses have been isolated from warts in humans (12). Whether these types are associated with specific clinical expression of wart virus is unknown. Nevertheless, the difference between polypeptides and antigen in these strains is greater than that between the JCV and BKV strains (18). It may, therefore, be appropriate to accept the suggestion of Orth et al that these wart virus strains be designated as HPV types I and II.

The virion of BKV has a diameter of approximately 40 nm and when negatively stained appears as an icosohedron with 72 capsomeres. Tubular forms have been observed in cultures of both BKV and JCV (14). The infectivity of BKV is resistant to chloroform, that of JCV withstood ether and heating to 50 C for 1 hr (14).

Although its original isolation was made in Vero cells, a continuous line of African green monkey kidney cells (14), BKV multiplies with extensive vacuolization in primary cultures of human fibroblasts, liver, lung, brain, and fetal kidney, the latter being the cell most widely employed for the growth assay of this agent. BKV did not grow in hamster, mouse, or rat cells, or, surprisingly, in monkey brain cells (14).

In contrast, JCV exhibits a narrow range of experimental pathogenicity, being cytopathic for only primary human fetal glial cell cultures in which it grows slowly, and morphologic changes may not be observed until 10–14 days after inoculation. Basophilic intranuclear inclusion bodies, easily stained with hematoxylin and eosin, are prominent in cultures of both BKV and JCV. The infectious virions of these agents hemagglutinate human, guinea pig, and chick erythrocytes (RBC) but not those of the monkey, sheep, mouse, or hamster (15). The agglutinins are stable at 56 C for 1 hr, resist inactivation by chloroform or ether, and are useful reagents for serologic diagnosis.

Laboratory diagnosis

The diagnosis of warts continues to be made primarily upon clinical grounds and the presence of characteristic inclusions in scrapings or biopsies of verrucous material. The latter procedure is often employed where malignant transformation is suspected. Inclusions are most readily found in deeply embedded plantar warts and may not be observable in superficial verruca (9).

The diagnosis of active BKV and JCV infections requires isolation of the agents in cell culture. Hemagglutination-inhibition (HAI), complement fixation (CF), neutralization (Nt), and FA procedures have been utilized for confirmation and in serologic surveys (14). The BKV agent, with one exception, has thus far been found only in the urinary tract and, particularly, in immunosuppressed individuals. No specific disease has been associated with BKV infection. In contrast, there is compelling evidence that JCV can cause rare, demyelinating, and often fatal, illness in humans. It has not been possible to transmit PML to animals (15).

Virus isolation

There is no satisfactory evidence that human and animal strains of wart viruses are infectious for another species. Attempts to repeat the cultivation of a virus from human warts in embryonated eggs as described in Bivins (3) have not been successful (17). However, there have been at least 6 reports of the cultivation of agents which resemble the papovaviruses in monolayers of human, simian, or murine cells (see Ref 17 for review). The cytopathology and presence of typical virions and immunofluorescence suggests that the agent has been successfully cultivated.

BKV grows very slowly in Vero cells (7). However, when supernatant fluid and sediment from infectious urine samples were centrifuged at 2,500 rpm for 10 min and inoculated into cultures of primary human embryonic kidney cells they developed cytoplasmic vacuolization and intranuclear inclusions within 4–5 weeks (14). The inclusions were composed of virions. These could be readily visualized by EM, were numerous in the culture fluid, and were occasionally observed in the original urine (6).

Thus far the JCV has only been cultivated in primary cultures of human fetal glial cells in which it produces a cytopathic effect (CPE) within 2 weeks after inoculation; primary isolates may grow more slowly. The preparation of glial cell cultures from fetal human brain tissue is described in detail by Padgett, Rogers, and Walker (15). JCV has failed to multiply in other human embryonic or animal cell cultures. Intranuclear inclusion bodies are visible in infected monolayers stained with acridine orange.

Serologic diagnosis of wart viruses

Wart virus and cell-associated antigens have been used as research reagents in the CF, immunodiffusion (ID), and FA procedures. There is increasing evidence that the status of antibody correlates with the clinical course and may be of prognostic value. CF antibody (IgG) is stimulated by wart virions and is found in approximately 20% of patients with warts. Its presence is reported as associated with rapid healing (16). IgM antibody, measured by ID, is found in 80% of patients with warts and appears to have limited prognostic value (17). The viral genome cannot be detected in all warts even by sensitive hybridization procedures (18).

Complement-fixation test. Virus-rich extracts of minced wart tissues may be used as crude or clarified supernatants or high-speed centrifuge pellets which are subsequently solubilized by sonication (17). Extracts of similarly prepared normal human skin serve as controls. Tests are conducted in microtiter plates with 2 full units of complement and 4 units of antigen. Incubation at either 5 C or 37 C is satisfactory.

Immunodiffusion test. Antigens similar to those used for the wart CF test are placed in the central well of a plate of 0.9% agarose buffered to pH 7.4 with phosphate. Dilutions of human or animal serum are placed in the outer wells. The precipitin bands may be stained with amido black. An inverse correlation between a positive ID reaction (IgG antibody) and the duration and number of tumors has been reported by Pyrhonen and Pentinnen (16).

Immunofluorescence test. Several workers have employed an indirect FA procedure to learn more about the distribution of antigen in regressing and static warts. Both rabbit and human antiwart sera were used with labeled sheep antirabbit globulin. Human papovaviruses are highly antigenic, and potent antiserum is readily prepared in rabbits with crude or purified extracts of wart tissues. Matthews and Shirodaria observed that regressing warts exhibited strongly positive fluorescence, primarily in the nuclei of cells in the granular region. They suggest that regression results in the release of large amounts of antigen into the circulation (10).

Serologic diagnosis of BK and JC viruses

Virus assays. Monolayers of human embryonic kidney cells were infected with BKV and kept for 2 hr at room temperature. These were then overlayed with minimal essential medium (MEM) + 10% tryptose phosphate broth plus 10% fetal calf serum and 0.8% agar. The cultures were incubated for 7 days, stained with neutral red 1:10,000, reincubated for 3 days, and the plaques counted (6). JCV was titrated by production of CPE in primary human glial cell tube cultures or by counting individual infected cells binding fluorescent antibody (15).

Virus neutralization. Human or animal hyperimmune rabbit or guinea pig serum against BKV was mixed with equal volumes of virus diluted to contain 2×10^3 or 2×10^2 plaque forming units (pfu)/0.2 ml. The mixtures were again incubated for 1 hr at 37 and 2 hr at 40 C. The neutralization index was calculated as number of plaques in control/number of plaques in antiserum.

Hemagglutination. The BKV and JCV agglutinate chicken, guinea pig, and human RBC, but not monkey or hamster RBC. Maximal hemagglutination (HA) of human, group O RBC occurred at 4 C in a range of 6.1–7.4; no HA was observed at 37 C (14). Inactivation of the virus by 0.1% β-propiolactone does not destroy its hemagglutinin.

Gardner et al used crude JCV-infected cell culture fluids, 0.25 ml, mixed with an equal volume of 0.5% human O RBC. Doubling dilutions of the infected culture were employed and the endpoints were read after 1 hr at 4 C (7).

Hemagglutination inhibition. This is the procedure of choice for measuring human papovavirus antibodies. Using the virus HA titration described above, complete HA is taken as representing 1 hemagglutinating unit (HAU). Because human serum frequently contains nonspecific inhibitors it is necessary to treat it by incubating overnight with broth culture filtrates of *Vibrio cholera* or $NaIO_4$ (14) followed by inactivation at 56 C for 1 hr and absorption with packed human O RBC. Two-fold dilutions of the serum are made in plastic plates in volumes of 0.25 ml, and an equal volume of antigen containing 4 HAU is added to each dilution. The mixtures are allowed to react at room temperature for 1 hr, and then 0.25 ml of a 0.5% suspension of human O RBC is added to each well, and the plates are incubated at 4 C for 1 hr. The highest serum dilution completely inhibiting HA is taken as the endpoint, and the antibody titer is expressed as the reciprocal of this dilution. These tests are adaptable to microtiter procedures.

Complement fixation. Gardner et al prepared JCV antigen from Vero cell cultures showing minimal CPE (7). However, antigen can also be prepared from suspensions of infected primary human embryonic kidney cells which have been clarified by slow-speed centrifugation. In either case, the cells should be frozen and thawed at least twice to release virions, and the suspension then clarified by centrifugation. The CF test is performed in plastic plates using 3 units of complement and overnight fixation at 4 C. Control antigens are prepared from uninfected cultures.

Immunofluorescence procedures. The uptake and replication of these viruses can be followed by means of FA staining of infected cells cultivated on coverslips (15). The latter are fixed in 10% acetone and stained for FA counting with specific human, monkey, or rabbit antigen. The appropriate fluorescein conjugated antiglobulins are then applied and the antigen containing cells are counted. A fluorescent cell reduction procedure was used by Padgett et al for the measurement of JCV Nt antibody (15).

References

1. ALMEIDA JD, HOWATSON AF, and WILLIAMS MG: Electron microscopic study of human warts, sites of virus production, and nature of the inclusion bodies. J Invest Dermatol 33:337–345, 1962
2. BLANK H and RAKE G: Warts. Chap 9 *In* Viral and Rickettsial Diseases of the Skin, Eye, and Mucous Membranes of Man, 1st edition, Little, Brown, Boston, 1955, pp 156–181
3. BIVINS JA: The growth in the developing chick embryo of a filtrable agent from verruca vulgaris. J Invest Dermatol 20:471–481, 1953

4. CIUFFO G: Innesto positiv con filtrate di verruca volgar. G Ital Mal Ven 48:12–18, 1907
5. COOPER A: Lectures on the Principles and Practice of Surgery, 8th edition, Cox and Port-wine, London, 1835, p 497–498
6. DOUGHERTY RM and DI STEFANO HS: Isolation and characterization of a papovavirus from human urine. Proc Soc Exp Biol Med 146:481–487, 1974
7. GARDNER SD, FIELD AM, COLEMAN DV, and HULME B: New human papovavirus (BK) isolated from urine after renal transplantation. Lancet I:1253–1257, 1971
8. HOWATSON AF and CRAWFORD LV: Direct counting of the capsomeres in polyoma and papilloma viruses. Virology 21:1–6, 1963
9. LYELL A and MILES JAR: The myrmecia: a study of inclusion bodies in warts. Br Med J 1:912–915, 1951
10. MATHEWS RS and SHIRODARIA PV: Study of regressing warts by immunofluorescence. Lancet I:689–690, 1973
11. MELNICK JL: Papova virus group. Science 135:1128–1130, 1962
12. ORTH G, FAVRE M, and CROISSANT O: Characterization of a new type of human papilloma-virus that causes skin warts. J Virol 24:108–120, 1977
13. PADGETT BL, WALKER DL, ZURHEIN GM, ECKROADE RJ, and DESSEL BH: Cultivation of papova-like virus from human brain with progressive multifocal leukoencephalopathy. Lancet I:1257–1260, 1971
14. PADGETT BL and WALKER DL: New human papovaviruses. Prog Med Virol 22:1–35, 1976
15. PADGETT BL, ROGERS CM, and WALKER DL: JC virus, a human polyomavirus associated with progressive multifocal leukoencephalopathy: additional biological characteristics and antigenic relationships. Infect Immun 15:656–662, 1977
16. PYRHONEN S and PENTINNEN K: Regression of warts: an immunological study. Lancet I:593–595, 1975
17. ROWSON KE and MAHY BW: Human papova (wart) virus. Bacteriol Rev 31:110–131, 1967
18. ZUR HAUSEN H, MEINHOF W, SCHEIBER W, and BORNKAMM GW: Attempts to detect virus-specific DNA in human tumors. Int J Cancer 13:650–655, 1974

Cat-scratch Disease

(Cat-scratch Fever, Nonbacterial Regional Adenitis, Cat-scratch Encephalitis, and Parinaud Oculoglandular Syndrome)

In 1947, Foshay (Cincinnati) and Debre (Paris) were impressed by the similarity of some bizarre illnesses associated with cat scratches in humans. By 1950 the presumptive identity of cases in the United States and abroad (4, 14) was established. Since then the disease has been recognized with increasing frequency (2, 3, 12, 16, 17).

Clinical aspects

Cat-scratch disease is a benign, self-limited, and nonfatal illness; the cardinal feature is subacute, granulomatous lymphadenitis which is sterile on culture. This is associated with fever and malaise. The primary lesion is generally at the site of the scratch, followed in 2–6 weeks by involvement of the regional lymph nodes. This can proceed to suppuration and an erythematous maculopapular or morbilliform eruption can also be present. Cases without a history of a scratch have been reported (17). Involvement of the CNS (cat-scratch encephalitis) with convulsions, respiratory paralysis, and coma can occur in rare instances (16); occasionally it is associated with thrombocytopenic purpura (8). Based upon positive skin-test reactions with cat-scratch disease antigen, it would appear that the agent of cat-scratch disease can produce Parinaud oculoglandular syndrome (1). Daniels and MacMurray (3) and Margileth describe the clinical findings in 205 cases (12). The disease has a worldwide distribution.

Mollaret et al (14) described transmission of the disease to monkeys by intradermal inoculations of lymph node suspensions from patients having the illness. At the inoculation site, small nodules developed which when passaged further in monkeys induced cutaneous nodules and generalized lymphadenopathy. Attempts to infect other laboratory animals were unsuccessful. Attempts to propagate the causative agent in a variety of tissue cultures have been negative (15, 17).

Description of the agent

The exact etiology of cat-scratch disease remains obscure. Mollaret suggested that cat-scratch disease may be caused by an agent of the psittacosis-lymphogranuloma venereum (LGV) group (14). This association is based upon clinical similarities of lymphoid hyperplasia, observations of bodies resembling the elementary bodies of the LGV agent in stained sections of infected human and monkey lymph nodes, and the finding of CF antibody to the chlamydial group antigen in approximately 50% of patients convalescent from cat-scratch disease. Opposed to this assumption are the observations that antibodies did not increase during convalescence, broad-spectrum antibiotics are useless in cat-scratch disease (12), and the findings of Emmons et al. who obtained inconclusive results when the serum of 50 patients was tested by CF and FA against 5 chlamydial group antigens (6). There were no reactions with feline leukemia virus. The presence of CF antibodies reacting with chlamydial antigens must be interpreted with caution since they may be the result of past or current, overt or subclinical infection with any of the agents of that group. Final interpretation of serologic tests requires the demonstration of significant and consistent ($\geq$ 4-fold) increases in antibody to chlamydial group antigen during the course of cat-scratch disease. The histologic appearance of the lymph nodes is a non-pathognomonic reticulum cell hyperplasia. Other etiologic possibilities to be ruled out include Hodgkin disease, lymphoma, tuberculosis, brucellosis, and tularemia (17). Kalter et al. observed herpes-like particles in lymph node biopsy material from 8 cases of cat-scratch disease (9). However, they were unable to detect antibody to Epstein-Barr virus in convalescent cases (10).

Laboratory diagnosis

This involves the exclusion of other lymphadenopathies and a positive dermal reaction to tested antigen.

Intradermal skin test. A specific intradermal skin test for cat-scratch disease similar to the Frei reaction for LGV was developed by Hanger and Rose (cited in Ref 1). The test is not generally recommended at this time but is sometimes done on an experimental basis. Intradermal inoculation of 0.1 ml of antigen gives rise in 48 hr to a papule 0.5–1.0 cm diam or to an area of erythema 1.5–6.0 cm diameter or both. Nearly all (95%) patients with cat-scratch disease exhibit a positive reaction. Reactions to the Frei antigen in these same patients are negative.

Skin-test antigen is not available commercially and is prepared from material obtained from cat-scratch disease patients; these should be selected to exclude hepatitis A and B, syphilis, LGV, tuberculosis, and other transmissible infections (3, 7). Details of antigen preparation and safety testing are found in the report of Kalter et al (11). In essence, pus from the affected, suppurating lymph nodes is aspirated aseptically. Macerated necrotic lymph node tissue is also a satisfactory antigen. The material is suspended by grinding in sufficient sterile physiologic saline solution to give a homogenous emulsion at a dilution of 1:5. This is autoclaved at 10 lb for 10 min, put in a vial, and sterility tested for bacteria and fungi under aerobic and anaerobic conditions. Kalter et al culture the antigen with monkey and human cells, and inoculate suckling mice as additional safety procedures to insure freedom from viable viruses (11). It is advisable to either add a preservative (for example, merthiolate in 1:10,000 final concentration) to the antigen or store it at 4 C where its potency is stable for years.

Since not all pus specimens yield satisfactory antigens, it is necessary to determine the potency by skin test in patients known to have had the disease. Such patients are lifelong reactors. The appropriate dilution to use can be selected after intradermal titration in serial 2-fold dilutions of antigen in patients known to react with a positive test to cat-scratch-test antigen. The standardized antigen must not produce reactions in normal persons. Isolation attempts in tissue culture have not been successful as a diagnostic procedure.

Serologic diagnosis. CF tests with chlamydial group antigens are sometimes done but the significance of results is uncertain. These are performed with serum obtained from patients at the onset of illness and at 2, 4, and 8 weeks thereafter. Antigen may be prepared in individual laboratories (15) or purchased from commercial sources. The technique for conducting the CF test is described in Chapter 1. Test results must be evaluated with caution, as discussed above. Hemagglutination of rabbit RBC by pus from affected lymph nodes and suggestive inhibition of the phenomenon has been described (5) but not confirmed.

References

1. ANONYMOUS: Cat scratch disease and Parinaud's oculoglandular syndrome. J Am Med Assoc 152:1717, 1953
2. BLATTNER RJ: Cat-scratch fever. J Pediatr 39:123–124, 1951
3. DANIELS WB and MACMURRAY FG: Cat scratch disease: nonbacterial regional lymphadenitis: a report of 60 cases. Ann Intern Med 37:697–713, 1952
4. DEBRE R, LAMY M, JAMMET ML, COSTIL L, and MOZZICONACCI P: La maladie des griffes du chat. Bull Mem Soc Med Hop Paris 66:76–79, 1950
5. DODD MC, GRABER CD, and ANDERSON G: Hemagglutination of rabbit erythrocytes by pus from cases of cat scratch fever. Proc Soc Exp Biol Med 102:556–558, 1959

6. EMMONS RW, RIGGS JL, and SCHACHTER J: Continuing search for the etiology of cat scratch disease. J Clin Microbiol 4:112–114, 1976

7. GREER WER and KEEFER CS: Cat-scratch fever: a disease entity. N Engl J Med 244:545–548, 1951

8. JIM RTS: Thrombocytopenic purpura in cat-scratch disease. J Am Med Assoc 176:1036–1037, 1961

9. KALTER SS, KIM CS, and HEBERLING RL: Herpes-like virus particles associated with cat scratch disease. Nature 224:190, 1969

10. KALTER SS, HEBERLING RL, and RATNER JJ: Titers of antibody to Epstein-Barr virus in patients with cat-scratch disease. J Infect Dis 125:464–465, 1972

11. KALTER SS, RODRIGUEZ AR, and HEBERLING RL: Cat-scratch disease skin test antigen preparation. Lancet 2:607, 1977

12. MARGILETH AM: Cat scratch disease. The study of 145 patients and review of the literature. Pediatrics 42:803–811, 1968

13. MOLLARET P, REILLY J, BASTIN R, and TOURNIER P: La decouverte du virus de la lymphoreticulose benigne d'inoculation. II. Inoculation experimentale au singe et colorations. Presse Med 59:701–704, 1951

14. MOLLARET P, REILLY J, BASTIN R, and TOURNIER P: Documentation nouvelle sur l'adenopathie regionale subaigue et spontanement curable decrite en 1950; la lymphoreticulose benigne d'inoculation. Presse Med 58:1353–1355, 1950

15. NIGG C, HILLEMAN MR, and BOWSER BM: Studies on lymphogranuloma venereum complement-fixing antigens. I. Enhancement by phenol or boiling. J Immunol 53:259–268, 1946

16. THOMPSON TE JR and MILLER KF: Cat scratch encephalitis. Ann Intern Med 39:146–151, 1953

17. WARWICK WJ: The cat scratch syndrome, many diseases or one disease. Prog Med Virol 9:256–301, 1967

*

Exanthem Subitum

(Roseola Infantum, Roseola Subitum, Roseola Infantilis, Pseudo Rubella, and Rose Rash of Infants)

and

Erythema Infectiosum

(Duke Disease, Fourth Disease, Fifth Disease, and Parascarlatina)

Exanthem subitum is an acute, benign, febrile, probably viral, illness of infants and young children characterized by abrupt onset, high fever of 3- to 5-day duration and a transient macular or maculopapular rash which appears concurrently with improvement (6). Upon defervescence, the exanthem appears on the neck, trunk, upper extremities, thighs, and buttocks. Desquamation is rare, pigmentation does not occur, and an exanthem of erythematous specks and streaks may develop on the soft palate. Meningismus can be present occasionally, and a marked leukopenia and relative or absolute lymphocytosis are characteristic, being most marked around the third day of high fever. Residual encephalopathy is a rare complication. Slight enlargement of the lymph nodes may be present (8). Most cases occur sporadically rather than in epidemics, in contrast to erythema infectiosum. Pathologic changes during the illness are unknown.

Reported attempts to recover exanthem subitum virus are few. Kempe et al (7), and Hellstrom and Vahlquist (5) transmitted the disease from one infant to another by inoculation of serum obtained aseptically early in the illness. Infectious serum also produced febrile disease in monkeys (7). Neva and Enders recovered an agent from stools of a child with an illness resembling exanthem subitum, and it subsequently shown to be type 3 adenovirus (9, 10). Infections with the recovered virus was established by demonstration of rising titers of Nt and CF antibodies. Its relation to exanthem subitum is highly questionable.

Erythema infectiosum occurs characteristically in children 4–12 years of age. The disease is recognized at the appearance of rash; fever and prodromal symptoms are minimal or absent. The sharply delineated rash appears initially on the cheeks and later on the limbs and trunk. Characteristically, it is fleeting and leaves no staining or desquamation (4). Epidemics in school children have been worldwide (2, 3).

Werner et al (11) described an agent recovered from stools of patients, related to their illness serologically, which produced giant, multinucleated cells and intranuclear inclusions in rhesus kidney cell cultures. These workers did not rule out the possibility that they were dealing with a simian virus contaminant.

Other minor exanthematous diseases in children are readily differentiated from roseola, rubella, exanthem subitum, and erythema infectiosum on epidemiologic and clinical grounds. They may be sporadic or epidemic and have been associated with simultaneous infection with coxsackieviruses and echoviruses (1), with certain adenoviruses, or with dengue (4). Attempts to identify the etiology of such infections should include search for these groups of viruses.

References

1. ASHKENAZI A and MELNICK J: Topics in microbiology. Enteroviruses: a review of their properties and associated diseases. Am J Clin Pathol 38:209–229, 1962
2. BLATTNER RJ: Exanthem subitum In Textbook of Pediatrics, Vaughan VC and McKay RJ (eds), WB Saunders, Philadelphia, 1975, pp 662–663
3. BURNSTINE RC and PAINE RS: Residual encephalpathy following roseola infantum. Am J Dis Child 98:144, 1959
4. GUTEKUNST RR and HEGGIE AD: Viremia and viruria in adenovirus infections. Detection in patients with rubella or rubelliform illness. N Engl J Med 264:374–378, 1961
5. HELLSTROM B and VAHLQUIST B: Experimental inoculation of roseola infection. Acta Paediat 40:189–197, 1951
6. KEMP CH: Exanthem subitum and erythema infectiosum, Chap 54 In Viral and Rickettsial Infections of Man, 4th edition, Horsfall FL Jr and Tamm I (eds), JB Lippincott, Philadelphia, 1965, pp 810–813
7. KEMPE CH, SHAW EB, JACKSON JR, and SILVER HK: Studies on the etiology of exanthem subitum (roseola infantum). J Pediatr 37: 561–568, 1950
8. McENERY JT: Postoccipital lymphadenopathy as a diagnostic sign in roseola infantum. Clin Pediatr 9:512–514, 1970
9. NEVA FA and ENDERS JF: Isolation of a cytopathogenic agent from an infant with a disease in certain respects resembling roseola infantum. J Immunol 72:315–321, 1954

10. Rowe WP, Huebner RJ, Hartley JW, Ward TG, and Parrott RH: Studies of the adenoidal-pharyngeal-conjunctival (APC) group of viruses. Am J Hyg 61:197–218, 1955
11. Werner GH, Brachman PS, Ketler A, Scully J, and Rake G: A new viral agent associated with erythema infectiosum. Ann NY Acad Sci 67:338–345, 1957

Encephalomyocarditis

(Columbia-SK Disease, MM-Virus Infection, Mengo Encephalomyelitis)

The encephalomyocarditis (EMC) viruses of the picornavirus group comprise a subgroup of closely related agents variously designated as the Columbia-SK, MM, EMC, Mengo, M, etc. (12, 13). Their mode of transmission is unknown, although arthropods very likely constitute one vector. Most strains of these viruses are highly pathogenic for rodents (mice, cotton rats, hamsters, guinea pigs) inoculated by the cerebral or peripheral routes, causing a fatal encephalitis which can be accompanied by myocardial and aortic lesions. Infected monkeys develop a poliomyelitis-like disease with myocarditis and often recover. EMC virus (EMCV) has been isolated from naturally infected human beings, chimpanzees, baboons, monkeys, mongooses, swine (9), and mosquitoes. Antibody to the agent is common in serum of wild caught rats (13), and these animals may constitute a reservoir for the disease (6).

The "M" variant of EMCV was found by Craighead and his associates to induce hyperglycemia and hypoinsulinemia in mice (3). Because the disease clinically resembles diabetes mellitus and is characterized by reduction in the number of islets of Langerhans and a deterioration of β cells, it has attracted considerable attention as a diabetes model (1). Although infection in the pancreas is short-lived (1–10 days), the elevated blood glucose persists for many months (1). The occurrence of the syndrome in mice is genetically influenced, and the host strain affects its course (2). Antibodies to EMCV have not been observed in the serum of patients with diabetes (3).

Proved EMCV infections in humans are rare. Warren lists 9 patients with CNS disease from whom EMCV was isolated; from 4 of these, virus was recovered from blood, brain, or spinal fluid (12). Smadel and Warren demonstrated increases in Nt antibody to EMCV in paired sera from an outbreak of a mild febrile disease called "Three Day Fever", which appeared in 1945 and 1946 among US Army troops in the Philippines (11). The patients presented syndromes of severe headache, moderately high fever lasting 2–3 days, pharyngitis, stiff neck, positive Kernig sign, and hyperactive deep reflexes. No cardiac symptoms were observed. The only notable laboratory finding was pleocytosis, principally lymphocytes, in the spinal fluid. Acute encephalitis occurred in a physician working in Uganda with the Mengo strain; the virus was isolated from his blood early in the disease, and an increase in Nt antibody level was demonstrated in the serum after recovery from the illness (5). In experimentally infected animals the lesions are most prominent in the CNS and in striated and cardiac muscles. Their extent and severity are related to the duration and route of infection.

Description of the agent

EMCV is a single-strand, cytocidal RNA virus of cubic symmetry with particle sizes of approximately 30 μ and made up of 12 capsomeres. Crystalline preparations are thin, rectangular wafers with an estimated molecular weight of 3.1×10^6. It is quite stable when stored at -70 C or in 50% glycerol; it does not retain infectivity when lyophilized and is inactivated by heating to 60 C for 30 min. EMCV is ether-resistant and lacks essential lipid. Strains of EMCV grow well in the embryonated egg and in cultured cells of primate and rodent origin. Cytopathogenicity, animal virulence, and plaque morphology vary between strains and with conditions of culture (8). EMCV are biologically similar to those of the group B coxsackieviruses. All strains are antigenically alike.

Laboratory diagnosis

Virus isolation. Little is known about distribution of the virus in human tissues, but it is widespread in the viscera of experimentally infected monkeys. Virus isolation should be attempted by intracerebral inoculation of white mice with spinal fluid or serum collected from the patient during the acute phase of the disease, or with clarified suspensions of brain, cord, myocardium, and spleen from fatal cases. Portions of the inocula should be retained at -70 C for corroborative reisolation and for inoculation of embryonated eggs and tissue cultures. Mice inoculated with small amounts of a neurotropic laboratory-adapted strain of the virus become lethargic within 2–3 days, develop a flaccid paralysis, and die in 3–4 days; given a large dose of virus, acute encephalitis develops without paralysis, and death occurs in 18-24 hr. On primary isolation, the incubation period is considerably longer. Several rodent cell systems are highly susceptible to EMCV, such as the BHK-21, murine L, and embryonic fibroblasts. These could be useful in attempted isolations of virus from suspect materials. Virus recovered from the patient is identified in Nt tests with known positive serum, as described below.

Serum neutralization test. Serum is obtained from patients at onset of illness and again 3–4 weeks later; acute- and convalescent-phase specimens should be titrated simultaneously in the same test. Because the mouse is highly susceptible, it has been used almost exclusively over tissue culture procedures.

Clarified suspension is prepared in 30% normal rabbit serum-saline solution from brains of inoculated mice with symptoms of EMCV infection. The LD_{50} titer of such preparations is usually $10^{-8.5}/0.03$ ml in intracerebral mouse titration, or $10^{-7}/0.1$ ml when the mouse intraperitoneal test (ip) is used.

Positive control serum for use in the diagnostic Nt test and for identification of newly recovered strains is prepared in young adult rabbits hyperimmunized at weekly intervals by 3 ip injections of 5 ml of the live virus preparation described above. The rabbits are bled 10 days after the last injection; the serum should neutralize 100,000 LD_{50} of EMCV when tested in mice inoculated ip or 1000 LD_{50} by the mouse intracerebral test.

The serum is mixed with equal volumes of the proper serial 10-fold dilutions of seed virus and, after incubation at 37 C for 1 hr, 0.1 ml of each mixture are inoculated ip into groups of 6 mice weighing 12–14 g each. Acute-phase patient serum is tested with 1, 10, 100, and 1000 LD_{50}, while the convalescent-phase serum is tested with 10, 100, 1000, and 10,000 LD_{50} of virus. A known positive control serum is included in the tests (hyperimmune animal serum is satisfactory), and a titration of the seed virus is performed simultaneously. The mice are observed for typical CNS signs for 14 days; the deaths are recorded. A positive test is one in which the convalescent-phase specimen neutralizes at least 2 $\log_{10}$ more virus than does the acute-phase sample.

Complement-fixation test. A 20% suspension of EMCV-infected mouse brain in physiologic saline solution is centrifuged for 10 min at 3000 rpm to remove large particles; the supernatant fluid is clarified by centrifugation for 1 hr at 13,000 rpm in the angle-head centrifuge. The supernatant fluid antigen must be water-clear and, since it is infectious, the usual precautions should be taken. The potency is preserved for several months when stored at -20 C in sealed glass vials. Control antigen is prepared in an identical manner from brains of normal mice of the same age. Infected hamster, mouse, and HeLa cell cultures may also be used as a source of antigen (4).

Convalescent-phase serum from EMCV-infected rats, hamsters, mice, or monkeys is employed. The animals are injected peripherally with sublethal amounts of virus grown in the same host and are bled after recovery from the illness.

The paired sera from patients are tested simultaneously with EMCV and control antigens using overnight incubation procedures described in Chapter 1. The endpoint is read as the highest initial dilution of serum which gives $\geq 3+$ fixation of complement. A ≥ 4-fold increase in antibody level in the patient serum during convalescence is diagnostic and is of greater significance than a positive test with a single specimen alone. Serum from persons with syphilis may react with the mouse brain component of the antigens; such reactivity may be reduced by inactivating the serum at 60 or 65 C instead of the usual 56 C temperature.

Hemagglutination-inhibition (HAI) test. Viruses of the EMC group hemagglutinate sheep RBC in the cold (5 C) but not at room temperature; this HA reaction is inhibited by specific antibody (4, 6, 10). Tube or plate tests to measure antibody in serum specimens can be carried out by the same HAI technique used for influenza virus (7). A clarified suspension of infected mouse brain or a centrifuged homogenate of infected HeLa cells in Eagle basic medium serves as HA antigen in the test. The HAI test has not been evaluated as a diagnostic tool with serum from individuals with EMCV infection. It should be noted, however, that a high percentage (27%) of serum from patients with CNS disease (paralytic or nonparalytic poliomyelitis, aseptic meningitis, or encephalitis) gave positive reactions in an HAI test devised for EMC by Gard and Heller (6). Since none of these same sera neutralized EMCV, the positive HAI findings may have been due to non-specific factors in the test.

References

1. BOUCHER DW and NOTKINS HL: Virus induced diabetes mellitus: 1. Hyperglycemia and hypoinsulinemia in mice infected with EMC virus. J Exp Med 137:1226-1239, 1973
2. CRAIGHEAD JE and HIGGINS DA: Genetic influences affecting the occurrence of a diabetes mellitus-like disease in mice infected with encephalomyocarditis virus. J Exp Med 139:414-426, 1974
3. CRAIGHEAD JE and McLANE MF: Diabetes mellitus: induction in mice by encephalo-myocarditis virus. Science 162:913, 1968
4. CRAIGHEAD JE and SHELOKOV A: Encephalomyocarditis virus hemagglutination-inhibition test using antigens prepared in HeLa cell cultures. Proc Soc Exp Biol Med 108:823-826, 1961
5. DICK GWA, BEST AM, HADDOW AJ, and SMITHBURN KC: Mengo encephalomyelitis, a hitherto unknown virus affecting man. Lancet 2:286-289, 1948
6. GARD S and HELLER L: Hemagglutination by col-MM-virus. Proc Soc Exp Biol Med 76:68-73, 1951
7. GARD GP, BATTY EM, and SABA HM: Microtiter HAI test for the detection of EMC virus antibodies. Appl Microbiol 27:272-273, 1974
8. LIEBERHABER H and TAKEMOTO K: The basis for the size differences in plaques produced by variants of encephalomyocarditis (EMC) virus. Virology 20:559-566, 1963
9. MURNANE TG, CRAIGHEAD JE, MONDRAGON H, and SHELOKOV A: Fatal disease of swine due to encephalomyocarditis virus. Science 131:498-499, 1960
10. OLITSKY PK and YAGER RH: Hemagglutination by Columbia-SK, Columbia MM, mengo encephalomyelitis and encephalomyocarditis viruses: experiments with other viruses. Proc Soc Exp Biol Med 71:719-724, 1949
11. SMADEL JE and WARREN J: The virus of encephalomyocarditis and its apparent causation of disease in man. J Clin Invest 26:1197, 1947
12. WARREN J: Chap 54 *In* Viral and Rickettsial Infections of Man, 4th edition, Horsfall FL Jr and Tamm I (eds), JB Lippincott, Philadelphia, 1965, p 1164
13. WARREN J, RUSS SB, and JEFFRIES H: Neutralizing antibody against viruses of the encephalomyocarditis group in the sera of wild rats. Proc Soc Exp Biol Med 71:376-378, 1949
14. WARREN J, SMADEL JE, and RUSS SB: The family relationship of encephalomyocarditis. Columbia-SK, MM, and mengo encephalomyelitis viruses. J Immunol 62:387-398, 1949

*

Foot-and-Mouth Disease

(Fievre Aphteuse, Maul-und-Klauenseuche, Aphthous Fever, Epizootic Stomatitis)

Foot-and-mouth disease (FMD) is a highly contagious, epidemic disease of cloven-hoofed animals, especially cattle, sheep, goats, and pigs (3). The disease is characterized by fever, increased salivation, and the appearance of fluid-filled vesicular lesions on the mucous membranes of the mouth, tongue, and lips, on the muzzle, between the claws, and on the teats and udder. The vesicular fluid and saliva is highly infectious (7). The disease is occasionally transmitted to humans, causing a self-limited, febrile illness characterized by pain in the limbs, excessive salivation, and the appearance of vesicular lesions on the buccal or lingual epithelium and on the skin of the hands, feet, and other parts of the body (6).

Humans can carry the virus for at least 24 hr in their nasopharynx and can transmit it to other humans or susceptible animals via infectious aerosols (10). The agent also multiplies in the nasopharyngeal tissue of immunized cattle in concentrations sufficient to decrease the titer of pre-existing, Nt antibodies (8). Considerable control of FMD has resulted from the systematic immunization of cattle and swine with inactivated vaccines. These are usually polyvalent, now grown mainly in cell cultures, concentrated, inactivated with formaldehyde or substituted ethyleneimines (1). Adjuvants, such as saponin, hydrocarbon oils, aluminum hydroxide gel, and DEAE-dextran, are generally added (12).

Description of the agent

FMD is caused by 7 different immunologic types and numerous antigenic subtypes of biologically similar viruses. These are geographically localized. It is a picornavirus containing RNA and several polypeptides. The virus is 20–25 μ in size and with a group-specific soluble antigen of 7 μ. It is ether-resistant, unstable at low pH, and inactivated by formaldehyde, saponin, and ethylene oxide. Bacharach and McKercher found that only substituted ethyleneimines were able to inactivate purified FMD virus in accordance with first order kinetics (1). The disease is readily transmitted to guinea pigs or suckling mice; less easily to poultry; rabbits, rats, adult mice, dogs, and cats are irregularly susceptible, and ferrets and horses are resistant. All strains produce a lytic infection in cell cultures of bovine, porcine, ovine, or rodent origin. The stable BHK-21 line of hamster cells is now widely used for the industrial manufacture of large volumes of virus which can be readily purified and concentrated by centrifugation and/or precipitation prior to its use as a vaccine (12).

Due to the rigid quarantine regulations of the Bureau of Animal Diseases, US Department of Agriculture, the United States has been free of FMD, and public law prevents importation of the virus for experimental purposes into the mainland of the United States. The Secretary of Agriculture has, however, established laboratories for research on FMD on Plum Island, NY.

In cattle, the rapid diagnosis of FMD and its differentiation from vesicular stomatitis is essential for the prevention of epidemic spread of this highly infectious virus. For diagnosis of cases in humans, vesicle fluid or scrapings of the underlying skin should be collected in sterile vials and immediately frozen for shipment to a *qualified* laboratory. Regional authorities should also be immediately notified.

Laboratory diagnosis

FMD may be diagnosed by recovery and identification of the virus from the vesicular fluid obtained from lesions in the patient or by demonstration of a rise in antibody titer in the patient serum during convalescence from the illness.

Virus Isolation. Young adult guinea pigs inoculated intradermally in the foot pads develop vesicular lesions at the site of injection in 24–48 hr; this is followed by the appearance of vesicles in the mouth 18–36 hr later. While the disease is usually not fatal in guinea pigs, the virus can be demonstrated in the blood at the time of appearance of the initial lesions. Suckling mice (7–14 days old) inoculated intracerebrally develop spastic muscular paralysis of the hind limbs 1–2 days after injection; this spreads to other parts of the body and death occurs within 12 hr after appearance of the initial signs of illness (11). Primary recoveries of field strains can also be made in goat, bovine, and hamster kidney cell cultures. Recovered viruses are identified by pathogenicity tests in animals and by cross-immunity or serologic procedures.

FMD in its natural hosts is clinically indistinguishable from two other vesicular diseases which occur in the United States—vesicular stomatitis (VSV) of horses and cattle and occasionally of humans (6), and vesicular exanthema (VE) of swine. For this reason, infectious material can also be inoculated intradermally into the tongue of the horse and cow, intramuscularly into the cow, and intradermally into the snout of the pig. Based on the development of vesicular disease in these animals, preliminary differentiation can be made. FMD is not infectious for horses; VSV will not cause illness in cows by the intramuscular route, and VE will not infect the cow by any route.

Several methods of identification and strain typing are available for diagnostic and research purposes. Based upon their speed and reliability, the following are recommended for the diagnosis of human or animal FMD.

Complement-fixation test. For practical purposes, there is no cross-reactivity between the major types; therefore, known specific antisera or antigens are required.

Homogenates of suspect vesicle tissue or infected mouse or guinea pig tissue are prepared in distilled water or physiologic saline. The vesicle fluid itself can also be employed as antigen. These are clarified by low-speed centrifugation and used in 2-fold dilutions. Two to 4 units of hyperimmune guinea pig serum and 2–5 exact units of complement are employed in either a tube or plate format (5). The mixtures are incubated for 1 hr at 37 C, sensitized RBC are added, followed by further incubation at 37 C for 45–60 min. The test may be set up and read in 4–6 hr (3).

Cell-culture-grown virus is commonly used as CF antigen for strain differentiation and diagnosis. The culture fluids are usually concentrated by centrifugation or precipitation with some suitable agent as polyethylene glycol (13). Antigens are used in a series of 2-fold dilutions to estabilsh the optimum range for maximal fixation. Dilutions of the inactivated serum are then tested in a grid-type protocol to determine their endpoints. For additional details, see references 5 and 2.

Hemagglutination-inhibition (HAI) test. In a comparison of the HAI and serum neutralization procedures with cattle serum, Booth et al found that both were of equal sensitivity for the detection of FMD antibody (2).

Concentrated viral antigens are mixed with guinea pig RBC and incubated at 37 C for 1 hr. One HA unit is the highest dilution of antigen yielding a pattern of complete agglutination. Inactivated bovine serum is absorbed with washed guinea pig RBC for 1 hr at 37 C followed by overnight refrigeration. The absorbed serum is then serially diluted, 2-fold, and 4 HAU added. The mixtures are incubated for 30 min at 37 C followed by the addition of RBC suspension. The HAI endpoint is read after continued incubation for 1 hr.

Serum neutralization test. The acute-and convalescent-phase sera (2–3 weeks after onset of illness) from the patient are tested by the usual Nt procedure using serum dilutions with representative viruses of the 7 basic immunologic types, or at least the prevalent types in the geographic region of the case. A convenient source of virus for such tests is vesicular fluid from infected guinea pigs, infected brain tissue from suckling mice, or infected cell culture fluids. Positive control antiserum for use in the tests is obtained from guinea pigs which are convalescent from the disease and which may be hyperimmunized by repeated intramuscular injections of the same infectious agent. The Nt tests are carried out in bovine or hamster cell cultures (3, 4) or, if these are not available, one may use intradermal inoculation into the foot pad of guinea pigs or intracerebral inoculation of baby mice or inoculation into the tongue epithelium of cattle. A positive test in humans is one in which the convalescent-phase serum from the patient neutralizes 2 $\log_{10}$ more of virus than the acute-phase specimen. In animal studies, a regression plot of serum titer against the actual test dose employed may be used to determine the antibody titers against exactly 100 $TCID_{50}$ of virus (2).

Additional serologic techniques, primarily used for research in FMD, include ID (13), indirect CF (4), and FA staining (9).

References

1. BACHARACH HL and MCKERCHER PD: Immunology of food and mouth disease in swine: Experimental inactivated-virus vaccines. J Am Vet Med Assoc 160:521–526, 1972
2. BOOTH JC, PAY TWF, HEDGER RS, and BARNETT IT: The use of the haemagglutination-inhibition test for detecting antibodies to type SAT 2 food and mouth disease viruses in cattle sera. J Hyg 74:115–121, 1975
3. COTTRAL GE: Diagnosis of bovine vesicular diseases. J Am Vet Med Assoc 161:1293–1298, 1972
4. DESIMONE F, LODETTI E, PANINA G, and NARDELLI L: Immunological responses of cattle vaccinated against foot and mouth disease under field conditions. Atti Soc Ital Sci Vet 24:580–583, 1970
5. FORMAN AJ: A study of foot and mouth disease virus strains by complement fixation. J Hyg 72:407–413, 1974
6. HANSON RP, RASMUSSEN AF JR, BRANDLY CA, and BROWN JW: Human infection with the virus of vesicular stomatitis. J Lab Clin Med 36:754–758, 1950
7. HYSLOP NS: Secretion of foot-and-mouth disease virus and antibody in the saliva of infected and immunized cattle. J Comp Pathol 75:111–117, 1965
8. MCVICAR JW and SUTMOLLER P: Growth of foot and mouth disease virus in the upper respiratory tract of non-immunized, vaccinated and recovered cattle after intranasal inoculation. J Hyg 76:467–481, 1976
9. MOHANTY GC and COTTRAL GE: Foot and mouth disease virus: rapid assay using the fluorescent antibody techniques. Arch Gesamte Virusforsch 32:348–358, 1970
10. SELLERS RF, HERNIMAN KJ, and MANN JA: Transfer of foot and mouth disease virus in the nose of man from infected to non-infected animals. Vet Rec 89:447–449, 1971

11. SKINNER HH: Propagation of strains of foot-and-mouth disease virus in unweaned white mice. Proc Roy Soc Med 44:1041–1044, 1951
12. TELLING RG, CAPSTICK PB, PAY TWF, MENARD FJ, TAYLOR JL, ONETTI RC, and BANDAU R: The large scale manufacture of FMD vaccines by the BHK cell deep suspension culture method In Proc Second International Congress for Virology, Budapest Melnick JL (ed), S Karger, Basel, 1972
13. WAGNER GG, COWAN KM, and MCVICAR JW: Screening of sera for antibodies to foot and mouth disease viral antigen by radial immunodiffusion. Infect Immun 5:227–231, 1972

Equine Infectious Anemia

Equine infectious anemia (EIA) is an infection of equidae, but rarely of humans, that is caused by an RNA virus. Because it can cause a lifelong persistent viremia in the presence of antibody, with or without recurring episodes of anemia and lymphoproliferative changes, the detection and eradication of EIA is a veterinary problem of major economic proportions.

Clinical aspects

Natural transmission occurs through the bite of insects, particularly, Tabanid flies. It has been experimentally transmitted to only equidae by any of the common parenteral routes permitting virus entrance into the blood stream. The disease in equines may be acute, subacute, chronic, or latent (symptom-free). EIA is primarily a degeneration of the reticuloendothelial tissues resulting in a prolonged anemia, emaciation, and paroxysmal fever. The fatality rate in the acute and chronic form may reach 80%. Horses often have a persistent, symptom-free, high viremia for years and, apparently, constitute the reservoir of infection (4, 5). Such latent cases cannot be distinguished from healthy horses, and this often necessitates the destruction of valuable equines.

The reported disease in humans was characterized by fever, anemia, renal pains, and diarrhea. A persistent viremia was demonstrable in one patient whose blood was reported as infective for horses over a period of 3 years (11).

Pathology

Pathologic changes occur primarily in the hematopoetic organs. Spleno- and hepatomegaly arise from parenchymatous degeneration, edema, and activation of RES cells accompanied by hemorrhage. A prolonged, sidero-leukocytosis is common in acute, but not chronic, EIA.

Description and nature of the agent

This RNA virus is an enveloped sphere, 80–140μ in diameter, which arises by budding at the cell membrane. It is sensitive to 5% ether and, in serum, is destroyed at 56 C for 1 hr (7). The virus resists trypsin, ribonuclease, and deoxyribonuclease. Its taxonomic position and chemical composition remain obscure. Nakajima et al (10) have suggested that its low density, obscure internal structure by electron microscopy, and surface projections resemble properties of the RNA tumor viruses.

This similarity is strengthened by the recent finding of an RNA-instructed polymerase and an RNA of high molecular weight in the virion. These properties led Archer et al to suggest that EIA be classified with the family *Retroviridae* (1).

Based upon Nt tests, Kono et al (6) were able to differentiate 8 strains in specimens from the United States, Germany, Australia, and Japan. These viruses were regionally associated. EIA induces a common CF antibody demonstrable by its reaction with antigen from EIA-infected horse leukocyte cultures (2, 4). Hemadsorption and HA or the occurrence of a soluble antigen have not been consistently demonstrable.

EIA virus can be propagated in cultures of horse leukocytes or bone marrow cells producing CPE within 7–10 days (7). High-titer virus, suitable for diagnostic purposes, was prepared in equine embryonic spleen and a line of embryonic dermal cells by Malmquist et al (9). Spleen suspensions from known infected horses have also been employed as a source of antigen (2).

Laboratory diagnosis

Direct examination of clinical material. The acute and subacute forms of EIA in horses can generally be diagnosed on the basis of fever and the hematologic and clinical signs described above. Examination of liver biopsy is often combined with serologic testing in latent cases.

Virus isolation. Although virus isolation can be made by the inoculation of suspect material into known, healthy horses or cultures of equine cells, these are usually research procedures not used in routine diagnosis. Commonly used techniques are CF, Nt, ID, and FA. These were not available for the study of the few reported human cases (11). This led Dreguss and Lombard to question whether EIA was capable of causing infection in humans (4). This question is apparently still unresolved.

Complement-fixation test. (See Ref 8 for details.) CF antibody, while group-specific, is usually detectable for only a few weeks after the first appearance of fever. The Wyoming strain of EIA is most widely used for the antigen which is prepared in monolayer cultures of equine leukocytes. Either macro- or microtiter systems are suitable.

Virus neutralization. (See Ref 8 for details.) Although Nt antibodies persist for years, they are strain specific, and virus isolates taken from infected horses at successive periods appear changed in their antigenicity, suggesting a concomitant shift in antibody specificity (7). Kono et al employ a constant amount of serum against dilutions of virus, and the endpoints are CPE in replicate horse leukocyte cultures. A Nt index of ≥1.3 is reported as positive.

Immunodiffusion test. (See Refs 2 and 9 for details.) This is currently the most widely used diagnostic procedure because it detects early precipitating antibody, is not strain specific, and is technically simple. However, false-negative reactions occasionally occur, particularly late in the disease and in chronic carriers. Antigens are prepared from centrifuged concentrates of cultured virus or from spleen suspensions of infected horses. The availability of a stable cell line of equine dermal cells provides a source of antigen which is free of the problem of herpesvirus contamination which is often present in primary, human leukocyte cultures (9).

Immunofluorescence test. (See Chapter 4 for details.) Both direct (3) and indirect (5) FA tests have been useful in the study of the site of virus replication *in vitro*. EIA antigen can be detected within 48 hr after the inoculation of horse leukocyte cultures with infectious material. Its concentration paralles that of the CF antigen titer. Immunofluorescence has not been used as a diagnostic procedure.

References

1. ARCHER BG, CRAWFORD TB, McGUIRE TC, and FRAZIER ME: RNA-dependent DNA polymerase associated with equine infectious anemia virus. J Virol 22:16–22, 1977
2. COGGINS L and NORCROSS NS: Immunodiffusion reaction in equine infectious anemia. Cornell Vet 60:330–335, 1970
3. CRAWFORD TB, McGUIRE TC, and HENSON JB: Detection of equine infectious anemia virus in vitro by immunofluorescence. Arch Gesamte Virusforsch 34:332–339, 1971
4. DREGUSS MN and LOMBARD LS: Experimental Studies in Equine Infectious Anemia. Univ Penn Press, Philadelphia 1954
5. ISHII S and ISHITANI R: Equine infectious anemia. Adv Vet Sci Comp Med 19:195–222, 1975
6. KONO Y: Viremia and immunological response in horses infected with equine infectious anemia virus. Natl Inst Anim Health Q 9:1–9, 1969
7. KONO Y, YOSHINO T, and FUKANAGA Y: Growth characteristics of EIA in horse leukocyte cultures. Arch Gesamte Virusforsch 30:252–256, 1970
8. KONO Y, KOBAYASHI K, and FUKANAGA Y: Antigenic drift of EIA virus in chronically infected horses. Arch Gesamte Virusforsch 41:1–10, 1973
9. MALMQUIST HA, BARNETT D, and BECVAR CS: Production of EIA antigen in a persistently infected cell line. Arch Gesamte Virusforsch 42:361–370, 1973
10. NAKAJIMA H, TANAKA S, and USHIMI C: Physiochemical studies of EIA virus. Arch Gesamte Virusforsch 26:395–397, 1970
11. PETERS JT: Equine infectious anemia transmitted to man. Ann Int Med 23:271–274, 1945

CHAPTER 32

PSITTACOSIS-LYMPHOGRANULOMA VENEREUM AGENTS/TRIC AGENTS

Julius Schachter and Chandler R. Dawson

Introduction

Chlamydiae appear to be virtually ubiquitous throughout the animal kingdom. They have been recovered from 130 avian species belonging to 12 orders (61). Avian infections are of greatest significance to human health because birds are the reservoirs of psittacosis. Most domestic animals may also be infected naturally by chlamydiae, and infections in feral species have been commonly reported. These features of chlamydial parasitism have been recently reviewed, as have the broad aspects of human chlamydial infections (97, 113).

Trachoma is among the human diseases recognized since antiquity, having been described in the Ebers papyrus. It also is the disease from which chlamydiae were first demonstrated. In 1907 Halberstaedter and Prowazek discovered the inclusions produced by chlamydiae in the conjunctiva (32). Shortly thereafter, the chlamydial infections of the human genital tract were also recognized (54). Because they are obligatory intracellular parasites, technologic problems restricted research on these organisms for many years. However, recent advances, particularly the development of an efficient and relatively simple tissue-culture isolation method, have spurred research on human chlamydial infections, and the clinical spectrum associated with these organisms has been expanding greatly in recent years.

Clinical aspects

Psittacosis. Psittacosis is a human respiratory disease caused by *Chlamydia psittaci* and contracted by exposure to infectious material (usually fecal droppings) from avian species (60). Infection is often subclinical although it may be very mild, resembling a common cold or a mild influenzal attack; however, severe and even fatal pneumonitis may occur. Pneumonia or fatal infection is more likely in individuals above the age of 50. The incubation period may range from 4 days to approximately 4 weeks but is usually between 7 and 14 days. The prodrome is usually associated with mild nonspecific symptoms such as general malaise, low-grade fever, and head-ache. Severe disease is characterized by fever and severe headache. Deliri-um is not rare. Despite extensive radiologic evidence of a pneumonic pro-cess, the cough is usually nonproductive. The clinical features are often sim-ilar to those of atypical pneumonia. Occasionally a severe, systemic, "toxic" disease develops in the absence of respiratory involvement. The pulse is often slow, particularly in view of the high fever. Hepatosplenome-galy may occur. The disease and the infection both respond to tetracycline (1 g/day for 21 days), but the clinical response may be variable, and recovery is often prolonged. While the disease is generally not communicated person to person, secondary cases have been noted, particularly in those attending severely ill or dying patients with productive coughs.

Lymphogranuloma venereum (LGV). This venereal disease, caused by certain *C. trachomatis* serotypes, is a systemic disease (112), generally de-scribed as having 3 stages. The primary lesion, a small and transient vesicle or ulcer, develops on the genitalia approximately 1–2 weeks after exposure. The secondary stage occurs a week or more after the primary stage and is characterized by the development of inguinal lymphadenopathy (buboes) in males. During this stage, fever and chills may occur. Often, women do not develop inguinal buboes. Apparently, the spread of the agent in the female through pelvic or retroperitoneal (rather than inguinal) lymph nodes deter-mines the sites involved in sequential development of disease. The tertiary stage (commonly called the anogenital syndrome) is characterized by inflam-mation of the anorectal canal, and fistulae and strictures are often present. Primary lesions and lymphadenopathy may occur elsewhere, depending on the primary site of infection. Implantation in the mouth or eye or through lesions on the fingers will result in the lymph nodes draining the sites in-volved. Systemic complications are recognized and may be common.

Trachoma. Trachoma is a chronic conjunctivitis caused by *C. tracho-matis*. It is still considered one of the leading causes of preventable blind-ness in the world. Blinding trachoma is a major public health problem in North Africa, sub-Saharan Africa, the Middle East, and Southeast Asia (20, 31, 45), and small pockets of blinding trachoma exist elsewhere in the world. In areas with endemic disease, trachoma is almost invariably as-sociated with infection by *C. trachomatis* serotypes A, B, Ba, or C (31). In blinding trachoma, superimposed bacterial infections play a significant role in the pathogenesis of the disease (20, 45).

It has been found that trachoma is essentially a disease of families (31). Most active disease is seen in relatively young children and usually results from direct person-to-person transmission among children. In areas with ho-loendemic disease, virtually none of the children under the age of 2 years are spared (20, 70). The natural course of uncomplicated trachoma appears to be relatively self-limiting in terms of active disease or inflammation due to infection. Unfortunately, in areas with endemic trachoma, reinfection is common, and secondary bacterial infections interfere with the tendency to-wards healing and prolong the inflammatory disease for years. The active disease eventually disappears (usually by 10–15 years of age) but may leave a residuum of permanent lesions that can lead to blindness. Conjunctival scars may shrink and cause the eyelid to turn inward so that lashes constantly abrade the cornea (entropion and trichiasis). This constant trauma may result in corneal ulceration and subsequent opacity ultimately causing blindness. Mild cases of trachoma are common and rarely lead to visual loss.

Adult inclusion conjunctivitis. Adult inclusion conjunctivitis is an acute follicular conjunctivitis, almost invariably acquired by exposure to infective genital-tract discharges (21, 43, 64, 107). Generally, the disease is considered to be benign and self-limited, but it may in some instances become chronic or result in scarring of the conjunctiva and corneal vascularization (pannus) that lead to a diagnosis of acute trachoma (31, 43). It is one of the more common forms of follicular conjunctivitis, particularly prevalent in sexually active young adults.

Genital-tract infections. C. trachomatis, now recognized as one of the most common sexually transmitted pathogens (31, 87, 96, 99), is a major cause of nongonococcal and postgonococcal urethritis (42, 74, 86). Cervical infections are also common, but cervicitis is not a necessary response to chlamydial infection since asymptomatic and subclinical cervical infections are common (31, 87, 96). Serious complications in the genital tract are recognized, and strong circumstantial evidence has implicated *Chlamydia* as a cause of epididymitis in males and salpingitis in females (36, 57).

Neonatal chlamydial infections. Inclusion conjunctivitis of the newborn (ICN), also known as inclusion blennorrhea, is a chlamydial infection acquired by the neonate during passage through the birth canal. The incubation period is usually 5–14 days. ICN is an acute mucopurulent conjunctivitis. The course is generally considered benign, and the disease tends to resolve spontaneously several weeks to several months after onset. In severe cases, pseudomembranes may form in the conjunctiva, and scarring may result. Corneal micropannus may develop (65). Persistent infection is known, and some cases have remained clinically active for years, resulting in a trachoma-like picture of the conjunctiva (31, 43, 64). Early treatment seems to prevent development of scars and corneal vascularization (65).

Pneumonitis had been reported as a sequela of ICN, but chlamydial infection in the newborn is now of greater concern in light of the recent observations by Beem and Saxon that *C. trachomatis* could be regularly recovered from nasopharyngeal and tracheobronchial aspirates collected from infants with a distinctive pneumonia syndrome (10, 102). This pneumonia was characterized by an afebrile course, chronic diffuse lung involvement, tachypnea, and elevated serum of immunoglobulins G (IgG) and M (IgM). Many of the infants had a distinctive cough, and some had a slight eosinophilia.

Mammalian chlamydiae. C. psittaci are common pathogens of lower mammals (113). Because they cause arthritis, pneumonitis, abortion, enteritis, conjunctivitis, and encephalomyelitis, these pathogens are of considerable economic import in domestic mammals. Many mammalian chlamydiae are harbored in the intestinal tract, and large numbers are shed in the feces. Preliminary results suggest that there are 2 major serotypes, one causing the arthritis-conjunctivitis complex of diseases and the other causing abortions (95). Tissue tropism appears to be consistent across species, as single strains seem to cause the same diseases in different host species. A major problem in this field (as in ornithosis) remains the elucidation of natural chains of infection. Interspecies transfer and insect vectors have been postulated but remain unproven (24, 79).

Mammalian chlamydiae are not known to be a significant threat to human health, however, a number of cases of human infection have been confirmed following laboratory exposure and, in a few instances, following normal exposure to infected mammals (8, 113). Circumstantial evidence has indicated that human abortions may have been associated with chlamydiae of mammalian origin (89). Cases of conjunctivitis associated with feline pneumonitis agent, documented in the United States and in England (S. Darougar, personal communication) are perhaps the most commonly known human infections with these agents (105). However, it is likely, considering the large amounts of C. psittaci present in discharges from infected mammals, that these agents are of relatively low communicability or pathogenicity for humans.

Pathology

Psittacosis. The lesions of human psittacosis are generally those of a severe pneumonitis. In severe cases large areas of lung consolidation are found, with alveoli filled with fibrin, erythrocytes (RBC), and mononuclear cells. Extensive polymorphonuclear neutrophil infiltrate often indicates secondary bacterial infection. Septal cell hyperplasia and marked phagocytic activity with macrophage infiltration is common. Bronchioles may be clear although there is often a desquamation of some of the mucosa. The spleen is usually congested, the sinuses are engorged, and much phagocytic activity is observed both in spleen and liver. Necrotic areas are common, particularly in the liver.

In birds the lesions of chlamydial infection are similar for most species, although with some infecting strains there appear to be differences (60). For example, myocardial involvement may be the major finding caused by some isolates from turkeys (78). Generally, the bird is wasted and may show signs of enteritis. A seropurulent exudate may coat thickened air sacs. Often, pericardial involvement with serofibrinous exudate occurs. The liver is usually swollen and engorged and may have many areas of focal necrosis. Also, the spleen is often enlarged. However, none of these signs are pathognomonic of psittacosis.

Lymphogranuloma venereum (LGV). The lesions of LGV, particularly of the lymph nodes are not pathognomonic. The inflammatory process largely involves mononuclear infiltration with many plasma cells. There may be focal necrosis with stellate abcesses.

Trachoma and inclusion conjunctivitis (TRIC). Acute active trachoma is characterized by lymphoid follicles with germinal centers in the conjunctiva. There is a cellular infiltration of plasma cells, and lymphocytes and polymorphonuclear cells are often present. With progressing disease the follicles become necrotic, and scar tissue is formed. In severe cases with considerable scar formation, the scars contract after a period of years resulting in inturning of the upper eyelid (entropion), and the eyelashes abrade the cornea (trichiasis) causing corneal ulcers and ultimately blindness. The pathology of adult inclusion conjunctivitis is much like that of acute trachoma.

Neonatal infections. In infants with ocular disease, the germinal centers and follicle formation are generally not seen until the third or fourth week of life. The pneumonia associated with *C. trachomatis* infection in neonates is characterized by significant airway damage with lesions similar to those found in necrotizing bronchiolitis. Disease results in marked infiltration by mononuclear cells into the alveoli, and the interstitial components appear to be secondary.

Microbiology

Common characteristics

The chlamydiae are obligatory intracellular parasites once considered to be large viruses sensitive to the action of some antimicrobials or antibiotics. However, a more sophisticated definition of viruses and bacteria has allowed the recognition that the chlamydiae are bacteria-like and definitely not viruses (67, 68). They differ from the viruses in having 2 nucleic acids and a discrete cell wall, quite analogous in structure and content to those of the gram-negative bacteria (56). The chlamydiae have a restricted metabolic capability and multiply within the host cell by binary fission; they undergo no eclipse phase. They are susceptible to antibiotics. The sole feature chlamydiae share with viruses is the obligatory intracellular nature of their parasitism. Chlamydiae are restricted to an intracellular milieu because they are incapable of synthesizing adenosine triphosphate (ATP) and may be considered energy parasites. In addition to being the sole source of the ATP required for the chlamydial metabolic reactions, the host cell supplies metabolites (from its pool rather than by degradation). Some of these metabolites, such as isoleucine, may be growth restricting (39). When chlamydiae infect the host cell, they divert its synthetic capabilities to their own metabolic requirements and prevent cell multiplication. All chlamydiae share a group antigen and, most significantly, a common and unique growth cycle.

Size, shape, and growth cycle

We do not yet fully understand the complex developmental cycle of the chlamydiae, which differentiates them from all other microorganisms. The length of the cycle is approximately 48 hr but can vary as a function of the infecting strain, cell type, and temperature. After attachment of the infectious elementary body (EB) to the surface of the susceptible cell, the particle enters the cell in a phagocytic vesicle. The EB remains intact and undergoes a reorganization so that within approximately 6–8 hr it has changed from an EB to an initial body. The noninfectious initial bodies are metabolically very active, whereas the EBs are not. They synthesize new material and divide by binary fission until approximately 18–24 hr after infection. During this stage of the developmental cycle, only initial bodies are seen. At approximately 18–24 hr after infection, the initial bodies stop multiplying and undergo another reorganization, during which they "condense" from an initial body of approximately 800 nm to an EB approximately 350 nm in size. Both particles are coccoid, with slight variability found in the initial bodies. Both particles are basophilic, the EB only slightly so while the initial body is more so. Throughout the cycle the inclusion (ultimately a microcolony) remains within the expanding phagocytic vesicle.

Chemical composition

Chlamydiae are as chemically complex as bacteria (68). The dry weights are approximately 35% protein, with a lipid content of approximately 40–50%. Nucleic acids are present [both ribonucleic (RNA) and deoxyribonucleic (DNA) acids] in both EBs and initial or reticulate forms, although the latter have higher quantities of RNA. The protein content of the particles is approximately 33% in both intact particles and cell walls. Of the common amino acids only arginine and histidine appear to be missing from the meningopneumonitis agent. The carbohydrate content ranges from 1% to 2%, the RNA content from 2% to 7%, and the DNA content from 3% to 4% (total nucleic acid content of the EB is approximately 5%). The DNA of chlamydial strains has a guanine plus cytosine ratio of approximately 45% for *C. trachomatis* and 41% for *C. psittaci*, although some workers after having tested a number of isolates have suggested that the range between these 2 extremes is actually a spectrum (25, 48).

The cell walls of the EBs are quite analogous in structure to the cell walls of gram-negative bacteria (56). There are very slight differences in amino acid content between chlamydial and *Escherichia coli* cell walls, while there are marked differences in amino acid content of gram-positive bacteria.

Resistance

As a group the chlamydiae are relatively unstable in normal laboratory conditions. Infectivity may be lost in 48 hr at 37 C, within 5 min at 56 C, and in a matter of weeks at 0 C. Chylamydiae can be inactivated with 0.1% formalin or 0.5% phenol in approximately 24 hr. The pH range of stability is narrow, and the rate of inactivation by ultraviolet irradiation is comparable to that of *E. coli*. Organic solvents are efficient inactivators; ether and ethanol destroy infectivity within 30 min at room temperature. The agents are best preserved by freezing of suspensions at −70 C or lower and, in some cases, by lyophilization. Frozen suspensions will maintain their titer for years.

Classification

Because of their unique developmental cycle, these agents have been placed in a separate order, the Chlamydiales (114). There is one genus, *Chla-*

mydia and two species, *C. psittaci* and *C. trachomatis* (77). The species are differentiated on the basis of inclusion type and sulfonamide sensitivity. *C. trachomatis*, which is sensitive to sulfa drugs, produces inclusions that stain with iodine because they contain glycogen. *C. psittaci* is usually sulfa-resistant, and its inclusions do not stain with iodine.

Antigenic composition

The major antigenic component of all chlamydiae is a heat-stable, group-specific complement-fixing (CF) antigen. This appears to be associated with the cell wall and can be detected throughout the growth cycle of the organisms (84). This ether-soluble, heat-stable antigen may be extracted or partially solubilized from chlamydial particles by boiling or treating with acid, alkali, deoxycholate, or ether. The antigen is inactivated by periodate, and it may be precipitated with acetone. There appear to be separable components within the group antigen, but it is not known whether this is a reflection of physical state or actual chemical structure. Lecithin may be a carrier since some of the purified antigens were inactive in the CF test until lecithin was added. Dhir and colleagues have further studied the antigen, purified the active moiety, and identified it as a 2-keto-3-deoxyoctanoic acid (22).

Some of the soluble group antigens have been used as CF antigens or in immunodiffusion (ID) tests. Species-specific antigens have also been demonstrated in solubilized chlamydial suspensions.

Although many studies have shown antigenic differences between strains, there is still no readily useful technique for differentiating *C. psittaci* strains on the basis of antigenic structure. Workers at the Hooper Foundation have tried to develop a serologic system for classification, and the results suggest that isolates of avian origin seem to have an antigenic pattern which reflects the species in which they naturally occur (5). Those isolates obtained from domestic mammals seem to be more restricted in antigenic structure, with the same two major serotypes being recovered from sheep, cattle, and other mammals (95).

The *C. trachomatis* strains may be immunotyped with much greater ease. This is largely owing to the efforts of Wang and associates in applying the microimmunofluorescence (micro-IF) test (121). This test, developed in 1970 by Wang and Grayston, has allowed identification of a number of related serotypes of TRIC and LGV strains. Currently, 11 TRIC types (designated A–K) and 3 serotypes of LGV strains (L-1, L-2, and L-3) are recognized (31). These antigens appear to be shared to some degree with serotypes reacting more or less in a manner reminiscent of the senior-junior antigenic evolution of the influenza viruses. None of these antigens has been identified biochemically. This test has not yet been applied systematically to the *C. psittaci* strains, but preliminary results show promise (46).

The chlamydiae also possess a murine toxin capable of killing mice within a few to 24 hr after intravenous (iv) inoculation. Antiserum has been shown to prevent toxic death and was utilized by Manire and Meyer to differentiate a variety of *C. psittaci* strains (55). In addition, the mice may be immunized, and this mouse-toxicity prevention test has been used as the basis for differentiating *C. trachomatis* strains (1, 11). However, the test has been supplanted by the micro-IF test, which appears to give identical groupings.

The chlamydiae produce a hemagglutinin during their growth cycle. This hemagglutinin appears to be related to the group antigen in both activity and physical properties (28). It was first described in infective allantoic fluids and reacts with murine RBC (41). It will also agglutinate hamster RBC and chicken RBC if the latter cells are susceptible to agglutination by vaccinia virus (7). These hemagglutination (HA) reactions can be inhibited by chlamydial antibodies, but this is not a useful diagnostic test. Neither have the indirect HA tests that have been described proven useful.

The chlamydiae do not share antigens with any other organism. One-way cross-reactions have been reported between chlamydial group antigen and an organism known as *Bacterium antitratum* and *Herrellea* species (111, 119). These bacterial antigens react with chlamydial antibodies, but antibodies against these bacterial antigens do not react with chlamydial antigens; therefore, there is no known cross-reaction that would interfere with serologic diagnosis of chlamydial infections.

Host range

Naturally occurring *C. psittaci* infections appear to be virtually ubiquitous throughout the animal kingdom (61, 113). Avian species and mammals are commonly parasitized. Many different diseases may be caused by chlamydial infection in single host species. For example, cattle are subject to the following diseases of chlamydial etiology: abortion, arthritis, conjunctivitis, encephalomyelitis, enteritis, pneumonitis, and seminal vesiculitis (113). Latent infections are common in all natural host species. Experimental host range tests in mice (by different inoculation routes), guinea pigs, and certain other mammalian and avian indicator hosts may be useful in identifying biotypes (62, 75). As far as is known, all human infections with *C. psittaci* are zoonotic.

On the other hand, humans are the sole natural host for *C. trachomatis* (with the exception of some rodent pneumonia isolates). The useful experimental host range for the TRIC isolates is limited to primates, while LGV strains will also grow in mice.

The only system capable of supporting the growth of all known chlamydiae is the yolk sac, although with the assistance of centrifugation they can be grown in cell cultures. Thus, these two host systems are the isolation methods of choice. Chlamydiae of avian origin may be readily recovered in mice, and some mammalian strains are highly lethal for guinea pigs.

Growth in cell culture

Chlamydial strains vary considerably in their infectivity for cell cultures and other laboratory hosts. The general rule of thumb for microbiologists has been that TRIC strains grow well only in the nonselective medium of the embryonated hen's egg. TRIC agents grow very poorly in cell cultures, although some have been adapted to serial growth in cell culture. The so-called fast TRIC strains, which are now recognized as being biologically identical to LGV agents (122), grow well in eggs and tissue culture systems and are infective for mice by the intracerebral and intranasal routes.

From the work of Gordon and Quan and that of Weiss and Dressler, it appeared that the major limitation in the ability of TRIC agents to infect cells was the efficiency of their attachment and penetration into the host cell (30, 125). Centrifugation to enhance the contact between the parasite and the cell increased the infectivity of a number of chlamydial isolates in both species. Although this technique was originally applied to normal cells, Gordon obtained better results centrifuging TRIC agents into irradiated McCoy cells. This system evolved into the first generally applicable tissue culture method for isolation of these agents. The refinements that have been made in the system have been reviewed (17). Alternate methods, such as use of iododeoxyuridine treatment as substitute for irradiation have also been developed (126). Harrison used pretreatment of cells with diethylaminoethyl (DEAE)-dextran to enhance the infectivity of an ovine chlamydial strain (38). DEAE-dextran is a positively charged macromolecule which has been shown to enhance the infectivity and transforming ability of a number of lytic and nonlytic viruses. It would appear that the key aspect of this pretreatment involves changing the surface charge of the cell to allow for greater attachment of the EB to the cell membrane. Presumably, this attachment is simply electrostatic. Becker, Hochberg, and Zakay-Rones have shown that treatment of EBs already absorbed onto the cell membrane with heparin (a negatively charged polysaccharide) causes very marked elution of a *C. trachomatis* agent from the cell surface, resulting in decreased infectivity (9). The enhancing effect of DEAE-dextran has been used in isolation procedures for TRIC agents. Thus, Rota and Nichols and Kuo et al found that DEAE pretreatment of tissue cultures enhanced inclusion counts when the infecting inoculum was centrifuged into either McCoy or HeLa cells (50, 91). Although DEAE-dextran enhanced the infectivity of the TRIC agents, it was apparent from the results of Rota and Nichols that centrifugation of inoculum is the most important single step for increasing infectivity, and that centrifugation at approximately 33 C represents the optimal system for inclusion production (92).

Kuo, Wang, and Grayston further investigated the effect of polycations, polyanions, and neuraminidase on the infectivity of TRIC agents and LGV organisms (49). These workers found that TRIC agents and LGV organisms differed significantly in the response to DEAE-dextran and neuraminidase in that the LGV organisms were not affected, while infectivity of the TRIC agents was enhanced by the DEAE-dextran treatment and inhibited by neuraminidase treatment. Thus, the authors considered that there may well be different receptor sites or points of attachment of LGV and TRIC agents. Further evidence was obtained for this viewpoint when they found that the TRIC agent's attachment could be specifically blocked by pretreatment of the cells with heat-inactivated TRIC organisms but not by heat-inactivated

LGV strains or influenza virus. The authors therefore concluded that, with respect to these 2 modes of cell treatment, it was possible that there might be 3 groups of chlamydiae: the TRIC strains enhanced by DEAE-dextran and inhibited by neuraminidase, the LGV isolates unaffected by either, and the single strain of psittacosis agent that was enhanced by DEAE-dextran pretreatment but unaffected by neuraminidase.

C. psittaci strains vary considerably in infectivity for laboratory animals, but most of these strains grow quite well in cell cultures. Differences in virulence for laboratory animals include variations by different routes of inoculation as well as for different animals. Thus, some isolates may kill mice (by any route of inoculation) and guinea pigs; other isolates may kill mice (by any route of inoculation) but are innocuous to guinea pigs; still other isolates may be lethal for mice after intracerebral infection but not after intraperitoneal (ip) infection. This variability appears to be relatively systematic and has been used in the past for identifying isolates on a crude basis by the use of pathogenicity patterns, pathogenicity indices, or pathotypes (62, 75).

Psittacosis strains have been shown to grow in a variety of cells. Their growth in mouse L cells, Chang human liver cells, fetal-mouse-lung cell cultures, and human diploid cells seems to be quite similar (73, 80). Officer and Brown studied psittacosis agents' growth in tissue culture (73). They used the 6 BC and Borg strains in Chang human liver cells and found that both cell lines supported the growth of the Borg strain at essentially the same level, but that the 6 BC strain was much more invasive for the liver line than for the fetal-mouse-lung line. They observed that attachment between the agent and the cell was a highly inefficient process and it required a high multiplicity of infection in order to initiate an observable reaction. Chlamydial absorption was the same at temperatures ranging from 22 C to 37 C and at pH values between 6.0 and 8.0. The morphologic development of the 6 BC strain and the Borg strain was the same in both cells but differed between agents.

Chlamydiae can be grown not only in cells in monolayers, but they can also be grown in suspended cells in spinner culture (110). Also, growth of the meningopneumonitis strain in L cells supported by a defined medium in spinner cultures has been reported (66). For chlamydial strains capable of continued multiplication in tissue culture, plaquing systems have been developed with L cells and chick fibroblasts (40, 82). A highly sensitive, reproducible method using L-929 cells has proven effective in assaying plaque-forming infectivity of a wide variety of C. psittaci isolates of avian and mammalian orgin and of LGV strains (4). This assay has been used in the development of a plaque-reduction system to measure neutralizing (Nt) antibodies. This system has allowed a relatively crude serotyping of chlamydial strains of avian and mammalian origin (5, 95).

Harrison found that absorption of chlamydiae (ovine origin) onto HEp-2 cells is more efficient at 37 C than at 30 C (38). The smaller the volume, the more efficient the inoculum's absorption. In the studies of Banks and colleagues, it was found that the efficiency of absorption had to be carefully counterbalanced with the inactivation of the agent (5). Longer periods of contact between inoculum and agent may, in some systems, yield higher plaque counts, but in other systems the titers may fall because of the thermo-lability of the agent. In some systems it has been found that serum thought to contain Nt antibody actually enhanced the concentration of the infecting agent. Further studies have shown that this enhancement is due to the pro-tective effect of the serum protein. When dilutions were made in normal serum or with addition of a protein diluent, the titers stabilized and the effect of immune serum in reducing plaque counts could be shown.

Preparation of Immune Serum

Human convalescent-phase serum is often useful as a source of chla-mydial antibodies. Both psittacosis and LGV cases may provide reagent for CF tests, and LGV convalescent-phase serum can be used in fluorescent-antibody (FA) tests for inclusions.

Highly potent immune serum for use as a reagent for FA or CF tests may be prepared in the guinea pig. Adult guinea pigs are inoculated ip with viable suspensions of chlamydiae. Boosters may be given at weekly inter-vals, and the animals exsanguinated after a 1-month rest period. Alternative-ly, purified chlamydial suspensions may be inoculated subcutaneously in in-complete Freund adjuvant. Intraperitoneal injection of aqueous suspensions is used for booster inoculations 3–4 weeks later, and the animals are bled 2–4 weeks after the booster. Similar schedules may be used to immunize rabbits for FA reagent, but rabbit antiserum is not as useful in CF tests.

Mouse antiserum is used for typing *C. trachomatis* isolates in the micro-IF test. The mice are inoculated iv with an agent grown in yolk sac or tissue culture; booster inoculations are given by the same route 7 days later, and the animals are bled 4 days after that.

Nt tests are not generally used with *Chlamydiae* because it is difficult to produce Nt antibodies. Irregular successes have been obtained with mam-malian antiserum. Rooster antiserum has been the best (but still a poor) source of Nt antibody.

Collection and Processing of Specimens for Laboratory Diagnosis

Precautions

Isolation of psittacosis agents should not be undertaken by laboratories lacking suitable isolation or containment facilities. Laboratory infections with these highly infectious human pathogens are common among even the most experienced laboratory workers. Avian specimens are most dangerous since they contain the largest amount of agent.

The *C. trachomatis* strains are less dangerous, but laboratory infections have occurred. Aseptic technique is required, and suitable disinfection pro-cedures should be followed.

Isolation of Chlamydiae

For practical purposes only three experimental systems need be considered for the isolation of chlamydiae. First, all known chlamydiae grow in the yolk sac of the embryonated hen's egg. Second, with centrifugation of the inoculum, it appears that all chlamydiae (with some variability) will grow in tissue culture; psittacosis and LGV agents are capable of serial growth in tissue culture without centrifugation. Third, the psittacosis agents will grow in mice after intracerebral, ip, and intranasal inoculation, and LGV agents after intracerebral and intranasal inoculation, although the latter route is rarely used. Mice are of no use in recovering TRIC agents.

The specimens to be tested include ocular and genital-tract epithelial-cell scrapings for TRIC agents, bubo pus and genital-tract specimens for LGV agents, and blood, sputum, and biopsied tissues for psittacosis.

General guidelines for handling specimens are listed below. The diluents and antibiotics used to control bacterial contamination will differ with the isolation system being used, resulting in some minor variations. For yolk sac procedures a suitable collection medium is nutrient broth containing streptomycin (2.5 mg/ml), neomycin (0.5 mg/ml), and nystatin (100 u/ml). For isolation in tissue culture, a useful collection medium is complete cell culture medium containing gentamicin (10 μg/ml), vancomycin (100 μg/ml), and fungizone (4 μg/ml). Either diluent may be used for mice. Other tissue culture collection media have been used, such as modifications of the sucrose-phosphate buffer solutions originally developed for rickettsiae (17). These, however, are toxic to the cells and must be replaced after inoculation. Fresh samples are preferred, but frozen material (-60 C) is acceptable.

Ocular and genital-tract specimens. For maximal results it is imperative that adequate specimens be collected. Since the object is to obtain a representative sample of epithelial cells, the specimens must be collected with some vigor. With genital-tract specimens the samples must be obtained (either by swabbing or scraping) from the transitional zone of the cervix or the endourethra (4–6 cm from the meatus). Culture of discharges or of urine is inadequate. The material is inoculated into yolk sac or tissue culture. Calcium alginate swabs are preferable to cotton or dacron if the material is to be inoculated into cell cultures.

Bubo pus. Grind the viscous material. Suspend in nutrient broth or tissue-culture medium to at least 20% of weight. Even when pus is not viscous, dilution is advisable. If the bubo is not fluctuant, sterile saline may be injected and aspirated for isolation attempts. Test for bacterial contaminants, treat with antibiotics, and inoculate the material into mice intracerebrally, into eggs by the yolk-sac route, or into cell cultures.

Blood. If there is a clot, grind it and add beef heart broth or tissue culture medium to make a 10% suspension.

Sputum or throat washings. Sputum is cultured for bacteria on blood agar plates. To prepare the emulsion, suspend sputum, depending on its consistency, in 2–10 times its volume of sterile antibiotic-containing broth (pH

7.2–7.4) or tissue-culture medium; emulsify thoroughly by shaking with glass beads in a sterile, tightly-stoppered container. Refrigerate the material for 18–24 hr at about 0–4 C to extract the chlamydiae, or inoculate into the isolation system after 1–2 hr of treatment with antibiotics at room temperature. It may be advisable to centrifuge extracts for 20–30 min at 100 × g to remove coarse material.

Pleural fluid or vomitus. Determine the extent of bacterial contamination of pleural fluid by culturing on blood agar plates. Treat it with an antibiotic solution, and then refrigerate the specimen until it is used for inoculation. When much vomitus is available, the coarse material is sedimented by centrifugation; the supernatant fluid is treated in the manner used for fecal specimens (see below).

Fecal samples. Cloacal or rectal swabs, the droppings from caged birds, or fecal pellets are suspended in antibiotic broth or medium. The suspension (approximately 20%) is shaken thoroughly. After centrifugation at 300 × g for 10 min, the supernatant fluid is removed. It may be further diluted (1:2 and 1:20) with antibiotic solution and held for 1 hr at room temperature prior to inoculation into tissue culture, yolk sac, or mice. More concentrated material may be used for ip inoculation of mice.

Another method has been recommended by Storz and associates (115). Fecal samples are collected from the rectum of sheep, cattle, or other mammals with use of a fresh, wooden tongue depressor for each animal. Immediately after collection, the samples are taken to the laboratory, ground, and brought to a 10% suspension in Earle balanced salt solution containing 0.5 mg of streptomycin/ml. The samples are centrifuged for 30 min at 1800 × g. Supernatant fluid is gently withdrawn, mixed with an equal amount of fresh diluent, and centrifuged again. This procedure is repeated once more. About 3 ml of supernatant fluid is then withdrawn, and 0.5 ml each of 1:40 and of 1:400 dilutions is inoculated into the yolk sacs of 7-day-old chicken embryos. Appropriate bacteriologic controls are also prepared.

Tissues. Frozen tissue is thawed in a refrigerator at about 4 C for 18–24 hr. The specimen is weighed, minced with sterile scissors, and ground to a paste. Grinding may be done with such equipment as a Ten Broeck tissue grinder; a 150- × 20-mm Pyrex test tube in which a narrower, but longer and stronger test tube (200 × 10 mm) with a roughened outer surface acts as a pestle (the risk of contamination is less with this device than with a mortar); a sterile mortar and sterile carborundum (size 60); a scissors for mincing; and a special metal container for grinding that can be hermetically closed and operated on a blender base. This last method is particularly useful for breaking up large pieces of organ, but there is greater potential for aerosolization.

After the tissue has been ground thoroughly, the volume of antibiotic-containing diluent required to make a 10–20% emulsion is added to the tube, and the suspension is thoroughly mixed. Plain nutrient broth (pH 7.2–7.4) may be used if the tissue is bacteriologically sterile. If testing is not urgent, holding the suspensions in the refrigerator for 18–24 hr is advisable, since this permits additional sedimentation and diffusion of the chlamydiae into the diluent for mouse or yolk-sac inoculation. For tissue culture, antibiotic-containing collection medium is used, and 10^{-1} and 10^{-2} dilutions are inoculated.

Before being refrigerated, a sample of the untreated emulsion is cultured on blood plates and on eosin-methylene blue plates to detect possible bacterial contamination.

Collection, storage, and processing for serodiagnosis

Human serum. Blood should be collected before treatment on the day the patient is first examined, and thereafter on the days 8, 16, 30, and 40—that is, throughout the illness and convalescence. The blood sample (10–15 ml) must be collected aseptically from a vein, usually the basilic or cubital, and allowed to clot. If it is to be shipped any distance, the serum should be left on the clot for at least 24 hr before it is removed asepticallly and sent by air mail. It should not be frozen. Handling the blood specimen aseptically permits the blood clot to be used for isolation of the chlamydiae while the serum furnishes antibody tests. The small volumes of blood obtained by puncturing the heel of neonates is adequate for micro-IF tests.

Human secretions. Tears or genital-tract secretions may be collected with precalibrated cellulose sponges or filter-paper strips. It is most convenient to place the collected material directly into diluent to yield a dilution of 1:10 and freeze for storage.

Avian serum. Blood samples of the larger birds (pigeons, parrots, cockatoos, conures, macaws, doves, turkeys, egrets, ducks) can be obtained easily with 2- to 5-ml syringe and a 24-gauge needle. The blood is usually taken from the wing vein. Parakeets may be bled from the jugular vein or from the heart before autopsy. To enable an assistant to hold the bird more easily while the blood is drawn, Amazon parrots, cockatoos, macaws, and other large birds may be put under light ether anesthesia.

If the blood is put into tubes prepared with a very thin, even coating of vaseline or embedding paraffin, the yield of clear serum will be greater. For shipping, carefully withdraw the serum into the prepared tube, cork tightly, label, and send by air express. The clots should also be submitted for isolation as they often yield chlamydiae from seropositive birds.

Mammalian serum. Puncturing the jugular vein is the most satisfactory means of obtaining blood samples from sheep, cattle, or goats. The radial or saphenous vein is chosen in the dog or cat. The blood should be treated as described for human serum.

Collection of specimens for microscopy

Light microscopy and IF examination. Fixation methods will vary according to the staining procedure to be followed. For cytologic studies in human oculogenital infections, the goal of specimen collection is to obtain an adequate amount of material (at least 1000 epithelial cells) and to distribute it on the slide in a manner that will facilitate microscopic examination. The specimen should be spread in a manner that minimizes heaping of cells and allows visualization of single cells. The scrapings are usually collected, after topical anesthesia, with a spatula (usually blunt, although some workers prefer sharp edges) and are spread on the slide. Specimens are usually collected from the upper formix in the case of trachoma and from the lower conjunctiva in inclusion conjunctivitis. Genital-tract specimens can be collected with spatulas (the Jones-Dunlop curettes are excellent) and are usually collected from 3 to 6 cm down the male urethra and from the transitional zone of the cervical epithelium.

If follicular expressions are particularly sought, the follicles can be removed with a curette or ring forceps, and the collected material spread on the slide.

Impression smears (touch preparations) are useful in diagnosis of some *C. psittaci* infections and are commonly used for microscopic identification of chlamydiae in experimental host systems.

Electron microscopy. Although inclusions have been demonstrated by electron microscopy (EM) in human ocular and genital-tract specimens, this technique is not useful in diagnosis.

Laboratory Diagnosis

Direct examination of clinical material

Human psittacosis can rarely be diagnosed on cytologic grounds. Occasionally, inclusions can be demonstrated in touch preparations and, in rare instances, in sections from involved sites studied at autopsy. The impression smears may be stained by the Giemsa, Gimenez, or Macchiavello techniques described below. These techniques are highly successful in experimental systemic chlamydial infections. For example, mice inoculated ip with psittacosis agents will yield spleen and liver smears rich in inclusions. Stained impression smears are occasionally helpful in detecting chlamydial infection in the tissues of infected birds.

Our experience with examining sections has shown that the thickness of the section is of paramount importance. Sections should be cut at $<4\mu$ (preferably 2μ) from tissues that have been fixed in Zenker, Bouin, Carnoy, or Schaudinn fixative. The recommended stains include Wolbach Giemsa stain and Noble stain: the reader should consult standard histopathology books or earlier editions of this book for procedures. Use of newer embedding materials (such as Epon) may improve results, but the search for inclusions is rarely rewarded, in part because of sampling problems. Histopathology is generally applied in experimental work. We never use this technique in routine diagnostic work, but only for retrospective testing when fixed tissue is available and a suggestion of chlamydial infection is made too late for other tests to be used.

FA procedures have been described for the diagnosis of *C. psittaci* infections in birds and experimental hosts (14, 23, 52). We do not find these techniques helpful in experimental systems, and they currently play no role in diagnosing human psittacosis.

It is rarely worth the effort to search for inclusions in pus aspirated from the buboes of LGV. Although chlamydial developmental forms have occasionally been shown, it is very difficult to recognize chlamydiae against the background of cell detritus and active phagocytosis in frank pus. Rarely, inclusions can be demonstrated in biopsy or necropsy material from late lesions of LGV, but none of these procedures can be recommended.

It is in the diagnosis of the ocular chlamydial infections, trachoma and inclusion conjunctivitis, that cytology has been most important. Visualization of the typical intracytoplasmic inclusion has been the classical method of diagnosis. The Giemsa stain has been the time-honored method to which all new techniques must be compared. The essential epidemiology of ocular and genital-tract TRIC agent infections was elucidated by this technique long before the agents were isolated.

Each of the three generally accepted methods (Giesma, FA, and iodine) for demonstrating TRIC agent inclusions in clinical specimens offers certain advantages, depending on the specific situation. The Giesma stain provides permanent preparations and allows the observer to assess the patient's inflammatory cell response (127). The inflammatory cells may be particularly helpful in the diagnosis of sporadic cases of adult inclusion conjunctivitis. These cases may be confused in the differential diagnoses with other forms of acute follicular conjunctivitis (primarily adenovirus and occasionally herpesvirus infections). Presumptive differentiation may be made on the basis of cell response, for the viral infections have a predominantly lymphocytic response while the chlamydial infection is typified by a mixture of polymorphonuclear leukocytes (PMN), lymphocytes, and other cells. Atopic conjunctivitis and vernal catarrh, which are sometimes confused with trachoma, may be recognized by the presence of eosinophilic leukocytes and free granules in smears.

The cell response in active trachoma may also be characterized. In addition to the PMN, there are also lymphocytes and macrophages. In active cases, with mature follicles, there may be many immature lymphoid cells and plasma cells together with necrotic material. Leber cells or giant macrophages containing phagocytosed material may be present. Inclusions (found in epithelial cells) may or may not accompany the typical cell population.

Experience has shown that slides with intact sheets of epithelial cells and few inflammatory cells do not reward long scrutiny. Moreover, severe trachoma is often complicated by secondary infections with bacteria that may also be identified by the Giemsa methods (127).

The necessity for close examination of slides is one of the drawbacks of the Giemsa stain. Scanning of slides is best left for only the most experienced microscopists. If slides are not examined under oil immersion (at 400X to 1000X), many inclusions can be missed. It is common to spend 30 min to 1 hour or more in examination of a single slide. Obviously, this is an arduous procedure for surveys. Another potential drawback to the use of this staining procedure is the presence of artifacts and cellular structures which may be confused with inclusions.

In neonates with severe inclusion conjunctivitis, who produce copious amounts of agent, Giemsa stain is as good as any technique for establishing the diagnosis—but virtually all tests will be positive (98, 106). Milder infections are more difficult to diagnose by cytology. In the adult form, inclusions are found in approximately 50% of those who can be proven infected by any means. In proven genital-tract infections, approximately 50% of the cervical scrapings and 15% of the urethral scrapings will show inclusions.

From our experience we cannot recommend routine use of Giemsa stain for genital-tract specimens, since it is relatively insensitive and time consuming. Cervical scrapings, in particular, are difficult to interpret because bacteria may obscure cells and appear intracellularly in forms that could be confused with inclusions.

The Giemsa stain is also used to demonstrate inclusions in histologic sections, impression smears, and tissue cultures. For *C. trachomatis* tissue culture isolation systems, this method is more time consuming than the iodine or FA stains. Screening of the coverslips may be speeded up by use of dark-field illumination of the Giemsa-stained monolayers.

The FA technique is the most sensitive cytologic method. It has been most successfully applied to the diagnosis of trachoma. In studies of severe endemic trachoma in Saudi Arabia, the FA method was more sensitive than Giemsa-staining and egg-isolation techniques (71). In the American Indian population, trachoma has become milder, apparently because of the combined effects of control measures and environmental improvement, and only FA techniques can demonstrate chlamydiae in this population (33, 100). Thus, it appears that the extreme sensitivity of the FA techniques may be useful in studies of severe trachoma and be required in studies of mild forms.

FA techniques have also been shown to be the most sensitive cytologic tools for studying chlamydial oculogenital infections (98, 106). FA added little to the diagnosis of severe inclusion blennorrhea (where all tests are likely to be positive) and was slightly more sensitive than Giemsa staining in diagnosing adult inclusion conjunctivitis or cervical infections, but it was much more sensitive than Giemsa staining in detecting chlamydial infections of the male urethra. It appears, then, that FA methods have an advantage in infections with small amounts of agent. In these studies on oculogenital infections, FA staining of smears was compared with isolation in eggs in the period before tissue culture isolation techniques became routine. Although there have been no large-scale comparative studies, it seems certain that the tissue culture method for isolation is the preferred method to detect chlamydial genital-tract infections (29).

The FA technique has several shortcomings. Even though it appears to be the most sensitive and specific cytologic procedure, it is very time consuming, requiring rigorous interpretation and criteria. In addition, the staining fades rapidly so smears cannot always be reexamined at a later date.

Giemsa-staining methods. This method gives excellent permanent preparations if a reliable brand of stain is used. In preparing the stain for use, dilutions can be made with neutral distilled water (orange with neutral red, or purple with hematoxylin), but buffered-water solution is more reliable. Prepare solution (a): M/15 Na_2HPO_4 using 9.5 g of the anhydrous salt in 1 liter of distilled water. Prepare solution (b): M/15 NaH$_2$PO$_4$ by dissolving 9.2 g of the salt in 1 liter of distilled water. To make buffered water of pH 7.2, mix 72 ml of (a) with 28 ml of (b) and 900 ml of distilled water.

Commercial cytologic buffers may also be used. Any pH between 6.8 and 7.2 is acceptable (although the more basic side is preferable) as long as it is kept constant to minimize tinctorial variation.

Giemsa stain is prepared by dissolving 0.5 g of powder in 33 ml of acetone-free absolute methanol. The solution is mixed thoroughly, allowed to sediment, and stored at room temperature for use as stock. Dilutions of this stock stain are made with neutral distilled water or buffered water, in a ratio of 1 part of stock Giemsa solution to 40 or 50 parts of diluent. There is some variability in currently available, prepared, stock Giemsa solutions, and these commercial products should be screened before being accepted for routine use.

The smear is air-dried, fixed with absolute methanol for at least 5 min, and dried again. It is then covered with the diluted Giemsa stain (freshly prepared the same day) for 1 hr. The slide is then rinsed rapidly in 95% ethyl alcohol to remove excess dye and to enhance differentiation; it is then dried and examined microscopically. Longer staining periods (1.5 hr) may be preferable with heavy tissue-culture monolayers. EBs stain reddish-purple. The initial bodies are more basophilic, staining bluish, as do most bacteria.

FA technique. Either direct or indirect methods are acceptable. The indirect method may be better suited for laboratories initiating such studies because staining reagents are commercially available and, theoretically, there may be some advantages in the sensitivity of the test.

Slides are air-dried, fixed with cold (−20 C) acetone, and stored at −20 C to −70 C before staining. The slides are overlaid with antiserum for 1 hr in a moist chamber; this antiserum ideally would include antibodies to the serotypes prevalent in the area. The alternative, and possibly more practical method would be use of a broadly reactive serum. At the WHO Collaborating Centre for Reference and Research on Trachoma and Other Chlamydial Infections, we use hyperimmune rabbit serum against an LGV strain (434B, Type L-2); high-titer human convalescent-phase LGV serum might be equivalent, but it is difficult to obtain. The slides are then washed twice with phosphate-buffered saline (PBS), pH 7.2–7.4, for 5 min each time, and stained for 1 hr with commercially prepared fluorescein-labeled goat anti-rabbit globulin. After being washed with PBS for 15 min, the slides are mounted in 90% glycerol in PBS and examined by dark-field fluorescence or interference microscopy with appropriate filters.

The reagents for the tests are most easily standardized against monolayers of HeLa or other susceptible cells infected with an LGV isolate. The cells are incubated at 35 C after being infected with an inoculum that produces inclusions in 30–90% of the cells. Maximal staining of inclusions is observed 40–42 hr after infection, before the inclusions become too large and the antigen concentration decreases. For a positive reaction the inclusions must stain brightly. The titers of both the rabbit and fluorescein-conjugated antirabbit serum are determined with these infected monolayers. The antisera used with clinical material are 4 times more concentrated than the dilution endpoint for bright staining of inclusions in the infected monolayers. For example, a serum specimen with an end point at 1:80 would be used at 1:20 as a reagent. Standard tests (blocking, staining of normal cells) are performed to prove the specificity of the reaction. In addition, the sera should be tested to assure that they stain inclusions of all known *C. trachomatis* immunotypes. The LGV antisera mentioned above meet this criterion, although there is some variation in the brightness of the inclusions of different immunotypes. Small quantities of these sera are available from the WHO Collaborating Centre to enable laboratories to initiate studies on *Chlamydia*.

The criteria for detecting chlamydial inclusions in a clinical specimen are based on the presence of a brightly fluorescing mass in the cytoplasm of an epithelial cell, preferably adjacent to the nucleus. Areas of the smears with heaped cells are difficult to interpret and must be excluded since all cells are not morphologically identifiable. General brightness or free fluorescing masses should be ignored.

Iodine stain: Rice found that chlamydial inclusions contained a glycogen-like material that could be stained with iodine, but the method has been applied only sporadically (85). It offers the advantages of simplicity and speed. It is easily the fastest staining procedure, and entire slides can be screened in a matter of minutes. Inclusions may also be recognized in the thick areas of the slide unsuitable for examination by other techniques. The iodine-stained slides can be maintained for permanent record or can be counterstained by the Giemsa method, and suitable cells reexamined for confirmation.

In a heavily infected preparation, the ease of reading slides can compensate for relatively poor sensitivity, for this is the least sensitive of the cytologic techniques. This is particularly true in testing for inclusion conjunctivitis (106). Also, the technique is not applicable to scrapings from the genital tract, since normal specimens may have glycogen-containing cells.

The iodine stain probably finds its greatest application today in the staining of monolayers employed in chlamydial isolation attempts. Here, speed is the requisite feature, and since many specimens can be screened, the occasional missed positive specimen is acceptable. This technique does not stain inclusions of *C. psittaci*, and the possibility that these organisms may be involved in the disease must be ignored if this stain is to be used.

The iodine-staining technique follows. Monolayers or scrapings are air-dried, fixed in absolute methanol, and stained with Lugol iodine or 5% iodine in 10% potassium iodide for 3–5 min. Slides are examined as wet mounts. The matrix of inclusions may appear as a reddish-brown mass recognizable under low magnification. The slides may be decolorized with methanol and restained with Giemsa stain.

Macchiavello and Gimenez stains. Any of the above mentioned techniques can be used to stain inclusions in impression smears. The Macchiavello and Gimenez stains are not used in routine diagnosis but are usually applied to impression smears.

These staining methods are generally used to detect EBs in yolk-sac smears. They may also be used to demonstrate inclusions in impression smears made from organs of infected birds or mammals. These methods are quite similar in principle, but the Gimenez is probably simpler for inexperienced workers. The Macchiavello stain gives similar results but may require greater attention to detail. Although the Giemsa method is occasionally used for detecting EBs in yolk-sac smears, it is not the method of choice; it requires considerable experience because the EBs do not stain in marked contrast to the yolk-sac material.

1. Modified Macchiavello's stain — This stain is prepared as follows:

Stock solutions

Basic fuchsin	0.25 g in 100 ml double-distilled water
Citric acid	0.5 g in 200 ml double-distilled water
Methylene blue	1.0 g in 100 ml double-distilled water

Prepare citric acid solution fresh daily.

After drying in air, the smear or impression preparation is fixed by heat. The basic fuchsin solution, first passed through filter paper in a small funnel, is dropped onto the film and left for 5 min before being quickly drained off. The slide is first washed in tap water and then dipped for a few seconds in the citric acid solution, which is best held in a Coplin jar. The slide is then washed thoroughly with tap water and stained with 1% methylene blue for 20–30 sec; it is washed again in tap water and dried.

The citric acid solution must be fresh. Exposure to citric acid for more than a few seconds decolorizes the chlamydiae, and they all stain blue. In a properly prepared slide, most EBs stain red against a blue background.

2. Gimenez modification of the Macchiavello technique

Stock solutions

1. 10% (wt/vol) basic fuchsin in 95% ethanol . . . . .100 ml
   4% (wt/vol) aqueous phenol . . . . .250 ml
   distilled water . . . . .650 ml
2. 0.1 M sodium PBS, pH 7.45 (mix 3.5 ml of 0.2 M NaH_2PO_4, 15.5 ml of 0.2 M Na_2HPO_4, and 19 ml of distilled water)
3. 0.8% aqueous malachite green oxalate

To prepare a working solution of carbol fuchsin, mix 4 ml of stock solution with 10 ml of buffer (pH 7.45); filter immediately and filter again before each staining. The working solution remains satisfactory for about 40 hr.

A very thin air-dried smear (heat fixation is not necessary for cytologic reasons but should be employed for safety) is covered with the filtered carbol basic fuchsin working solution and held for 1–2 min. After a thorough washing in tap water, it is covered with the malachite green solution for 6–9 sec and washed again in tap water. The slides are finally dried with absorbent paper. EBs stain red; the background greenish.

Chlamydial isolation

Isolation in mice. The mice to be used should be proven susceptible to chlamydiae because there are some genetic variations in this regard. Mice should be obtained from a colony shown to be free of latent chlamydial infection. There have been at least 7 reports of subclinical chlamydial infections in mouse colonies. These agents have been identified as *C. psittaci* as well as *C. trachomatis,* and some have been viscerotropic while others were pneumotropic (3, 27, 72). These infections were revealed by persistent blind passage of "normal" mouse tissue.

1. Intraperitoneal injection—Most psittacine, turkey, and egret isolates will be revealed by inoculation by the ip route; those from pigeons, chickens, some turkeys, or ducks may produce significantly enlarged spleens and ascitic fluid but do not regularly cause death.

Administer 0.5 ml of the prepared 10% or 20% sterile emulsion. Virulent material from parrots, parakeets, humans, and some turkeys, injected by the ip route in this amount causes death of the mouse in 3–30 days, usually within 3–10 days. Some animals recover. Death of the animals within 2 or 3 days after infection indicates the presence of high concentrations of a virulent toxic isolate, such as certain turkey or egret isolates.

If mice die within 2 or 3 days, little that is abnormal can be seen with the naked eye; spleen and liver may look normal in size and architecture. Some animals may show signs of vascular damage. Quite characteristic, and often the only sign, is a bloated duodenum covered with a thin viscous exudate. In some animals the surface of the liver and intestines may be moist and covered with a thin, sticky exudate that contains abundant endothelial cells packed with chlamydial particles.

When death occurs within 5–15 days, the spleen is enlarged, and early necrotic lesions of the liver can be seen. Microscopically, hemorrhages and necrosis are common in the liver; the phagocytic cells of liver and spleen may be packed with chlamydiae. The abdominal cavity may be filled with stringy, turbid, fibrinous exudate.

If animals survive until day 21, they should be sacrificed, and further blind passage of emulsions of their spleen and liver made. In our experience if chlamydiae are not found by the third passage, they cannot be isolated no matter how many more passages are made. Mice that recover and are sacrificed 3 weeks after infection have few gross lesions. In general, the intestines are slightly distended and pale. Exudate may be present in the abdominal cavity. The spleen is conspicuously enlarged, the liver friable and mottled, and the kidneys grayish. EBs are sparse in tissue smears, but animal passage has shown that they may exist as long as 300 days after initial infection. Most survivors have an infection immunity.

This technique offers the advantages of simplicity, reliability, and large inocula. If it is desired, the animals may receive multiple (at daily intervals) inoculations from the original specimen. In addition, the mice may "filter" out bacteria that have not been controlled by antibiotics or centrifugation and dilution.

2. Intracranial injection—Tissue specimens from humans, sterile exudates from the pericardial or air sacs of birds, or peritoneal fluid and suspensions prepared from infected mice may be safely infected by this route, which may furnish excellent specimens for rapid histologic diagnosis. Inoculate 0.03 ml of a 10% emulsion. Somnolence and paralysis often develop within 24–48 hr, and death follows within 3–5 days. Blind passage is performed at 10 days.

This route has the advantage of not involving the respiratory tract, precluding the possibility of activating latent mouse pneumonitis. Smears made from the dura teem with chlamydiae. A relatively fast and sensitive method for isolating psittacosis and ornithosis agents, this technique is somewhat less effective with LGV. This route of inoculation suffers a disadvantage in terms of small volume of inoculum and in the susceptibility of the mice to bacteria that may contaminate the specimen.

3. Intranasal instillation—Instill 0.03–0.05 ml of a 10% tissue suspension, with the mouse under light anesthesia (ether is suitable). If the material inoculated is virulent or if isolates have been established, signs of infection—hunched posture, apathy, and increasingly labored respiration—develop rapidly, and death follows within 2–20 days. Bacterial contamination must be ruled out. In typical successful isolation attempts, death may take place between days 8 and 16 if the agent is present in high concentration. However, with less virulent material all symptoms may gradually disappear; in such cases blind passage should be performed 21 days after inoculation. Blind passage is usually required. Segments or entire lobes of the lung may be extensively consolidated. Discrete foci of pneumonia are manifested as limiting infective dilutions are approached. These areas, which are gray, almost translucent, and 1–3 mm in diameter, lie in apparently normal lung.

Fewer EBs are seen in smears from lungs infected for more than 10 days, and there may be difficulty finding them in old lesions. Repassage may furnish excellent material for microscopy.

Isolation in embryonated eggs. The yolk-sac method, long used in psittacosis work, was shown by Wall to be the method of choice in isolating LGV agents (120). It was used by T'ang et al in the first isolation of the trachoma agent (116). Until tissue-culture procedures were developed, the yolk-sac technique was the only practical way to culture TRIC agents.

The yolk-sac technique is not particularly sensitive for isolating TRIC agents because it may require many EBs to produce 1 egg mean lethal dose (LD_{50}). With more virulent psittacosis strains, a single particle may be lethal. This system is much more sensitive for the recovery of *C. psittaci* strains, in general. The technique is cumbersome, making it difficult to screen large numbers of specimens. In addition, it can be quite time consuming, taking anywhere from 1 to 6 weeks to obtain a definitive result.

The eggs to be used must be derived from a flock fed an antibiotic-free diet. They should be free from mycoplasma.

The yolk-sac isolation technique follows: The specimen, in an appropriate antibiotic broth, is held for 1 hr at room temperature before inoculation of 0.25 ml into the yolk sac with a 1.5-inch, 22-gauge needle. Prior to inoculation, the fertile eggs are incubated at 38.5–39 C in a moist atmosphere. When 7 days old, embryonated hens' eggs are candled for viability, and the location of air sacs and embryos marked with a pencil. The shell over the air sac is painted with tincture of iodine, and a hole is gently punched. The specimen is inoculated at a slight angle away from the embryo; we recommend that 3 or 4 eggs be used for each specimen. The eggs are labeled with a pencil or marking pen. After inoculation, the shell is again swabbed with iodine, and the hole sealed (with glue or tape). The eggs are then incubated in a moist environment at 35 C and candled daily for 13 days. Embryos that die in the first 3 days after inoculation are discarded.

The yolk sacs of eggs with dead embryos thereafter are harvested. This procedure entails painting the shell with iodine, cracking and removing the shell over the air sac, dissecting the shell and chorioallantoic membranes away, and removing the yolk sac with forceps. Excess yolk material may be stripped away. It is important that all instruments are sterile and that fresh instruments are used for each specimen. Impression smears are made and stained (Gimenez or the modified Macchiavello method). Sterility tests are performed on yolk sac with thioglycolate broth. If the embryos are still viable 13 days after inoculation, the eggs are chilled for several hours, and yolk sacs are harvested, ground in nutrient broth, centrifuged lightly, and passaged to another group of four 7-day-old embryonated hens' eggs (1 ml 50% yolk sac/egg). After 2 blind passages, attempts are terminated as negative.

The generally acceptable criteria for isolation are the finding of EBs in the impression smears, serially transmissible egg mortality, the presence of group antigen in the yolk sac, and the absence of contaminating bacteria (93).

The clinical specimens should not be held at ambient temperature for more than 2–3 hr. They may be refrigerated for up to 18 hr (with significant loss of infectivity) and should be frozen at -70 C (or in liquid nitrogen) for longer storage.

The specimens can be collected with a scraper or a swab. If swabs are used, they should be of a pretested type that will not inactivate TRIC agents.

Psittacosis isolation attempts may be positive within 5–10 days of the first passage. Some isolates require more adaptation but, once adapted, will often reach concentrations of 10^8 or 10^9 egg LD_{50}/g. In titrations these strains will kill eggs within 8–9 days at limiting dilutions, and surviving embryos are rarely infected.

Successful attempts to isolate LGV strains usually become apparent in the latter part of the first passage or early in the second passage. The adaptation process is slower, and usually more than 5 passages are required before the peak concentrations ($>10^7$ LD_{50}/g) are obtained. Surviving embryos in these early passages are often infected. Until peak levels are reached, the isolated LGV agents may not possess all the properties usually attributed to LGV strains. For example, LGV and TRIC agents are generally stated to differ on the grounds that LGV agents will kill mice by the intracranial route, while TRIC agents will not. This is not true in early-passage LGV isolates (103). These LGV isolates do not kill mice because it apparently requires in excess of 10^5 LD_{50} to kill a mouse, and these levels are not obtained in early passage in eggs.

With TRIC strains there is considerable variation, but the successful isolation attempt usually results in egg lethality in the second week of the second passage. Rarely will specific lethality occur in the first passage, although occasionally EBs are seen at blind passage. Egg infectivity titers greatly exceed egg lethality titers with $ID_{50}:LD_{50}$ ratios as high as 10^4 or 10^5. These TRIC agent isolates often require much adaptation and display great variability in their behavior *in ovo*. After 4 or 5 passages, the isolates often stabilize at 10^6-10^7 LD_{50}/g: they kill the eggs more slowly than psittacosis or LGV agents, with specific lethality commencing on day 6–7 and continuing to day 12 or 13. Some isolates never develop a regular pattern of egg lethality.

Although tissue-culture procedures may be preferred, the yolk-sac technique will continue to be used by many laboratories. It still results in yields of agent that cannot be matched in tissue-culture systems. It will continue to be used for isolation of chlamydiae, particularly in laboratories that are not using tissue culture regularly or that have problems in obtaining tissue-culture reagents.

Isolation in tissue culture. Psittacosis and LGV agents have been successfully propagated in cell-culture systems for several decades. The irradiated McCoy cell technique for isolation of TRIC agents was introduced by Gordon, and it has been adapted for the isolation of psittacosis agents (30, 51, 109). But it has been largely the work of the group at the Institute of Ophthalmology in London that has led to the refinement of the techniques for the procedures that are generally used today. The changes from the original techniques involved the routine use of swabbing, rather than scraping, for collecting specimens and the use of high temperatures (35–38 C) and higher forces of centrifugation ($2700 \times g$) (18, 19). It is apparent that there is no difference in the collection methods, and swabbing is easier from the viewpoint of patient comfort and maintenance of patient-physician relationship.

Wentworth and Alexander simplified the isolation system by introducing the use of 5-iodo-2-deoxyuridine (IUDR) treatment of cells as a substitute for irradiation (126). They found that cells pretreated with IUDR were equally as effective in recovering and propagating chlamydial strains. The obvious advantage of this widely used system is that it allows tissue culture isolation techniques to be performed in areas where irradiation facilities are not available. A recently described procedure, using cycloheximide, may simplify the cell culture isolation method (88). This antimetabolite acts on the cells but does not affect the chlamydiae (2). This technique offers the advantage of not requiring pretreated cells to be available.

Kuo et al have used DEAE-treated HeLa cells for isolating chlamydiae from cervical scrapings (50). They found their system to be as sensitive as the irradiated McCoy cells. Croy, Kuo, and Wang found that the HeLa-229 cell line was the most sensitive of the eleven they tested and that it supported growth of some chlamydial serotypes better than the IUDR-treated McCoy cells (16).

There is no clearly superior cytologic staining method for screening tissue cultures for isolates. The options are largely limited to iodine, Giemsa, and FA techniques. It appears that there may be some difference depending on cell type. For example, the HeLa cells do not lend themselves to routine use of the iodine-staining procedure because they occasionally have light iodine-staining material in the cytoplasmic background. The iodine stain is somewhat limited by being positive for a relatively short time within the developmental cycle of the inclusion. Since different isolates may have slightly different growth rates, any set incubation time is a compromise. On the other hand, the iodine stain offers an obvious advantage in giving good contrast with the background and lends itself to rapid scanning. Iodine will not stain *C. psittaci* inclusions.

The Giemsa stain is probably slightly more sensitive than the iodine but requires more time to interpret. The use of Giemsa stain followed by dark-field microscopy avoids this problem; when the EBs within the inclusion are viewed by dark-field illumination, they are bright yellow and contrast sharply with the background cells (17). Unfortunately, there appears to be some variability in this procedure, and not all preparations of stain and coverslips work well in a dark-field system. The reason for this variation is not known.

The FA staining procedure obviously presents problems in reagents. While it appears to be a quick method, it probably offers no advantages in terms of sensitivity. Kuo and colleagues compared Giemsa and direct FA staining methods to demonstrate inclusions in a HeLa cell isolation system and found that results were essentially the same, although the FA slides took only 5-10 min to interpret, whereas the Giemsa coverslip took 20-30 min to interpret (50).

For the tissue culture technique, many cell lines are suitable. The McCoy cells are most commonly used. Confluent monolayers of the cells are grown in the standard growth medium (10% fetal calf serum in Eagle minimal essential medium supplemented with glutamine and 30 μM/ml glucose). The cells are irradiated (5000 r), and 1-7 days later the cells are seeded onto coverslips. Round coverslips (12 mm in diameter) placed in short, 15-mm diameter, disposable flat-bottom vials are especially suitable. Each tube receives approximately 125,000 cells, and they may be used 1-7 days after planting. If many specimens are tested routinely, it is preferable to prepare fresh cells twice each week. The number of cells transferred should be sufficient to obtain light, confluent monolayers.

As a replacement for irradiation, the cells may be treated with IUDR. The light monolayers are treated for 3 days with medium containing 25 μg/ml IUDR or cells are planted with the drug. The medium containing the antimetabolite is then removed, and the cells are washed and inoculated.

A third method involves the infection of normal cell monolayers with a collection medium containing 1 μg/ml of cycloheximide. The rest of the procedure is the same.

The cells in the test specimen should be treated to release chlamydiae. Although sonication of specimens may be preferred, a simple and satisfactory method for dispersing the specimen is to have 2 or 3 sterile glass beads in each collection tube; these tubes are then shaken mechanically for 30-60 sec before inoculation. The inoculum (0.25-0.5 ml) is placed into 2-4 vials containing the cell monolayers on coverslips. The vials are then centrifuged at 2700-3000 $\times g$ at 33-35 C for 1 hr. Depending on the clinical source, the inoculum is either replaced after 2 hr at 37 C with 1 ml of growth medium, or medium is added to reach that volume. The tubes are then incubated at 37 C (5% CO_2 atmosphere may be required if loose caps are used) for 65 hr. At that time 1 coverslip is stained with iodine (after methanol fixation) and examined microscopically for inclusions. The coverslip may be stained and examined after 40-48 hr of incubation. The inclusions are not seen as easily as after 65 hr but can usually be identified. At least 90% of isolates are obtained in the first passage. If isolation is to be attempted (or if blind passage is being done), the remaining tubes are shaken vigorously and passed at day 3 or 4 to fresh tubes by the same method. Alternatively, the other coverslips may be stained and examined for inclusions. If the specimen had few infectious particles only one of the coverslips may be positive.

With trachoma, inclusion conjunctivitis, and the genital-tract infections, the technique is exactly as described above. In LGV the aspirated bubo pus is diluted (10^{-1} and 10^{-2}) and treated as above. Second passages are always made because detritus from the inoculum may make it difficult to interpret the slides. In an alternate procedure which we have used for LGV and use routinely for *C. psittaci* isolation attempts, the inoculated monolayers are incubated for 10 days, with routine examination at 5 and 10 days or whenever a CPE is noted (109). The cells are stained by the Giemsa method and examined for inclusions. Blind passage may be performed at 10 days. This technique has yielded isolates in cases of psittacosis (including avian specimens), ornithosis, human infections with feline pneumonitis agents, and chlamydial infections in cats and other mammals.

As the clinical spectrum of human chlamydial infections expands, and the isolation procedures are simplified, there will be a greater demand for patients to be tested. A problem with interpretation of the tissue culture isolation procedures could develop because diagnosis is often completely based on the results of a single staining method applied to a single monolayer. The individual reading the slides not only has to be familiar with the staining characteristics of chlamydial inclusions throughout the growth cycle, but also must appreciate the staining artifacts and detritus from the clinical specimens that may be confused with inclusions. In order to minimize the possibility of false-positive results, minimal criteria, such as passage of the isolate in addition to some immunologic identification, should be established to assure that chlamydiae are actually present.

Serologic diagnosis

Techniques available. There are no wholly satisfactory serologic methods for diagnosing human chlamydial infections, and no single test that is generally applicable. A test that is useful for diagnosing one of the diseases may be totally useless for diagnosing some of the other infections. At best, the current status of chlamydial diagnostic serology leaves much to be desired. Problems stem from inadequate antibody response for certain tests, inability to obtain appropriately paired sera because of long incubation periods or inapparent infections, and high background reactor rates in high-risk populations (94). Because human chlamydial infections do not necessarily result in immunity, reinfection is common in exposed individuals.

For practical purposes only two serologic methods can be recommended. These are the CF test and the Wang micro-IF technique (121). The CF test is most useful in diagnosing psittacosis and LGV (systemic infections), considerably less helpful in diagnosing TRIC-agent oculogenital infections, and virtually useless in diagnosing trachoma, a wholly superficial infection (98, 104, 108). Because serum from some avian species does not fix guinea-pig complement, several modifications of the CF test, most notably the indirect CF test, have been developed to allow use of the test with avian serum (47). The recently developed micro-IF test has not been used in the routine diagnosis of psittacosis, although it may be adapted to this use in the future, but it is most useful in the diagnosis of chlamydial oculogenital infections and trachoma (46). Neither of these tests is as useful in diagnosing *C. trachomatis* infections as serologic tests may be for routine diagnosis of other microbial infections. Both tests are more useful in serologic surveys than in the diagnosis of individual infections.

The CF test is a group-specific test. It measures antibodies to an antigenic determinant common to all chlamydiae. In contrast, the micro-IF test measures specific antibodies that are not detected by the CF test. Wang and Grayston initially introduced the micro-IF in 1970 for serotyping *C. trachomatis*, but further studies from the same and other laboratories found it also to be a highly sensitive and specific indicator of chlamydial antibodies (31, 35, 44, 81, 83).

The CF tests and micro-IF tests when applied to individual serum samples are generally carried through an appropriate dilution range to allow determination of end points against the antigens. In survey work it may be possible to simplify testing by screening sera at the specific dilutions that are considered to be indicative of significant titers, in order to determine prevalence of chlamydial antibodies.

Complement-fixation test

Preparation of CF antigen. There is no commercially available source of highly potent antigen. Therefore, the antigens must be prepared in the laboratory. Several available methods produce suitable antigens. The deoxycholate-extracted group antigen or the ether-extracted (and acetone-precipitated, if preferred) group antigens are perfectly satisfactory (90, 118). Partially purified EB suspensions can also be used.

Virtually any chlamydial strain can be used to prepare a group antigen, as it appears to be the major antigenic component for all strains. However, comparative tests have shown that some strains or isolates are to be preferred over others; for instance, the psittacosis antigens have been superior to the LGV antigens, even with LGV serum (13). The 6BC strain that has been used at the Hooper Foundation for many years is available from the American Type Culture Collection or the WHO Collaborating Centre for Reference and Research on Trachoma and Other Chlamydial Infections at the Hooper Foundation. This strain is a fully virulent psittacosis strain and appropriate precautions must be taken.

The technique of preparation involves inoculation of a 7-day-old embryonated hen's egg via the yolk sac with a standardized inoculum (0.25 ml containing approximately 10^5 egg LD_{50}), which kills most of the embryos in approximately 96 hr. Embryos dying before 72 hr are discarded. When approximately 50% of the embryos are dead, all the eggs are refrigerated for 3–24 hr. The yolk sacs are harvested and examined microscopically (with use of Gimenez or Macchiavello stain) for EBs. If rich in particles, they are pooled and weighed. Yolk sacs are then ground thoroughly with sterile sand (or homogenized), and a 20% suspension in nutrient broth (pH 7.0) is prepared. Sterility tests are performed, and the material is refrigerated for 6 weeks. During this period the antigen preparation is occasionally shaken. The suspension is then centrifuged lightly (200 × g for 30 min) to remove coarse tissue debris and then is steamed at 100 C for 30 min. After cooling, phenol is added to a final concentration of 0.5%. This antigen is dispersed in working volumes and stored in the refrigerator until use. The titer of the solution should be at least 1:256, and if stored properly and protected from contamination by use of aseptic technique, the antigen will be stable for years. Small quantities of CF antigen are available from the WHO Collaborating Centre for Reference and Research on Trachoma and Other Chlamydial Infections for reference purposes. The normal yolk-sac control is prepared in a similar manner from uninfected embryos.

CF test procedures. The CF test may be performed in either the tube system or the micro system. We strongly prefer the standardization of reagents in the tube system, regardless of which system is being used for the test. We find the microtiter systems most useful in screening large numbers of sera but prefer to retest all positive specimens in the tube system. We occasionally find that serum specimens with titers in the 1:4–1:8 range in the micro system are positive at 1:16 (which we consider the significant level) in the tube system. The micro system uses standard plates and one-tenth the volumes used in the tube test. The CF test is performed on serum specimens heated at 56 C for 30 min (preferably acute- and convalescent-phase paired sera tested together). In each test a positive control serum specimen of high titer is included together with a known negative serum specimen.

The reagents for the CF test are standardized by the Kolmer technique and include special buffered saline, group antigen, antigen (normal yolk sac) control, the positive serum, the negative serum, guinea-pig complement, rabbit anti-sheep hemolysin, and sheep RBC. The guinea-pig complement should be carefully tested for chlamydial antibodies since many herds are enzootically infected with a chlamydial agent, guinea-pig inclusion conjunctivitis (69). The hemolytic system is titrated and the complement unitage is determined. The test may be performed by either the water-bath technique or the overnight (icebox) technique, although the former is preferred. Doubling dilutions of the serum (from 1:2) are made in a 0.25-ml volume of diluent. The serum is also tested for reactivity to normal yolk-sac antigen and for anticomplementary activity. The antigen is added at 4 units (0.25 ml), and 2 exact units of complement (0.5 ml) are added. Standard reagent controls are always included. The normal yolk-sac control is used at the same dilution as the group antigen. The tubes are shaken well and incubated in a water bath at 37 C for 2 hr, after which 0.5 ml of sensitized sheep RBC are added and the tubes shaken and placed in the water bath for another hour. The tubes are rated for hemolysis on a scale of 1+ to 4+, roughly equivalent to 25–100% inhibition of RBC lysis. The endpoint of the serum is considered the highest dilution producing less than 50% (2+) hemolysis after complete inhibition of hemolysis has been observed. It is general practice in our laboratory to shake the tubes to resuspend the settled cells and then to refrigerate the tubes overnight and recheck the results the following morning.

Micro-immunofluorescence test

Preparation of micro-IF antigens. The antigens for the micro-IF are Eb suspensions. The chlamydiae may be propagated in yolk sac or tissue culture although the former usually provides a richer suspension. The yolk-sac antigens are not commercially available and must be prepared in the laboratory. For a complete battery of tests, antigen types A, B, Ba, C, D, E, F, G, H, I, J, and K and LGV antigens L-1, L-2, and L-3 must be included. For routine screening of human serum a simplified antigen pattern involving fewer antigen dots is useful. Closely related antigens may be pooled; for example, D and E, L-1 and L-2, G and F, and C and J (124).

Some workers have suggested that single broadly reactive strains (LGV type L-2 or immunotype E) may be adequate for serologic surveys on sexually transmitted *C. trachomatis* (117). An alternate method uses infected cell culture monolayers as antigen and inclusion fluorescence is determined (10, 87).

The yolk sacs are inoculated with suspensions of chlamydiae titrated to kill the embryos in approximately 7 days. In some instances more time may be required. When 50% of the embryos are dead, the rest of the eggs are chilled, and the yolk sacs are harvested.

Micro-IF test procedure. The individual yolk sacs are selected microscopically for EB richness and are pretitrated to give an even distribution of particles. It is generally found that a 1–3% yolk-sac suspension (PBS, pH 7) is satisfactory. The working dilution of antigen is stored frozen in appropriate volumes, and after thawing, they are mixed well in a Vortex mixer before use. Thawed suspensions should be used within 1–2 weeks. Antigen dots are placed on a slide in a specific pattern, with separate pen points for each antigen. Up to 9 clusters of dots that include all the antigenic types to be tested can be conveniently placed on each slide. The antigen dots are air-dried and fixed on slides with acetone (15 min at room temperature). Slides may be stored frozen. When thawed, water may condense on the slides, but they can be conveniently dried with a portable hair dryer set for blower only (i.e., no heat).

For the test, serial dilutions of serum (or tears or exudate) are placed on the individual clusters. The clusters of dots are sufficiently separated to avoid the running of serum from cluster to cluster. After the serum dilutions have been added, the slides are incubated for 30–60 min in a moist chamber at 37 C. They are then placed in a buffered saline wash for 5 min, followed by a second 5-min wash. The slides are then dried and stained with fluorescein-conjugated antihuman globulin. These conjugates are pretitrated in a known positive system to determine appropriate working dilutions. This reagent may be prepared against any class of globulin being considered (IgA or secretory piece for secretions, IgG or IgM). Counter stains such as bovine serum albumin conjugated with rhodamine may be included. The slides are then washed twice again, dried, and examined by standard fluorescence microscopy. Use of a monocular tube is recommended to allow greater precision in determining fluorescence for individual EB particles. The endpoints are read as the dilution giving bright fluorescence clearly associated with the well-distributed EBs throughout the antigen dot. Identification of the type-specific response is based upon dilution differences reflected in the end-points for different prototype antigens (44, 123).*

Application and interpretation of CF and micro-IF results. With either CF or micro-IF it is clear that a ≥4-fold rise in titer will support the diagnosis of chlamydial infection in the clinical syndrome being considered. Unfortunately, this is usually not observed, and often the clinician must simply use a single titer, which must be interpreted in terms of the patient's disease and the background prevalence of antibody titers.

The percentage of "normal" persons with antibody against the chlamydiae (normal background) reflects the diseases prevalent in the community and varies depending upon the geographic area where tests are performed and the specific population group to be tested. In the CF test, for example, 2–3% of the general population in the San Francisco area shows a 1:16 titer (Table 32.1). However, if one were testing veterinarians one would find between 10% and 20% with significant CF levels depending on the type of practice. Among sexually active young adults, the background is approximately 5% for men and 15–20% for women. CF titers of 1:64 or higher are rarely seen in the normal population and are uncommon in sexually active males, although they do occur more often in sexually active females. CF titers of this level are common with psittacosis or lymphogranuloma venereum. Among patients with Reiter syndrome, 10% have CF titers over 1:64, and another 15% have titers over 1:16.

There has not been similar broad experience with the micro-IF test, but the published results together with unpublished data from the Hooper Foundation indicate no problem with group-specific cross-reactions. For example, we have tested psittacosis convalescent-phase sera with CF titers of 1:512 and found them completely nonreactive against heterologous agents in the micro-IF test. But there is a substantial prevalence of seroreactors with this test. For example, among sexually active young adults, we find 25% of men and 60–70% of women with detectable micro-IF titers (94). In Seattle 60% of patients attending a venereal disease (VD) clinic were seropositive compared with 25% of controls (31). Thus, as a diagnostic test a single positive titer could again only be used to determine previous exposure. In epidemiologic studies type-specific reactions could be of considerable interest in detecting predominant serotypes, transmission chains, patterns of clustering, etc. IgM antibodies in the micro-IF test may give greater support for a diagnosis of active or recently acquired infection; however, experience indicates that only 28–33% of patients with active infections have these antibodies, and some patients who have IgM antibodies detected by micro-IF do not have demonstrable chlamydial infection (81, 83). Better results have been obtained in studies on men having first attacks of urethritis; in these studies 80% of men with chlamydial infection had IgM antibodies (12). Unfortunately, many of these infections tend to be chronic, and the best estimate is that the IgM antibody response may last for approximately one month

---

*Monotypic A reactions, at least in the United States, must be interpreted with caution. Most, perhaps all, apparently reflect antibody response to a cross reacting nonchlamydial antigen. This type of response is commonly found in infants and occasionally in V.D. clinic patients.

TABLE 32.1—CHLAMYDIAL ANTIBODIES IN SELECTED POPULATIONS TESTED AT THE HOOPER FOUNDATION

GROUP	Complement fixation ≥1:16	Micro-immunofluorescence ≥1:8
SCREENING STUDIES	(%)	(%)
Normal adults, all ages	2–3	25–45
Pediatric serum	<1	10
Trachoma-endemic population	5–15	>80
Males, VD study, young adults without disease	5–10	20–25
Males, symptomatic, attending VD clinic	10	60
Females, VD study, young adults	15–20	50–70
Prostitutes	30–60	≥85
Women with cervical atypia	20	75
PROVEN CHLAMYDIAL INFECTIONS**		
Lymphogranuloma venereum	100	100
Psittacosis	100	ND*
Adult inclusion conjunctivitis	50	100
Male, urethritis	15	90
Female, cervical infection	45	99

* Not determined

after infection (123). In the pediatric population we have found approximately 10% of children with micro-IF titers. Infants with natally acquired systemic chlamydial infections tend to have high antibody levels (10).

Patients with LGV tend to have high CF titers and very high, broadly reactive micro-IF antibody responses (81, 108, 123). We often find that LGV patients have CF titers of 1:128 or 1:256 and micro-IF titers ≥1:4000. The highest micro-IF titers we have observed have been in sera obtained from prostitutes; these titers have been as high as 1:16,000–1:32,000 and have not correlated with CF titers as well as have those of LGV sera.

The CF test should be used routinely whenever LGV is considered in the differential diagnosis, such as in the case of young men being examined for inguinal lymphadenopathy, with or without systemic complications.

For LGV the disadvantages of the CF test are not its lack of specificity (for there are no known, defined cross-reactions), but rather the ubiquitous nature of some of the chlamydial parasites and the group specificity of the test. There will be high rates of low-titer reactors in VD clinic populations. Thus, the positive serologic result may support a diagnosis of LGV but cannot prove it. Serologic proof of the diagnosis would be based on demonstration of a rise in titer (a >4-fold difference in the titers of paired acute- and convalescent-phase sera), but in most cases the patient has had the chlamydial infection for too long before the test is performed. Even in acute lymphadenopathy in the male, there is usually a 3- to 4-week period from infection to presentation. Since it may be necessary to rely on a single titer, higher CF titers are more suggestive of LGV (≥1:64, even though any titer above the

1:8 or 1:16 range is considered significant). The titers in men take on greater meaning than those in women, because the common chlamydial infections causing nongonococcal urethritis in the male tend not to produce either as high a rate or as high a titer of antibody as do the genital-tract infections in women (cervicitis). It is uncommon to find a man with simple chlamydial urethritis having a CF titer above 1:16. Any patient tested for LGV should also have a serologic test for syphilis. Some patients will have both diseases, and VDRL-reactive serum may react with both LGV and normal yolk-sac antigens.

The CF test should be performed whenever a diagnosis of psittacosis is considered. Pneumonitis, a persistent influenzal disease, or any acute or chronic febrile disease following exposure to birds would be clinical indications that psittacosis should be considered in the differential diagnosis. Here the CF test is much more satisfactory for diagnosis, since acute- and convalescent-phase sera can be obtained and often demonstrate a rise in titer. In fact, in our experience the great majority of psittacosis cases may be diagnosed in this manner. The diagnosis may have to be based upon a single high titer if the patient has a persistent or relapsing disease, but such a titer would clearly support the clinical impression. The problems of cross-reactions and previous exposure to other chlamydiae are clearly the same as discussed earlier. High seroreactor rates may be found for individuals with occupational or other long-term contact with birds. In general, psittacosis infections produce high CF antibody levels ($\geq$1:64). If a patient has had early and persistent treatment with tetracycline, the antibody levels may be suppressed. There have been a number of human infections (proven by agent isolation) in which no serologic response has occurred because of early therapy (63).

The CF test has not been useful in the diagnosis of trachoma (104). Nor is it particularly useful in the diagnosis of oculogenital infections since, at best, only 50% of individuals with eye and genital-tract infections will have significant ($>$1:16) CF titers (101). In the uncomplicated genital-tract infections such as urethritis or cervicitis, the CF reactor rates are even less. The CF test is almost useless for diagnosing urethritis, since only 15% of men with proven urethritis caused by chlamydiae have shown significant CF levels. However, approximately 40% of the women with chlamydial cervicitis have significant CF levels (101). CF titers in the background populations, i.e., sexually active men and women, show a similar distribution to that of reactor rates. Women have a higher background rate of CF reactors than men.

The micro-IF test measures specific antibodies to antigenic determinants present in the cell walls of the EB particles. It is much more sensitive than the CF test (81). For example, in 1 series of 55 isolate-positive patients, we found only 29 with significant CF reactions, while all 55 were positive by micro-IF. The respective geometric mean titers were 1:12 and 1:164. The micro-IF test can be applied to patients with LGV or TRIC-agent ocular or oculogenital infections. The presence of a reaction in a single serum specimen simply reflects previous exposure. A rise in titer may be seen in patients who are examined relatively early in the course of an infection, but patients are seldom seen at this time. One advantage of the micro-IF is that information on the specific serotype responsible for the infection may be obtained. The micro-IF offers the added advantage of determining the immunoglobulin class of the reactive antibodies.

Another advantage of the micro-IF test is that it may be used to test secretions for antibody activity. Thus, the demonstration of chlamydial antibody in tears may support a diagnosis of chlamydial infection (34, 58). Undoubtedly this test will be applied in the future to genital-tract secretions (59).

The major disadvantage of this test is that its results reflect the high prevalence of chlamydial infection in certain groups (99, 101). In other words, appropriate populations may have very high reactor rates from previous exposure to the chlamydiae. These micro-IF antibodies may persist for life, although in some patients they disappear spontaneously, possibly reflecting brief antigenic exposure (101, 123).

Other tests. A variety of other serologic techniques have been used for research projects. Some of these tests have not been tried in the routine diagnosis of human infections, while others have been found to be ineffective. For example, the microagglutination tests once used in diagnosing avian chlamydial infections were found successful only with serum from certain avian species. While agglutination tests are standard in some laboratories, they have not been applicable to human serum in our experience. The radioisotope immune precipitation test has been applied in specialized serologic surveys and appears to be considerably more sensitive than the CF test, although it is of similar specificity (26, 83). The long-range usefulness of this test has not been determined, but it will probably be limited because it is expensive and group reactive.

Chlamydiae produce a hemagglutinin (for certain avian and murine RBC), and both direct and indirect HA techniques have been described (6, 53). The ID tests that have been described appear to be relatively group specific (although enhanced specificity has been demonstrated in some tests), and the sensitivity of the ID technique currently offers no advantages with human serum but may be more useful with avian serum (15, 76).

The Nt tests that have been described have no role in diagnosing chlamydial infections. Nt antibodies are rarely found.

References

1. ALEXANDER ER, WANG S-P, and GRAYSTON JT: Further classification of TRIC agents from ocular trachoma and other sources by the mouse toxicity prevention test. Am J Ophthalmol 63:1469–1478, 1967
2. ALEXANDER JJ: Separation of protein synthesis in meningopneumonitis agent from that in L cells by differential susceptibility by cycloheximide. J Bacteriol 95:327–332, 1968
3. ATA FA, STEPHENSON EH, and STORZ J: Inapparent respiratory infection of inbred Swiss mice sulfadiazine-resistant, iodine-negative chlamydiae. Infect Immun 4:506–507, 1971
4. BANKS J, EDDIE B, SCHACHTER J, and MEYER KF: Plaque formation by *Chlamydia* in L cells. Infect Immun 1:259–262, 1970
5. BANKS J, EDDIE B, SUNG M, SUGG N, SCHACHTER J, and MEYER KF: Plaque reduction technique for demonstrating neutralizing antibodies for *Chlamydia*. Infect Immun 2:443–447, 1970

6. BARRON AL and RIERA MC: Studies on hemagglutination by *Chlamydia*. Proc Soc Exp Biol Med 131:1087–1090, 1969

7. BARRON AL, ZAKAY-RONES Z, and BERNKOPF H: Hemagglutination of chicken erythrocytes by the agent of psittacosis. Proc Soc Exp Biol Med 119:377–381, 1965

8. BARWELL CF: Laboratory infection of man with virus of enzoötic abortion of ewes. Lancet 2:1369–1371, 1955

9. BECKER Y, HOCHBERG E, and ZAKAY-RONES Z: Interaction of trachoma elementary bodies with host cells. Isr J Med Sci 5:121–124, 1969

10. BEEM MO and SAXON EM: Respiratory-tract colonization and a distinctive pneumonia syndrome in infants infected with *Chlamydia trachomatis*. N Engl J Med 296:306–310, 1977

11. BELL SD, SNYDER JC, and MURRAY ES: Immunization of mice against toxic doses of homologous elementary bodies of trachoma. Science 130:626–627, 1959

12. BOWIE WR, WANG S-P, ALEXANDER ER, FLOYD J, FORSYTH PS, POLLOCK HM, LIN J-SL, BUCHANAN TM, and HOLMES KK: Etiology of nongonococcal urethritis. Evidence for *Chlamydia trachomatis* and *Ureaplasma urealyticum*. J Clin Invest 59:735–742, 1977

13. BUCCA MA: Comparison of CF and HI tests on psittacosis-LGV serums. Public Health Rep 73:461–464, 1958

14. BUCKLEY SM, WHITNEY E, and RAPP F: Identification by fluorescent antibody of the developmental forms of psittacosis virus in tissue cultures. Proc Soc Exp Biol 90:226–230, 1955

15. COLLINS AR and BARRON AL: Demonstration of group- and species-specific antigens of chlamydial agents by gel diffusion. J Infect Dis 121:1–8, 1970

16. CROY TR, KUO CC, and WANG S-P: Comparative susceptibility of eleven mammalian cell lines to infection with trachoma organisms. J Clin Microbiol 1:434–439, 1975

17. DAROUGAR S, JONES BR, KINNISON JR, VAUGHN-JACKSON JD, and DUNLOP EMC: Chlamydial infection. Advances in the diagnostic isolation of *Chlamydia*, including TRIC agent from the eye, genital tract and rectum. Br J Vener Dis 48:416–420, 1972

18. DAROUGAR SJ, KINNISON R, and JONES BR: Simplified irradiated McCoy cell culture for isolation of chlamydiae *In* Trachoma and Related Disorders Caused by Chlamydial Agents, Nichols RL (ed), Excerpta Medica, Amsterdam, 1971, pp 63–70

19. DAROUGAR S and JONES BR: Conjunctival swabbing for the isolation of TRIC agent (*Chlamydia*). Br J Ophthalmol 55:585–590, 1971

20. DAWSON CR, DAGHFOUS T, MESSADI M, HOSHIWARA I, and SCHACHTER J: Severe endemic trachoma in Tunisia. Br Ophthalmol 60:245–252, 1976

21. DAWSON CR and SCHACHTER J: TRIC agent infections of the eye and genital tract. Am J Ophthalmol 63:1288–1298, 1967

22. DHIR SP, HAKOMORI S, KENNY GE, and GRAYSTON JT: Immunochemical studies on chlamydial group antigen (presence of a 2-keto-3-deoxycarbohydrate as immunodominant group). J Immunol 109:116–122, 1972

23. DONALDSON P, DAVIS DE, WATKINS JR, and SULKIN SE: The isolation and identification of ornithosis infection in turkeys by tissue culture and immunocytochemical staining. Am J Vet Res 19:950–954, 1958

24. EDDIE B, MEYER KF, LAMBRECHT FL, and FURMAN DP: Isolation of ornithosis bedsoniae from mites collected in turkey quarters and from chicken lice. J Infect Dis 110:231–237, 1962

25. GERLOFF RK, RITTER DB, and WATSON RO: DNA homology between the meningopneumonitis agent and related microorganisms. J Infect Dis 116:197–202, 1966

26. GERLOFF RK and WATSON RO: The radioisotope precipitation test for psittacosis group antibodies. Am J Ophthalmol 63:1492–1498, 1967

27. GERLOFF RK and WATSON RO: A *Chlamydia* from the peritoneal cavity of mice. Infect Immun 1:64–68, 1970

28. GOGOLAK FM: The mouse erythrocyte hemagglutinin of feline pneumonitis virus. J Infect Dis 95:220–225, 1954

29. GORDON FB, HARPER IA, QUAN AL, TREHARNE JD, DWYER R STC, and GARLAND JA: Detection of *Chlamydia* (Bedsonia) in certain infections of man. I. Laboratory procedures: comparison of yolk sac and cell culture for detection and isolation. J Infect Dis 120:451–462, 1969

30. GORDON FB and QUAN AL: Isolation of the trachoma agent in cell culture. Proc Soc Exp Biol Med 118:354–359, 1965
31. GRAYSTON JT and WANG S-P: New knowledge of chlamydiae and the diseases they cause. J Infect Dis 132:87–105, 1975
32. HALBERSTAEDTER L and VON PROWAZEK S: Zur atiologie des trachoms. Dtsch Med Wochenschr 33:1285–1287, 1907
33. HANNA L: An evaluation of the fluorescent antibody technic in the diagnosis of trachoma and inclusion conjunctivitis. Rev Int Trach 4:345–359, 1968
34. HANNA L, JAWETZ E, BRIONES OC, KESHISHYAN H, HOSHIWARA I, OSTLER HB, and DAWSON CR: Antibodies to TRIC agents in tears and serum of naturally infected humans. J Infect Dis 127:95–98, 1973
35. HANNA L, JAWETZ E, NABLI B, HOSHIWARA I, OSTLER B, and DAWSON C: Titration and typing of serum antibodies in TRIC infections by immunofluorescence. J Immunol 108:102–107, 1972
36. HARNISCH JP, ALEXANDER ER, BERGER RE, MONDA G, and HOLMES KK: Aetiology of acute epididymitis. Lancet 1:819–821, 1977
37. HARRISON MJ: Enhancing effect of DEAE-dextran on inclusion counts of an ovine *Chlamydia (Bedsonia)* in cell culture. Aust J Exp Biol Med Sci 48:207–213, 1970
38. HARRISON MJ: Conditions for growth of an ovine *Chlamydia (Bedsonia)* in cell culture. Aust J Exp Biol Med Sci 50:447–466, 1972
39. HATCH TP: Competition between *Chlamydia psittaci* and L cells for host isoleucine pools. A limiting factor in chlamydial multiplication. Infect Immun 12:211–220, 1975
40. HIGASHI N and TAMURA A: A plaque assay for meningopneumonitis virus in monolayers of strain L cells. Virology 12:578–588, 1960
41. HILLEMAN MR, HAIG DA, and HELMOLD RJ: The indirect complement fixation, hemagglutination and conglutinating complement absorption tests for viruses of the psittacosis-lymphogranuloma venereum group. J Immunol 66:115–130, 1951
42. HOLMES KK, HANDSFIELD HH, WANG S-P, WENTWORTH BB, TURCK M, ANDERSON JB, and ALEXANDER ER: Etiology of nongonococcal urethritis. N Engl J Med 292:1199–1206, 1975
43. JONES BR: Ocular syndromes of TRIC virus infection and their possible genital significance. Br J Vener Dis 40:3–18, 1964
44. JONES BR: Laboratory tests for chlamydial infection. Their role in epidemiological studies of trachoma and its control. Br J Opthalmol 58:438–454, 1974
45. JONES BR: Prevention of blindness from trachoma. Trans Ophthalmol Soc UK 95:16–33, 1975
46. JONES BR and TREHARNE JD: Micro-immunofluorescence type-specific serological tests for chlamydial infection applied to psittacosis, ornithosis, lymphogranuloma venereum, trachoma, paratrachoma and 'nonspecific' urethritis. Proc R Soc Med 67:735–736, 1974
47. KARRER H, MEYER KF, and EDDIE B: The complement fixation inhibition test and its application to the diagnosis of ornithosis in chickens and in ducks I. Principles and technique of the test. J Infect Dis 87:13–23, 1950
48. KINGSBURY DT and WEISS E: Lack of deoxyribonucleic acid homology between species of the genus *Chlamydia*. J Bacteriol 96:1421–1423, 1968
49. KUO C-C, WANG S-P, and GRAYSTON JT: Effect of polycations, polyanions and neuraminidase on the infectivity of trachoma-inclusion conjunctivitis and lymphogranuloma venereum organisms in HeLa cells. Sialic acid residues as possible receptors for trachoma-inclusion conjunctivitis. Infect Immun 8:74–79, 1973
50. KUO C-C, WANG S-P, WENTWORTH BB, and GRAYSTON JT: Primary isolation of TRIC organisms in HeLa 229 cells treated with DEAE-dextran. J Infect Dis 125:665–668, 1972
51. LEWIS VJ and THACKER WL: Susceptibility of McCoy cells to infection by *Chlamydia psittaci*. Can J Microbiol 19:617–621, 1973
52. LEWIS VJ, THACKER WL, and CACCIAPUOTI AF: Detection of *Chlamydia psittaci* by immunofluorescence. Appl Microbiol 24:8–12, 1972
53. LEWIS VJ, THACKER WL, and ENGELMAN HM: Indirect hemagglutination test for chlamydial antibodies. Appl Microbiol 24:22–25, 1972
54. LINDNER K: Gonoblennorrhöe, Einschlussblennorrhoe, und trachoma. Graefe's Arch Ophthalmol 78:380, 1911

55. Manire GP and Meyer KF: The toxins of the psittacosis-lymphogranuloma group of agents III. Differentiation of strains by the toxin neutralization test. J Infect Dis 86:241–250, 1950

56. Manire GP and Tamura A: Preparation and chemical composition of the cell walls of mature infectious dense forms of meningopneumonitis organisms. J Bacteriol 94:1178–1183, 1967

57. Mardh P-A, Ripa T, Svensson L, and Weström L: *Chlamydia trachomatis* infection in patients with acute salpingitis. N Engl J Med 296:1377–1379, 1977

58. McComb DE and Nichols RL: Antibodies to trachoma in eye secretions of Saudi Arab children. Am J Epidemiol 90:278–284, 1969

59. McComb DE, Nichols RL, Semine DZ, Evrard JR, Alpert S, Crockett VA, Rosner B, Zinner SH, and McCormack NM: Antibody to *Chlamydia* in the genital secretions of women as an indicator of infection. Presented at the Sixteenth Interscience Conference on Antimicrobial Agents and Chemotherapy, Chicago, October 29, 1976

60. Meyer KF: Ornithosis *In* Diseases of Poultry, 5th edition, Biester HE and Schwarte LH (eds), The Iowa State University Press, Ames, Iowa, 1965, pp 675–770

61. Meyer KF: The host spectrum of psittacosis-lymphogranuloma venereum (PL) agents. Am J Ophthalmol 63:1225–1246, 1967

62. Meyer KF and Eddie B: Human pneumonitis viruses and their classification. Arch Gesamte Virusforsch 4:579–590, 1952

63. Meyer KF and Eddie B: The influence of tetracycline compounds on the development of antibodies in psittacosis. Am Rev Tuberc Pulm Dis 74:566–571, 1956

64. Mordhorst CH: Studies on oculogenital TRIC agents isolated in Denmark. Am J Ophthalmol 63:1282–1288, 1967

65. Mordhorst CH and Dawson C: Sequelae of neonatal inclusion conjunctivitis and associated disease in parents. Am J Ophthalmol 71:861–867, 1971

66. Morrison SJ and Jenkin HM: Growth of *Chlamydia psittaci* strain meningopneumonitis in mouse L cells cultivated in a defined medium in spinner cultures. In Vitro 8:94–100, 1972

67. Moulder JW: The Psittacosis Group as Bacteria (CIBA Lectures in Microbial Biochemistry, 1963, Wiley, New York, 1964

68. Moulder JW: The relation of the psittacosis group (*Chlamydiae*) to bacteria and viruses. Annu Rev Microbiol 20:107–130, 1966

69. Murray ES: Guinea pig inclusion conjunctivitis virus. I. Isolation and identification as a member of the psittacosis-lymphogranuloma-trachoma group. J Infect Dis 114:1–12, 1964

70. Nichols RL, Bobb AA, Haddad NA, and McComb DE: Immunofluorescent studies of the microbiologic epidemiology of trachoma in Saudi Arabia. Am J Ophthalmol 63:1372–1408, 1967

71. Nichols RL, McComb DE, Haddad NA, and Murray ES: Studies on trachoma. II. Comparison of fluorescent antibody, Giemsa, and egg isolation methods for detection of trachoma virus in human conjunctival scrapings. Am J Trop Med Hyg 12:223–229, 1963

72. Nigg C and Eaton MD: Isolation from normal mice of a pneumotropic virus which forms elementary bodies. J Exp Med 79:497–510, 1944

73. Officer JE and Brown A: Growth of psittacosis virus in tissue culture. J Infect Dis 107:283–299, 1960

74. Oriel JD, Reeve P, Thomas BJ, and Nicol CS: Infection with *Chlamydia* group A in men with urethritis due to *Neisseria gonorrhoeae*. J Infect Dis 131:376–382, 1975

75. Page LA: Comparison of "pathotypes" among chlamydial (psittacosis) strains recovered from diseased birds and mammals. Bull Wildl Dis Assoc 3:166–175, 1967

76. Page LA: Application of an agar gel precipitin test to the serodiagnosis of avian chlamydiosis. Proceedings from the Seventeenth Annual American Association of Veterinary Laboratory Diagnostician Meeting, Roanoke, Virginia, October 15, 1974, pp 51–61

77. Page LA: Order II. Chlamydiales storz and page 1971. Part 18. The Rickettsias, *In* Bergey's Manual of Determinative Bacteriology, 8th edition, Buchanan RE and Gibbons NE (eds), Williams and Wilkins, Baltimore, 1974, pp 914–928

78. PAGE LA, DERIEUX WT, and CUTLIP RC: An epornitic of fatal chlamydiosis (ornithosis) in South Carolina turkeys. J Am Vet Med Assoc 166:175–178, 1975

79. PAGE LA and ERICKSON K: Serologic evidence of natural and experimental transfers of *Chlamydia psittaci* between wild and domestic animals. Proceedings of the Annual Conference, Bull Wildl Dis Assoc 5:284–290, 1969

80. PEARSON JW, DUFF JT, GEARINGER NF, and ROBBINS ML: Growth characteristics of three agents of the psittacosis group in human diploid cell cultures. J Infect Dis 115:49–58, 1965

81. PHILIP RN, CASPER EA, GORDON FB, and QUAN AL: Fluorescent antibody responses to chlamydial infections in patients with lymphogranuloma venereum and urethritis. J Immunol 112:2126–2134, 1974

82. PIRAINO F and ABEL C: Plaque assay for psittacosis virus in monolayers of chick embryo fibroblasts. J Bacteriol 87:1503–1511, 1964

83. REEVE P, GERLOFF RK, CASPER E, PHILIP RN, ORIEL JD, and POWIS PA: Serological studies on the role of *Chlamydia* in the aetiology of non-specific urethritis. Br J Vener Dis 50:136–139, 1974

84. REEVE P and TAVERNE J: Some properties of the complement-fixing antigens of the agents of trachoma and inclusion blennorrhoea and the relationship of the antigens to the developmental cycle. J Gen Microbiol 27:501–508, 1962

85. RICE CE: Carbohydrate matrix of epithelial-cell inclusion in trachoma. Am J Ophthalmol 19:1–8, 1936

86. RICHMOND SJ, HILTON AL, and CLARKE SKR: Chlamydial infection. Role of *Chlamydia* subgroup A in non-gonococcal and post-gonococcal urethritis. Br J Vener Dis 48:437–444, 1972

87. RICHMOND SJ and SPARLING PF: Genital chlamydial infections. Am J Epidemiol 103:428–435, 1976

88. RIPA KT and MARDH P-A: New simplified culture technique for *Chlamydia trachomatis In* Non-Gonococcal Urethritis and Related Infections, Holmes KK and Hobson D (eds), Am Soc Microbiol, Washington, D.C., 1977, pp 323–327

89. ROBERTS W, GRIST NR, and GIROUD P: Human abortion associated with infection by ovine abortion agent. Br Med J 4:37–39, 1967

90. ROSS MR and JENKIN HM: Cell wall antigens from members of the psittacosis group of organisms. Ann NY Acad Sci 98:329–336, 1962

91. ROTA TR and NICHOLS RL: Infection of cell cultures by trachoma agent: enhancement by DEAE-dextran. J Infect Dis 124:419–421, 1971

92. ROTA TR and NICHOLS RL: *Chlamydia trachomatis* in cell culture. I. Comparison of efficiencies of infection in several chemically defined media, at various pH and temperature values, and after exposure to diethylaminoethyl-dextran. Appl Micribiol 26:560–565, 1973

93. SCHACHTER J: Recommended criteria for the identification of trachoma and inclusion conjunctivitis agents. J Infect Dis 122:105–107, 1970

94. SCHACHTER J: Chlamydiae *In* Manual of Clinical Immunology, Am Soc for Microbiol, Washington, DC, pp 494–499, 1976

95. SCHACHTER J, BANKS J, SUGG N, SUNG M, STORZ J, and MEYER KF: Serotyping of *Chlamydia*: isolates of bovine origin. Infect Immun 11:904–907, 1975

96. SCHACHTER J, CAUSSE G, and TARIZZO ML: Chlamydiae as agents of sexually transmitted diseases. Bull WHO 54:245–254, 1976

97. SCHACHTER J and DAWSON CR: Human Chlamydial Infections, Publishing Sciences Group, Inc. Littleton, MA, 1978

98. SCHACHTER J, DAWSON CR, BALAS S, and JONES P: Evaluation of laboratory methods for detecting acute TRIC agent infection. Am J Ophthalmol 70:375–380, 1970

99. SCHACHTER J, HANNA L, HILL EC, MASSAD S, SHEPPARD CW, CONTE JE JR, COHEN SN, and MEYER KF: Are chlamydial infections the most prevalent venereal disease? J Am Med Assoc 231:1252–1255, 1975

100. SCHACHTER J, HANNA L, TARIZZO ML, and DAWSON CR: Relative efficacy of different methods of laboratory diagnosis in chronic trachoma in the United States *In* Trachoma and Related Disorders Caused by Chlamydial Agents, Nichols RL, (ed), Excerpta Medica, Amsterdam, 1971, pp 469–475

101. SCHACHTER J, HILL EC, KING EB, COLEMAN VR, JONES P, and MEYER KF: Chlamydial infection in women with cervical dysplasia. Am J Obstet Gynecol 123:753–757, 1975

102. SCHACHTER J, LUM L, GOODING CA, and OSTLER B: Pneumonitis following inclusion blennorrhea. J Pediatr 87:779–780, 1975

103. SCHACHTER J and MEYER KF: Lymphogranuloma venereum II. Characterization of some recently isolated strains. J Bacteriol 99:636–638, 1969

104. SCHACHTER J, MORDHORST CH, MOORE BW, and TARIZZO ML: Laboratory diagnosis of trachoma. A collaborative study. Bull WHO 48:509–515, 1973

105. SCHACHTER J, OSTLER HB, and MEYER KF: Human infection with the agent of feline pneumonitis. Lancet 1:1063–1065, 1969

106. SCHACHTER J, ROSE L, DAWSON CR, and BARNES M: Comparison of procedures for laboratory diagnosis of oculogenital infections with inclusion conjunctivitis agents. Am J Epidemiol 85:453–458, 1967

107. SCHACHTER J, ROSE L, and MEYER KF: The venereal nature of inclusion conjunctivitis. Am J Epidemiol 85:445–452, 1967

108. SCHACHTER J, SMITH DE, DAWSON CR, ANDERSON WR, DELLER JJ JR, HOKE AW, SMARTT WH, and MEYER KF: Lymphogranuloma venereum. I. Comparison of Frei test, complement fixation test, and isolation of the agent. J Infect Dis 120:372–375, 1969

109. SCHACHTER J, SUGG N, and SUNG M: Psittacosis—the reservoir persists. J Infect Dis 137:44–49, 1978

110. SCHECHTER EM: Synthesis of nucleic acid and protein in L cells infected with the agent of meningopneumonitis. J Bacteriol 91:2069–2080, 1966

111. SHIMIZU Y and BANKOWSKI RA: The nature of the cross-reactions between a bacterium of the genus *Herellea* and the ornithosis virus in complement fixation. Am J Vet Res 24:1283–1290, 1963

112. SIGEL MM: *Lymphogranuloma venereum*. Epidemiological, Clinical, Surgical and Therapeutic Aspects Based on a Study in the Caribbean, The Univ Miami Press, Coral Gables, FL, 1962, pp 21–29

113. STORZ J: *Chlamydia* and *Chlamydia*-Induced Diseases, Charles C. Thomas, Springfield, Ill, 1971, pp 5–358

114. STORZ J and PAGE LA: Taxonomy of the chlamydiae. Reasons for classifying organisms of the genus *Chlamydia*, family *Chlamydiaceae*, in a separate order, *Chlamydiales* ord nov. Int J Sys Bacteriol 21:332–334, 1971

115. STORZ J, SHUPE JL, MARRIOTT ME, and THORNLEY WR: Polyarthritis of lambs induced experimentally by a psittacosis agent. J Infect Dis 115:9–18, 1965

116. T'ANG F-F, CHANG H-L, HUANG Y-T, and WANG K-C: Trachoma virus in chick embryo. Natl Med J China 43:81–86, 1957

117. THOMAS BJ, REEVE P, ORIEL JD: Simplified serological test for antibodies to chlamydia trachomatis. J Clin Microbiol 4:6–10, 1976

118. VOLKERT M and CHRISTENSEN PM: Two ornithosis complement-fixing antigens from infected yolk sacs. Acta Path Microbiol Scand 37:211–218, 1955

119. VOLKERT M and MATTHIESEN M: An ornithosis related antigen from a coccoid bacterium. Acta Path Microbiol Scand 39:117–126, 1956

120. WALL MJ: Isolation of the virus of lymphogranuloma venereum from twenty-eight patients. Relative value of the use of chick embryos and mice. J Immunol 54:59–64, 1946

121. WANG S-P and GRAYSTON JT: Immunologic relationship between genital, TRIC, lymphogranuloma venereum, and related organisms in a new microtiter indirect immunofluorescence test. Am J Ophthalmol 70:367–374, 1970

122. WANG S-P and GRAYSTON JT: Studies on the identity of the 'fast' egg-killing chlamydia strains *In* Trachoma and Related Disorders Caused by Chlamydial Agents, Nichols RL (ed), Excerpta Medica, Amsterdam, 1971, pp 322–336

123. WANG S-P and GRAYSTON JT: Human serology in *Chlamydia trachomatis* infection with microimmunofluorescence. J Infect Dis 130:388–397, 1974

124. WANG S-P, GRAYSTON JT, ALEXANDER ER, and HOLMES KK: A simplified microimmunofluorescence test with trachoma-lymphogranuloma venereum (*Chlamydia trachomatis*) antigens for use as a screening test for antibody. J Clin Microbiol 1:250–255, 1975

125. WEISS E and DRESSLER HR: Centrifugation of rickettsiae and viruses onto cells and its effect on infection. Proc Soc Exp Biol Med 103:691–695, 1960
126. WENTWORTH BB and ALEXANDER ER: Isolation of *Chlamydia trachomatis* by use of 5-iodo-2-deoxyuridine-treated cells. Appl Microbiol 27:912–916, 1974
127. YONEDA C, DAWSON CR, DAGHFOUS T, HOSHIWARA I, JONES P, MESSADI M, and SCHACHTER J: Cytology as a guide to the presence of chlamydial inclusions in Giemsa-stained conjunctival smears in severe endemic trachoma. Br J Ophthalmol 59:116–124, 1975

CHAPTER 33

THE RICKETTSIAE

Bennett L. Elisberg and F. Marilyn Bozeman

Introduction

The etiologic agents of the rickettsial diseases of humans constitute a biologically distinctive group of microorganisms within the family *Rickettsiaceae*. A listing of the diseases, the etiologic agents, taxonomic classification, and other pertinent ecologic information is presented in Table 33.1. Based upon similarities of antigenic composition and other common attributes, the human pathogens included within the tribe Rickettsieae are classified into three different genera. Within the genus *Rickettsia* are three biotypes: the Typhus Group, the Spotted Fever Group, and the Scrub Typhus Group. The newly created genus *Rochalimaea* includes the agent of trench fever, and the agent of Q fever is within the genus *Coxiella* (25).

All of the causative agents have in common an association with certain arthropods and, with the exception of epidemic typhus and trench fever, all have well-documented infection cycles in nature that involve vertebrate hosts other than humans. Endemicity of the diseases is maintained by the cyclic transmissions of the rickettsial agents from infected arthropod to uninfected arthropod through the medium of a vertebrate reservoir. Transovarial transmission in the tick- and miteborne rickettsioses is an additional important mechanism for perpetuation of rickettsial species. Recently, epidemic typhus rickettsiae were isolated from flying squirrels (*Glaucomys volans volans*) trapped in the eastern United States (33), and the organism isolated from Canadian voles (*Microtus pennsylvanicus*) in 1943 (11) has been shown to be a strain of *Rochalimaea quintana,* the etiologic agent of trench fever (225). Until the public health implications of these findings have been determined, in epidemic typhus and trench fever the human body louse is considered to be the most important vector, and humans, its preferred host, the reservoir of the infection. For Q fever the important reservoirs are cattle, sheep, and goats, and transmission of *Coxiella burnetii* among these domestic animals occurs independently of tick vectors.

Illness develops in humans usually as the result of an accidental encounter with an infected arthropod or, as is the case with Q fever, principally by inhalation of an infectious aerosol. Infection in the tick- and miteborne rickettsioses occurs by direct inoculation through the mouth parts of the arthro-

TABLE 33.1—RICKETTSIAL DISEASES OF HUMANS

BIOTYPE	ETIOLOGIC AGENT*	DISEASES AND SYNONYMS	TRANSMISSION TO HUMANS	INCU-BATION (DAYS)	GEOGRAPHIC DISTRIBUTION	NATURAL INFECTION CYCLE	
						ARTHROPOD VECTOR	VERTEBRATE HOST
TYPHUS GROUP	*Rickettsia prowazekii*	Epidemic typhus, louse-borne typhus, exanthematous typhus	Infected louse feces into broken skin or inhaled	6–15	Worldwide except Australia	Body louse, squirrel louse, and flea	Humans; flying squirrel (USA)
	R. prowazekii	Brill-Zinsser disease, sporadic typhus, recrudescent typhus	Reactivation of latent infection years after primary epidemic typhus		Worldwide	—	
	R. typhi	Murine typhus, endemic typhus, urban typhus, shop typhus, flea-borne typhus	Infected flea feces into broken skin	6–14	Worldwide	Rat flea	Commensal rats
SPOTTED FEVER GROUP	*R. rickettsii*	Rocky Mountain spotted fever, fiebre manchada, Sao Paulo typhus, tobia fever	Tick bite	3–12	Western Hemisphere	Tick	Small and medium-sized wild mammals, birds, dogs
	R. conorii	Boutonneuse fever, Marseilles fever, South African tickbite fever, Kenya tick typhus, Indian tick typhus	Tick bite	5–7	Mediterranean countries, Africa, India	Tick	Small wild animals, dogs

BIOTYPE	ETIOLOGIC AGENT*	DISEASES AND SYNONYMS	TRANSMISSION TO HUMANS	INCUBATION (DAYS)	GEOGRAPHIC DISTRIBUTION	NATURAL INFECTION CYCLE	
						ARTHROPOD VECTOR	VETEBRATE HOST
	R. australis	Queensland tick typhus	Tick bite	7–10	Australia	Tick	Small wild rodents, marsupials
	R. sibirica	Siberian tick typhus, North Asian Tick-borne rickettsiosis	Tick bite	2–7	Siberia, Mongolia	Tick	Wild and domestic animals, birds
	R. akari	Rickettsialpox, vesicular rickettsiosis	Mite bite	7–10	Northeast USA, USSR	Gamasid mite	House mouse
SCRUB TYPHUS GROUP	*R. tsutsugamushi*	Scrub typhus, tsutsugamushi disease, mite-borne typhus, tropical typhus, rural typhus	Chigger bite	6–21	Asia, Australia Pacific Islands	Trombiculid mite	Small wild rodents, birds
TRENCH FEVER	*Rochalimaea quintana*	Trench fever, Wolhynian fever, five-day fever	Infected louse feces into broken skin	9–17	Europe, Middle East, North Africa, Mexico	Body louse	Humans
Q FEVER	*Coxiella burnetii*	Q fever, Balkan grippe	Inhalation of infected aerosol	7–17	Worldwide	Tick	Small wild mammals
						Cattle, sheep, goats without arthropod vector	

*Order, Rickettsiales; Family, *Rickettsiaceae*; Tribe, Rickettsieae pod at the time of feeding. With louse- and fleaborne diseases, infection results when the arthropod's feces containing the rickettsiae are rubbed or scratched into abraded skin or into the conjunctiva.

After a variable incubation period, the diseases usually begin suddenly with fever and severe headache. At the time of onset of illness, a primary lesion or eschar may be evident at the site of the bite in scrub typhus, and in all of the Spotted Fever Group infections except Rocky Mountain spotted fever. Although the basic pathologic lesion in rickettsial infection is a diffuse endangiitis, there are important differences in the clinical manifestations and severity of the diseases that are dependent on the distribution and extent of the vascular involvement. A characteristic cutaneous eruption is seen in all rickettsial diseases, except Q fever. Maculopapular eruptions are evident in murine typhus and scrub typhus; a vesicular rash is seen in rickettsialpox; and in epidemic typhus, Rocky Mountain spotted fever, and other tickborne Spotted Fever Group infections, the skin lesions are usually petechial or frankly hemorrhagic. The rash in tickborne Spotted Fever Group infections appears first on the extremities and spreads to the trunk, whereas the reverse is generally true in epidemic, murine, and scrub typhus. About 50% of Q fever patients have signs and symptoms of primary atypical pneumonia, and the remainder manifest only fever with few other distinguishing features. Rarely, in Q fever chronic infection in the form of a subacute rickettsial endocarditis or granulomatous liver disease may develop. Recrudescence of an epidemic typhus infection may occur after a prolonged period of latency, thereby causing Brill-Zinsser disease. The clinical manifestations of the classical rickettsial diseases, when present, are sufficiently distinctive to permit the physician to differentiate them from viral, bacterial, and other infectious diseases endemic in the same geographic region. However, in the majority of the cases of suspected rickettsial disease, it is an understanding of the basic ecology and epidemiology of the diseases and a history of known or possible exposure to infected arthropods that lead to a correct clinical diagnosis (72).

Epidemic typhus, Rocky Mountain spotted fever, and scrub typhus are among the most severe infectious diseases, and mortality rates in untreated cases have ranged from 20% to 40%. In order of decreasing severity, the remaining rickettsial infections follow: the tick typhuses, murine typhus, Q fever, rickettsialpox, and trench fever. The last three illnesses have virtually no mortality in uncomplicated cases. All rickettsial infections respond dramatically to adequate treatment with tetracycline antibiotics or chloramphenicol supplemented with intensive supportive measures.

Infectious Agents

General characteristics

Species of *Rickettsia* are rod-shaped, ellipsoidal, coccoid, diplococcoid, or occasionally filamentous microorganisms about 0.3–0.6 μm in diameter and 0.8–2.0 μm in length. They give a gram-negative staining reaction. *C.*

burnetii, a gram-positive species (87), is somewhat smaller in size, and some forms are capable of passing through filters that retain other rickettsiae (66, 126). Although there are definite differences in the morphologic appearance of the various species, these features are rarely of value in their identification. Recent electron microscopic examinations of ultrathin sections have revealed additional structural resemblances to gram-negative bacteria.

In most electron micrographs of rickettsiae, a trilaminar cell wall and an underlying trilaminar plasma membrane are seen, but with better resolution a 5-layered cell wall has been demonstrated. Internally, ribosomes and deoxyribonucleic acid (DNA) strands are evident, but a well-defined nuclear area is rarely seen. A superficial, external, capsule-like layer has been observed in some species (5, 6, 104, 150, 161, 162, 196). The known similarities of *Rickettsieae* to bacteria follow: a) both divide by binary fission (184); b) both contain ribonucleic acid (RNA) and DNA (2) and the size of the genome has been estimated at 1.5×10^6 nucleotide pairs, which is comparable to that of other microorganisms of similar size (117); c) the cell walls of rickettsiae contain muramic acid, an essential component of mucopeptide characteristically found in the cell walls of all bacteria studied (165); d) diaminopimelic acid, limited to the mucopeptide of all bacteria except gram-positive cocci, has been demonstrated also in 4 rickettsial species studied (148); e) both exhibit endotoxic activity (9, 47, 236). Chemical analyses of purified rickettsial suspensions and cell walls derived from them have demonstrated carbohydrate, protein, and lipid components and complexes resembling the composition of gram-negative bacteria (26, 185, 248). Small but distinct differences in the DNA base composition (molar percentages of guanine plus cytosine) have been found that differentiate the biotypes of the *Rickettsieae* (213). All *Rickettsieae* are obligate intracellular parasites with the single exception of *Ro. quintana,* which has been cultivated on a cell-free medium (216). However, numerous enzymatic activities involving several systems have been identified in the intact organisms (82, 223) in a cell-free environment. There are significant differences among the rickettsial species in the ability to utilize glutamate, glutamine, pyruvate, and succinate, and characterization of the metabolic activities may provide information on the phylogeny of these microorganisms (228). Rickettsiae cultivated in cell cultures (99, 124) and inoculated intravenously into experimental animals induce interferon, but the microorganisms are relatively insensitive to its action both *in vitro* and *in vivo* (110). Viable *Rickettsia prowazekii* and *R. typhi* lyse the erythrocytes (RBC) of several species of mammals (202), and the mechanism of adsorption and the nature of the receptor site on the cell membrane has been described (177–179, 233, 234). More details about the characteristics of rickettsiae can be found in recent review articles (156, 223).

The organisms within the genus *Rickettsia* are relatively labile and are readily inactivated in the laboratory by unfavorable conditions. They are killed quickly by 8% formaldehyde, 1% phenol, sodium hypochlorite (50–500 ppm available chlorine) disinfectants, 70% ethyl alcohol, and ultraviolet irradiation. At temperatures of 56 C or above, viability is lost within 30 min.

Infectivity titers of suspensions of rickettsiae in buffered physiologic saline solution decline rapidly after several hours at room temperature and after 24 hr at 0–4 C. The optimal pH for survival is about 7, but little difference is noted over the range 6.5–7.4. On the other hand, *C. burnetii* is considerably more resistant to physical and chemical agents. For example, the organism will tolerate 1% formalin for 24 hr and heating to 63 C for 30 min (180) and has survived in dried tick feces at room temperature for at least 586 days (166). Its ability to withstand desiccation, heat, and exposure to ultraviolet irradiation plays an important role in the ecology and epidemiology of Q fever.

Many different types of media have been recommended from time to time for use as diluents to preserve the biological activity of different species of rickettsiae during isolation attempts, preparation of seed suspensions, purification procedures, and measurement of infectivity and toxicity titers, as well as for studies of metabolic activities. Sucrose PG diluent containing sucrose, high potassium ion concentration, and glutamate, which has been used widely, generally preserves infectivity titers of rickettsial suspensions for several hours at room temperature and for almost a week at 0–4 C and protects against inactivation caused by freezing and thawing (28). The formula for this solution is as follows:

Sucrose PG Diluent (Snyder II)

Sucrose	0.218 M
KH_2PO_4	0.0376 M
K_2HPO_4	0.0071 M
Potassium glutamate	0.0049 M

Sterilize by autoclaving for 20 min at 10–12 lb pressure. Final pH should be 7. If L-glutamic acid is used instead of potassium glutamate, adjust pH with 10 N KOH.

Owing to the high potassium content, this diluent may be toxic for small animals, particularly if given intravenously; when animal inoculations are contemplated, Snyder I solution (107) should be used. This is an earlier version of sucrose PG solution and is identical except that Na_2HPO_4 (0.0086 M) is substituted for K_2HPO_4 and, when L-glutamic acid is used, the pH is adjusted with 10 N NaOH. The protective capacity of both sucrose PG and Snyder I diluents can be enhanced by the incorporation of bovine serum albumin to give a final concentration of 1%.

Recently, the relative effectiveness of sucrose PG and other types of diluents in maintaining rickettsial infectivity was reassessed with use of a plaque assay system. Seed suspensions of selected members of the Typhus and Spotted Fever Groups diluted in brain-heart infusion broth gave consistently higher plaque titers than with the other diluents (231, 232).

Infectivity of rickettsial suspensions in sucrose PG diluent is maintained for long periods by storage at temperatures of −65 C or below. However, such material should be frozen rapidly, in a dry ice-alcohol bath prior to storage and thawed quickly at 35–37 C at the time of use. Manifold lyophilization of suspensions in ampules at room temperature has not been a wholly satisfactory means of preservation. The freeze-drying process results in at least 100-fold loss in infectivity, but in the dried state the residual activity remains unchanged for at least 1 year.

Classification and antigenic composition

Typhus and Spotted Fever Group rickettsiae. In addition to the rickettsiae in the Typhus and Spotted Fever Groups responsible for human illnesses, other antigenically related rickettsial agents have been isolated from arthropods or rodents but are not known to produce disease (Table 33.2). The Typhus Group comprises *R. prowazekii,* the etiologic agent of both epidemic typhus and Brill-Zinsser disease; *R. typhi,* the cause of murine typhus; and *R. canada.* The last-mentioned was recovered from *Haemaphysalis leporispalustris* ticks removed from indicator rabbits in the vicinity of Richmond, Ontario, Canada (140). Although serologic evidence of presumed infection of humans has been reported (31), information on the geographic distribution, the natural infection cycle, and direct causal relationship to human disease is not yet available. Strain Madrid E (52), which has been under evaluation for use as an attenuated living vaccine (81), is a variant of *R. prowazekii* with reduced virulence but immunologically unaltered.

The Spotted Fever Group currently includes 10 different species, 5 of which are not known to cause disease in man: *R. parkeri,* previously known as Maculatum agent and originally isolated from *Amblyomma maculatum* ticks (163); avirulent rickettsiae including *R. montana,* isolated from ticks from eastern Montana (16), and the Western Montana U strain (175); and the JC-880 and TT-118 strains isolated from ticks collected in West Pakistan and Thailand, respectively (182) (see Table 33.2). The Spotted Fever Group agents can be divided into 5 subgroups on the basis of immunologic differences (130, 182). Recently, other strains of Spotted Fever Group rickettsiae have been isolated from patients and from *Rhipicephalus sanguineus* ticks in Israel (92) and from *Rh. sanguineus* ticks in the United States (44); these rickettsiae show some antigenic differences from selected established members of the biotype. Further studies are required to determine if they are sufficiently distinctive to be considered new species.

Classification into either the Typhus or Spotted Fever Group is based upon group-specific, soluble, complement-fixing antigens that are released from the rickettsiae during treatment with diethyl ether. These antigens are common to all species in the respective biotypes. Heating Typhus and Spotted Fever Group organisms in an alkaline solution releases an erythrocyte-sensitizing substance (ESS) which is readily adsorbed onto sheep or human group O RBC and exhibits group-specific serologic reactivity (48–50). The ESS does not react in the complement fixation (CF) or precipitation test; furthermore, it appears to differ from the antigens responsible for the Weil-Felix reaction. Members of the Typhus and Spotted Fever Groups share common antigens with certain *Proteus* bacilli. Epidemic and murine typhus infections evoke *Proteus* OX_{19} agglutinins in humans and responsive animals, and infections with the human pathogens of the Spotted Fever Group, with the exception of *R. akari,* elicit agglutinins for *Proteus* OX_{19} or *Proteus* OX_2, or both.

TABLE 33.2—CLASSIFICATION AND ANTIGENIC COMPOSITION OF *RICKETTSIEAE*

BIOTYPE AND SUBGROUP	SPECIES*	IMMUNO-TYPES (NUMBER)	SOLUBLE COMPLEMENT FIXING (CF)	ERYTHOCYTE-SENSITIZING SUBSTANCE	CF	CORPUSCULAR MICRO-IF	CORPUSCULAR AGGLUTINATION	TOXIN	WEIL-FELIX PROTEUS AGGLUTININ
TYPHUS GROUP	*Rickettsia prowazekii*	1§	GS*	GS	SS†	SS	SS	SS	OX$_{19}$
	R. typhi	1	GS	GS	SS	SS	SS	SS	OX$_{19}$
A	*R. canada*	1	GS	ND	SS	SS	SS	SS	ND
A	*R. rickettsii*	1	GS	GS	SS	SS	ND	SS	OX$_{19}$ or OX$_2$
A	*R. sibirica*	1	GS	ND	SS	SS	SS	SS	OX$_{19}$ or OX$_2$
A	*R. conorii*	1	GS	GS	SS	SS	ND	SS	OX$_{19}$ or OX$_2$
SPOTTED FEVER GROUP B	*R. parkeri*	1	GS	ND	SS	SS	SS	SS	ND
C	*R. akari*	1	GS	GS	SS	SS	SS	None	None
C	*R. australis*	1	GS	ND	SS	ND	ND	None	OX$_{19}$ or OX$_2$
D	*R. montana*	1	GS	ND	SS	ND	ND	None	ND
D	Western Montana U	1	GS	ND	SS	ND	ND	None	ND
E	Pakistan JC-880	1	GS	ND	ND	ND	ND	SS	ND
E	Thai TT-118	1	GS	ND	ND	ND	ND	SS	ND
SCRUB TYPHUS GROUP	*R. tsutsugamushi*	At least 8	SS	None	SS	SS	ND	3 strains only	OXK
TRENCH FEVER	*Rochalimaea quintana*	Unknown	SS	None	SS	ND	ND	None	None
Q FEVER	*Coxiella burnetii*	2 phases	None	None	SS	SS	ND	None	None

*Group specific.
†Species specific.
§Strain Madrid E is a variant with reduced virulence but is immunologically unaltered.
ND=Not done.

There are minor antigenic relationships between the Typhus and Spotted Fever Group rickettsiae that are indicated by similarities of the Weil-Felix *Proteus* OX_{19} antibody response and by a certain degree of cross-reactivity between soluble CF antigens and preparations of ESS. Animals infected with epidemic and murine typhus occasionally will exhibit minimal immunity against infection with spotted fever strains but not *vice versa*. However, when cross-reactions are encountered, great differences in the magnitude of the respective reactions distinguish homologous from inter-group reactivity.

Species within the Typhus and Spotted Fever Groups can be differentiated by CF and agglutination tests employing suspensions of washed, highly purified rickettsial organisms as antigens, as well as by indirect immunofluorescence. Polyacrylamide gel electrophoresis (153, 214) and radionuclide-labeling techniques (71) have been used recently to begin to define more critically the nature and source of the soluble group-specific antigen, as well as other subcellular protein fractions of selected members of the Typhus and Spotted Fever Groups. Isoelectric focusing and analysis of specific enzymatic activities have been used to compare cell-free extracts of strains of *R. prowazekii* of human origin, including the E strain, with those isolated from flying squirrels, as well as with a strain of *R. typhi* (64). Continued development of this technology and its application to rickettsiae can be expected to provide another means for the definitive identification of new strains, and a better understanding of the structural components of the etiologic agents and their immunogenic and biochemical properties.

Highly concentrated suspensions of viable *R. prowazekii* (210), *R. typhi* (85), *R. canada* (140), *R. rickettsii, R. sibirica, R. conorii,* and *R. parkeri* (18, 20), as well as of the JC-880 and TT-118 strains (182), inoculated intravenously into white mice cause death within a few hours. This phenomenon, erroneously attributed to a "toxin," cannot be dissociated from the living rickettsiae. The toxic effect is due to a diffuse alteration in the permeability of capillary endothelium with widespread loss of plasma into the interstitial spaces causing shock and death (151, 220). The toxicity of the rickettsial suspensions can be neutralized specifically by immune serum which serves to differentiate the species immunologically (20, 95, 140, 182). The source of the immune serum is an important consideration because, in humans and 3 species of monkey, serum from certain normal individuals will nonspecifically neutralize the toxicity of *R. typhi* suspensions. In humans, the neutralizing property was associated with β-lipoprotein (17, 18).

Scrub Typhus Group rickettsiae. In contrast to the species of *Rickettsia* in the Typhus Group and Spotted Fever Group, where each is represented by a single immunotype, strains of the Scrub Typhus Group display a marked degree of antigenic heterogeneity. Definitive identification of *R. tsutsugamushi* is dependent upon close intragroup relationships displayed in mouse cross-immunity tests (212, 252); i.e., mice convalescent from infection with one strain resist challenge with heterologous scrub typhus strains. Soluble CF antigens prepared by ether treatment are generally strain-specific in reactivity (22, 23, 211), and the levels of antibody detected are 16- to 64-fold lower than those found with corpuscular antigens. Owing to the fragility of scrub typhus organisms, satisfactory corpuscular antigens cannot be prepared by methods used with other species of rickettsiae. Studies using suspensions of *R. tsutsugamushi* purified partially with a cation exchange resin (123, 191, 250) have demonstrated the presence of strain-specific antigens, as well as common intragroup antigens. On the basis of CF reactivity of the particulate antigens, 3 immunotypes have been recognized in Japan, represented by the Karp, Gilliam, and Kato strains (192). In addition to these scrub typhus immunotypes, 5 others have been identified in Thailand (74). Antigenic analyses of the 8 immunotypes using indirect immunofluorescence suggested that these strains are comprised of a mosaic of different antigens and differ in the relative concentrations of the dominant and minor components (75). The full extent of the antigenic diversity among scrub typhus organisms is not known. An ESS has not been recovered from *R. tsutsugamushi*. The toxic effect of viable rickettsial suspensions for mice can be demonstrated consistently with the Gilliam strain (201), which grows well in embryonated eggs. With the poorer growing Karp and Kato strains, 20–40% suspensions of infected yolk sacs are required (121). As with other species the activity can be specifically neutralized by immune serum. Scrub typhus infection in some patients elicits development of antibodies that will agglutinate suspensions of *Proteus mirabilis* OXK.

Q fever agent. In addition to the innate hardiness of the organism, there are important biologic features of *C. burnetii* that distinguish it from *Rickettsia:* a) it is gram-positive when alcoholic iodine is used as the mordant, b) soluble CF antigen is not released by extraction with ether, c) an ESS is not recovered by treatment with heat and alkali, and d) viable suspensions do not have toxic effects.

Unlike the Typhus, Spotted Fever, and Scrub Typhus Group organisms, which maintain their antigenic integrity irrespective of the host employed for cultivation, Q fever rickettsiae undergo a phase variation similar to the smooth → rough changes observed with *Streptococcus pneumoniae* (205). The changes are host-dependent and are associated with alteration of antigenic structure and serologic reactivity. Strains recovered from naturally infected ticks, wild or domestic animals, and humans are in phase I and remain in this state if propagated in susceptible laboratory animals. However, when phase I organisms are cultivated serially in the yolk sac of embryonated chicken eggs, conversion to phase II occurs gradually after a variable number of passages. Egg-cultivated phase II organisms are transformed back to phase I by passage through susceptible animals. Guinea pigs, irrespective of the phase of the infecting Q fever organism, first develop CF antibodies that react only with phase II antigens. About 4 weeks after infection, antibodies are produced which react with phase I CF antigens. Thus, guinea pig serum collected "early" after infection contains phase II antibodies, while specimens obtained "late" have both phase I and phase II antibodies. The same phenomenon can be demonstrated with phase I and phase II antigens in microagglutination (78) and indirect immunofluorescence tests (89). Minor differences in antigenic composition of strains of *C. burnettii* recovered from different geographic regions have been encountered that are not related to phase variation (206). Owing to the marked stability of *C.*

burnetii, highly purified suspensions of organisms can be prepared readily. Corpuscular phase I antigens are employed in CF and in a variety of agglutination tests. Phase II antigens are used extensively in CF tests, but cannot be used in agglutination tests because of their tendency to agglutinate spontaneously. However, the phase I antigen can be removed from the phase I rickettsiae by extraction with trichloroacetic acid (78) or destroyed with sodium periodate (186) to produce phase II antigens that perform equally well in agglutination and CF tests. With polycationized ferritin as a cytochemical probe, electron microscopic examination showed anionic binding sites on the cell membranes of phase II organisms but not on phase I rickettsiae (129). Ultrasonic disruption of phase I organisms releases a phase I antigenic fraction which will adsorb onto normal sheep RBC. A small amount of this fraction has been detected in ultrasonic extracts of phase II organisms by sensitive hemagglutination-inhibition (HAI) techniques (10).

Trench fever agent. Specific CF antigens have been prepared from *Ro. quintana* cultivated on a supplemented blood agar. Ether treatment of suspensions of trench fever organisms releases a soluble antigen in low concentration (217). The organism has been grown also in a liquid medium (136, 147, 149). An ESS has not been isolated, and toxic effect is unknown. No information is available about antigenic differences among strains of this microorganism.

Animal pathogenicity and host range

A variety of arthropods and animals serve as natural hosts of the species of *Rickettsieae* (Table 33.1). The infection cycle may be relatively simple as in epidemic typhus and trench fever, which involves principally the body louse and humans, or it may be very complex as in some of the other rickettsioses. Ecologic studies of Rocky Mountain spotted fever in the eastern United States, for example, have implicated *Dermacentor variabilis, H. leporispalustris, Amblyomma americanum,* and *Ixodes dentatus* ticks as arthropod vectors. Among the vertebrate hosts are 15 different species of mammals included in 5 different orders (Rodentia, Lagomorpha, Marsupialia, Carnivora, and Artiodactyla) as well as 18 species of birds belonging to 3 different orders (Passeriformes, Ciconiiformes, and Piciformes) (34). In the western United States (40, 101) and other parts of the Western Hemisphere where Rocky Mountain spotted fever is endemic, other species of ticks and mammals not indigenous to the eastern United States are involved. Thus, the arthropod vectors and vertebrate hosts for a specific rickettsial agent may differ markedly from one geographic area to another. *C. burnetii* infects at least 38 species of ixodid and argasid ticks within 10 different genera in nature throughout the world (8). It is not within the scope of this text to describe fully the ecology of rickettsial diseases. The reader interested in more details of vectors and vertebrate hosts is referred to the pertinent chapters of *Viral and Rickettsial Infections of Man,* 4th edition (edited by F. L. Horsfall and I. Tamm, Philadelphia, J. B. Lippincott, 1965).

A variety of species of monkeys, white rats, cotton rats, inbred and outbred mice, deer mice, voles, gerbils, ferrets, squirrels, guinea pigs, rabbits, hamsters, dogs, sheep, goats, cattle, swine, donkeys, and other animals, as well as a variety of arthropods have been successfully infected experimentally with one or more of the different rickettsial organisms. That all the species of *Rickettsieae*, except *Ro. quintana*, could be readily propagated in the yolk sac of the developing chick embryo (61, 62) obviated the need for the majority of these laboratory hosts. Currently, the guinea pig and the white mouse are employed extensively for isolation and identification studies, while the other animals are used only rarely or for special investigations and as models for the human disease. Meadow voles (*Microtus pennsylvanicus*) reared in the laboratory have been successfully employed in attempts to isolate *R. prowazekii* (35, 158), *R. rickettsii*, and other Spotted Fever Group organisms (43, 44) and are more susceptible than guinea pigs.

Growth in tissue culture

Representative species of the *Rickettsieae* have been propagated in various primary and continuous cell lines derived from mammalian, avian, and insect tissues. In the early days of tissue culture, epidemic typhus rickettsiae were grown in tissue explants and later in Maitland-type cultures of minced tissues. These procedures were crude, and quantitation of rickettsiae was subjective. Later, when cell culture technology became more refined and continuous cell lines became important tools in the laboratory, quantitation and sequential examination of cell populations infected with rickettsiae became possible (32, 54, 97, 98, 128, 184). In recent years, the application of the improved cell culture systems to rickettsial research has led to significant advances, but the real value of this technology to the routine diagnostic laboratory has yet to be proven. The development of a plaque assay system permitted enumeration of rickettsiae in seed suspensions, studies of the effects of media and diluents, determination of antibiotic sensitivity, and purification of strains by cloning (127, 137, 138, 157, 221, 231, 232). The plaque assay system also has been used to isolate rickettsiae from blood and tissues of infected guinea pigs (143, 230) and monkeys (69, 113) and from tick hemolymph (230). Primary chicken embryo cells have been employed most extensively for plaque assay, but Vero (60), WI-38, DBS-FRhL-2, HeLa (160), L-929 (152, 160), and *Aedes albopictus* mosquito (59, 251) cell lines have been used in studies of selected strains of rickettsiae. In general, members of the Spotted Fever Group produce plaques in the chick cell system within 5–6 days, *C. burnetii* within 8–10 days, species of the Typhus Group in 11–12 days, while strains of *R. tsutsugamushi* require 17–19 days of incubation.

Rickettsiae multiply only in actively metabolizing cells or in the viable cytoplasm of enucleated cells at a relatively slow rate, increasing about 3-fold in 24 hr (32, 207, 243). Thus, when primary isolation of rickettsiae is attempted from inocula containing relatively few organisms, routine cell cultures maintained in liquid medium have to be held for several weeks or longer before infection can be detected. The susceptibility of most of the rickettsiae to penicillin and streptomycin or other antibiotics (245) precludes the routine use of antimicrobials in the medium to control bacterial contamination.

Tissue cultures have been used infrequently thus far for cultivation of rickettsiae for preparation of antigens for serologic tests (12, 193), and attempts to demonstrate *in vitro* neutralization with antiserum have been almost totally unsatisfactory (13, 193). Cultures of a variety of cell types used for studying the infection cycle of several species of *Rickettsia* have yielded much information on penetration, growth kinetics, and other rickettsia-host cell interaction in phagocytic and nonphagocytic cells (6, 32, 54, 125, 184, 237, 243, 244), including the influence of strain virulence, antibody, and other factors related to humoral and cellular immunity on the fate of rickettsiae in infected cells (14, 15, 83, 84, 96, 111, 118, 120, 235, 238, 239, 240, 242).

Metabolic studies have been carried out in irradiated host cells (226, 227). In the past, cell culture was rarely used to propagate rickettsiae for the preparation of experimental vaccines (171). Recently, Rocky Mountain spotted fever vaccines prepared from infected duck and chick embryo cell cultures were reported to be more immunogenic for experimental animals than the commercial product made from infected yolk sacs (112, 115, 116).

Collection and Preparation of Specimens for Isolation and Serologic Diagnosis

Precautions

Virtually every laboratory conducting research on Typhus, Spotted Fever, and Scrub Typhus Group rickettsiae and *C. burnetii* has experienced accidental infection of laboratory personnel. In addition, infections have occurred in administrative, secretarial, and maintenance staffs, as well as in visitors (108, 109, 208). In many laboratories, infections occur with such regularity that the majority have not been documented in the medical literature. When rickettsial diagnostic or research work is to be initiated, it is imperative to be aware of the hazards that have been encountered in rickettsial laboratories and how they have been minimized (198, 222). Avoidance of laboratory infections, barring the overt accident, depends upon the skill of the worker and his meticulous attention to details, the adequacy of laboratory techniques and equipment, and the architectural design of the laboratory. The small laboratory lacking the experience and equipment to handle highly infectious agents should avoid attempts to establish a rickettsial diagnosis by isolation of the causative agent. Generally, definitive information about the etiology of suspected rickettsial diseases can be obtained more rapidly and with less expense and effort by serologic procedures using noninfectious antigens than by isolation studies. Since the majority of the infections acquired in the laboratory cannot be related to obvious accidents, it is mandatory that all persons at risk report directly to a responsible physician whenever fever and headache develop. If these complaints increase in severity or persist unabated for 48–72 hr, the patient should be presumed to have a rickettsial infection. After the appropriate specimens necessary to establish an etiologic diagnosis have been collected, specific therapy should be instituted.

The effectiveness of vaccines against epidemic typhus and Rocky Mountain spotted fever which are currently available from commercial sources have been questioned. However, highly effective experimental vaccines have been made against Q fever.

Human disease

Rickettsemia occurs in humans during the febrile period of all of the diseases. Blood collected early in the course of illness before administration of antibiotics is the most suitable material for isolation attempts. When the specimen is obtained during the first week of illness, heparinized (0.2 mg or 20 units per ml) or defibrinated whole blood may be used for isolation. Alternatively, blood is collected and allowed to coagulate.

After centrifugation, the serum is removed and stored for serologic testing. The clot is ground, and a 20–50% suspension prepared in Snyder I diluent or brain-heart infusion broth is inoculated into suitable laboratory hosts or a cell culture system. The chances of recovering the agent from whole blood collected later than the first week of disease are much reduced, and the clot should be used for isolation attempts. Separation of the serum from the clot removes inhibitory antibodies that might be present. If more than 1 hr is expected to elapse between the time the blood is collected and inoculation can be done, the clot and serum, after separation, should be frozen rapidly in an alcohol-dry ice bath and kept frozen on dry ice or liquid nitrogen until processed. Frozen specimens are thawed rapidly in a 37 C water bath or warm tap water, promptly processed, and inoculated. A sample of the inoculum is preserved at −65 C or lower temperatures for additional isolation studies if required. All diluents are chilled to 4 C before use, and all suspensions are kept on ice.

On occasion, it is necessary to carry out isolation attempts on tissues obtained at autopsy. Ideally, 1- to 2-cm cubes of each of the visceral organs and the brain should be obtained aseptically, placed individually in suitable sterile screw-cap containers and frozen rapidly as previously described. In most instances the tissues received in the laboratory are heavily contaminated. If the specimens were not collected aseptically, all exposed surfaces are sliced off, and an inner portion of the tissue is obtained. The tissues are processed individually, or equal amounts are combined and inoculated as a pool. A 20% tissue suspension is prepared in Snyder I diluent or brain-heart infusion broth. If bacterial contamination is suspected, before inoculation a portion is treated for 30 min at room temperature with 100–1000 units of penicillin per ml of inoculum and, depending upon the laboratory host to be used, 100–500 μg of streptomycin. Penicillin and streptomycin can be used to prepare material for inoculation of mice and embryonated eggs but not for inoculation of cell cultures or guinea pigs. These concentrations of antibiotics inhibit the growth of most of the rickettsiae in cell cultures, and the cited concentrations of streptomycin are toxic for guinea pigs. The broad spectrum antibiotics, chloramphenicol and tetracycline, cannot be used to suppress the bacteria because of rickettsiostatic effect. Gentamicin sulfate may be inhibitory for rickettsiae even at a concentration of 50 μg/ml (229).

Serologic diagnosis of a rickettsial disease depends upon the demonstration of a significant increase in titer of specific antibodies in the serum during the course of illness and convalescence. To accomplish this, blood should be collected as early in the course of the disease as possible, again on day 10-14, when antibodies may first be present, and later on day 21-28 after onset, when significant titers should be demonstrable. If intensive antibiotic therapy is initiated during the first few days of illness, the development of antibodies may be delayed. In rare circumstances, it may be necessary to obtain a fourth specimen after 2-3 months in order to demonstrate a significant level of antibody.

On each occasion at least 5 ml of blood are collected aseptically with a dry needle and syringe to minimize hemolysis. The specimen is placed in a screw-cap or rubber-stopper sterile tube without anticoagulant. After the blood has coagulated, the clot is separated from the wall of the tube with a sterile applicator stick, and the specimen is placed at 4 C for 6-18 hr to allow retraction of the clot. After centrifugation, the serum is removed from the clot and stored without chemical preservatives in a screw-cap or rubber-stopper glass or tightly sealed plastic container. If the processing is delayed longer, serum specimens may develop anticomplementary activity. The serum may be stored at 4 C until tested; however, at this temperature there is a slow deterioration of antibody. If serum is to be retained for an extended time, it should be stored frozen at -20 C or lower. Evaluation of the stability of the different immunoglobulin classes of rickettsial antibody in blood stored on filter-paper disks in the dried state showed that the IgM antibody activity declined rapidly and the IgG activity was relatively constant over a 4-month period at -20 C (53).

Arthropods and animal reservoirs

Research and public health laboratories concerned with ecologic and epidemiologic investigations have resources that generally are not available to the clinical diagnostic laboratory. Field studies require the collective services of entomologists, mammalogists, and epidemiologists, who know which potential arthropod vectors and reservoir hosts should be investigated, as well as how to collect and handle them. These specimens should be processed in the field in a manner which will provide the laboratory worker with materials that are best suited to obtain information about possible infection with rickettsial agents.

With few exceptions, inoculation of laboratory hosts with suspensions freshly prepared from living specimens provides the best opportunity for the recovery of rickettsial agents. This may be accomplished by processing the material and inoculating mice and guinea pigs in a field station or, as is usually the case, at the base laboratory upon receipt of the specimens. Lice, fleas, ticks, larval trombiculid mites, and gamasid mites have different requirements for temperature and humidity for survival. A variety of containers have been devised for shipping live arthropods. These are made of clear plastic or glass, partially filled with a mixture of plaster of Paris and charcoal, and stoppered with a screw-cap or cotton plug. Desiccation of the arthropods is prevented by moistening the plaster with water before use. Lice, fleas, chiggers, and mites will survive at least several days and ticks for longer if extremes of temperature are avoided by shipping them in an insulated container. When the base laboratory is too remote from the field activity for the lice, fleas, chiggers, and mites to arrive alive, the arthropods should be identified and sorted into pools of uniform composition as they are collected. A representative sample, 10-20%, should be preserved in 70% alcohol for subsequent definitive identification by an entomologic taxonomist. The remainder are preserved for isolation studies by rapidly freezing the intact arthropods in a tightly sealed container in a dry ice-alcohol bath, or in liquid nitrogen, and maintaining the material at -65 C or lower. Engorged ticks are processed in the same manner as the other arthropods, but unfed ticks should receive special handling. When attempting to recover *R. rickettsii* from unengorged ticks, incubation at 37 C for 2-3 days in a humid atmosphere or feeding the ticks on laboratory animals is necessary to reactivate the microorganisms (203). It is not known whether this is necessary for the recovery of other Spotted Fever Group agents from their respective tick vectors. Nevertheless, it is recommended that unfed ticks be incubated as described before processing to improve the chances of recovery.

Small rodents and other small- and medium-sized mammals captured by live-trapping are handled in the following manner. The animal is transferred from the trap to a strong white linen or muslin bag, which is securely tied to prevent loss of arthropods that might be present. After being lightly anesthetized with ether, the animal is combed or brushed, and the unattached arthropods are collected. The cloth bag is carefully inspected for detached arthropods. Under anesthesia, the animal is exsanguinated, and serum separated from the blood is kept for serologic studies. The spleen and a piece of the liver and kidney, removed aseptically, provide suitable material for isolation studies. A suspension of tissues is prepared and inoculated immediately, or the unprocessed tissue is quickly frozen and stored at -65 C or lower until processing. The animal is then examined again, and all attached arthropods of interest are removed.

Laboratory hosts are inoculated with a suspension prepared by grinding the living arthropods or freshly harvested tissues in Snyder I diluent or brain-heart infusion broth. If the specimens are frozen, the material is thawed rapidly immediately before processing. Large particles are removed by light centrifugation ($100-400 \times g$), and the supernatant fluid is the inoculum.

When animals are to be used for isolation studies, it is rarely necessary to treat the arthropods before grinding to reduce the number of bacteria contaminating the exterior surface. Many arthropods have a natural intestinal flora that is difficult to eliminate without destroying rickettsiae that may be present. Mice and guinea pigs tolerate moderate amounts of bacterial contaminants when inoculated intraperitoneally. In special studies in which attempts are made to recover rickettsiae from arthropods by inoculation of embryonated eggs, preliminary decontamination and washing is mandatory. Usually the arthropods are immersed in a 1:1000 solution of merthiolate for about 1 hr at room temperature. Thereafter, the arthropods are washed thoroughly in several changes of sterile distilled water or buffered saline. Penicillin alone (100–1000 u/ml), or in combination with dihydrostreptomycin (100–500 μg/ml), may be added to the bath as well as to the diluents used for preparing the suspension. Although the use of antibiotics may decrease the chance of successful recovery, without it the isolation attempt will probably be invalid because of death of the embryos from bacterial growth. *R. rickettsii* has been isolated directly from tick hemolymph by a plaque assay technique in primary chick embryo tissue culture (230).

Laboratory Diagnosis

Direct examination of specimens

The concentration of rickettsiae in the blood of patients during the acute phase of illness is relatively low, and it is virtually impossible to identify the microorganisms with any degree of certainty in leukocytes or monocytes in blood films stained by standard aniline dyes or immunofluorescence techniques. In 2 patients with classical Rocky Mountain spotted fever, *R. rickettsii* organisms stained with specific fluorescein-labeled antibody were identified in sections of the macular lesion obtained by a full-thickness biopsy of the skin performed on the third and eighth day of disease, respectively (249). Although fluorescent-antibody (FA) techniques have been used satisfactorily to demonstrate rickettsial organisms in tissues of experimentally infected animals during the early stages of disease (164), it is futile to examine smears of spleen or other tissues from wild animals suspected of being vertebrate hosts. When preparations of the tissues of various noninfected arthropods are stained with aniline dyes, structures are found which morphologically are indistinguishable from pathogenic rickettsiae. Direct FA staining techniques have been used to identify *R. rickettsii* in experimentally and naturally infected *Dermacentor andersoni* ticks (38, 188) and *R. prowazekii* in human body lice (57). Ticks infected with *R. rickettsii* can be rapidly differentiated from those that are not by use of immunofluorescent staining to examine hemolymph obtained by amputating the distal portion of one or more legs (39). This hemolymph test proved to be a valuable adjunct in a public health educational campaign to alert the public and medical personnel to the seriousness of Rocky Mountain spotted fever (41). A highly reproducible method for counting rickettsiae has proven useful in quantitating the organism content of seed suspensions, purified corpuscular antigens, and experimental vaccines (195).

Rickettsia isolation

Although both the plaque assay system (see above) and cultivation of autogenous circulating monocytes (see below) have proven useful for rapid isolation and identification of certain species of rickettsiae present in the blood of experimental animals early in the course of infection, successful application of the procedures to diagnosis of the respective diseases in humans has yet to be reported. The available data indicate that these procedures, as now refined, have a sensitivity equal to and, at times, greater than the susceptibility of other laboratory hosts. However, these techniques have not been evaluated systematically with all the species of *Rickettsieae* known to infect humans.

The adult male guinea pig and the adult white mouse are the animals of choice for use in the primary isolation of all known species of *Rickettsieae* (Table 33.3) except *Ro. quintana,* which can be cultivated on artificial medium. Although all of the rickettsiae except the trench fever organism have been adapted to propagation in eggs, with rare exceptions to be explained later, this host is not used for primary isolation.

Typhus and Spotted Fever Group infections and Q fever in guinea pigs. A certain amount of variation in susceptibility to rickettsial infection can be expected among guinea pigs from random-bred colonies. Increased resistance may be manifested by lack of the expected clinical response, an antibody response of low magnitude, and in some instances a complete absence of clinical or serologic evidence of infection. Generally, mature animals weighing 550–650 g tend to respond more uniformly, but animals within the range of 450–750 g can be used. A specimen of blood should be obtained from all guinea pigs and tested for serologic reactivity. If the serum displays anticomplementary activity or fixes complement nonspecifically in the presence of rickettsial or normal tissue antigens, the animal should be discarded. To compensate for the expected differences in response, a minimum of 3 guinea pigs should be inoculated intraperitoneally. The volume of the inoculum depends on the amount and nature of the specimen. Although guinea pigs can be injected safely with as much as 5 ml, usually 2–4 ml of blood from the febrile patient is inoculated into each animal. Daily observations are made for signs of illness for 14 days. Rectal temperatures are taken at the same time each day, preferably in the morning, and before feeding the guinea pigs vegetable greens. Temperatures of 40 C (104 F) and higher are indicative of fever. Successful recovery of the rickettsial agent from blood of patients infected with members of the Typhus and Spotted Fever Groups and the Q fever agent is almost invariably accompanied by the appearance of fever in the guinea pig. However, the time of onset after injection and the duration of the febrile response depend on the infectivity titer of the inoculum, and these findings do not provide information on the possible identity of the agent. With the exception of certain strains of *R. rickettsii* and *C. burnetii,* the infections caused by the numbers of organisms present in isolation specimens are self-limiting, and the animals recover without sequelae. Convalescence is associated with the development of specific antibodies, which can be demonstrated by appropriate serologic procedures. The finding of a scrotal reaction is of some help in preliminary identification. In general, after infection with *R. typhi* and members of the Spotted Fever Group, the scrotal reaction manifested by edema and erythema appears coincidentally with fever or shortly thereafter. The scrotum becomes swollen, inflamed, and taut, and the testes cannot be pushed back readily into the abdominal cavity. Epidemic typhus and Q fever infection are not associated with a visible scrotal reaction.

TABLE 33.3—PRIMARY ISOLATION OF *RICKETTSIEAE* IN LABORATORY ANIMALS

ETIOLOGIC AGENT	PREFERRED HOST	INCUBATION PERIOD (DAYS)	CLINICAL MANIFESTATIONS	EXPECTED MORTALITY	TISSUES HARVESTED FOR PASSAGE
Rickettsia prowazekii	Male guinea pig	5–12	Fever	None	Spleen or Brain
R. typhi	Male guinea pig	3–10	Fever, scrotal edema, and erythema	None	Spleen Tunica
R. rickettsii	Male guinea pig	3–10	Fever, scrotal edema, erythema, hemorrhage, and necrosis	Frequent	Spleen Blood Tunica
R. conorii	Male guinea pig	3–6	Fever, scrotal edema, and erythema	Rare	Spleen Tunica
R. australis	Male guinea pig	4–5	Fever, scrotal edema, and erythema	None	Spleen Tunica
R. sibirica	Male guinea pig	5–10	Fever, scrotal edema, and erythema	None	Spleen Tunica
	Adult white mouse	6–9	Inactivity, rough fur	Usual	Spleen
R. akari	Male guinea pig	3–7	Fever, scrotal edema, and erythema	Rare	Spleen Tunica
R. tsutsugamushi	Adult white mouse	6–18	Inactivity, rough fur, ascites	Usual	Spleen
Coxiella burnetii	Male guinea pig	5–12	Fever	Rare	Spleen

R. rickettsii strains have been classified on the basis of virulence for guinea pigs. R-type strains evoke fever and a severe scrotal reaction with typical hemorrhagic and necrotic lesions, which occasionally involve also footpads and ears. Infection invariably results in death. S strains cause fever and scrotal reactions but are not fatal, and T strains produce only a febrile disease. Infection with U strains is evidenced only by serologic conversion, and these strains cannot be propagated serially in guinea pigs (176). Isolation and cultivation of U strains require the use of embryonated hens' eggs. R, S, and T strains have been associated with serious illnesses in humans, but U strains have been recovered only from naturally infected ticks and small mammals.

On the second or third day of illness, one guinea pig in the group is sacrificed; tissues are harvested for passage, and smears are made for microscopic examination. Under ether anesthesia, 10–15 ml of blood are collected aseptically by cardiac puncture, heparinized, and kept at 4 C until passaged. Postmortem examination reveals few abnormalities other than those associated with a mild peritonitis; i.e., a thin fibrinous exudate covers the surface of the visceral peritoneum. When a scrotal reaction is evident, the tunica vaginalis is exposed by applying traction to the spermatic cord retracting the testes into the abdominal cavity. The tunica is hyperemic, edematous, and occasionally hemorrhagic. Smears prepared from the peritoneal surface of the spleen and from the tunica vaginalis are stained and examined microscopically for presence of rickettsiae. The spleen, whole blood, and the tunica, if inflamed, are ground with an abrasive or homogenized, with Snyder I diluent or brain-heart infusion broth used to make a 10-20% tissue suspension; this is lightly centrifuged to sediment heavy particles. The supernatant fluid serves as the inoculum for injection of additional guinea pigs. Since this material also may be used to initiate egg lines, it is important to adhere to strict aseptic techniques. Serum should be obtained from all animals, including asymptomatic guinea pigs, 21-28 days after inoculation and tested serologically for evidence of infection. Guinea pigs becoming ill in the second passage are processed as described above, and the agent is passaged successively in guinea pigs until it is well established. A portion of tissue suspension from each passage is stored at −65 C for future reference. In the absence of overt disease in the first-passage guinea pigs, routine blind passage is generally valueless except in C. burnetii infection. Newly isolated strains of this agent, which do not evoke a febrile response, may be serially propagated in guinea pigs.

Scrub typhus and rickettsialpox in mice. Although certain strains of *R. akari* and some strains of *R. tsutsugamushi* will cause overt signs of illness in guinea pigs, the white mouse is the preferred laboratory host. A group of 4-6 mice, each weighing 14-16 g, is injected intraperitoneally with 0.2-0.5 ml of the specimen under study. Mice infected with virulent strains of these rickettsiae develop signs of illness at the end of the first or during the second week. The animals become less active, the fur roughens, and ascites develops. Prior to death, respiration becomes rapid and labored. Moribund animals are sacrificed, and an autopsy is performed under aseptic conditions. Pathologic changes are minimal in animals that die between the sixth and ninth day and are limited to slight accumulation of a serofibrinous exudate. If seriously ill animals survive for 14 days or longer, the pathology is more striking. At necropsy subcutaneous edema and lymphadenitis are evident. Several milliliters of a serofibrinous hemorrhagic exudate are present in the peritoneal cavity. The spleen is enlarged. Smears prepared from the surface of the spleen and from the parietal peritoneum are stained and examined microscopically for presence of rickettsiae. A 10-20% spleen suspension is used for inoculation of additional mice, or for adaptation to cultivation in eggs. In the event that none of the animals manifest overt illness by day 14 after inoculation, all mice are sacrificed, and a 10-20% suspension is prepared from a pool of their spleens. This suspension is injected intraperitoneally into 15-20 additional mice. Animals becoming ill in the second passage are processed as described above, and the agent is passaged serially until it is established in the host. If none of the animals become ill by the end of the second week, 4 or 5 of the group are sacrificed, and the spleens are harvested, frozen rapidly, and stored at −65 C. These specimens can be used to initiate additional passages if indicated. The surviving animals are challenged 28–35 days after inoculation: one-half with 1,000 LD_{50} of *R. tsu-tsugamushi* and the other half with a comparable dose of *R. akari*. Survival of the mice indicates prior infection.

Strains of *R. tsutsugamushi* vary markedly in their virulence for mice irrespective of whether they are recovered from patients, wild animals, or trombiculid chiggers. Strains that produce no visible evidence of infection in mice have been isolated from seriously ill patients.

Practically all newly recovered strains of *R. typhi* and *C. burnetii* may produce in mice minimal changes that are apparent at the time the animal is sacrificed for blind passage on day 14. Some strains of *R. typhi* have killed mice at the time of primary isolation. It is important to be alert to the possible recovery of these agents in mice. This is particularly true of *C. burnetii*, which is excreted in the urine and feces of mice with subclinical infections, thereby constituting an unrecognized hazard to laboratory personnel and animal caretakers. In addition, *C. burnetii* may infect other animals caged in the same room. It may be recovered inadvertently in other isolation lines, or it may contaminate other experiments.

Plaque assay and autogenous monocyte culture. A step-by-step procedure for the preparation of primary monolayer cultures of chick embryo cells and their use for plaque assays and cloning of rickettsiae can be found in the *Tissue Culture Association Manual* (157). The plaque assay procedure has been used to quantitate the level of rickettsemia in guinea pigs infected with *R. rickettsii* (230) and *R. typhi* (143), as well as in monkeys infected with *R. rickettsii* (69, 113). If this assay system proves to be equally sensitive for the primary isolation of the other *Rickettsieae,* the advantages over the guinea pig and the mouse are obvious. However, its usefulness as a means for early definitive diagnosis of human disease would be limited by the time required for plaques to appear. Another procedure which may have greater promise in this regard, but for which there is even less information about its utility, is the cultivation of autogenous monocytes circulating in the peripheral blood. In guinea pigs infected with *R. rickettsii* (36, 37) and in monkeys infected with the same organism (37, 69), rickettsiae could be visualized in the monocyte cultures by immunofluorescent staining within 2–5 days after their initiation.

Trench fever. Ro. quintana cannot be cultivated serially in the guinea pig, mouse, or embryonated egg. Previously, the etiologic agent could be recovered only by use of lice and xenodiagnosis. It is now known that *Ro. quintana* can be propagated with ease on blood agar incubated at 37 C in a moist atmosphere of 5% CO_2 in air. The basic medium consists of Difco blood agar base (beef heart infusion, tryptose, NaCl, and agar), 6% horse serum inactivated at 56 C for 30 min, and 4% horse RBC washed 3 times with phosphate-buffered saline solution (pH 7.2) and hemolyzed with either distilled water or by rapid freezing to −60 C and rapid thawing at 37 C (216). *Ro. quintana* has been recovered from freshly collected heparinized blood and from specimens previously stored at −60 C. Organisms were present in the blood during the stage of acute illness as well as during asymptomatic periods. Twelve to 14 days after inoculation of the surface of the medium (in 60-mm × 15-mm plastic Petri dishes) by streaking 0.05 ml of blood, minute colonies 65 μm-200 μm in diameter can be seen on the surface under 20X magnification. Subculture is carried out after emulsification of the colonies in sucrose PG diluent (Snyder II). Growth on subculture becomes apparent within 3-5 days. In the solid medium, crystalline hemoglobin or hemin can be used instead of the lysed RBC, and bovine albumin or a colloidal "detoxifying agent" such as starch or charcoal can replace serum (147). Liquid medium has been developed that can be used for subcultivating strains isolated on solid medium and for preparing antigens (136, 149). The morphologic appearance of the organisms can be confirmed by examining smears stained by Giemsa or Giménez techniques. Identity is confirmed either by demonstrating specific fixation of complement with hyperimmune rabbit serum and antigens prepared from the organisms grown on agar or in the liquid medium or by immunofluorescent staining by the direct or indirect method.

Rickettsia identification

Microscopic examination. At autopsy of sick laboratory animals, smears of infected tissues are prepared by lightly touching the uncut surface of the mouse or guinea pig spleen, the tunica vaginalis of the guinea pig, or the parietal peritoneum of the mouse to a clean glass slide. Plaques seen in chick embryo cell cultures can be aspirated and smeared on glass slides. Several slides with smears of each of the tissues are prepared. One set of smears may be stained by the Giemsa method, which stains intracytoplasmic rickettsiae bluish-purple. However, the Macchiavello or Giménez (86) stains usually are preferred; with the former the rickettsiae are bright red against a contrasting blue background, and with the latter red rickettsiae are seen against a greenish background. For immunofluorescent staining, the slides are fixed in acetone at room temperature for 10 min. If not processed the same day, these slides should be stored at -20 C or lower. Survival of *C. burnetii* in cell monolayers fixed in acetone at -60 C for periods up to 4 hr has been reported (93). Materials and procedures for preparing these stains are described below.

Macchiavello Stain

Reagents

1. Basic fuchsin *stock solution;* 5% in alcohol: Grind 5 g basic fuchsin in 100 ml 95% ethyl alcohol. Filter and store in a tightly sealed bottle at room temperature.

2. Basic fuchsin *working solution;* 0.25%: Dilute 5 ml stock solution with 95 ml freshly boiled, cold, distilled water. Store at 4 C.

3. Citric acid; 0.25% in distilled water, prepared fresh.

4. Methylene blue; 1% in distilled water: Grind 1 g methylene blue in 100 ml distilled water. Filter and store at 4 C.

Procedure

1. *Lightly* heat-fix slide. Smears should be processed soon after preparation and not allowed to remain at room temperature unstained.

2. Filter basic fuchsin *working solution* onto smear, and let stand for 5-6 min.

3. Pour fuchsin off, quickly dip slide into freshly prepared citric acid solution, and then rinse in running tap water. (In practice if the tap water is acidic, satisfactory results can be obtained by omitting the citric acid treatment and rinsing the slides thoroughly in tap water only.)

4. Filter methylene blue solution onto slide, and let stand for 10-15 sec.

5. Rinse in running tap water. Blot dry and examine.

(This method satisfactorily stains Typhus and Spotted Fever Group rickettsiae and

C. burnetii in smears prepared from infected yolk sacs and animal tissues and cell cultures. The Macchiavello technique stains *R. tsutsugamushi* poorly, and the Giemsa stain is employed regularly for this agent.)

Giménez Stain

Reagents

1. Carbol basic fuchsin *stock solution:* Mix 100 ml 10% basic fuchsin in 95% ethanol (10 g basic fuchsin in 100 ml 95% ethyl alcohol), 250 ml 4% aqueous phenol (10 ml phenol in 250 ml distilled water), and 650 ml distilled water. Incubate at 37 C for 48 hr before use.

2. Stock buffers: 0.2 M NaH_2PO_4 (2.84 g in 100 ml distilled water) and 0.2 M $Na_2 HPO_4$ (2.76 g in 100 ml distilled water).

3. Carbol basic fuchsin *working solution:* 4 ml carbol basic fuchsin stock and 10 ml 0.1 M sodium phosphate buffer solution, pH 7.45. The buffer solution is prepared by mixing 3.5 ml 0.2 M NaH_2PO_4, 15.5 ml 0.2 M Na_2HPO_4, and 19 ml distilled water. Filter immediately and again before each use. Remains suitable for use for about 48 hr.

4. Malachite green oxalate: 0.8% solution in distilled water.

5. Fast green FCF: 0.5% solution in distilled water.

6. Ferric nitrate: 4% $Fe(NO_3)_3 \cdot 9H_2O$ in distilled water.

Procedure for all rickettsiae except R. tsutsugamushi

1. Air dry smear, and fix by passing slide through flame.
2. Filter *working* carbol basic fuchsin onto slide and let stand 1-2 min.
3. Wash thoroughly under tap water.
4. Cover smear with malachite green for 6-9 sec.
5. Wash thoroughly under tap water.
6. Cover smear again with malachite green for 6-9 sec.
7. Wash thoroughly under tap water.
8. Blot dry and examine.

Procedure for scrub typhus rickettsiae

1. Air dry smear and fix by passing slide through flame.
2. Filter *working* carbol basic fuchsin onto slide and let stand 1-2 min.
3. Wash thoroughly under tap water.
4. Add 4-6 drops ferric nitrate solution and wash off immediately under tap water.
5. Cover smear with fast green for 15-30 sec.
6. Wash thoroughly under tap water.
7. Blot dry and examine.

The Giménez technique is superior to the standard Macchiavello procedure, but neither method gives selective staining of rickettsiae, and certain bacteria will retain the red color. Differentiation of rickettsiae from bacteria must be made on the basis of morphologic appearance and culture techniques. All suspensions prepared during the course of rickettsial studies should be cultured routinely for contaminating bacteria by inoculation of blood agar slants and tubes of thioglycollate broth.

Rickettsiae are usually scarce in smears of tissues from first passage animals, and additional passages may be required before organisms can be recognized with certainty. The rickettsiae are most readily found intracytoplasmically in cells of the serosa. The presence of rickettsiae in the nucleus is a diagnostic feature of Spotted Fever Group species. An exception to this rule is the growth of *R. canada,* a member of the Typhus Group, in the nucleus of a variety of tissues of infected ticks including the hemocytes (42).

When sufficient numbers of rickettsiae are found in smears stained with aniline dyes, immunofluorescence techniques can be used to identify the organism (Fig 33.1). Experience with the 2-step indirect procedure, with use of human, mouse, or guinea pig convalescent-phase serum (51, 73, 90) and the corresponding antiglobulin conjugated with fluorescein

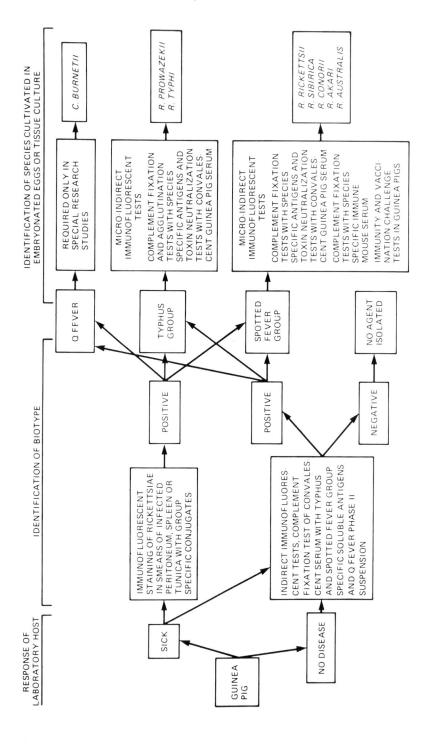

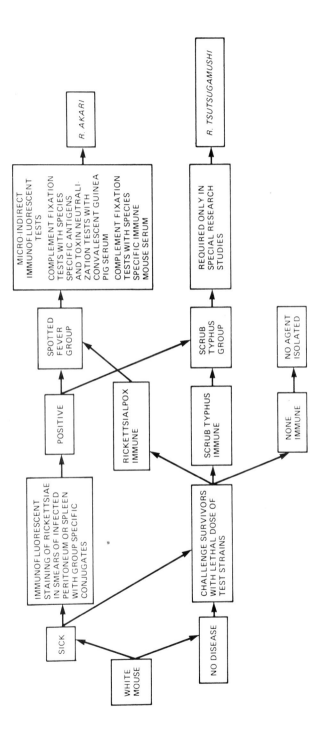

Figure 33.1—Schematic summary of procedures for isolation and identification of *Rickettsieae* known to infect man

isothiocyanate, indicates that the reaction is group-specific and cannot be used to identify species or strains of rickettsiae within a group. Thus, a newly recovered agent can be shown to be a member of the Typhus, Spotted Fever, or Scrub Typhus Group or the Q fever agent. Specific conjugates for direct staining of *R. tsutsugamushi* have been prepared that will distinguish among antigenically distinctive strains (102). However, additional studies must be carried out to determine whether specific rickettsial antibody-fluorescein conjugates can be prepared that will distinguish the different species within the Typhus and Spotted Fever Groups.

Agents recovered in guinea pigs. Information about the identity of the rickettsiae isolated in guinea pigs is obtained from CF tests, or from micro-indirect immunofluorescence (micro-IF) tests (see below) performed with the serum collected about 28 days after inoculation. With the CF test the antigenic category can be identified by tests employing group-specific soluble antigens prepared from Typhus and Spotted Fever Group rickettsiae and a Q fever antigen comprised of a suspension of phase II organisms (Fig 33.1). When Typhus or Spotted Fever Group antibodies are demonstrated, a presumptive identification of the intragroup species can be made on the basis of the geographic location of the patient and pertinent epidemiologic and ecologic factors associated with the occurrence of disease. The finding of Q fever antibodies in guinea pig serum is sufficient evidence to identify the agent as *C. burnetii,* and further studies are not required.

Definitive identification of a member of the Typhus Group can be established by CF and agglutination tests with specific corpuscular rickettsial antigens (172) and by toxin neutralization (Nt) tests in mice (95) with *R. prowazekii, R. typhi,* and *R. canada.* In these serologic procedures the homologous antibody titer of guinea pig serum is significantly higher than the level of heterologous antibodies. Cross-protection (immunity-challenge) tests do not contribute greatly since guinea pigs convalescent from infection with one species have a considerable degree of immunity against the other members of the group. Although guinea pigs immunized with formalin-inactivated vaccines are protected principally against the homologous strain, vaccination challenge tests are not employed routinely.

Owing to close immunologic relationships among the members of the Spotted Fever Group, a variety of serologic procedures must be employed to differentiate the species. Furthermore, in most instances the newly recovered agent must be cultivated in embryonated eggs to obtain the concentrations of rickettsiae required for infectious challenge and preparation of toxin and CF antigens. The procedures employed in the past included CF tests with guinea pig antiserum and washed rickettsial suspensions (173), cross-protection (immunity-challenge) tests in guinea pigs (67, 130), toxin Nt tests in mice (21), and vaccination of mice against toxic challenge (21). More recently, Spotted Fever Group species have been differentiated by CF tests with immune mouse serum which is species-specific and does not react with soluble cross-reacting antigens of heterologous species (170). This technique readily differentiated *R. akari, R. australis,* and *R. montana.* However, to induce type-specific antibody against *R. conorii* and *R. sibirica,* extremely large concentrations of organisms equivalent to 1–2 LD_{50} of toxin were required. Most attempts with *R. rickettsii* failed to evoke CF antibody even though doses that killed more than 50% of the mice within 7 days were administered.

Alternatively, the convalescent-phase serum from the guinea pigs can be examined with the micro-IF test using as antigens smears of rickettsial suspensions of each of the members of the Typhus and Spotted Fever Groups and *C. burnetii* (phase II). Although intragroup and, to a certain degree, intergroup cross-reactivity between the agents in the Typhus and Spotted Fever Groups can be expected, the titer with the homologous species will predominate.

Agents recovered in mice. The identity of the rickettsia recovered in mice can be established by mouse cross-protection tests. Convalescent animals will withstand homologous challenge with more than 1000 LD_{50} of established strains of *R. akari* (105) or *R. tsutsugamushi* (252). Although relationship of a newly recovered organism to *R. akari* may be established by cross-protection tests, definitive identification should depend upon procedures described in the preceding section, which differentiate the Spotted Fever Group species. On the other hand, with scrub typhus rickettsiae only mouse immunity-challenge tests are required. This procedure, which demonstrates intragroup relationship among antigenically dissimilar strains of *R. tsutsugamushi*, provides definitive identification of newly recovered strains. When highly lethal strains are encountered, immune mice can be obtained by providing the animals with drinking water containing chloramphenicol (2.5 mg/ml) for 3 weeks (106).

Inapparent infections of mice with *Encephalitozoon cuniculi* (142) and *Histoplasma capsulatum* (183) effectively increase the resistance of the animals to scrub typhus infection. Both of these microorganisms may be encountered inadvertently during attempts to recover rickettsiae from tissues of wild animals or, as is often the case with the protozoa, latent infections may exist in the mouse colony. Although mice infected with these agents may resist about 100 LD_{50} of the challenge strain, it is rare that protection would be afforded against more than 1000 LD_{50}.

Antigenic relationship of isolates to the prototype Gilliam, Karp, or Kato strains, or to other distinctive strains that undoubtedly exist, is most readily demonstrated by the CF test. In this procedure, serum from guinea pigs infected by intracerebral inoculation of the newly recovered agents are tested with antigens comprised of partially purified suspensions of whole rickettsial organisms (192). Studies employing highly strain-specific CF antigens indicated that a significant proportion of strains of *R. tsutsugamushi* recovered from wild animals, from *Leptotrombidium* chiggers, and from patients were mixtures of two or more antigenically different types (74, 76). This method of classification distinguishes strains on the basis of the major antigen component. However, strain-specific CF antigens are difficult to produce. Indirect immunofluorescence offers a more practical method of determining the relationship of new strains to the prototype strains. The major and minor antigens of the prototype strains have been defined, but further studies are required to determine whether wild strains of *R. tsutsugamushi* with the same major antigens as the standard strains also have the same secondary antigens (75).

Agents recovered in tissue cultures. Strains of rickettsiae isolated either by use of the plaque assay system or by the cultivation of autogenous mono-cytes can be identified by the application of procedures already described. The most direct method is immunofluorescent staining smears of infected cells with reagents of defined specificity. If only the biotype can be deter-mined by this process, then the species of the strain can be identified with tests carried out with immune serum produced by inoculation of either guin-ea pigs or mice, as indicated, and the appropriate antigens prepared from infected embryonated eggs or tissue cultures.

Cultivation of rickettsiae in embryonated eggs. Occasionally the strain or species of rickettsiae cannot be identified because of reduced virulence for laboratory animals, or the serologic procedures outlined above fail to provide the desired differentiating results. Adaptation of the agent to cultiva-tion in embryonated hens' eggs is necessary if direct serologic and immuno-logic comparisons to standard rickettsiae are to be made. This process is usually difficult and tedious and must be carried out with strict aseptic tech-nique. Bacteriologically sterile suspensions of spleen, blood, and tunica vag-inalis from infected guinea pigs, or spleen suspensions from infected mice, or suspensions of infected cell cultures are inoculated into the yolk sac of 5- to 7-day-old embryonated hens' eggs (see Chapter 1). If the rickettsial sus-pensions prepared from tissues of guinea pigs or mice are contaminated with bacteria, the extraneous organisms usually can be eliminated by harvesting the brain of the infected animal. Most bacterial contaminants remain local-ized in the peritoneal cavity while the rickettsiae are disseminated through-out the body. A brain suspension is injected intraperitoneally into additional animals. After the onset of disease, the usual tissues are harvested for in-oculation of eggs. Depending upon the species, strain of rickettsia, and the time of death of the chick embryos, serial passages of yolk sac suspensions prepared from the remaining living eggs are made at 6- to 12-day intervals. Adaptation of the rickettsiae with resulting luxuriant growth may occur after a few passages, but occasionally many months of intensive effort are re-quired. Experience has shown that concentrations of approximately 10^6 rick-ettsiae per gram of tissue must be attained before the organisms are readily demonstrable in stained smears of yolk sac. Furthermore, yolk sacs contain-ing greater than 10^7–10^8 rickettsiae per gram are required for the preparation of potent CF antigens and suspensions with toxic activity. Excellent detailed descriptions of the exacting requirements for cultivation of rickettsiae in em-bryonated eggs have been published (200). Also, information about the dy-namics of rickettsial growth in eggs has been summarized (223). Note should be made of the special conditions for optimal growth of members of the Spotted Fever Group (204).

Preparation of immune serum

Immune serum for use as a positive control in CF tests and for the identification of newly recovered agents is readily obtained from con-valescent guinea pigs. The illness caused by almost all rickettsial organisms is self-limiting. If highly lethal strains of *R. rickettsii, C. burnetii,* or others are encountered, the dose can usually be diluted sufficiently or administered subcutaneously so that infection does not result in death. The infectious inoculum for production of immune serum with members of the Typhus Group, Spotted Fever Group, and Q fever rickettsiae consists of spleen and other tissues harvested from guinea pigs. Mouse spleen serves as the immunizing antigen for scrub typhus-immune serum. The details describing selection of tissues, time of harvest, and method of processing are the same as given in "Rickettsia Isolation."

A preimmunization blood specimen is obtained from the guinea pig and tested; if the serum has anticomplementary activity or reacts nonspecifically with rickettsial or normal tissue antigens, the animal is discarded. Guinea pigs are inoculated intraperitoneally with infected tissue suspensions of Typhus and Spotted Fever Group organisms and intracerebrally with scrub typhus rickettsiae. The animals are exsanguinated 4 weeks later when maximal antibody titers should be present. In the case of Q fever, serum collected 2 weeks after infection contains moderate levels of only phase II CF antibody. After 50 days, significant levels of both phase I and II antibodies are present. If groups of guinea pigs are inoculated, each serum specimen is tested individually and pools are prepared by combining only specimens with satisfactory titers.

Rabbits are not satisfactory for the production of CF antibodies although high titers are obtained after rickettsial infection. Sera from unimmunized animals frequently react nonspecifically with rickettsial antigens derived from infected yolk sacs.

Serologic Diagnosis

Diagnosis of the etiology of rickettsial diseases can be accomplished most easily and rapidly by demonstrating a significant increase in specific antibodies in the serum of the patient during the course of infection and convalescence. Although a variety of serologic procedures have been developed, the laboratory that cannot prepare the needed reagents is limited to techniques which can be carried out with antigens available from commercial sources. At the present time, because of the small demand for the products, only materials for the Weil-Felix test and certain CF antigens can be obtained commercially.

In the United States, serum specimens from patients suspected of having rickettsial diseases can be sent to the local or state health department or to the Center for Disease Control (CDC), Atlanta, GA, where the appropriate routine diagnostic tests can be carried out. When specialized testing is needed, the CDC will refer the specimens to one of the few research laboratories where the procedure is carried out. The Rocky Mountain Laboratory, Hamilton, MT, and the Department of Microbiology, University of Maryland School of Medicine, Baltimore, MD, both serve as a World Health Organization Collaborating Center for Rickettsial Reference and Research.

Weil-Felix reaction

In rickettsial infections the Weil-Felix reaction depends upon the development of antibodies that agglutinate certain strains of nonmotile *Proteus* organisms. Serial 2-fold dilutions of serum are mixed with equal portions of suspensions of *P. vulgaris* OX_{19} and OX_2, and *P. mirabilis* OXK. The procedure (187) has been carried out both as a tube test and as a slide test. The former is more accurate and is preferred for use in the laboratory, while the latter is of value in field operations. The tube test is incubated at 37 C for 2 hr followed by storage overnight in the refrigerator, or at 52 C for 16–18 hr. The latter procedure is preferred because it intensifies the agglutination, and the test is easier to read. To be certain that the antigens are performing as expected, the controls for the test should include known positive human sera from proven cases of rickettsial disease, as well as negative human serum. Antigens from different commercial sources may vary markedly in specificity and sensitivity. Aging sometimes causes the antigens to react nonspecifically giving false-positive results. Paired sera are included in the same test, i.e., a specimen obtained as soon as possible after onset of disease and another obtained during convalescence. The test is considered positive if the antibody titer of the second specimen is ≥4-fold than that of the first specimen. The classic reactions obtained are summarized in Table 33.4.

Weil-Felix agglutinins, if they do develop, may appear as early as day 5 or 6 after the onset of disease, but they are usually present by day 12. Peak titers are evident during early convalescence, and the antibody levels then decline rapidly over the next several months. In murine typhus the *Proteus* agglutinins have been identified as IgM immunoglobulin (77). The test is nonspecific and provides only presumptive serologic evidence for the occurrence of rickettsial infection. The absence of a Weil-Felix response does not exclude a rickettsial etiology because patients with rickettsialpox, Q fever, or trench fever infection never develop *Proteus* agglutinins, and those with Brill-Zinsser disease only rarely do. Also, there have been patients with other Typhus Group and Spotted Fever Group infections who did not develop OX_{19} or OX_2 agglutinins. Outbreaks of scrub typhus have occurred in which none of the patients developed OXK agglutinins. False-positive reactions have been obtained with serum from patients with *Proteus* urinary tract infections, leptospirosis, *Borrelia* infections, and severe liver disease due to a variety of causes.

TABLE 33.4—WEIL-FELIX REACTION

	MAGNITUDE OF ANTIBODY RESPONSE		
	Proteus ANTIGENS		
RICKETTSIAL DISEASE	OX_{19}	OX_2	OXK
Epidemic typhus (primary)	+ + + +	+	0
Murine typhus	+ + + +	+	0
Rocky Mountain spotted fever	+ + + +	+	0
Other tickborne SFG infections*	+	+ + + +	0
Rickettsialpox	0	0	0
Scrub typhus	0	0	+ + + +
Q fever	0	0	0
Trench fever	0	0	0

*Spotted Fever Group

Complement-fixation test

Typhus and Spotted Fever Group-specific soluble CF antigens have been prepared by a variety of methods, all of which employ ether extraction of saline solution suspensions of infected yolk sacs (204, 211, 247). The procedure in current use in our laboratory is as follows (34):

A 50% wt/vol suspension of infected yolk sacs in McIlvaine buffered saline solution, pH 7.6, is centrifuged at 4 C for 30 min at 16,300 × g. The supernatant fluid and floating fat are discarded, and the sediment is resuspended in 1 ml of sterile distilled water for each gram of original yolk sac tissue. After storage at 4 C for 10–14 days, the suspension is extracted with 2 volumes of anesthetic ether or with a mixture of 9 parts absolute ether and 1 part 95% ethyl alcohol. The aqueous layer is extracted again with 1 volume of anesthetic ether or the ether-alcohol mixture. Residual ether is removed under partial vacuum, and the suspension is clarified by centrifugation at 365 X g for 10 min. For each 100 ml of antigen, 0.85 g NaCl is added. The final product is stored at −20 C when not in use. A control antigen is prepared in the same manner from yolk sacs of uninfected 14- to 16-day-old embryonated eggs.

Irrespective of the method of preparation or commercial source, soluble CF antigens will vary considerably with respect to species- and group-specificity. Before initial use, the degree of intragroup reactivity of an antigen should be assayed in grid- or block-type tests with immune guinea pig serum and, if possible, with human convalescent-phase serum representing each member of the group.

Highly purified suspensions of rickettsiae for use as species- or type-specific CF or agglutinating antigens have been obtained from infected yolk sac tissues by many different methods. No single procedure is applicable to all *Rickettsieae,* and the methods that have been used do not give uniformly satisfactory preparations.

Type-specific washed rickettsial antigens have been obtained with rickettsiae in the Typhus, Spotted Fever, and Scrub Typhus Groups and with *C. burnetii* by a series of differential centrifugations supplemented with ether extraction (63, 122, 172, 200), adsorption with celite (241), cation exchange resins (amberlite series) (250), and anion exchange resins (diethyl-amino-ethyl and ECTEOLA) (79); precipitation with bovine serum albumin (27, 70); use of hypertonic salt solutions (55, 154, 181); treatment with proteolytic enzymes (228, 241); and Genetron extraction (70) to remove extraneous host tissue components. In addition, anion exchange resins in chromatographic columns (100), density gradient sedimentation in sucrose (3, 4, 45, 181, 194, 248), glycerol-potassium tartrate (214), and Renografin-76 (65, 224) have provided highly purified rickettsial suspensions which have been used in studies of antigenic composition, immunogenicity, and metabolic activities.

Phase II Q fever organisms and suspensions of Typhus and Spotted Fever Group rickettsiae must be stored at 4 C; freezing and thawing potentiates spontaneous agglutination of Q fever rickettsiae, and the latter groups of organisms deteriorate, rendering the antigens less species-specific. Indeed, after relatively short periods of storage at 4 C, the Typhus and Spotted

Fever species-specific antigens often develop group-reactivity and must be reprocessed and restandardized before use.

The diagnosis of disease can be confirmed with use of group-soluble or species-specific corpuscular antigens when the convalescent-phase serum has a level of CF antibodies 4-fold greater than the titer of the acute-phase specimen. The finding of a significant level of antibodies or a sustained high titer in a series of convalescent-phase specimens should be considered only a presumptive diagnosis.

The CF test has been used widely for serologic detection of infection in domestic and wild animals for ecologic studies. Since both soluble and type-specific washed antigens satisfactory for use with human serum may react nonspecifically with animal serum, positive results do not always indicate the presence of specific antibodies (167). Although the mode of action has yet to be defined, the nonspecific reactivity of animal serum may be eliminated by treatment with dry ice (103). The serum to be tested is diluted 1:10 with sterile distilled water, and a small piece of dry ice is added. When bubbling has ceased, the precipitate that has formed is removed by centrifugation at 2000 rpm. To each 0.9 ml of the supernatant fluid is added 0.1 ml of 8.5% saline solution. Prior to CF testing the treated specimen is heat-inactivated in the standard manner. Also, anticomplementary reactivity may be reduced by inactivating the initial serum dilution at 60 C for 30 min.

Typhus and Spotted Fever Group infections. Identification of the etiologic agent as a member of the Typhus or Spotted Fever Group of rickettsiae is readily obtained by using respective group-specific soluble CF antigens. Owing to the distinctive differences in geographic distribution and ecology of these rickettsial diseases, information about circumstances of possible exposure to known arthropod vectors often permits a presumptive diagnosis. Definitive identification of the causative agent requires the use of species-specific washed corpuscular antigens.

CF antibodies generally appear in the patient's serum toward the end of the second week after onset of disease, attain peak titers during the succeeding 2 weeks, and decline slowly thereafter over the next 8-11 months. Low levels of antibody may persist in certain individuals for years, particularly after primary epidemic typhus infection. The antibody response of the patient who receives specific antibiotic therapy early in the course of disease may be delayed, and the titers diminished (199). However, it is unlikely that early treatment would prevent completely the development of antibodies. The extensive experience of the CDC with use of soluble antigens prepared with members of the Typhus and Spotted Fever Groups for diagnosing rickettsial diseases in the United States during the period 1971-1974 has been summarized (189).

Serologic diagnosis of primary epidemic typhus or murine typhus infection when the patient has not been vaccinated can be established by using the respective species-specific CF antigens. The higher antibody titer corresponds to the causative agent. Difficulties may be encountered in serologic diagnosis of Brill-Zinsser disease and when epidemic or murine typhus occurs in an individual who has been immunized previously with epidemic typhus vaccine. In contrast to the findings in primary epidemic typhus, the antibodies in Brill-Zinsser patients appear during the first week after onset and usually attain peak titers between the eighth and tenth day. Further-more, the CF antibodies in recrudescent typhus are principally IgG, whereas in primary typhus the antibodies are IgM (144, 146). If the serum is treated with ethanethiol or heated to 60 C for 30 min, it is possible to distinguish between the two classes of immunoglobulins simply and rapidly in a CF test (145). In contrast, after murine typhus infection, CF antibodies detected by soluble and corpuscular antigens on the thirteenth day were both IgM and IgG, and after 90 days the serologic reactivity present was only in the IgG immunoglobulin (77).

If an individual was vaccinated with epidemic typhus vaccine, it is gen-erally not possible to differentiate between a subsequent epidemic typhus or murine typhus infection by the CF test because antibody titers with the spe-cies-specific antigens are not significantly different. However, when these same antigens are used in agglutination tests, diagnostic results are ob-tained (197).

Scrub typhus. CF tests utilizing soluble antigens obtained by ether ex-traction of suspensions of infected yolk sacs have not been satisfactory for routine diagnostic use. Although positive findings in tests with soluble anti-gens provide an etiologic diagnosis, failure to demonstrate antibodies in con-valescent-phase serum does not exclude scrub typhus infection because of the strain-specific reactivity displayed by these preparations and the marked antigenic diversity that exists among strains. Partially purified antigens of whole rickettsiae prepared from yolk sacs infected with Karp, Kato, and Gilliam prototype strains have been used for laboratory diagnosis of acute disease and for seroepidemiologic surveys for past and inapparent infections in Japan (191). However, since these antigens tend to be anticomplementary and to react nonspecifically with human serum, it is difficult to detect low levels of antibody (76, 123). More recently, antigens derived from BS-C-1 cell cultures infected with the prototype strains have given satisfactory re-sults (12), but these reagents must be evaluated further before they can be accepted for routine diagnostic use. At the present time, indirect immuno-fluorescent staining is the preferred method for serologic diagnosis of scrub typhus infection.

Q fever. After *C. burnetii* infection, antibodies which fix complement in the presence of suspensions of phase II rickettsiae are present in about 65% of patients in the second week after onset of disease and in more than 90% by the fourth week (132). In uncomplicated illness, phase I CF antibodies are found infrequently. In the absence of prior vaccination, the presence of high levels of phase I CF antibody is considered diagnostic of past or current chronic Q fever infection. This finding is of particular value in the recogni-tion of subacute Q fever endocarditis (141, 174).

Indirect fluorescent-antibody test

Indirect FA staining employing smears of rickettsial organisms as anti-gens can be used for the serologic diagnosis of rickettsial infections of hu-mans (73). However, positive FA reactions identify only the antigenic group to which the causative agent belongs and not the rickettsial species. Thus, infections with Typhus Group, Spotted Fever Group, Scrub Typhus Group, and Q fever rickettsiae can be distinguished from each other. Epidemic and murine typhus infections have been differentiated by indirect immuno-fluorescence by antibody absorption methods using soluble antigens (91). It is possible also with the indirect FA test to determine the immunoglobulin class of the rickettsial antibodies directly by using specific anti-immunoglobulin conjugates without having to pretreat the serum as is necessary with the CF test. However, more experience with the use of this refinement must be gained before its value in the laboratory diagnosis of disease can be assessed. A variation of the indirect FA staining procedure in which complement, bound to a rickettsial antigen-antibody reaction, was stained by an anti-guinea pig serum fluorescein conjugate has been described (90), but the technique has been difficult to duplicate and has not been widely used. More recently, a micro-IF test was developed which has been shown to be a highly specific and sensitive method for serologic diagnosis and epidemiologic studies of the trachoma-inclusion conjunctivitis (TRIC) and lymphogranuloma venereum (LGV) chlamydiae (218), as well as for the immunologic classification of the TRIC-LGV organisms (219). The micro-IF test, which has the important technical advantage over other FA procedures of being able to react the same drop of diluted serum with 9 different antigens simultaneously, has been used for serologic studies of patients with Rocky Mountain Spotted Fever and Typhus Group infections (168, 169) and with epidemic typhus (159).

The indirect FA test has its greatest value in the specific diagnosis of *R. tsutsugamushi* infection (29, 30). At present, the Karp, Kato, and Gilliam strains of the Scrub Typhus Group are used as antigens, but other strains may be found in the future which should be included to cover the spectrum of antigenically diverse strains that exist within the group. On the basis of information available to date, approximately 60% of 65 patients experiencing their first scrub typhus infection had antibodies detected with one or more of the antigens as early as day 5 or 6 after onset. The number of positive reactors increased during the succeeding days, and between days 18 and 20, patients had significant levels of antibody. Peak titers were observed during the fourth week and declined slowly over a period of months. Significant titers ($\geq 1:40$) were present after 6 months, and 73% of the patients still had positive titers 12–19 months after onset of the disease. In patients who had experienced more than one scrub typhus infection, significant levels of antibodies persisted for as long as 12.5 years after the last illness.

Diagnosis depends on the demonstration of an $\geq$8-fold increase in antibody titer when 4-fold serial dilutions of the specimen are tested. This should be possible in all instances if the acute-phase serum is drawn on or before the fourth day of disease and the convalescent-phase serum is collected during the fourth week. However, as in the serologic diagnosis of other rickettsial diseases, it is possible in many instances to show significant increases in antibody levels when the first specimen is obtained at the end of the first week and the second specimen at the end of the second week. Second and third attacks of scrub typhus occur, and antibodies persisting from a previous infection may be detected at significant levels with one of the antigens early in the course of the current disease. Nevertheless, it should be possible to demonstrate diagnostically significant increases in antibody titer in later specimens with the other antigens.

Agglutination tests

With highly purified rickettsial suspensions used as antigens, agglutination tests have been employed to diagnose epidemic and murine typhus and Rocky Mountain spotted fever. If the patient has been vaccinated previously with epidemic typhus, the agglutination test is often the only serologic procedure that differentiates between epidemic and murine typhus infections. In Q fever studies agglutination tests have been used for detection of past and current infections in humans and in domestic and wild animals, as well as for investigation of the antibody response following vaccination. The procedure has been used only rarely with Spotted Fever Group organisms. Currently, the antigens are prepared from infected yolk sacs (see above), but satisfactory materials have been obtained in the past from lungs of intranasally infected mice (46). Because the antigens are difficult to prepare and cannot be obtained from a commercial source, the rickettsial agglutination test has not been adopted for routine serologic diagnosis in clinical laboratories.

A variety of methods of performing agglutination tests has been developed. Macroscopic tests with Typhus Group antigens in which the reaction is visible to the unaided eye have been carried out in special conical-shaped tubes (172), as well as with reduced volumes of reagents mixed and incubated on glass slides (46, 80). A more sensitive method for detecting Q fever (7) and other rickettsial antibodies (88) is the microscope slide agglutination test. In this test, the occurrence of agglutination after incubation is evaluated by microscopic examination of the antigen-serum dilution mixture on the slide after it has dried and has been stained. In this procedure it is often difficult to differentiate specific agglutination from artifact produced by drying. The capillary tube agglutination test employing *C. burnetii* antigen stained with hemotoxylin (133), which facilitates reading, was developed as a seroepidemiologic tool to detect Q fever antibody in bovine serum and milk (135) and has had limited use for examining sera from humans, guinea pigs, and sheep (134). In the Q fever agglutination-resuspension test (155), the test serum, diluted in a 25% bovine serum-saline diluent, is mixed with antigen and is centrifuged after incubation. The presence of agglutination is determined by observing the state of the antigen when the pellet is resuspended.

Recently the microtiter technique has been adapted for use in a microagglutination test for Q fever, epidemic and murine typhus (78, 159), and Rocky Mountain spotted fever (168). A highly purified suspension of phase I *C. burnetii* stained with hematoxylin is used to detect phase I antibody. Because of the tendency to agglutinate spontaneously, phase II organisms cannot be used in agglutination tests. Trichloroacetic acid treatment of phase I organisms removes phase I antigen. Organisms treated in this manner react as phase II antigens in CF and agglutination tests. These antigens can be stained, are stable, and can be used in the microagglutination test. Highly purified *R. prowazekii* and *R. typhi* suspensions become unstable when stained with hematoxylin and are unsuitable for agglutination reactions. These antigens are therefore used unstained, and reading of the test is facilitated by addition of acridine orange after incubation. The agglutination tests carried out in this manner show a high degree of specificity and sensitivity.

The agglutination test is more sensitive than the CF test and somewhat less so than the micro-IF test. Rickettsial agglutinins generally can be detected earlier in the course of disease and persist longer after convalescence than do CF antibodies. In primary epidemic typhus (146), the agglutinins demonstrated from day 11 through day 58 were identified as IgM immunoglobulin. Similarly, in murine typhus the agglutinating activity was associated with the same class of immunoglobulin (77). In Brill-Zinsser disease the rickettsial agglutinin was identified as IgG immunoglobulin (146).

With the exception of the Q fever capillary tube agglutination test (133) and the agglutination-resuspension test (155), which employ phase I antigens, the phase status of the antigens used in prior studies of the antibody response following natural infection has not been documented. With antigens of known phase activity, phase II agglutinins appear toward the end of the first week after onset and attain maximal titer 2 weeks later. Phase I agglutinins are found toward the end of the second week and are significantly lower in titer than the phase II agglutinins (78). The immunoglobulin identity of the respective agglutinins has not been reported.

Other serologic procedures

Other serologic procedures have been employed in the past for detection of rickettsial antibodies, and from time to time there is a resurgence of interest in them. The latest-reported new addition to the list of serologic procedures is an enzyme-linked immunosorbent assay (ELISA) using soluble group-specific antigens prepared from *R. prowazekii* and *R. typhi* (94). The ELISA titers are higher by 1 or 2 orders of magnitude and somewhat more type-specific than those obtained with CF with the same soluble antigens. The applicability of the assay to detection of antibodies induced by other species of the *Rickettsieae* and its utility in the serologic diagnoses of human disease remain to be established. In the main the tests have not been used extensively for diagnosing disease but have been of value in basic research.

Q fever antiglobulin sensitization tests. These procedures are based on the principles of the test used for the detection of incomplete Rh antibodies. The original antiglobulin sensitization test, which employed washed suspensions of *C. burnetii*, was specific and considerably more sensitive than direct agglutination (56). The sensitivity of the technique was increased by tagging the Q fever phase I organism with radioactive iodine (^{131}I). In the radioisotope precipitation (RIP) test, the radiolabeled antigen is added to serial dilutions of the serum specimens under investigation, and the antigen-antibody complex is agglutinated by the corresponding antiglobulin. Low-speed centrifugation is used to sediment the agglutinated rickettsiae, and if the residual radioactivity of the supernatant fluid is less than 50% of the original, the test is positive (131, 209). The RIP test has been used for epidemiologic studies (68, 139) and for evaluation of the response of humans to vaccination.

Toxin neutralization test. The ability of concentrated suspensions of rickettsiae belonging to the Typhus Group, certain members of the Spotted Fever Group, and the Gilliam, Karp, and Kato strains of the Scrub Typhus Group to kill mice within a few hours after intravenous inoculation has been described in earlier sections. Although specific antibodies that neutralize the toxic phenomenon appear in the serum of patients during the second week after infection and may persist for years, the test has not been used as a diagnostic procedure because of technical difficulties. The nonspecific neutralization of the toxic effect of *R. typhi* suspensions by a normal β-lipoprotein component in the serum of some people and monkeys has also been described. The test has been used principally in the identification and classification of Typhus and Spotted Fever Group rickettsial strains and in the evaluation of potency and effectiveness of epidemic typhus vaccines. It is used less frequently as a seroepidemiologic tool.

Indirect hemagglutination (IHA) test. Untreated human group O and sheep RBC sensitized with ESS obtained by heat and alkali treatment of Typhus and Spotted Fever Group rickettsiae are agglutinated by antibodies in the serum of patients convalescing from the corresponding disease (48–50). Glutaraldehyde-treated sheep RBC can be used also (190). The antibodies are first detected during the second week of illness, attain peak titers during the third week, and disappear in 3-6 months. In murine typhus the ESS agglutinin is associated with the IgM immunoglobulin (77). Comparison of the relative sensitivity and specificity of the IHA test with the CF and Weil-Felix tests for the diagnosis of Rocky Mountain Spotted Fever and Typhus Group infections (190), as well as with the CF, micro-IF, and micro-agglutination tests for the diagnosis of Rocky Mountain spotted fever (168) have been carried out. Positive results indicate only the group identity of the infecting organism. Although the test was considered more sensitive, economical, technically simpler, and as reliable as CF, the procedure has not been utilized as a diagnostic tool.

In a limited experience with 7 cases, an IHA test for trench fever employing sonicated antigen adsorbed onto tanned sheep RBC detected antibody as early as 4 days after the onset of primary disease. Persistence of antibody varied from 4 to 24 months in primary disease and for as long as 12 months after relapse. Although antibodies belonging to both IgM and IgG classes were detected, the major reactive antibody was IgG (58).

Neutralization test. This test, in which antibody is added to a suspension of organisms and the mixture is injected into susceptible animals, has not generally given as clear-cut results with rickettsiae as has been obtained with certain viral agents. The procedure has been used as an extremely sensitive means of detecting serologic evidence of Q fever infection in epidemiologic surveys (1) and for antigenic characterization of strains of the Scrub Typhus Group (24). Tissue culture has not been used to any great extent for plaque reduction or other types of Nt tests. The early experience indicated that the technique would not be suitable for diagnostic purposes (13, 54). Typhus-immune serum, with or without complement, has no direct rickettsiocidal action on *R. prowazekii* or *R. typhi* and does not prevent infection of chicken embryo cells in culture and subsequent rickettsial growth (246). However, specific plaque reduction correlated to rickettsial antibody concentration was demonstrated when a goat antimonkey immuno-globulin was added to the mixture of rickettsiae and immune monkey serum before inoculation of chicken embryo cell cultures (114).

Acknowledgement

We express our sincere appreciation to Mr. Charles F. Needy and Mrs. Naomi I. Stocks for their assistance in the bibliographic research and to Mrs. Carol C. Lee for her efforts in the preparation of the manuscript.

References

1. ABINANTI FR and MARMION BP: Protective or neutralizing antibody in Q fever. Am J Hyg 66:173–195, 1957
2. ALLISON AC and BURKE DC: The nucleic acid contents of viruses. J Gen Microbiol 27:181–194, 1962
3. ANACKER RL, GERLOFF RK, THOMAS LA, MANN RE, and BICKEL WD: Immunological properties of *Rickettsia rickettsii* purified by zonal centrifugation. Infect Immun 11:1203–1209, 1975
4. ANACKER RL, GERLOFF RK, THOMAS LA, MANN RE, BROWN WR, and BICKEL WD: Purification of *Rickettsia rickettsi* by density gradient zonal centrifugation. Can J Microbiol 20:1523–1527, 1974
5. ANACKER RL, PICKENS EG, and LACKMAN DB: Details of the ultrastructure of *Rickettsia prowazekii* grown in the chick yolk sac. J Bacteriol 94:260–262, 1967
6. ANDERSON DR, HOPPS HE, BARILE MF, and BERNHEIM BC: Comparison of the ultra-structure of several rickettsiae, ornithosis virus, and mycoplasma in tissue culture. J Bacteriol 90:1387–1404, 1965
7. BABUDIERI B: Studies on the microscopic slide-agglutination test for Q fever. Bull WHO 19:981–994, 1958
8. BABUDIERI B: Q fever: a zoonosis. Adv Vet Sci 5:81–182, 1959
9. BACA OG and PARETSKY D: Partial chemical characterization of a toxic lipolysaccharide from *Coxiella burneti*. Infect Immun 9:959–961, 1974
10. BAKEMEIER RF: A study of phase variation in *Coxiella burnetii* employing hemagglutina-tion tests. J Immunol 95:880–886, 1965
11. BAKER JA: A rickettsial infection in canadian voles. J Exp Med 84:37–51, 1946
12. BARKER LF and PATT JK: Production of rickettsial complement-fixing antigens in tissue culture. J Immunol 100:821–824, 1968
13. BARKER LF, PATT JK, and HOPPS HE: Titration and neutralization of *Rickettsia tsutsuga-mushi* in tissue culture. J Immunol 100:825–830, 1968
14. BEAMAN L and WISSEMAN CL JR: Mechanisms of immunity in typhus infections. V. Dem-onstration of *Rickettsia mooseri*-specific antibodies in convalescent mouse and hu-man serum cytophilic for mouse peritoneal macrophages. Infect Immun 14:1065–1070, 1976
15. BEAMAN L and WISSEMAN CL JR: Mechanisms of immunity in typhus infections. VI. Differential opsonizing and neutralizing action of human typhus *Rickettsia*-specific cytophilic antibodies in cultures of human macrophages. Infect Immun 14:1071–1076, 1976
16. BELL EJ, KOHLS GM, STOENNER HG, and LACKMAN DB: Non-pathogenic rickettsias related to the spotted fever group isolated from ticks, *Dermacentor variabilis* and *Dermacentor andersoni* from eastern Montana. J Immunol 90:770–781, 1963
17. BELL EJ, LACKMAN DB, ORMSBEE RA, and PEACOCK M: Neutralization of murine typhus toxin by serum of normal human beings and monkeys. Am J Trop Med Hyg 18:559–572, 1969

18. BELL EJ, MUNOZ JJ, PEACOCK M, and COLE RL: Murine typhus toxin: studies on identification of the neutralizing factor present in normal human serum. Infect Immun 6:232–239, 1972

19. BELL EJ and PICKENS EG: A toxic substance associated with the rickettsias of the spotted fever group. J Immunol 70:461–472, 1953

20. BELL EJ and STOENNER HG: Immunologic relationships among the spotted fever group of rickettsias determined by toxin neutralization tests in mice with convalescent animal serums. J Immunol 84:171–182, 1960

21. BELL EJ and STOENNER HG: Spotted fever vaccine: potency assay by direct challenge of vaccinated mice with toxin of *Rickettsia rickettsii*. J Immunol 87:737–746, 1961

22. BENGTSON IA: Apparent serological heterogeneity among strains of tsutsugamushi disease (scrub typhus). Public Health Rep 60:1483–1488, 1945

23. BENGTSON IA: A serological study of 37 cases of tsutsugamushi disease (scrub typhus) occurring in Burma and the Philippine Islands. Public Health Rep 61:887–894, 1946

24. BENNETT BL, SMADEL JE, and GAULD RL: Studies on scrub typhus (tsutsugamushi disease). IV. Heterogeneity of strains of *R. tsutsugamushi* as demonstrated by cross-neutralization tests. J Immunol 62:453–461, 1949

25. Bergey's Manual of Determinative Bacteriology. The Rickettsias. 8th edition, BUCHANAN RE and GIBBONS NE (eds), Williams and Wilkins Company, Baltimore, 1974, pp 882–893.

26. BOVARNICK MR: Incorporation of acetate-1-C^{14} into lipids by typhus rickettsiae. J Bacteriol 80:508–512, 1960

27. BOVARNICK MR and MILLER JC: Oxidation and transamination of glutamate by typhus rickettsiae. J Biol Chem 184:661–676, 1950

28. BOVARNICK MR, MILLER JC, and SNYDER JC: The influence of certain salts, amino acids, sugars, and proteins on the stability of rickettsiae. J Bacteriol 59:509–522, 1950

29. BOZEMAN FM, and ELISBERG BL: Serological diagnosis of scrub typhus by indirect immunofluorescence. Proc Soc Exp Biol Med 112:568–573, 1963

30. BOZEMAN FM and ELISBERG BL: Studies of the antibody response in scrub typhus employing indirect immunofluorescence. Acta Med Biol 15(Suppl):105–111, 1967

31. BOZEMAN FM, ELISBERG BL, HUMPHRIES JW, RUNCIK K, and PALMER DB JR: Serologic evidence of *Rickettsia canada* infection of man. J Infect Dis 121:367–371, 1970

32. BOZEMAN FM, HOPPS HE, DANAUSKAS JX, JACKSON EB, and SMADEL JE: Study on the growth of rickettsiae. I. A tissue culture system for quantitative estimations of *Rickettsia tsutsugamushi*. J Immunol 76:475–488, 1956

33. BOZEMAN FM, MASIELLO SA, WILLIAMS MS, and ELISBERG BL: Epidemic typhus rickettsiae isolated from flying squirrels. Nature 255:545–547, 1975

34. BOZEMAN FM, SHIRAI A, HUMPHRIES JW, and FULLER HS: Ecology of Rocky Mountain spotted fever. II. Natural infection of wild mammals and birds in Virginia and Maryland. Am J Trop Med Hyg 16:48–59, 1967

35. BOZEMAN FM, WILLIAMS MS, STOCKS NI, CHADWICK DP, ELISBERG BL, SONENSHINE DE, and LAUER DM: Ecological studies on epidemic typhus infection in the eastern flying squirrel, *In* Rickettsiae and Rickettsial Diseases, Kazar J, Ormsbee RA, and Tarasevich IN (eds) VEDA, Bratislava, 1978, pp 493–504

36. BUHLES WC, JR, HUXSOLL DL, and ELISBERG BL: Isolation of *Rickettsia rickettsi* in primary bone marrow cell and circulating monocyte cultures derived from experimentally infected guinea pigs. Infect Immun 7:1003–1005, 1973

37. BUHLES WC, HUXSOLL DL, RUCH G, KENYON RH, and ELISBERG BL: Evaluation of primary blood monocyte and bone marrow cell culture for the isolation of *Rickettsia rickettsii*. Infect Immun 12:1457–1463, 1975

38. BURGDORFER W: Evaluation of the fluorescent antibody technique for the detection of Rocky Mountain spotted fever rickettsiae in various tissues. Pathol Microbiol 24(Suppl):27–39, 1961

39. BURGDORFER W: Hemolymph test: a technique for detection of rickettsiae in ticks. Am J Trop Med Hyg 19:1010–1014, 1970

40. BURGDORFER W: A review of Rocky Mountain spotted fever (tick-borne typhus), its agent, and its tick vectors in the United States. J Med Entomol 12:269–278, 1975

41. BURGDORFER W, ADKINS TA, JR, and PRIESTER LE: Rocky Mountain spotted fever (tick-borne typhus) in South Carolina: an educational program and tick/rickettsial survey in 1973 and 1974. Am J Trop Med Hyg 24:866-872, 1975

42. BURGDORFER W and BUNTON LP: Intranuclear growth of *Rickettsia canada,* a member of the typhus group. Infect Immun 2:112-114, 1970

43. BURGDORFER W, COONEY JC, and THOMAS LA: Zoonotic potential (Rocky Mountain spotted fever and tularemia) in the Tennessee Valley region. II. Prevalence of *Rickettsia rickettsi* and *Francisella tularensis* in mammals and ticks from land between the lakes. Am J Trop Med Hyg 23:109-117, 1974

44. BURGDORFER W, SEXTON DJ, GERLOFF RK, ANACKER RL, PHILIP RN, and THOMAS LA: *Rhipicephalus sanguineus:* Vector of a new spotted fever group rickettsia in the United States. Infect Immun 12:205-210, 1975

45. CANONICO PG, VAN ZWEITEN MJ, and CHRISTMAS WA: Purification of large quantities of *Coxiella burnettii* rickettsia by density gradient zonal centrifugation. Appl Microbiol 23:1015-1022, 1972

46. CASTAÑEDA MR: Differentiation of typhus strains by slide-agglutinative tests. J Immunol 50:179-183, 1945

47. CHAN ML, McCHESNEY J, and PARETSKY D: Further characterization of a lipopolysaccharide from *Coxiella burneti.* Infect Immun 13:1721-1727, 1976

48. CHANG RS-M: A serologically active erythrocyte-sensitizing substance from typhus rickettsiae. I. Isolation and titration. J Immunol 70:212-214, 1953

49. CHANG RS-M, MURRAY ES, and SNYDER JC: Erythrocyte-sensitizing substances from rickettsiae of the Rocky Mountain spotted fever group. J Immunol 73:8-15, 1954

50. CHANG RS-M, SNYDER JC, and MURRAY ES: A serologically active erythrocyte-sensitizing substance from typhus rickettsiae. II. Serological properties. J Immunol 70:215-221, 1953

51. CHERRY WB, GOLDMAN M, CARSKI TR, and MOODY MD: Fluorescent antibody techniques in the diagnosis of communicable diseases. Public Health Service Publication No. 729, US Government Printing Office, Washington, DC, 1961

52. CLAVERO G and PEREZ GALLARDO F: Estudios sobre la cepa e de *Rickettsia prowazeki* viva en la immunizacion humana. Rev Sanid Hig Publica 17:547-560, 1944

53. COHEN AB, HATGI JN, and WISSEMAN CL JR: Storage stability of different antibody species against arbovirus and rickettsial antigens in blood dried on filter paper discs. Am J Epidemiol 89:345-352, 1969

54. COHN ZA, BOZEMAN FM, CAMPBELL JM, HUMPHRIES JW, and SAWYER TK: Study on growth of rickettsiae. V. Penetration of *Rickettsia tsutsugamuchi* into mammalian cells in vitro. J Exp Med 109:271-292, 1959

55. COLTER JS, BROWN RA, BIRD HH, and COX HR: The preparation of a soluble immunizing antigen from Q-Fever rickettsiae. J Immunol 76:270-274, 1956

56. COOMBS RRA and STOKER MGP: Detection of Q fever antibodies by the antiglobulin sensitization test. Lancet 2:15-17, 1951

57. COONS AH, SNYDER JC, CHEEVER FS, and MURRAY ES: Localization of antigen in tissue cells. IV. Antigens of rickettsiae and mumps virus. J Exp Med 91:31-38, 1950

58. COOPER MD, HOLLINGSDALLE MR, VINSON JW, and COSTA J: A passive hemagglutination test for diagnosis of trench fever due to *Rochalimaea quintana.* J Infect Dis 134:605- 609, 1976

59. CORY J and YUNKER CE: Rickettsial plaques in mosquito cell monolayers. Acta Virol 18:512-513, 1974

60. CORY J, YUNKER CE, ORMSBEE RA, PEACOCK M, MEIBOS H, and TALLENT G: Plaque assay of rickettsiae in a mammalian cell line. Appl Microbiol 27:1157-1161, 1974

61. COX HR: Cultivation of rickettsiae of Rocky Mountain spotted fever, typhus and Q fever groups in the embryonic tissues of developing chicks. Science 94:399-403, 1941

62. COX HR: Use of yolk sac of developing chick embryo as medium for growing rickettsiae of Rocky Mountain spotted fever and typhus groups. Public Health Rep 53:2241-2247, 1938

63. CRAIGIE J: Application and control of ethyl-ether-water interface effects to the separation of rickettsiae from yolk sac suspensions. Can J Res, Sect E 23:104-114, 1945

64. DASCH GA, SAMMS JR, and WEISS E: Biochemical characteristics of typhus group rickettsiae with special attention to the *Rickettsia prowazekii* strains isolated from flying squirrels. Infect Immun 19:676-685, 1978

65. DASCH GA and WEISS E: Characterization of the Madrid E strain of *Rickettsia prowazekii* purified by renografin density gradient centrifugation. Infect Immun 15:280-286, 1977

66. DAVIS GE and COX HR: A filter-passing infectious agent isolated from ticks. I. Isolation from *Dermacentor andersoni*, reactions in animals, and filtration experiments. Public Health Rep 53:2259-2267, 1938

67. DAVIS GE and PARKER RR: Comparative experiments on spotted fever and boutonneuse fever. Public Health Rep 49:423-428, 1934

68. DEIBEL R, OSTERHOUT G, and CULVER J: Immune globulins to *Coxiella burneti* in man determined by radioisotope precipitation technic. Am J Epidemiol 90:262-268, 1969

69. DESHAZO RD, BOYCE JR, OSTERMAN JV, and STEPHENSON EH: Early diagnosis of Rocky Mountain spotted fever. J Am Med Assoc 235:1353-1355, 1976

70. DUBOIS DR, CUTCHINS EC, BERMAN S, LOWENTHAL JP, and TIMCHAK RL: Preparation of purified suspensions of *Coxiella burneti* by genetron extraction followed by continuous-flow ultracentrifugation. Appl Microbiol 23:841-845, 1972

71. EISEMANN CS and OSTERMAN JV: Proteins of typhus and spotted fever group rickettsiae. Infect Immun 14:155-162, 1976

72. ELISBERG BL: The Rickettsial Diseases *In* Current Diagnosis, 3rd edition, Conn HF and Conn RB Jr (eds). WB Saunders Co, Philadelphia 1971, pp 151-164

73. ELISBERG BL and BOZEMAN FM: Serological diagnosis of rickettsial diseases by indirect immunofluorescence. Arch Inst Pasteur Tunis 43:193-204, 1966

74. ELISBERG BL, CAMPBELL JM, and BOZEMAN FM: Antigenic diversity of *Rickettsia tsutsugamushi:* epidemiologic and ecologic significance. J Hyg Epidemiol Microbiol Immunol 12:18-25, 1968

75. ELISBERG BL, NEEDY CF, and BOZEMAN FM: Antigenic interrelationships among strains of *Rickettsia tsutsugamushi. In* Rickettsiae and Rickettsial Diseases, Kazar J, Ormsbee RA, and Tarasevich (eds), VEDA, Bratislava, 1978, pp 253-262

76. ELISBERG BL, SANGKASUVANA V, CAMPBELL JM, BOZEMAN FM, BODHIDATTA P, and RAPMUND G: Physiogeographic distribution of scrub typhus in Thailand. Acta Med Biol 15(Suppl):61-67, 1967

77. ELISBERG BL, WOOD WH JR, and BELLANTI JA: Serologic properties of immune globulins in human murine typhus. (Abstr) Fed Proc 29:420, 1967

78. FISET P, ORMSBEE RA, SILBERMAN R, PEACOCK M, and SPIELMAN SH: A microagglutination technique for detection and measurement of rickettsial antibodies. Acta Virol 13:60-66, 1969

79. FISET P and SILBERMAN R: Purification des rickettsies au moyen d'echangeur d'ions. Arch Inst Pasteur Tunis 43:231-236, 1966

80. FITZPATRICK FK: Studies on rickettsial agglutination in typhus. J Lab Clin Med 30:577-586, 1945

81. FOX JP, MONTOYA JA, JORDAN ME, CORNEJO UBILLUS JR, GARCIA JL, ESTRADA MA, and GELFAND HM: Immunization of man against epidemic typhus by infection with avirulent *Rickettsia prowazeki* (Strain E) V. A brief review and observations during a $3^{1}/_{2}$ year period as to the occurrence of typhus among vaccinated and control populations in the Peruvian Andes. Arch Inst Pasteur Tunis 36:449-479, 1959

82. FULLER HS: Biologic properties of pathogenic rickettsiae. Arch Inst Pasteur Tunis 36:311-338, 1959

83. GAMBRILL MR and WISSEMAN CL JR: Mechanisms of immunity in typhus infections. II. Multiplication of typhus rickettsiae in human macrophage cell cultures in the nonimmune system: influence of rickettsial strains and of chloramphenicol. Infect Immun 8:519-527, 1973

84. GAMBRILL MR and WISSEMAN CL JR: Mechanisms of immunity in typhus infections. III. Influence of human immune serum and complement on the fate of *Rickettsia mooseri* within human macrophages. Infect Immun 8:631-640, 1973

85. GILDEMEISTER E and HAAGEN E: Fleckfieberstudien I Mitteilung: nachweis eines toxins in Rickettsien-Eikulturen (*Rickettsia mooseri*). Dtsch Med Wochenschr 66:878-880, 1940

86. GIMÉNEZ DF: Staining rickettsiae in yolk-sac cultures. Stain Technol 39:135–140, 1964

87. GIMÉNEZ DF: Gram staining of *Coxiella burnetii.* J Bacteriol 90:834–835, 1965

88. GIROUD P and GIROUD ML: Agglutination des rickettsiaes, test de séroprotection et réaction d'hypersensibilité cutanée. Bull Soc Pathol Exot 37:84–93, 1944

89. GOLDWASSER RA and HALEVY M: Differentiation of phase I and phase II *Coxiella burnetii* by means of fluorescent antibody techniques. Israel J Med Sci 8:583–587, 1972

90. GOLDWASSER RA and SHEPARD CC: Staining of complement and modification of fluorescent antibody procedures. J Immunol 80:122–131, 1958

91. GOLDWASSER RA and SHEPARD CC: Fluorescent antibody methods in the differentiation of murine and epidemic typhus sera; specificity changes resulting from previous immunization. J Immunol 82:373–380, 1959

92. GOLDWASSER RA, STEIMAN Y, KLINGBERG W, SWARTZ T, and KLINGBERG MA: The isolation of strains of rickettsiae of the spotted fever group in Israel and their differentiation from other members of the group by immunofluorescence methods. Scand J Infect Dis 6:53–62, 1974

93. HAHON N and ZIMMERMAN WD: Intracellular survival of viral and rickettsial agents in acetone at −60 C. Appl Microbiol 17:775–776, 1969

94. HALLE S, DASCH GA, and WEISS E: Sensitive enzyme-linked immunosorbent assay for detection of antibodies against typhus rickettsiae, *Rickettsia prowazekii* and *Rickettsia typhi.* J Clin Microbiol 6:101–110, 1977

95. HAMILTON HL: Specificity of the toxic factors associated with epidemic and murine strains of typhus rickettsiae. Am J Trop Med 25:391–395, 1945

96. HINRICHS DJ and JERRELLS TR: In vitro evaluation of immunity to *Coxiella burnetii.* J Immunol 117:996–1003, 1976

97. HOPPS HE, JACKSON EB, DANAUSKAS JX, and SMADEL JE: Study on the growth of rickettsiae. III. Influence of extracellular environment on the growth of *Rickettsia tsutsugamushi* in tissue culture cells. J Immunol 82:161–171, 1959

98. HOPPS HE, JACKSON EB, DANAUSKAS JX, and SMADEL JE: Study on the growth of rickettsiae. IV. Effect of chloramphenicol and several metabolic inhibitors on the multiplication of *Rickettsia tsutsugamushi* in tissue culture cells. J Immunol 82:172–181, 1959

99. HOPPS HE, KOHNO S, KOHNO M, and SMADEL JE: Production of interferon in tissue cultures infected with *Rickettsia tsutsugamushi.* (Abstr) Bact Proc 1:115, 1964

100. HOYER BH, BOLTON ET, ORMSBEE RA, LEBOUVIER G, RITTER DG, and LARSON CL: Mammalian viruses and rickettsiae. Science 127:859–863, 1958

101. HUGHES LE, CLIFFORD CM, GRESBRINK R, THOMAS LA, and KEIRANS JE: Isolation of a spotted fever group rickettsia from the Pacific Coast tick, *Ixodes pacificus,* in Oregon. Am J Trop Med Hyg 25:513–515, 1976

102. IIDA T, KAWASHIMA H, and KAWAMURA A: Direct immunofluorescence for typing of tsutsugamushi disease rickettsiae. J Immunol 95:1129–1133, 1965

103. IMAM IZE and ALFY L: The elimination of the anticomplementary reactions of the sera by CO_2. J Egypt Public Health Assoc 41:33–36, 1966

104. ITO S and VINSON JW: Fine structure of *Rickettsia quintana* cultivated in vitro and in the louse. J Bacteriol 89:481–495, 1965

105. JACKSON EB, DANAUSKAS JX, COALE MC, and SMADEL JE: Recovery of *Rickettsia akari* from the Korean vole *Microtus fortis pelliceus.* Am J Hyg 66:301–308, 1957

106. JACKSON EB, DANAUSKAS JX, SMADEL JE, FULLER HS, COALE MC, and BOZEMAN FM: Occurrence of *Rickettsia tsutsugamushi* in Korean rodents and chiggers. Am J Hyg 66:309–320, 1957

107. JACKSON EB and SMADEL JE: Immunization against scrub typhus. II. Preparation of lyophilized living vaccine. Am J Hyg 53:326–331, 1951

108. JOHNSON JE and KADULL PJ: Laboratory-acquired Q fever. A report of fifty cases. Am J Med 41:391–403, 1966

109. JOHNSON JE and KADULL PJ: Rocky Mountain spotted fever acquired in a laboratory. N Engl J Med 277:842–847, 1967

110. KAZAR J, KRAUTWURST PA, and GORDON FB: Effects of interferon and interferon inducers on infections with a nonviral intracellular microorganism, *Rickettsia akari.* Infect Immun 3:819–824, 1971

111. KELLY MT: Activation of guinea pig macrophages by Q fever rickettsiae. Cell Immunol 28:198–205, 1977

112. KENYON RH, ACREE WM, WRIGHT GG, and MELCHIOR FW JR: Preparation of vaccines for Rocky Mountain spotted fever from rickettsiae propagated in cell culture. J Infect Dis 125:146–152, 1972

113. KENYON RH, CANONICO PG, SAMMONS LS, BAGLEY LR, and PEDERSEN CE JR: Antibody response to Rocky Mountain spotted fever. J Clin Microbiol 3:513–518, 1976

114. KENYON RH and McMANUS AT: Rickettsial infectious antibody complexes: detection by antiglobulin plaque reduction technique. Infect Immun 9:966–968, 1974

115. KENYON RH and PEDERSEN CE JR: Preparation of Rocky Mountain spotted fever vaccine suitable for human immunization. J Clin Microbiol 1:500–503, 1975

116. KENYON RH, SAMMONS LS, and PEDERSEN CE: Comparison of three spotted fever vaccines. J Clin Microbiol 2:300–304, 1975

117. KINGSBURY DT: Estimate of the genome size of various microorganisms. J Bacteriol 98:1400–1401, 1969

118. KISHIMOTO RA, VELTRI BJ, CANONICO PG, SHIREY FG, and WALKER JS: Electron microscopic study on the interaction between normal guinea pig macrophages and *Coxiella burnetii*. Infect Immun 14:1087–1096, 1976

119. KISHIMOTO RA, VELTRI BJ, SHIREY FG, CANONICO PG, and WALKER JS: Fate of *Coxiella burnetii* in macrophages from immune guinea pigs. Infect Immun 15:601–607, 1977

120. KISHIMOTO RA and WALKER JS: Interaction between *Coxiella burnetii* and guinea pig peritoneal macrophages. Infect Immun 14:416–421, 1976

121. KITAOKA M and TANAKA Y: Rickettsial toxin and its specificity in 3 prototype strains, Karp, Gilliam, and Kato, of *Rickettsia orientalis*. Acta Virol 17:426–434, 1973

122. KOBAYASHI Y, NAGAI K, and TACHIBANA N: Purification of complement-fixing antigens of *Rickettsia orientalis* by ether extraction. Am J Trop Med Hyg 18:942–952, 1969

123. KOBAYASHI Y and TACHIBANA N: Purification of complement-fixing antigen of *Rickettsia orientalis*. J Immunol 95:412–417, 1965

124. KOHNO S, KOHASE M, SAKATA H, SHIMIZU Y, HIKITA M, and SHISHIDO A: Production of interferon in primary chick embryonic cells infected with *Rickettsia mooseri*. J Immunol 105:1553–1558, 1970

125. KOKORIN IN: Biological peculiarities of the development of rickettsiae. Acta Virol 12:31–35, 1968

126. KORDOVÁ N: Study of antigenicity and immunogenicity of filterable particles of *Coxiella burneti*. Acta Virol 4:56–62, 1960

127. KORDOVÁ N: Plaque assay of rickettsiae. Acta Virol 10:278, 1966

128. KORDOVÁ N and BREZINA R: Multiplication dynamics of phase I and II *Coxiella burneti* in different cell cultures. Acta Virol 7:84–87, 1963

129. KRAUSS H, SCHIEFER H-G, and SCHMATZ H-D: Ultrastructural investigations on surface structures involved in *Coxiella burnetii* phase variation. Infect Immun 15:890–896, 1977

130. LACKMAN DB, BELL EJ, STOENNER HG, and PICKENS EG: The Rocky Mountain spotted fever group of rickettsias. Health Lab Sci 2:135–141, 1965

131. LACKMAN DB, GAYLE G, and PHILIP RN: Application of the radio-isotope precipitation test to the study of Q fever in man. Health Lab Sci 1:21–28, 1964

132. LENNETTE EH, CLARK WH, JENSEN FW, and TOOMB CJ: Q fever studies XV development and persistence in man of complement-fixing and agglutinating antibodies to *Coxiella burnetii*. J Immunol 68:591–598, 1952

133. LUOTO L: A capillary agglutination test for bovine Q fever. J Immunol 71:226–231, 1953

134. LUOTO L: A capillary tube test for antibody against *Coxiella burnetii* in human, guinea pig and sheep sera. J Immunol 77:294–298, 1956

135. LUOTO L and MASON DM: An agglutination test for bovine Q fever performed on milk samples. J Immunol 74:222–227, 1955

136. MASON RA: Propagation and growth of *Rickettsia quintana* in a new liquid medium. J Bacteriol 103:184–190, 1970

137. McDADE JE and GERONE PJ: Plaque assay for Q fever and scrub typhus rickettsiae. Appl Microbiol 19:963–965, 1970

138. McDADE JE, STAKEBAKE JR, and GERONE PJ: Plaque assay system for several species of *Rickettsia*. J Bacteriol 99:910–912, 1969

139. McKiel JA and Millar AM: Serodiagnosis in Q fever with special emphasis on the radio-isotope precipitation test. Can J Microbiol 14:721–726, 1968

140. McKiel JA, Bell EJ, and Lackman DB: *Rickettsia canada.* A new member of the typhus group of rickettsiae isolated from *Haemaphysalis leporispalustris* ticks in Canada. Can J Microbiol 13:503–510, 1967

141. Marmion BP: Subacute rickettsial endocarditis: an unusual complication of Q fever. J Hyg Epidemiol 6:79–84, 1962

142. Morikawa M: Studies on the antagonistic phenomenon *in vivo* between *Rickettsia orientalis* and *Encephalitozoon cuniculi.* Ochanomizu Igaku Zasshi 7:2888–2898, 1959 (In Japanese)

143. Murphy JR, Wisseman CL Jr, and Snyder LB: Plaque assay for *Rickettsia mooseri* in tissue samples. Proc Soc Exp Biol Med 153:151–155, 1976

144. Murray ES, Gaon JA, O'Connor JM, and Mulahasanovic M: Serologic studies of primary epidemic typhus and recrudescent typhus (Brill-Zinsser disease). I. Differences in complement-fixing antibodies: high antigen requirement and heat lability. J Immunol 94:723–733, 1965

145. Murray ES, O'Connor JM, and Gaon JA: Differentiation of 19S and 7S complement fixing antibodies in primary *versus* recrudescent typhus by either ethanethiol or heat. Proc Soc Exp Biol Med 119:291–297, 1965

146. Murray ES, O'Connor JM, and Gaon JA: Serologic studies of primary epidemic typhus and recrudescent typhus (Brill-Zinsser disease). II. Differences in immunoelectrophoretic patterns, response to 2-mercaptoethanol and relationships to 19S and 7S antibodies. J Immunol 94:734–740, 1965

147. Myers WF, Cutler LD, and Wisseman CL Jr: Role of erythrocytes and serum in the nutrition of *Rickettsia quintana.* J Bacteriol 97:663–666, 1969

148. Myers WF, Ormsbee RA, Osterman JV, and Wisseman CL Jr: The presence of diaminopimelic acid in the rickettsiae. Proc Soc Exp Biol Med 125:459–462, 1967

149. Myers WF, Osterman JV, and Wisseman CL Jr: Nutritional studies of *Rickettsia quintana:* nature of the hematin requirement. J Bacteriol 109:85–95, 1972

150. Myers WF, Provost PJ, and Wisseman CL Jr: Permeability properties of *Rickettsia mooseri.* J Bacteriol 93:950–960, 1967

151. Neva FA and Snyder JC: Studies on the toxicity of typhus rickettsiae. III. Observations on the mechanism of toxic death in white mice and white rats. J Infect Dis 97:73–87, 1955

152. Oaks SC Jr, Osterman JV, and Hetrick FM: Plaque assay and cloning of scrub typhus rickettsiae in irradiated L-929 cells. J Clin Microbiol 6:76–80, 1977

153. Obijeski JF, Palmer EL, and Tzianabos T: Proteins of purified rickettsiae. Microbios 11:61–76, 1974

154. Ormsbee RA: A method of purifying *Coxiella burnetii* and other pathogenic *Rickettsiae.* J Immunol 88:100–108, 1962

155. Ormsbee RA: An agglutination-resuspension test for Q fever antibodies. J Immunol 92:159–166, 1964

156. Ormsbee RA: Rickettsiae (as organisms). Ann Rev Microbiol 23:275–292, 1969

157. Ormsbee RA and Peacock MG: Rickettsial plaques assay and cloning procedures. Tissue Culture Assoc. Manual 2:475–478, 1976

158. Ormsbee RA, Peacock MG, Bell EJ, and Burgdorfer W: Experimental infections of lambs with *Rickettsia prowazeki.* Am J Trop Med Hyg 20:950–957, 1971

159. Ormsbee R, Peacock M, Philip R, Casper E, Plorde J, Gabre-Kidan T, and Wright L: Serologic diagnosis of epidemic typhus fever. Am J Epidemiol 105:261–271, 1977

160. Osterman JV, and Parr RP: Plaque formation by *Rickettsia conori* in WI-38, DBS-FRhL-2, L-929, HeLa, and chick embryo cells. Infect Immun 10:1152–1155, 1974

161. Palmer EL, Mallavia LP, Tzianabos T, and Obijeski JF: Electron microscopy of the cell wall of *Rickettsia prowazeki.* J Bacteriol 118:1158–1166, 1974

162. Palmer EL, Martin ML, and Mallavia L: Ultrastructure of the surface of *Rickettsia prowazeki* and *Rickettsia akari.* Appl Microbiol 28:713–716, 1974

163. Parker RR, Kohls GM, Cox GW, and Davis GE: Observations on an infectious agent from *Amblyomma maculatum.* Public Health Rep 54:1482–1484, 1939

164. Pedersen CE Jr, Bagley LR, Kenyon RH, Sammons LS, and Burger GT: Demonstration of *Rickettsia rickettsii* in the rhesus monkey by immune fluorescence microscopy. J Clin Microbiol 2:121–125, 1975

165. PERKINS HR, and ALLISON AC: Cell-wall constituents of rickettsiae and psittacosis-lymphogranuloma organisms. J Gen Microbiol 30:469–480, 1963

166. PHILIP CB: Observations on experimental Q fever. J Parasitol 34:457–464, 1948

167. PHILIP CB, LACKMAN DB, PHILIP RN, SCHENONE H, and COSCARON S: Serological evidence of rickettsial zoonoses in South American domestic animals. Acta Med Biol 15(Suppl):53–60, 1967

168. PHILIP RN, CASPER EA, MacCORMACK JN, SEXTON DJ, THOMAS LA, ANACKER RL, BURGDORFER W, and VICK S: A comparison of serologic methods for diagnosis of Rocky Mountain spotted fever. Am J Epidemiol 105:56–67, 1977

169. PHILIP RN, CASPER EA, ORMSBEE RA, PEACOCK MG, and BURGDORFER W: Microimmunofluorescence test for the serological study of Rocky Mountain spotted fever and typhus. J Clin Microbiol 3:51–61, 1976

170. PICKENS EG, BELL EJ, LACKMAN DB, and BURGDORFER W: Use of mouse serum in identification and serologic classification of *Rickettsia akari* and *Rickettsia australis*. J Immunol 94:883–889, 1965

171. PLOTZ H, BENNETT BL, and REAGAN RL: Preparation of an inactivated tissue culture scrub typhus vaccine. Proc Soc Exp Biol Med 61:313–317, 1946

172. PLOTZ H, BENNETT BL, WERTMAN K, SNYDER MJ, and GAULD RL: Serological pattern in typhus fever. I. Epidemic. Am J Hyg 47:150–165, 1948

173. PLOTZ H, REAGAN RL, and WERTMAN K: Differentiation between fièvre boutonneuse and Rocky Mountain spotted fever by means of complement fixation. Proc Soc Exp Biol Med 55:173–176, 1944

174. POWELL OW, and STALLMAN ND: The incidence and significance of phase I complement-fixing antibody in Q fever. J Hyg 60:359–364, 1962

175. PRICE WH: The epidemiology of Rocky Mountain spotted fever. I. The characterization of strain virulence of *Rickettsia rickettsii*. Am J Hyg 58:248–268, 1953

176. PRICE WH: A quantitative analysis of the factors involved in the variations in virulence of rickettsiae. Science 118:49–52, 1953

177. RAMM LE, and WINKLER HH: Rickettsial hemolysis: adsorption of rickettsiae to erythrocytes. Infect Immun 7:93–99, 1973

178. RAMM LE and WINKLER HH: Rickettsial hemolysis: effect of metabolic inhibitors upon hemolysis and adsorption. Infect Immun 7:550–555, 1973

179. RAMM LE and WINKLER HH: Identification of cholesterol in the receptor site for rickettsiae on sheep erythrocyte membranes. Infect Immun 13:120–126, 1976

180. RANSOM SE and HUEBNER RJ: Studies on resistance of *Coxiella burnetii* to physical and chemical agents. Am J Hyg 53:110–119, 1951

181. RIBI E and HOYER BH: Purification of Q fever rickettsiae by density-gradient sedimentation. J Immunol 85:314–318, 1960

182. ROBERTSON RG and WISSEMAN CL JR: Tick-borne rickettsiae of the spotted fever group in West Pakistan. II. Serologic classification of isolates from West Pakistan and Thailand: evidence for two new species. Am J Epidemiol 97:55–64, 1973

183. SALVIN SB and BELL EJ: Resistance of mice with experimental histoplasmosis to infection with *Rickettsia typhi*. J Immunol 75:57–62, 1955

184. SCHAECHTER M, BOZEMAN FM, and SMADEL JE: Study on the growth of rickettsiae. II. Morphological observations of living rickettsiae in tissue culture cells. Virology 3:160–172, 1957

185. SCHAECHTER M, TOUSIMIS AJ, COHN ZA, ROSEN H, CAMPBELL J, and HAHN FE: Morphological, chemical and serological studies of cell walls of *Rickettsia mooseri*. J Bacteriol 74:822–829, 1957

186. SCHRAMEK S, BREZINA SR, and URVOLGYI J: A new method of preparing diagnostic Q fever antigen. Acta Virol 16:487–492, 1972

187. SHAFFER JG and GOLDIN M: Serodiagnostic test in diseases other than syphilis *In* Clinical Diagnosis by Laboratory Methods 13th edition, Davidsohn I and Wells BB (eds) WB Saunders, Philadelphia, 1965, pp 889–890

188. SHEPARD CC and GOLDWASSER RA: Fluorescent antibody staining as a means of detecting Rocky Mountain spotted fever infection in individual ticks. Am J Hyg 72:120–129, 1960

189. SHEPARD CC, REDUS MA, TZIANABOS T, and WARFIELD DT: Recent experience with the complement fixation test in the laboratory diagnosis of rickettsial diseases in the United States. J Clin Microbiol 4:277–283, 1976

190. SHIRAI A, DIETEL JW, and OSTERMAN JV: Indirect hemagglutination test for human antibody to typhus and spotted fever group rickettsiae. J Clin Microbiol 2:430–437, 1975

191. SHISHIDO A: Identification and serological classification of the causative agent of scrub typhus in Japan. Jpn J Med Sci Biol 15:308–322, 1962

192. SHISHIDO A: Strain variation of *Rickettsia orientalis* in the complement fixation test. Jpn J Med Sci Biol 17:59–72, 1964

193. SHISHIDO A AND HIKITA M: Study on complement fixing antigens of *Rickettsia tsutsugamushi* from tissue culture sources. Acta Virol 12:58–62, 1968

194. SHISHIDO A, HIKITA M, SATO T, and KOHNO S: Particulate and soluble antigens of *Rickettsia tsutsugamushi* in the complement fixation test. J Immunol 103:480–490, 1969

195. SILBERMAN R and FISET P: Method for counting rickettsiae and chlamydiae in purified suspensions. J Bacteriol 95:259–261, 1968

196. SILVERMAN DJ, BOESE JL, and WISSEMAN CL JR: Ultrastructural studies of *Rickettsia prowazeki* from louse midgut cells to feces: search for "dormant" forms. Infect Immun 10:257–263, 1974

197. SMADEL JE: Complement fixation and agglutination reactions in rickettsial diseases *In* Rickettsial Diseases of Man, Moulton FR (ed), American Association for the Advancement of Science, Washington, DC, 1948, pp 190–197

198. SMADEL JE: The hazard of acquiring virus and rickettsial diseases in the laboratory. Am J Public Health 41:788–795, 1951

199. SMADEL JE: Influence of antibiotics on immunologic responses in scrub typhus. Am J Med 17:246–258, 1954

200. SMADEL JE and JACKSON EB: Rickettsial infections *In* Diagnostic Procedures for Viral and Rickettsial Diseases, 3rd edition, Lennette EH and Schmidt NJ (eds), Amer Public Health Assoc, Inc, New York, 1964, pp 755–757

201. SMADEL JE, JACKSON EB, BENNETT BL, and RIGHTS FL: A toxic substance associated with the Gilliam strain of *R. orientalis*. Proc Soc Exp Biol Med 62:138–140, 1946

202. SNYDER JC, BOVARNICK MR, MILLER JC, and CHANG RS: Observations on the hemolytic properties of typhus rickettsiae. J Bacteriol 67:724–730, 1954

203. SPENCER RR and PARKER RR: Rocky Mountain spotted fever: experimental studies on tick virus. Public Health Rep 39:3027–3040, 1924

204. STOENNER HG, LACKMAN DB, and BELL EJ: Factors affecting the growth of rickettsias of the spotted fever group in fertile hens' eggs. J Infect Dis 110:121–128, 1962

205. STOKER MGP, and FISET P: Phase variation of the Nine Mile and other strains of *Rickettsia burnetii*. Can J Microbiol 2:310–321, 1956

206. STOKER MGP, PAGE Z, and MARMION BP: Problems in the diagnosis of Q fever by complement-fixation tests. WHO Bull 13:807–827, 1955

207. STORK E and WISSEMAN CL JR: Growth of *Rickettsia prowazeki* in enucleated cells. Infect Immun 13:1743–1748, 1976

208. SULKIN SE and PIKE RM: Survey of laboratory-acquired infections. Am J Public Health 41:769–781, 1951

209. TABERT GG and LACKMAN DB: The radioisotope precipitation test for study of Q fever antibodies in human and animal sera. J Immunol 94:959–965, 1965

210. TOPPING NH, BENGTSON IA, HENDERSON RG, SHEPARD CC, and SHEAR MJ: Studies of typhus fever. Nat Inst Health Bull No. 183, 1945

211. TOPPING NH and SHEPARD CC: The preparation of antigens from yolk sacs infected with rickettsiae. Public Health Rep 61:701–707, 1946

212. TRAUB R, JOHNSON PT, MIESSE ML, and ELBEL RE: Isolation of *Rickettsia tsutsugamushi* from rodents from Thailand. Am J Trop Med Hyg 3:356–359, 1954

213. TYERYAR FJ JR, WEISS E, MILLAR DB, BOZEMAN FM, and ORMSBEE RA: DNA base composition of rickettsiae. Science 180:415–417, 1973

214. TZIANABOS T, PALMER EL, OBIJESKI JF, and MARTIN ML: Origin and structure of the group-specific, complement-fixing antigen of *Rickettsia rickettsii*. Appl Microbiol 28:481–488, 1974

215. VAN DER SCHEER J, BOHNEL E, and COX HR: Diagnostic antigens for epidemic typhus, murine typhus and Rocky Mountain spotted fever. J Immunol 56:365–375, 1947

216. VINSON JW: *In Vitro* cultivation of the rickettsial agent of trench fever. Bull WHO 35:155–164, 1966

217. VINSON JW and CAMPBELL ES: Complement fixing antigens from *Rickettsia quintana*. Acta Virol 12:54–57, 1968
218. WANG S-P: A micro immunofluorescence method. Study of antibody response to TRIC organisms in mice *In* Trachoma and Related Disorders Caused by Chlamydial Agents, Nichols RL (ed), Excerpta Medica, Amsterdam, 1971, pp 273–288
219. WANG S-P and GRAYSTON JT: *op. cit.*, pp. 305–321.
220. WATTENBERG LW, ELISBERG BL, WISSEMAN CL JR, and SMADEL JE: Studies of rickettsial toxins. II. Altered vascular physiology in rickettsial toxemia of mice. J Immunol 74:147–157, 1955
221. WEINBERG EH, STAKEBAKE JR, and GERONE PJ: Plaque assay for *Rickettsia rickettsii*. J Bacteriol 98:398–402, 1969
222. WEDUM AG: Bacteriological safety. Am J Public Health 43:1428–1437, 1953
223. WEISS E: Growth and physiology of rickettsiae. Bacteriol Rev 37:259–283, 1973
224. WEISS E, COOLBAUGH JC, and WILLIAMS JC: Separation of viable *Rickettsia typhi* from yolk sac and L cell host components by renografin density gradient centrifugation. Appl Microbiol 30:456–463, 1975
225. WEISS E, DASCH GA, WOODMAN DR, and WILLIAMS JC: Vole agent identified as a strain of the trench fever rickettsia, *Rochalimaea quintana*. Infect Immun 19:1013–1020, 1978
226. WEISS E, GREEN AE, GRAYS R, and NEWMAN LM: Metabolism of *Rickettsia tsutsugamushi* and *Rickettsia rickettsi* in irradiated host cells. Infect Immun 8:4–7, 1973
227. WEISS E, NEWMAN LW, GRAYS R, and GREEN AE: Metabolism of *Rickettsia typhi* and *Rickettsia akari* in irradiated L cells. Infect Immun 6:50–57, 1972
228. WEISS E, REES, HB JR, and HAYES JR: Metabolic activity of purified suspensions of *Rickettsia rickettsii*. Nature 213:1020–1022, 1967
229. WHITE LA, HALL HE, TZIANABOS T, and CHAPPEL WA: Effect of gentamicin on growth of viral, chlamydial, and rickettsial agents in mice and embryonated eggs. Antimicrob Agents Chemother 10:344–346, 1976
230. WIKE DA and BURGDORFER W: Plaque formation in tissue culture by *Rickettsia rickettsi* isolated directly from whole blood and tick hemolymph. Infect Immun 6:736–738, 1972
231. WIKE DA, ORMSBEE RA, TALLENT G, and PEACOCK MG: Effects of various suspending media on plaque formation by rickettsiae in tissue culture. Infect Immun 6:550–556, 1972
232. WIKE DA, TALLENT G, PEACOCK MG, and ORMSBEE RA: Studies of the rickettsial plaque assay technique. Infect Immun 5:715–722, 1972
233. WINKLER HH: Inhibitory and restorative effects of adenine nucleotides on rickettsial adsorption and hemolysis. Infect Immun 9:119–126, 1974
234. WINKLER HH and RAMM LE: Adsorption of typhus rickettsiae to ghosts of sheep erythrocytes. Infect Immun 11:1244–1251, 1975
235. WISSEMAN CL JR: Interaction of rickettsiae and phagocytic host cells. II. Chemotactic action of typhus rickettsiae on human polymorphonuclear leukocytes *in vitro*. J Immunol 87:468–471, 1961
236. WISSEMAN CL JR: Some biological properties of rickettsiae pathogenic for man. Zentralbl Bakteriol Parasitenk Infektionskr Hyg Abt 206:299–313, 1968
237. WISSEMAN CL JR, EDLINGER EA, WADDELL AD, and JONES MR: Infection cycle of *Rickettsia rickettsii* in chicken embryo and L-929 cells in culture. Infect Immun 14:1052–1064, 1976
238. WISSEMAN CL JR, FISET P, and ORMSBEE RA: Interaction of rickettsiae and phagocytic cells. V. Phagocytic and opsonic interactions of phase 1 and phase 2 *Coxiella burnetii* with normal and immune human leukocytes and antibodies. J Immunol 99:669–674, 1967
239. WISSEMAN CL JR, GAULD JR, and WOOD JG: Interaction of rickettsiae and phagocytic host cells. III. Opsonizing antibodies in human subjects infected with virulent or attenuated *Rickettsia prowazekii* or inoculated with killed epidemic typhus vaccine. J Immunol 90:127–131, 1963

240. WISSEMAN CL JR, GLAZIER J, and GRIEVES MJ: Interaction of rickettsiae and phagocytic host cells. I. *In vitro* studies of phagocytosis and opsonization of typhus rickettsias. Arch Inst Pasteur Tunis 36:341-360, 1959

241. WISSEMAN CL JR, JACKSON EB, HAHN FE, LEY AC, and SMADEL JE: Metabolic studies of rickettsiae. I. The effects of antimicrobial substances and enzyme inhibitors on the oxidation of glutamate by purified rickettsiae. J Immunol 67:123-136, 1951

242. WISSEMAN CL JR, and TABOR H: Interaction of rickettsiae and phagocytic host cells. IV. Early cellular response of man to typhus rickettsiae as revealed by the skin window technique, with observations on *in vivo* phagocytosis. J Immunol 93:816-825, 1964

243. WISSEMAN CL JR and WADDELL AD: In vitro studies on rickettsia-host cell interactions: intracellular growth cycle of virulent and attenuated *Rickettsia prowazeki* in chicken embryo cells in slide chamber cultures. Infect Immun 11:1391-1401, 1975

244. WISSEMAN CL JR, WADDELL AD, and SILVERMAN DJ: In vitro studies on rickettsia-host cell interactions: lag phase in intracellular growth cycle as a function of stage of growth of infecting *Rickettsia prowazeki*, with preliminary observations on inhibition of rickettsial uptake by host cell fragments. Infect Immun 13:1749-1760, 1976

245. WISSEMAN CL JR, WADDELL AD, and WALSH WT: In vitro studies of the action of antibiotics on *Rickettsia prowazekii* by two basic methods of cell culture. J Infect Dis 130:564-574, 1974

246. WISSEMAN CL JR, WADDELL AD, and WALSH WT: Mechanisms of immunity in typhus infections. IV. Failure of chicken embryo cells in culture to restrict growth of antibody-sensitized *Rickettsia prowazekii*. Infect Immun 9:571-575, 1974

247. WOLFE DM, VANDERSCHEER J, CLANCY CF, and COX HR: A method for the preparation of complement-fixing antigens in a study of experimental tsutsugamushi disease (scrub typhus). J Bacteriol 51:247-255, 1946

248. WOOD WH JR and WISSEMAN CL JR: The cell wall of *Rickettsia mooseri*. I. Morphology and chemical composition. J Bacteriol 93:1113-1118, 1967

249. WOODWARD TE, PEDERSEN CE JR, OSTER CN, BAGLEY LR, ROMBERGER J, and SNYDER MJ: Prompt confirmation of Rocky Mountain spotted fever: identification of rickettsiae in skin tissue. J Infect Dis 134:297-301, 1976

250. YAMAMOTO T, KAWAMURA A, HARA H, and AIKAWA K: Partial purification of rickettsiae with a cation exchange resin I Method of purification. Japan J Exp Med 28:329-336, 1958

251. YUNKER CE: Arthropod tissue culture in the study of arboviruses and rickettsiae: A review. Curr Top Microbiol Immunol 55:113-126, 1971

252. ZARAFONETIS CJD, SNYDER JC, and MURRAY ES: Immunity following para-aminobenzoic acid therapy in experimental tsutsugamushi disease (scrub typhus). Proc Soc Biol Med 61:240-242, 1946

INDEX

A

Accidental infections (*see* Laboratory infections)

Acid-citrate-dextrose reagent, 796

Acute gingivostomatitis due to herpes simplex virus, 309, 311

Acute hemorrhagic conjunctivitis, association with enterovirus infection, 472, 473

Acute hemorrhagic cystitis due to adenovirus, 231

Acute mesenteric lymphadenitis, association with adenovirus, 231

1-Adamantanamine, effect on rubella virus, 732

Adenitis due to the agent of cat-scratch disease, 1005

Adenoviridae family, (table) 233

Adenoviruses, 229–255
  antigenic composition, 234–236
    hemagglutinating antigens, 236
    immunotypes, 234, (table) 235
    viral and soluble antigens, 234, 236
  characteristics, 232–233
    chemical composition, 233
    size and shape, 232
    stability, 233
  classification, 233–234
    based on hemagglutination properties, 233, (table and figure) 234
    hosts and cryptograms (table), 233
  direct examination of specimens, 241
  growth in tissue, culture, 236–238
  history, 229
  identification of isolates, 242–247
    by complement fixation, 244–245
    by hemagglutination and hemagglutination-inhibition, 245–246
    by neutralization, 246
  in etiology of human gastroenteritis, 942, 943
  infections due to, 229–231
  isolation in tissue cultures, 236–238, 241–242
  pathogenicity for animals, 236
  preparation of complement-fixing antigen, 113

preparation of immune serum, 238–239
schematic representation of (figure), 232
serologic tests, 247–248
  alternative procedures, 248
  complement fixation, 247–248
  hemagglutination-inhibition, 248
  neutralization, 248
specimen collection, 239–240
  for microscopy, 240
  for serodiagnosis, 240
  for virus isolation, 239–240
  precautions, 239

Aerosols as source of infections, 52

African Burkitt lymphoma, Epstein-Barr virus in etiology of, 441, 452–453

African hemorrhagic fever (*see* Ebola virus)

Agar gel diffusion test
  for arenaviruses, 831
  for hepatitis B antigens, 893, 911–912

Agglutination techniques in serologic diagnosis, general principles, 25–26

Agglutination tests for rickettsiae, 1095–1096

Allantoic route of egg inoculation, (figure) 45, 47

Alphaviruses, arboviruses classified as, (table) 770

Alsever solution, 796

Alsever solution, modified
  for complement fixation test, 35
  for rubella hemagglutination-inhibition test, 747

Amniotic inoculation technique, 43–46

Anemia, equine infectious (*see* Equine infectious anemia)

Animal hosts of rickettsiae, (table) 1072–1073

Animals, experimental
  safety precautions in handling, 56–57
  treatment of monkey bites, 368

Antibiotics
  effect on rickettsiae, 1064, 1072, 1074
  use in cell culture media, 75–76, 81, 127–128

Antibodies, antiviral and peroxidase-labeled, sources of, 166–167

Antifungal agents, use in cell culture media, 76, 81, 127

Arthralgia
  as a complication of rubella, 728
  as a sign of hepatitis B infection, 885
Arthritis
  as a complication of rubella, 728
  due to arboviruses
    clinical aspects, 768
    viruses causing, (table) 770-772
Arthropod-borne viruses (*see* Arboviruses)
Athropod vectors of rickettsial disease, (table) 1072-1073
Arthropods as probable vectors of encephalomyocarditis viruses, 1010
Aseptic meningitis
  association with enterovirus infection, 472, 473
  due to herpes simplex virus, 310, 312
  due to lymphocytic choriomeningitis virus, 817
Asthma, exacerbation by respiratory syncytial virus, 696
Astroviruses in etiology of human gastroenteritis, 942
Aviadenovirus hosts and cryptograms, (table) 233
Avian infections
  due to chlamydiae (*see* Psittacosis)
  due to influenza virus, 585
  due to Newcastle disease virus, 655
Avian infectious bronchitis virus, classification, 712

B

Bacteriological media as components of cell culture media, 73
Balanced salt solutions
  composition, 128
  use in cell culture media, 73-74
Bead-in-tube cultures for maintaining established cell lines, 93-94
Bell's palsy, as a complication of infectious mononucleosis, 443
Biological safety cabinets, classes of, 55-56
Biosafety, Office of, reporting laboratory accidents to, 49
BK virus
  characteristics, 1001
  history, 1000-1001
  isolation, 1002
  serologic diagnosis, 1003-1004
Blood transfusion, cytomegalovirus infection following, 402

BME, Eagle basal medium
  development of, 74-75
  formulation source, 74
Bolivian hemorrhagic fever (*see* Machupo virus)
Brill-Zinsser disease (*see* Typhus group)
Bronchiolitis
  as a complication of measles, 667
  due to parainfluenza virus, 612
  due to respiratory syncytial virus, 695-696
Bronchitis
  exacerbation by respiratory syncytial virus, 696
  exacerbation by rhinoviruses, 536
Bunyaviruses, arboviruses classified as, (table) 771-772
Burkitt lymphoma, Epstein-Barr virus in etiology of, 441, 452-453

C

Caliciviruses in etiology of human gastroenteritis, 942
California State Department of Health CF test, 35-42
Canine distemper virus, relation to measles virus, 670, 671
Carcinoma, nasopharyngeal, Epstein-Barr virus in etiology of, 441-442, 452-453
Carcinoma of the cervix, association with herpes simplex virus, 310, 319-320
Cat-scratch disease, 1005-1008
  characteristics of agent, 1006
  clinical aspects, 1005-1006
  history, 1005
  intradermal skin test for, 1006-1007
  serologic diagnosis, 1007
Cell cultures (*see also* Tissue cultures), 65-139
  apparatus for, 123-127
  cell dispersing agents for, 129-130
  cell dispersing techniques for, 76-80
  definitions of kinds, 65-67
  detection of virus replication in, 67-70
  enumeration of cells in, 80-81
  handling and storage of fresh tissues for, 76
  media and reagents for
    biological materials as components, 72-73
    chemically defined media, 73-76
    composition and preparation, 81-85, 116-118, 127-134
    mycoplasma contamination of, 115-123
    neutralization tests in, 104-111

I

J

M

X-Y-Z